Ursula H. Hübner
Gabriela Mustata Wilson
Toria Shaw Morawski · Marion J. Ball
Editors

Nursing Informatics

A Health Informatics, Interprofessional and Global Perspective

Fifth Edition

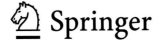
Springer

Editors
Ursula H. Hübner
University of Applied Sciences (UAS)
Osnabrück
Osnabrück, Niedersachsen
Germany

Gabriela Mustata Wilson
The University of Texas at Arlington
(UTA)
Arlington, TX
USA

Toria Shaw Morawski
Healthcare Information and
Management Systems Society (HIMSS)
Chicago, IL
USA

Marion J. Ball
The University of Texas at Arlington
(UTA)
Arlington, TX
USA

ISSN 1431-1917   ISSN 2197-3741   (electronic)
Health Informatics

ISBN 978-3-030-91236-9   ISBN 978-3-030-91237-6   (eBook)
https://doi.org/10.1007/978-3-030-91237-6

This Springer imprint is published by the registered company Springer Nature Switzerland AG
The registered company address is: Gewerbestrasse 11, 6330 Cham, Switzerland

Health Informatics

This series is directed to healthcare professionals leading the transformation of healthcare by using information and knowledge. For over 20 years, Health Informatics has offered a broad range of titles: some address specific professions such as nursing, medicine, and health administration; others cover special areas of practice such as trauma and radiology; still other books in the series focus on interdisciplinary issues, such as the computer based patient record, electronic health records, and networked healthcare systems. Editors and authors, eminent experts in their fields, offer their accounts of innovations in health informatics. Increasingly, these accounts go beyond hardware and software to address the role of information in influencing the transformation of healthcare delivery systems around the world. The series also increasingly focuses on the users of the information and systems: the organizational, behavioral, and societal changes that accompany the diffusion of information technology in health services environments.

Developments in healthcare delivery are constant; in recent years, bioinformatics has emerged as a new field in health informatics to support emerging and ongoing developments in molecular biology. At the same time, further evolution of the field of health informatics is reflected in the introduction of concepts at the macro or health systems delivery level with major national initiatives related to electronic health records (EHR), data standards, and public health informatics.

These changes will continue to shape health services in the twenty-first century. By making full and creative use of the technology to tame data and to transform information, Health Informatics will foster the development and use of new knowledge in healthcare.

More information about this series at https://link.springer.com/bookseries/1114

Ursula H. Hübner
Gabriela Mustata Wilson
Toria Shaw Morawski • Marion J. Ball
Editors

Nursing Informatics

A Health Informatics, Interprofessional and Global Perspective

Fifth Edition

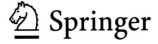 Springer

Editors
Ursula H. Hübner
University of Applied Sciences (UAS)
Osnabrück
Osnabrück, Niedersachsen
Germany

Gabriela Mustata Wilson
The University of Texas at Arlington
(UTA)
Arlington, TX
USA

Toria Shaw Morawski
Healthcare Information and
Management Systems Society (HIMSS)
Chicago, IL
USA

Marion J. Ball
The University of Texas at Arlington
(UTA)
Arlington, TX
USA

ISSN 1431-1917   ISSN 2197-3741   (electronic)
Health Informatics

ISBN 978-3-030-91236-9   ISBN 978-3-030-91237-6   (eBook)
https://doi.org/10.1007/978-3-030-91237-6

This Springer imprint is published by the registered company Springer Nature Switzerland AG
The registered company address is: Gewerbestrasse 11, 6330 Cham, Switzerland

This book is dedicated to the next generation of scientists and practitioners working in nursing and health informatics and beyond.

—Ursula H. Hübner

This book is dedicated to my FAMILY and all the STRONG WOMEN in my life who have inspired me along the way. Their elegance, intelligence, and diplomacy on how to deal with challenges in life remind me that even though inside they might have been broken, they continued to walk tall and with grace because they never stopped believing in themselves.

—Gabriela M. Wilson

I dedicate this book to my three main pillars of support: My husband Michał Morawski, mother Victoria Shaw, and best friend Heather Walsh. To my beloved family and friends, sheroes, mentors, and ancestors who opened the doors of possibility: Thank you for the unconditional love and support every step of the way!

—Toria Shaw Morawski

I dedicate this book to my beloved brother Dr. Peter Jokl who has stood by me throughout my life—always giving love and support.

—Marion J. Ball

Foreword

I am delighted to have been given the honor to write the Foreword to the fifth edition of this very important textbook. For us at the Healthcare Information and Management Systems Society (HIMSS), informatics and its deployment in clinical practice is our lifeblood and indeed enshrined within our mission, which is to reform the global health ecosystem through the power of information and technology.

Informatics and its applicability and deployment have come of age, and we are now entering an era where digital transformation continues to accelerate, and the digital modalities have now become part of the normal methods of communication with patients and citizens.

The journey to where we are now has been anything but proportionate and predictable. For many years, we have been waiting for the power of information and its application to start to transform the interactions between clinicians and patients, and until late 2019, the levels of deployment were still far short of what we all aspired to. Then we had the COVID-19 pandemic, which largely outpaced the ability of health and care systems to manage its effects, and suddenly we achieved as much in weeks as we had previously achieved in decades. Digital transformation had suddenly come of age and has been adopted globally.

The challenges we are now facing, as a result, is to ensure that our workforce is in a position to be able to exploit the myriad of advantages that this digital transformation brings. This book is part of that journey because the world we are all operating in is very different to the one which existed in the previous decade.

This new world is one where information and its deployment is everyone's business from the nursing information officer to the nurse on the hospital ward or in the emergency room or even in the community. How else can we best care for people, be working using the appropriate personal pathways, from the same version of the medical record? Also, how else can we ensure that the patient receives the most optimal transfer of care between caring institutions when we know this is the time when most of the adverse effects happen? Finally, how else can we assist the patient in reducing their risk factors through behavior change unless all our decisions are based on data, not conjecture? The use of information has become as important as the essential part of the nursing process. It is now indeed every health carer's business.

There are many other potential improvements to care we can now use. Modern health and care have increasingly become more precise, and personalized and care pathways have also become more complex and individual. The adoption of personalized clinical digital support can assist us in ensuring we follow the right pathway at the right time and with the right patient, thus decreasing medical and nursing errors and improving care.

In a similar vein, in the care of people with noncommunicable diseases, we can be sure we offer patients every opportunity at the right time to reduce the impact of any risk factors they may exhibit.

The comfort that we are working from the same version of a health record should also reduce the chances of adverse events, missed opportunities to deliver care, and medical errors.

So, what should we say to those among us who are perhaps less enamored with this new way of working and hark back to the analogue days? It is certainly the case that the tempo of care delivery has increased in recent years, also exacerbated by the fact that as people age, the levels of multimorbidity increase, and the numbers of pathways and actions follow. However, the power of digital transformation has the potential to alleviate some of this pressure by automating tasks like data entry and utilizing data-driven decision-making to reduce duplication, specifically around investigations.

The most significant opportunity, however, is around allowing the health carer to devote more time to assist the patient in behavior modification and to care for the patient as a person and not as a group of diseases that inhabit a patient.

Nursing has made significant advances over the last few years. As well as being a full and contributing member of all high functioning transformation boards, nursing is now taking on and implementing transformational leadership roles in informatics.

What is notable about these developments is the retention of what is at the heart of what constitutes modern nursing—which is holistic care for patients as people, taking all aspects of a person into consideration when delivering care. The appropriate use of informatics and skillful deployment of digital modalities gives every opportunity to strengthen this vital aspect of what constitutes the core of modern nursing care.

Finally, there is a significant convergence of values we need to highlight. The vision that drives modern nursing is compassion and caring for people, to evidence-based approaches to continuously improve the quality of patient care. The vision for HIMSS as a global not-for-profit membership organization is to realize the full health potential of every human, everywhere.

We are all trying to deliver the same outcome, and given the magnitude of the task, no one person or organization can do this alone, given the scale of the challenge. This book is uniquely placed to equip nurses and health professionals with what they need to deliver the best of care.

HIMSS   Charles Alessi
Chicago, IL, USA

Foreword

I have been fortunate in my career to see our wonderful and peculiar discipline of nursing informatics evolve. Over 30 years ago, as a young Registered Nurse, I was curious about the green monochrome monitors that sat consuming space and electricity, but which remained largely unused on the nurses' station (the early desktop systems did not have a mouse—perhaps we were all waiting for this essential piece of hardware to be delivered!). While these early information systems sought mainly to automate patient administration (holding demographic information and summary details about contact with services), visionary researchers were already exploring the potential of information technology for nursing, and had been doing since the very early days of computing. Seeing this potential contributed to my own decision to seek further training in computer science and embark on my lifetime (second) career in nursing informatics.

I have worked with some incredible nurses and have seen them rise to informatics leadership positions at the very highest levels, thereby placing nursing on an equal footing with other professions. I have also worked with some incredible people from other disciplines, and have experienced first-hand the warm collegiality that characterizes our field. Everyone who has a positive contribution to make is welcome—and everyone's contribution is valued. Nursing informatics is very often singled out as being highly productive, perhaps due to (a) its focus on the needs of citizens, (b) a shared sense of purpose, and (c) an unfailing commitment to succeed. The success of nursing informatics, and of nursing itself, is reliant on the willingness (and enthusiasm) of its constituents to collaborate and share what they know with others—and it is reliant also on the hunger in those others to learn.

I have enjoyed seeing the different approaches that nurses around the world take to delivering the best possible care for people in their communities. This diversity in practice serves to ensure that practice around the world remains relevant, with no single system of nursing asserting inappropriate dominance over others. In addition to the differences, I have also enjoyed seeing the commonalities in nursing practice and nursing informatics practice, in very different settings. Nursing globally provides a living laboratory that, together with the willingness to collaborate and share, ensures that we remain a learning profession with an evolving knowledge base. Nursing informatics is no different in this regard.

This important book embodies this ethos. It builds on previous editions, and shares local case studies to facilitate learning and further demonstrate the positive global impact of informatics. The book effectively serves as the fifth edition of the hugely popular text *Nursing Informatics: Where Technology and Caring Meet*. The title *Nursing Informatics: A Health Informatics, Interprofessional and Global Perspective* sets a new tone that better reflects contemporary priorities. The distinguished and experienced team of Editors exudes inter-professionality. Nurses rarely practice in isolation from other health workers, and, through almost 50 chapters, the text illustrates how different professional groups interface and interrelate via technology—and puts the patient or citizen center stage, thereby revealing the seldom-seen "softer" side of informatics.

The COVID-19 pandemic, which comes in the wake of a number of previous global health emergencies, has provided another sobering reminder that local concerns are also very often global concerns. The pandemic has also re-asserted (a) the pressing need for an adequate nursing workforce; (b) the vital importance of good nursing care; and (c) the outstanding need for a robust informatics infrastructure for nursing. As with previous editions, this book represents essential reading for both the present and the future, with experts in the field covering important topics such as innovation, application, transformation, education, regulation, standards, leadership, collaboration, and many more.

As a profession, nursing now finds itself in a very interesting position. There have been very many major gains over the past several decades that have served to computerize aspects of nursing practice. However, I believe we need to do more if we are to stand any chance of meeting current and future needs. Without the engagement, involvement, and active participation of nursing itself, I believe that we, as members of the nursing informatics community, run the risk of stepping into a space where incremental gains—small steps—are all we can possibly hope for. I believe it is time for nursing to look at itself—to really look at itself—and to reinterpret fundamentally its own informatics practice for an electronic context, rather than to continue to shoehorn existing manual approaches into a rather uncomfortable ill-fitting boot.

I believe that this book, along with other related texts, provides both a springboard and a catalyst that will facilitate positive transformation in nursing and nursing informatics practice that will benefit both nurses and the people and communities they care for.

School of Human and Health Sciences   Nicholas Hardiker
University of Huddersfield,
Huddersfield, UK

Foreword

It is an honor to have the opportunity to provide this message and to introduce this timely, innovative contribution to the informatics literature. This fifth edition of *Nursing Informatics* challenges the field to integrate new technology, new knowledge regarding informatics, data analytics, and tools to solve the challenges that have been exacerbated by the COVID-19 pandemic. This book is being published less than a year into the pandemic where we have seen every health care provider discipline, healthcare agency, business, and government entity, be challenged to maximize their use of information and technology, particularly online and distant connections, to deliver their service. For individuals and families, this has often meant receiving health care through "telehealth" visits, completing documentation and payment electronically, and reducing face-to-face contact in the receipt of care. Many of us in our professional lives and personal lives have been challenged to adopt new technology and complete our daily activities supported by increased use of informatics. This transformation provides the opening for maximizing the influence of health informatics in the delivery of health and nursing care. This book provides the latest information to guide nurses, doctors, public health leaders, administrators, computer scientists, information technology specialists, and all members of the interprofessional care team, in building on the progress made to date while capitalizing on the positive experiences of many who have become more familiar with, and dependent on, technology and informatics to maintain their health and well-being during this crisis to create innovations to advance health care in the future.

The fifth edition of this *Nursing Informatics* book series focuses on both interprofessional and global perspectives. It builds on the editors' internationally recognized expertise and wisdom gained through on-going leadership of successful health informatics initiatives in education, research, and service. I am particularly pleased that two of the editors, Dr. Marion Ball and Dr. Gabriela Mustata Wilson, have chosen to extend their influence on the health and nursing informatics community by joining the University of Texas at Arlington to develop and lead the Multi-Interprofessional Center for Health Informatics, with tenure in the College of Nursing and Health Innovation where I am a dean. This center will provide a catalyst for the development of innovative educational and research initiatives building on the knowledge shared in this latest edition of *Nursing Informatics*. The focus on interprofessional collaborations in the fifth edition of *Nursing Informatics* provides insights into stakeholders' perspectives through description of roles and perspectives of the multiple disciplines who need to work together as a team to maximize the use of information and data both efficiently and effectively to provide patient centered health care. Too often in the past, organizations have not included all disciplinary perspectives in the development and planning of an initiative; the focus on the ultimate objective of promoting better and better quality health care can be stifled without effective collaboration among stakeholders. Readers will gain insights into many perspectives other than their own disciplinary perspective throughout this book. The field is still challenged to have seamless interoperable systems across different health care and provider agencies. There are still challenges in making individuals' health care data readily available to them and challenges in integrating data from smart mobile assistants with data generated from use of the formal health care system. These issues will be advanced by incorporating ideas explored in the text in innovative solutions.

This book could not have been timelier in taking a global perspective. Any perception that the health of individuals is not affected by global health challenges and solutions should have been shattered by the occurrence of the pandemic which highlighted the interdependency of people, countries and of scientific findings and breakthroughs. The section on global developments will take you around the world to understand the different approaches and contributions to health informatics and will allow you to gain insights into opportunities for collaboration. An innovative focus examines patient safety through a global lens. The fifth edition is forward thinking in incorporating a focus on population health. Many technology improvements have started within our largest of companies, hospitals, and smaller health agencies, health departments, rural health clinics, and small provider groups which have been delayed in obtaining the newest health informatics solutions. A change to a philosophy of promoting population health through integrated health informatics solutions provides an opportunity to enhance the contributions of informatics to increasing the health of communities and over-coming the social determinants of health that serve as barriers to health and too often not addressed within current health care ecosystems. With the rapid speed of technology and informatics innovations in recent years, the health care communities are now challenged to build on this foundation and develop health and nursing informatics solutions that are shared and connect colleagues across the world in collaborations to improve the health of populations.

The fifth edition of *Nursing Informatics* provides the basis for students of all disciplines to gain a broad knowledge of informatics. Experienced professionals, whether in practice or returning to seek a higher level educational degree, will be challenged to use their new informatics knowledge to integrate with their existing background to identify how they can leverage informatics to improve care and health. Educators are challenged to review their curricula and integrate the use of data to create information and solve health care problems at all levels of education.

While the subject of informatics can be complex, the authors' style will allow you to enjoy learning about the latest in health and nursing informatics. The book concludes with a focus on emerging technologies and future for health informatics careers. I challenge you to think about your role in the future and contributions you can make through incorporating health and/or nursing informatics into your daily practice or into your contributions toward improving the health of populations. Informatics will advance the future of interprofessional connections and global health.

College of Nursing and Health Innovation   Elizabeth I. Merwin
University of Texas at Arlington
Arlington, TX, USA

Preface: Transforming Healthcare Through Learning

This book aims to contribute toward equipping students, adult learners, and the nursing and healthcare workforce with the necessary knowledge of how data and digitalization can support in making the best decisions and achieving optimal health outcomes. Due to the wide range of nursing informatics within the context of health informatics, this book includes the interprofessional perspective, inviting other health professions and students/adult learners to learn from the different topics of the individual chapters or the book as a whole. At the same time, this book strives to share a global perspective and learning across regions, countries, and continents to broaden the foundation of health informatics knowledge. The goal is to plant the seeds of understanding how health information and technology have succeeded abroad, how things can be changed at home, and how international alliances can be forged in science and industry alike.

The structure of this book and its chapters are entrenched in the previous editions and the vast contributions of a global network of authors as well as a series of projects at the local and international levels. These projects served and continue to serve as hubs to reach out to international stakeholders and collaborators worldwide to bring together as many experts as possible to gather unique and invaluable perspectives on nursing and health informatics education.

Guided by the global projects referenced above, two main publications have also shaped this book: first the *"Technology Informatics Guiding Education Reform—TIGER—An International Recommendations Framework of Core Competencies in Health Informatics for Nurses"* [1], shortly referred to as the TIGER Recommendations Framework 1.0, and *"Towards the TIGER International Framework for Recommendations of Core Competencies in Health Informatics 2.0: Extending the Scope and the Roles"* [2], referred to as the TIGER Recommendations Framework 2.0. While the previous Framework 1.0 targets nursing, Framework 2.0 encompasses the competency needs of the full bandwidth of healthcare professionals, inclusive of physicians, nurses, pharmacists, therapists, health information managers, clinical and administrative chief executive officers, clinical and technical chief information officers, engineers, scientists, and educators. Their opinions on the relevant competency areas in nursing and health informatics were empirically captured through surveys and case studies to form the foundation of each recommendation framework cohesively. These frameworks were extensively informed by previously published work on nursing and health informatics education, in particular, the "*Recommendations of the International Medical Informatics Association (IMIA) on Education in Biomedical and Health Informatics*" [3] and the "*Global Academic Curricula Competencies for Health Information Professionals*" [4] and the two recommendations of the American Medical Informatics Association (AMIA), "*AMIA Board white paper: definition of biomedical informatics and specification of core competencies for graduate education in the discipline*" [5] and and "*AMIA Board White Paper: AMIA 2017 core competencies for applied health informatics education at the master's degree level*" [6].

Organization of the Book

Drawing on the structure of competency areas in nursing and health informatics from the two TIGER Recommendation Frameworks and from the American Association of Colleges in Nursing [7], this book is organized into the following ten parts:

    I. Introduction
   II. The 360° Stakeholder Perspective
  III. Using Data and Information to Generate Knowledge
  IV. Interoperable Systems
   V. Safe Systems and Patient Safety
  VI. Privacy, Security, Confidentiality and Ethics in Healthcare
 VII. Managing Technology and People
VIII. Health Informatics Education for the 21st Century
  IX. Global Perspectives in Health Informatics
   X. Future Trends in Health Informatics

It thereby emphasizes the role of data, information, and knowledge that are fueled by the multi-stakeholder expectations and their active contributions. To obtain high-quality and up-to-date data from different sources, interoperable, safe, and secure technical systems have to be in place. As increased personal data is also captured outside the clinical setting, privacy, confidentiality, and ethics come to the forefront and are considered if a system can be actually used for a given purpose. Therefore, it needs leaders and champions to make the right decisions, not only on the grounds of legal and ethical requirements but from the entire canon of needs voiced by interprofessional teams. These leaders must address both the technology and people applying the technology to arrive at a meaningful digital health system. Digital literacy through appropriate education and training is the leverage to raise awareness in leaders, champions, users, and decision-makers at all levels. As a result, competency-based education and training establish the foundation on which we can build and shape digital workflows, participate in designing systems, be on alert for privacy and confidentiality issues, know about implications of poor communication and data sharing, be aware of the quality of data and the consequences when artificial intelligence (AI) methods are employed, and most importantly, know what serves the patient best.

Awareness-raising and education work best when looking out of the box. This is the reason for including the global perspective. Finally, education is no means to corroborate the status quo; it serves as the engine to go forward in with a vision focused on the future.

Following the Introduction (**Part I**), which includes two chapters, **Part II** "The 360° Sakeholder Perspective" sets the stage for all subsequent chapters incorporating the view of many different stakeholders, including the patient, on health IT and informatics methods. Beyond the patient's view (Chap. 3), this part comprises chapters reflecting the nurse's view (Chap. 4), the physician's (Chap. 5), the pharmacist's (Chap. 6), the chief information officer's (CIO's) (Chap. 7), the chief nursing information officer's (CNIO's) (Chap. 8), the chief medical information officer's (CMIO's) (Chap. 9), the health information manager's (HIM's) (Chap. 10), and the educator's view (Chap. 11). It thus yields an overview of the many voices within the interprofessional team.

Part III is dedicated to "Using Data and Information to Generate Knowledge," referencing the notion that nurses and other health professionals are knowledge workers acting in a world of a swiftly changing landscape of facts and evidence. Laying the foundation, the first chapter of this part describes the concepts and data-driven mechanisms of a learning health system (LHS) working at the junction of practice and research (Chap. 12). This part displays the opportunities of employing electronic health record (EHR) data to monitor ICU patients and alert providers, hereby automatically exploiting data beyond the human capacity (Chap. 13). The following two chapters (Chaps. 14 and 15) delineate the use of clinical documentation in EHRs, capitalizing on structured data and standardized terminologies. Besides use in patient care, they emphasize the opportunity of helping nursing management allocate human and other resources reusing this data. Often internal EHR data need to be supplemented by community data to allow for a correct diagnosis or therapy plan that is sensitive to the fact that many diseases and health conditions possess underlying social determinants (Chap. 16). Additional data sources, e.g., biomarkers and sensors, need to be developed, particularly providing data captured by citizens as Chap. 17 explains. Likewise, social media is gaining importance as a citizen-generated data source to predict health events (Chap. 18). This part of chapters is rounded up by showing how data of different provenance can be analyzed and visualized (Chap. 19).

Part IV is focused on "Interoperable Systems" displaying an overview of systems capable of capturing, storing, analyzing, and communicating data, information, and knowledge. Chapter 20 demonstrates the essence of interoperability as a fundamental prerequisite for exchanging, sharing, and interpreting data. The following chapters provide examples of systems and their support of nurses, physicians, and other interprofessional team members to provide better care. Chapter 21 gives insights into how clinical decision support systems work in general and how they can be integrated in nursing. While such a system could work within a single organization or in a network of provider organizations, telehealth, as described in Chap. 22, reaches out beyond the confines of an individual institution to connect patients and providers and providers and their peers. Chapter 23 goes a step further, addressing the entire population to display how health reporting to public health authorities benefits from digital connectivity.

Innovative and successful health IT systems need be not only interoperable but also safe—for their own purpose (IT security) and for the sake of the patients (patient safety). **Part V** is therefore devoted to the wide field of "Safe Systems and Patient Safety." Chapter 24 comprehensively sketches the opportunities of digital systems to enable and improve patient safety while also outlining the risks to safe care arising from the use of digital technology. Chapter 25 continues where Chap. 24 ends showing how to curb these risks through employing systematic management techniques and education. Technologies can become unsafe to a patient and, thus, can jeopardize the work of an entire organization when being attacked. Chapter 26, therefore, is concerned with raising the awareness of these attacks and with countermeasures to cyberattacks, thereby ensuring confidentiality and data integrity while also allowing for the availability of data. Another threat originates in health IT systems and mainly apps on smart devices that present wrong information to app users through wrong algorithms or wrong data. Chapter 27 describes these problems and provides a solution to build trustful mHealth applications.

"Privacy, Security, Confidentiality and Ethics in Healthcare" were already touched upon in the previous part and are now fully fleshed out in **Part VI** from the perspective of the USA (Chap. 28) and Europe (Chap. 29). Further details are provided in Chap. 30. which looks specifically at EHRs in the context of legal requirements, access, ownership, and patient rights. Many legal topics, e.g., privacy and confidentiality, also overlap with ethical areas concerning patients, providers, and systems. Chapter 31 provides an introduction into ethical principles, demonstrating how important ethical issues become when system boundaries between care and research and between patients and providers are blurring.

In **Part VII** "Managing Technology and People," the focus is shifting from the data, information, and technology clusters to the people and their contributions who make health IT applications successful. Chapter 32 sets the stage describing management principles and providing real-world examples to prove how these principles have been applied. Two chapters on strategic alignment and leadership follow Chap. 33, focusing on strategic information management, and Chap. 34 on interprofessional strategic leadership, both of which illustrate the need for strategy to achieve change and innovation. Chapter 35 reveals that innovation is no smooth transition from one stage to another but is inherently accompanied by disruption. Apart from strategic leadership, sound skills in project management (Chap. 36) and process management (Chap. 37) warrant the success of new digital workflows and procedures.

Managing people leads to education, which is the primary topic of **Part VIII**, "Health Informatics Education for the 21st Century." Its chapters plead for interprofessional health informatics education as the foundation for modern interprofessional care. Focusing on the TIGER (Technology Informatics Guiding Education Reform) initiative, Chap. 38 yields an overview of its first years as a mainly nursing-centered grassroots initiative. TIGER's expansion is presented via its two global Health Informatics Recommendation Frameworks focused on furthering global workforce development. Also, Chap. 39 resumes methods and tools for preparing the healthcare workforce particularly addressing the health informatics workforce and providing a personal account of a career in this field. Only if the healthcare professionals are ready to face the complexity and continuous challenges, health IT applications can be employed to care for patients. Thus, health IT can be developed and applied so that it is driven by patient care needs. Health informatics education is more than workforce development; it embraces all levels of academic education and training, as presented in Chap. 40. Building upon connectivity and information exchange, Chap. 41 capitalizes on one of the essentials of health informatics, demonstrating how information sharing among different health professionals can be imparted, trained practically, and translated into daily work. Finally, health informatics education can also make use of informatics methods and tools. Online teaching approaches and advanced concepts to develop digital courses are covered in detail within Chap. 42.

Part IX, "Global Perspectives in Health Informatics," incorporates international experiences and hereby links to the core theme of this book. This part starts with an account of how telehealth is harnessed to implement a portable health clinic in Bangladesh (Chap. 43); the second chapter in this part gives an overview on health IT adoption in Brazil (Chap. 44) and shows how structured nursing data can be (re-)used to inform healthcare practice. The third chapter reports on a comparison of the healthcare systems and their IT adoption in Finland, Germany, and the USA (Chap. 45). The next chapter shares Nigeria's global health informatics journey, inclusive of the challenges and health informatics methods leveraged along the way (Chap. 46). Finally, Chap. 47 describes how Saudi Arabia transformed its healthcare system through digitalization. At the end of the book, Part X, "Future Trends in Health Informatics," strives to provide glimpses into the future of the field. Chapter 48 focuses on emerging technologies for surgery and Chap. 49 on what data-driven medicine and healthcare promise to offer in the future.

The large majority of the chapters include a series of review questions that can be used to assess the learners' understanding of the content presented. In addition, this book yields many good healthcare examples of informatics milestones illustrated through real examples. This perspective is expanded by showing how health IT is successfully adopted, implemented, and used throughout the various case studies that encourage critical thinking and additional learning.

It is the hope of the editors that this book will contribute to transforming healthcare through learning to prepare the health workforce so that it can meet the challenges of today and tomorrow.

Osnabrück, Germany	Ursula H. Hübner
Arlington, TX	Gabriela Mustata Wilson
Chicago, IL	Toria Shaw Morawski
Arlington, TX	Marion J. Ball

References

1. Hübner U, Shaw T, Thye J, Egbert N, de Fatima Marin, Chang P, O´Connor S, Day K, Honey M, Blake R, Hovenga E, Skiba D, Ball MJ. Technology informatics guiding education reform—TIGER—an international recommendations framework of core competencies in health informatics for nurses. Methods Inf Med 2018;57(Open 1):e30–42. https://doi.org/10.3414/ME17-01-0155
2. Hübner U, Thye J, Shaw T, Elias B, Egbert N, Saranto K, Babitsch B, Procter P, Ball MJ. Towards the TIGER international framework for recommendations of core competencies in health informatics 2.0: extending the scope and the roles. Stud Health Technol Inform. 2019;264:1218–22. https://doi.org/10.3233/SHTI190420
3. Mantas J, Ammenwerth E, Demiris G, Hasman A, Haux R, Hersh W, Hovenga E, Lun KC, Marin H, Martin-Sanchez F, Wright G. Recommendations of the International Medical Informatics Association (IMIA) on Education in Biomedical and Health Informatics. Methods Inf Med. 2010; 49:105–20.
4. Global Health Workforce Council (GHWC), Global Academic Curricula Competencies for Health Information Professionals, Chicago: The AHIMA Foundation. http://www.ahima.org/about/global/global-curricula
5. Kulikowski CA, Shortliffe EH, Currie LM, et al. AMIA Board white paper: definition of biomedical informatics and specification of core competencies for graduate education in the discipline. J Am Med Inform Assoc. 2012;19(6):931–8. https://doi.org/10.1136/amiajnl-2012-001053
6. Valenta AL, Berner ES, Boren SA, et al. AMIA Board White Paper: AMIA 2017 core competencies for applied health informatics education at the master's degree level. J Am Med Inform Assoc. 2018;25(12):1657–68. https://doi.org/10.1093/jamia/ocy132
7. American Association of Colleges of Nursing. The essentials: core competencies for Professional Nursing Education. April 6th, 2021. https://www.aacnnursing.org/Portals/42/AcademicNursing/pdf/Essentials-2021.pdf

Acknowledgments

Special Acknowledgement

We would like to acknowledge the outstanding contribution of Dr. Marion J. Ball, the globally renowned scholar and educator, to the health informatics arena and her and continuing inspiration. Her foundational work on this book and all editions that followed have become standard texts in nursing schools across North America and around the world, and established a new way of training nurses to enable them to respond rapidly, safely, and efficiently to the needs of the patient by using data, information, knowledge, and technology.

Dr. Ball's reputation is grounded in her long-standing and remarkable contributions to the international scientific community. She was the first American and first woman to be elected President of the International Medical Informatics Association (IMIA), the globally most influential association in biomedical and health informatics. Dr. Ball is one of the very few experts in health informatics worldwide who has gained unprecedented recognition and acceptance. In her early work dating back to the 1970s, she introduced landmark developments such as the importance of computer training, having nurses present in the decision-making process, as well as the involvement of health professionals from all disciplines to integrate informatics with the ultimate goal of improving patient care. These developments seem self-evident to us today, but we also know these highly relevant processes were cutting edge in previous decades.

In January 2005, a core group of prominent nursing leaders, dubbed the "*TIGER* Team" for *T*echnology *I*nformatics *G*uiding *E*ducational *R*eform, agreed that "utilizing informatics" is a core competency for healthcare professionals in the twenty-first century as cited by the Institute of Medicine (IOM) in Health Professions Education: A Bridge to Quality. There was also agreement that the majority of nurses lacked IT skills and the use of informatics competencies in their roles. Dr. Ball served as the catalyst for the global TIGER Initiative coming into existence as she is a founding member of this grassroots effort. This initiative formally began in 2006 within the nursing community and received support from over 70 contributing organizations and financial support from the Robert Wood Johnson Foundation. TIGER was formed to engage and prepare the nursing workforce in using technology and informatics to improve the delivery of patient care. In 2014, TIGER transitioned into the Healthcare Information and Management Systems Society (HIMSS), a global nonprofit organization with the mission to "reform the global health ecosystem through the power of information and technology." With this transition came a shift to a new interprofessional, competency-based approach. Dr. Marion J. Ball continues to play an essential role by mentoring and providing leadership to the next generation of "TIGERs." Nearly 15 years after TIGER's founding, 29 countries are represented by over 60 volunteers from all over the world.

The HIMSS TIGER Interprofessional community has a membership base of over 3,000 and growing. Today, the spirit of TIGER continues to support a learning health system that maximizes the integration of technology and informatics into seamless practice, education, research, and resource development.

Dr. Ball has received numerous coveted academic, national, and international awards for her contribution to the medical and information technology industry. In 1993, she was the recipient of the Distinguished Service Award from the American Health Information Management Association (AHIMA).

In 2002, she received the Morris F. Collen Lifetime Achievement Award from the American College of Medical Informatics (ACMI)/the American Medical Informatics Association (AMIA). In 2003, she was made an honorary member of Sigma Theta Tau International, and in 2008, she was inducted as Honorary Fellow of the American Academy of Nursing (AAN). In 2010, Dr. Ball received the Award of Excellence, an IMIA Lifetime Achievement award. In 2011, she was selected as one of the 50 most influential IT professionals by the HIMSS over the last 50 years, and in February 2014, she was given the Lifetime Membership Award by HIMSS for 30 years of service and significant contributions to the field of health informatics. In 2017, she was recognized by HIMSS as one of the Most Influential Women in Health IT. Also, in 2017, she was named one of the Most Powerful Women in Healthcare IT by Health Data Management.

Dr. Ball's innovative ideas are continuously inspiring—moving people and projects forward with passion, grace, and extraordinary results. Not only is she an exceptional leader, teacher, and mentor, she is an exceptional human being who is kind, inclusive, and incredibly giving to all who cross her path. Through her brilliant influence, vision, and courage that led to profound changes, Dr. Marion J. Ball has categorically impacted the global health IT/informatics field for decades to come.

Ursula H. Hübner
Gabriela M. Wilson
Toria Shaw Morawski

Contribution by members of the Technology Informatics Guiding Education Reform (TIGER) Initiative

The fifth edition of *Nursing Informatics* was significantly shaped by members of the Technology Informatics Guiding Education Reform (TIGER) initiative. Through their contributions, this book features the interprofessional, intergenerational, and global perspective, which is TIGER's core vision. Learning and teaching health and nursing informatics across professions, regions, countries, and continents is the motivation that unites the diverse group of TIGER's health informatics specialists with their varied backgrounds.

The editors, therefore, wish to give special credit to the authors who are members of the global TIGER network. The following table highlights the chapters that reflect their broad knowledge, engagement, and innovative thinking.

Authors	Chapters
Hübner, Wilson, Shaw Morawski, Ball	Nursing Informatics through the Lens of Interprofessional and Global Health Informatics
Wilson, Obasanya	Principles of Health Informatics
Reich	The Physician's View: Healthcare Digital Transformation Priorities
Franky, Fung	The Pharmacist's View: Patient-Centered Care through the Lens of a Pharmacist
Schleyer	The Chief Nursing Informatics Officer's (CNIO) View: Strategic Nursing Leadership for Informatics-Power Health and Healthcare
Abdelhak, Händel	The View of Health Information Managers (HIM): Strategic Insights through Data Analytics
Shaw Morawski, Thye, Liston	The Educator's View: Global Needs for Health Informatics Education
Rauch, Hübner	Learning Health System: Concepts, Principles and Practice for Data-Driven Health
Herasevich, Lipatov, Pickering	EHR Data: Enabling Clinical Surveillance and Alerting
Saranto, Kinnunen, Liljamo, Mykkänen, Kuusisto, Kivekäs	Interprofessional Structured Data: Supporting the Primary and Secondary Use of Patient Documentation
Hinton-Walker, Walker	Citizen Generated Data: Opening new Doors in Health IT Research and Practice
Ozkaynak, Skiba	Data Analytics, Artificial Intelligence and Data Visualization
Sensmeier	Interoperability: There is no Digital Health without Health IT Standards
DuBose-Morris, Chike-Harris, Garber, Shimek, Stroud	Telehealth: Reaching out to patients and providers
Händel, Abdelhak	Practice and Legal issues: Clinical Documentation, Data Ownership, Access and Patient Rights
Hübner, Egbert, Schulte	Ethical Issues: Patients, Providers and Systems
Troseth, Christopherson	Innovative Strategies for Interprofessional Leadership
Elias, Stephens, Pitts	Disrupting Healthcare through Innovations in Information and Communications Technology
Shaw Morawski, Liang	The TIGER Initiative: Global, Interprofessional Health Informatics Workforce Development
Klinedinst	Preparing the Health Informatics Workforce for the Future
Thate, Brookshire	Health Informatics Education: Standards, Challenges, and Tools
Delaney, Peisja, Brandt	Interprofessional Practice and Education: Core Data Set and Information Exchange Infrastructure
Marin, Ciqueto Peres	Brazil: Information Communication and Technology for nurses and patient care delivery
Akindele, Okuzu, Olaniran	Nigeria: Interprofessional Health Informatics Collaboration
Justinia	Saudi Arabia: Transforming Healthcare with Technology

Many other renowned contributors are featured in this edition. These authors infuse their rich and interdisciplinary expertise in the field of health informatics through their unique experiences and impressive backgrounds to seamlessly augment the TIGER perspective throughout this textbook.

Contents

About the Authors

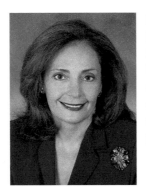

Mervat Abdelhak, PhD, MSIS, RHIA, FAHIMA Emeritus Professor Department of Health Information Management (HIM), University of Pittsburgh, USA, after having served as Chair since 1986, spearheaded the development of one of the first master's degree program as well as doctoral degree studies for HIM and Health professionals.

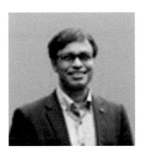

Ashir Ahmed, PhD is Associate Professor at the Faculty of Information Science and Electrical Engineering in Kyushu University Japan. His research aims to produce technologies to achieve social goals. After receiving PhD from Tohoku University in 1999, he worked with Avaya Labs (former Bell Labs), and NTT Communications, Japan.

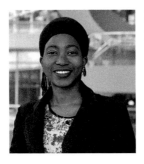

Bilikis J. Oladimeji, MD, MMCi, CPHIMS is a physician and healthcare informatics professional with experience in clinical medicine, Clinical Research, Pharmaceutical and Life Sciences. She obtained her medical degree from the College of Medicine, University of Lagos, Nigeria, in 2010 and a Master in Management in Clinical Informatics from Duke University, Fuqua School of Business, in 2013, USA. She currently serves as the Senior Director Health Informatics at Optum.

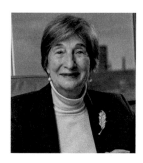

Marion J. Ball, EdD, FACMI, FAAN, FIAHSI, FHIMSS is the Raj and Indra Nooyi Endowed Distinguished Chair in Bioengineering and Presidential Distinguished Professor and Executive Director of the Multi-Interprofessional Center for Health Informatics (MICHI) at the University of Texas at Arlington, USA. She is Professor Emerita at Johns Hopkins University in the School of Nursing and has a joint appointment in the Division of Health Sciences Informatics in the Johns Hopkins University School of Medicine. She is a member of the National Academy of Medicine (NAM), served on the Board of Health on the Net (HON) in Geneva, Switzerland, and was elected as member of the IBM Industry Academy. Currently, Dr. Ball works both nationally and internationally on patient safety, nursing informatics, the electronic health record, and enabling technologies as it applies to clinical point of care initiatives.

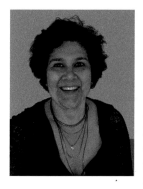

Sayonara de Fatima F. Barbosa, RN, PhD is an Associate Professor at the Federal University of Santa Catarina, Brazil, with a post-doctorate in nursing informatics at the University of Michigan School of Nursing. She teaches different courses in Undergraduate and Graduate Programs in Nursing. She is Vice-Coordinator of Professional Master's Program in Health Informatics. She is currently developing research in health informatics applications to improve patient safety, with interest in predictive modeling, Internet of things, and social network analysis.

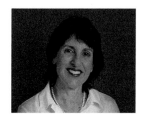

Haya Barkai, MBA is the Deputy CIO and Director of the Clinical Application and Digital Services Department in the Division of Health Information Technology at Maccabi Healthcare Services, Israel. She is responsible for electronic health record applications, tele-radiology, and telemedicine communication applications at Maccabi. She manages the development of organizational portals, the interactive patient website, and application where members can access their personalized health information, interact with their clinician, and make appointments.

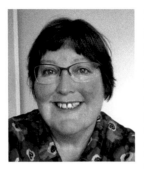

Nessa Barry, RGN, BSc is the Knowledge Exchange Manager, with the International Engagement Team, Technology Enabled Care and Digital Healthcare Innovation, Digital Health and Care Directorate, Scottish Government, UK. Prior to joining the team in 2019, Nessa worked with the national Scottish Centre for Telehealth and Telecare (SCTT). Nessa originally trained as a Registered General Nurse (London) before undertaking a Health Science BSc.

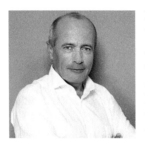

Dieter Baumberger, RN, NEd, MNS, PhD works as head of development and research at LEP AG, Switzerland. Key areas of knowledge and experience are the design of classification systems according to different purposes and principles, the linking of health interventions in the care and treatment process, mappings between classification systems of health interventions, the multipurpose use of data from electronic patient documentation, payments per case, and performance-based care financing.

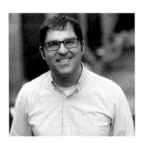

Andrew F. Beck, MD is Associate Professor at the University of Cincinnati College of Medicine and an attending physician in the Divisions of General and Community Pediatrics and Hospital Medicine at Cincinnati Children's Hospital Medical Center, USA. He received his BA in Anthropology from Yale University, his MD from the University of Pittsburgh School of Medicine, and his MPH from Harvard University, USA. He completed residency and fellowship training at Cincinnati Children's. Dr. Beck's research aims to equitably improve child health outcomes by addressing key social determinants of health. Dr. Beck has a lead role in the hospital's Community Health Initiative which strives to, together with families and the community, help Cincinnati's kids to stay and become healthy.

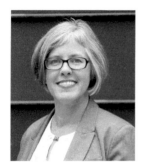

Marianne Behrends, PhD is a senior researcher at the Peter L. Reichertz Institute for Medical Informatics of TU Braunschweig and Hannover Medical School in Hannover, Lower Saxony, Germany. She has led the research group "e-learning for technology enhanced teaching and learning." Since 1997 she has developed a series of e-learning applications for facilitating learning processes through computer technologies and conducted research in the field of digital skills in medical education and integration of digital learning into nursing workflows.

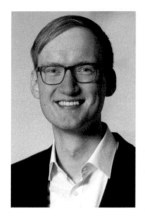

Nils-Hendrik Benning, MSc is a research associate at the Institute of Medical Biometry and Informatics at Heidelberg University Hospital, Germany. His research focuses on using patient-generated data, especially from wearables, for research and care. Prior to his affiliation with Heidelberg University, he worked in a product management department of a company producing cardiology documentation software. He received his master's degree in medical informatics at Heidelberg University.

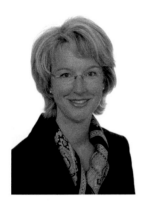

Hendrike Berger, MA, MSc, PhD is a professor for Health Economics at Osnabrück University of Applied Sciences, Germany.Ever since studying abroad herself and working in the international project management of a pharmaceutical company, she has been particularly interested in international comparisons and what healthcare systems and citizens can learn from other countries. Each year since 2010, she has been conducting binational seminars, merging students from Osnabrück and US students from partner University of Southern Indiana, for summer/winter schools on healthcare system comparison involving collaborative study, health facilities tours, and cultural experiences.

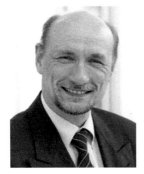

Oliver J. Bott, PhD   received his PhD in Medical Informatics from Technical University of Braunschweig, Germany. He is Professor of Medical Informatics of the University of Applied Sciences and Arts in Hannover (HsH). He was the founding director of the E-Learning Services Center and Chief Information Officer/Vice President for research, IT, and information management at the HsH. His research and lecturing focuses on information systems in healthcare and clinical research, especially architectural concepts and methods and tools for analyzing, developing, and managing such systems, and on e-learning in medicine and medical informatics.

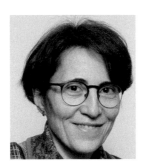

Célia Boyer, PhD   As a widely recognized specialist in the quality assessment of online medical information, Célia Boyer from Switzerland is on expert panels for international medical conferences and working groups and is active in European Union research activities as well as collaborates on project internationally in the USA and other countries. She is the author of over 70 scientific publications in peer-reviewed scientific journals and author of several chapters in books, including *eHealth: Legal, Ethical and Governance Challenges*.

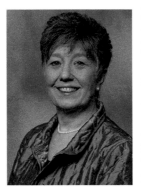

Barbara Fifield Brandt, PhD, EdM, FNAP   is the Founding Director of the National Center for Interprofessional Practice and Education at the University of Minnesota (UMN), USA. Established in 2012, the National Center is a public–private partnership funded and founded by a cooperative agreement with the Health Resources and Services Administration in addition to grants and contracts from the Josiah Macy Jr. Foundation, the Robert Wood Johnson Foundation, and the Gordon and Betty Moore Foundation. Dr. Brandt is a tenured professor in the UMN College of Pharmacy, Department of Pharmaceutical Care and Health Systems.

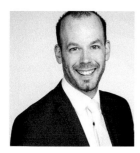

Bernhard Breil, PhD is a medical computer scientist and psychologist and professor for health informatics in the Faculty of Health Care at the Hochschule Niederrhein. In teaching, he is primarily active in the Medical Informatics program and teaches lectures such as clinical IT systems, system integration, and IT project management. His research focuses on the socio-technical aspects at the interface between humans and IT, where, in addition to technical aspects, the effects of these aspects on humans are also investigated. Further research topics are the networking of medical information systems and the acceptance of eHealth applications.

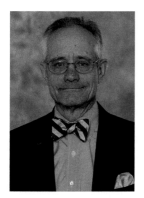

Robert G. Brookshire, PhD is Director of the Master of Health Information Technology Program at the University of South Carolina, USA. He holds a PhD from Emory University and has previously taught at the University of North Texas, James Madison University, the University of Virginia, and New York University USA.

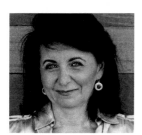

Shawna Butler, RN, MBA is a nurse economist and the EntrepreNURSE-in-Residence at Radboud University Medical Center, the Netherlands. She is part of the Exponential Medicine team at Singularity University. Her portfolio of projects includes implementing an enterprise-wide digital radiology solution and creating an international emergency medicine training rotation between a US medical school and a New Zealand hospital system. Her clinical nursing experience includes emergency, cardiac, critical care, international medical flight transport, and workplace wellness.

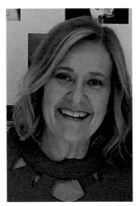

Heloisa Helena Ciqueto Peres, RN, MA, PhD is a Full Professor at the School of Nursing, University of São Paulo, and was the Director of the Department of Nursing, University Hospital, University of São Paulo, Brazil. She is the leader of the Research Group on Information Technology in Nursing at the National Council for Scientific and Technological Development- Brazil. She also serves as a nursing counselor of the Regional Council of Nursing—São Paulo, Brazil.

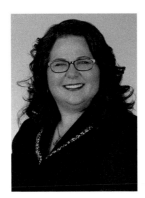

Katherine E. Chike-Harris, BS, BSN, MSN, DNP holds degrees in chemistry (BS 1991) and nursing [BSN 2007, MSN (pediatrics) 2009, and DNP 2011. She is currently an assistant professor at the Medical University of South Carolina (MUSC), USA, College of Nursing, where she teaches in the Doctor of Nursing Practice program and is leading the integration of telehealth education into its nursing curriculum. In addition to teaching, Dr. Chike-Harris is a practicing certified pediatric nurse practitioner with the MUSC Center for Telehealth's school-based health clinics, providing acute care to children across the state of South Carolina in the school setting using synchronous telehealth.

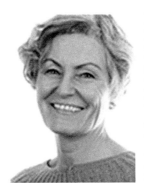

Bente Christensen, RN Cand Nursing Science, PhD, holds a position as Senior Adviser on E-health at the Norwegian Nurses Organisation, and as Associate Professor at the Faculty of Nursing and Health Sciences at Nord University in Norway. Her main working field is in terminologies and structuring of nursing documentation. She has been working as a clinical nurse mainly on an orthopedic surgery ward, where she later had positions as head nurse and head of department. Her PhD is from the Artic University of Norway, Tromsø, and is on the user's role in the developing and scaling an information infrastructure for healthcare based on the openEHR specification.

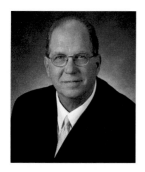

Charles E. Christian, LFCHIME, LFHIMSS, CHCIO, is the Vice President of Technology and CTO for Franciscan Alliance, a thirteen-hospital system serving Indiana and Illinois.Previously, he served as the Vice President of Technology and Engagement at the Indiana Health Information Exchange. He also served as the VP/Chief Information Officer of St. Francis Hospital, a position he held for 2.5 years. Before his role at St. Francis, Mr. Christian served as the VP/CIO for Good Samaritan Hospital, in Vincennes, Indiana, a position he held for 24 years. Mr. Christian started his career in healthcare as a Registered Radiologic Technologist, serving in various roles for 14 years.

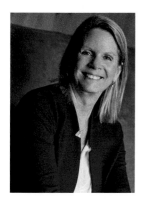

Tracy Christopherson, PhD-c, MS, BAS, RRT is the cofounder of MissingLogic, a US-American consulting and coaching company. She is an advocate for interprofessional collaborative practice and has mentored/coached healthcare leaders across North America to develop and sustain interprofessional collaborative practice work environments. She is also a doctoral candidate in Interprofessional Healthcare Studies at Rosalind Franklin University of Medicine and Science in North Chicago, IL, USA.

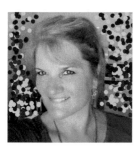

Grace T. M. Dal Sasso, RN, PhD is an Associate Professor at the Federal University of Santa Catarina Brazil, with a background in health informatics and as a post-doctorate in medical informatics at the School of Health Information Sciences at Houston—USA. She serves as the coordinator of the Professional Master's Program in Health Informatics.

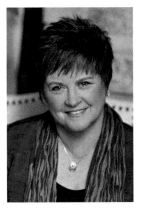

Connie White Delaney, PhD, RN, FAAN, FACMI, FNAP serves as Professor NS Dean, School of Nursing, University of Minnesota, Minneapolis, MN, USA. She is the Knowledge Generation Lead for the National Center for Interprofessional Practice and Education located at the University of Minnesota. She serves as an adjunct professor in the Faculty of Medicine and Faculty of Nursing at the University of Iceland, where she received the Doctor Scientiae Curationis Honoris Causa (Honorary Doctor of Philosophy in Nursing) in 2011. She holds a BSN with majors in nursing and mathematics, MA in Nursing, and PhD Educational Administration and Computer Applications.

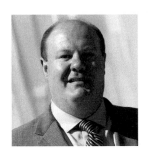

Brian E. Dixon, PhD, MPA is the Director of Public Health Informatics, Regenstrief Institute, Inc., and an Associated Professor at the Indiana University Richard M. Fairbanks School of Public Health at IUPUI. Dr. Dixon's research focuses on applying informatics methods and tools to improve population health in clinical as well as public health organizations. His work leverages clinical and administrative data in electronic health records to measure population health, better understand the determinants of health, examine information flow in the health system, and improve outcomes in individuals and populations. Dr. Dixon also teaches informatics courses to future clinical as well as public health leaders, and he regularly mentors junior informatics professionals.

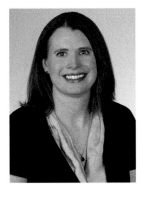

Ragan DuBose-Morris, PhD is an Associate Professor at Medical University of South Carolina USA (MUSC) and the Director of Telehealth Education at the Center for Telehealth, where she is responsible for implementing telehealth services through virtual, distance, and in-person systems while developing educational programs for healthcare students and professionals. She holds an EdS and PhD in Computing Technology in Education from Nova Southeastern University, USA.

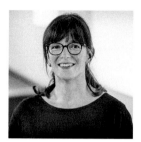

Nicole Egbert, MA is a research fellow in the Health Informatics Research Group at Osnabrück University of Applied Sciences, Germany. Her research focuses on competency development of health professionals in the context of medical and health informatics to improve information continuity and patient safety in healthcare through online-based continuing education. Prior to her academic work, she studied Business Management in the Health Sector and Healthcare Management, also at the Osnabrück University of Applied Sciences.

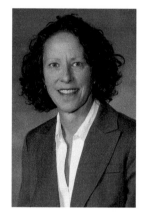

Beth L. Elias, PhD, MS, FHIMSS completed her PhD in Instructional Technology at the Curry School of Education at the University of Virginia (UVA) with a research focus on user satisfaction with healthcare information systems. Dr. Elias also received an MS in the Management of Information Technology from the McIntire School of Commerce at UVA and a BS in Computer Science from the State University of New York Institute of Technology. Prior to returning to graduate school, she worked as a computer systems and information engineer primarily in healthcare and biomedical research. Her research interests include the effective use of information technology in healthcare such as point-of-care testing devices and electronic medical records.

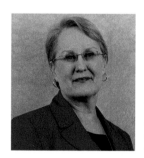

Susan H. Fenton, PhD, RHIA, CPHI, FAHIMA is an Associate Professor and Associate Dean for Academic and Curricular Affairs at the University of Texas School of Biomedical Informatics in Houston, TX. She is responsible for their certificate, master's, and doctoral degree programs. Dr. Fenton recently led the development of a practice doctorate in health informatics(DHI). She received the UT Regents' Outstanding Teacher Award and the Texas Health Information Management Association Legacy Award in 2019. In 2020, Dr. Fenton was inducted into the UT Shine Academy of Master Teachers and named a Distinguished Teaching Professor. Dr. Fenton has received $7 million in grant funding and serves on a variety of regional and national committees. Dr. Fenton has more than 30 years' experience in health informatics and information management. She holds a BS in health information management from UTMB in Galveston, an MBA from the University of

Houston, and a PhD in health services research from Texas A&M.

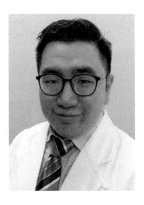

Franky is a practicing pharmacist who has previously worked at Woodlands Health Campus, Singapore, and was involved in implementing electronic health records within the country's public healthcare system. He received his Bachelor of Pharmacy (Honors) from Monash University, Australia. He is currently pursuing the Master of Health Care (Digital Health) at the Savonia University of Applied Sciences, Finland. Franky is board certified in geriatric pharmacy.

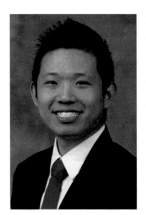

Brian K. Fung, BS, PharmD, MPH is a Medication Management Informaticist at Mayo Clinic and a former Graduate Student Intern at the Office of the National Coordinator for Health Information Technology (ONC). At Mayo, he was responsible for the implementation of the Antimicrobial Stewardship and Infection Control programs into the Epic electronic health record. He received his BS in Human Nutrition and PharmD from the University of Florida and his MPH from the Johns Hopkins Bloomberg School of Public Health, USA. Brian is board certified in pharmacotherapy and has also received additional training in antimicrobial stewardship through MAD-ID. Brian holds academic appointments as an Instructor of Pharmacy at the Mayo Clinic School of Health Sciences and a Clinical Assistant Professor at the University of Florida College of Pharmacy, USA.

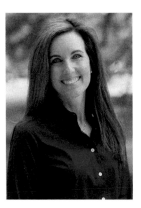

Kelli Garber, MSN, APRN, PPCNP-BC is the Lead Advanced Practice Provider and Clinical Integration Specialist for the Medical University of South Carolina Center for Telehealth, USA. In addition to overseeing the clinical operations of the Medical University of South Carolina (MUSC) School-Based Health Program (USA), she provides care via telehealth to children across the state of South Carolina. She also provides telehealth education and consultative services to healthcare providers as they implement telemedicine in their respective disciplines. Kelli Garber is Co-Chair of the National Health Policy Committee.

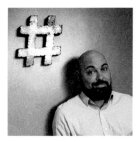

Michael A. Gaspar, BA is a Social Media Program Manager at the Health Information Management Systems Society (HIMSS) based in Chicago, IL, USA. In this role, he manages end-to-end social media programming—including website optimization, program and content strategy, social advertising, program execution oversight, outcome analysis, and innovation initiatives—to engage and delight health IT audiences across the nonprofit and media sides of the business.

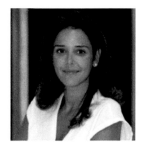

Nadine Hachach-Haram, MD, FRCS, BEM is an NHS surgeon, lecturer, and clinical entrepreneur. Nadine founded Proximie, an augmented reality platform that improves access to expert care and scales clinical expertise. Nadine was the recipient of the British Empire Medal in the Queen's Birthday Honours for 2018. She is a member of the Royal College of Surgeons' Commission on the Future of Surgery, which aims to investigate the advances that will transform surgery over the next 20 years. She is also the Clinical Lead for Innovation at Guy's and St. Thomas' NHS Foundation Trust, London, UK.

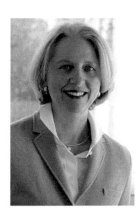

Angelika Haendel, MA holds a bachelor's degree in applied health sciences and a master's degree in healthcare management. Her field of work comprises clinical documentation and health information management, DRG controlling, quality management, and integrated care projects at the University Hospital of Erlangen, Germany. Between 2013 and 2016, she was president of the International Federation of Health Information Management Associations (IFHIMA) and has been serving on the Global Health Workforce of the American Health Information Management Association (AHIMA).

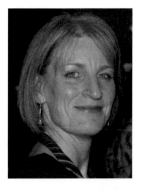

Donna Lesley Henderson, DipCOT, SROT is the Head of the International Engagement Team in the Technology Enabled Care & Digital Healthcare Innovation Division of the Digital Health and Care Directorate, Scottish Government, UK. She has been a Coordinator of the European Innovation Partnership on Active and Health Ageing B3 Action Group on Integrated Care since 2012. Donna is Chair of the Digital Health Network of the Assembly of European Regions (AER).

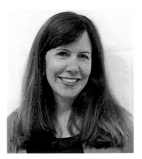

Adrienne W. Henize, JD manages partnerships between health clinics and community partners at Cincinnati Children's Hospital Medical Center, USA, including the Child Health-Law Partnership (Child HeLP). Her work focuses on building, implementing, and sustaining partnerships with community organizations and evaluating their impact on child health. She also actively assists with resident physician education around issues related to social determinants of health and poverty. She earned a law degree from Washington University in St. Louis and a journalism degree from Boston University, USA.

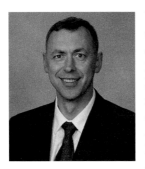

Vitaly Herasevich, MD, PhD, MSc is Professor of Anesthesiology and Medicine in the Department of Anesthesiology and Perioperative Medicine, Division of Critical Care, Mayo Clinic, Rochester, Minnesota, USA. He has been involved in medical informatics for over 20 years, with a specific concentration on applied clinical informatics in critical care. He codirects the Clinical Informatics Intensive Care laboratory that works to decrease complications and improve outcomes for critically ill patients through applied clinical informatics and quality improvement.

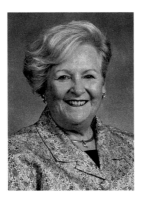

Patricia Hinton Walker, PhD, RN, FAAN, MCC, CBCC is an accomplished coach at MentorCoach, LLC, in Bethesda, MD, USA, and teaches informatics, leadership, and health promotion in national schools of nursing. Pat served as a dean and recently as Dean in the Graduate School of Nursing then later as university Vice President at Uniformed Services University, in the Department of Defense, USA, where she is Professor Emeritus. As former Dean of the School of Nursing at the University of Colorado, USA, she was instrumental in advancing online education and the use of technology to improve quality and safety in healthcare.

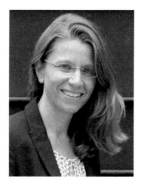

Ina Hoffmann, MSc is a medical computer scientist and research associate at the Peter L. Reichertz Institute for Medical Informatics of TU Braunschweig and Hannover Medical School in Hannover, Germany. Her research interests are in the field of health information systems and of competencies needed by medical professionals in a digitalized healthcare system.

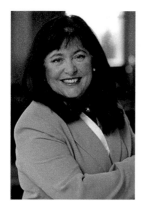

Krysia W. Hudson, RN, DNP, BC is a leader in informatics practice and education and Assistant Professor working at Johns Hopkins School of Nursing Baltimore MD USA. She is a member of the innovative team that has implemented a bedside computer system at Johns Hopkins Hospital (SICU) and configured an electronic health record system (EHR) for use in the school baccalaureate program, the first in the USA. In addition, she created the Electronic Teaching Assistant (TA), an online supplemental educational resource, and helped co-create the first completely online class for nursing students. Her work has had practical application for students and public health nurses alike.

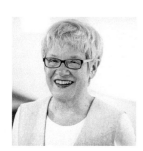

Ursula H. Hübner, PhD, FIAHSI is a professor of medical and health informatics and quantitative methods at the University of Applied Sciences, Osnabrück, Germany, where she also serves as academic dean for digitalization and the promotion of young scientists. She is head of the Health Informatics Research Group that focuses on health IT maturity, adoption and diffusion studies, recommendations for health informatics education, development of IT standards for continuity of care, and clinical decision support systems. Prior to returning to academia, she had worked in the research department of an international computer company with headquarters in Paris, France. Ursula received her PhD from the Department of Natural Sciences and Mathematics Düsseldorf University, Germany, on a thesis combining informatics and neuroscience.

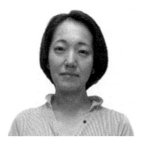

Rieko Izukura, PhD is an Assistant Professor/ Registered nurse of Medical Information Center at Kyushu University Hospital, Japan. She received PhD in nursing at Kyushu University after nursing experiences in cancer medicine and intensive care field. Her research interest is health promotion and patient-reported outcomes (PROs)/quality of life (QOL) for cancer patients/survivors.

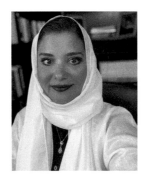

Taghreed Justinia, PhD is the founding Regional Director IT Services, Technology & Health Informatics Department at King Saud bin Abdulaziz University for Health Sciences (KSAU-HS), Saudi Arabia, where she is also (Joint Appointment) Assistant Professor of Health Informatics and Director for the Master's in Health Informatics Program in the Western Region. Taghreed Justinia holds a PhD in Health Informatics and an MSc in Healthcare Management from Swansea University, UK. She studied Computer Science in the USA as an undergraduate, and has maintained a career in the IT field that spans almost 20 years in executive IT positions in healthcare, including senior IT roles at the Saudi Arabian Ministry of Health and the Ministry of National Guard, Health Affairs.

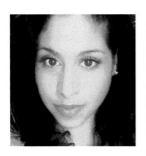

Jamila S. Karim, BM, BMedSc served as the Head of Research & Strategic Development at Proximie, an augmented reality platform. She is a UK-based physician with a background in trauma and orthopedic surgery and clinical trials research. She undertook a research mentorship at the University of Toronto and an internship at the IBM Toronto Software Laboratory, Canada. Among others, her research focuses on applying simulation models to assess the effectiveness of quarantine measures on disease spread.

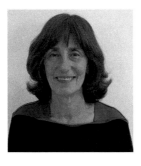

Rachelle Kaye, PhD is the International Projects Coordinator for Assuta Medical Centers, Israel, as well as a member of the core team for implementing digitally enabled integrated care. She was the Deputy Director of the Medical Department (1984–2003) of Maccabi Healthcare Services, Israel's second largest HMO, where she was actively involved in the implementation of Health IT from the start. She established and directed the

Maccabi Institute for Health Services Research until 2013. Dr. Kaye is a member of the Board of Directors of EHTEL (the European Health Telematics Association) and acts as a consultant to a number of Israeli and European Organizations, particularly in the area of integrated care and eHealth.

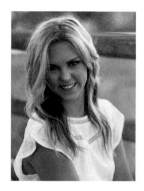

Grace Kennedy is a young consumer advocate on a mission to put health information in the hands of the consumer. Grace is actively engaged in creating awareness on the importance of the use of personal health information (PHI) to support continuity of care and improve health outcomes. She has presented at conferences in France, Sweden, and the USA. Grace is a former Blue Cross Blue Shield, Louisiana Quality Forum "My Health My Way" winner.

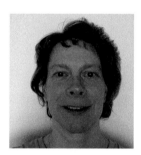

Joan M. Kiel, PhD, CHPS is Chairman, University HIPAA Compliance and Professor of Health Management Systems, Duquesne University, Pittsburgh, PA, USA. She is coeditor of the book *Healthcare Information Management Systems*, now in its fifth edition. Previously, Dr. Kiel worked at Lutheran Medical Center, Brooklyn, New York, and the Pittsburgh Mercy Health System, Pittsburgh, Pennsylvania, USA.

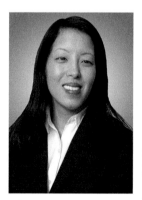

Lee Kim, JD, CISSP, CIPP/US, FHIMSS is the Director of Thought Advisory at the Healthcare Information and Management Systems Society (HIMSS), USA. Lee serves as an analyst with the United States Department of Homeland Security Analytic Exchange Program (AEP). She is a licensed attorney and registered patent attorney. Lee is an AV Preeminent peer review rated attorney. Lee also holds cybersecurity and information privacy certifications: CISSP and CIPP/US. She authors domestic and international works on topics that include information privacy, cybersecurity, law, and public policy.

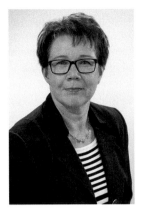

Ulla-Mari Kinnunen, PhD, RN is Adjunct Professor and Senior Lecturer in Health and Human Services Informatics at the University of Eastern Finland. Her experience is in terminology development, evidence-based practice (EBP), and informatics competencies. She is a core staff member of the Finnish Centre for Evidence-Based Health Care: A Joanna Briggs Institute (JBI) Centre of Excellence, a member of the Centre´s review panel, and an accredited trainer of JBI comprehensive systematic review training program.

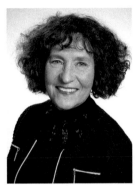

Eija Kivekäs, PhD, RN is a nurse manager (Primary Health Care) and postdoctoral researcher in Health and Human Services Informatics at the University of Eastern Finland, Department of Health and Social Management. Dr. Kivekäs has coordinated several clinical development projects and worked as a project manager for several years. Her research interest is the role of patient safety in electronic health records as well as competencies and management issues in information system implementation.

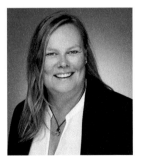

Andrea Diana Klausen, RN, Dipl.-Päd worked as a registered nurse for 14 years in the intensive care area of cardiothoracic and vascular surgery at Hannover Medical School, Germany. After studying education at the University of Hannover, Germany, she worked as a language educator in a practice and clinic before moving into teaching nursing. In 2020, she changed from the Carl-von-Ossietzky University Oldenburg, where she had worked since 2016, to the Institute for Medical Informatics at the University Hospital RWTH Aachen, Germany.

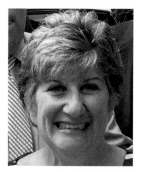

JoAnn Klinedinst, MEd, CPHIMS, PMP, CPTD, LFHIMSS, FACHE As vice president of professional development for the Health Information Management Systems Society (HIMSS), based in Chicago, IL, USA, JoAnn W. Klinedinst defines strategies that attribute to the lifelong learning, continuing engagement, and professional development for health information and technology professionals globally. A lifelong learner, she holds a master's in adult education from the Pennsylvania State University, USA. Ms. Klinedinst volunteers her time and serves on various boards nationally that promote the transformation of healthcare information and technology initiatives.

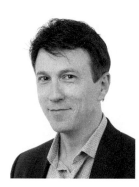

Daniel Kraft, MD is a physician-scientist, inventor, entrepreneur, and innovator and serves as the XPRIZE Pandemic Alliance Task Force Chair. With over 25 years of experience in clinical practice, biomedical research, and healthcare innovation, Kraft has chaired the Medicine for Singularity University since its inception in 2008, and is founder and chair of Exponential Medicine, a program that explores convergent, rapidly developing technologies and their potential in biomedicine and healthcare. Following undergraduate degrees from Brown University and medical school at Stanford, Daniel was board certified in both internal medicine and pediatrics after completing a Harvard residency at the Massachusetts General Hospital and Boston Children's Hospital, USA, and fellowships in hematology, oncology, and bone marrow transplantation at Stanford.

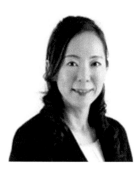

Kimiyo Kikuchi, PhD is a lecturer at the Faculty of Medical Sciences, Kyushu University, Japan. She received her PhD in Health Science. Her specialty areas are global health, HIV infection, and maternal and child health. She studied at the Graduate School of Medicine, University of Tokyo. Worked as a consultant of official development in the Japan International Cooperation Agency projects on maternal health, school health, and water and sanitation in Africa and the Middle East. She launched a project to improve the continuum of care on maternal and child health in Bangladesh using a telemedicine system by collaborating with Grameen Communications.

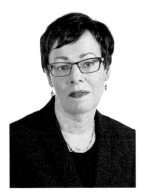

Anne Kuusisto, PhD, RN is a postdoctoral researcher. Her dissertation research was related to securing the continuity of patient care by means of an electronic nursing discharge summary. Her present research topics are continuity of care and advanced care planning.

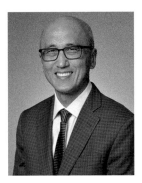

John Lee, MD is an emergency physician by training. He was initially drawn into health IT as a subject matter expert in the implementation of his hospital's emergency department information system in 2006. The combination of his physician and technical skills eventually led him to be appointed as chief medical information system at Edward-Elmhurst Health. Currently, he serves as the Chief Medical Information Officer at Allegheny Health Network, Pittsburgh, USA.

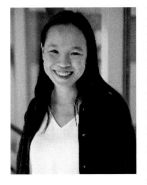

Man Qing Liang, Pharm D, MSc is pursuing a Master of Biomedical Informatics at Harvard Medical School. Previously, she obtained her Master of Health Services Administration from the Université de Montréal School of Public Health (Montréal, Canada) and served as the international TIGER Scholars Informatics Intern 2020–21. Her research focuses on studying technologies to optimize medication use, such as computerized provider order entry systems. Man Qing obtained her Doctorate of Pharmacy (Pharm D) from the Université de Montréal.

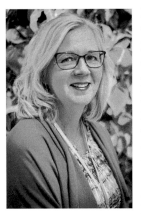

Pia Liljamo, PhD, RN postdoctoral researcher, works as a development manager at the national Health Village portal coordinating the planning of e-health services and the development of digital patient care paths at Oulu University Hospital, Finland. She has three decades of experience in patient care and the development of various healthcare services. Her dissertation research is focused on the agreement between clinical and administrative nursing data, and her postdoctoral research interests include nursing terminology and reuse of patient data, as well as the digitization of patient care and e-health services.

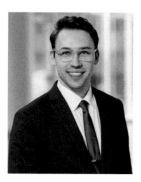

Kirill Lipatov, MD is a clinical pulmonary medicine and critical care fellow at the Mayo Clinic in Rochester, Minnesota, USA. He has an interest in applied critical care informatics with a focus on surveillance, monitoring, and early recognition.

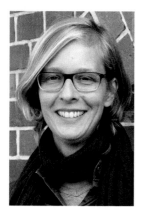

Myriam Lipprandt, PhD studied computer science specializing in medical informatics at the University of Hamburg, Germany. After finishing her doctoral thesis at the division of automation and measurement technology at the Carl von Ossietzky University, Oldenburg, Germany, she was an interim professor at the Jade University of Applied Sciences and post-doc scientist at the Department of Medical Informatics at the Carl von Ossietzky University of Oldenburg. She is currently deputy of the institute of medical informatics at the University Hospital RWTH Aachen, Germany, and head of the department for "Medical Software Engineering (MSE)."

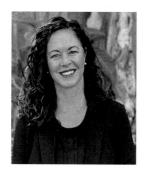

Jessica Liston, DNP, MS, RN-BC, CNOR, CPHIMS is the Clinical Informatics Coordinator for Sutter Health at the campuses of California Pacific Medical Center in San Francisco, California, USA. She completed her Master's in Nursing Administration from the Valley Foundation School of Nursing at San Jose State University and received her Doctor of Nursing Practice from the CSU Northern California Consortium. Her works continue to focus on optimizing nurse workflow, quality improvement, and decreasing documentation burden for clinicians.

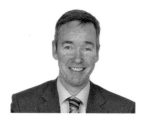

Thomas Lux, PhD is a professor for process management in healthcare at the Niederrhein University of Applied Sciences, Germany, where he founded the Competence Center eHealth. He holds a master's degree in business administration and economics from Ruhr University of Bochum, Germany, and received his PhD in the field of business informatics. His research is on various areas of process management and business intelligence in healthcare. He conducted research at Tongji University Shanghai, China. Furthermore, he is a member of the supervisory board of a hospital group.

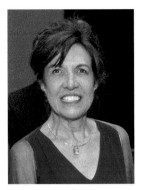

Heimar Marin, PhD, FACMI, FAAN, FIAHSI is the Editor-in-Chief of the *International Journal of Medical Informatics*, Elsevier. She is an Alumni Professor in Nursing and Health Informatics at the Federal University of Sao Paulo and the coordinator of the Certificate Program in Health Informatics at the Hospital Sirio Libanês, Sao Paulo, Brazil.

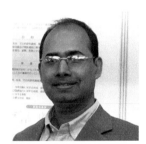

Rafiqul Islam Maruf, PhD is working as an Associate Professor at Medical Information Center of Kyushu University Hospital under Kyushu University, Japan. Besides, he has been working as a Director of Global Communication Center, the ICT-based R&D wing of Grameen Communications, Bangladesh, since 2009. Earlier Dr. Maruf worked in Japanese IT industries for 12 years after completing his PhD in Information Engineering in 1997 from Hokkaido University, Japan.

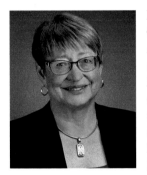

Ruth Metzger, PhD is retired faculty from the Center for Health Informatics, University of Texas, Arlington, USA. Her interests and research center on policy and practice surrounding substandard housing and its impact on population health. She continues to work as a consultant and advocate for safe, affordable housing in her home community of Evansville, Indiana, where she co-chairs the housing work group for Evansville's Promise Zone. Dr. Metzger earned her BA and MBA at Indiana University, Bloomington, her BSN at the University of Southern Indiana, and her PhD in Public Policy and Administration from Walden University, USA.

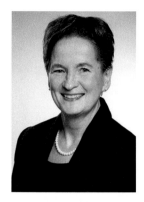

Minna Mykkänen, PhD, RN   is the Director of Nursing at Kuopio University Hospital, Finland. She has been involved in the implementation of the electronic patient record system (EPR), and she has been developing the EPR together with clinicians and the information system provider. She has worked as a development manager in the introduction of structured nursing documentation and nursing summary in the hospital. Her dissertation research focused on modeling the structural knowledge of nursing documentation and developing the primary and secondary use of this knowledge.

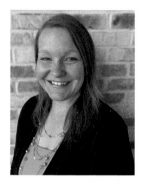

Rebecca Nally, **MHA, PMP** has worked in the healthcare field for over 15 years and is currently a Project Manager in Healthcare IT focusing on implementing and integrating the electronic medical record systems. She graduated with a bachelor's degree in health services and a master's in health administration at the University of Southern Indiana, USA. She earned her PMP after beginning work as a project manager.

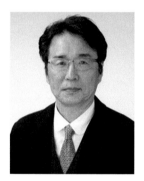

Naoki Nakashima, MD, PhD is the Director/ Professor (2014–) of the Medical Information Center of Kyushu University Hospital, and also Vice CIO of Kyushu University, Japan. He has been a specialist of diabetes mellitus for more than 30 years and simultaneously worked as a specialist of medical informatics for 18 years. Dr. Nakashima focuses on the disease management methodology and patient-engagement promotion of chronic diseases including among others personal health record (PHR) and telemedicine.

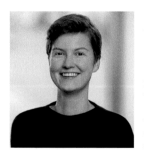

Laura Naumann, MA   is working as a research fellow and lecturer at the University of Applied Science Osnabrück at the Health Informatics Research Group. She has a background in management for health services. She is a PhD candidate at University Osnabrück/ Osnabrück University of Applied Sciences working on a dissertation thesis on "IT-Innovation in health care from an international perspective: Comparing health care." Her research field is national and international eHealth policy.

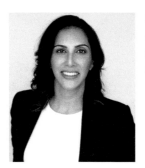

Geeta Nayyar is the General Manager Healthcare & Life Sciences and Executive Medical Director for Salesforce, a US-American software company.

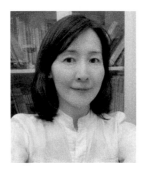

Mariko Nishikitani, BS, MS, MPH, PhD is a public health professional recognized by the Japanese Society of Public Health. She received her PhD in social medicine, BS and MS in food science, and MPH in public health. Throughout her career, her primary research interest was occupational health, mainly occupational injury, overtime work, workers' stress and mental health, health checkups, women's health, and social security system for workers. Dr. Nishikitani serves as a faculty at the Medical Information Center of Kyushu University Hospital, Japan, as a visiting scholar of Weatherhead East Asian Institute of Columbia University, USA, and as an Adjunct Associate Professor in the Erickson School of Aging Studies, University Maryland, Baltimore County, USA.

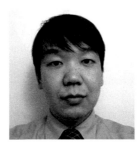

Yasunobu Nohara, PhD is an Associate Professor of Kumamoto University, Japan. He has a PhD of Engineering from Kyushu University and joined Kyushu University Hospital from 2010. He has been involved in Portable Health Clinic project from the beginning as informatician.

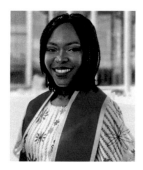

Mercy Obasanya is a graduate student in Public Health Epidemiology at the University of Texas at Arlington, USA. She is a Graduate Research Assistant at the Multi-Interprofessional Center for Health Informatics. Mercy Obasanya's research interests are in data analysis and public health research, maternal and child health research, and social determinants of health. Mercy Obasanya is a member of the Texas Public Health Association and strives to continue to gain research and data analysis skills to advance in public health and address health disparities in minority communities.

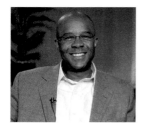

Okey Okuzu, BS, MBA holds a bachelor's degree in economics from the University of Lagos, Nigeria, and an MBA in Finance and Strategy from Columbia Business School, New York, USA. He founded InStrat Global Health Solutions in 2010 to focus on global health innovation by identifying and deploying technology-based healthcare solutions to underserved markets.He was a Strategy and Innovation lead at Novartis Pharmaceuticals Corp. where he was responsible for identifying opportunities to innovate its strategic Managed Markets business models. Prior to Novartis, Okey spent approximately ten years in leadership positions at Pfizer Inc's worldwide headquarters in New York developing business strategy for its lead division.

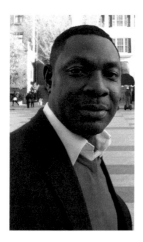

Oluwaseun Olaniran, MD is a family physician and health informaticist with over 13 years of clinical and health informatics experience. He is currently furthering his postgraduate training at the Department of Integrated Information Technology, University of South Carolina, Columbia, USA, where he is also a teaching assistant.

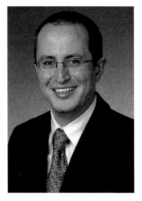

Mustafa Ozkaynak, PhD, FHIMSS is an associate professor at the University of Colorado (CU), College of Nursing, USA. His research interests include work systems in clinical and non-clinical health settings and the organizational and social consequences of health information technologies. He has utilized artificial intelligence and machine learning approaches to examine asthma treatment in pediatric emergency departments. He teaches courses on clinical decision support systems, system development life cycle, foundation of health informatics, knowledge management, and quantitative methods.

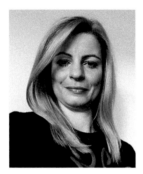

Andrea Pavlickova, PhD is the International Engagement Manager, TEC and Digital Healthcare Innovation Division, Digital Health and Care Directorate, Scottish Government, UK. She has managed the EU Public Health Programme funded projects SCIROCCO and SCIROCCO Exchange. Andrea is on the Board of the Network of European Regional and Local Health Authorities (EUREGHA).

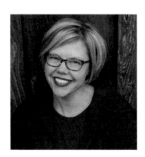

Laura Pejsa, PhD is the Director of Evaluation and Organizational Learning for the National Center for Interprofessional Practice and Education at the University of Minnesota, USA. Dr. Pejsa also serves as the lead evaluator on HRSA grants with the University of Minnesota Department of Family Medicine and Southern Illinois University-Edwardsville School of Nursing, USA. Dr. Pejsa holds a PhD in Educational Policy and Administration—Evaluation Studies from the University of Minnesota, USA.

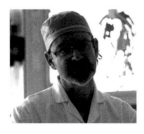

Brian W. Pickering, MD, MSc, FFARCSI is Associate Professor of Anesthesiology in the Department of Anesthesiology—Division of Critical Care, Mayo Clinic, Rochester, USA. Dr. Pickering was born in Dublin, Ireland. He completed his medical education at Trinity College, Dublin, prior to his residency and fellowship training in anesthesiology and critical care at the College of Anesthetists, Royal College of

Surgeons, Ireland. Dr. Pickering's primary research area is focused on application of clinical informatics to the task of improving patient health and outcomes while reducing medical costs. His group has developed bedside informatics tools for the intensive care patient population.

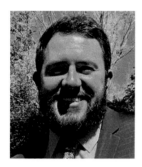

Jonathan Pitts, MSN, RN, CPHIMS is critical care RN and has been working as a nurse for over six years. He is a recent graduate from the University of North Carolina (UNC) at Chapel Hill, USA, where he earned his Master of Nursing Science in Health Care Systems and Informatics. He has been employed as a staff and charge nurse for UNC Rex Health Care in the Cardiac Intensive Care Unit in Raleigh, NC, USA. At UNC Rex, he also serves as the current chair of the Quality Improvements nursing committee.

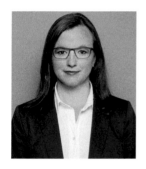

Renate Ranegger, RN, BSc, MSc, PhD works as Nursing Scientist at the Institute of Research and Development at LEP AG, Switzerland. Her scientific interests include clinical coding systems with a focus on health interventions in the care and treatment process, nursing workload measurement systems, grade mix in nursing care, clinical data reuse, and implementation projects of electronic health records. In addition, she is an associated researcher at the Institute of Biomedical Computer Science and Mechatronics at the Private University for Health Sciences, Medical Informatics and Technology (UMIT) Hall, Austria.

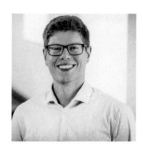

Jens Rauch, PhD studied psychology and computer science at the University of Bremen and the Carl von Ossietzky University of Oldenburg, Germany. He received his PhD in Health Informatics from the University of Osnabruck. He is a postdoctoral researcher and lecturer at the Health Informatics Research Group, Osnabrück University of Applied Sciences, Germany. His research interests include health data analytics, information systems, and learning health systems.

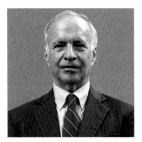

Joel Reich, MD is a health tech advisor/consultant and faculty teaching graduate level population health at the Jefferson College of Population Health and University of New Haven, USA. Previously, he was Chair of Emergency Medicine, Medical Director of EMS, and Chief Medical Officer of Eastern Connecticut Health Network, a community healthcare system, and interim Chief Medical Officer of Commonwealth Care Alliance, a unique nonprofit Medicare-Medicaid dual eligible "Social ACO" organization. Dr. Reich has master's degrees in medical management, health and medical informatics, and technology and human affairs. His special interests include population health, innovative care and payment models, healthcare system transformation, care management, complex populations, and health technology applications including telehealth/remote patient monitoring.

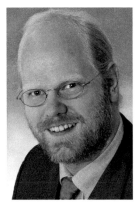

Rainer Röhrig, MD worked in the Department for Anaesthesiology and Intensive Care Medicine at the University Hospital Giessen, Germany, for 14 years after having studied computer science and medicine. In addition to his work as a physician, he led a scientific working group Medical Informatics in Anaesthesiology and Intensive Care Medicine. In 2014, he accepted the appointment to the professorship of Medical Informatics at the Carl von Ossietzky University, Oldenburg. In 2019, he moved to RWTH Aachen University, Germany, as director of the Institute of Medical Informatics.

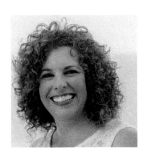

Reut Ron, MSc is a research analyst in the Assuta Health Services Research Institute, Israel. Reut holds a degree in epidemiology from Tel Aviv University, and she has experience in promoting, designing, and conducting research. Prior to her position in Assuta, Reut was a research coordinator in the Department of Child and Women's Health at the Gertner Institute for Epidemiology and Health policy research.

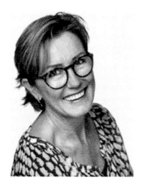

Ann Kristin Rotegård, RN, Cand Nursing Science, PhD has a candidacy in nursing science didactics. Her doctoral thesis in nursing science is on health assets (people's strengths, resources, and empowerment). Her background is in pediatric nursing, where she has been working as a head nurse, nurse coordinator, research and development nurse, and editor. Currently, she is the manager of VAR Healthcare, Norway.

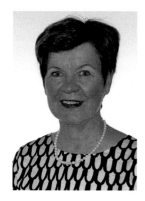

Kaija Saranto, PhD, RN, FACMI, FAAN, FIAHSI Professor in Health and Human Services Informatics at the University of Eastern, Finland. Dr. Saranto has launched the first master's and doctoral degree programs in health and human services informatics in Finland following the international development in the field. She is an experienced educator in continuing education and in-service training in healthcare. Dr. Saranto also acts as the Deputy Director at the Finnish Centre for Evidence-Based Health Care, a JBI Centre of Excellence. She is currently leading research groups focusing on data analytics, impacts of eHealth, virtual care, and patient safety.

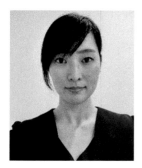

Yoko Sato, MSN is an Assistant Professor of Department of Health Science, Faculty of Medical Sciences, in Kyushu University, Japan. She is nationally certified as a nurse, public health nurse, and midwife. She obtained master's in nursing at Kyushu University while she worked at the Comprehensive Maternity and Perinatal Care Center, Kyushu University Hospital. Ms. Sato teaches midwifery education to master's students and maternity nursing to bachelor's students.

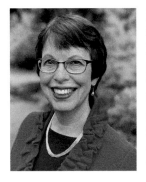

Ruth Schleyer, MSN, RN-BC, COI serves as Chief Nursing Informatics Officer for Legacy Health, Portland, Oregon, USA, where, in dyad partnership with Legacy's CMIO, she collaborates with nursing and interprofessional teams to ensure health information technology and communication solutions are designed and implemented to improve safety, quality, efficiency, and patient and clinician experience across care settings. Throughout her 30-year nursing informatics career, Ruth has held multiple roles, including Chief Nursing Informatics Officer (CNIO) in multiple health systems, and has helped implement the electronic health record in over 30 hospitals. Ruth led development of the online Applied Health Informatics Certificate Program at the University of Providence, USA, where she continues as faculty.

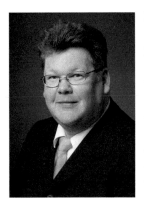

Bernd Schütze, PhD, LL.B. studied computer science, medicine, and law. In addition, he completed training as a medical product integrator. Since 1995, he has been dealing with data protection aspects within the healthcare sector. He qualified as a data protection officer and successfully completed his training as a data protection auditor. Dr. Schütze has more than 10 years of clinical experience and has been familiar with questions regarding the use of IT in hospitals and with data protection issues for more than 20 years.He has also worked as a lecturer at various universities in Germany.

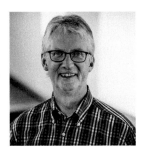

Georg Schulte, RN, PhD is a nurse and nursing manager who had worked in the clinical setting for more than 30 years. He received his PhD in health informatics from Osnabrück University in cooperation with the University Applied Sciences Osnabrück, Germany. His work embraces among others the analysis of ethical issues in the context of digital communication across settings. He holds a postdoctoral position at the Health Informatics Research Group, at the Osnabrück University of Applied Sciences, Germany.

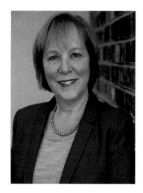

Joyce Sensmeier, MS, RN-BC, FHIMSS, FAAN is the Senior Advisor, Informatics for HIMSS, a nonprofit organization focused on reforming the global health ecosystem through the power of information and technology. In this role, she provides thought leadership in the areas of clinical informatics, interoperability, and standards programs and initiatives. Sensmeier served as Vice President Informatics at HIMSS. She is president of IHE USA, a nonprofit organization whose mission is to improve our nation's healthcare by promoting the adoption and use of IHE and other world-class standards, tools, and services for interoperability.

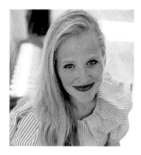

Janae Sharp, BA is the founder of the Sharp Index, a nonprofit dedicated to reducing physician suicide and burnout. After her former husband died by suicide, she noted the disconnect with physician burnout. If our healers are not able to be healthy, our health system will fail. With a background in healthcare IT and patient engagement, she decided to start contributing to the solution. The Sharp Index addresses solutions to help healthcare systems quantify and fix organizational problems that lead to physician burnout.

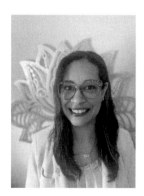

Toria Shaw Morawski, MSW serves as the Senior Manager of Professional Development and TIGER Staff Liaison for the Healthcare Information and Management Systems Society (HIMSS). In this role, she directs all programs, activities, resources, volunteer efforts, and research for the advancement of health informatics and global workforce development efforts aligned with the TIGER Initiative and TIGER's Virtual Learning Environment (VLE). Prior to HIMSS, Toria had 10 years of experience working in countries throughout Africa, the Caribbean, and Europe focused on global health and international development initiatives. In 2009, she co-created Global Implementation Solutions (GIS), a nonprofit organization with a mission to provide customized sustainable solutions that support the strengthening of healthcare systems worldwide. Tori serves as the President of the GIS Board of Directors. She obtained her Master of Social Work from the

University of Illinois at Chicago's Jane Addams College of Social Work.

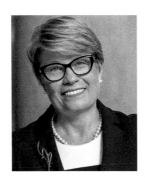

Gabriela Mustata Wilson, PhD, MSc, FHIMSS, SNAI is Professor and Co-Director, at the Multi-Interprofessional Center for Health Informatics at The University of Texas at Arlington, USA and an internationally recognized health informatics expert. For the past twenty years, she educated and trained in various settings, conducted research in industry and academia, participated in team projects, and led partnerships across industry, academic institutions, and the community. Before joining the University of Texas at Arlington, Dr. Wilson served as the founding Chair of Health Informatics and Information Management at the University of Southern Indiana, USA, where she developed a comprehensive competency-based curriculum. Dr. Wilson is Fellow Member of HIMSS bestowed in recognition of service, professional participation, job experience, publications, and presentations. She is also Senior Member of the National Academy of Inventors (NAI), a distinction given to individuals who demonstrate a high degree of innovation through US patents that have brought real impact on the welfare of society.

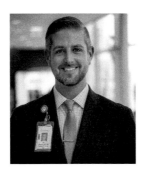

Aric M. Shimek, BSN, RN, CPN is a Telehealth Program Manager at Ann & Robert H. Lurie Children's Hospital of Chicago, USA. He is experienced in both pediatric intensive care and pediatric emergency medicine disciplines. In his current role, Mr. Shimek leads telehealth projects aimed at improving both the access to and the quality of pediatric care for patients across Illinois and the Lurie Children's domestic and international partner institutions. He holds a BA in International Relations from the University of Wisconsin-Madison and a BS of Nursing from Resurrection University, USA.

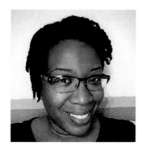

Danielle Siarri, MSc is a global health technology writer and publisher, focused on medical database innovation and management. Danielle has a Master of Science in Nursing Informatics and is a registered nurse with experience ranging from transplants to trauma hospital settings. In addition, Danielle previously worked as a case manager in a corporate environment. She serves as the Lead Publisher at InnoNurse.info.

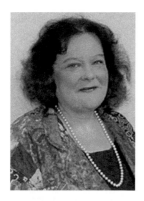

Diane Skiba, PhD, FACMI, ANEF, FAAN is a Professor Emerita at the University of Colorado (CU) College of Nursing, USA. She previously served as the CU's director of the healthcare informatics graduate program that received numerous accolades as one of the top ten online graduate programs throughout its long 25-year history. She taught nurses about informatics since 1982, and was the editor for Emerging Technologies Column for the journal *Nursing Education Perspectives* for 14 years.

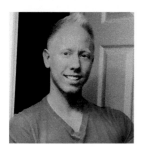

Cory Stephens, MSN, RN is an ANCC Board-Certified Informatics Nurse Specialist (RN-BC) and a Senior HIMSS Member who holds a BSN from Indiana University, USA, an MSN in Nursing Informatics from Walden University, USA, and the CPHIMS certification. Cory is an Informatics Nurse Consultant in the Department of Clinical Research Informatics at the National Institutes of Health Clinical Center and a virtual academic coach and tutor for many high school and college students across the country.

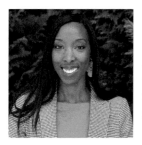

Kelli Stroud, BSN, MSN, DNP obtained her BSN from Winston Salem State University, USA, and MSN and DNP from the University of South Alabama, USA. She is board certified in informatics nursing from the ANCC. She currently works full-time in informatics at a large healthcare organization and is an adjunct faculty at a university.

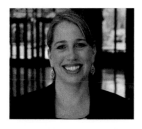

Jennifer Thate, BSN, MSN, DNP is Assistant Professor and Chair of the Baldwin Nursing Program at Siena College in Albany, New York, USA. She holds a PhD from Villanova University and a BSN and MSN from the Johns Hopkins University School of Nursing, USA. She also completed a Research Training Practicum in Clinical Informatics at Partners eCare, Brigham & Women's Hospital, Boston, Massachusetts. She has been a nurse educator for 17 years and teaches health informatics to nursing students and those pursuing careers in the health professions. Her primary area of research has been focused on formats and structures that support interprofessional communication and shared decision-making through the electronic health record and the use of nursing documentation.

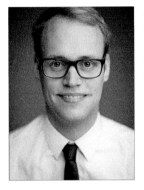

Johannes Thye, PhD is a research fellow at the Health Informatics Research Group at the Osnabrück University of Applied Sciences, Germany. He researches in the areas of health information management and IT adoption and diffusion. He holds a bachelor's degree in business management in the health sector and a master's degree in healthcare management from the Osnabrück University of Applied Sciences, Germany. He received his PhD from the University Osnabrück in cooperation with the Osnabrück University of Applied Sciences.

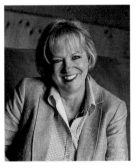

Michelle Troseth, MSN, RN, FNAP, FAAN is the cofounder of MissingLogic, a US-American consulting and coaching company. She is also a founding member of the West Michigan Kidney Foundation and the immediate past president of the National Academies of Practice (NAP) representing 14 different health professions to advance interprofessional care in the USA.

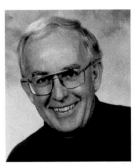

John M. Walker, MA has an undergraduate degree in psychology and a master's in social science. John was an evaluator, a teacher, a staff officer and director of operations for general officers while in the USAF, and a commander. As an Air Force retiree, John was a programmer, and was recruited to the inaugural role of Senior Administrator and Assistant Dean for HR, finance, information systems, and environmental manager for two nationally recognized academic health center schools of nursing.

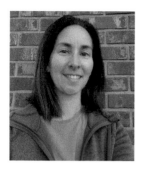

Ginny Waters, BSc, MSc received her BSc from the University of Evansville and her MSc from Indiana University Bloomington, USA. She has worked in various roles throughout the healthcare industry for the past 25 years and most recently spent the past 12 years implementing electronic medical record (EMR) systems into outpatient clinical care facilities, including workflow development and end user training, and seeing the improvement in patient care coordination that can occur post-stabilization.

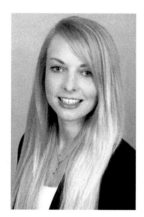

Marie-Louise Witte, MA is a research assistant at the Hannover University of Applied Sciences, Germany. She is engaged in the development of teaching modules for data analysis and data quality in the context of medical research at the University Hospitals Heidelberg, Göttingen, and Hannover and the German Centre for Cancer Research.

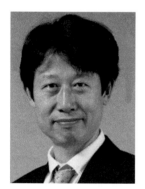

Fumihiko Yokota, PhD is currently a lecturer at the Institutes of Decision Science for a Sustainable Society at Kyushu University, Japan. He received a Master of Public Health at the University of California, Los Angeles, in 2001 and PhD in Public Health & Tropical Medicine at Tulane University in the USA in 2007. Dr. Yokota has more than 15 years of epidemiological research experience in over 10 countries including Indonesia, India, Bangladesh, Thailand, China, Malaysia, Papua New Guinea, and the USA.

Part I

Introduction

Nursing Informatics Through the Lens of Interprofessional and Global Health Informatics

Ursula H. Hübner, Gabriela Mustata Wilson,
Toria Shaw Morawski, and Marion J. Ball

Learning Objectives
- Learn the meaning of nursing informatics within the field of health informatics, to understand its interprofessional nature
- Understand the breadth of the field "from cells to populations" on the micro level (individuals) to the meso level (organizations) and the macro level (countries)
- Understand the role of each individual as a healthcare stakeholder
- Recognize the areas where informatics, nursing, and health informatics have aligned to reached milestones
- Comprehend why a global informatics perspective is essential
- Understand the importance of the interprofessional and global aspects, as well as training and curricula development tied to competency attainment in nursing informatics

Key Terms
- Nursing informatics
- Health informatics
- Inter- and multi-professionalism
- Global health informatics
- Connectivity
- Knowledge generation
- Democratization of knowledge
- Transparency
- Visualization
- Cognitive support
- Mobility
- Data
- Information
- Knowledge
- Data analytics
- Interoperable systems
- Safe systems
- Patient safety
- Privacy
- Confidentiality
- Security
- Ethics
- Management
- Leadership
- Education
- Global case studies
- Future
- Vision

U. H. Hübner (✉)
University of Applied Sciences (UAS) Osnabrück,
Osnabrück, Niedersachsen, Germany
e-mail: u.huebner@hs-osnabrueck.de

G. Mustata Wilson · M. J. Ball
Multi-Interprofessional Center for Health
Informatics, The University of Texas at Arlington,
Arlington, TX, USA
e-mail: Gabriela.wilson@uta.edu; marion.ball@uta.edu

T. Shaw Morawski
Healthcare Information and Management Systems
Society (HIMSS), Chicago, IL, USA
e-mail: tori@torism44.com

© Springer Nature Switzerland AG 2022
U. H. Hübner et al. (eds.), *Nursing Informatics*, Health Informatics,
https://doi.org/10.1007/978-3-030-91237-6_1

Introduction

Nursing informatics has evolved significantly since the first edition of *Nursing Informatics: Where Caring and Technology Meet* was published by Marion J. Ball and colleagues in 1988. More editions followed in 1995 and 2000 [1] and the fourth in 2011 [2]. Nursing informatics continues to address how enabling technology can advance patient care from a nursing perspective. However, as increasing practical evidence from implementations is available, the focus has shifted toward added value in care and research seen through an interprofessional lens.

The International Medical Informatics Association (IMIA) defines nursing informatics as the science and practice that *"integrates nursing, its information and knowledge and their management with information and communication technologies to promote the health of people, families, and communities worldwide"* [3]. This definition was first coined in 1998, updated in 2009, and is still relevant today.

From the nursing perspective, healthcare is always a multifaceted, multidisciplinary activity. Many nurses manage overall care processes and serve as a focal point of information exchange between patients and providers. This circumstance has led nurses to become an integral part of the multi-professional team of caregivers. Likewise, nursing informatics—rooted in nursing data, information, and knowledge—considers not only nursing data but all data to render the full picture of the patient. This might be one of the reasons why nursing informatics as a discipline has incorporated all aspects of health informatics.

For this reason, a textbook on nursing informatics must include core topics that reflect not only nursing but also health and biomedical informatics, such as data modeling; designing standards, artificial intelligence (AI), data analytics, decision support, and interoperable and safe systems; ensuring patient safety; managing the technology and the people to provide valuable systems and enable the workforce to use them properly; and so much more. Therefore,

there are no clear boundaries between nursing and health informatics although nursing informatics has retained a unique core dedicated to nursing via its alliance with nursing education. This association has shown to be extremely beneficial over the years; its impact is reflected by the increasing number of nursing informatics courses at all academic levels and in continuing education. This phenomenon is witnessed around the globe that parallels the political and professional call for "digitalization of nursing and healthcare." This digitalization is meant to enable, advance, and transform nursing and interprofessional practice. For example, to realize the continuity of care through digital networks by reaching remote and underserved populations through telecare and to shape the patient-provider relationship as a new bond that guides self-management of diseases via wearables and personal health records. This transformation process also impacts nursing and health science in the sense that more and more up-to-date patient data become available digitally, leveraging new research designs to find their way into nursing science that make use of new AI methods. At the same time, discussions about the role of observational data to accrue nursing and health evidence and discourses about the ethics of big data in nursing and healthcare cannot be neglected. They are an integral part of this transformation process. The digitalization process will continue to influence the transformation of nursing and interprofessional education significantly. Online learning and teaching are now the new normal, accelerated as a consequence of the COVID-19 pandemic. Finally, nursing management will continue to change too as more data about care processes become digitally available. These new data streams must be converted into intelligence that drives evidence-based decisions. These are just a few examples illustrating how digitalization affects and changes the nursing realm in a significant way and, likewise, touches the entire health domain.

Although there are differences in the adoption of health IT and informatics around the world, the health informatics language is virtually the same.

International health IT standards, including terminologies and classifications as well as data and information models, are an integral part of this language. Building on these foundations, health IT applications share many common features and IT vendors are operating worldwide. Driven by the sciences, nursing and health informatics is shaped by experts who share their experiences and studies on the global level at conferences and through their membership of international societies, such as the International Medical Informatics Association (IMIA), the European Federation of Medical Informatics (EFMI), and the Healthcare Information and Management Systems Society (HIMSS). All of them embrace nursing informatics as a field of science and practice and weave it into the health informatics agenda. TIGER, the Technology Informatics Guiding Education Reform initiative [4], took a leading role by establishing a structure for bringing together international experts in the field of nursing and health informatics from all continents to learn from each other and to build a network of common resources, research projects, and educational events. TIGER is a living example of global health informatics, which will be extensively described in various chapters of this book.

As transformed practice environments emerge under the changes in the healthcare industry as a result of globalization and the economics of quality care, healthcare practice demands that all practitioners be skilled in working collaboratively with other disciplines. The marketplace demands these skills, in addition to professions-specific skills, creating the urgent need for educators to shift from focusing solely on profession-specific skills to preparing students for the realities of communicating and working with other healthcare professions in practice. The need for an interprofessional, competency-based, global approach sets the stage for this fifth edition of nursing informatics as a textbook that covers the many complex aspects of (nursing) informatics from the perspective of all health professionals, with the patient as the focal point of care.

Breadth of the Field

The breadth of health informatics translates to nursing informatics and covers all topics of the health sciences from a nursing and interprofessional perspective. It embraces the entire field from cells to populations. It integrates science and practice at the micro, meso, and macro levels meaning that individuals, organizations, and societies are both the target groups and the actors within nursing informatics. Whatever the specific direction is, the patient stays at the center of nursing and personal healthcare focus in a hospital, in a clinic, or at home. This is the yardstick for the quality of all nursing and interprofessional endeavors. The patient is also the one whose role has changed from somebody who is cared for to someone who directly participates in the care process and decides, together with all integrated healthcare providers, about the next steps in a co-created manner. The sovereignty of the patient guides the activities in nursing and, thus, is a core focus in nursing and health informatics too. This is not only a shift in the paradigm of healthcare but also of nursing; while serving as healthcare providers, nurses must now integrate the patient as a central member of the healthcare team. However, this empowerment entails a series of questions that need to be answered by nursing and health informatics related to the following:

- Proper data access via interoperable systems
- Data sharing, in conformity with local law, and with the patient's and the provider's intent
- Context of the data for adequate interpretation
- Mechanisms to manage flexible data storage
- Communication
- Analysis that transforms data into intelligence that all members of the health team can understand

Mobile technologies, inclusive of wearables, social media, and apps, have paved the way toward lowering the threshold to use (health) IT by virtually anybody. This fact comes along with great promises but also great risk as hurdles still exist. The digital divide of society can leave the frail and poor, the vulnerable, and those with poor digital health literacy behind. Patient and citizen education is, therefore, crucial and is needed more than ever. Educators, nurses, and all clinicians must be capable of understanding informatics methods and tools, not only how to use them but also how to teach these mechanisms and their implications for the patient, the organization, the profession, and society. By taking on this role, nurses and nurse informatics specialists are building bridges between different worlds that require a set of core digital competencies. Nurses and healthcare providers must speak their professional language. At the same time, they also need to communicate and negotiate with people in the field of data and technology, such as bioengineers, computer scientists, statisticians, bioinformaticians, data science experts, epidemiologists, economists, and healthcare managers. This seems complicated and hard to achieve, but it is not impossible with an adequate education. The informatics avenue is rewarding as new professional opportunities arise for nurses, physi-cians, pharmacists, and the entire interprofessional team. Therefore, this textbook will cover many pressing topics within the informatics fields (from a discipline perspective) and provide a clear picture of how competencies translate into potential professional careers in this continuously evolving field.

Milestones of Informatics

Current nursing informatics education stands on the shoulders of significant achievements in informatics. Health and biomedical informatics are on the verge of revolutionizing healthcare and health sciences even further. Figure 1.1 provides an overview of these monumental achievements and illustrates the fundamental advancements of digitalization. These achievements allow us to see the essence of informatics and digitalization as it shapes the healthcare environment. It is clear that nursing and health informatics touch the very foundational aspects of our lives as health professionals, patients, and citizens. It is also obvious that digital competencies go much further than

Fig. 1.1 Milestones of digitalization

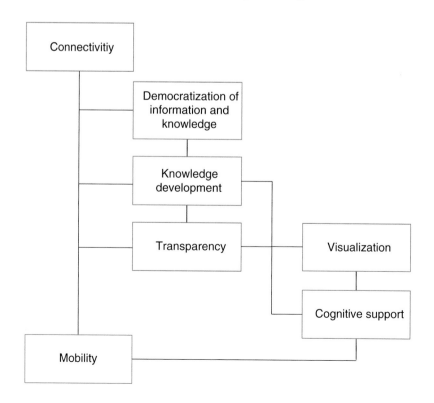

knowing how to operate a specific software application.

Digitalization has become inherently intertwined with the notion of **connectivity**. This is not surprising as the term information and communication technology (ICT) reflects networks such as the Internet protocol, the World Wide Web, and Internet applications like social media. Connectivity encloses the connection between machines as well as between man and machines, indicating that the opportunity to connect digitally facilitates social interactions in a very similar way. Connectivity promises the crossing of space and time but also of hierarchies and professions. In healthcare, telemedicine and telehealth have already shown great potential during the COVID-19 pandemic [5], as well as before that in countries with a large territory and rural regions, such as shown in studies from Australia, Canada, and the United States [6]. Another classic use case of connectivity is patient discharge management that bridges different settings, including clinical professions [7]. Without digital technology, information cannot be easily shared across various healthcare settings. However, connectivity can hold its promises only in an interoperable environment in which systems can exchange signals, data, and information in a meaningful manner. Without health IT standards, such interoperable connectivity is not achievable. Connectivity comes with other challenges as well—first and foremost, IT security as connectivity also opens the door to cyber-attacks. This is why the connectivity of health IT systems is still an endeavor that requires research, knowledge, and intentional efforts to implement them against all the odds.

Due to the pervading nature of connectivity, informatics is all about distributing and sharing particular knowledge at a universal level. This fact has caused, to a great extent, the **democratization of information and knowledge** (such example is the development of Wikipedia). Knowledge—previously physically confined in libraries with limited access—has been opened and is now available 24/7/365. In healthcare, the National Library of Medicine (NLM) has contributed to this megatrend with the PubMed portal and its arsenal of tools [8]. Other databases with a similar focus are CINAHL for nursing, research, and the allied health sciences [9], as well as the Cochrane Library [10] for high-quality, evidence-based medicine—to name a few. Medicine, nursing, and healthcare are fortunate to have such resources at their fingertips. The democratization of knowledge was further fueled by open access publications that have gained increasing popularity in the last decade by attaining support through networks like the global alliance of the Open Access Initiative 2020 (OA2020) [11], through open data initiatives like the Human Genome Project [12], and freely documented development projects such as the Corona-Warn-App development in GitHub [13]. Democratization starts with the broad availability of scientific data and knowledge—across the globe—and continues by gaining benefit through increased literature reviews as well as meta-analyses, paving the way toward evidence across the healthcare system(s). Democratization also encompasses more transparency, diffusion of knowledge, and learning across borders, for example, worldwide massive open online courses (MOOCS) [14], and practicing global classrooms at universities [15].

Knowledge development has been given particular emphasis due to the electronic availability of large amounts of patient data in electronic health records (EHRs) and the availability of data from citizens via social media or other means. The principles of Learning Health Systems (LHS) [16] have been devised based on the notion that practice can contribute to the development of evidence through large amounts of observational data and speed up the cycle of obtaining valid results. This concept of practice-based evidence is meant to complement the classical route of evidence-based practice relying on high-quality randomized and controlled studies. In the same way, precision medicine and precision healthcare data-driven approaches build upon massive amounts of data to identify subgroups of patients who react differently to treatments or have a different profile of their genotype and phenotype [17]. This leads the way to specific knowledge and individualized interventions.

While interoperability is the foundation of achieving connectivity, it is also the key to reaching **transparency**, yet another milestone of digitalization. It is closely linked with the democratization mentioned above. Transparency is a feature that sheds light on previously enclosed and impassable areas. It builds on the availability of up-to-date, relevant, and high-quality data from all sources necessary and spans across multiple time points. Through transparent data, nursing can manifest its vast contributions to healthcare [18], and it is self-evident that these requirements cannot be achieved without digital media.

Notwithstanding, transparency does not come as a by-product of any sort of digitalization. To analyze the data in response to specific questions, the data must be comparable across units within one organization, across organizations and regions or countries, and over time. This kind of comparability is rooted in a shared understanding of what this data should express, which is achieved through the use of standardized terminologies. Healthcare has a long tradition of using classifications, first and foremost, the International Classification of Disease (ICD) codes for medical diagnoses [19]. However, nursing can also look back at a history of different terminologies that have been successfully implemented. Examples for successful implementation include NANDA for nursing diagnosis, the Nursing Intervention Classification (NIC) and the Nursing Outcome Classification (NOC), the International Classification of Nursing Practice (ICNP), the OMAHA system, and the Clinical Care Classification (CCC)—to name a few [20]. At the level of multi-professional classifications, SNOMED CT (Systematized Nomenclature of Medicine—Clinical Terms) has been gaining popularity and acceptance entailed by use in many countries. It has been mapped with several nursing classifications, but further work is needed for integration into nursing practice [21]. Transparency also demands flexible analytics capacities, including proper data storage and advanced statistics.

Transparency makes use of another great accomplishment of digitalization, i.e., **visualization** of data, which can be attributed to both the physical and virtual worlds. The complexity of data and data analyses can be reduced by visualization (such as color-coded heatmaps, examples see [22]) so that the results become more comprehensible and the message becomes more understandable. Healthcare, nursing, and medicine have benefited from digital visualization, not only in 2D, 3D, and 4D diagnostic imaging and signal processing, but also when it comes to learning anatomy and using anatomy for various purposes, such as the Visible Human Project [23]. Recently, augmented reality (AR) has enabled the blending of digital objects with physical reality, and virtual reality (VR) has extended the horizon of what is possible through visualization. Applications in therapy, such as motor training of patients with paresis, and education via simulation or serious games [24], are available.

Aside from visualization, any **cognitive support** can be leveraged by digitalization. Memory support is a trivial example that has penetrated our life through calendar reminders, storage of important information, and easy retrieval through intelligent search machines. Clinical decision support systems (CDSS) are another way of cognitive support, helping to remember a myriad of facts and drawing conclusions from them. Early on, clinical decision support systems—also in nursing—demonstrated their use to leverage patient safety [25]. These systems may come as a light version of supporting clinical workflows with intelligent information logistics, i.e., providing the right information at the right time to the right person, or as highly advanced systems with very little human input, with the "healthcare provider in the loop" [26].

Cognitive support not only affects the work of healthcare professionals, including nurses, but is also a means for patients to manage disabilities and improve cognition.

Mobility is transforming healthcare by enabling providers to deliver better care. The increasing use of mobility in healthcare improves efficiencies, enhancing the patient experience both inside and outside the hospital, optimizing communication and collaboration between patients and healthcare providers as well as providers and their peers. Mobility is not just empowering health organizations with mobile devices and apps but also significantly enhancing the patient-provider relationship. Due to the digital connectivity, data, information, and knowledge are highly mobile and underpin the motto of telenursing and telemedicine of "move the data, not the patient," which proves valuable in the case of immobile patients. Likewise, teleservices allow health professionals to use their time in the office to communicate with the patients remotely instead of traveling long distances [27]. At the same time, mobile devices such as smartphones and tablets enable health professionals, patients, and citizens to access relevant information at the point of care wherever this happens to be. Digitalization can also support health professionals either staying where they are or moving around, giving them the freedom of choice. In the case of patients with limited sensory-motor or cognitive resources, mobility can be achieved by utilizing intelligent devices, including smartphones and tablets, which can guide people to better orientate themselves.

AI-empowered systems increasingly influence all these fields by data and algorithms and their practice. AI may, as a result of this, appear in an "embodied manner," such as is true for intelligent devices and robots or, in a "disembodied manner," like the use of data analytics to build new knowledge, enable transparency, and better visualization. Supporting humans in various ways is the mode of action whereby the focus is on the augmentation of human capabilities rather than on automation and replacement of people [28]. The more data is captured outside the confines of healthcare organizations, the fuzzier the boundaries become between care and research, and the more ethical issues arise. Have the patients given their consent in an adequate manner, is the context of the data clear, is the data unbiased, and are the AI results understandable for health professionals and patients? These are only a few questions that are coming to the forefront through new AI techniques.

These milestones demonstrate that digitalization is not merely a technological topic but also a process that impacts our lives in manifold and fundamental ways. Nursing and health informatics touches not only the daily routine of nurses but of all health professionals in an all-encompassing fashion. For this to happen reasonably and adequately, digitalization needs to be shaped so that its tools, methods, and implementations work according to various needs in a usable, meaningful, legal, and ethical manner. Workforce development and patient education for digital literacy are, therefore, indispensable prerequisites.

Reference of This Book to the Informatics Milestones

Digitalization has changed our society and world, as witnessed by everyone in our daily lives. In contrast to previous generations, students nowadays experience what connectivity, mobility, visualization, and cognitive support mean to them as consumers when using social media apps on mobile devices or relying on the navigation system when driving a car. They can see that open access to knowledge matters to them at the university, and they can comprehend that transparency of data and facts have a significance for governing an organization and a national healthcare system, as we all witnessed during the COVID-19 pandemic.

While these experiences can help us better understand what digital health signifies, they are not sufficient enough to translate digital options into the complex reality of nursing and healthcare practice. This book, therefore, aims to motivate nursing students and nurses, as well as other healthcare providers, educators, and students, to explore and deepen the understanding of nursing and interprofessional health informatics and what digitalization implies for patient care in detail. It is a field of significant importance as it shapes and transforms how nursing and healthcare are performed in an unprecedented manner to better patient care. In order for nurses and the interprofessional health team to play an active part in the new digital world, they must speak the informatics language and have a comprehensive understanding of the principles of digitalization and what consequences it has. Far beyond making paper electronic, digitalization opens new avenues while also requiring proper and careful planning to avoid adverse events due to health IT.

This book also makes reference to the milestones of informatics as presented above. *Connectivity* of systems, organizations, and humans are golden threads woven throughout the book, which are already prepared by Part II "360° Stakeholder Perspective," where the voices of the many professions are orchestrated to build the interprofessional backdrop of this book. There is no fully fledged interprofessional care without *Connectivity* that enables people to communicate and share data. From a technical point of view, *Connectivity is* significantly covered in Part IV "Interoperable systems," which highlights intramural, intermural, and population-wide connectivity through interoperable systems. While *Connectivity* is often discussed with a positive connotation, as an enabler, it also comes along with new threats in the form of cyber-attacks, which is addressed in Part V "Safe Systems and Patient Safety" and with new legal and ethical challenges as presented in the Part "Privacy, Security, Confidentiality and Ethics in Healthcare." *Connectivity* and data sharing lay the foundation to accrue data in EHRs, data warehouses, and data lakes to be used for data-driven and open *Knowledge Development* at various levels. While *Connectivity* has been presented as the golden thread of this book, there is data (re-)use as another major strand that characterizes this book. It is not only in Part II "Using Data and Information to Generate Knowledge" that the various sources of data and analytical methods are described, this theme is resumed in the last Part, "Future Trends in Health Informatics" discussing the future of data-driven medicine and healthcare. Learning health systems (LHS), the meta-concept that combines data provision, analysis, and the dissemination of the results under one roof, is at the core of *Knowledge Development*, and extensively presented in this book. LHS are also mechanisms—

particularly if at a regional, national, and supranational level—for broad dissemination of the findings that contribute to the *Democratization of Knowledge and Science*. It is no longer the academic institutions alone that generate knowledge through scientific studies, each hospital in a region, country, or worldwide can contribute data, prediction models, and knowledge. Further *Democratization* takes place when citizens themselves actively collect data and becomes part of the scientific process, as shown in one of the chapters.

Concomitantly with data-driven knowledge development, *Transparency* as an outcome of applying informatics methods in up-to-date and relevant data is similarly addressed by several chapters in this book to allow for a transparent skills-based allocation of human resources, to meet the requirements of customers for more cost and quality transparency, to build trust in information through a transparent manner of how applications work and trust in the digital transformation process through making data transparent.

Visualization of data and aggregated findings, yet another milestone of informatics also in healthcare, accompanies many health informatics tools to make an abundance of data and highly abstract findings tangible, as illustrated in chapters of Part II "Using Data and Information to Generate Knowledge." For example, in the case of merging and geospatial mapping of health and community data to identify social determinants of health or in the case of a Tower Control dashboard to visualize clinical cases and alert the care providers. As explained in this section, visualization techniques aim to support human cognition and perception to direct attention to the most important statements. Interestingly the authors refer to the historical example of Florence Nightingale, who was the first to visualize statistical findings from the Crimean War in coxcomb or polar area diagrams. Also in the future, *Visualization* will play a predominant role, e.g., in the form of AR in surgery, as shown in Part X "Future Trends in Health Informatics." How to achieve further *Cognitive Support* not only is described in the in Part III "Interoperable systems" when focusing on decision support systems, but resonates virtually in all chapters of Part II "Using Data and Information to Generate Knowledge."

Finally, the last informatics milestone, *Mobility*, is reflected through the chapters on telemedicine and mHealth in various sections following the idea of moving the data not the patients who can, for example, stay in their community and still receive the same high-quality care or allowing for portable clinics in low-resource areas that are connected with hubs. Mobility is also mirrored by the myriad of apps on mobile devices that allow data from social media to be collected directly from citizen scientist donors that can ensure patient safety, but that must also be tested for trustfulness before being used to empower their users.

Summary

By the end of this book, readers will gain substantial knowledge that will help them understand the importance of health informatics and how to apply it to nursing and other health professions. Through the variety of topics described, readers will obtain an overview and the necessary terminology to better communicate with individuals from other disciplines, make decisions and direct health IT projects, and become champions in their own organizations toward better use of data, information, and knowledge. They will also gain a clear understanding that connectivity and interprofessionalism belong to each other, serving as the catalyst for becoming proficient in transforming patient care through enhanced cooperation and coordination. In addition, readers will also have obtained insights into the active role of patients and citizens in a digital world and that the digital divide in our society needs to be addressed sooner than later if we want to address health disparities at the local and global levels. Readers will also discover how health IT entails risks, develops an understanding of the ethical dimension, and becomes aware of the legal constraints. Above all,

readers will not only become more knowledgeable but also responsibly minded.

Conclusions and Outlook

The book serves as a compass for global citizens seeking a professional career in nursing and health informatics practice and science. It also serves as a source for nurses and health professionals to upgrade their knowledge and enlarge their professional radius of action. Encompassing the interprofessional and global perspective of nursing informatics adds a new dimension and opens the door to further developing the field. It is within our reach to enact change if only we reach for it.

Review Questions
1. Why is healthcare always a multifaceted, multidisciplinary activity from the nursing point of view?
2. What are the milestones of informatics, health, and nursing informatics?
3. What is meant by the breadth of the field?

Appendix: Answers to Review Questions

1. Why is healthcare always a multifaceted, multidisciplinary activity from the nursing point of view?

Very often nurses serve as focal points in sharing and exchanging information among the providers and also between the providers and the patients and their relatives. Nursing—though rooted in nursing data, information, and knowledge—considers not only nursing data but all data to render the full picture of the patient.

2. What are the milestones of informatics, health, and nursing informatics?

Connectivity, mobility, democratization of information and knowledge, knowledge development, transparency, visualization, cognitive support, and assistance/ambient assisted living.

3. What is meant by the breadth of the field?

Nursing informatics covers all topics of the health sciences from a nursing perspective. It embraces the entire field from cells to populations. It integrates science and practice at the micro, meso, and macro levels meaning that individuals, organizations, and societies are both the target groups and the actors within nursing informatics. As educators, nurses must be capable of understanding informatics methods and tools, not only how to use them but also how to teach the mechanisms and their implications for the patient, the organization, the profession, and society. Nurses and healthcare providers must speak their professional language. At the same time, they also need to communicate and negotiate with people in the field of data and technology, such as bioengineers, computer scientists, statisticians, bioinformaticians, data science experts, epidemiologists, economists, and healthcare managers.

References

1. Ball MJ, Hannah KJ, Newbold KS, Douglas JV. Nursing informatics: where caring and technology meet. New York: Springer; 1988. (1st edition), 1995 (2nd edition) and 2000 (3rd edition)
2. Ball MJ, Douglas JV, Hinton Walker P, DuLong D, Gugerty B, Hannah KJ, Kiel J, Newbold SK, Sensmeier J, Skiba DJ, Troseth M. Nursing informatics: where technology and caring meet. New York, London: Springer; 2011. (4th edition)
3. International Medical Informatics Association – Special Interest Group on Nursing Informatics. https://imianews.wordpress.com/2009/08/24/imia-ni-definition-of-nursing-informatics-updated/. Accessed 16 Oct 2020.
4. TIGER International Task Force page. https://www.himss.org/tiger. Accessed 16 Oct 2020.
5. Annis T, Pleasants S, Hultman G, et al. Rapid implementation of a COVID-19 remote patient monitoring program. J Am Med Informatics Assoc. 2020; https://doi.org/10.1093/jamia/ocaa097.
6. Speyer R, Denman D, Wilkes-Gillan S, Chen YW, Bogaardt H, Kim JH, Heckathorn DE, Cordier R. Effects of telehealth by allied health professionals and nurses in rural and remote areas: a systematic review and meta-analysis. J

Rehabil Med. 2018;50(3):225–35. https://doi.org/10.2340/16501977-2297.
7. Bowles KH, Chittams J, Heil E, Topaz M, Rickard K, Bhasker M, Tanzer M, Behta M, Hanlon AL. Successful electronic implementation of discharge referral decision support has a positive impact on 30- and 60-day readmissions. Res Nurs Health. 2015;38(2):102–14. https://doi.org/10.1002/nur.21643.
8. Lindberg DA, Humphreys BL. Rising expectations: access to biomedical information. Yearb Med Inform. 2008;3(1):165–72.
9. The Cumulative Index to Nursing and Allied Health Literature. https://health.ebsco.com/products/the-cinahl-database. Accessed 16 Oct 2020.
10. Cochrane Library. https://www.cochranelibrary.com/. Accessed 16 Oct 2020.
11. The Open Access Initiative 2020. https://oa2020.org/. Accessed 16 Oct 2020.
12. National Human Genome Research Institute. Human Genome Project. https://www.genome.gov/human-genome-project. Accessed 12 Jan 2022.
13. Corona Warn App Solution Architecture. 2020. https://github.com/corona-warn-app/cwa-documentation/blob/master/solution_architecture.md. Accessed 16 Oct 2020.
14. Jia M, Gong D, Luo J, Zhao J, Zheng J, Li K. Who can benefit more from massive open online courses? A prospective cohort study. Nurse Educ Today. 2019;76:96–102. https://doi.org/10.1016/j.nedt.2019.02.004.
15. Indiana University. Global Classroom. https://global.iu.edu/education/internationalization/classroom/index.html. Accessed 16 Oct 2020.
16. Friedman C, Rubin J, Brown J, Buntin M, Corn M, Etheredge L, Gunter C, Musen M, Platt R, Stead W, Sullivan K, Van Houweling D. Toward a science of learning systems: a research agenda for the high-functioning learning health system. J Am Med Inform Assoc. 2015;22(1):43–50. https://doi.org/10.1136/amiajnl-2014-002977.
17. Fu MR, Kurnat-Thoma E, Starkweather A, Henderson WA, Cashion AK, Williams JK, Katapodi MC, Reuter-Rice K, Hickey KT, Barcelona de Mendoza V, Calzone K, Conley YP, Anderson CM, Lyon DE, Weaver MT, Shiao PK, Constantino RE, Wung SF, Hammer MJ, Voss JG, Coleman B. Precision health: a nursing perspective. Int J Nurs Sci. 2019;7(1):5–12. https://doi.org/10.1016/j.ijnss.2019.12.008.
18. Ameel M, Kontio R, Junttila K. Nursing interventions in adult psychiatric outpatient care. Making nursing visible using the nursing interventions classification. J Adv Nurs. 2019;75(11):2899–909. https://doi.org/10.1111/jan.14127.
19. World Health Organization. The International Statistical Classification of Diseases and Related Health Problems. https://www.who.int/classifications/icd/icdonlineversions/en/. Accessed 16 Oct 2020.
20. The Office of the National Coordinator of Health Information Technology. Standard nursing terminolo-

gies: a landscape analysis. 2017. https://www.heal-thit.gov/sites/default/files/snt_final_05302017.pdf. Accessed 16 Oct 2020.

21. Kim J, Macieira TGR, Meyer SL, Ansell Maggie M, Bjarnadottir Raga RI, Smith MB, Citty SW, Schentrup DM, Nealis RM, Keenan GM. Towards implementing SNOMED CT in nursing practice: a scoping review. Int J Med Inform. 2020;134:104035. https://doi.org/10.1016/j.ijmedinf.2019.104035.

22. Barter RL, Yu B. Superheat: an R package for creating beautiful and extendable heatmaps for visualizing complex data. J Comput Graph Stat. 2018;27(4):910–22. https://doi.org/10.1080/10618600.2018.1473780.

23. National Library of Medicine. The Visible Human Project. https://www.nlm.nih.gov/research/visible/visible_human.html. Accessed 16 Oct 2020.

24. Buijs-Spanjers KR, Harmsen A, Hegge HH, Spook JE, de Rooij SE, Jaarsma DADC. The influence of a serious game's narrative on students' attitudes and learning experiences regarding delirium: an interview study. BMC Med Educ. 2020;20(1):289. https://doi.org/10.1186/s12909-020-02210-5.

25. Ball MJ, Weaver C, Abbott PA. Enabling technologies promise to revitalize the role of nursing in an era of patient safety. Int J Med Inform. 2003;69(1):29–38. https://doi.org/10.1016/s1386-5056(02)00063-1.

26. O'Sullivan S, Nevejans N, Allen C, Blyth A, Leonard S, Pagallo U, Holzinger K, Holzinger A, Sajid MI, Ashrafian H. Legal, regulatory, and ethical frameworks for development of standards in artificial intelligence (AI) and autonomous robotic surgery. Int J Med Robot. 2019;15(1):e1968. https://doi.org/10.1002/rcs.1968.

27. Bashshur RL, Shannon GW, Smith BR, Alverson DC, Antoniotti N, Barsan WG, Bashshur N, Brown EM, Coye MJ, Doarn CR, Ferguson S, Grigsby J, Krupinski EA, Kvedar JC, Linkous J, Merrell RC, Nesbitt T, Poropatich R, Rheuban KS, Sanders JH, Watson AR, Weinstein RS, Yellowlees P. The empirical foundations of telemedicine interventions for chronic disease management. Telemed J E Health. 2014;20(9):769–800. https://doi.org/10.1089/tmj.2014.9981.

28. Davenport TH, Glover WJ. Artificial intelligence and the augmentation of health care decision making. New England Journal of Medicine Catalyst. 2018. https://catalyst.nejm.org/ai-technologies-augmentation-healthcare-decisions/. Accessed 16 Oct 2020.

Principles of Health Informatics

2

Gabriela Mustata Wilson and Mercy Obasanya

Abbreviations

3D	Three Dimensional
AI	Artificial Intelligence
AMIA	American Medical Informatics Association
ARRA	American Recovery and Reinvestment Act of 2009
BMI	Biomedical Informatics
CDSS	Clinical Decision Support System
CMS	The Centers for Medicare & Medicaid Services
CPOE	Computerized Provider Order Entry system
CT	Computerized Tomography
EHR	Electronic Health Records
EMR	Electronic Medical Records
HIE	Health Information Exchange
HIMSS	Healthcare Information and Management Systems Society
HIPAA	Health Insurance Portability and Accountability Act
HITECH	Health Information Technology for Economic and Clinical Health Act
ML	Machine Learning
MPI	Master Patient Index
MRI	Magnetic Resonance Imaging
PACS	Picture Archiving and Communication System
PPACA	Patient Protection and Affordable Care Act
PPRL	Privacy-Preserving Record Linkage
VR	Virtual Reality

Learning Objectives
- Define and describe health informatics, information management, and information systems
- Explain the basic principles that underlie informatics practice
- Understand major professional roles and skills of health informaticians
- Discuss emerging trends in information technology and examine the challenges presented by them

Key Terms
- Definition and role of Health Informatics and Information Management
- Role of data, information, and knowledge in healthcare
- Informatics drivers
- The concept of Information Systems
- Role of Health Information Exchange and Interoperability
- Emerging trends in Health Information Technology
- Health Intelligence

G. M. Wilson (✉) · M. Obasanya
The University of Texas at Arlington,
Arlington, TX, USA
e-mail: gabriela.wilson@uta.edu;
mercy.obasanya@uta.edu

© Springer Nature Switzerland AG 2022
U. H. Hübner et al. (eds.), *Nursing Informatics*, Health Informatics,
https://doi.org/10.1007/978-3-030-91237-6_2

Health Informatics

What Is Health Informatics?

Health Informatics is a multidisciplinary field applied to healthcare to manage healthcare information using technology [1]. As we know it now, the field of Health Informatics emerged when computer technology became refined enough to handle large amounts of data. However, it was not until the 1960s that Health Informatics began to standardize as a field of study.

While various informatics definitions have been published, two have been selected as significant to the field. The first definition comes from the American Medical Informatics Association (AMIA) [2], a non-profit organization "committed to the vision of a world where informatics transforms people's care." According to their website, "Informatics is the intersection between the work of stakeholders across the health and healthcare delivery system who seek to improve outcomes, lower costs, increase safety and promote the use of high-quality services" [3].

The second definition, crafted by Marion J. Ball, emphasizes Health Informatics as an evolving discipline at the intersection of data science, health information technology, health information management, and data analytics, which is focused on improving health and healthcare by bringing theory into practice through enabling technologies [4].

With the expansion of technology and innovations, informatics has become an integral part of healthcare. When you think of informatics, you think of computers, but it is much more than that. **Health Informatics** is the integration of healthcare sciences, computer science, information science, and cognitive science to assist in managing healthcare information. There is a critical need to develop information systems that lead to more effective decisions and greater efficiency within the healthcare industry. Health Informatics meets this need through an interdisciplinary collaboration of scholars and knowledgeable practitioners from medicine, nursing, pharmacy, public health, social work, dentistry, library science, etc. Health Informatics promotes the effective and efficient use and analysis of information to improve society's health, well-being, and economic functioning.

Brief History of Health Informatics

Florence Nightingale (1820–1910) is credited with being the founder of modern nursing. She might also be considered the first health informatician as she made use of information and its organization to improve the care of patients to suggest how health professionals, not just nurses, might collect and analyze data for improved patient care [5].

The development of Health Informatics is generally traced to the first use of computers in healthcare in the 1950s. In 1960s, the French term "informatique" (i.e., informatics) began to appear in French literature. In 1966, François Grémy recognized the key role played by information sciences in medicine and the need to join Medicine and Informatics, which resulted in the birth of "Informatique Médicale/Medical Informatics" as a new scientific discipline [6].

It was not until the 1970s when computers started being used in actual patient care that Health Informatics developed into a discipline [7]. Much earlier to the 1970s, many strands of activities and innovation were started in the world of information and technology. Over the years, Health Informatics has evolved as both a discipline and an area of specialization within the health professions to support healthcare delivery and improve health for all (Fig. 2.1).

The Field of Informatics

Biomedical and Health Informatics are interdisciplinary, scientific fields that study and pursue the practical uses of biomedical data, information, and knowledge for scientific inquiry, problem-solving, and decision making, motivated by efforts to improve human health [8]. Biomedical and Health Informatics apply computer and information science principles to the advancement of life sciences research, health

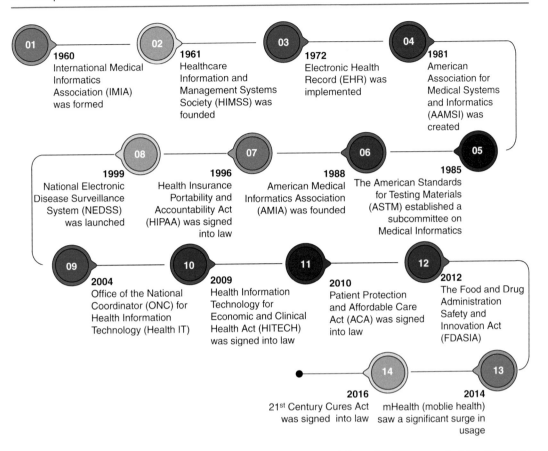

Fig. 2.1 Highlights of main initiatives that advanced the field of Health Informatics (US perspective) [7] (Copyright belongs to Gabriela Mustata Wilson, PhD, MSc, FHIMSS, SNAI) (2021))

professions education, public health, and patient care. They build bridges to healthy communities by establishing informatics as a bridge to accelerate the translation of discoveries to improve individual patients' health and translate the science of healthcare delivery for better population health.

Direct applications are:

- Develop and apply theories, methods, and processes for the generation, storage, retrieval, use, and sharing of biomedical data and information
- Build on computing, communication, and information sciences and technologies
- Investigate and support reasoning, simulation, experimentation, and translation from molecules to populations, dealing with a variety of biological systems, bridging clinical research practice and the healthcare enterprise
- Draw upon the social and behavioral sciences to inform the design and evaluation of technical solutions and the evolution of complex systems

In response to dramatic changes in healthcare, the discipline of Biomedical and Health Informatics has rapidly expanded to include a much larger number of components under the umbrella of "Health Informatics," and that number continues to grow (Fig. 2.2).

Medical Informatics is a term that covers the use of information and communication technologies to process, generate, and communicate medical information and knowledge [9]. It is the subdiscipline of Health Informatics that

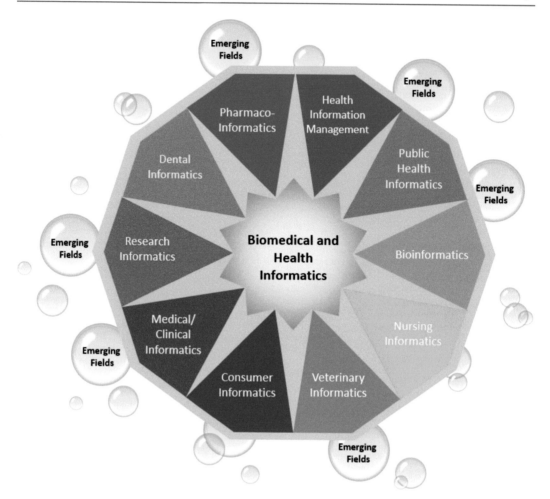

Fig. 2.2 The Health Informatics discipline and sub-domains. (Copyright belongs to Gabriela Mustata Wilson, PhD, MSc, FHIMSS, SNAI) (2021)

directly impacts the patient-physician relationship. It focuses on the information technology that enables the effective collection of data using technology tools to develop medical knowledge and facilitate the delivery of patient medical care. Medical informatics aims to ensure access to patient medical information at the precise time and place it is needed to make medical decisions [9]. Medical informatics also focuses on the management of medical data for research and education.

Nursing informatics is the specialty that integrates nursing science with information and analytical sciences to identify, define, manage, and communicate data, information, knowledge, and wisdom in nursing practice [9].The application of nursing informatics knowledge is empowering for all healthcare practitioners in achieving patient-centered care.

Core areas of work include [9]:

- Concept representation and standards to support evidence-based practice, research, and education
- Data and communication standards to build an interoperable national data infrastructure
- Research methodologies to disseminate new knowledge into practice
- Information presentation and retrieval approaches to support safe patient-centered care

- Information and communication technologies to address interprofessional workflow needs across all care venues
- Vision and management for the development, design, and implementation of communication and information technology
- Definition of healthcare policy to advance the public's health

Pharmaco-informatics is the discipline where technology is used with any aspect of drug delivery, from the basic sciences to the clinical use of medications in individuals and populations [9]. It is a combination of informatics, technology, and medical management for efficient and safe patient care. It involves:

- Prescribing—using clinical decision support to facilitate rational ordering
- Verifying & Dispensing (Perfecting)—interpreting, translating, and perfecting medication orders, including using informatics and technology in the dispensing process
- Administering—information flow and clinical decision support in the electronic medication administration process, including documentation and checking the "5 rights" (right patient, drug, dose, form, time)
- Monitoring—relating to the use of ADE surveillance/prevention, pharmacoepidemiology, pharmacovigilance, and Pharmacoeconomics to enhance patient outcomes
- Educating—promoting professional and patient education

Consumer Informatics analyzes consumers' needs for information, studies, and implements methods for making information accessible to consumers, and models and integrates consumers' preferences into health information systems [9]. It is patient-focused informatics, health literacy, and consumer education. The focus is on information structures and processes that empower consumers to manage their own health, such as health information literacy, consumer-friendly language, personal health records, and Internet-based strategies and resources.

Dental Informatics is a multidisciplinary field in Health Informatics that seeks to improve healthcare by applying computer and information science to dental practice, delivery, research, education, and management [9]. The primary objective of dental informatics is to improve patient care and increase administrative efficiency through the use of information technology. It also advocates for the adoption of standards that can benefit dentists and their patients. Dental Informatics is a newly emerging field within informatics and has the potential to bridge the gap between clinical care delivery in dental and medical settings [9].

Research Informatics involves the use of informatics to discover and manage new knowledge relating to health and disease. It is the use of informatics to facilitate biomedical and health research, which incorporates the area of *clinical research informatics* that is widely used to describe informatics applications in clinical research [9]. It includes the management of information related to research trials and involves informatics related to secondary research use of clinical data.

Bioinformatics is a subdiscipline of biology and computer science concerned with the acquisition, storage, analysis, and dissemination of biological data, most often DNA and amino acid sequences. It is the use of informatics in microbiology, biochemistry, physiology, and genetics, describing data from biological experiments [9]. It also uses computer programs for a variety of applications, including determining gene and protein functions, establishing evolutionary relationships, and predicting the three-dimensional shapes of proteins. The main components of bioinformatics are the development of software tools and algorithms and the analysis and interpretation of biological data by using a variety of software tools and particular algorithms [9].

Imaging Informatics, sometimes referred to as radiology informatics or medical imaging informatics, describes how medical images are used and exchanged throughout complex healthcare systems. It relates to computational methods targeting tissues and organs. Imaging informatics focuses on improving patient outcomes through the effective use of images and imaging-derived information in research and clinical care [9]. The field has implications in diagnosing disease, optimizing treatment, tracking disease response, and predicting outcomes. Virtually every healthcare clinical discipline depends on imaging informatics.

Clinical informatics focuses on the application of informatics and information technology to deliver healthcare services [9]. It is concerned with information use in healthcare settings by clinicians. Clinical informatics includes a wide range of topics ranging from clinical decision support to visual images (e.g., radiological, pathological, dermatological, ophthalmological), from clinical documentation to provide order entry systems, and from system design to system implementation and adoption issues. It can be applied in various healthcare settings, including hospitals, physician's practices, and military.

Public Health Informatics is the effective use of data, information, computer science, and technology to improve population health outcomes through health practices, research, and learning. It is the application of informatics in public health areas, including surveillance, prevention, preparedness, outbreak management, health promotion, and electronic laboratory reporting [9]. Public Health Informatics (can also be called population Health Informatics) uses information

science and technology to promote population health rather than each individual's health.

Data, Information, Knowledge, and Wisdom

To better understand informatics, one needs to learn the differences between data, information, knowledge, and wisdom (Fig. 2.3). **Data** are simple symbols, isolated facts, and measurements. When such data are processed, put into a context, and combined within a structure, information emerges [10]. **Information** is meaningful data or facts from which conclusions can be drawn. It provides the answers to "who, what, when, and where." According to Claude Shannon, information is "thought of as a set of possible messages, where the goal is to send these messages over a noisy channel and then to have the receiver reconstruct the message with a low probability of error, despite the channel noise" [11]. Basically, information is thought of as the resolution to uncertainty. When information is given meaning by interpreting it, that is, there is an application of data, information becomes knowledge. **Knowledge** is information that is justifiably considered to be true. It answers the "how" questions. Finally, **wisdom** is the critical use of knowledge to make intelligent decisions. It is

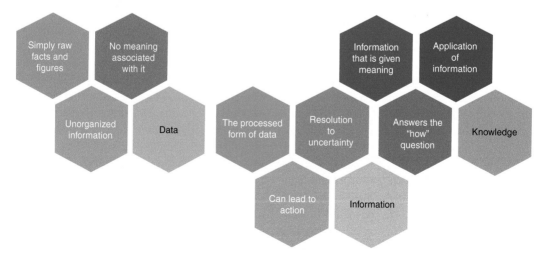

Fig. 2.3 Data vs. Information vs. Knowledge. (Copyright belongs to Gabriela Mustata Wilson, PhD, MSc, FHIMSS, SNAI) (2021)

evaluated understanding and answers the "why" questions [10]. Central to informatics is the processing of data, so it becomes meaningful.

Informatics Drivers

Drivers are factors that affect the performance of something, which has a big impact on whether things go well or not. There are multiple motivations driving the adoption of informatics. These include [12]:

Technological advancements: One example will be the use of a Health IT framework that aligns organization's resources with its goals and objectives for accountable care. The framework emphasizes:

- Information sharing among clinicians, patients, and authorized entities
- Data collection and integration from multiple clinical, financial, operational, and patient-derived sources
- Supporting patient safety and strong privacy protections

Policy: Both the Patient Protection and Affordable Care Act (PPACA) and the Health Information Technology for Economic and Clinical Health (HITECH) Act, a part of the American Recovery and Reinvestment Act of 2009 (ARRA), acknowledge the importance of health IT in improving the quality and cost-efficiency of healthcare. Another policy is the National eHealth Strategy, which provides a toolkit of framework and method for the development of a national eHealth vision, action plan, and monitoring framework [13]. It is a "practical, comprehensive, step-by-step guide, directed chiefly toward the most relevant government departments and agencies, particularly ministries of health and ministries of information technology and communication" [13]. The advantage of the toolkit is that it can be applied by all governments around the world regardless of their current level of eHealth advancement.

Privacy and security: With information stored online, it makes data vulnerable to cyber-attack and hacking. Strategies should be used to ensure the privacy and security of health data.

Information governance: This involves implementing policies, structures, controls, and other procedures to ensure an organization's data assets are handled appropriately. It optimizes health data extraction abilities while also mitigating risk and ensuring that compliance guidelines are met.

Interoperability: This is the ability of computer software or systems to communicate and exchange information in a way that the data is understandable to the user.

Data analytics: Raw data does very little to impact healthcare, so numbers must first be analyzed to ensure that the information is appropriately leveraged. It also helps with decision-making processes and cut down on administrative costs. Data analysis can be qualitative or quantitative in nature.

Other drivers are the need to:

- Increase the efficiency of healthcare (improve physician, nurse, and overall healthcare productivity)
- Improve the quality (patient outcomes) of healthcare, resulting in improved patient safety
- Reduce healthcare costs
- Improve healthcare access with technologies such as telemedicine
- Improve communication, coordination, and continuity of care
- Improve medical education for clinicians and patients
- Standardization of medical care

Theory of Informatics

Theories are a collection of thoughts that represents reality. It comprises abstraction and interpretation of research findings. Theory in Health Informatics can provide a helpful framework for evaluation, design, or implementation [14]. They include concepts that can inform and provide a framework for informatics, essential for Health Informatics teaching and research and evidence-based practices. There are so many theories surrounding Health Informatics. These theories are *Information Value Chain Theory, Activity Theory, Unified Theory of Acceptance and Use of Technology (UTAUT), Actor-Network Theory, Collective Mindfulness Theory, Deterioration Communication Management Theory, Social Learning Theory, Social Cognitive Theory, Planned Behavior Theory, Control Theory, Normalization Process Theory, and Shannon's Information Theory* [15].

A few of these theories are highlighted below.

Change Theory: Computerization of information systems involves change, for example, moving from a paper-based environment to a completely paperless environment [16]. It can be a minor or major change depending on the previous system's maturity, most notably the information system users.

An example of change theory is Lewin's Change Theory (planned change). As indicated in Fig. 2.4, this theory occurs in three stages [16]:

- *Unfreezing:* It involves finding ways to overcome the resistance to change and conformity, introducing the mentality of change to a group. An example is when a documentation system is replaced with an electronic system in a healthcare system. Users may struggle and be resistant to change. To get past this, professionals have to agree to the new requirements for change. One has to transition

through this stage smoothly, or they cannot move to the next step.

- *Cognitive:* It involves bringing the organization into choosing a new level of thoughts and behaviors toward the change. An example is nurses having to be computer literate and forgo the old methods of recording the patient's information (i.e., clinical documentation). To get through this stage, the user has to be convinced that the new approach is safer and better than the old and have a change in behavior to give space for the new process, which is evident by learning how to use the electronic system.
- *Refreezing:* It involves establishing the introduced methods to ensure that it becomes the standard operating method. An example will be continuous rewards, support, and leadership maintained for those using the new electronic system.

Chaos Theory: This theory says that things are loosely associated. It states that within the randomness of a chaotic complex system, there are underlying interconnectedness, self-organization, and a dominant oscillator that can reset the chaotic system [17]. It helps us to better understand behaviors occurring in systems that are not random and that there is an attractor causing the behavior. For example, a nurse has many protocols and standardization in their approach but then add patients to this mix; this can create chaos. Some patients do not follow protocols, have different backgrounds and understandings, or there is miscommunication or problems with coordination. When you start introducing so many different pieces to healthcare, then it starts to become disorganized and very chaotic. This is when chaos theory steps in. With an understanding of this theory, a nurse, or any health professional, can step in as a reorganization force, someone who can redirect everyone's attention and energy efficiently.

Cognitive Science Theory: It includes mental models, skills acquisition, perception, and problem-solving that explain how the brain perceives and interprets a computer screen.

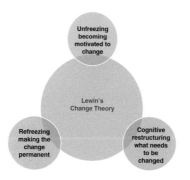

Fig. 2.4 Lewin's Change Theory. (Copyright belongs to Gabriela Mustata Wilson, PhD, MSc, FHIMSS, SNAI) (2021)

Cognitive theory can be related to input, output, and processing. This theory helps to understand human cognitive processes and apply computing procedures. Understanding this theory is helpful to informatics because design engineers can develop usable, efficient, and appropriate technology interfaces for clinical information systems and transform healthcare practices such as nursing [18]. When a system is appropriately designed, it can reduce the clinician's cognitive load using the interface and allow the user to focus energies on higher-order thinking skills rather than on using the interface.

General Systems Theory: This is a concept that systems cannot be reduced to a series of parts functioning in isolation, but that, to understand the whole, one must understand the interrelations between these parts [19]. This theory is characterized by different parts that continuously interact with each other, and these are confined within some form of a boundary. For example, the human body is considered the system as it houses the different body organs of humans. Since Health Informatics is multidisciplinary, general systems theory is important. For example, having different healthcare professionals in a team enhances patient care because different elements and units, large or small, affect the way care is provided to patients. Understanding general systems theory helps healthcare providers to be system thinkers.

Sociotechnical Theory: This theory focuses on how to improve the interaction between the information system and the organizational culture adopting the innovation [20]. The theory finds the best fit for an organization adopting a new system. Understanding this theory helps technology designers create a system that aligns with the organization's financial needs. A poor fit can lead to implementation failures such as bypassing system functions, failure to use system functions, and systems used in unintended ways. This can change the way healthcare is delivered or when there are no improvements in the quality of patient care. Sociotechnical fit means the system was designed and developed by an organization for its own use, which achieves the healthcare outcomes intended when the system was created and developed.

Health Information Systems

The Concept of Information Systems

When people think of information, they think of data; however, **information** consists of data that has been organized and cleaned to help solve problems or give answers to a question. An **information system** is defined as the combination of hardware, software, and other components to collect, organize, and analyze data in a useful way. In simple terms, it turns raw data into useful information. The typical components of information systems can be described using a three-layer graph-based meta-model ($3LGM^2$). The model can effectively describe health information systems by hospital functions, application systems, and physical data processing components [21]. The three layers are the physical instrument layer (hardware), the logical instrument layer (software), and the functional layer (processes). **Hardware** is for computer-based information systems and includes processors, monitors, keyboards, and printers. **Software** is the program used to organize, process, and analyze data. **Database** is where the system organizes data into tables and files for storage. **Network** is different elements connected so that different people in an organization can use the same information system. **Procedure** is how specific data are processed and analyzed in order to get the answers which the information system is designed for.

Different Categories of Information Systems

Organizations employ different types of information systems that help healthcare professionals deliver care to patients, from electronic medical records (EMRs) to electronic patient records, electronic health records, and personal health records. The overview of various healthcare information systems is highlighted in Table 2.1 [22].

Table 2.1 Healthcare information systems. (Copyright belongs to Gabriela Mustata Wilson, PhD, MSc, FHIMSS, SNAI) (2021)

Medical practice management system	Electronic health records (EHR)	Medical billing software	Patient portal	Urgent care applications	Master Patient Index (MPI)
An integral part of the healthcare system geared toward a facility's clerical work, such as managing various documents, scheduling appointments, and more.	It is concerned about the patient's medical information. It can be accessed instantly using a mobile or computer and also enables doctors to easily share data across different departments, allowing them to provide quick and accurate treatment.	It is the most integral type of health management system and most time-consuming processes. Billing software makes it easy by automatically generating medical bills and handling the entire workflow.	It provides a platform where patients can access their health-related data using any device. It includes all the information stored in an EHR, such as patients' medical history, treatments, and other medications previously taken.	A type of health management information system that keeps track of patients that might require immediate attention. It enables patients to skip the waiting room and get the care instantly. It provides patients with knowledge about health-related queries, informative health articles, and even let them track their medical care status.	A crucial part of the hospital management system as it aims at connecting patient records from more than one database. It is generally used by hospitals or large clinics whereby they enter data regarding their patients. Once stored, it can be used for future references by any institute sharing the database.
By automating routine clerical tasks, it allows you to concentrate more on the quality of patient care. It gives you easy access to healthcare data. You can view all the documents online.	EHR increases efficiency by eliminating paperwork and giving immediate access to patients' data. It improves the quality of patient care as the same information is shared across all departments, avoiding any medical errors.	Besides patient billing, the software also takes care of insurance claims and verification, payment tracking, and processing.	It also allows users to schedule appointments, view bills, and make payments online. They can use their personal devices, including smartphones, tablets, or computer to access it.	It increases patients' satisfaction rate as urgent care app provides quick service to them. Urgent care apps provide medical help 24/7 hours a day.	The main purpose of MPI is to reduce duplication of patient records and also to avoid inaccuracy of information that can result in wrong treatment.
Example: eClinicalWorks https://www.eclinicalworks.com/	Example: CureMD https://www.curemd.com/	Example: It sends out alerts for late payments or if there is any pending bill from the hospital's end.	Example: MedFusion https://www.medfusion.com/	Example: HealthTap https://www.healthtap.com/	Example: MPI creates an index of all medical records for a specific patient, which is easily accessible by all departments.

Examples of other healthcare information systems include **E-Prescribing Software,** which enables doctors to generate prescriptions electronically; **Clinical Decision Support System (CDSS)**, which combines information about a diagnosis, drug interactions, and patients to assist healthcare professionals in making decisions; **Picture Archiving and Communication System (PACS),** which manages the acquisition, communication, and storage of medical images inside a radiology department; and **Computerized Provider Order Entry system (CPOE),** which allows providers to electronically prescribe medication and submit admission, laboratory, referrals, radiology, and procedure orders. These systems increase efficiency and reduce clinical errors. Information systems can also help deliver care remotely. These types include **Remote Patient Monitoring** that reads body functions and sends data from anywhere to healthcare professionals at the facility, **teleradiology** provides remote medical imaging diagnosis, teledermatology that diagnoses skin disease,

and **telesurgery**. They are mainly used to reach underserved communities.

At the population level (**Public Health**), information systems are used to provide solutions that influence the population as a whole. They are used for health promotion, disease outbreak surveillance and management, disease prevention, and electronic reporting. At the consumer level (**Consumer Health**), information systems are tools, such as apps, available to individuals committed to promoting health (mental and physical) and assisting in chronic disease management.

Health Information Exchange and Interoperability

Health information exchange (HIE) allows doctors, nurses, pharmacists, other healthcare providers, and patients to appropriately access and securely share a patient's vital medical information electronically, improving the speed, quality, safety, and cost of patient care [23] (Fig. 2.5).

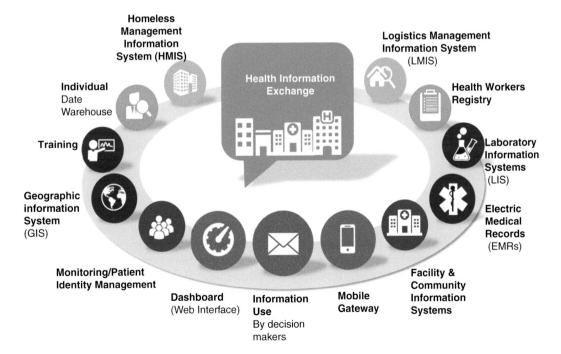

Fig. 2.5 Health Information Exchange with application to healthcare (Figure created with SketchBubble www.sketchbubble.com). (Copyright belongs to Gabriela Mustata Wilson, PhD, MSc, FHIMSS, SNAI) (2021)

While electronic health information exchange cannot replace provider-patient communication, it can significantly improve patient's records, as past history, current medications, and other information are jointly reviewed during visits. Appropriate, timely sharing of vital patient information can better inform decision making at the point of care and allow providers to avoid readmissions, avoid medication errors, improve diagnoses, decrease duplicate testing.

Benefits of HIE include [23]:

- Provides a means for improving the quality and safety of patient care by reducing medical errors
- Encourages patients' involvement in their own healthcare
- Increases efficiency by eliminating unnecessary paperwork
- Provides caregivers with clinical decision support tools for more effective care and treatment
- Eliminates unnecessary testing
- Improves public health reporting and monitoring
- Facilitates efficient deployment of emerging technology and healthcare services
- Provides a basic level of interoperability among electronic health records (EHRs) maintained by individual physicians and organizations
- Reduces health-related costs

Although described in detail in a separate chapter, three types of health information exchange [23] are worth mentioning here:

Directed exchange is used by providers to quickly and securely send patient information such as laboratory orders and results, patient referrals, or discharge summaries directly to another healthcare professional. For example, a primary care provider can directly send electronic care summaries that include medications, problems, and lab results to a specialist when referring their patients. Directed exchange is also being used to send immunization data to public health organizations or report quality measures to the Centers for Medicare & Medicaid Services (CMS).

Query-based exchange is used by providers to search and discover accessible clinical sources on a patient. This type of exchange is often used when delivering unplanned care. The two examples below are very relevant:

- Emergency room physicians who can utilize the query-based exchange to access patient information—such as medications, recent radiology images, and problem lists—might adjust treatment plans to avoid adverse medication reactions or duplicative testing.
- Suppose a pregnant patient goes to the hospital. In that case, a query-based exchange can assist a provider in obtaining her pregnancy care record, allowing them to make safer decisions about the patient's care and her unborn baby.

Consumer-mediated exchange provides patients with access to their health information, allowing them to manage their healthcare online in a similar fashion to managing their finances through online banking. Patients can actively participate in their care coordination by:

- Providing other providers with their health information
- Identifying and correcting wrong or missing health information
- Identifying and correcting incorrect billing information
- Tracking and monitoring their own health

Exchanging individual and population health data involves a common language that can enable information to flow between state and federal databases and allow access to extensive health data pools for research purposes [24]. In this way, the information exchanged can give a complete and accurate depiction of health issues affecting communities [25]. Patients participate in research by providing information through various Health IT applications, which is essential to guarantee the maximum amount of pertinent data are shared for research purposes [24]. Emergent technologies are used to analyze individual and population health data to drive research looks to improve outcomes, patient safety, and patient care. Data analyses classify IT opportunities to encourage data sharing expediently to identify disease patterns at the national and global levels [24].

As indicated in Fig. 2.5, to be able to exchange health information, different information technology systems and software applications need to be able to communicate, exchange data, and use the information that has been exchanged. It is called **interoperability**. **Interoperability** is defined as the ability of health information systems to work together within and across organizational boundaries to advance the health status of and the effective delivery of healthcare for individuals and communities [26].

There are four levels of interoperability [27].

- **Foundational (Level 1)**: Establishes the inter- connectivity requirements needed for one sys- tem or application to securely communicate data to and receive data from another.
- **Structural (Level 2)**: Defines the format, syn- tax, and organization of data exchange, includ- ing at the data field level for interpretation.
- **Semantic (Level 3)**: Provides for standard underlying models and codification of the data, including the use of data elements with standardized definitions from publicly avail- able value sets and coding vocabularies, pro- viding shared understanding and meaning to the user. This level of interoperability is pos- sible via potentially disparate electronic health record (EHR) systems, business-related infor- mation systems, medical devices, mobile technologies, and other systems to improve wellness, as well as the quality, safety, cost- effectiveness, and access to healthcare delivery.
- **Organizational (Level 4)**: Includes gover- nance, policy, social, legal, and organizational considerations to facilitate the secure, seam- less, and timely communication and use of data both within and between organizations, entities, and individuals. These components enable shared consent, trust, and integrated end-user processes and workflows.

The Health Informatics Team

Every profession has its own roles, skills, and responsibilities, contributing to efficient prac- tices in managing patient care. However, these professionals cannot work in isolation to the benefit of the patient/service user without the collaboration of other healthcare professionals that make up the multidisciplinary team. Benefits of interprofessional collaboration include fewer medical errors, reduced health- care costs, and improved relationships across disciplines.

The Health Informatics team is highly multi- disciplinary and interprofessional, composed of experts with a variety of backgrounds:

- Technical background (e.g., network specialists, database specialists, systems administration)
- Health background (e.g., nurses and physi- cians, public health specialists)
- Data science background (e.g., data analyst, health information manager)
- Administrative background (e.g., finance/ accounting)

The Health Informatics field is interprofes- sional. Team diversity is critical to get the best ideas on the table to achieve the best results. Each member contributes their unique knowledge and experiences to the team, and only through this level of teamwork and collaboration can profes- sionals be successful in the highly complex field of Health Informatics.

Roles, Skills, and Responsibilities of Members of the Health Informatics Teams

Members of Health Informatics teams use their knowledge of healthcare, information systems, databases, and information technology security to gather, store, interpret, and manage the massive amount of data generated when care is provided to patients. They are typically respon- sible for [28]:

- Selecting and customizing health information systems
- Planning, designing, and defining functional requirements for health information systems
- Managing health IT projects
- Analyzing data and processes to help facilitate decisions
- Evaluating the application and impact of information systems in support of health goals
- Developing data-driven solutions to improve patient health
- Using data standards to support interoperability of data between systems
- Ensuring confidentiality, security, and integrity standards
- Creating, maintaining, or facilitating new ways for medical facilities and practices to implement and maintain electronic health records (EHRs)
- Improving communication between healthcare providers and facilities to ensure the best patient outcomes
- Being knowledgeable about health data standards, sources, and meaningful use of health data
- Facilitating the communication of regulatory and IT requirements between departments

Health informaticians use information technology to process data into information and knowledge through the following direct applications:

- **Biostatistics and Informatics:** translate data into meaningful information that can then be used to make logical and beneficial clinical and public health decisions.
- **Clinical Informatics and Health Quality Assurance:** analyze the application of information technology in clinical settings to improve efficiency and quality (e.g., study the safety and efficacity of a medical device in a hospital setting).
- **Predictive Modeling:** This area of Health Informatics is closely associated with biostatistics. It involves using computer modeling in a predictive fashion, for example, using predictive modeling to diagnose health conditions in a clinical environment and recognizing common problems related to known drug interactions, prior health conditions, and past injuries or illnesses.
- **Human-Computer Interaction:** For example, assess current interfaces and propose the development of more efficient and intuitive user interfaces, allowing medical professionals to access relevant information more quickly than they otherwise might. These can be developed in collaboration with computer scientists, etc.
- **Organizational Development:** Examines the various needs, uses, and consequences of information in organizational contexts, such as organizational types and characteristics, functional areas and business processes, information-based products and services, the use of and redefining role of information technology, the changing character of work-life and organizational practices, sociotechnical structures, and the rise and transformation of information-based industries.
- **Process Management:** Defines the healthcare organization's business approach by allowing people, systems, and information to interact with greater consistency. Process Management can essentially change how healthcare functions, with less waste, cost savings, streamlined processes, increased compliance, and better patient care.
- **Health Intelligence:** Digital metrics with real-time streams from multiple social media channels analyzed by AI algorithms, local adaptation to disease, digital disinformation campaigns, website traffic, human movement through anonymized cell phone data, and anonymized financial transactions. These multiple data streams are incorporated and fused into a single data visualization tool, allowing us to understand the patterns of movement and behavior that might influence the spread of a virus, disease, etc.

Health Informatics can significantly improve care by developing standardized processes, improved communication, evaluation of performance measures, establishing accountability, and strong care coordination. Integration of Health

IT applications such as workflow improvement, error reduction, data quality, preventive care, and chronic disease management is necessary, and it has the potential to compare the effectiveness of new approaches to traditional approaches to increase patient safety and prevent complications/hospital readmissions. As a result, there is a need for adaptable training programs and the competencies needed to improve and coordinate care, develop, and sustain a data infrastructure essential for value-based payment models.

Academic institutions worldwide have started to address this need by creating new programs that support this transformation and the demand for higher educational standards. These competencies require knowledge in data and information (information sciences), clinical and health terminologies, data analysis and management, and communication skills [29, 30]. Health Informatics competency-based education and training are necessary to improve patient safety and catalyze collaborative interprofessional research and practice initiatives that will impact healthcare and public health at the local, regional, national, and international domains.

Emerging Trends in Health Information Technology

Managing one's health today involves an app, a "smart" device, or a patient portal. The way of delivering healthcare through digitally enabled technologies is moving fast and furious, creating both opportunities and risks. Nevertheless, the positives outweigh the negatives, and the impact of this technology-driven era provides more analytics, accountability, and accessibility.

Some of the emerging technologies that are changing the way we deliver healthcare and impact the field of Health Informatics are as follows:

Artificial Intelligence (AI) is a technology designed to mimic human cognitive processes. AI can be used to mine medical data to improve how hospitals and healthcare professionals deliver care to patients [31]. It can also be used to rapidly and accurately identify cancerous and healthy tissues on CT and MRI scans of patients with head and neck cancer for more targeted radiotherapy treatment.

Machine Learning (ML) is a subset of AI through which computers learn by themselves when they face new data, with minimal human supervision. It is the fastest-growing field in computer science, with application to healthcare due to the benefits of improved medical diagnoses, disease analyses, and pharmaceutical development. Machine learning is a data analysis approach that automates analytical model building through algorithms that iterate over the supplied data and then produce reliable, repeatable decisions and results. Successful application of machine learning in healthcare needs a multidisciplinary effort among experts ranging from computer and data science to biomedical informatics and health sciences.

Biosensors embedded in clothing that include tissue, thermal, DNA, and immuno-sensors are significant innovations in the healthcare field that will continue to evolve [32]. The sensors incorporated into clothing aid in sensing biological activity in the body by measuring broadrange markers, including sweat and skin debris and temperature ranges. This type of innovation is a game-changer due to its ability to blend with regular physical activity and day-to-day life. Virtual health appointments are a common practice in the conventional world. From applications that offer medical diagnoses to interventions, it is evident that virtual arrangements are the future trends regarding the management of common illnesses [33].

Blockchain Technology is a distributed, public ledger, recording transactions, tracking assets, and immutability is guaranteed by a peer-to-peer network of computers, not by any centralized authority [32]. Blockchain technology is expected to improve medical record management and the insurance claim process, accelerate clinical and biomedical research, and advance biomedical and healthcare data ledger [34]. These are based on blockchain technology's key aspects, such as decentralized management, immutable audit trail, data provenance, robustness, and improved security and privacy.

Virtual Reality (VR) is steadily changing the way we live and significantly contributes to improving our daily well-being and health. It involves using computer technology to create a simulated environment placing the user inside the virtual experience by simulating different senses like vision, hearing, smell, or even touch and other actions. VR has been assessed in mental health conditions for the rehabilitation of patients with schizophrenia, the treatment of post-traumatic stress disorder symptomatology, or the management of phobic disorders. Exposing patients to VR allows therapy delivery in a form that they may find it easier to accept. They can control the unexpected, making it safer for specific fears that may be difficult to reproduce in real situations [35].

Robotics is the design, engineering, and use of robotic machines to perform partially or fully automated physical and cognitive functions [31]. An example of its use in healthcare is a robot-assisted surgical system controlled by a surgeon that uses minimally invasive surgical instruments and 3D high-definition visuals to enhance accuracy and control. In informatics, robotics enables the autonomous collection of data, providing accurate and continual data for professionals.

3D Bioprinting prints solid, 3D objects from a digital file with an additive process using different materials such as liquid metals, polymers, ceramics, or living cells. It can be used to print living human tissue using stem cell bio-ink and reduce the shortage of organs for transplants [31]. Three-dimensional bioprinting furthers the study and research of the molecular basis of disease through 3D-printed human tissue cells for testing.

Nanomedicine utilizes nanotechnology for developing precise devices to advance biomedical research and clinical practice [31]. An example of how it is used in healthcare is injecting nanorobots into a patient's bloodstream for drug delivery and disease monitoring. In informatics, nanomedicine is necessary for integrating large data sets at the nano level for research.

Cloud computing enables the delivery and access to computing resources and services over the Internet. Virtual resources are servers, storage, networking, databases, and analytics [31]. It can be used for high-volume storage of data at lower costs for healthcare organizations. Health Informatics relies on access to extensive medical data and EHRs; cloud computing enables safe and affordable storage data with mobile access to professionals.

Challenges Presented by Emerging Trends

Having described various trends in information technology, what challenges do these emerging technologies present? They include privacy and security concerns, liability risk, lack of law or legislation governing the boundaries, lack of payment for engagement, frequent updates, and healthcare providers' resistance [36].

- **Privacy and confidentiality:** The Health Insurance Portability and Accountability Act (HIPAA) of 1996 was created initially for the portability, privacy, and security of personal health information (PHI) that was largely paper based. HIPAA regulations were updated in 2009 and again in 2013 to better cover the electronic transmission of PHI (ePHI) [37]. To satisfy this requirement, the US Department of Health and Human Services (HHS) published what are commonly known as the *HIPAA Privacy Rule* [38] and the *HIPAA Security Rule* [39]. The Privacy Rule, or Standards for Privacy of Individually Identifiable Health Information, establishes national standards to protect certain health information. Many governmental institutions are addressing this through the privacy-preserving record linkage (PPRL), which eliminates the need to expose identifiers, so data are shared securely, safely, and privately [40].

- **Ethical issues:** Every aspect of Health Informatics is affected by ethical and legal concerns finding a way to balance the need to protect patient information security with the potential for better care and outcomes associated with greater interoperability and improved ability to share patient information among healthcare entities. Similarly, the growing interest and use of social media platforms in healthcare research [41], as well as the use of wearable technology for data collection, has generated several ethical questions, including concerns about disclosure of data collection, the selling of data, manipulation of insurance premiums, different ways of interpreting data, and worries about data loss due to poor cybersecurity. The patient can be in a vulnerable position if there is no appropriate balance between ethically justified ends and otherwise reasonable means.

- **High cost to adopt:** Technologies such as picture archiving and communications systems (PACS) and EHRs are expensive solutions to adopt by a healthcare organization.
- **Inadequate time:** Providers do not have enough time to learn how to utilize new technologies and adopt them.
- **Legal issues:** The Stark and Anti-kickback Laws prevent hospital systems from providing or sharing technology such as computers and software with referring physicians. Exceptions were made to these laws in 2006 for hospitals to share EHRs and e-prescribing programs with clinician's offices.

Other challenges to new technologies are usability, processes by which health information systems are analyzed and designed.

Case Study

Liberty Health was lagging in technological advances. The not-for-profit business model was not structured to purchase new technology or software programs and had no workforce or time to implement an EMR system. The practice sees about 30 patients a day from ages 2 to 75. The majority of patients live below the poverty level. These patients consume a large share of American healthcare services, which has increased the demand on the healthcare system for this population. One of the significant issues Liberty Healthcare is experiencing is providing a wide

range of skills and services to meet this population's future needs.

Manual record keeping has caused significant problems and threatened to decrease the clinic's efficiency in healthcare delivery and compromise care delivery. In the past, Liberty Health performed all documentation on paper, including patient information, details of each patient's visit, vitals, and patient history. The practice also utilized other billing services from private insurers. The practice began seeing a trend of mistakes in the paperwork as well as inefficient work practices. Also, patients wanted easier access to their health information, and this became time-consuming for employees. Duplication of procedures to replace lost or missing test results jeopardized patients' health and left the practice at risk of adverse medical events. Duplication of unnecessary procedures also contributed to delayed results and created potentially harmful situations for patients; it was also a needless expense. Liberty Health attempted numerous ways to improve its workflow process, but unfortunately the efforts were not successful, and the problems were multiplying.

The practice comprises two full-time physicians, one nurse practitioner, and four full-time registered nurses. Liberty Health has been in the area for about eight years. The not-for-profit practice recently received a generous donation from a local doctor who appreciated how effective this practice is and the positive effect it has on the surrounding community. The practice saw an opportunity to make some significant changes with the donation and collectively decided there was an urgency to increase efficiency and improve patient satisfaction by implementing an electronic medical record system.

Liberty Health approached Your Care Consulting for an internal assessment of its current workflow, recommendations on selecting an electronic medical record (EMR), and the most effective ways to implement the EMR. Liberty Health is also asking Your Care Consulting to develop an improved workflow to be utilized in the practice (see description of the solution in Appendix).

Summary

This chapter provides an introduction to the world of Health Informatics along with its different fields, theories, systems, interoperability, and emerging trends. **Health Informatics** integrates healthcare sciences, computer science, information science, and cognitive science to assist in managing healthcare information. The development of Health Informatics is generally traced to the first use of computers in healthcare in the 1950s. Some of the different fields in Health Informatics are biomedical, nursing, public health, consumer, medical, and pharmaco-informatics. Knowing the differences between data, information, knowledge, and wisdom is key to understanding informatics. Different theories such as chaos theory, change theory, and cognitive science theory can provide a helpful framework for evaluation, design, or implementation in Health Informatics. Many healthcare organizations utilize different information systems such as Electronic Health Record (EHR) to help deliver care to patients. Therefore, interoperability is critical. This is achieved through Health Information Exchange (HIE), in which different healthcare providers and patients can appropriately access and securely share a patient's vital medical information electronically, improving the speed, quality, safety, and cost of patient care. With advances in technology, the world of Health Informatics sees emerging trends that are changing the way we deliver healthcare. Some of them are artificial intelligence, blockchain technology, and cloud computing. As the world of Health Informatics continuously evolves, it will continue to play an essential role in developing solid care coordination between different fields and best practices for patient care.

Conclusions and Outlook

Healthcare is an information-rich industry. Health Informatics plays a significant role in improving care by developing standardized processes, improved communication, evaluation of performance measures, the establishment of accountability, and strong care coordination. Integration of Health IT applications is necessary to compare the effectiveness of new approaches to traditional ones, increase patient safety, and prevent complications/hospital readmissions. Nevertheless, technology alone cannot solve the problems: community-wide initiatives and multi-interprofessional and multidisciplinary collaborations are crucial to improving healthcare services, patient health outcomes, and population health. Training in Health Informatics needs to integrate interprofessional learning models across platforms through research and idea incubation, nurturing innovation, and outreach and engagement. The expectation to collaborate, partner, and innovate with the community in mind is the formula for sustainable change.

Useful Resources

1. American Medical Informatics Association https://www.amia.org/
2. Healthcare Information and Management Systems Society https://www.himss.org/
3. HealthCare IT News https://www.healthcare-itnews.com/
4. HealthIT.gov https://www.healthit.gov/
5. International Journal of Medical Informatics https://www.journals.elsevier.com/international-journal-of-medical-informatics
6. International Medical Informatics Association https://imia-medinfo.org/wp/
7. Journal of the American Medical Informatics Association https://academic.oup.com/jamia
8. Journal of Biomedical Informatics https://www.journals.elsevier.com/journal-of-biomedical-informatics/
9. The State of Health Care Quality: How Good is Care? http://www.hcqualitycommission.gov

Review Questions

1. What is the major characteristic of Biomedical and Health Informatics?
2. How health informaticians use information technology to process data into information and knowledge?

3. Use each stage of Lewin's Change Theory to explain the transition from paper-based records to an EMR in a small dental clinic.
4. Which type of health information exchange should be used to send data to public health organizations? Directed Exchange or Consumer-Mediated Exchange?
5. What are the ethical concerns associated with the use of wearable devices?

Appendix: Answers to Review Questions

1. What is the major characteristic of Biomedical and Health Informatics?

Biomedical and Health Informatics are interdisciplinary, scientific fields that study and pursue the practical uses of biomedical data, information, and knowledge for scientific inquiry, problem-solving, and decision making, motivated by efforts to improve human health. Biomedical and Health Informatics apply computer and information science principles to the advancement of life sciences research, health professions education, public health, and patient care. They build bridges to healthy communities by establishing informatics as a bridge to accelerate the translation of discoveries to improve individual patients' health and translate the science of healthcare delivery for better population health.

2. How health informaticians use information technology to process data into information and knowledge?

Health Informaticians use information technology, such as computers, to retrieve information from the data and then generate knowledge. While computers are used to store data, health informaticians find meaning in the data by using methods and computer-generated models to extract the knowledge from information.

3. Use each stage of Lewin's Change Theory to explain the transition from paper-based records to an EMR in a small dental clinic.

The three stages of Lewin's Change Theory are Unfreezing, Cognitive, and Refreezing.

Unfreezing: During this stage, the benefits that a basic digital charting program can provide to the dental practice should be highlighted (Examples: Improved quality and patient safety; Increased security; Reduced paperwork and storage issues; Increased efficiency and productivity; Reduced operational costs such as transcription services and overtime labor; E-prescribing and clinical documentation capabilities; More efficient patient billing process; Increased accuracy, etc.).

Cognitive: The users would need to be convinced that the new approach is safer and better than the old and have a change in behavior to give space for the new process, which is evident by learning how to use the EMR.

Refreezing: The leadership and implementation team should offer rewards and support to those transitioning from the paper-based system to the EMR.

4. Which type of health information exchange should be used to send data to public health organizations? Directed Exchange or Consumer-Mediated Exchange?

Directed Exchange is being used to send immunization data to public health organizations or report quality measures to The Centers for Medicare & Medicaid Services (CMS).

5. What are the ethical concerns associated with the use of wearable devices?

The ethical concerns associated with the use of wearable devices include disclosure of data collection, the selling of data, manipulation of insurance premiums, different ways of interpreting data, and worries about data loss due to poor cybersecurity.

Case Study: Electronic Medical Record Implementation at Liberty Health

(Conceptualized by graduate-level Health Informatics students at the University of Southern Indiana)

Liberty Health was lagging in technological advances. The not-for-profit business model was not structured to purchase new technology or software programs and had no workforce or time to implement an EMR system. The practice sees about 30 patients a day from ages 2 to 75. The majority of patients live below the poverty level. These patients consume a large share of American health care services, which has increased the demand on the healthcare system for this population. One of the significant issues Liberty Healthcare is experiencing is providing a wide range of skills and services to meet this population's future needs.

Manual record keeping has caused significant problems and threatened to decrease the clinic's efficiency in healthcare delivery and compromise care delivery. In the past, Liberty Health performed all documentation on paper, including patient information, details of each patient's visit, vitals, and patient history. The practice also utilized other billing services from private insurers. The practice began seeing a trend of mistakes in the paperwork as well as inefficient work practices. Also, patients wanted easier access to their health information, and this became time-consuming for employees. Duplication of procedures to replace lost or missing test results jeopardized patients' health and left the practice at risk of adverse medical events. Duplication of unnecessary procedures also contributed to delayed results and created potentially harmful situations for patients; it was also a needless expense. Liberty Health attempted numerous ways to improve its workflow process, but unfortunately, the efforts were not successful, and the problems were multiplying. **YourCare Consulting** was asked to help Liberty Health address the following:

- Internal assessment of the current workflow of the practice
- Recommend an EMR that best suits the needs of the healthcare facility
- Develop best practices and plans on how to implement the EMR in the most efficient way

Workflow Requirements

Patient Appointment Workflow

It is crucial to have an effective workflow process to increase productivity and understand protocols and tactical procedures. This allows team members involved to quickly comprehend what is expected and needed to complete a job successfully. Figure 2.6 illustrates the workflow process that will be utilized with the implementation of the new EMR. This workflow, consisting of approximately ten steps in the process, would benefit from checking-in a patient and placing them in an exam room because it records every step and saves documentation for future appointments. A nurse or doctor can recall the patient's medical history with a few clicks. This improves patients' flow during the day and, if used correctly, could increase the number of patients seen daily.

The main goal of implementing new technology in a small to medium size practice is to provide complete and accurate records of patient information. This ensures the quality and safety of patient care. Nevertheless, providers may have concerns about how computer-driven systems will affect their role as caregivers or if using such a system will impact the patient-provider relationship. Providers may also be concerned about challenges while adapting to new technology. One of the most significant concerns surrounding the EMR is whether it will positively or negatively affect patient satisfaction. Patients may be hesitant at the beginning of the transition due to data confidentiality. However, formal evaluations of EMR rarely address patients' views of the quality of care after implementation. Measurement of patient satisfaction is an essen-

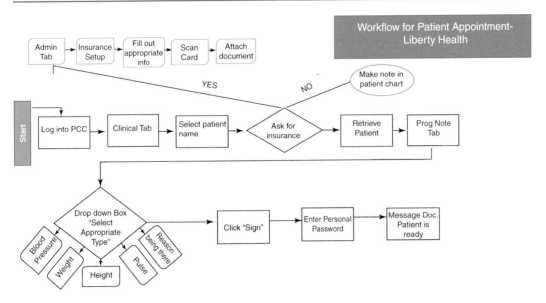

Fig. 2.6 Workflow for patient appointment—Liberty Health

tial tool for research for any size organization. Administration and planning to ensure the practice receive the best feedback after implementation is vital.

Providers and healthcare professionals will need time to become familiar with the selected EMR system properly. The extent to which the chosen EMR system can operate, exchange, and interpret healthcare data is critical for successful implementation. Liberty Health desires an EMR system that can work within and across the boundaries of the healthcare organization. Adopting an EMR system could reduce rework by healthcare professionals and improve the exchange of new medical knowledge among physicians throughout the practice and other entities. Interoperability is essential because it decreases the cost of electronic medical records and makes it feasible for an individual or small group of providers to acquire and adopt these systems.

Implementing an EMR Solution

The implementation of an EMR solution will enable clinical staff to conduct cost/benefit analyses, trend clinical information to improve care

and financial information to contain costs, target clinical quality indicators, and retrospectively analyze information for strategic and tactical decision making [42, 43]. The EMR will generate a unique patient identifier, thereby reducing the potential for duplicate patient records. Care coordination has improved as a result of the EMR system. Legible, accurate, timely information that can be simultaneously accessed allows the clinicians to work more efficiently as a team.

Liberty Health's implementation of an EMR system would potentially solve the major issues with their paper system. These issues have impacted the practice's ability to bill for services properly and therefore, has impeded its revenue stream. The proper EMR will increase revenue and decrease billing time. Reducing medical errors will help the practice provide better care to patients and decrease the risk of a serious complication due to a medical error. Also, with the implementation of the EMR system, patients will be able to look at their medical history and current course of treatment online. Overall, the implementation of an EMR system will significantly benefit Liberty Health and the benefits listed below will far outweigh the cost.

As a health care practice, it is crucial to manage risks and stay ahead of unexpected challenges that might arise; the recommended EMR solution provides those tools. Managing patient and staff risk is an important aspect of quality care and the recommended EMR solution will continuously allow focus on quality improvements. It will also provide management of incident reports by collecting information and records data for analysis. Having access to such reports will allow for high compliance monitoring resulting in improved quality care. To ensure that the practice is compliant, the staff and care team need to be informed regularly. By implementing the recommended EMR solution, the practice will have access to various learning and teaching resources.

Documentation is vital but often a demanding task when managing patient risk. There are specific documentation requirements that must be followed. Accurate filing, documenting, and collecting patient information is more straightforward with the proposed EMR solution.

EMR Vendor Selection

An EMR that is user friendly and has the ability to operate efficiently and effectively is vital. Usability can pose a barrier toward implementation; thus, all staff must learn how to use EMR effectively. Lack of technical training and support from vendors has been reported as a barrier to the adoption of EMRs in the past by providers; therefore, it is vital to choose a vendor that offers outstanding, extensive training programs and allows for a pilot demonstration before implementation. To prevent gaps in data transfers and losses, all systems should be password-protected and connected to a secure server that can protect and improve the organization's internal processes.

The following questions can be used to identify the desired characteristics of vendors

- What is the market share this vendor maintains?
- What is the vendor's reputation?
- How long has the vendor been around?
- Does the vendor have CCHIT certification?

- Does the vendor offer any additional services (i.e., web design)?
- Does the vendor provide functionality updates for each stage of meaningful use?
- Does the vendor provide support in helping to obtain the maximum incentive payment?

In conclusion, YourCare Consulting recommends that Liberty Health purchase an EMR system that aligns with the practice needs, which will result in raising revenues, improving patient care, enhancing documentation, and providing easier access to data. Usability is a critical factor, and choosing an EMR system that is integrated with a practice management system made by the same vendor would be most beneficial.

The most important benefit Liberty Health would see after the implementation of an EMR would be the reduction of errors in the workplace. Issues with misplaced records, errors because of illegible handwriting, and other staff mistakes would be eliminated with an Electronic Medical Records program. EMR would also expedite testing processes, reduce the number of errors in diagnostic testing, and eliminate duplicate testing. The need for staff to assemble, file, and retrieve charts would also be eliminated, creating a more efficient use of staff time.

Another issue EMR would address is low patient satisfaction scores in terms of patients accessing medical information. Currently, patients call the practice to request information, and a staff member searches through paper records for that information. Staff is pulled away from other tasks to retrieve the information; also, the information may not even be current because of the time it takes to add information to paper files. After implementing the EMR system, patients will be able to seamlessly access their medical records online or via an app on mobile phones, recent lab tests, and prescriptions. Liberty Health should expect to see an increase in patient satisfaction scores. Because patients will feel more involved in their own care, overall, patients' health will likely improve and reduce readmissions or repeat visits to the healthcare facility.

References

1. Sweeney J. Healthcare informatics. Online J Nurs Inform. 2017;2(1). https://www.himss.org/resources/healthcare-informatics.
2. American Medical Informatics Association. 2020. www.amia.org. Accessed 5 Nov 2020.
3. American Medical Informatics Association. Why informatics? 2020. https://www.amia.org/why-informatics. Accessed 5 Nov 2020.
4. Ball MJ. Better health through informatics: managing information to deliver value. In: Public Health Informatics and Information Systems. Basingstoke: Springer Nature; 2003. p. 39–51. https://doi.org/10.1007/0-387-22745-8_3.
5. Betts H, Wright G. Was Florence nightingale the first nursing informatician. Berlin: Research Gate; 2003. p. 20–5. https://www.researchgate.net/publication/233380253_Was_Florence_Nightingale_the_First_Nursing_Informatician
6. Degoulet P, Fieschi M, Goldberg M, Salamon R. François Grémy, a humanist and information sciences pioneer. Yearb Med Inform. 2014;9:3–5. https://www.ncbi.nlm.nih.gov/pmc/articles/PMC4287063/
7. Jain A. Milestones of public health informatics. 2020. https://www.timetoast.com/timelines/milestones-of-public-health-informatics. Accessed 23 Oct 2020.
8. American Medical Informatics Association. What is biomedical and health informatics? 2011. https://www.amia.org/sites/default/files/What-is-Informatics-Fact-Sheet-040811.pdf. Accessed 23 Oct 2020.
9. American Medical Informatics Association. Informatics area. 2020. https://www.amia.org/. Accessed 23 Oct 2020.
10. Robert EH, Hersh WR. Health informatics: practical guide. 7th ed. Singapore: Informatics Education; 2018.
11. Collins GP. Claude E. Shannon: founder of information theory. Scientific American. 2002. https://www.scientificamerican.com/article/claude-e-shannon-founder/. Accessed 11 Nov 2020.
12. University of Illinois Chicago. Current trends in the health information management field. 2017. https://healthinformatics.uic.edu/blog/current-trends-in-the-health-information-management-field/. Accessed 23 Oct 2020.
13. World Health Organization. National eHealth strategy toolkit. 2012. https://www.who.int/ehealth/publications/overview.pdf. Accessed 11 Nov 2020.
14. Scott P, Briggs J, Wyatt JC, Georgiou A. How important is theory in Health informatics? A survey of UK academics. Stud Health Technol Inform. 2011;169:223–7. https://www.researchgate.net/publication/51621327_How_important_is_theory_in_health_informatics_A_survey_of_UK_academics
15. Scott P, Keizer N, Georgiou A. Applied interdisciplinary theory in health informatics: a knowledge base for practitioners. Studies in health technology and informatics. Amsterdam: IOS Press; 2019.
16. Peptiprin A. Lewin's change theory. 2020. https://nursing-theory.org/theories-and-models/lewin-change-theory.php. Accessed 23 Oct 2020.
17. Krienheder M. Chaos theory in nursing. 2017. https://drmattk.com/chaos-theory-in-nursing/. Accessed 23 Oct 2020.
18. Mastrian K, McGonigle D. Cognitive informatics: an essential component of nursing technology design. Am Acad Nurs. 2008;56:332–3. https://doi.org/10.1016/j.outlook.2008.09.010
19. Cordon CP. System theories: an overview of various system theories and its application in healthcare. Am J Syst Sci. 2013;2:13–22. https://www.researchgate.net/publication/263039164_System_Theories_An_Overview_of_Various_System_Theories_and_Its_Application_in_Healthcare
20. Borycki EM, Kushniruk AW. Towards and integrative cognitive-socio-technical approach in health informatics: analyzing technology-induced error involving health information systems to improve patient safety. Open Med Inform J. 2010;4:181–7. https://doi.org/10.2174/2F1874431101004010181.
21. Winter A, Brigl B, Funkat G, Häber A, Heller O, Wendt T. 3LGM2-modeling to support management of health information systems. Int J Med Inform. 2007;76(2–3):145–50. https://doi.org/10.1016/j.ijmedinf.2006.07.007.
22. Shrushti. 8 types of health information technology & healthcare software systems. 2020. https://www.softwaresuggest.com/blog/types-of-health-information-technology-and-healthcare-software/#:~:text=%20Different%20Types%20of%20Healthcare%20Information%20System%20,software%20is%20a%20beneficial%20technology%20as...%20More%20. Accessed 18 Nov 2020.
23. Health IT. Health information exchange. 2020. https://www.healthit.gov/topic/health-it-and-health-information-exchange-basics/what-hie. Accessed 23 Oct 2020.
24. Impact Insights. 2020-2025 federal health IT strategic plan 2020. https://www.impact-advisors.com/regulatory/federal-health-it-strategic-plan/2020-2025-federal-health-it-strategic-plan-what-you-need-to-know/. Accessed 11 Nov 2020.
25. Haque SM, Shellery Ebron M, Bailey R, Barry Blumenthal M. Using health information exchange to support community-based innovations. Perspect Health Inf Manag. 2018. https://www.perspectives.ahima.org.
26. Healthcare Information and Management Systems Society. Dictionary of healthcare information technology terms, acronyms and organizations. 3rd ed. Chicago, IL: HIMSS; 2013. p. 75.
27. Healthcare Information and Management Systems Society. Interoperability in healthcare. 2020 https://www.himss.org/resources/interoperability-healthcare. Accessed 11 Nov 2020.

28. University of South Florida. The job of a health informatics professional. 2020. https://www.usfhealthonline.com/resources/career/a-day-in-the-life-of-health-informatics-professional/#:~:text=Health%20informatics%20professionals%20use%20their,care%20is%20provided%20to%20patients.&text=Developing%20data%2Ddriven%20solutions%20to%20improve%20patient%20health. Accessed 23 Oct 2020.

29. Thye J. Understanding health informatics core competencies. 2020. https://www.himss.org/resources/health-informatics. Accessed 18 Nov 2020.

30. Kulikowski CA, Shortliffe EH, Currie LM, Elkin PL, Hunter LE, Johnson TR, Kalet IJ, Lenert LA, Musen MA, Ozbolt JG, Smith JW, Tarczy-Hornoch PZ, Williamson JJ. AMIA board white paper: definition of biomedical informatics and specification of core competencies for graduate education in the discipline. J Am Med Inform Assoc. 2012;19(6):931–8. https://doi.org/10.1136/amiajnl-2012-001053

31. University of Illinois Chicago. 5 emerging technologies and their impact on health informatics. https://health-informatics.uic.edu/blog/5-emerging-technologies-and-their-impact-on-health-informatics/. Accessed 23 Oct 2020.

32. Mehrotra P. Biosensors and their applications–a review. J Oral Biol Craniofac Res. 2016;6(2):153–9. https://doi.org/10.1016/j.jobcr.2015.12.002

33. Wu H, Lu N. Online written consultation, telephone consultation, and offline appointment: an examination of the channel effect in online health communities. Int J Med Inform. 2017;107:107–19. https://doi.org/10.1016/j.ijmedinf.2017.08.009

34. Yoon H. Blockchain technology and healthcare. Healthc Inform Res. 2019;25(2):59–60. https://doi.org/10.4258/hir.2019.25.2.59

35. Clus D, Larsen ME, Lemey C, Berrouiguet S. The use of virtual reality in patients with eating disorders: systematic review. J Med Internet Res. 2018;20(4):e157. https://doi.org/10.2196/jmir.7898.

36. Bath PA. Health informatics: current issues and challenges. J Inf Sci. 2008;34:501. https://doi.org/10.1177/2F0165551508092267.

37. Health and Human Services. Summary of the HIPAA security rule. 2013. https://www.hhs.gov/hipaa/for-professionals/security/laws-regulations/index.html. Accessed 18 Nov 2020.

38. Health and Human Services. The HIPAA privacy rule. 2020. https://www.hhs.gov/hipaa/for-professionals/privacy/index.html. Accessed 18 Nov 2020.

39. Health and Human Services. The security rule. 2020. https://www.hhs.gov/hipaa/for-professionals/security/index.html. Accessed 18 Nov 2020.

40. Kum HC, Krishnamurthy A, Machanavajjhala A, Reiter MK, Ahalt S. Privacy preserving interactive record linkage (PPIRL). J Am Med Inform Assoc. 2013;21(2):212–20. https://doi.org/10.1136/amiajnl-2013-002165

41. Azer SA. Social media channels in health care research and rising ethical issues. AMA J Ethics. 2017;19(11):1061–9. https://journalofethics.ama-assn.org/sites/journalofethics.ama-assn.org/files/2018-05/peer1-1711.pdf

42. Health IT. How much is this going to cost me? 2020. https://www.healthit.gov/faq/how-much-going-cost-me. Accessed 30 Oct 2020.

43. Health IT. Why adopt EHRs? 2020. https://www.healthit.gov/topic/health-it-basics/benefits-ehrs. Accessed 30 Oct 2020.

Part II

The 360° Stakeholder Perspective

The Patient's View: The Patients as "Editor-in-Chief" of Their Data

3

Grace Kennedy

Learning Objectives
- Learn the effects of health informatics on the implementation of patient-centered care
- Appreciate the transparency health informatics provides patients and the effects it has on patient engagement
- Understand the effects of patient-centered care on health outcomes

Key Terms
- Autonomy critical to patient compliance
- Access to your own data
- Patient-provider relationship is partnership with dual responsibilities
- Transparency and education on the part of the physician
- Shared decision making
- Health informatics tools to access data
- Health literacy
- Patient safety and errors of commission
- Modification of lifestyle
- Proactive disease and health management

Introduction

The introduction of health informatics (HI) has allowed healthcare practitioners (HCPs) the chance to work more quickly and consequently increase their patient load. The benefits HI integration poses on the efficiency of HCPs, especially via electronic charting, placing orders, and viewing results of laboratory tests, are undeniable. Not only does the use of HI make the job of healthcare providers more efficient, but it also allows for more patient autonomy, increasing the role of the patient in their own health management. This almost directly relates to better compliance to prescribed treatment regimens. HI also aids in preventing miscommunication between specialists and ensures that all parties involved in the care of the patient are working cohesively and minimizing treatment risks. Many, if not all, of these efforts ultimately result in a reduced financial burden on the US economy by lowering the costs of managing chronic disease states.

Health informatics is defined as a scientific discipline concerning the cognitive, informative-processing, and communication tasks of healthcare practice and education [1]. This includes the information science and technology utilized to support those responsibilities [2]. One particularly impactful use of HI is the electronic health record (EHR). The integration of the EHR in patient care has allowed HCPs to streamline charting patient encounters and placing orders while managing patient care, allowing these systems to work more effectively in the sometimes unpredictable field of medicine. The EHR also gives patients unprecedented access to information regarding their care, making it the primary

G. Kennedy (✉)
Summerfield, LA, USA

© Springer Nature Switzerland AG 2022
U. H. Hübner et al. (eds.), *Nursing Informatics*, Health Informatics,
https://doi.org/10.1007/978-3-030-91237-6_3

focus of this chapter. We will explore the expanded role of the patient as a result of EHRs, the challenges patients and their care teams often face, and how the use of EHRs can present solutions to those challenges and further benefit the field of healthcare.

The Role of the Patient

In the 360-stakeholder perspective, the patient is at the core of the healthcare system. The patient is responsible for presenting the chief complaint, around which HCPs center their thought process in order to develop differential diagnoses with the help of health informatics. In this thought, without the patient there would be no chief complaint to study, no therapeutic goals, and no role for HCPs. As the core of the care team, the patients are responsible for education surrounding their condition, communication, and expression of concerns shared decision making and implementation of their autonomy, advocacy, and self-care, which involves compliance to treatment regimens [3]. Because autonomy is so critical to patient compliance, the need for patient consent is vital for the physician to be able to diagnose and treat patients. This concept is essential for the patient's right to accept or decline treatment and/or clinical evaluation and participate in developing their care goals [4].

The relationship between the patient and the physician is a true partnership with dual responsibilities. The physician is responsible for educating patients on their disease states and informing them on how to achieve health and wellness. The role of the patient is to take initiative on the information given by the physician and to use it to their best health interest [5]. The only way to ensure harmony among both parties is effective communication and transparency. Patient compliance is reliant on three things: transparency and education on the part of the physician, expressed autonomy of the patient in shared decision making of treatment regimens, and access to the information discussed during that encounter after the fact. This is where HI further expands the role of the patient in healthcare.

After the integration of HI, the patient is no longer simply a vessel carrying a potential diagnosis but is now a team player actively participating in the achievement of therapeutic goals. This expansion of the role for educated, decision-making patients is a central theme of healthcare reform along with responsive care teams of HCPs [6]. Studies have proven that patient anxiety levels increase during office visits, explaining white coat phenomenon. This increased anxiety can have an effect on how accurately patients absorb new information regarding their care. Giving patients limited access to their health records electronically allows them to thoroughly review all that was discussed during their visit, new therapeutic goals, and any educational materials referenced by their physician during their visit in a relaxed setting in which they can absorb material more completely. This allows patients to act more intentionally in their daily lives with their health goals in mind.

Challenges Facing the Patient

The beginning stages of healthcare reform highlighted the challenges faced by the patient in the 360-stakeholder view. There have not always been clearly defined roles in the patient-physician partnership, taking away some of the patient's autonomy and, as a result, their compliance as well. This manifests as a lack of transparency between healthcare workers, limited access to HCPs, and medical information that is recorded inaccurately. More barriers patients face include limited access to advanced technology, narrow scope of health literacy, and miseducation to the benefits of treatment regimen and personal interventions. These are just a few of the obstacles that often lead to poor patient engagement, compliance, and retention. Unfortunately, a traditional health system is not prepared to overcome these hurdles and facilitate improved patient engagement [4]. As healthcare reform highlights more of these challenges, it is critical that our healthcare system evolves to meet those needs.

The need for transparency in healthcare has never been more evident than now. Patients not only want to be involved in decision making, they want to know all of their options and the risks that come with them in order to make informed decisions. This desire for information mixed with the expansive information available in a web search can lead to patient miseducation and physician distrust. This is why it is imperative for physicians to be fully forthcoming in their encounters with patients, putting an emphasis on patient education. In relation to risks of treatments, patients are of course concerned with health risks, but they are also concerned with the financial risk treatment options come with. Unfortunately, in our current healthcare system physicians are not always aware of the cost implications of interventions, or whether or not a patient's insurance will cover all of the presented options. Transparency in this regard requires a collaborative approach between the physician, patient, and billing specialists.

Placing a stronger focus on patient education and taking a more collaborative approach may sound like a simple fix to many; however, a traditional health system complicates this potential fix. Inadequate staff and resources can afflict clinical facilities deeply, resulting in the development of counterproductive practices, like inaccurate record keeping and HCP burnout. Take, for example, an adult patient admitted to the hospital for four days. Research shows that this patient may very well interact with nearly 50 different employees during their stay [7]. With each shift change and increase in patient load, the likelihood that each new physician or nurse is obtaining a full HPI from the patient diminishes, meaning the success of the patient rests heavily on accurate documentation in their health record. Any inaccuracy documented by any party on the patient's care team can lead to a misdiagnosis or unnecessarily prolonged hospital stay. This not only has implications on the patient's health and personal finances, but also adds to the ever-rising healthcare management costs.

If we want solutions to the challenges our patients face, we need to prioritize patient education and safety. This can be achieved only with successful healthcare reform centered around exhibiting improved quality of care through the development of more efficient systems for HCPs [8]. This may look like additional resources for some or expanded staff for others. But for everyone, total reform requires the continued integration of health informatics into the practice of modern medicine. The success of the patient relies on it.

Solutions Health Informatics Presents

The use of tools developed to better utilize HI is key in the future of healthcare reform. Not only it is crucial for increased HCP efficiency, but it has profound benefits for the patient, both directly and indirectly. While these tools, like EHRs, are great in improving efficiency in patient encounters, some of these tools can also be used to increase patient safety, improve patient engagement, and enhance patient outcomes in chronic disease management.

History shows that the use of big data is one of the most common ways in a field to improve the efficiency of the workplace. The healthcare field is no different; in fact, even small changes in the healthcare field can have huge impacts on patient outcomes. Reducing discrepancies in practices and procedures by streamlining these practices into as few platforms as possible is one of many ways to increase efficiency in a healthcare setting [9]. The integration of HI in patient care has already given us widespread use of the EHR, which has minimized errors in record keeping and allowed HCPs to focus on the more meaningful work they do and communicate more effectively with other professionals in the field. This is a critical point as ineffective interprofessional communication in healthcare is one of the major causes of medical error leading to patient harm according to current research [10].

In regard to medical errors, we have seen a reduction in the number of errors of commission, specifically, with the use of EHRs. Errors of commission are the result of wrong actions taken. An example would be administering a medication to which your patient has a known allergy [11]. With the use of EHRs, HCPs must place an order for each medication they intend to give their patients. If the EHR recognizes you've ordered a drug to which your patient is allergic, it alerts you to that error. As fast paced as the medical field is, errors of commission aren't uncommon. The use of HI in medical practice serves as a second set of eyes to reduce unintentional human error in patient care. Fewer errors allow for more effective and timely prescription of treatment regimens and reduced healthcare costs for the patient.

The collaborative approach between physicians, allied health professionals, billing specialists, and the patient in the decision-making process can also be assisted with the use of HI. Some EHR applications allow HCPs to quickly order a consultation with an available social worker or billing specialist before the patient is discharged or shortly after their visit to allow for more transparency and informed consent to treatment. This along with improved patient education leads to improvements in the patient-physician relationship that relate directly to improved patient engagement and compliance [12].

EHRs have also integrated an education component into each patient encounter by adding clearly written informational sheets to discharge instructions, which ensures patients have access to critical information regarding their diagnosis and care instructions at home. Efforts like this increase transparency between HCPs and patients and give patients more power to make conscious decisions to improve their personal health. This increased transparency during physician interactions not only improves patient engagement, but also improves the patient's trust in their physician and allows them to disclose pertinent information more freely, which is a key component to patient safety.

Patient safety is defined as the avoidance, prevention, and correction of adverse outcomes or injuries stemming from the processes of healthcare [13]. In order to improve patient outcomes in the healthcare industry, practitioners must be able to identify problems sooner rather than later [9]. There are several barriers preventing early detection of health problems. One of those is the lack of transparency previously discussed in this chapter. Others include inefficient scheduling procedures, distrust of HCPs, and general fear of poor health. The integration of HI gives the patient access to their medical records, physician-approved education materials, and online appointment scheduling and messaging connecting them to their practitioner seamlessly. It also gives the patient a sense of control over their own health and engages the patient in unparalleled ways.

We have mentioned patient engagement so much in this chapter because it is a multi-stage journey that dictates how the patient interacts with, or maneuvers through, the healthcare system. The stages have been defined as awareness, help, care, treatment, behavioral and lifestyle changes, and ongoing care and proactive health, with the latter being the most engaged stage of them all [4]. Awareness is defined as a self-assessment of presenting symptoms, which leads to the help stage which is the initial contact between the patient and an HCP via phone or email. The care stage is in-person assessment of symptoms, which is followed by the treatment stage, which consists of follow-up care. Once the patients have a greater sense of control over their health, they enter the lifestyle modification stage, which is ultimately followed by the proactive health stage [4]. The integration of HI is directly linked to the achievement of this proactive health stage physicians long for their patients to reach. At this point, the patient has been enabled to better manage their own care through continued commitment of the physician to patient education and encouragement. This is made possible only by the integration of big data into the healthcare field. The time that EHRs free up for physicians allows ample time to educate their patients thoroughly, discuss personal roadblocks the patient may face, and help discover solutions to allow them to be more proactive in their own health.

As far as a collaborative effort is concerned with the 360-stakeholder model, HI integration prioritizes clear understanding of needs disclosed during patient encounters amid all parties involved [14]. This encourages interprofessional teamwork between healthcare specialists, which is extremely important in the management of chronic disease processes, and a more hands-on approach on the part of the patient regarding their own care. It is well known that the incorporation of everyone's perspective—from the physician, allied health professionals, social workers, nutritionists, and most importantly the patient—will result in the best possible outcomes for the patient's health. The answer to the question how we achieve this collaborative effort in an efficient manner is continued healthcare reform driven by the integration of HI.

Summary

Health informatics allows room for a collaborative approach to patient care where not only the HCPs have all of the information needed to establish a plan of care, but the patient also has access to the same data and can make more informed decisions. The use of EHR, specifically, has improved the transparency in the patient-provider relationship and improved patient engagement and compliance. The patient is allowed to take on the role of "editor-in-chief" and ensure that everything recorded in their record is accurate with the utilization of apps.

The role of the patient is one of the most important roles in healthcare. In the 360-stakeholder perspective, the patient is at the core of the ever-evolving healthcare system. The success, or lack of success, of treatment regimens is completely dependent upon the engagement of the patient in their own care. The patient is accountable for voicing their concerns, participating in the decision-making process with their physician, implementation of treatment regimens, advocacy, and prolonged self-care.

The beginning stages of healthcare reform highlighted the challenges faced by the patient in the 360-stakeholder view. The lack of transparency, limited access to advanced technology, and inaccurate record keeping are just a few challenges the patient face. It is critical that our healthcare system evolves and meets the needs of the patient, particularly in regard to patient education to increase patient engagement and reduce healthcare costs. Now more than ever, the need

for transparency is evident. Traditional healthcare systems complicate the potential fix of a collaborative approach on patient education. However, prioritizing the patient's education and safety is one of many solutions to the challenges patients face.

The key to the future of healthcare reform is the use of tools developed to better utilize HI. Big impacts on patient outcomes are initiated by not only the major changes in the healthcare field but even the small ones. The use of EHRs has helped the number of errors of commission to decrease. Loss of patient information and incomplete transfer of data between specialists for those patients with a disease process that consists of multiple organ systems have also been prevented by EHRs. With the decrease in errors, the prescription of treatment regimens has become more efficient and timely. HI integration prioritizes clear and complete understanding of the patient's needs among all parties involved. How we achieve the collaborative effort in a timely manner is continued in healthcare reform driven by integration of HI.

Conclusions and Outlook

Health informatics has led the change of healthcare reform. Increased integration of HI has increased HCP efficiency and created more space in healthcare for patient education. A collaborative health system that recognizes the importance of patient-generated health data is critical to a patient's care. The results of this are, of course, increased patient engagement but also better health outcomes, especially in the management of chronic disease processes. The impact this has on the economy, as far as decreasing the burden of health costs and reducing the number of sick days our patients need to use, is undeniable.

As the field of medicine has evolved, we've found that medical records are useful to more than just HCPs and billing specialists/insurance companies. The use of EHRs gives patients access to their own visit charts and test results, which gives them a greater sense of control over their medical care. It also gives patients greater access to their HCPs by allowing them to communicate as needed via an online inbox and schedule their own appointments online. This increased access correlates directly with the timeliness of that initial medical encounter and improves patient safety vastly.

Today, medical records are used by doctors, teachers, and more importantly by the patient. The more patient-centered approach to healthcare we see today \\has been spearheaded by the integration of HI. This approach recognizes that a collaborative approach to patient care health information where and when you need it is not just changing lives, it is saving them.

Review Questions

1. What is health informatics?
2. What is the role of the patient in healthcare?
3. What are some challenges that patients might face in the healthcare system?
4. Why is the need for transparency between healthcare professionals important?
5. What are the stages of patient engagement?

Appendix: Answers to Review Questions

1. What is health informatics?

Health informatics is a scientific discipline concerning the cognitive, informative-processing, and communication tasks of healthcare practice and education.

2. What is the role of the patient in healthcare?

The patient is at the core of the healthcare system. The success, or lack of success, of treatment regimens is completely dependent upon the engagement of the patient in their own care. The patient is responsible for voicing their concerns, participating in the decision-making process with their physician, implementation of treatment regimens, advocacy, and prolonged self-care.

3. What are some challenges that patients might face in the healthcare system?

A few challenges that patients might face in the healthcare system include lack of transparency, limited access to advanced technology, and inaccurate record keeping. It is critical that our healthcare system evolves and meets the needs of the patient, particularly in regard to patient education to increase patient engagement and reduce healthcare costs.

4. Why is the need for transparency between healthcare professionals important?

A traditional health system complicates the potential fix to taking a more collaborative approach to placing a stronger focus on patient education. The development of counterproductive practices, like inaccurate record keeping and HCP burnout, is a result inadequate staff and resources can afflict clinical facilities. Any inaccuracy documented by any party on the patient's care team can lead to a misdiagnosis or unnecessarily prolonged hospital stay. Increased transparency during physician interactions not only improves patient engagement, but also improves the patient's trust in their physician and allows them to disclose pertinent information more freely, which is a key component to patient safety.

5. What are the stages of patient engagement?

The stages of patient engagement are awareness, help, care, treatment, behavioral and lifestyle changes, and ongoing care and proactive health. Awareness is defined as a self-assessment of presenting symptoms, which leads to the help stage, which is the initial contact between the patient. The care stage is in-person assessment of symptoms, which is followed by the treatment stage, which consists of follow-up care. Once the patients have a greater sense of control over their health, they enter the lifestyle modification stage, which is ultimately followed by the proactive health stage.

References

1. HI and HIM what is the difference [internet]. Cahiim.org. https://www.cahiim.org/accreditation/health-information-management. Accessed 6 Aug 2020.
2. AHIMA Work Group. Defining the basics of health informatics for HIM professionals - retired. J AHIMA. 2014;85(9):60–6.
3. https://www.rheumatology.org/I-Am-A/Patient-Caregiver/Health-Care-Team/Role-of-a-Patient
4. Evariant.com. https://www.evariant.com/faq/what-is-patient-engagement. Accessed 6 Aug 2020.
5. https://www.ncbi.nlm.nih.gov/pmc/articles/PMC5242136/
6. Nih.gov. https://www.ncbi.nlm.nih.gov/pmc/articles/PMC3270921/. Accessed 6 Aug 2020.
7. https://www.ncbi.nlm.nih.gov/books/NBK2637/
8. https://library.ahima.org/doc?oid=107443#.XxHJVi3MxQJ
9. https://healthinformatics.uic.edu/blog/the-power-of-health-informatics-in-improving-patient-outcomes/
10. https://www.ncbi.nlm.nih.gov/books/NBK43663/
11. https://www.ncbi.nlm.nih.gov/books/NBK499956/
12. https://www.healthcatalyst.com/Key-Overcoming-Challenges-Transparency-in-Healthcare
13. https://www.ncbi.nlm.nih.gov/pmc/articles/PMC5787626/
14. https://www.ncbi.nlm.nih.gov/pmc/articles/PMC5830162/

The Nurse's View: Stakeholders, Challenges, and Innovation During COVID-19 Pandemic

Krysia W. Hudson

Learning Objectives
- Who are the stakeholders?
- What is the traditional role of nurses?
- What are challenges, opportunities, and innovations identified by stakeholders?
- Who are the new stakeholders?
- In consideration of the new challenges posed by COVID-19 pandemic, what are opportunities for collaboration?

Key Terms
- Health IT
- 360° Perspective
- Stakeholder
- Nurse as patient advocate
- Direct and indirect patient care
- Emerging new roles and new stakeholders
- Telemedicine and telemonitoring
- Crisis as a chance
- Innovation
- Change

Introduction

Healthcare has always been a critical component in daily life. However, the Coronavirus-19 (COVID-19) pandemic has forced nursing to re-

K. W. Hudson (✉)
Johns Hopkins University School of Nursing, Baltimore, MD, USA
e-mail: khudson2@jhu.edu

evaluate its 360° view of healthcare. Additionally, the pandemic has rocked the many things that consumers take for granted: working, traveling, shopping, and performing daily activities. Local, statewide, national, and international impacts have occurred related to this healthcare issue. With this in mind, this chapter will address re-evaluating the 360° perspective of informatics.

Definition and Role of Nurses in Healthcare

Traditional Perspective

Nursing has long been considered the premier bedside advocate and patient advocate in all healthcare settings. Perhaps due to the nature of patient advocacy, the first certification of informatics was created for nurses in 1992, and American Nurses Association soon provided certification for this specialty [1]. As a trusted profession, nursing has long advocated for the protection, provided direct care, and ensured well-being of patients. Nurses are primary stakeholders of the care of the patient. For the purpose of this chapter, a stakeholder is anyone who contributes to the well-being of the patient or healthcare consumer. There are many stakeholders that provide either direct or indirect care to patients or healthcare consumers (Please see Fig. 4.1) [2]. This chapter will expand the concept of

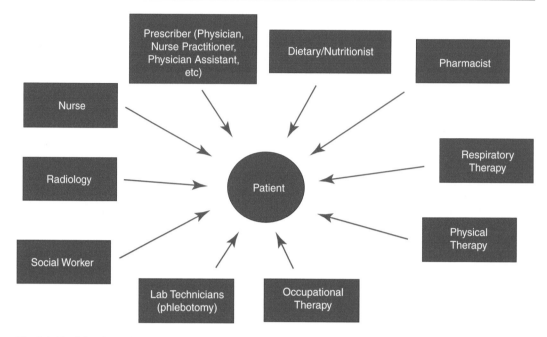

Fig. 4.1 Traditional stakeholders

stakeholders from the traditional professions (like nurses and physicians) that directly affect patient care to consider other roles that also impact patient well-being.

What Is the 360° Perspective?

The 360° perspective is a perspective from all angles or viewpoints from many stakeholders. Singular perspective would involve the view from the role of the nurse, as the patient advocate. Nursing has long enjoyed the reputation as a respected profession [3], and in fact, the World Health Assemble declared 2020 "The Year of the Nurse and the Nurse Midwife" [4]. But this chapter is devoted to re-evaluating the 360° perspective. In reviewing this perspective, this chapter may create more questions than answers. The interprofessional care team (in an acute care facility—hospital) has traditionally resembled Fig. 4.1. This team can be further divided into direct and indirect care. Direct care is being defined as where the individual must enter a patient room and interview, interact, or physically assess a patient and their significant others. Indirect care may be defined as professions that provide a direct service (e.g., pharmacists) but

may not directly enter the patient room and interact with the patient in a face-to-face manner. Interaction obviously changes per setting. For instance, once a patient moves to a home setting, the pharmacist provides face-to-face interaction, counsels patients, and makes recommendations.

Instead, this chapter will identify challenges and some innovations identified by healthcare stakeholders while facing the COVID-19 pandemic. This pandemic highlights the need to redefine and reassess the emerging perspectives of many stakeholders in healthcare.

Challenges of All Professions in State-of-the-Art Care Delivery: COVID-19 Pandemic

The Coronavirus-19 (COVID-19) pandemic posed many unique challenges to the world. This pandemic is caused by a highly contagious virus; it is generally transmitted by airborne droplets via the infected person and causes severe acute respiratory syndrome. This disease has many similarities to severe acute respiratory syndrome (SARS) and Middle East respiratory syndrome (MERS) [5–8]. Additionally, if the infected person coughs, the droplets may also land on a surface creating fomites [8]. An uninfected individual can touch the contaminated surface and transmit the virus by touching his/her face, eyes, nose, or mouth [5, 8]. Infected persons with COVID-19 can have either mild symptoms, such as cough, fever chills, sore throat, fatigue, headache, or runny nose, or they can present with more severe symptoms, such as shortness of breath or chest pain [9]. This virus poses a unique issue for the healthcare system in that more severe cases require extensive supportive care (respirators and/or intensive care beds) for a considerable amount of time. This extended supportive care utilizes multiple specialty intensive care beds, hence leaving scarce beds for emergent or elective care. Populations most vulnerable to COVID-19 include those with pre-existing diseases (e.g., diabetes, obesity) and those with an immunocompromised state (e.g., elderly) [9].

The COVID-19 pandemic has caused a variety of issues other than increasing the burden on the healthcare industry. As of January 2021, as per the Johns Hopkins Coronavirus Tracking Center, there are over 423,000 American deaths attributed to COVID-19 virus and over 2,149,000 deaths internationally [10]. The pandemic has crippled the American economy—with many Americans out of work. Compared to the Great Recession where unemployment spiked at 10% in October 2009, the COVID-19 pandemic caused 14.8% unemployment in April 2020 [11]. The hardest hit portion of the American economy is in leisure and hospitality where the unemployment rates marked 39.3% in April 2020 [11]. Besides fostering critical economic stability, this pandemic has changed every aspect of daily life. In sum, individuals have to reconsider, reimagine, and re-engineer how to work, play, celebrate, and interact.

Health Informatics Priorities from the Perspective of Nurses: Traditional Stakeholders' Challenges and Need for Innovations

Nurses are a primary stakeholder in an acute care facility. Even prior to the epidemic, challenges were numerous. The COVID-19 pandemic changed the nursing landscape dramatically. Due to the extensive amount of PPE (personal protective equipment) necessary, the main goal is to "group tasks" and minimize contact with the infected COVID-19 patient—minimizing exposure to the virus. Gone are the days where a nurse pops in and "rounds" on their patients due to infectious nature of this disease. Instead, some propose [12] the use of telemedicine (via robotic carts) within hospital units and within acute care units to monitor patients. This technology will allow the nurses to remotely peer into rooms without donning equipment. Education is necessary to optimize this new telemonitoring technology. Other enabling technologies that provide remote monitoring include the use of smart watches, rings, bracelets, or monitors [13, 14]. Cleaning of these devices is key—ultraviolet sterilization has been successfully used [15]. Additionally, if devices, like robots, travel from one room to another, cleaning is also necessary before entering other patient rooms [15]. One large challenge is the human factor. Many nurses express the grief in not being able to allow family to stay with patients [16]. Nurses have bridged this gap via the use of mobile devices to communicate with loved ones (e.g., iPad) [16]. Another challenge is the lack of therapeutic touch or recognition. Patients have difficulty in identifying healthcare members due to the amount of PPE worn. Hoods, caps, N95 masks obstruct the faces of caregivers. Patients are fearful and often confused as to who is entering their room. One simple innovation is the use of a plastic wrapped smiling picture of the caregiver [16]. As one nurse mentioned, "A smile is universal."

Physicians too struggle with the challenge of COVID-19 patients. These infectious patients consume many critical care beds—making bed availability a challenge for most facilities. In smaller facilities where intensivists are not present, the use of telecritical care is an option [17, 18]. This innovation prevents hospital transfer and decreases exposure to others. In the early portion of the pandemic, some facilities ran out of critical care beds, hence non-critical care units were hosting critical patients until beds were available. This required oversight by intensivists and training of floor nurses who have never managed a critical ventilated patient for an extended period of time. Some literature [19] also suggests a "tiered telemonitoring system" where an experienced critical care physician monitors and consults multiple non-ICU physicians and non-ICU nurses. Additionally, Scott [19] also suggests a low-contact, communication and isolation model. Here, physicians use a "paired tablet" approach. Any patient with COVID-19 or any patient "under investigation" for COVID-19 is given a tablet in a dedicated room and then the other tablet is in the provider room. As always, clinicians must learn how to use enabling technologies while conveying a caring disposition while interacting with a scared individual.

Respiratory therapists face a daunting challenge with COVID-19. These healthcare professionals are focused on the respiratory status of patients. Principally, the most critical patients with COVID-19 infection display acute respiratory distress related to the virus and require respiratory therapist care. Consequently, the demand for respiratory therapists is skyrocketing [20]. Additionally, the workload of the respiratory therapist has also doubled during this pandemic [20]. Specifically, respiratory therapists ensure the proper utilization of ventilators and other respiratory devices or treatments. Since these patients require long-term ventilator use related to complications of COVID-19, ventilators are in short supply. To combat this, an interprofessional team of physicians and respiratory therapists have incorporated a few new strategies at University of Pennsylvania. First, they began using a CPAP helmet, which is used extensively in Europe to prevent intubation [21]. The helmet encloses the head which also helps to contain the virus. Second, they incorporated the use of E-Lert [21]. The E-Lert system uses high-quality cameras in each patient room and is manned by certified respiratory therapists. This system remotely monitors all acutely ill patients, minimizes exposure to patients, and quickly identifies patient issues (like disconnected oxygen) [21].

Many traditional stakeholders that only have to interview clients (i.e., dieticians, pharmacists, social workers) can also use the "paired tablet approach" to minimize the use of PPE and minimize contact with the patient [19]. Challenges do apply, with COVID-19; many patients who are in the acute care facility may be short of breath. This could minimize the ability to communicate via the paired tablet approach. Additionally, patients if unable to speak will need to be able to type responses. Last, this also requires that patients know how to use mobile devices (literacy). In sum, these "paired interactions" may necessitate the mediation or operation by a nurse or a nursing assistant—negating the use of the innovation.

Health Informatics Priorities in Collaboration with Other Professions: The New Stakeholders

In looking at a 360° view, let us consider new stakeholders (in green) due to this COVID-19 pandemic, their challenges and potential innovations (See Fig. 4.2). By no means is this list conclusive, but in consideration of this pandemic, these emerging stakeholders have taken an increasing role in contributing to improved patient outcomes.

Veterinarians have not traditionally been a stakeholder in the health of consumers. However, the last few coronavirus outbreaks (e.g., severe acute respiratory syndrome [SARS] and Middle East respiratory syndrome [MERS]) are zoonotic viruses that have been identified in animals. These viruses have acquired the ability to transmit from person to person [22–24]. Due to this connection and the ability for these treacherous viruses to travel from animals or pets to humans, veterinarians have become a new stakeholder in combatting new diseases. Their input into disease transmission is critical to halting epidemics—like COVID-19.

Chaplains are another stakeholder that has emerged during the COVID-19 pandemic. This disease, by nature, is very isolating. This stakeholder can offer the "emotional connection" that many isolated COVID-19 patients require. Chaplains can offer emotional or spiritual support via in-person visits or via virtual telehealth visits. Some chaplains are able to also connect, provide support groups or gaming via zoom or other means like through Calm™ or Vennly™ [25]. Moreover, the chaplains can further support

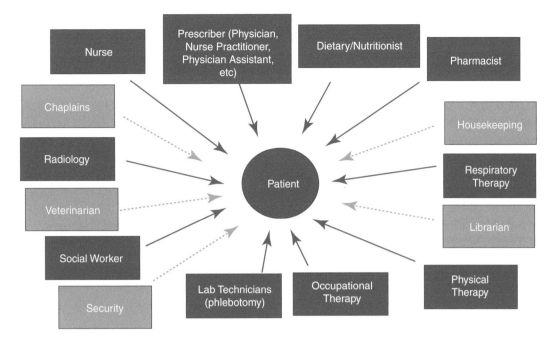

Fig. 4.2 New stakeholders

the staff caring for such sick populations. Healthcare providers have long expressed a burn-out related to the COVID-19 crisis and need the psychological support [26].

Housekeepers have long since supported direct patient care. The main goal of the house-keeper is to maintain and improve the environment of the patient and healthcare providers. In lieu of the COVID-19 pandemic, this profession has been key in providing a safe space. As mentioned prior, the use of UV light has been very successful in sterilizing equipment [15]. Robots, like LightStrike™ equipped with UV light technology, can also be deployed to disinfect an unoccupied operating room in 12 minutes, compared to 90 minutes via a human counterpart [27, 28]. Human assistance is necessary in that the partnered housekeeper can flip furniture mattresses, etc., to allow for cleaning of surfaces not previously reached. Although this technology is quick, the price is steep, and they must operate in an unoccupied space. Additionally, the machines are not easily suited to clean all areas, often getting stuck [27]. Last, the human factor is also an issue. Housekeepers provide an element of normalcy and human connection. Since these stakeholders routinely visit each room, this interaction is valued by patients [29].

Security is another stakeholder not previously mentioned. As the COVID-19 pandemic evolves, there is a need to contain the virus. A necessary stakeholder in any acute care facility is the physical gatekeeper or hospital security. These professionals help squelch the influx of anxious visitors and must be able to turn away individuals. At the most basic level, they are protecting outsiders from contamination and virus spread. Some apps, like Prodensity™, have been deployed to also ensure the health safety of individuals as well. Individuals who work in the healthcare facility must log into their app daily, answer specific health-check, and Prodensity™ can provide a green pass—which is shown to security as they enter the building [30]. Downside of this app is that data is self-reported. Individuals with COVID-19 are infectious up to two days prior to being symptomatic [31]; hence, self-reporting will not identify those who may already be infectious. A newer app, to help identify post exposure is MD COVID Alert ™, which uses Bluetooth technology to notify individuals if they have exposure to those identified as having COVID-19 for 15 minutes or more [32].

The healthcare librarian or informatist is an under-represented stakeholder in the COVID-19 pandemic. This stakeholder can be key in finding new tools in fighting new outbreaks and sharing the information in a contextual manner. The thirst for knowledge and success was very evident in the COVID-19 pandemic. New therapies and trends were brought to light like the possible role of vitamin D [33], preventative effects of aspirin in preventing coagulopathy [34], guidelines for multisystem inflammatory syndrome in children [35], and the challenges of proning with COVID-19 patients [36]. Informaticists need to be brought into the frontlines to find new therapies and discourage detrimental therapy and disseminate to the healthcare team.

Summary

In summary, the healthcare landscape is changing as realized by the current COVID-19 pandemic. As identified by the challenges and innovations above, each stakeholder has reconfigured its workplace and its perspective based on this pandemic. This needs to continue. It is only via collaboration and open communication with other stakeholders that we can tackle the mounting healthcare needs of the future.

Conclusions and Outlook

After reflection of the traditional and new stakeholders in the COVID-19 pandemic, there are a few common themes when operating. First, the main goal is to provide optimal care while minimizing the spread of the virus. Stakeholders need the latest information to optimize care guidelines and improve outcomes. Every member of the healthcare system plays a vital role in optimizing care. Second, COVID-19 is highly contagious, and it is hard to communicate with empathy and caring when in extensive PPE. Patients are isolated and terrified. When in isolation, the only human interaction is via healthcare stakeholders. The use of technological innovation must allow for empathy and caring. Third, many of the innovations/guidelines require interprofessional discovery and operationalization, stakeholders can

no longer work in silos. Considering that there is a national shortage of critical care beds (and professionals to operate them), there is a call for future development of a National Emergency Telecritical Care Network utilizing the mobile and remote monitoring technologies in a private/public partnership [19].

Useful Resources
1. Remote Telehealth Policy: https://www.cch-pca.org/resources/search-telehealth-resources#
2. Center for Care Innovation: https://www.care-innovations.org/resources/
3. COVID-19 Resource Wiki: https://wiki.care-innovations.org/Main_Page
4. Chaplain Innovation Lab: https://chaplaincy-innovation.org/

Review Questions
1. How would you define a stakeholder?
2. After review of this chapter, please identify and defend which stakeholder should have increased input in healthcare delivery?
3. Name some practical considerations of using remote technology. MARK ALL THAT APPLY.
   (a) Sterilizing the remote technology
   (b) Validating data of remote technology
   (c) Providing education of remote technology
   (d) Offering alternate manners of collecting data
4. Thanks to the COVID-19 pandemic, what are some scarce resources identified? MARK ALL THAT APPLY.
   (a) Patients
   (b) ICU nurses
   (c) Intensivists
   (d) ICU beds
   (e) Groceries
   (f) PPE
5. What is the practical consideration when using mobile technology to communicate with patients? MARK ALL THAT APPLY.
   (a) Literacy of the patient
   (b) Technological literacy of the patient
   (c) Physical ability to operate the mobile device
   (d) The Wi-Fi stability of the environment

Appendix: Answers to Review Questions

1. How would you define a stakeholder?

A stakeholder is a role where the individual has a vested interest in the positive outcome of a patient. This could be a nurse, pharmacist, prescriber, etc.

2. After review of this chapter, please identify and defend which stakeholder should have increased input in healthcare delivery?

A new stakeholder is someone that is not a traditional stakeholder. This person could be a chaplain, a veterinarian, a housekeeper, a unit secretary, a dentist. These new stakeholders must be sought out in healthcare or in the health of the consumer. In lieu of the COVID-19 pandemic, COVID patients living at home need the grocery delivery or pharmaceutical delivery. These non-traditional roles must be explored and incorporated into collaboration to optimize consumer health.

3. Name some practical considerations of using remote technology. MARK ALL THAT APPLY.
   (a) Sterilizing the remote technology
   (b) Validating data of remote technology
   (c) Providing education of remote technology
   (d) Offering alternate manners of collecting data

4. Thanks to the COVID-19 pandemic, what are some scarce resources identified? MARK ALL THAT APPLY.
   (a) Patients
   (b) ICU nurses
   (c) Intensivists
   (d) ICU beds
   (e) Groceries
   (f) PPE

5. What is the practical consideration when using mobile technology to communicate with patients? MARK ALL THAT APPLY.
   (a) Literacy of the patient
   (b) Technological literacy of the patient
   (c) Physical ability to operate the mobile device
   (d) The Wi-Fi stability of the environment

References

1. Cummins MR, Gundlapalli AV, Murray P, Park HA, Lehmann CU. Nursing informatics certification worldwide: history, pathway, roles, and motivation. Yearb Med Inform. 2016;(1):264–71. https://doi.org/10.15265/IY-2016-039.
2. Hoffman J, Sullivan N. Medical surgical nursing: making connections to practice. 2th ed. Duxbury, VT: FA Davis; 2019.
3. American Hospital Association. For the 17th year in a row, nurses top Gallup's poll of most trusted profession. https://www.aha.org/news/insights-and-analysis/2019-01-09-17th-year-row-nurses-top-gallups-poll-most-trusted-profession. Accessed 20 Jan 2021.
4. World Health Organization. Year of the nurse and the midwife 2020. https://www.who.int/campaigns/year-of-the-nurse-and-the-midwife-2020. Accessed 20 Jan 2021.
5. Cascella M, Rajnik M, Cuomo A, Dulebohn SC, Di Napoli R. Features, evaluation and treatment coronavirus (COVID-19). Treasure Island, FL: StatPearls; 2020.
6. Luo L, Liu D, Liao X, Wu X, Jing Q, Zheng J, et al. Modes of contact and risk of transmission in COVID-19 among close contacts (pre-print). MedRxiv. 2020; https://doi.org/10.1101/2020.03.24.20042606.
7. World Health Organization. Infection prevention and control of epidemic-and pandemic-prone acute respiratory infections in health care. Geneva: World Health Organization; 2014. https://apps.who.int/iris/bitstream/handle/10665/112656/9789241507134_eng.pdf;jsessionid=41AA684FB64571CE8D8A453C4F2B2096?sequence=1
8. World Health Organization. (2020). Modes of transmission of virus causing COVID-19: implications for IPC precaution recommendations: scientific brief, 27 March 2020. World Health Organization. https://apps.who.int/iris/handle/10665/331601. License: CC BY-NC-SA 3.0 IGO.
9. Centers for Disease Control. Symptoms of coronavirus. https://www.cdc.gov/coronavirus/2019-ncov/symptoms-testing/symptoms.html. Accessed 20 Jan 2021.
10. Johns Hopkins University Coronovirus Resource Center. COVID-19 dashboard. https://coronavirus.jhu.edu/map.html. Accessed 28 Jan 2021.
11. Congressional Research Service. Unemployment rates during the COVID-19 pandemic: in brief. 2021.

https://fas.org/sgp/crs/misc/R46554.pdf. Accessed 28 Jan 2021.

12. Kapoor A, Guha S, Das MK, Goswami KC, Yadav R. Digital healthcare: the only solution for better healthcare during COVID-19 pandemic? Indian Heart J. 2020;72(2):61–4. https://doi.org/10.1016/j.ihj.2020.04.001.

13. Hornyak T. What America can learn from China's use of robots and telemedicine to combat the coronavirus. https://www.cnbc.com/2020/03/18/how-china-is-using-robots-and-telemedicine-to-combat-the-coronavirus.html. Accessed 28 Jan 2020.

14. Verillo SC, Cvach M, Hudson K, Winters BD. Using continuous vital sign monitoring (cVSM) to detect early deterioration in adult postoperative inpatients. J Nurs Care Qual. 2019;34(2):107–13. https://doi.org/10.1097/NCQ.0000000000000350.

15. Yang G-Z, Nelson BJ, Murphy RR, Choset H, Christensen H, Collins SH, Dario P, Goldberg K, Ikuta K, Jacobstein N, Kragic D, Taylor RH, McNutt M. Combating COVID-19—The role of robotics in managing public health and infectious diseases. Sci Robotics. 2020;5:eabb5589.

16. M Health. The person behind the PPE: nurse uses smiling photo to break down barrier. 2020. https://www.mhealth.org/blog/2020/may-2020/the-person-behind-the-ppe-nurse-using-smiling-photo-to-break-down-barriers. Accessed 28 Jan 2021.

17. Subramanian S, Pamplin JC, Hravnak M, Hielsberg C, Riker R, Rincon F, Laudanski K, Adzhigirey LA, Moughrabieh MA, Winterbottom FA, Herasevich V. Tele-critical care: an update from the society of critical care medicine tele-ICU committee. Crit Care Med. 2020;48:553–61.

18. Lilly CM, Greenbard B. The evolution of tele-ICU to tele-critical care. Crit Care Med. 2020;48:610–1.

19. Scott B, Miller G, Fonda S, Yeaw R, Gaudoen J, Pavliscsak H, Quinn MT, Pamplin J. Advanced digital health technologies for COVID-19 and future emergencies. Telemed J E Health. 2020;26(10):1–7. https://doi-org.proxy1.library.jhu.edu/10.1089/tmj.2020.01

20. D' Ambrosio A. Respiratory therapists play critical role in COVID-19 Pandemic. 2020. https://www.medpagetoday.com/infectiousdisease/covid19/86302. Accessed 27 Jan 2021.

21. Sapega S. Respiratory therapists lend special expertise to keep COVID patients breathing easier. 2020. https://www.pennmedicine.org/news/internal-newsletters/system-news/2020/july/a-moment-to-shine-respiratory-therapists-emerge-as-heroes-from-covid-crisis. Accessed 27 Jan 2021.

22. Gilbert GL. Commentary: SARS, MERS and COVID-19—new threats; old lessons. Int J Epidemiol. 2020;49(3):726–8. https://doi.org/10.1093/ije/dyaa061

23. Wang LF, Eaton BT. Bats, civets and the emergence of SARS. Curr Top Microbiol Immunol. 2007;315:325–44.

24. Zumla A, Hui DS, Perlman S. Middle east respiratory syndrome. Lancet. 2015;386:995–1007.

25. Multifaith Chaplaincy Learning. Chaplaincy innovation lab shares resources for chaplains encountering coronavirus. 2020. https://www.multifaithchaplaincy.org.au/2020/03/22/chaplaincy-innovation-lab-shares-resources-for-chaplains-encountering-coronavirus/. Accessed 28 Jan 2020.

26. Lagasse J. Healthcare workers experiencing burnout, stress due to COVID-19 pandemic. 2020. https://www.healthcarefinancenews.com/news/healthcare-workers-experiencing-burnout-stress-due-covid-19-pandemic#:~:text=Nurses%20reported%20having%20a%20higher,have%20emotional%20support%20(45%25). Accessed 28 Jan 2020.

27. Lerman R. Robot cleaners are coming, this time to wipe up your coronavirus germs. The Washington post. 2020. https://www.washingtonpost.com/technology/2020/09/08/robot-cleaners-surge-pandemic/. Accessed 28 Jan 2021.

28. Xenex. Destroy deadly pathogens to improve safety & peace of mind. 2021. https://xenex.com/. Accessed 28 Jan 2021.

29. Burke D. He was a Covid-19 patient. She cleaned his hospital room. Their unexpected bond saved his life. 2020. https://www.cnn.com/2020/06/11/health/orlando-hospital-coronavirus-patient-housekeeper-wellness/index.html. Accessed 28 Jan 2021.

30. Prodensity. ProDensity: JHU needs U. 2021. https://prodensity.jh.edu/welcome. Accessed 27 January 2021.

31. WHO. Coronavirus disease (COVID-19): how is it transmitted? 2020. https://www.who.int/emergencies/diseases/novel-coronavirus-2019/question-and-answers-hub/q-a-detail/coronavirus-disease-covid-19-how-is-it-transmitted. Accessed 27 January 2021.

32. MD COVID Alert. COVID alert. 2021. https://covidlink.maryland.gov/content/mdcovidalert/. Accessed 28 Jan 2021.

33. Rubin R. Sorting out whether vitamin D deficiency raises COVID-19 risk. JAMA. 2021;325(4):329–30. https://doi.org/10.1001/jama.2020.24127.

34. Haque S, Jawed A, Akhter N, Dar SA, Khan F, Mandal RK, Areeshi MY, Lohani M, Wahid M. Acetylsalicylic acid (Aspirin): a potent medicine for preventing COVID-19 deaths caused by thrombosis and pulmonary embolism. Eur Rev Med Pharmacol Sci. 2020;24(18):9244–5. https://doi.org/10.26355/eurrev_202009_23005.

35. Henderson LA, Canna SW, Friedman KG, Gorelik M, Lapidus SK, Bassiri H, Behrens EM, Ferris A, Kernan KF, Schulert GS, Seo P, Fson MB, Tremoulet AH, RSM Y, Mudano AS, Turner AS, Karp DR, Mehta JJ. American College of Rheumatology Clinical Guidance for multisystem inflammatory syndrome in children associated with SARS-CoV-2 and hyperinflammation in pediatric COVID-19: version 1. Arthritis Rheumatol. 2020;72(11):1791–805. https://doi.org/10.1002/art.41454.

36. Cotton S, Zawaydeh Q, LeBlanc S, Husain A, Malhotra A. Proning during covid-19: challenges and solutions. Heart Lung. 2020;49(6):686–7. https://doi.org/10.1016/j.hrtlng.2020.08.006.

The Physician's View: Healthcare Digital Transformation Priorities and Challenges

5

Joel Reich

Learning Objectives
- Identify the characteristics of the medical profession
- Examine physicians' use of clinical informatics and digital technologies
- Describe the role of physicians in health care informatics leadership
- Explain the role of interprofessional teams in clinical informatics
- Assess physicians' health informatics priorities and challenges

Key Terms
- Electronic health records (EHR)
- Triple/Quadruple Aim
- Profession of medicine
- Leadership
- Population health
- Value-based payment/care
- Interoperability
- Interprofessional teams
- Burnout
- Artificial intelligence (AI)
- Health Systems Science (HSS)
- Continuing medical education (CME)
- Natural language processing (NLP)

J. Reich (✉)
Thomas Jefferson University, Philadelphia, PA, USA

Frank H. Netter School of Medicine, North Haven, CT, USA

University of New Haven, West Haven, CT, USA

Introduction

In contrast to the discovery of penicillin, x-rays, and immunotherapy, clinical informatics is not usually thought of as a "medical breakthrough". Yet, it has profoundly changed medicine forever. What began 30 years ago as a "solution" for illegible medical records, medication errors, duplication of orders, clinical variation, and unavailability of data, has largely reshaped health care's clinical, business, communication, and research processes. While much has been accomplished, many challenges remain.

"Clinical informatics is not simply 'computers in medicine' but rather is a body of knowledge, methods, and theories that focus on the effective use of information and knowledge to improve the quality, safety, and cost-effectiveness of patient care as well as the health of both individuals and populations" [1]. Concurrent with the advancement of clinical informatics, health care systems have been evolving from the individual disease-based model to a population-based model in response to increasing prevalence of chronic disease, aging populations, and limited resources. Population health layers management of the population's health on top of the care of the individual and recognizes the profound influence the social determinants of health (SDoH) play in health outcomes. Population health management goals are concisely summarized by the Institute for Healthcare Improvement's (IHI) Triple Aim

© Springer Nature Switzerland AG 2022
U. H. Hübner et al. (eds.), *Nursing Informatics*, Health Informatics,
https://doi.org/10.1007/978-3-030-91237-6_5

which has become the unofficial *mantra* of the changing healthcare system. The Triple Aim highlights the relationship between the health of the population, the patient's experience (including patient safety and quality outcomes), and the cost of care. The Triple Aim has been amended to the "Quadruple Aim" with the addition of provider experience, in recognition of the importance of clinician well-being [2].

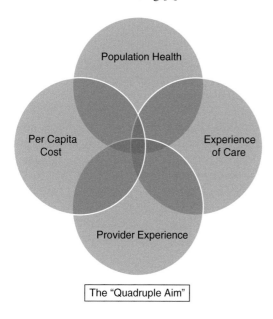

The "Quadruple Aim"

Clinical informatics plays an integral role in attaining the Triple Aim by enabling "patient-centered" care, supporting communication, using data to improve patient outcomes and financial management, and improving the physician experience through technology. The Aims were an integral part of the health care policy driven by passage of the Patient Protection and Affordable Care Act (PPACA or ACA) in 2010. The ACA has advanced population health in the U.S. with new care and payment models transforming payment from "fee-for service" to "value-based". In value-based payment reimbursement for each individual, healthcare service is replaced by population-based payment based upon linkage of quality performance and payment to increase value. Value-based payment and the accompanying care processes are highly dependent on clinical informatics and technology.

Clinical informatics impacts every aspect of the practice of medicine. Although there are considerable differences in health care business models, health care systems share a common need for patient orders, record-keeping, communication, and collecting, analyzing, applying, and sharing data. Physicians have frequent interaction with electronic health records (EHRs), using them for order entry, documentation, test results, and patient information retrieval. Although nearly all hospitals and physicians have EHRs, most EHRs have been designed for individual encounters and defined episodes of care, rather than the longitudinal view necessary for population health management [3].

In addition to the EHR, physicians regularly encounter other types of information technology, including email, texting, telehealth, mobile apps, and analytics and population health management systems. In an ideal world all of these technologies would have a common access point ("single sign-on"), a similar user environment ("common feel"), seamless interoperability, and a single data repository. Unfortunately, this is not the common real-world experience. Clinical, financial, and care management functions, are often in different EHR modules, and sometimes in different EHR systems. The majority of is in the form of free text rather than structured data which presents significant challenges to sharing and using the data. Design and functional deficiencies in clinical informatics result in workarounds and dependence on outdated technologies such as the fax machine, earning healthcare recognition as the "last bastion" of the fax machine. This presents substantial challenges as the system changes to population health management and value-based payment and care. Population health management strategies are heavily data-dependent and require data systems to collect, aggregate, analyze, report, and risk stratify data, as well as to support timely care management, coordination, and communication for care, business, and patient engagement.

It has become increasingly difficult to remember the *good ole' days* of handwritten paper patient charts, separate sections for physician nursing notes; lost orders and lost test results;

unreconciled medication lists; and, near-total separation of patients' medical records in a structure akin to "parallel universes". Technology has enabled us to address many of these, but not without creating a new set of challenges including altered workflow, staff burnout, and perceived and real barriers between patients and clinicians. As we approach the brink of widely applied data analytics, artificial intelligence, and mobile applications for remote care, despite the shortcomings of technology there is no going back.

Definition and Role of the Profession in Health Care

The profession of medicine is built upon a defined body of knowledge, accepted practices, and standards. Government confers the authority to practice medicine through licensing, laws, and regulations. Medicine, along with other professions, has the responsibility to develop and enforce performance standards through self-governance; if it fails to properly manage this delegated authority, government retains the power to intervene and mandate change.

Professions have a degree of autonomy delegated along with the responsibility to provide care in a responsible and ethical manner. The degree of autonomy varies considerably from country to country. Prestige and political influence, historical precedents, health system governance, practice structure and payment, changing science, cultural and societal beliefs, and laws and regulations affect the powers and authority delegated to the profession. While clinical practices in different regions and countries are often shared, there are substantial differences in health system governance. In countries with centralized health system governance and/or a preponderance of employed physicians there tends to be less autonomy. U.S. physicians historically enjoyed high prestige and autonomy. However, in the twenty-first century there has been a decline in physician autonomy due to physicians leaving independent practice for employment, driven by new practice complexities such as Meaningful Use and value-based contract requirements.

Proliferation of interprofessional care teams may present a challenge to physician autonomy. However, well-deployed teams with clear-cut roles and responsibilities, that enable all team members to concentrate their duties "at the top of their license", leaving the more complex functions to the physician team lead, may actually strengthen the physician role.

The manner by which clinical informatics and EHRs are designed, implemented, utilized, and governed has a material effect on system function and the physician role. National health care systems can be classified based upon governance authority, standards of care, and finance models. Governance is characterized as, "top-down" centralized national government-driven; "bottom-up" locally driven; and, "middle-out" under which local healthcare providers change their system to comply with national system standards. The United Kingdom has a centralized governance and payment structure. The United States (US) has gravitated from "bottom-up" toward "middle-out". Due to its uniquely structured healthcare finance structure, the US is different from most other countries in its extensive reliance of the EHR for financial processes [3, 4].

Leadership

Physicians are responsible for direct patient care as well as attaining high value through maximization of quality outcomes while minimizing expenditures, all of which is dependent upon clinical informatics. As the focus on population health and value-based payment and care has intensified the need for strong physician leadership in healthcare has moved to the forefront. Physicians want and expect to be actively involved in clinical informatics leadership, including roles in policy, system design, equipment selection, function, implementation, optimization, and oversight. Physician roles range from clinical team leadership, committee, and workgroup participation, to titled leadership roles at the department and executive team levels. Effective clinical informatics leadership requires high level cooperation between clinical leaders, administrators, and information technology leaders. Administrators who prioritize physician involvement through appointment and support for non-clinical time are viewed as demonstrating a true commitment to physician participation.

There is no "single best" model for clinical informatics leadership. The organization's structure, size, governance, and business model determine the leadership structure. Effective leaders possess clinical, business, and informatics skills. Clinical informatics leadership experience and skill requirements vary based upon factors such as centralized or. decentralized governance, health system or freestanding hospital, and physician group size. Clinical informatics responsibilities and functions cross many domains, including information technology, clinical care, quality, and analytics. Population health management and value-based payment's linkage of clinical and financial interests has generated development of new cross-disciplinary roles. Common high level leadership roles include the Chief Information Officer, Chief Medical officer, Chief Clinical Officer, Chief Nursing Officer, Chief Nursing Information officer, Chief Integration Officer, and Chief Population Health Officer. As health care systems evolve the roles, functions, and organizational reporting relationships of these roles is constantly changing driving the need for clear leadership authority and accountability, particularly while going through organizational changes.

Training, Education, Certification, and Licensing

Initially driven by EHR training, clinical Informatics has become an integral part of medical school, post-graduate, and continuing medical education. Medical schools in the U.S. and other countries have incorporated Health Systems Science (HSS) into their curriculum as the "Third Pillar" of medical education [5, 6]. HSS includes healthcare finance and economics, leadership, interprofessional teams, quality and performance, research, value-based payment, and population health.

In the US, clinical informatics is a recognized physician subspecialty, open to physicians, board certified in their primary specialty. The Accreditation Council for Graduate Medical Education (ACGME) has defined clinical informatics as "… the subspecialty of all medical specialties that transforms health care by analyzing, designing, implementing, and evaluating information and communication systems to improve patient care, enhance access to care, advance individual and population health outcomes, and strengthen the clinician-patient relationship." [7] Requirements for certification eligibility mandate residency training and successful completion of a certification exam [1].

The growth of clinical informatics and remote care technologies creates challenges to licensing and regulatory policies. Licensing has been traditionally controlled at a national level in some countries, and at the state level in the U.S., with variable levels of reciprocity across jurisdictional boundaries. The emergency declarations allowing cross-jurisdictional practice issued during the COVID-19 pandemic demonstrated the value of flexibility and highlighted the constraints imposed by traditional restrictions.

Challenges of the Profession in State of the Art Care Delivery

Healthcare system transformation is expanding the physician's role from the traditional doctor-patient relationship to additional responsibilities including managing quality and financial benchmarks, leading teams, and helping patients manage their SDoH. Many aspects of medical care are changing simultaneously which makes it difficult to distinguish individual effects. While clinical informatics can be extremely helpful in providing patient care, if not managed skillfully, unintended effects may actually diminish the doctor-patient relationship. For example, the positioning of the exam room computer may divert the physician from the usual face-to-face patient interaction. While telehealth encounters have been generally well-accepted, there are generational differences at both ends of the encounter that may result in varying degrees of satisfaction. Additional risks may be associated with "templated" medical records which may fail to capture the essence of the patient's story.

While it is easy to focus on EHRs consuming as much as 50% of clinician time [8] and other problems created or exacerbated by EHRs, much has been accomplished to improve patient care. EHR implementation has enabled real-time availability of test results, sharing of records among the care team, e-prescribing, Clinical Decision Support (CDS), care pathways, and uniform order sets, readily available data for quality/performance improvement and population health management. The original drivers of EHR adoption: illegible records, drug interactions, and totally siloed medical records, have been largely addressed. Most physicians, if given the choice, would not go back to hand-written records. However, there is a strong desire to change EHR design and function to improve usability, and workflow, reduce mouse clicks and the number of screens required to navigate to the desired data, and overall time spent at the computer, and improve interoperability. Many question, "Why am I sitting here at midnight typing patient care notes into the EHR?", "Is this information for reimbursement, regulations, or truly for patient care?", or, "Am I documenting to protect myself from legal issues?" Although most physicians and hospitals have implemented EHRs, there are, and will be, continuing implementations as the result of system replacements and upgrades, addition of population health management software, integration AI and telehealth, and increased system interoperability.

Physicians, as a group, have at times been labeled as "tech phobic", sometimes related to broad assumptions about generational differences. While it has been a more natural process for "digital natives" to adopt new technology, for others much of the resistance emanates from frustration with non-intuitive design, suboptimal implementation, and disruption of workflow. Physicians are big users of technology in everyday practice and have been for most of the last century. However, they approach new technology cautiously to protect patients from negative outcomes as they have experienced with new drugs

and errors that they have encountered related to EHR use. Physicians demonstrated their willingness to innovate and accept new technology in their response to the COVID-19 pandemic, as seen with telehealth.

Physician Practice Structure

While helping drive the U.S. out of the great recession, the 2010 HITECH (Health Information Technology for Economic and Clinical Health) $30 billion funding succeeded in increasing hospital and physician EHR adoption. However, the cost and complexity of "going digital" contributed to health system and physician practice consolidation into larger health systems with stronger financial resources and technological expertise. At present, more than half of U.S. physicians have become employed, and the trend is continuing. Billing, compliance, and other requirements have set the U.S. quite apart from other countries' health systems and the manner in which they configure and use EHRs.

Interoperability

One of the great promises of EHRs was to make patient data readily available at "the right time and place". Inaccessible data prevents the physician from seeing the entire patient "picture" which increases the risk of medical errors and duplicate testing, both barriers to high value health care. Lack of interoperability hampers clinical and public health data-sharing as the experience in the COVID-19 pandemic showed. It also results in workarounds, such as unsecured texting and faxing. U.S. physicians are less likely to receive information from specialists, emergency departments/urgent care centers, and hospitals. Primary care physicians in the US and some other countries are not routinely exchanging data outside of their practices. In Europe the majority of health care facilities exchange data with hospitals, but considerably less with primary care [9].

There has been considerable finger pointing and casting of blame in the U.S. regarding the role of EHR vendors, health care systems, and government in addressing interoperability. There are multiple factors that contribute to the lack of interoperability, including system design, vendor and health system competitive forces, politics, and lack of regulatory standards. The U.S. government programs, Meaningful Use and the Quality Payment Program, have applied substantial financial incentives and penalties to promote and advance interoperability. These efforts have improved interoperability within physician groups, health systems, and entire countries connected through a common EHR platform. However, interoperability with outside entities and between multiple different physician EHRs is lacking. In some regions Health Information Exchanges (HIEs) have made it possible for participating healthcare organizations to share select data.

Physician Burnout

"Burnout is a long-term stress reaction marked by emotional exhaustion, depersonalization, and a lack of sense of personal accomplishment" [10]. Burnout severely disrupts physicians personal and professional lives, leading to loss of productive members of the physician workforce. It also presents a clear risk to patient and staff safety and well-being [11]. Studies have shown that more than half of U.S. physicians suffer from burnout, as do medical students and residents [8]. Job burnout among physicians in low-income and middle-income countries has been reported as 32% [12].

Too many bureaucratic tasks (documentation, coding, billing, paperwork), too many hours at work, lack of respect, increasing computerization of practice all contribute to burnout. Although burnout has multifactorial causes, the EHR is frequently identified as a major factor. It is difficult to separate EHR design from workflow factors, but clearly, they add up to a huge consumption of time. These low-value tasks include excessive data entry requirements, long cut-and-pasted notes, inaccessibility of data, notes geared toward billing, interference with work-life balance, and problems with posture and pain attributed to

computer use [13]. Physicians gave usability of current EHR systems a grade of F [14].

U.S. Physicians spend two hours on EHR and desk work for every clinical hour. In the exam room, about half of the time is spent in direct clinical "face time" and about one third on EHR and desk work. The inability to complete clinical record-keeping during clinical hours has led to a new term, "pajama time", the time needed to finish these tasks into the night hours. In other countries clinical documentation is far briefer, containing only relevant clinical information, and omitting much of the compliance and reimbursement documentation. U.S. physicians using the same EHR enter a lot of "low-value" administrative data, with clinical notes four times longer and total documentation doubling since the MU Program began. Physicians in other countries using the same EHR with lesser documentation requirements report higher satisfaction and believe the EHR improves efficiency [15–18].

Technology Integration

The US has become the world's health technology innovation center and largest market for clinical informatics and health care digital development and adoption. New technologies are being introduced at an unprecedented rate, including telehealth, smart speakers/chatbots/smartbots, mobile apps, and multiple AI applications. When properly designed, implemented, and integrated, technology can significantly enhance physician practice. If not thoughtfully deployed, it can be disruptive to work, and can result in an increase in siloed data, and create additional cognitive load. The COVID-19 pandemic demonstrated the power of rapid innovation with technology in addressing epidemiologic as well as clinical needs. However, many new technologies have been developed as freestanding devices and/or applications and they will require integration with existing systems to maximize value. In addition, the data report content, volume, format, timing, and reporting mode must be carefully designed with physician input to maximize the information availability and use.

Artificial Intelligence (AI)

AI applications offer solutions for clinical care, research, business functions, personalized medicine, and medical education. Clinical applications with demonstrated efficacy include augmented diagnosis, enhanced clinical decision support, and predictive analytics, e.g., pandemic spread, emergency department and hospital (re) admissions, and overall clinical and financial risk. Other AI applications hold considerable promise for simplification of tasks that will relieve physicians from the burden of low-value tasks such as prescription refills and prior authorizations. Teams benefit from AI applied to care management/coordination, and clinical and financial risk calculators. The covid-19 pandemic demonstrated the power of AI to identify patient risk, track patients, predict the course of disease, and monitor populations for outbreaks on social media. AI is supporting research as it refocuses from traditional random controlled trials to medicine-based evidence used to guide decision-making for an individual patient by profiling the patient's clinical features and then finding approximate matches. Medical education benefits from virtual training ranging from problem-based case studies to surgical procedures.

Several AI-related concerns need to be addressed. Experience and time will give an indication of how well physicians will generally accept "black box" AI applications, for which they accept responsibility and liability but cannot view the details of the software decision-making algorithms. They must also remain vigilant to avoid decision-making and interventions based upon AI-perpetuated bias. Physicians will need experience and time to become "comfortable" with interpretation of predictive analytics data and with how to avoid confusing predictive analytics data associations with correlations to avoid incorrect conclusions. Another concern is the potential loss of physician jobs particularly in medical imaging related to the early success of AI image interpretation. An alternative perspective is that AI will help address projected manpower shortages by relieving physicians of time-consuming tasks to concentrate on decision-making and more complex tasks. How well humans will accept machines that mimic empathy and other human emotional responses is still to be determined.

Privacy and Security

Physicians are affected in multiple ways by privacy and security concerns in both the clinical and business aspects of practice. These include breach of patient records, disclosure of confidential physician-patient communication, and EHR hacking for ransom. Privacy and security risks may increase as health system networks increase their size, number of employees, and locations. Other additive factors include increased interoperability, storage, sharing, and movement of larger datasets, increased patient access to medical records, absence of a secure texting solution, telehealth and mobile health utilization, and hackers becoming more aggressive and adept at their craft. Although most healthcare organizations have developed clear-cut policies regarding social media use by physicians, its pervasive use presents ongoing concerns including patient privacy and appropriate physician-patient interactions.

Legal

The expanded use of clinical informatics is reflected in new legal risks. Expanding health systems, new care models, and population health management drive the larger networks, teams, and new applications. As care shifts from solo to team-based care, there needs to be clarity in policy and procedures that assign responsibility for delegated tasks such as test results follow-up and clinical alerts. Lack of interoperability contributes to the risk that data may fail to transfer from one system to another. For example, the patient portal or telehealth system encounter or message data may not be integrated into the EHR, resulting in risk that critically needed patient data may not be readily available to the clinical team.

Workarounds such as "copy & paste" risk perpetuating inaccurate information as well as making the medical record unnecessarily long which might result in missing important details. All of these increase the risk of liability and malpractice actions, particularly in the U.S., but growing risk in other countries such as U.K. In the U.S. there is the added risk that documentation issues may lead to fraud, e.g., "copy forward" may document inaccurate information that gets coded in the billing process.

Patient safety issues arising directly from the EHR are difficult to assess. While some organizations have tracking systems, there is no central repository that tracks incidents on a large scale. There also may be EHR contract "gag clauses" that block public disclosure and discussion of patient safety issues.

Health Informatics Priorities from the Perspective of This Profession

Physicians' most important priority is having meaningful input in clinical informatics. Lessons learned from the past should drive organizations to truly engage physicians in *all* stages of planning, system selection, implementation, user acceptance, optimization, and leadership. Failure to involve physicians entails significant risk that physician burnout and lack of productivity will adversely affect organizations, and the organization may fail to derive the full value of the system [4]. Clinical Informatics and leadership education should be incorporated into the curriculum of all medical schools and residency programs as well as Continuing Medical Education (CME) programs, to ensure that physicians are prepared to fulfill these roles.

Physicians want improved user-friendliness and functionality that supports their work rather than creating additional burden. This is supported by the U.S. government's *twenty-first Century Act* which requires a plan of action to reduce regulatory and administrative burden relating to the use of health IT and EHRs. Physician priorities include ready access to complete patient data including data generated from within their practice, organization, health system as well as data generated by other healthcare organizations. The population health focus on SDoH has added the challenge of making data from outside of the traditional healthcare system available. Application Programming Interfaces (APIs) and Fast Healthcare Interoperability Resources (FHIR) are increasingly being adopted to enable data exchange between organizations.

There are many strategies for addressing physician burnout, including workload and workflow modification, healthier lifestyle programs, and resiliency training. When usability is improved, the burnout rate declines for each 1% increase in EHR usability, clinician burnout decreases 3% [14]. Considerable improvements can be derived from relatively simple changes. These include integration of technologies such as single sign-on and telehealth into the EHR, reduction of clicks, number of screens, and interrupt messages. New technology offers solutions to free the physician from the EHR screen, including voice-enabled transcription and NLP via smart speakers/chatbots/smartbots to enable face-to-face interaction with patients, while producing a contextualized visit note. Other improvements to the physician experience include using AI to directly route physician emails to other team members and using the EHR to remind staff about follow-ups and screenings. Physicians also want to know that patient safety issues resulting from EHR functions are investigated, tracked, and used to make improvements. The absence of a uniform process and centralized repository for collecting informatics related errors results in considerable uncertainty regarding the scope of the problem and creates a barrier to addressing it.

As the use of mobile monitoring devices proliferates, and population health management advances, data reporting will become increasingly challenging. Robust analytics will produce both more retrospective and real-time reports. Serious attention needs to be given to the volume of data, reporting formats, timing of reports, and directing of alerts to the most appropriate team member. In a similar manner, communication tools and devices need to be simplified with AI applications so that communication is timely and appropriately routed to the right team member but not overwhelming.

Health Informatics Priorities in Collaboration with Other Professions

The shared quest of the Quadruple Aim creates great opportunity for physicians and other healthcare professionals to collaborate. Shared priorities include improved EHR usability, workflow, data availability, and communication, while improving patient safety and protecting privacy and security. All health professions benefit by addressing burnout causative factors.

Most U.S. medical schools require interprofessional education to develop teamwork skills early in the educational process [19]. Interprofessional team models are widely used in population health management to address increasingly complex chronic disease issues, as well as the SDoH. These teams include physicians, nurses, pharmacists, physician assistants, social workers, paramedics, care managers/coordinators, coaches, community health workers, and others in information systems and other business functions. Interprofessional teams strive to have all members function "at the top of their license", to drive maximum value. This affords a great opportunity to expand evidence-based practice and CDS by distributing responsibilities across the team. However, EHRs are generally not designed for strong interprofessional team collaboration and they will require modifications to effectively support team structure. Mobile and remote devices have considerable potential to monitor patients as well as improve team communication and function, but require team design structure, and definition and clarification of individual roles, expectations, and functions.

Interprofessional team leadership does not "come naturally" to most teams. Physician leaders need to reconcile whether this is relinquishing authority, or actually extending leadership over a broader-based team and freeing up the physician for more complex tasks and decision-making. Transitioning from the model of autonomous "solo" physician to interprofessional team structure creates challenges including considerable modification of the traditional healthcare power dynamics. Some physicians prefer the model they were trained in and successfully used in practice, while others appreciate the team model and the opportunity to collaborate with others. This presents an opportunity for dyad or triad leadership models. Sharing the leadership role with another clinician or administrator can be very effective in managing the medical, social, financial, and informatics aspects of care. Clinical informatics supports teams by enabling access to data, information sharing, and enabling communication. This was widely experienced in the COVID-19 pandemic when teams became the most effective way to manage the sudden demands on health care systems throughout the world.

The High Reliability Organization (HRO) patient safety program is a prototype for how the health professions working collaboratively can affect meaningful and sustainable change. HRO is an excellent example of the powerful cultural changes and performance improvement that can result from the professions working in interprofessional teams. HRO has significantly advanced patient safety while bringing professionals into better working relationships. Clinical informatics has played a pivotal role in HRO by addressing data analytics needs, development of CDS programs to prevent serious safety events (e.g., identification of sepsis protocols), promotion of technologies like medication barcoding to prevent medication errors, and improvement of interprofessional communication through the use of structured protocols including site-of-care transitions, patient "handoffs", and opioid management.

Summary

In 30 years, clinical informatics has profoundly changed the practice of medicine across the entire international spectrum. As physicians and their healthcare colleagues address an aging population with extensive chronic disease, clinical informatics will continue to play an integral role in patient-centered, team-based, population health management.

However, we cannot neglect the human side of medicine, as such must address the unintended consequences of technology so that we can take full advantage of the efficiencies, decision-making enhancements, that AI, NLP, and mobile communications devices bring to medicine.

Conclusions and Outlook

Physicians dependence on reliable clinical informatics will continue to evolve and grow in importance as world-wide health systems seek ways to effectively manage an aging population with high chronic disease prevalence. While clinical informatics technology has addressed many problems, it has unintentionally created or exacerbated others. Given the right organizational and government support and effective leadership, it has the potential to address these and enable progress to continue moving forward, but only if we listen to the voice of physicians and make thoughtful decisions. Much remains to be done to optimize clinical informatics.

Useful Resources
1. HIMSS Physician Community https://www.himss.org/membership-participation/physician
2. Association of Medical Directors of Information Systems www.amdis.org
3. AMIA www.amia.org
4. International Medical Informatics Association www.imia-medinfo.org/

Review Questions
1. What changes can we implement to optimize EHRs for physicians?
2. How can clinical informatics and technology enhance interprofessional team function and performance?
3. How can engage and support physicians in clinical informatics' leadership?
4. What are the greatest clinical informatics challenges facing physicians?

Appendix: Answers to Review Questions

1. What changes can we implement to optimize EHRs for physicians?

Changes to optimize EHRs for physicians include interoperability, more intuitive functions and interfaces, reduction of screens and mouse clicks, increased CDS, reduction of alerts and interrupts, single sign-on, real-time data, and integration of telehealth.

2. How can clinical informatics and technology enhance interprofessional team function and performance?

Clinical informatics and related technology can improve interprofessional team function by improving real-time communications, routing alerts and messages to the most appropriate team member and improving interoperability between EHRs and population health/care management information systems.

3. How can engage and support physicians in clinical informatics' leadership?

Physicians can be best supported in clinical informatics leadership by involving giving them a genuine "voice" in decision-making, system selection, adoption, implementation, optimization, and oversight, and by supporting dedicated time away from clinical duties to perform clinical informatics functions.

4. What are the greatest clinical informatics challenges facing physicians?

The greatest clinical informatics' challenges include burnout, lack of interoperability, EHR design and function, rapid system change, introduction of new technology (e.g., AI), patient safety, and privacy and security.

References

1. Detmer DE, Shortliffe EH. Clinical informatics: prospects for a new medical subspecialty. JAMA. 2014;311(20):2067–8.
2. Bodenheimer T, Sinsky C. From triple to quadruple aim: care of the patient requires care of the provider. Ann Fam Med. 2014;12(6):573–6.
3. eHealth trend barometer: annual European eHealth survey 2019 [Internet]. HIMSS analytics - Europe. 2019. https://europe.himssanalytics.org/europe/ehealth-barometer/ehealth-trend-barometer-annual-european-ehealth-survey-2019. Accessed 21 Jan 2020.
4. Fragidis LL, Chatzoglou PD. Implementation of a nationwide electronic health record (EHR). Int J Health Care Qual Assur. 2018;31(2):116–30.
5. Health Systems Science Review - 9780323653701 | US Elsevier health bookshop [Internet]. https://www.us.elsevierhealth.com/health-systems-science-review-9780323653701.html. Accessed 26 Feb 2020.
6. Gonzalo JD, Dekhtyar M, Starr SR, Borkan J, Brunett P, Fancher T, et al. Health systems science curricula in undergraduate medical education: identifying and defining a potential curricular framework. Acad Med J Assoc Am Med Coll. 2017;92(1):123–31.
7. Common program requirements.pdf [Internet]. https://www.acgme.org/Portals/0/PFAssets/ProgramRequirements/381_ClinicalInformatics_2019_TCC.pdf?ver=2019-03-27-084451-767. Accessed 22 Jan 2020.
8. Download: taking action against clinician burnout: a systems approach to professional well-being | The National Academies Press [Internet]. https://www.nap.edu/download/25521. Accessed 8 Jan 2020.
9. Doty MM, Tikkanen R, Shah A, Schneider EC. Primary care physicians' role in coordinating medical and health-related social needs in eleven countries. Health Aff (Millwood). 2019;39(1):115–23.
10. Physician burnout [Internet]. http://www.ahrq.gov/prevention/clinician/ahrq-works/burnout/index.html. Accessed 26 Feb 2020.
11. Physician burnout is a public health crisis: a message to our fellow health care CEOs | Health Affairs [Internet]. https://www.healthaffairs.org/do/10.1377/hblog20170328.059397/full/. Accessed 9 Jan 2020.
12. Indicators associated with job morale among physicians and dentists in low-income and middle-income countries: a systematic review and meta-analysis | Global Health | JAMA Network Open | JAMA Network [Internet]. https://jamanetwork.com/journals/jamanetworkopen/fullarticle/2758470. Accessed 21 Feb 2020.
13. Kroth PJ, Morioka-Douglas N, Veres S, Babbott S, Poplau S, Qeadan F, et al. Association of electronic health record design and use factors with clinician stress and burnout. JAMA Netw Open. 2019;2(8):e199609.
14. Melnick ER, Dyrbye LN, Sinsky CA, Trockel M, West CP, Nedelec L, et al. The association between perceived electronic health record usability and professional burnout among US physicians. Mayo Clin Proc [Internet]. 2019. https://www.mayoclinicproceedings.org/article/S0025-6196(19)30836-5/abstract. Accessed 10 Jan 2020.
15. Downing NL, Bates DW, Longhurst CA. Physician burnout in the electronic health record era: are we ignoring the real cause? Ann Intern Med. 2018;169(1):50.
16. Tai-Seale M, Olson CW, Li J, Chan AS, Morikawa C, Durbin M, et al. Electronic health record logs indicate that physicians split time evenly between seeing patients and desktop medicine. Health Aff Proj Hope. 2017;36(4):655–62.
17. Burnout in healthcare workers: the elephant in the room [Internet]. ECRI Institute. https://www.ecri.org/components/HRC/Pages/RMRep1216.aspx. Accessed 9 Jan 2020.
18. Getting rid of stupid stuff reduce the unnecessary daily burdens for clinicians [Internet]. https://edhub.ama-assn.org/steps-forward/module/2757858. Accessed 21 Jan 2020.
19. Interprofessional education requirements at US medical schools [Internet]. AAMC. https://www.aamc.org/data-reports/curriculum-reports/interactive-data/interprofessional-education-requirements-us-medical-schools. Accessed 21 Feb 2020.

The Pharmacist's View: Patient-Centered Care Through the Lens of a Pharmacist

6

Franky and Brian K. Fung

Learning Objectives

- *Identify* priorities of pharmacy informaticians in the use and integration of data, information, knowledge, and technology involved with medication use processes to improve outcomes.
- *Describe* challenges faced by pharmacy informaticians in the application of emerging technologies.
- *Develop* an understanding of strategies to be employed to upskill the pharmacy workforce.

Key Terms

- Medication use process
- Artificial intelligence
- Natural language processing
- Machine learning
- RxNorm
- Dictionary of medicines and devices (dm+d)
- Australian Medicines Terminology (AMT)
- Singapore Drug Dictionary (SDD)
- Fast Healthcare Interoperability Resources (FHIR)
- e-Iatrogenesis

Introduction

Historically, the pharmacy industry has been an early adopter of technology and automation [1]. The first telephone exchange in history happened when the American Capital Avenue Drugstore was connected with 21 local physicians in the late 1970s, serving as a precursor to telemedicine [2]. Hence, it is not surprising that when medical informatics received recognition as a health science discipline, pharmacy informatics eventually emerged as one of the sub-specialties in both pharmacy practice and medical informatics.

As a subset of medical informatics, pharmacy informatics is concerned over the use of medication and pharmacy-related data to improve patient care and outcomes. At the same time, as pharmacy informatics emerged from the use of technology in pharmacy practice, the medication use process remains the primary focus of the discipline. This chapter will discuss the role of informatics pharmacists in health care and how the profession can spearhead efforts to tackle future challenges in medication use processes and beyond.

Franky (✉)
Institute of Mental Health, Singapore, Singapore
e-mail: frankybpharm@gmail.com

B. K. Fung
Mayo Clinic, Rochester, MN, USA
e-mail: brian@briankfung.com

© Springer Nature Switzerland AG 2022
U. H. Hübner et al. (eds.), *Nursing Informatics*, Health Informatics,
https://doi.org/10.1007/978-3-030-91237-6_6

Definition and Role of the Profession in Health Care

The American Society of Health-System Pharmacists (ASHP) defines pharmacy informatics as a subspecialty that focuses on "the use and integration of data, information, knowledge, technology, and automation in the medication use process for the purpose of improving health outcomes" [3]. Conventionally, informatics pharmacists are involved in the configuration of computerized prescriber order entry (CPOE), clinical decision support systems (CDSS), electronic prescribing, automated dispensing system (ADS), and barcode-assisted medication administration (BCMA) within health-system settings. Figure 6.1 shows how different health information technologies can support steps in the medication use process. In recent years, there has been an expansion of the informatics pharmacists' role to take on more diverse projects, from supporting antimicrobial stewardship programs [4] and

pharmacy practice initiatives [5] to manage clinical data [6]. Informatics pharmacists have evolved to become key players in the exploration of new frontiers within health care delivery.

Challenges of the Profession in the State of the Art Care Delivery

The emergence of artificial intelligence (AI) in a data-rich, healthcare environment serves as a major technological disruption presenting both opportunities and challenges for the pharmacy profession. The ability of AI to sift through large volumes of data and detect patterns can provide new insights into how we approach patient care. Conversely, there is an ongoing fear of AI in that it could result in the loss of pharmacy jobs. These considerations led to the 2019 ASHP publication, *Impact of artificial intelligence on healthcare and pharmacy practice* that examined the impact of AI on the pharmacy practice [8, 9]. Given its

Fig. 6.1 Medication use process and technology examples [2, 7]

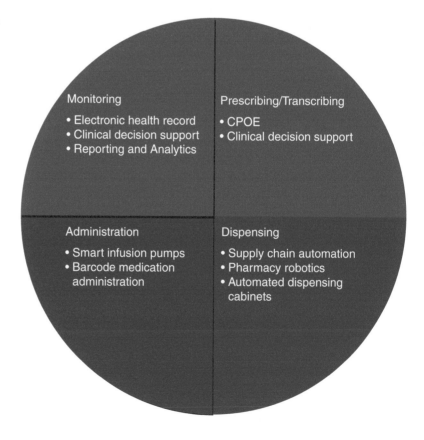

wider influence on healthcare, the National Academy of Medicine (NAM) recently consolidated AI literature into their 2020 report, *Artificial Intelligence in Health Care: The Hope, the Hype, the Promise, the Peril*, in an effort to inform the medical community at large on how best to proceed [10].

Currently, the application of AI to the practice of medicine falls into two categories: machine learning (ML) and natural language processing (NLP) [8]. ML is a method of AI that analyzes large data sets to identify patterns while NLP interprets and converts unstructured data (e.g., clinical notes) into structured data [8]. For pharmacists, these functions are attractive due to their potential to promote safe and effective medication use by, as the proverbial saying goes, "finding a needle in a haystack". Whether it's reviewing drug interactions, drug indications, or weighing the benefits and risks of a drug's side effects, it is not difficult to conjure up the various ways in which these technologies can augment the role of a pharmacist. In fact, following review of current literature, the different applications for AI in the pharmacy profession include:

- Use ML methods to recognize inappropriate electronic prescriptions by using two sequential processes—learning data patterns and applying learned patterns to classify and detect new cases [11].
- Develop a computerized decision support system (CDSS) that utilized ML algorithms to identify and intervene in possible medication prescription errors in real-time [12].
- Design a ML system that is capable of showing, by means of an automated classification, who is and who is not likely to encounter serious adverse reactions from a given drug, thus helping in therapy selection [11].
- Apply ML using algorithms to integrate and analyze patient and drug usage data to help predict drug par values for inventory management [11].
- Leveraging the use of NLP in the pharmacovigilance systems to evaluate data from various sources and predict adverse drug events or adverse drug reactions [13].

- Use ML algorithms to improve the decision-making processes of drug safety professionals by enabling a more effective and reliable review of reported incidents [14].
- Integrating conventional computational methods with ML techniques and current internal pharma repositories to improve speed and accuracy of predictions during the drug development and approval process [15].

Though, despite its potential utility, AI experts urge the healthcare community to proceed with caution [10]. There are numerous challenges with AI, which may be more than its benefits that should be discussed. The first challenge is the reliance of AI on data and the importance of data provenance. Large amounts of data, with some estimates of tens of thousands of records [11], are required to adequately train models for success. This makes the origin of the data extremely critical, as it will influence the outputs generated by the AI model [10]. For example, data quality issues from electronic health records (EHRs) and other operational databases that manifest in the form of missing data, duplicate data, and incorrectly generated data, can lead to incorrect assumptions and estimates about medication adherence [16]. This segues into concerns related to bias, regulation, and ethics. As the saliency of how social determinants of health (SDOH) can impact population health, regulation of this technology, and evaluation of it from an ethical perspective should occur simultaneously with its development. Documented examples of biased AI models deployed in hiring practices, administration of social services, and overall justice should serve as prime examples of what unintended consequences can occur if the data is not appropriately scrutinized [17]. Last, but not least, disruptive technology is usually coupled with a mismatch in the workforce, in both its efficiencies and training required to harness it. This manifests into two challenges: fear of job loss and a lack of individuals trained to deploy and use AI. In 2013, an estimated 47% of jobs in the United States (U.S.) were at risk of being automated [14]. Albeit, there is also a large opposing viewpoint in that AI will lead to the creation of many new types of jobs. Nevertheless, the one certainty is the fact that there is a large gap and consequent need for education and workforce development to fully leverage AI [10].

Health Informatics Priorities from the Perspective of This Profession

Pharmacists' priorities should always be dictated by patients' needs and safety. The continued digitalization of the healthcare environment, in light of AI, easily drives priorities toward upskilling the pharmacy workforce and creating high-quality, medication-related data. As suggested in the challenges section, data will continue to increase in importance over time and the ability to manage its growing volume in a scalable and tenable way needs to be addressed.

Adoption and implementation of medication-related standards is a key component to enriching information systems, both internally and externally. As it currently stands, commonly used data sources such as EHRs are still largely inadequate for training AI models with respect to both data quantity and dimensionality [10, 18]. Further, sufficient and appropriate representation of data, for the purposes of AI, will likely only be achieved through the exchange of data across multiple organizations [11]. With the advent of Health Level-7 (HL7)'s Fast Healthcare Interoperability Resources (FHIR) standard, widespread interoperability between organizations can be achieved and exposure of commonly used clinical standards to the FHIR standard can assist with semantic preservation. While some standards (e.g., Logical Observation Identifiers Names and Codes (LOINC), Systemized Nomenclature of Medicine—Clinical Terms (SNOMED CT)) have been adopted internationally, medication standards may differ from country to country [19]. For example, RxNorm is largely used in the United States, but equivalent medication

standards also exist in other countries such as the United Kingdom's Dictionary of medicines and devices (dm+d), the Australian Medicines Terminology (AMT), and Singapore's Drug Dictionary (SDD) [19, 20]. As medication experts, informatics pharmacists are well-positioned to lead the charge in maturing the RxNorm standard to accurately represent the intricacies of medication concepts.

RxNorm is a standardized naming system for generic and branded drugs produced by the National Library of Medicine (NLM) to support an efficient and unambiguous exchange of data between drug terminologies and pharmacy knowledge base systems [21]. When various health information technology (HIT) systems use several different sets of drug names, it can be difficult for one system to communicate with another. To overcome this challenge, RxNorm offers standardized names and specific identifiers for drugs available in the United States. RxNorm also implements relationships to link drug concepts (e.g., the active ingredient, dose form, brand name), enabling users to easily navigate through related drug identifiers [21]. Figure 6.2 shows an example representation of Cetirizine (a drug used in allergy rhinitis) using the RxNorm medication standard.

Prioritizing pharmacy informatics education should also occur in parallel as technology advancements currently outpace the supply of the global informatics workforce. There is not only a gap in informatics education in the doctorate of pharmacy programs (PharmD) in the U.S., but there is also a gap in the health informatics training programs overall [2, 22]. Moreover, the skill sets required to ethically and effectively deploy AI will further widen these gaps and likely lead to increased healthcare costs and lower value care [10]. Priorities regarding education should focus on both the clinical and informatics pharmacists. While clinical pharmacists validate data models that are being developed, informatics pharmacists can upskill as trainers, explainers, and sustainers of AI [10].

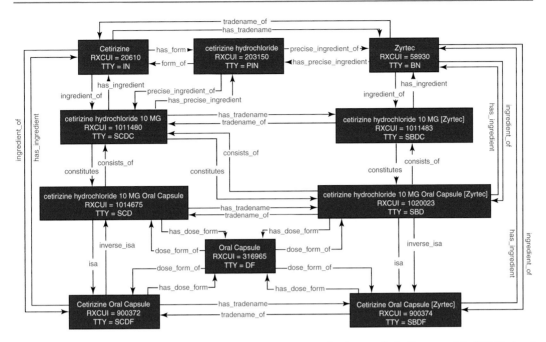

Fig. 6.2 Example Representation of Cetirizine using the RxNorm medication standard. *Courtesy of the U.S. National Library of Medicine* [21]

Health Informatics Priorities in Collaboration with Other Professions

Informatics pharmacists have moved beyond building technology infrastructures to supporting day-to-day pharmacy operations to work alongside other healthcare professionals to improve patient care through HIT [1]. More importantly, the medication use process underpins the importance of collaboration between pharmacists and other healthcare professionals to achieve a closed-loop medication management system to reduce human error and maintain consistency in delivering high-quality patient care. In the following sections, specific examples within the medication use process in which collaboration is critical will be highlighted.

As informatics pharmacists are familiar with standards representing medication information and configuration of medication records in EHRs, they can play a significant role in the development of CPOE systems. In particular, informatics pharmacists are concerned about the design of the CPOE interface (i.e., how the clinicians inter-

act with the system). The right interface should not contribute to the commission of e-iatrogenesis, which is an error caused in part by the use of HIT [23]. Instead, the system should guide clinicians to prescribe medications safely and improve patient care [24]. The partnership between informatics pharmacists and provider users will yield effective functional and usable HIT to prevent e-iatrogenesis.

A poorly designed system has been identified as one of the contributing factors to e-iatrogenesis that occurs during prescribing. One of the characteristics of a poorly designed CPOE interface would be variations in how drug names are displayed in the system. An analysis performed by Quist et al. [25] of 10 different CPOE systems across six health institutions discovered an inconsistency in the display of brand and generic drug names. There are even systems where drug names are displayed differently on the same screen. Quist et al. concluded that the variability in drug display names poses a risk for potential drug duplication errors [25]. Informatics pharmacists can work alongside physicians to standardize drug display names across the CPOE system to prevent medication errors, using existing guidelines, such as the Institute for Safe Medication Practices (ISMP) Guidelines for Safe Electronic Communication of Medication Information [26].

A deficit understanding of human-computer interaction can also lead to a poorly designed CPOE interface. In 2006, an auto-completion functionality within an electronic prescribing system had caused several physicians in the United Kingdom to unintentionally prescribe Viagra (a medication indicated to treat erectile dysfunction) for patients who should receive Zyban (a medication indicated to support smoking cessation) [27]. To prevent such errors from happening, ASHP recommends pharmacists to be essential members of the CPOE project team. Pharmacists are likely to have experience with electronic pharmacy systems which are equipped with order entry functionality. Hence, they can provide insights into human factors issues surrounding human-computer interaction [28].

Apart from physicians, informatics pharmacists also work closely with nurses, primarily on the configuration of bar coded medication administration (BCMA) and the integration between smart infusion pumps and EHRs. Vermeulen et al. [29] reported that a pharmacist-led implementation of a smart pump–EHR interoperability program at a hospital in the U.S. had improved intravenous medication safety measurably. During the implementation, pharmacists worked alongside various stakeholders, including nursing staff, to harmonize smart-pump data sets and EHR medication formulary. This exercise is necessary to ensure infusion information transmitted by the EHR accurately prepopulates infusion devices, leading to a reduced need for nursing staff to manually enter the information in the pumps and decreased risks for manual programming errors [29].

Summary

Informatics pharmacists play a significant role in curating medication-data, as they are well-versed in medication standards and concepts. At present, consistent electronic medication records (EMRs) are needed to ensure a safe and effective medication use process in EHRs. Not only that, but as we move into the future, good-quality medication data are also crucial in the configuration of AI in healthcare.

Conclusions and Outlook

In conclusion, AI is arguably the most pressing challenge for the profession of pharmacy at this time. It is imperative that pharmacy leaders identify how this profession can best train, augment, and ethically deploy the use of AI in practice. The profession could begin this process by identifying use-cases, establishing a data standard framework, and finally, preparing the global workforce required to support the new model of care [30].

Useful Resources

1. Informatics—ASHP [Internet]. [cited 2020 Jul 9]. Available from: https://www.ashp.org:443/Pharmacy-Practice/Resource-Centers/Informatics
2. Pharmacoinformatics | AMIA [Internet]. Pharmacoinformatics. [cited 2020 Jul 9]. Available from: https://www.amia.org/programs/working-groups/pharmacoinformatics
3. Pharmacy informatics [Internet]. Pharmacy informatics. [cited 2020 Jul 9]. Available from: https://www.rpharms.com/resources/pharmacy-guides/pharmacy-informatics
4. Pharmacy Informatics | Canadian Society of Hospital Pharmacists [Internet]. Pharmacy Informatics. [cited 2020 Jul 9]. Available from: https://cshp.ca/pharmacy-informatics
5. Vermeulen LC, Swarthout MD, Alexander GC, Ginsburg DB, Pritchett KO, White SJ, Tryon J, Emmerich C, Nesbit TW, Greene W, Fox ER. ASHP Foundation Pharmacy Forecast 2020: Strategic Planning Advice for Pharmacy Departments in Hospitals and Health Systems. American Journal of Health-System Pharmacy. 2019 Dec 5.
6. Oddis JA. Executive summary of the 2019 ASHP Commission on Goals: Impact of artificial intelligence on healthcare and pharmacy practice. American Journal of Health-System Pharmacy.

7. ASHP Practice Advancement Initiative 2030: New recommendations for advancing pharmacy practice in health systems. Am J Health Syst Pharm. 2020 Jan 8;77 (2):113–21.
8. Matheny ME, Whicher D, Israni ST. Artificial Intelligence in Health Care: A report from the National Academy of Medicine. Jama. 2020 Feb 11;323 (6):509–10.
9. Goundrey-Smith S. Information Technology in Pharmacy: An Integrated Approach. Springer Science & Business Media; 2012 Oct 5.
10. Dumitru D. The Pharmacy Informatics Primer. first ed. Bethesda, MD: American Society of Health-System Pharmacists (ASHP); 2008. 264 p.
11. Fox BI, Thrower MR, Felkey BG, American Pharmacists Association. Building core competencies in pharmacy informatics. Washington, DC: American Pharmacists Association. 2010.

Review Questions

1. Which of the following scenarios has AI been studied as an application within the practice of pharmacy?
   (a) Detection of adverse drug events
   (b) Drug discovery
   (c) Drug selection
   (d) Inventory management
   (e) All of the above
2. Which of the following are important considerations in the development and deployment of AI?
   (a) Training AI models with limited data sets to avoid complexity.
   (b) Trusting the prediction outcomes, as algorithms have proven to outperform humans.
   (c) Data provenance and validation of data used to train AI models.
   (d) Mismatch of demand and supply in AI deployment due to a surplus of trained individuals.
3. Which of the following clinical standards is NOT a medication standard?
   (a) AMT
   (b) LOINC
   (c) RxNorm

   (d) dm+d
   (e) SDD
4. True or False: Existing standards coupled with EHRs are sufficient for the widespread deployment of AI.
   (a) True
   (b) False
5. Which of the following will unlikely lead to e-iatrogenesis?
   (a) Designing poor user interfaces for CPOE.
   (b) Configuring medication records with different display names to ensure variability within the EHR.
   (c) Coordinating with stakeholders to harmonize data sets between smart pumps and EHR medication formularies.
   (d) Designing workflows and tools to be fully automated to avoid human-computer interaction altogether.

Appendix: Answers to Review Questions

1. Which of the following scenarios has AI been studied as an application within the practice of pharmacy?
   (a) Detection of adverse drug events
   (b) Drug discovery
   (c) Drug selection
   (d) Inventory management
   (e) All of the above

Explanation: All of the following have been studied as an application of AI in pharmacy.

2. Which of the following are important considerations in the development and deployment of AI?
   (a) Training AI models with limited data sets to avoid complexity.
   (b) Trusting the prediction outcomes, as algorithms have proven to outperform humans.
   (c) Data provenance and validation of data used to train AI models.
   (d) Mismatch of demand and supply in AI deployment due to a surplus of trained individuals.

Explanation: (a) is incorrect as training models require large data sets that can be upwards of tens of thousands of records; (b) is incorrect as data quality issues can lead to incorrect assumptions and should be appropriately scrutinized; (d) is incorrect as there is a shortage of trained individuals to effectively deploy AI.

3. Which of the following clinical standards is NOT a medication standard?
   (a) AMT
   (b) LOINC
   (c) RxNorm
   (d) dm+d
   (e) SDD

Explanation: LOINC is a terminology standard for health measurements, observations, and documents. It is not a medication standard.

4. True or False: Existing standards coupled with EHRs are sufficient for the widespread deployment of AI.
   (a) True
   (b) False

Explanation: Further maturation of existing infrastructure, especially as it pertains to enriching data quality and representation, is needed before we can achieve widespread deployment of AI. Moreover, near-term solutions should be focused on augmented intelligence rather than full automation. See the article from the National Academy of Medicine for further reading.

5. Which of the following will unlikely lead to e-iatrogenesis?
   (a) Designing poor user interfaces for CPOE.
   (b) Configuring medication records with different display names to ensure variability within the EHR.
   (c) Coordinating with stakeholders to harmonize data sets between smart pumps and EHR medication formularies.
   (d) Designing workflows and tools to be fully automated to avoid human-computer interaction altogether.

Explanation: all of the choices except (c) were listed as examples that could lead to e-iatrogenesis. Only (c) was an example of how to avoid e-iatrogenesis.

References

1. Pitre M, Thickson N. Should pharmacy informatics officer positions be based in, and report to, the pharmacy department, rather than the health information technology department? Can J Hosp Pharm. 2011;64(6):459–61.
2. Fox BI, Flynn AJ, Fortier CR, Clauson KA. Knowledge, skills, and resources for pharmacy informatics education. Am J Pharm Educ. 2011;75(5):93.
3. ASHP. Statement on the pharmacist's role in clinical informatics. Am J Health Syst Pharm. 2016;73(6):410–3.
4. Dustin Waters C. Pharmacist-driven antimicrobial stewardship program in an institution without infectious diseases physician support. Am J Health Syst Pharm. 2015;72(6):466–8.
5. Fox BI, Pedersen CA, Gumpper KF. ASHP national survey on informatics: assessment of the adoption and use of pharmacy informatics in US hospitals—2013. Am J Health Syst Pharm. 2015; 72(8):636–55.
6. Woodhead V. Why pharmacists should consider clinical data management as a career [Internet]. The Pharmaceutical Journal. 2003. https://www.pharmaceutical-journal.com/news-and-analysis/features/why-pharmacists-should-consider-clinical-data-management-as-a-career/20008578.article?firstPass=false. Accessed 11 Apr 2020.
7. Vest TA, Gazda NP, Schenkat DH, Eckel SF. Practice-enhancing publications about the medication use process in 2017. Am J Health Syst Pharm. 2019;76(10):667–76.
8. Executive summary of the 2019 ASHP Commission on Goals: impact of artificial intelligence on healthcare and pharmacy practice. Am J Health Syst Pharm. 2019;76(24):2087–92.
9. Vermeulen LC, Swarthout MD, Alexander GC, Ginsburg DB, Pritchett KO, White SJ, et al. ASHP Foundation pharmacy forecast 2020: strategic planning advice for pharmacy departments in hospitals and health systems. Vermeulen LC, Zellmer WA, editors. Am J Health Syst Pharm. 2020;77(2):84–112.
10. Matheny M, Israni ST, Whicher D. Artificial intelligence in health care: the hope, the hype, the promise, the peril [Internet]. National Academy of Medicine. 2019; p. 269 (The Learning Health System). https://nam.edu/wp-content/uploads/2019/12/AI-in-Health-Care-PREPUB-FINAL.pdf. Accessed 5 Mar 2020.

11. Flynn A. Using artificial intelligence in health-system pharmacy practice: finding new patterns that matter. Am J Health Syst Pharm. 2019;76(9):622–7.

12. Segal G, Segev A, Brom A, Lifshitz Y, Wasserstrum Y, Zimlichman E. Reducing drug prescription errors and adverse drug events by application of a probabilistic, machine-learning based clinical decision support system in an inpatient setting. J Am Med Inform Assoc. 2019;26(12):1560–5.

13. Wong A, Plasek JM, Montecalvo SP, Zhou L. Natural language processing and its implications for the future of medication safety: a narrative review of recent advances and challenges. Pharmacotherapy. 2018;38(8):822–41.

14. Danysz K, Cicirello S, Mingle E, Assuncao B, Tetarenko N, Mockute R, et al. Artificial intelligence and the future of the drug safety professional. Drug Saf. 2019;42(4):491–7.

15. Maharao N, Antontsev V, Wright M, Varshney J. Entering the era of computationally driven drug development. Drug Metab Rev. 2020;21:1–16.

16. Galozy A, Nowaczyk S, Sant'Anna A, Ohlsson M, Lingman M. Pitfalls of medication adherence approximation through EHR and pharmacy records: definitions, data and computation. Int J Med Inf. 2020;136:104092.

17. Matheny ME, Whicher D, Israni ST. Artificial intelligence in health care: a report from the National Academy of Medicine. JAMA. 2020;323(6):509–10.

18. Maddox TM, Rumsfeld JS, Payne PRO. Questions for artificial intelligence in health care. JAMA. 2019;321(1):31–2.

19. Bodenreider O, Cornet R, Vreeman DJ. Recent developments in clinical terminologies—SNOMED CT, LOINC, and RxNorm. Yearb Med Inform. 2018;27(1):129–39.

20. Integrated Health Information Systems (IHiS). Integrated Health Information Systems (IHiS) Standards [Internet]. 2018. https://cms.ihis.com.sg/Standards/Pages/Default.aspx. Accessed 29 Apr 2020.

21. RxNorm overview [Internet]. U.S. National Library of Medicine. https://www.nlm.nih.gov/research/umls/rxnorm/overview.html. Accessed 30 Apr 2020.

22. Khairat S, Sandefer R, Marc D, Pyles L. A review of biomedical and health informatics education: a workforce training framework. J Hosp Adm. 2016;5(5):10.

23. Weiner JP, Kfuri T, Chan K, Fowles JB. "e-Iatrogenesis": the most critical unintended consequence of CPOE and other HIT. J Am Med Inform Assoc. 2007;14(3):387–8.

24. Dumitru D. The pharmacy informatics primer. 1st ed. Bethesda, MD: American Society of Health-System Pharmacists (ASHP); 2008. p. 264.

25. Quist AJL, Hickman T-TT, Amato MG, Volk LA, Salazar A, Robertson A, et al. Analysis of variations in the display of drug names in computerized prescriber-order-entry systems. Am J Health Syst Pharm. 2017;74(7):499–509.

26. ISMP guidelines for safe electronic communication of medication information [Internet]. Institute for Safe Medication. Practices (ISMP). 2019. https://www.ismp.org/node/1322. Accessed 17 Apr 2020.

27. Cramb A. Giving up smoking? Take a Viagra. The Telegraph [Internet]. 2006. https://www.telegraph.co.uk/news/uknews/1536890/Giving-up-smoking-Take-a-Viagra.html. Accessed 17 Apr 2020.

28. ASHP Section of Pharmacy Informatics and Technology. ASHP guidelines on pharmacy planning for implementation of computerized provider-order-entry systems in hospitals and health systems. Am J Health Syst Pharm. 2011;68:e9–31.

29. Biltoft J, Finneman L. Clinical and financial effects of smart pump–electronic medical record interoperability at a hospital in a regional health system. Bull Am Soc Hosp Pharm. 2018;75(14):1064–8.

30. Dentzer S. Creating the future of artificial intelligence in health-system pharmacy. Am J Health Syst Pharm. 2019;76(24):1995–6.

The Chief Information Officer's (CIO) View: Observations, Perspective, and Opinions

Charles E. Christian

Learning Objectives
- Discuss the space Clinical Informatics occupies with People, Process, and Technology
- Discuss the early years of clinical automation and the contributing event
- Review the impacts of automating a paper-based process
- Identify the appropriate skill sets required for the clinical informatics team, from the chair of the CIO

Key Terms
- Intersection of technology and healthcare
- People
- Process
- Technologies
- Staff skill set
- Collaboration of care silos
- CIO as partner

Introduction

Over the last 30–40 years, the role of Healthcare Information Technology (HIT) has evolved and continuously impacted the care delivery and business processes of healthcare. In the early 1970s, healthcare operations and clinical pro-cesses were all paper-based (at least in most hospitals). With the changes around how care is reimbursed, the advent of employer-provided healthcare, and an ever-increasing regulatory burden, the business side of healthcare was one of the first areas that applied information technology to automate the processes of patient registration, revenue cycle, and order management. These changes began with the introduction of Diagnostic Related Groups or DRGs as they are referred to affectionally.

For someone working in Radiology, before DRGs, the first introduction to information technology was in an early attempt to automate the patient study history index that was then kept on 4×6 index cards. As many can well imagine in a bustling Radiology department, there were a significant number of index cards that were updated each day, with a percentage of them getting misfiled. This type of record-keeping just begged for a more efficient and accurate process; however, the opportunity costs were very high due to the current state of computer automation availability. Mainframe computers were costly, and mini-computers were just beginning to arrive at a somewhat affordable price point. Only as a historical marker, Intel was founded in 1968 and announced the 4004 microprocessor in 1971.

C. E. Christian (✉)
Franciscan Alliance, Indianapolis, IN, USA
e-mail: chuck.christian@franciscanalliance.org

© Springer Nature Switzerland AG 2022
U. H. Hübner et al. (eds.), *Nursing Informatics*, Health Informatics,
https://doi.org/10.1007/978-3-030-91237-6_7

CIO's Role at the Intersection of Technology and Healthcare

Clinical Informatics lives at the intersection of People, Process, and Technology (Fig. 7.1).

The **people** equate to our patients, the providers, and other members of the care team, not just the physicians and nursing, but the ancillary departments with direct and indirect patient care responsibilities. The **processes** equate to those that impact the care processes and workflows, quality improvement, best medical evidence/clinical practice, and data/terminology standardization. Last but not least, the **technology** equates to our electronic systems, such as the Electronic Health Record (EHR), ancillary process systems (i.e., Pharmacy, lab, radiology, etc.), which may be part of an integrated EHR solution, and the directly connected medical devices (i.e., IV pumps, O_2 sensors, physiological monitors, etc.). The clinical informatics professional navigates within the space where these intersect, understanding the role, actions, and workflows of the individual while having experienced the related workflows and then leverages the technology tools to engage the people and streamline/improve the processes. The informaticist needs to possess experience in clinical disciplines. They also need to have more than a working knowledge of the care processes they are expected to support and/or improve and need to possess a clear understanding of the technology they hope to leverage in the process.

In the early years of healthcare automation, we were striving to automate data capture and quickly found that the acquired data's usefulness required standardization of both the discrete data and the associated coding methods. Even today, the data's value is directly related to how well it is defined/described, and standardized, not only across a single healthcare system/enterprise but also across all healthcare settings and healthcare providers.

During this same period, the standardization of the data was complicated by the fact that there were no solutions/applications that encompassed all of the departments of a healthcare organization; there were hundreds of "best-of-breed," department-specific applications that were

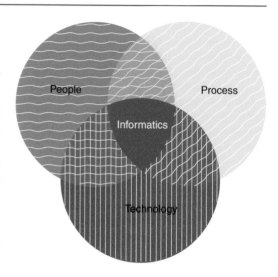

Fig. 7.1 The three components of informatics

designed and built without a great deal of consideration given to the need to communicate and share data/information with other departmental based systems. Of the two most widely implemented EHR solutions in use today, one was born out of the automation of the laboratory and the other out of the ambulatory/physician practice EHR market. Both are far more robust in the fact that the integration is internal to all applications, rather than the IT departments having to create and maintain the required level of integration; however, none of the solutions/systems truly contains functionality that every healthcare system requires for their clinical or business processes.

While the field of informatics has come a long way and is a very valuable tool in our quest to deliver higher quality care, at a lower cost point; it is not a panacea; it is the discipline that is expected to help delivery clarity where people, processes, and technology collide.

Challenges of the Profession Through the Eyes of My Early Experience with Health Care Automation and the Migration to the Digital Clinical Era

With the introduction of DRGs, the focus shifted to automating patient registration processes, including capturing the patient's employer-provided insurance information required to bill for the services provided. With the insurance information being captured in a timelier manner and hopefully more accurately, the processes of charge capture and billing were the next logical step. The manual process of charge capture and posting in an automated system leads to creating the data processing departments, which employed data-entry clerks. As the charge processes became more complex and numerous, the next target for automatization was order entry and communication. Most procedures in the care process required some level of a physician's order, either written or procedurally standard. Moving from a paper-based solution to communicate orders to an automated solution that would capture the charge as a by-produce of delivering the order increased the billing process's efficiency and decreased the amount of manual data entry required, reducing the need for, or eliminating the data-entry staff. One could say that the introduction of DRGs launched many electronic boats or processes.

While many individuals in leadership roles in the clinical disciplines welcomed the electronic assistance for the routine but required order management and billing processes, these business function systems had little impact on healthcare's core purpose: patient care. Nevertheless, the order management process did speed diagnostic and procedural processes. They allowed for an early level of data analytics but did little to assist in either augmenting the direct patient care processes or removing the related documentation burdens. In essence, most of the clinical processes took a backseat to the business office focused processes.

Entering the Digital Clinical Era

Just as DRGs launch the automation of the business side of healthcare, there was a similar catalyst for clinically focused automation; that was the seminal report from the Institute of Medicine (IOM), "To Err is Human: Building a Safer Health System," published in 2000 [1] and followed by "Cross The Quality Chasm: A New Health System for the 21st Century" [2]. The first of these publications created a laser focus on the fact that too many people are dying due to medical errors in our country, especially calling out those deaths caused by medication errors. The IOM explained the current understanding of why these errors occurred and asked the primary question; can we learn from these mistakes.

In this report, the IOM offered recommendations for improving patient safety and decreasing the number of error-related deaths; many were leadership and process-related (note: people and process), while others pointed toward the use of automation in the direct patient care setting (note: technology).

In the second publication, "Crossing the Quality Chasm," the IOM recommendations were around evidence-based best practices and the use of clinical information systems. Both IOM reports were escorting in the role of the clinical informaticist and providing a prescription for decreasing the number of medical error-related deaths and a path to bridge the quality chasm.

One of the critical areas that the IOM reports mentioned was the use of data/information in helping to correct many of the issues that were called into question. However, data/information alone is not the ultimate solution, but part of it. The solution needs to cover all three areas: people, processes, and technology. The clinical informaticists' role and expertise are critical in the realization of a much-improved healthcare system.

The healthcare system is being asked (some would say required) to always move from the volume-based reimbursement models toward a value-based or quality-based one. In a sense, the business of "healthcare," is more a business of "sick care." We are currently reimbursed for the encounters of care and not for the outcome of the care encounter. It is similar to paying your automobile mechanic for a visit even if they could not correct the issue you were having. This might sound like a bad example, as cars are much easier to repair than humans; however, we do perform parts replacement on all models.

Suppose we hope to correct the shortcomings identified in the IOM reports. In that case, it requires the skills and discipline of the clinical informaticists, who can bring their years of clinical knowledge combined with their systems expertise, married with analytical skills, standard project management processes, and continuous quality improvement technique to bear.

The Impact Automation on a Previously Paper-Based Process

Automation alone is not an all-encompassing solution. To err is human, but you can use a computer and still create a mess. The great thing about computerized systems is that once sent into motion, outcomes are typically standard and predictable; this translates that you can create errors in rapid succession.

In the IOM report mentioned earlier [1], one of the causes for patient harm came from the medication ordering/administration processes. There were those that felt that the solution was to rapidly implement Computerized Physician/Provider Order Entry or CPOE in conjunction with a level of Clinical Decision Support (CDS), which would be based upon Evidence-Based Medicine and/or standard protocols or Care Plans. As part of the process stream of ordering medications and administrating them to the patient, there is an array of primary and secondary processes that need to occur correctly for the medication to be delivered accurately and safely to the patient.

There were others that were concerned that even if the task of ordering the medication was automated, there were still ample opportunities for an adverse drug event when the medication was administrated to the patient. Automated medication administration systems utilized by nursing, would be required to close the process loop. However, when implementing solutions, one needs to be sure to consider all of the other systems and/or processes that feed into the primary process. Below is a real case describing the implementation of an electronic medication administration system, which, in the end, was very successful; however, it did not begin on that path. Even in the world of the computerized medication loop, there are several key divisions of labor and processes that need to be given consid-

eration related to how they interact; ordering physicians/providers, Pharmacy, and Nursing.

In the late 1990s, our organization embarked on implementing a closed-loop medication admiration system that was integrated into our EHR (electronic health record) and Pharmacy management system. I use the word "integrated" loosely; in 1998, there were no truly integrated solutions; these were stand-alone applications that were "integrated" by way of internal, custom interfaces that required a great deal of care and feeding. Although they were purchased from the same EHR vendor, these applications were assets from separate software acquisitions that were interfaced to appear as if they were integrated.

The Pharmacy Management system had been implemented years earlier, and the pharmacy department, not unlike other department-based application implementations, designed process workflows that were specific to their methods and procedures. That is not to say that they ignored the requirements of the nursing staff, only that they were in a position to electronically influence or be first to configure frequencies, schedules, abbreviations, and so on. The Medication Administration Records (MARs) were the paper-based document that nursing utilized for medication rounds and documentation; however, I learned that just because the administration times and schedules were printed on the MAR did not mean that nursing was following those schedules.

After the implementation team spent countless hours to ensure that the processes would provide the right medication to the right patient at the right time in the correct dose and the exact route, we still have multiple documented medication adverse events. After a great deal of analysis, it was determined that the grand majority of the adverse events were related to medication administration timing. At the request of the quality committee, the Pharmacy adjusted the administration schedule times that would populate the electronic MARs; unfortunately, that did not resolve the issue; it only exacerbated it. The clinical informatics team worked to identify the root causes of the increased adverse events. They found that the underlying causes were related more to a nursing process than an actual system issue. We learned that medication administration adherence to the Pharmacy established schedules varied depending upon the nursing unit type. Before the implementation of the electronic MAR, when the paper-based MARs were received on the nursing units (one per patient per shift), the nurse assigned to each patient would manual adjust (write-in) a medication administration schedule that was customized to the needs and/or activities of each patient.

Another finding of the clinical informatics team was that due to the difficulty in identifying early or late dose administration times with a paper-based process, there were really no prior metrics to benchmark against. With the implementation of the electronic MAR and the system's ability to establish standard administration time windows, the system could easily identify and report the early, last, and missed doses as adverse medication events.

With the administration times established in the pharmacy management system and these being entirely out of the control of nursing, a great deal of conversation and departmental friction ensued. During these conversations, it was learned that the administration times established by Pharmacy were really driven around another Pharmacy process; medicine cart fill times, which was driven by staffing, and so on.

To improve the process of medication delivery to patients, the clinical informatics team had to start at the beginning to establish the process drivers and what the future state needed to be. The process redesign encompassed moving the Pharmacy to a unit dose system, which allowed Pharmacy to utilize automation for a high percentage of their daily fill process, moving the patient medications from the centralized medicine carts to secured sections of the in-room nurse-serve closets to allow the appropriate medications to be readily available at the patient's bedside. With the medication fill and patient medication storage processes resolved, the Pharmacy could modify the administration schedules as appropriate to better accommodate the nursing workflow processes; however, in a standardized manner. These modifications

allowed nursing to concentrate on the proper administration workflows and provide additional support and education for the nursing staff, which precipitated a significant drop in the associated adverse drug events.

Importance of Appropriate Staff Skill Set

In most Information Systems (IS) or Information Technology (IT) departments, most of the staff had skill sets that were very technical in focus: mainframe or mini-computer operations, terminal wiring (real early), networking, and so on. Later came the client computing era, which required skills around server clusters, redundancy, high availability, and/or fault tolerance, and then there was networking, both local and wide-area. There were also those that understood and practiced the art and science of project management and, in some cases, utilized those skills as change managers.

In the early years, the IS or IT department leadership was very much technically focused to successfully implement and support the computer and network environments that were the plumbing of the systems they oversaw and managed. Early on in the healthcare automation, the technical teams and leadership could more easily adapt and understand the processes and workflows required for implementing the financial and back-office solutions.

Most of the teams led by a Chief Information Officer (CIO) who were technically focused did their best work when they could apply their skills on the inert equipment that were part of their environment; few had good people-skills required to implement and support clinically focused applications. It is no secret that most technically oriented individuals do not make good clinical informaticists. This is not because they lack a lot of the soft skills, but because they lacked the knowledge and understanding that one can only acquire by training and working experience in the clinical areas.

As the saying goes, "one cannot lead others to a place they have never been." It can be interpreted in several different ways; it is related to learned experiences in this instance. It is also related to having or earning the trust of those you would lead in a project, who understand that your personal credentials are like their own.

Clinical processes and workflows must be experienced to understand them fully. That full understanding of their interconnected natures is required, especially when one's job is to attempt to modify and/or automate them. An informaticist cannot hope to provide expert guidance in the level of process change that is required unless they can speak with the confidence, language, and knowledge one only acquires from hands-on experience.

In the very late 1990s, our organization realized that we had failed to provide a level of automation for our core business process of patient care. As we planned for that possibility, it was painfully apparent that a different skill set was needed to navigate various clinical processes. If we were to be successful, the IT leadership would need to engage with Nursing and Physician leadership, identity those who had in-depth clinical process knowledge and a willingness to participate, if not led, the change processes. We felt that the technical skills could be better taught to experienced clinicians more appropriately than attempting to teach clinical process knowledge to the technically oriented teams.

Once the staffing was set, the next question was, whom this new team should report to. Both IT and Nursing believed the clinical informatics team should report within their structures; both were right, and both were wrong. We found that the appropriate reporting structure was within the IT department during the initial implementation phase. Once the implementation phase was complete (the applications were in place), the process change management required that the clinical informatics team move to within the Nursing leadership structure, which provided the need for clinical process change management that would be necessary. The majority of the process change was related to nursing processes, which impacted physician processes; these change initiatives were not IT-focused; therefore, nursing leadership was better suited for the challenges that were ahead.

Once this phase of implementation and change management was addressed, the clinical infor-matics group moved into implementation, change management, and SME (subject matter expert) roles, and these are best managed within the framework of the IT department. The work really never changed, and the internal business partnerships never changed; only the organizational reporting relation changed.

The change management/leadership can be summed up in one focused statement. The changes must be, "Clinically Focused, Organization Led, and Technology-Enabled." This type of thinking always helps understand that technology is a tool, not the solution.

Collaboration Among the Care Silos

Before it became the industry standard, many CIOs were a proponent of using an integrated approach to application implementation. The integration was around core functions such as patient management (registration, revenue, and order management), financial management, and clinical management. However, over the last decade, it has become apparent that all these functions are so tightly interrelated that implementing a solution that does not require external integration or interfacing provides the most efficient and effective solution.

As a CIO. it is important to understand how the various departments/service areas within a healthcare organization must function to provide the highest level of patient care possible. Some organizations have mastered the necessary symbiosis level, and others have not. There is not one single healthcare department that can function as a process island; there are always interdependencies that can be easily identified.

Communication and coordination among the various care teams are just one of the areas when the clinical informaticists are critical to the success of any organization's ability to provide the best possible outcome for the patient populations that they serve. Information can be viewed as the fuel for the engine of health care, and the quality of that fuel determines patient outcomes.

We find ourselves in need of gathering, recording, and presenting information as part of the normal care process. However, each patient is an individual, and his or her care should be individualized. That is not to say that best practices should be ignored, only that variations between patients should be taken into consideration.

As indicated in the earlier example about the Medication Administration Record (MAR), attempting to automate a paper-based and/or manual process really does not end well; integrated processes and unique information demands require us to consider, with fresh eyes, the inputs and outputs of any processes that are under review/consideration for automation. Patient care is not only in the hospital and physician practice realm. Patient care now occurs in many different and varied care settings. The information/data from those care encounters must be made available and it must be shared among all care encounters if each patient is to receive the most complete and appropriate care possible.

What May the Future Hold?

Many have been predicting the future state of healthcare for years. Unfortunately, healthcare predictions are similar to predictions of a technology-enabled future society, such as predicting that by the year 2000, all of us should have all had cars without wheels that drove themselves. While we are moving closer and closer to driver-assisted technologies, we still have a long way to go.

With the recent response to the COVID-19 virus, we can now see the impact of the technologies that we have been implementing for decades. We can see the effects of the clinical process changes that have been discussed at many different levels. Unfortunately, it took a global pandemic to cause the healthcare industry to begin providing care in a more patient-focused and coordinated manner.

The process change in the clinical settings has required tightly coordinated efforts between the clinical and technical teams, utilizing the skills and knowledge of the clinical informatics professionals, those individuals who have the in-depth process knowledge necessary to implement the required process change quickly.

From virtual visits being conducted to provide routine and follow up care in the ambulatory care settings to "communal rounding" where one or two clinicians are in a patient's room, and others are observing and interacting utilizing a variety of video-enabled and enhanced tools, we have witnessed virtual family visits, virtual patient rounding in both the acute and post-acute care settings. Of more importance is the ability to provide a timelier and coordinated patient discharge process, where all of a patient's care team can interact simultaneously, regardless of where they may be physically located. These are the clinical process improvements that the industry has been predicting for years that will and can have a permanent impact on the way we coordinate and provide care.

The clinical informatics journey has been designed to help the healthcare industry. It utilizes now a tremendous amount of clinical knowledge and technical expertise to continue to usher in the next visions of coordinated patient care.

Summary

Over the last 30–40 years, the role of Healthcare Information Technology (HIT) has evolved and continuously impacted the care delivery and business processes of healthcare. In the early 1970s, healthcare operations and clinical processes were all paper-based (at least in most hospitals). With the changes around how care is reimbursed, the advent of employer-provided healthcare, and an ever-increasing regulatory burden, the business side of healthcare was one of the first areas that applied information technology to automate the processes of patient registration, revenue cycle, and order management. As the digital clinical era was entered clinical processes and workflows had to be understood and the skill set of the staff had to be adjusted to these needs. Communication and coordination among the various care teams are just one of the areas where the clinical informaticists are critical to the success and outcome of patient care. Chief information officers serves as the bridge builder who brings technology, processes and people together.

Conclusions and Outlook

The CIO should function as a partner with the clinical areas to utilize automation as an effective tool in providing patient care. It is imperative to identify the staff with the appropriate clinical expertise and experience to help lead the required changes during the introduction of new tools into the clinical workflows. Within the responses to the COVID-19 crisis, it became apparent that clinical informatics was key in the creation of new and innovative methods of providing high-quality care to our patients in a rapidly changing and stressful environment. The future for the clinical informaticists continues to be written, where the boundaries of technology and innovations will continue to be tested.

Useful Resources

1. "Gartner: Healthcare Provider CIOs" Build Clinical Informatics Leadership to Succeed in Digital Clinical Transformation. March 2020. ID G00464608 https://www.gartner.com/document/3982713
2. HealthManagement.org: Developing the Role of CIO in Healthcare Management: From "then IT Guy" to CIO. Volume 17–Issue 1, 2017 http://healthmanagement.org/c/healthmanagement/issuearticle/developing-the-role-of-cio-in-healthcare-management-from-the-it-guy-to-cio
3. CIO Review: Clinical Informatics and the Promise of Advanced Technologies. https://healthcare.cioreview.com/cxoinsight/clinical-informatics-and-the-promise-of-advanced-technologies-nid-23638-cid-31.html
4. Harvard School of Public Health: The Changing Role of Health IT Leaders: Positioning for Success Moving Forward. https://www.hsph.harvard.edu/ecpe/changing-role-health-cio-leaders/

Review Questions

1. Clinical Informatics lives in the overlap created in the Venn diagram where:
   (a) People, Process, and Information merge
   (b) Technology, Decision Support, and Evidence-Based Medicine intersect
   (c) People, Process, and Technology intersect
   (d) Process, Information, and Clinical Practice interact
2. In the early IOM (Institute of Medicine) reports, which of the following was identified as a leading cause of medical errors:
   (a) Medication ordering and administration processes
   (b) Medication dispensing
   (c) Poor handwriting
   (d) Inability to follow physician orders
3. The CIO's role is to ensure that clinical staff has access to technology.
   (a) True
   (b) False

Appendix: Answers to Review Questions

1. Clinical Informatics lives in the overlap created in the Venn diagram where:
   (a) People, Process, and Information merge
   (b) Technology, Decision Support, and Evidence Based Medicine intersect
   (c) People, Process and Technology intersect
   (d) Process, Information, and Clinical Practice interact

2. In the early IOM (Institute of Medicine) reports, which of the following was identified as a leading cause of medical errors:
   (a) Medication ordering and administration processes
   (b) Medication dispensing
   (c) Poor handwriting
   (d) Inability to follow physician orders

3. The CIO's role is to ensure that clinical staff has access to technology.
   (a) True
   (b) False

References

1. Wakefield M. To err is human: an institute of medicine report. Prof Psychol Res Pract. 2000;31(3):243–4. https://doi.org/10.1037/h0092814
2. Institute of Medicine (US) Committee on Quality of Health Care in America. Crossing the quality chasm: a new health system for the 21st century. Washington, DC: National Academies Press (US); 2001.

The Chief Nursing Informatics Officer's (CNIO) View: Strategic Nursing Leadership for Informatics-Powered Health and Healthcare

Ruth Schleyer

Learning Objectives:
- Discuss the CNIO role and the value it brings to health and healthcare.
- Assess the CNIO's health informatics challenges and priorities.
- Summarize key opportunities for and potential impacts of CNIO collaboration with interprofessional partners.

Key Terms:
- Strategy
- Leadership
- Visionary change agent
- Clinical communication and collaboration
- Administration
- Research and quality
- Education
- Patient engagement

Definition and Role of the Profession in Health Care

Introduction

CNIOs save lives. At first read, one might be challenged to connect such a bold statement with the role of the Chief Nursing Informatics Officer (CNIO). Perhaps it's not such a stretch when reflecting on how Florence Nightingale, acclaimed as the first nursing informaticist, documented nursing processes and care outcomes, gathering, analyzing and interpreting data for meaningful improvements in patient care delivery and population health [1]. Like Nightingale, today's CNIOs are transformational nurse leaders, who bring unique informatics expertise to their strategic and operational focus on promoting and improving health and healthcare.

Since the term nursing informatics (NI) was coined, descriptions of the specialty evolved from an early emphasis on the impact of computers and information technologies in healthcare through multiple models and frameworks with more conceptual orientations [2]. Twenty-first century definitions capture the breadth and impact of the specialty's science and practice on health and healthcare—and the transformative potential of the NI specialist role [2–4].

In United States (U.S.), the American Nurses Association (ANA) recognized informatics as a unique nursing specialty in 1992, followed in 1995 by the American Nurses Credentialing Center (ANCC) introduction of specialty board certification [5]. By the early twenty-first century in the U.S., nation-wide implementation of the electronic health record (EHR) ignited an explosion of NI roles, fueled by a 2004 Presidential Executive Order [6] and 2009 federal law providing financial incentives for mandatory EHR adoption and meaningful use [7]. The U.S.-based

R. Schleyer (✉)
Legacy Health, Portland, OR, USA
e-mail: rschleye@lhs.org

© Springer Nature Switzerland AG 2022
U. H. Hübner et al. (eds.), *Nursing Informatics*, Health Informatics,
https://doi.org/10.1007/978-3-030-91237-6_8

Healthcare Information and Management Systems Society (HIMSS) 2017 Nursing Informatics Workforce Survey captured 473 unique NI role titles, a reported increase from 308 in 2014 [8]. Similar focus on health informatics role expansion has echoed around the globe as EHR expansion has become nearly omnipresent [9].

NI specialists are critical to EHR implementation and adoption success, coupling their patient-centered focus and clinical practice knowledge with information systems technology skill to support efficient clinical workflows and operational goals [10, 11]. They are equally critical in bridging today's value-based, outcomes-driven focus on individual and population health and the world of disruptive, innovative technologies that enable it [10–12]. Beyond healthcare organizations, NI's unique skill set is in demand by academic institutions, technology vendors, consulting firms, government agencies, and entrepreneurial startups (sometimes their own) [4, 13].

Why the CNIO?

As health and healthcare models and related information and communication technologies (ICT) have evolved over the past decade, so have nursing and NI roles. According to the 2020 World Health Organization (WHO) report, *State of the World's Nursing*, 27.9 million nursing workforce members account for nearly 60% of all health professions, making them the largest global healthcare workforce sector [14]. Many in this massive sector use health ICT today and more will in the future. Although sheer numbers may call for NI leadership of healthcare's largest group of ICT users, they don't tell the whole story.

In their foundational 2012 position paper, the American Organization of Nurse Executives (AONE) makes the case for the CNIO/nursing informatics executive's (NIE) transformational value and impact [15]. AONE describes a role uniquely qualified to define and operationally lead vision and strategy by leveraging deep clinical experience and technical knowledge and skills with informatics expertise. The CNIO/NIE is a senior nursing leader positioned for impact from the bedside to the boardroom, from individuals to communities and beyond. Their role scope ranges from support of direct care delivery and clinical efficiency to a focus on safety, quality, operational, and financial outcomes. AONE portrays the CNIO/NIE as providing "guidance to organizations that will bridge practice, education, and research ... leveraging ... data and evidence for improving clinical practice, patient outcomes and population health" [15, p. 3].

U.S. CNIO/NIE role prevalence was first reported in the HIMSS 2014 Nursing informatics Workforce Survey with 30% of respondents indicating presence of the role in their organizations [16]. Multiple authors [10–13, 17] have detailed the strategic and operational importance of the emerging CNIO/NIE role and its responsibilities and qualifications. The role's interprofessional value was highlighted by its inclusion as a top Chief Clinical Informatics Officer (CCIO) candidate in the 2016 *American Medical Informatics Association (AMIA) Task Force Report on CCIO Knowledge, Education, and Skillset Requirements* [18]. The number of senior NI leaders continues to grow. In 2020, 41% of HIMSS 2020 Nursing Informatics Workforce Survey respondents reported their organization had a CNIO/NIE as compared with 32% in 2017 [19].

The CNIO role impact is recognized internationally. Remus and Kennedy [20] touted the value of the emerging Canadian CNIO role in 2012 and five years later, the CNIO role was recognized as an evidence-based implementation recommendation for Canada's health information technology (IT) strategic advancement [21]. CNIOs are playing a critical role in the United Kingdom's (UK) National Health Service (NHS) EHR implementations. NHS CNIOs' testimonials capture their energy and commitment to EHR-enabled care transformation that benefits patients and clinicians. They describe serving as a translator and liaison between nursing and IT, leading implementation and adoption, and driving a digital healthcare revolution [22, 23]. This value is echoed in a 2019 Australian College of Nursing (ACN) position statement advocating urgent expansion of the CNIO/Chief Nursing and Midwifery Information Officer (CNMIO) role across the continent as a strategic imperative in support of Australia's digital health transformation [24].

Who Is the CNIO?

A review of role descriptions and professional organization position statements provides a glimpse into the knowledge, skills, and experience that CNIOs bring to their jobs and the key functions for which they are responsible [10–12, 15, 25, 26]. In 2014, Sengstack [17] described a list of foundational CNIO/NIE responsibilities including expert informatics consultation and engagement in multiple areas. These key concepts are reflected in the 2016 *CNIO Job Description* published by the HIMSS Nursing Informatics Executive Workgroup [25] and were incorporated in the American Nursing Informatics Association (ANIA) 2018 position statement advocating for the CNIO [26]. The HIMSS CNIO job description provides a standardized industry reference for the competencies, qualifications, and reporting structure for a CNIO/NIE. It includes thirty-five key responsibilities organized into categories including strategy/leadership, quality, patient safety, policy and procedure, and technology. These responsibilities emphasize the role as a visionary, strategic liaison and change agent who represents and supports health professional and patient/citizen information and communication management and technology needs [25].

What skills do CNIOs need to meet this long list of responsibilities? Landi [12] cites a 2016 Witt/Kieffer survey of senior U.S. healthcare leaders that identified collaboration and consensus building and knowledge of NI as the top essential skills for CNIO success, followed by people management, team development, and emotional intelligence. Vision and creativity, system implementation, business and finance were ranked as very important skills [12]. Today's CNIO/NIE expertly demonstrates these skills and manages the polarities of clinical practice and

technology. Putting people first, they represent the voices and needs of patients/citizens, nurses, and the entire interprofessional team, co-creating quality, safety, and value in a technology-rich, digitally-enabled health and healthcare delivery environment.

The CNIO is a tenured healthcare leader with 5–10 years minimum relevant clinical, informatics and/or leadership experience at the director or executive role. CNIOs hold advanced educational degrees, with doctoral education in nursing/informatics preferred. Professional certification such as professional board-certification in informatics through the ANCC (U.S.) or Certified Professional in Healthcare Information and Management Systems (CPHIMS) is often expected [13].

CNIO role reporting structure varies in healthcare organizations. Although direct reporting to the organization's Chief Nursing Officer (CNO) or Chief Information Officer (CIO) is most common [19], it is the informal (and sometimes formal) matrixed reporting to both clinical and technical senior leadership that underscores the CNIO's value as an expert bridging both worlds. With matrixed/dual reporting comes the opportunity to participate in senior leadership teams, to represent the nursing and interprofessional clinical perspective to IT, and share technical insights and opportunities with the clinical world. Senior leadership team presence and participation is expected and is critical to CNIO role success. The ANIA 2018 position statement describes the CNIO as a "full member of the executive team providing strategic vision and leadership to drive transformation in health care delivery through the use of data, information, knowledge and wisdom" [26, p. 1].

The CNIO role is inherently interprofessional [4] and its effectiveness is multiplied by cultivating a network of trusted relationships and building teams. One of the CNIO's most critical relationships is dyad partnership with the organization's Chief Medical Informatics Officer (CMIO). As clinical informatics leaders for the organization, the two roles share accountability for high level strategic alignment and team-based, operational development, delivery, and measurement of clinical informatics services and value [27]. Other primary executive-level partners include the CNO and the CIO and evolving roles such as the Chief Clinical Officer (CCO) and the Chief Clinical Informatics Officer (CCIO) [18, 19, 28].

A true connector, the CNIO develops collaborative partnerships within and beyond the organization's boundaries. Multidisciplinary clinical specialties, information services and technology, quality and patient safety, privacy and security, health information management (HIM), research, analytics, performance excellence, organizational development and training, library services, project management, health and digital literacy, patient/citizen experience and education, home care, hospice, social care and community well-being, academia, vendors, professional organizations … the list of potential partners seems never-ending. Each day brings new opportunities for creative collaboration, integration, and steps toward healthcare improvement and transformation—and concomitant challenges and lessons in pragmatism, perseverance, and prioritization (see Fig. 8.1).

Challenges of the Profession in State of the Art Care Delivery & Health Informatics Priorities from the Perspective of this Profession

CNIO Challenges and Opportunities

Faced with multiple opportunities and challenges, where do CNIOs focus their energy, and expertise? How can they best leverage their unique knowledge, skills, and abilities for state-of-the-art care delivery in an uncertain and evolving healthcare ecosystem? What initiatives will have the largest impact on patient/citizen and clinician health and well-being?

Focus on the basics is a powerful starting point. The CNIO is first, and always, a professional nurse. As senior nursing leaders, CNIOs are responsible for improving nursing practices and patient care by leveraging ICT used throughout the healthcare continuum. CNIOs bring a nursing perspective, creatively and strategically integrating ICT to extend professional nurses'

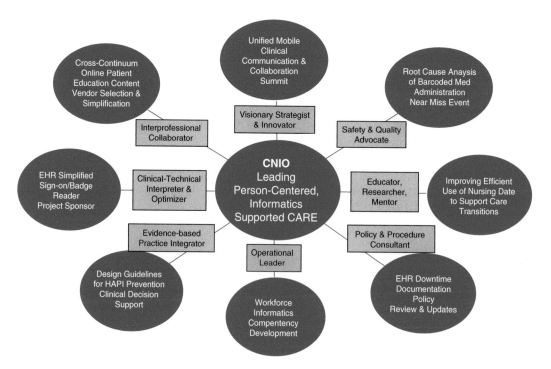

Fig. 8.1 CNIO: Snapshot from a Week in the Life

capacity for providing the best quality, safest, evidence-based patient care as efficiently as possible.

CNIOs pragmatically recognize that technology and tools alone are not the complete answer. One brief item in the HIMSS CNIO position description sets a large stage as the CNIO "ensures a competent, technology-enabled workforce" [25, p. 2]. The importance of informatics competencies for every healthcare professional has long been recognized [29] and the CNIO is a standard-bearer for their contribution to patient and clinician safety in today's complex healthcare environments.

The importance of nursing workforce informatics competency and competency inclusion in nurses' education has been described in multiple countries [4, 13, 30, 31], setting a growing expectation that *every nurse is an informatics nurse*. In the U.S., informatics competencies are considered requisite for all registered nurses and "select nursing informatics competencies are now required in all prelicensure, undergraduate, graduate, and doctoral nursing curricula" [4, p. 37]. Challenges beyond the academic setting persist as many nurses' professional education predates this requirement. CNIOs can help close that gap in the operational setting through support of informatics knowledge and skill acquisition for the entire nursing workforce, including nurse leaders. Recent international work focused on nursing and interprofessional health informatics competencies, provides role and domain-specific context and tools available for CNIOs' use in their organizations [32, 33]. Perseverance prevails as the CNIO fosters an informatics and data-aware frontline nursing culture, continually linking informatics competency concepts to the nursing process.

While the EHR is the most ubiquitous system, today's nurses may use ICT in multiple aspects of their varied professional roles. Managing this ever-expanding and frequently updated EHR/ICT portfolio (see Fig. 8.2) can contribute to nurses'

CARE Organizing Framework: Nursing
Health Information & Communication Technology Portfolio

- **C**linical & **C**ommunication/**C**ollaboration
  - EHR Documentation & Review; Medication Management (BCMA, IV infusion pump integration, etc.)
  - Data Acquisition Systems (hemodynamic monitors; vital signs, etc.)
  - Clinical Decision Support
  - Care Planning, Care Coordination & Transitions
  - Voice & Text Clinical Communication (nurse call, handheld mobile device, electronic whiteboard, etc.)
  - Virtual Care & Remote Monitoring

- **A**dministrative
  - Workforce Management (Staffing, Scheduling, Time & Attendance)
  - Workload Intensity/Patient Classification
  - Financial Management & Budgeting
  - Email, Intranet, Personal Productivity and Team Collaboration Tools
  - Real Time Tracking & Location Systems (RTLS)

- **R**esearch & Quality
  - Nursing Knowledge Creation; Big Data Science
  - Clinical & Administrative Reporting & Analytics
  - Dashboards & Scorecards

- **E**ducation & **E**ngagement/**E**xperience
  - Nurse: Learning Management System, On-line References & Resources, Rounding Tools
  - Patient/Citizen: Portals, Health Education Content, Interactive Patient Care Systems

R. Schleyer 2020

Fig. 8.2 CARE Organizing Framework: Nursing HICT Portfolio

cognitive burden and burnout risk [27, 34]. The 2019 National Academy of Medicine report *Taking Action Against Clinician Burnout: A Systems Approach to Supporting Professional Well-Being* identified the high personal and economic costs of clinician burnout, a phenomenon reported by 35–54% of nurses and physicians [34]. Several contributing factors were linked to inadequate, poorly designed technology and documentation burden, findings all too familiar to many CNIOs.

Needs for system improvements and changes must be weighed against the risks of added burden and unintended negative consequences. Results of the HIMSS 2020 Nursing Informatics Workforce Survey indicate that systems implementation (44%) and utilization/optimization (41%) continue to be top job responsibilities for NI specialists [19]. CNIOs approach optimization opportunities with a blend of strategy and tactics. They apply knowledge of human factors usability and human-centered design to engage frontline clinicians in identifying and addressing unmet care needs and challenges [35]. Keeping a laser focus on patient and clinician safety, CNIOs ensure optimization initiatives are prioritized by principles-guided, clinically-led governance that supports standards-driven evidence, practice integration, and streamlined operational workflows.

CNIOs are ideally positioned to sponsor and lead initiatives that improve nurses' EHR experience by enabling mastery and building competencies in efficient, standardized use of the system to its full potential. In partnership with nursing leaders, CNIOs work to clarify nursing documentation expectations by communicating the 'why' and to decrease nurses' documentation burden by focusing on evidence-supported, essential data that simultaneously reflect nursing care, support nurses' clinical decisions, and capture measurement of nursing's value and unique contribution to patient outcomes [36].

The HIMSS sample job description calls out multiple CNIO role connections to evidence-based practice, nursing and informatics research, and analytics and reporting [25]. These role responsibilities guide CNIO advocacy for use of terminology standards for nursing and interprofessional EHR documentation. Use of terminology standards and adoption of a unique nursing identifier are aligned with the Nursing Knowledge: Big Data Science (NKBDS) initiative's "vision of better health outcomes resulting from the standardization and integration of the information nurses gather in electronic health records and other information systems, which is increasingly the source of insights and evidence used to prevent, diagnose, treat and evaluate health conditions" [37, p. 1]. At the local level, CNIOs lead nurses' development of personal accountability for data quality, their competency in using transformed data through workflow-imbedded tools (e.g., decision support, predictive analytics, and dashboards), and recognition of the multi-faceted impacts of shareable, comparable, actionable data.

Health Informatics Priorities in Collaboration with Other Professions

What's Now (and Next) for the CNIO and Interprofessional Partners?

The CNIO shares many health informatics priorities with a collaborative team of clinical, operational, and technical interprofessional partners. As joint enablers of current and future care delivery models they support health and social care and well-being. The team brings a shared patient/citizen focus, collective understanding of each member's unique role and expertise, and awareness of their data, information, and knowledge management needs—including those of the patient/citizen. The importance of informatics competencies for all health professionals sets a shared foundation for success [29, 33, 34].

Together, the team evolves beyond an EHR implementation and optimization focus to leverage data captured in the EHR and other systems. Big data science extends beyond nursing and gets even bigger in the interprofessional team context, including patient/citizen-generated data. Related concepts such as decision support, analytics, machine learning, and artificial intelligence are of deep interest to the entire team in their quest to drive quality and safety, personalize care, and support patient engagement in shared decision-making.

Shared health informatics priorities derive from shared goals and creation of a shared roadmap that supports the overall organization's vision and strategy. Clinical, technical, and operational partners are all engaged in roadmap creation. One example priority may include investment in solutions that help provide a seamless patient/citizen and interprofessional clinician experience. A cross-setting experience is one in which the patient/citizen's story is known by all care team members, the longitudinal plan of care is co-created, and shared documentation elements support integrated data and information visualization and reporting. It is an experience in which the patient/citizen's digital and health literacy are proactively addressed so that their portal access to health records and education materials is useful and usable. It is also an experience that includes enabling technologies and workflows to improve team communication and collaboration in highly mobile and virtual environments. An experience that puts resources at patients', citizen's, and clinicians' fingertips when and where needed—an experience of connected health that occurs everywhere.

The CNIO and their collaborative partners must balance ICT innovations for that seamless experience (or other selected strategies) with cost effectiveness. From chatbots to robots; from interactive patient care systems to virtual visits; from smartphone apps to remote novice-to-expert nurse consultation and patient monitoring; from smart hospital rooms to smart homes; from patient-generated data to social determinants of health—ideas and opportunities to connect health, clinical and social care, and technology abound. But resources are limited. The interprofessional team members share the operational reality and priority to ensure initiatives align with strategy and, ideally, deliver a return on investment (ROI) that helps bend the healthcare cost curve while improving patient/citizen and clinician experience.

Summary

Chief Nursing Informatics Officers (CNIOs) are transformational nurse leaders, who bring unique informatics expertise to their strategic and operational focus on promoting and improving health and healthcare. This chapter describes CNIO role development and the evolving profile of CNIO role expectations and key functions. Challenges and opportunities faced by CNIOs and the role's impact in support of patients/citizens, nurses, and the health and social care team are explored. Emphasis on the CNIO role as inherently interprofessional provides the foundation for a discussion of health informatics priorities the CNIO shares with a collaborative team of clinical, technical, and operational partners. As the CNIO role gains global prominence and strategic importance, the outlook for its continued growth is bright.

What Is the Outlook for the CNIO?

The CNIO/NIE role continues to gain prominence globally. 43% (40 of 94) of non-U.S. respondents to the HIMSS 2020 Nursing Informatics Workforce Survey indicated the presence of a senior NIE/CNIO in their organizations (Email communication, T. Kwiatkoski, May 19, 2020). Mirroring U.S. trends, the role is often launched concomitantly with major EHR implementations [20, 23]. As global EHR use matures, the CNIO's role focus is also maturing and evolving.

A critical transition to a truly strategic, transformational CNIO role is underway today [13, 27, 28, 35, 38]. Long-noted in position descriptions, the role of CNIO as strategist has been overshadowed by their tactical, albeit necessary, focus on EHR-related activities. The CNIO's strategic focus anticipates the impacts of evolving healthcare delivery paradigms and leverages knowledge that crosses team boundaries and multiple industry sectors. CNIOs see beyond the hospital walls. They identify the connections, care transitions, and health and social care-related data, information and knowledge needs of patients/citizens and the care team in all settings. CNIOs help ensure nurses have informatics competencies to safely practice wherever they are.

Nagle et al. [13] describe the evolving role of the NI leader related to data science and use of data; it is moving from capturing data to using data to derive new nursing knowledge and then applying that practice-based evidence to inform quality and safety improvement initiatives. Recent health informatics research trends reveal a shift from clinical documentation to patient-focused knowledge generation and support of informed decisions with a focus on patient benefit creation [39]. Who better than CNIOs to engage in this strategic research focus?

As more CNIOs hold doctoral degrees, published performance improvement projects and formal informatics research led by CNIOs will increase, including measuring the value and impact of NI contributions to health outcomes. To date, measurement of NI value has been challenging and somewhat elusive. In a 2019 Health Management Academy (HMA) survey of 19 large U.S. health system CNIOs, 84% indicated they did not have quantitative measurement of NI value at their organization and 68% worried that C-Suite-level understanding of the NI value proposition remains inconsistent [28]. The HMA survey findings are consistent with those of an international survey with respondents from 46 countries that reported, "perceived mediocre environmental support for NI as a discipline" [31, p. 228] and created the platform for increasing visibility and measuring the impact and value of NI [31]. Data will be critical to NI and CNIO role development, continued viability, and impact measurement on a global scale.

As senior NI leaders, CNIOs model professional development in their field and often serve as mentors or preceptors for aspiring early informatics careerists and students. CNIOs are positioned to build academic-industry partnerships that provide mutually beneficial outcomes. They can support nursing faculty incorporation of informatics essentials in the curriculum by sharing their experiences and can influence student acquisition of workforce-required informatics competencies. Beyond consultation, CNIOs are ideal candidates to serve as adjunct faculty where their visibility as informatics experts, change leaders, and advocates for policy engagement at the local, state/regional, and federal levels will inspire students. CNIOs will continue to help shape the way for nursing's future.

Conclusions and Outlook

Who is the CNIO? The CNIO is a transformative, inspiring, resilient nurse leader. She or he is a model for professional nursing practice and patient/citizen advocate. A visionary strategist, influencer, and operational tactician. An interprofessional collaborator, team-builder, and change agent. A researcher and data scientist and translator. A clinical practice-technology polarity manager and creative connector for innovative solutions. A wisdom-holder and force for health and well-being.

The CNIO/senior nursing informatics executive continues Florence Nightingale's legacy as an advocate and exemplar for the power and possibilities of informatics to transform global health and healthcare. Using data, information, knowledge, and wisdom for safety and global health, CNIOs do, indeed, save lives.

Useful Resources

1. American Organization of Nurse Executives. Position paper: Nursing informatics executive leader. 2012. https://www.aonl.org/sites/default/files/aone/informatics-executive-leader.pdf.
2. Australian College of Nursing. Leading digital health transformation: The value of Chief Nursing Informatics Officer (CNIO) roles [Position Statement]. Oct 2019. https://www.acn.edu.au/wp-content/uploads/position-statement-leading-digital-health-transformation-value-cnio-roles.pdf.
3. HIMSS Nursing Informatics Community. CNIO job description. 2016. https://www.himss.org/sites/hde/files/d7/himss-cnio-job-description.pdf.
4. Ventura R. The role of the Chief Nursing Informatics Officer: Position statement of the American Nursing Informatics Association

Board of Directors. 27 Nov 2018. https://www.ania.org/assets/documents/position/cnioPosition.pdf.

Review Questions

1. The CNIO role has gained global prominence over the past decade. Healthcare organizations are investing in this senior nursing informatics executive position because:
   (a) EHR optimization is nearing completion and other nursing informatics roles are being eliminated.
   (b) The nursing workforce is the smallest sector in healthcare and CNIOs are critical to nurse recruitment and retention.
   (c) The CNIO's clinical knowledge and informatics expertise make them uniquely qualified to represent nursing, health professional, and patient/citizen ICT needs.
   (d) The nursing application portfolio is shrinking and CNIO strategic direction is needed to reduce organizational focus on nursing workforce informatics competencies.

2. You work as a front-line clinician in an integrated healthcare delivery system. One of your biggest challenges is finding information needed to identify and communicate patients' shared goals for their health outcomes. You contact the CNIO to share your concerns because you know they collaborate with the interprofessional team as a:
   (a) Quality and safety advocate.
   (b) Clinical-technical integrator and translator.
   (c) Business intelligence consultant.
   (d) Strategic and operational leader.
   (e) All the above.

Appendix: Answers to Review Questions

1. The CNIO role has gained global prominence over the past decade. Healthcare organizations are investing in this senior nursing informatics executive position because
   (a) EHR optimization is nearing completion and other nursing informatics roles are being eliminated. *(EHR optimization is never-ending; nursing and clinical informatics roles continue to play a critical role in EHR adoption and ongoing improvement.)*
   (b) The nursing workforce is the smallest labor sector in healthcare and CNIOs are critical to nurse recruitment and retention. *(The nursing workforce is the largest healthcare labor sector; CNIOs contribute to nurse retention through initiatives to reduce cognitive burden and decrease risk of HICT/EHR-related burnout.)*
   (c) The CNIO's clinical knowledge and informatics expertise make them uniquely qualified to represent nursing, health professional, and patient/citizen ICT needs.
   (d) The nursing application portfolio is shrinking and CNIO strategic direction is needed to reduce organizational focus on nursing workforce informatics competencies. *(The nursing application portfolio continues to expand bringing a critical need for improved nursing workforce informatics competencies.)*

2. You work as a front-line clinician in an integrated healthcare delivery system. One of your biggest challenges is finding information needed to identify and communicate patients' shared goals for their health outcomes. You contact the CNIO to share your concerns because you know they collaborate with the interprofessional team as a
   (a) Quality and safety advocate
   (b) Clinical-technical integrator and translator
   (c) Business intelligence consultant
   (d) Strategic and operational leader
   (e) All the above

References

1. Betts H, Wright G. Was Florence Nightingale the first nursing informatician? In: de Fatima Marin H, Pereira Margues E, Hovenga E, Goossen W, editors. Proceedings of the 8th International Congress in Nursing Informatics: E-health for

all: designing a nursing agenda for the future. Rio de Janeiro, Brazil: E-papers Serviços Editorias Ltd; 2003. https://www.researchgate.net/publication/233380253_Was_Florence_Nightingale_the_First_Nursing_Informatician. Accessed 2 Apr 2020.

2. Staggers N, Thompson CB. The evolution of definitions for nursing informatics: a critical analysis and revised definition. J Am Med Inform Assoc. 2002;9(3):255–61. https://doi.org/10.1197/jamia.m0946.

3. International Medical Informatics Association. IMIA-NI definition of nursing informatics updated. 2009. https://imianews.wordpress.com/2009/08/24/imia-ni-definition-ofnursing-informatics-updated/. Accessed 2 Apr 2020.

4. American Nurses Association. Nursing informatics: scope and standards of practice. 2nd ed. Silver Spring, MD: Nursesbooks.org; 2015.

5. Bickford CJ. The professional association's perspective on nursing informatics and competencies in the US. Stud Health Technol Inform. 2017;232:62–8. https://doi.org/10.3233/978-1-61499-738-2-62.

6. Bush GW. Executive order 13335—incentives for the use of health information technology and establishing the position of the National Health Information Technology Coordinator. 2004. https://www.govinfo.gov/content/pkg/WCPD-2004-05-03/pdf/WCPD-2004-05-03-Pg702.pdf. Accessed 25 May 2020.

7. Health Information Technology for Economic and Clinical Health Act of 2009, P.L. no.111-5, § 123 stat. 227. 2009. https://www.hhs.gov/sites/default/files/ocr/privacy/hipaa/understanding/coveredentities/hitechact.pdf. Accessed 23 May 2020.

8. Healthcare Information and Management Systems Society. HIMSS 2017 nursing informatics workforce survey. 2017. https://www.himss.org/sites/hde/files/d7/2017-nursing-informatics-workforce-full-report.pdf. Accessed 23 May 2020.

9. Marc D, Butler-Henderson K, Dua P, Lalani K, Fenton SH. Global workforce trends in health informatics & information management. Stud Health Technol Inform. 2019;26(4):1273–7. https://doi.org/10.3233/SHTI190431.

10. Kirby SB. Informatics leadership: the role of the CNIO. Nursing. 2015;45(4):21–2. https://doi.org/10.1097/01.nurse.0000462394.23939.8e.

11. Mitchell MB. We save lives: an informatics perspective on innovation. Nursing. 2015;45(2):20–1. https://doi.org/10.1097/01.NURSE.0000459593.78396.c4.

12. Landi H. CNIOs go strategic. Healthcare Innovation. 2016. https://www.hcinnovationgroup.com/population-health-management/article/13027622/cnios-go-strategic. Accessed 1 May 2020.

13. Nagle LM, Sermeus W, Junger A. Evolving role of the nursing informatics specialist. Stud Health Technol Inform. 2017;232:212–21. https://doi.org/10.3233/978-1-61499-738-2-212.

14. World Health Organization. State of the world's nursing 2020: executive summary. 2020. https://apps.who.int/iris/bitstream/handle/10665/331673/9789240003293-eng.pdf. Accessed 12 May 2020.

15. American Organization of Nurse Executives. Position paper: nursing informatics executive leader. 2012. https://www.aonl.org/sites/default/files/aone/informatics-executive-leader.pdf. Accessed 15 Apr 2020.

16. Anderson C, Sensemeier J. Nursing informatics: a specialty on the rise. Nurs Manag. June 2014;45(6):16–8. https://doi.org/10.1097/01.NUMA.0000449768.37489.ac.

17. Sengstack PP. Chief nursing informatics officer: strategic partner for health care organizations. AONE Voice of Nursing Leadership. 2014:12–4.

18. Kannry J, Sengstack P, Thyvalikakath TP, Poikonen J, Middleton B, Payne T, et al. The chief clinical informatics officer: AMIA task force report on CCIO knowledge, education, and skillset requirements. Appl Clin Inform. 2016;7(1):143–76. https://doi.org/10.4338/ACI-2015-12-R-0174.

19. Healthcare Information and Management Systems Society. HIMSS nursing informatics workforce survey. 2020. https://www.himss.org/resources/himss-nursing-informatics-workforce-survey. Accessed 23 May 2020.

20. Remus S, Kennedy MA. Innovation in transformative nursing leadership: nursing informatics competencies and roles. Nursing Leadership. 2012;25(4):14–26. https://doi.org/10.12927/cjnl.2012.23260.

21. Canadian Nurses Association and Canadian Nursing Informatics Association. Joint position statement: nursing informatics. 2017. https://www.cna-aiic.ca/-/media/cna/page-content/pdf-fr/nursing-informatics-joint-position-statement.pdf. Accessed 15 Apr 2020.

22. Postelnicu L. How one CNIO is preparing staff for the digital future. Healthcare IT News. 2019. https://www.healthcareitnews.com/news/how-one-cnio-preparing-staff-digital-future. Accessed 2 Apr 2020.

23. DHI News Team. A reflection on the state of the art by a CNIO. Digital health. 2019. https://www.digitalhealth.net/2019/11/a-reflection-on-the-state-of-the-art-by-a-cnio/. Accessed 2 Apr 2020.

24. Australian College of Nursing. Leading digital health transformation: the value of chief nursing informatics officer (CNIO) roles [position statement]. 2019. https://www.acn.edu.au/wp-content/uploads/position-statement-leading-digital-health-transformation-value-cnio-roles.pdf. Accessed 24 Apr 2020.

25. HIMSS Nursing Informatics Community. CNIO job description. 2016. https://www.himss.org/sites/hde/files/d7/himss-cnio-job-description.pdf. Accessed 2 Apr 2020.

26. Ventura R. The role of the chief nursing informatics officer: position statement of the American Nursing Informatics Association Board of Directors. 2018. https://www.ania.org/assets/documents/position/cnioPosition.pdf. Accessed 13 Jan 2020.

27. Scottsdale Institute. Scottsdale Institute 2019 chief nursing information officers and chief medical information officers summit report: care standardization: why and how to make this work. 2019. https://scottsdaleinstitute.org/wp-content/uploads/SI-2019-CMIO-CNIO-Summit-Report.pdf. Accessed 28 Mar 2020.

28. Cheung J, Stahl M. Quick-hitting survey: role of the CNIO. The Health Management Academy. 2019. https://academynet.com/sites/default/files/quick-hit-roleofcnio.pdf. Accessed 27 Jan 2020.

29. Institute of Medicine (IOM). Health professions education: a bridge to quality. 2003. http://www.nap.edu/openbook.php?isbn=0309087236. Accessed 27 Jan 2020.

30. Murphy J, Goossen W. Introduction: forecasting informatics competencies for nurses in the future of connected health. In: Weber P, Murphy J, Goossen W, editors. Forecasting informatics competencies for nurses in the future of connected health: proceedings of the nursing informatics post conference 2016, 2017. Amsterdam: IOS Press.

31. Peltonen LM, Pruinelli L, Ronquillo C, Nibber R, Perezmitre EL, Block L, et al. The current state of nursing informatics: an international cross-sectional survey. Finnish J eHealth eWelfare. 2019;11(3):220–31. https://doi.org/10.23996/fjhw.77584.

32. Hubner U, Shaw T, Thye J, Egbert N, Marin HDF, Chang P, O'Connor S, Day K, Honey M, Blake R, Hovenga E, Skiba D, Ball MJ. Technology Informatics Guiding Education Reform – TIGER: an international recommendation framework of core competencies in health informatics for nurses. Methods Inf Med. 2018;57(S 01):e30–42. https://doi.org/10.3414/ME17-01-0155.

33. Hubner U, Thye J, Shaw T, Elias B, Egbert N, Saranto K, Babitsch B, Proctor P, Ball MJ. Towards the TIGER international framework for recommendations of core competencies in health informatics 2.0: Extending the scope and the roles. Stud Health Technol Inform. 2019;264:1218–22. https://doi.org/10.3233/SHTI190420.

34. National Academies of Sciences, Engineering, and Medicine. Taking action against clinician burnout: a systems approach to professional well-being. Washington, DC: The National Academies Press; 2019. https://doi.org/10.17226/25521.

35. McCleerey M. Vendor support of the expanded role of the CNIO. Online J Nurs Inform. 2019;23(1) http://www.himssorg/ojni. Accessed 4 Apr 2020

36. Collins S, Couture B, Kang MJ, Dykes P, Schnock K, Knaplund C, Chang F, Cato K. Quantifying and visualizing nursing flowsheet documentation burden in acute and critical care. AMIA Annu Symp Proc. 2018;2018:348–57.

37. Nursing Knowledge 2019 Big Data Science. Conference proceedings. 2019. https://www.nursing.umn.edu/sites/nursing.umn.edu/files/2019_big_data_science_proceedings.pdf. Accessed 22 May 2020.

38. Jackson T, Ross H. From tactician to strategist: the evolving role of the CNIO. HealthsystemCIO.com. 2019. https://healthsystemcio.com/2019/05/13/from-tactician-to-strategist-the-evolving-role-of-the-cnio/. Accessed 1 May 2020.

39. Hackl WO, Hoerbst A. Managing complexity. From documentation to knowledge integration and informed decision findings from the clinical information systems perspective for 2018. Yearb Med Inform. 2019;28(01):95–100. https://doi.org/10.1055/s-0039-1677919.

The Chief Medical Informatics Officer's (CMIO) View: Clinical, Technical and Leadership Acumen

9

John Lee

Learning Objectives

- Learn about the origins of the CMIO position.
- Discover the history and changing responsibilities of the CMIO.
- Discuss how the CMIO position interfaces and interacts with the rest of the provider and administrative team.
- Illuminate the future of the CMIO role and other clinical informaticist professions.

Key Terms

- HITECH Act
- Meaningful use
- Clinical informatics
- Socio-technical gap
- System and terminology standardization
- Patient safety and quality
- Clinical process optimization
- User experience and usability

Introduction

The profession of the Chief Medical Information (or Informatics) Officer (CMIO) is a relatively new one. Many see this role as the "geek doctor" or the person to call if the electronic medical record (EMR) is not meeting the needs of the clinical staff. While these characterizations may be true, it helps to understand why the CMIO profession has experienced such a dramatic growth in the past decade.

The delivery of modern healthcare has become increasingly difficult because of the amount of data, information, and knowledge that a clinician needs to consume and act upon. Ultimately, the role is not meant to make physicians less unhappy with the EMR or to develop cool decision support tools. It is to save lives.

We are reminded of the tragedy of Dr. Ignaz Semmelweis. In the nineteenth century, he tried to convince his physician colleagues to wash their hands. He was castigated and eventually died alone in a mental institution. To this day, despite enormous evidence, physicians still struggle with the task of getting front-line providers to perform this simple life saving task.

More recently, the tragedy of Ms. Grant, a 68-year-old patient is emblematic of the problem doctors are trying to solve. She underwent coronary bypass surgery. After the surgery, in the intensive care unit (ICU), her arterial line became clogged. Her nurse responded with a heparin flush. Soon thereafter, she became unresponsive and started seizing. The treatment team discovered that her blood sugar was undetectable. The nurse had inadvertently given her insulin instead of heparin. She remained in a coma for seven weeks until her family decided to withdraw life support and she died.

J. Lee (✉)
Allegheny Health Network, Pittsburgh, PA, USA

© Springer Nature Switzerland AG 2022
U. H. Hübner et al. (eds.), *Nursing Informatics*, Health Informatics,
https://doi.org/10.1007/978-3-030-91237-6_9

There is an explosion of medical knowledge (Fig. 9.1). It is increasingly and exponentially impossible for any single provider to keep up with the new knowledge needed to deliver up to date, evidence-based healthcare [1].

The Institute of Medicine's (IOM) "To Err is Human" described the toll that systematic error has on our medical system. Nearly 100,000 people die a year because of such errors. These errors occur not because medical professionals lack skill or competence. Instead, they occur because the system is rigged against our human-ness. The situation that resulted in Ms. Grant's death was not a result of an incompetent nurse. It was a result of the systematic complexity of medical systems. This complexity simply overwhelms the capacity of our human brains. The authors suggested that the solution is not to make healthcare providers better but to create a system better able to accommodate our human fallibility [2].

Onto this backdrop, those in medicine began to accelerate the journey into the world of information technology (IT) in the late 1990s. There was a recognition that tension was developing between the "traditional" centers of IT power and influence, the Chief Financial Officer (CFO), Chief Informatics Officer (CIO) and academics, and the clinical operations who were being tasked to use these technologies to facilitate day-to-day care of the patient [3]. The development of computer technology resulted in a growing number of physicians who "design, select and build infrastructure to enhance patient care and ensure that optimum systems are selected for each medical activity." [4] As these tensions increased, some organizations took it upon themselves to cultivate a new type of physician professional: the chief medical information officer. This role took on the task of relieving this tension. In this confluence of increasing cognitive load and technological capabilities, Drs. Lucian Leape and Donald Berwick cited implementing electronic health records (EHRs) as one of four key elements to solving the systematic issues [5].

Earlier, the chief information officer (CIO) earlier matured from the back-office nerd who kept the network and email working to a key stra-

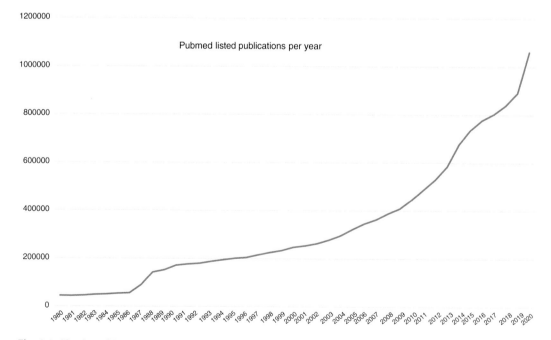

Fig. 9.1 Number of Pubmed listed publications per year from 1980 to 2020 based on the search for the keywords "health" or "nurs*" or "medic*" or care (search performed by Ursula Hübner)

tegic role player in most organizations. Businesses eventually realized that maintenance of the digital and information infrastructure is too important to be relegated to such a back-office role. The CMIO has made the same transition. There is a fundamental gap between the information that can potentially positively alter a patient's (and population's) clinical course and the information that is immediately available to the clinical decision makers who can affect such a positive change. Organizations have recognized that "information processing has been at the very core of medical practice" and we need to solve the literal life-threatening crisis that results from the asymmetric delivery of medical data, information and knowledge [6].

Who Is the Chief Medical Information Officer?

The American Medical Informatics Association (AMIA) has defined the CMIO: "Clinical informaticians transform health care by analyzing, designing, implementing, and evaluating information and communication systems that enhance individual and population health outcomes, improve patient care, and strengthen the clinician-patient relationship." [7] In other words, the CMIO's role is to remove the asymmetry in information delivery. As a result, the CMIO find themselves at the nexus of almost every decision that is made in our health system.

The legislation known as the Health Information Technology for Economic and Clinical Health Act (HITECH Act) markedly increased the profile of the CMIO. However, even before HITECH, the concept of a "Chief Medical Information Officer" began to take hold. Some healthcare organizations started to understand that the medical knowledgebase and the technology needed to optimally deliver healthcare were both exceedingly complex on their own. Together, their combined complexity was exponentially greater. This then spawned the need of a new skilled professional. This was someone who understood the medicine, the technology, and the novel workflows that would be

required to meld them together. These early CMIOs had varying levels of mandate and authority. They most often lacked formal authority, budget, and support staff. However, what they did bring to the table was advocacy for their front-line clinical colleagues [8].

These early CMIOs recognized the previously mentioned asymmetry that plagued our healthcare systems. They saw the potential for digital technology to make physicians more efficient and effective. The data that results from the delivery of healthcare can yield insights that can improve operational efficiency, reduce systemic mistakes, and develop new insights [6].

In 2009, the United States (U.S.) Congress and the Obama administration passed the HITECH Act. Although it was couched as a "voluntary" program, it effectively mandated that all healthcare organizations in the U.S. "meaningfully use" electronic medical records (EMRs). There was widespread optimism that this legislative act was a significant step forward [9].

Critically, as lofty and laudable as were the goals of the HITECH Act, the details of how to achieve "meaningful use" was left out the legislation. The regulations and specific definition of "meaningful use" was left to a follow up regulatory process that took years to mature. In fact, the aftermath of this process is still maturing to this day. One result of this uncertainty was the rise of the CMIO, on whom healthcare organizations increasingly depended to guide them on the yellow brick road to "Meaningful Use."

Simultaneously, the regulations were just a small piece of a very complex puzzle. Strict focus on the regulatory definitions of "Meaningful Use" often distracted from true, effective, real world *meaningful use* of EMRs. This nuanced dance between medical knowledge, real world workflows, and regulatory compliance required a unique skill set.

As we entered the twenty-first century, information technology (IT) had radically transformed our personal lives and business operations outside of the House of Medicine. Products and business services were delivered at a lower cost, better quality with an improved consumer experience. The IT that the HITECH Act's authors anticipated would be inoculated into our healthcare operations would likewise would facilitate the goal of achieving this "triple aim" of reduced cost, improved quality, and improved patient experience. The critical competencies to achieve the triple aim were bundled together by CMIOs in the discipline of clinical informatics, which "is not simply 'computers in medicine' but rather is a body of knowledge, methods, and theories that focus on the effective use of information and knowledge to improve the quality, safety, and cost-effectiveness of patient care as well as the health of both individuals and populations" [10].

Challenges and Opportunities

As one looks at the opportunities presented by clinical informatics in general and specifically after enactment of the HITECH Act, it was easy to become excited at the prospect of truly transforming healthcare. However, the reality of the triple constraints of time, cost, and scope soon blunted the exuberance. CMIOs soon realized that achieving the triple aim was going to require hard work and a very nuanced strategy [11].

The authors of the HITECH Act had a notion that digitizing the messy landscape of the then paper-based healthcare landscape would result in dramatic results. Similarly, healthcare business leaders often had (and have) grandiose sense of what a CMIO should be or do. Even CMIOs are often naive about the task and are often bewildered by the obstacles they face.

Regulatory

Prior to the HITECH Act, many physicians who worked with electronic systems in the healthcare environment, typically focused on niche, specialty-specific platforms and their work often did not have an enterprise-wide impact. HITECH changed that.

Ironically, though, one of the handcuffs that bound CMIOs the most was the HITECH Act itself. The act triggered an enormous external incentive to rapidly mobilize IT resources but also consumed enormous resources to comply with a changing, wide-ranging list of requirements that the Act mandated.

For years before HITECH (and afterward as well), CMIOs have been tasked with "playing the game" better. Billing constructs such as E/M coding, case mix indices, diagnosis-related groups (DRGs), as well as the reporting of complications, often necessitated manipulating workflows instead of addressing underlying systemic problems. The HITECH Act, in many ways, massively accentuated and magnified this effort [12].

Technical

Healthcare is full of specialization and silos of knowledge. As we try to transform healthcare systems, the importance of cross functional knowledge is becoming increasingly important. A non-IT example was highlighted in a recent publication that underscored how our obsession with specialization negatively impacted the response to the recent U.S. COVID crisis [13].

If we then consider healthcare and IT, the siloing of skills into "clinician" and "IT" buckets results in miscommunication and missed opportunities. As noted previously, the raison d'etre of the CMIO and clinical informaticists in general originates from the complexity that is exponentially created by combining two extremely complex disciplines: healthcare and IT. The socio-technical gap exists because experts who sit in each of these disciplines exclusively of the other do not have a good understanding of the other. The physician does not understand the technology and what it can and cannot accomplish. The IT professional may understand the technology but may have difficulty understanding how the technology fits into healthcare and how it can solve key problems.

Because of this, a core competency of a good CMIO is this ability to bridge the socio-technical gap [14]. It is certainly true that the ideal CMIO needs to have strong clinical skills and a clinician-first mentality. They are physicians with IT skills, not an IT professional who knows about medicine [15]. However, physicians who can maintain their "clinician first" mindset but still become steeped in the technology create exponential value. For instance, a special breed of physicians have developed the technical skills to directly mold and configure the clinical systems can "bend the system to the will" of physicians. Instead of the physician serving the EHR master, the EHR becomes an invaluable tool for the clinician. Physicians with such clinical tools understand and can speed development of clinician friendly tools because they can "cut to the chase" to identify the real reason for a request. Moreover, they often can see optimization opportunities that others who only have clinical or IT skill sets cannot see [16]. As we now move on from HITECH and the initial implementation phase of our digital healthcare landscape, there are competencies even more technical such as analytics and artificial intelligence (AI) that will come into play.

Inertia and Change

Healthcare is well known for its resistance to change. Much has been made of the imperative to change our financial, data, and delivery models. The U.S. simply cannot sustain the current models. In spite of this, U.S. delivery models have largely stayed intact with only incremental advances in the directions that it needs to go in [17].

Despite the inertia that is endemic to the U.S. healthcare system, we must continue to try to achieve the triple aim. We simply cannot stop trying. IT is a critical piece of this effort. As we continue to attempt to make these changes, what are the key characteristics of a CMIO that help facilitate these changes?

A 2003 study showed that the single most important factor in the implementation of advanced information systems in clinical settings was a high level of clinical leadership [18]. This fits with the general theme that a CMIO is a physician and healthcare executive first and an IT professional second.

CMIOs were initially considered the geeky doctor with a few EHR tricks up their sleeves. The first generation of CMIOs had a single primary task: address physician colleagues' resistance to the EMR [19]. A 2003 report stressed the importance of clinical leadership in computer provider order entry (CPOE) initiatives [20]. As recently as 2006, CMIOs were only officially part of healthcare systems' leadership teams about 30% of the time. By 2012, 75% of healthcare systems had CMIOs [21]. This corresponded with the imperative of complying with HITECH.

After the HITECH Act, though, it became increasingly clear that healthcare was fundamentally changed and organizations needed someone with a special skill set to meld the complex world of healthcare with the equally complex world of healthcare software. Since then, this special administrative role has transformed.

In 2008, the CMIO's role was described as a clinical leader and liaison. In 2014, the primary focus was compliance with Meaningful Use. By 2017, the key words in a CMIO's job description were data, analytics, and optimization [22]. Over a period of ten years, the role has fundamentally changed. Most CMIOs' initial responsibility was to implement an EHR and attest to HITECH Act's Meaningful Use. Eventually, the role evolved and morphed so that any enterprise organizational quality or process improvement project required the expertise of a skilled clinical informatician and CMIO [21, 23].

Differing Landscapes

This evolution of the CMIO from a "super-user" to a critical member of the strategic team started to require a different skill set and a different sort of CMIO. Overall, the position has become far more strategic and less operational or tactical. The CMIO needed to be a visionary to "understand the interactions between the complex areas within a health system including everything from operations, analytics, research, informatics, finance and IT." A new "chief health information officer" (or CHIO) which grew from the CMIO but that had less focus on the EMR and more on use of data to change decision making [24]. CMIO 1.0 evolved from to CMIO 2.0 and the new CHIO role. "It's a much broader skill set than the CMIO 1.0 and requires an informatics leader who can interact not solely with the front-line clinicians and technology team but also senior leadership and boards of directors." CMIOs are no longer individual contributors and have increasingly larger teams. Additionally, this evolution is starting to bleed into advanced technologies such as AI and data science. "The second-generation CMIO has gone from being the doctor who liked technology to a true strategic partner at the highest executive level. The current work in digital optimization will only amplify this further as we now begin to talk about what the CMIO 3.0 will look like." [25] This increasing level of strategic responsibility has led to a trend of some CMIOs becoming CIOs themselves [26–28].

The new strategic roles require the CMIO to extend beyond the initial flurry of EMR technology and fundamental healthcare delivery. This evolution is requiring an expansion into other skill sets. CMIOs needs to extend their views of the healthcare landscape. This will include developing expertise in finance, safety, quality, nursing, and other system operations. The job will not be just making the EMR work better for physicians. As previously noted, as a nation, the U.S. healthcare system (as well as many other global healthcare systems) needs to change. To a large extent, healthcare systems are not changing quickly enough. The organizations that are able to change successfully will be the ones that survive and thrive. The CMIO will be front and center in affecting this change and will need change management skills. The CMIO will need to deepen relationships with key stakeholders across the healthcare system. This will help in the traditional job of enlisting better buy-in. However, just as importantly, it will also create resources to help the CMIO anticipate the future needs of the healthcare organization. Increasingly, the CMIO needs to know where "the puck is going" rather than just facilitating the status quo. They will need to be students of new digital technologies. In short, the CMIO needs to need turn into a futurist [23].

Priorities

While there is a need for change, the CMIO will also need to be a key person to invoke discipline. Otherwise, organizations will be attracted to an avalanche of shiny objects. Doing so will dilute the limited resources that will create the changes we so desperately need.

Mission Statement

Technology is complex. Healthcare is complex. Assuming that one can just overlay technology on a broken healthcare system and assume that it will work is a fallacy. There is large variability in the tasks that a CMIO performs in differing organizations. However, the basic premise is that there is a socio-technical gap [14]. The digital transformation we desire will require a key physician leader to facilitate and fully leverage these new digital tools by asking the simple question, "What is the problem you are trying to solve?" [29] This helps to create a North Star and mission statement without which the technology can overwhelm the senses.

Ultimately, all CMIOs have a mission to facilitate delivery of the right information and data to the right person at the right time and in a way that it is immediately actionable (even if the action is to take no action). Our previous paper systems and, in different ways, our current electronic systems deliver data and information highly inefficiently. The methodologies have been very blunt hammers. We need the precision of a surgeon's scalpel.

Death of a Thousand Cuts

The HITECH Act effectively imposed a digital foundation for healthcare delivery. Unfortunately, this transition was far from being a panacea for the ills that ailed our healthcare system. Physicians and other users complained, with good justification, about poor and many times nonsensical workflows. Moreover, poorly designed EMR workflows have been linked with the increasingly difficult problem of physician burnout [30, 31].

More concerning was that the EMR, a promised savior from the scourge of medical error, seemed to actually create a burgeoning class of error itself. In fact, about a fifth of medication errors were caused by the EMR. In comparison, paper-based errors caused less than half the number. In the aftermath of the study, a physician was quoted, "I didn't go through all my training to have my ability to take care of patients destroyed by devices that are an impediment to medical care." [32] It is upon this backdrop that skilled informaticists and CMIOs can smooth the rough edges of EMRs by leveraging their technical skillset and melding it with their clinical and organizational skills [8, 33]. This ongoing struggle by providers and other clinical users of electronic systems has spawned a fourth "aim" to add to the triple aim—the provider experience. The now quadruple aim is a recognition that, without addressing the provider and clinical usability, we will be unable to achieve the other goals of cost reduction, improved quality, and patient experience.

Financial vs. Clinical Quality

As has been noted, health IT implementation has fallen short of lofty expectations. Beyond the widespread subjective narrative that our electronic systems have had a qualitatively negative impact on physician workflow, there is objective evidence that there has been a negative impact on financial productivity [34]. In spite of this, there is hope that two components of the triple and quadruple aim will improve: financial and clinical quality improvement. Intuitively, they have been couched as opposites and at constant tension. After all, how can one create better outcomes without spending more money? However, a key premise in our healthcare reform strategies is that our systems are fraught with systematic error, waste, and inefficiencies. This fact makes the system ripe for using IT to root out these problems and accomplish both improved costs and quality [1, 2]. In particular, the partnership between the traditionally more business minded CIO and the quality minded CMIO can create a powerful synergy that would "uncover the real value provided, both quality and cost." [35].

HITECH and the broader strategies' mindsets were that implementation of a digital healthcare environment would create value by improving quality at a lower cost by using key digital tools. Electronic clinical documentation would facilitate information transmission and retrieval. Electronic result review and other information delivery would democratize and speed delivery of results and other key clinical information. Computerized provider order entry (CPOE) of diagnostic tests, therapeutics, consultations and nursing and ancillary orders would facilitate accuracy, transparency, and reduce mistakes. Finally, the ultimate digital accomplishment would be accurate decision support delivered in the electronic clinical workflow that would guide clinicians to avoid harm and promote beneficial actions.

The end goal was a patient centered medical home (PCMH). The concept was to unify the fragmented health care system and have the system and health data circulate around the patient rather than the other way around [36].

Health Informatics Priorities in Collaboration with Other Professions

The CMIO cannot do his work in a vacuum. Certainly, this is the case when the team reporting to the CMIO is small and the team clearly needs to lean on others to do much of the work. However, even in situations where the CMIO is given substantial budgetary and human resources, the very nature of the complexity our healthcare and IT systems requires a strong streak of collaboration.

Interprofessional Teams

Clinical informatics is a young discipline with fluid roles and responsibilities based on the organization. It is quite difficult to create a one-size fits all model of optimal team structure. However, a few prominent themes will always apply.

Any good physician will relate innumerable times their hide was saved by an astute nurse. Likewise, first and foremost, collaboration with the nursing staff and nursing informaticists is of prime importance to a CMIO.

Beyond the intuitive sense that it makes sense to make sure nursing workflows are addressed, the practical matter is that nurses are in our electronic system far more than the physicians. One physician informaticist related, "Keep your nurses happy. They are in the EMR 24/7. It needs to work for them or you'll never sell it to your docs." [11].

More pointedly, two key organizations, the Robert Wood Johnson Foundation and the IOM recognized that healthcare reform could not occur without nursing leadership, particularly since nurses are the largest workforce in healthcare [37]. In a similar way as CMIOs, the CNIO has come to be part of many healthcare organizations' leadership. Nursing staff need the same

sort of bridging and translational advocate as physicians [21]. Also, in 2012, American Organization of Nurse Executives (AONE) recognized the importance of the CNIO in attaining quality, safety, and financial goals [38]. Optimization efforts focused solely on physicians yield poor results on this effort. A train can go only as fast as its slowest car. Thus, a holistic approach addressing not only physicians, but also nurses and support staff, synergistically improves all stakeholders' efficiency and job satisfaction [39]. The principle of cross domain collaboration is particularly important since leadership positions are typically lumped together by profession (i.e.: physician and nurses) at the top of the hierarchy but their executable decisions are integrated across professions within a single clinical domain (e.g.: emergency department (ED), operating room (OR), intensive care unit (ICU)) on the front lines of care (see Fig. 9.2 illustrating the various interprofessional partnerships). Therefore, it is critical to have effective communication across professional leadership roles such as the chief nursing information officer, the CIO and the CMIO as well as across clinical disciplines.

Most of the principles and competencies that make a good CMIO also apply to non-physician

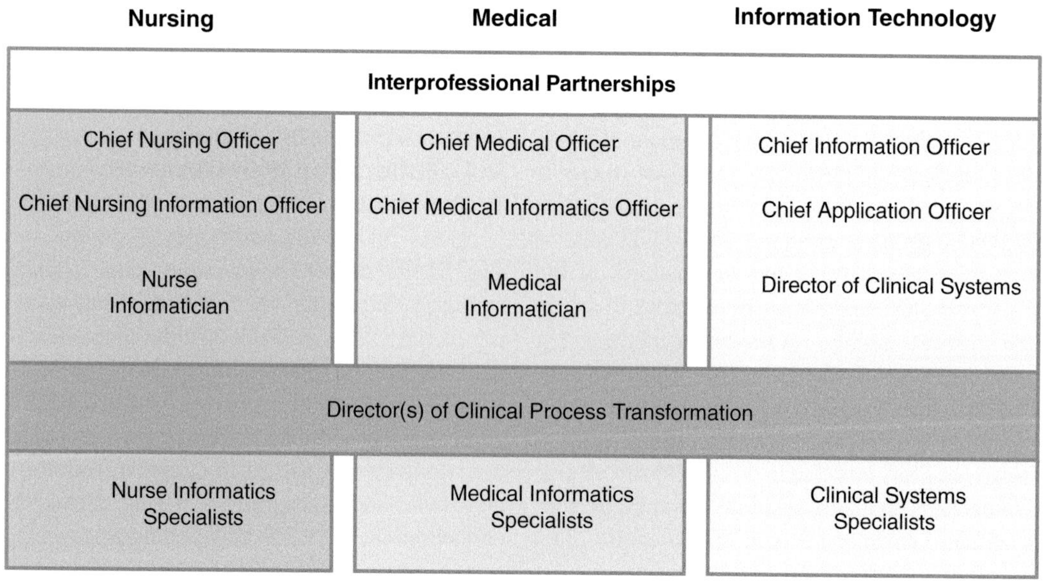

Nursing	Medical	Information Technology
Interprofessional Partnerships		
Chief Nursing Officer	Chief Medical Officer	Chief Information Officer
Chief Nursing Information Officer	Chief Medical Informatics Officer	Chief Application Officer
Nurse Informatician	Medical Informatician	Director of Clinical Systems
Director(s) of Clinical Process Transformation		
Nurse Informatics Specialists	Medical Informatics Specialists	Clinical Systems Specialists

Fig. 9.2 Interprofessional partnerships (see also [40] for additional information)

Fig. 9.3 Model of clinical informatics governance (see also [40] for additional information)

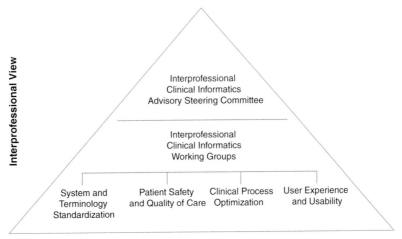

roles in the clinical IT work stream. In particular, one needs staffs who are both clinically astute and have the technology chops to understand how to appropriately use the technology and come up with novel ways to fully leverage the technology.

On the other side of the equation, the CMIO's relationship with the CIO is critically important. CIO and CMIO need to function as two halves of the same IT/clinical team [15, 41].Without the CIO, the CMIO will be unable to deliver the necessary tools. Without the CMIO, the CIO will be delivering tools without focus and likely, without the buy-in and acceptance by the front-line clinical staff [42, 43]. As we move from fee-for-service (FFS) to value and quality, we need to fully leverage data. We will only be able to accomplish this if we have a synergistic "partnership between CIO and CMIO, and an overlapping grasp of each other's realm." [35].

Operational Communication

All these cross functional teams require skills beyond that of a physician or technologist.

The CMIO needs to have a role as both IT representative to clinical operations and clinical representative to IT operations. These bridges, informal networks, and the ability to influence colleagues, peers and leadership, is increasingly

a critical piece of a good CMIO's armamentarium [8]. A structure that enhances and encourages cross discipline and interprofessional communication and collaboration is really a necessary key to success (Fig. 9.3 illustrates an example of an interprofessional informatics governance structure).

There are many headwinds and many naysayers. However, in spite of the negative publicity, even early implementations had success stories. This sort of success had far less to do with technical acumen and more to do with culture, relationships, and leadership [44].

Summary

We are at a crossroads in the delivery of healthcare in the U.S. It is simply too expensive and too many systematic errors are eroding our economy and harming too many patients. The situation is in a critical state now and we must fix the issues. We have the misfortune of tremendous inefficiency and systematic errors and both need serious effort and attention to fix.

At the same time, the fix for cost and quality cannot be a draconian blunt knife. We must also preserve and improve the patient and provider experience, completing the four components of the quadruple aim. The only way we will be able to accomplish this is by appropriately using IT to efficiently deliver the right information to the right person at the right time to facilitate the right decision.

Given the results of the national experiment with the HITECH Act and meaningful use, the job of a CMIO or any clinical informaticist for that matter, can be clouded by a wide variation of experiences. Thus, this quote seems appropriate: "It's not what you know any more. It's what you do with what you know that really makes the difference." [45] There are many really smart people out there trying to make a difference but intelligence and technical acumen is only (a very small) piece of the puzzle. The mark of an effective CMIO will depend on clinical, technical, and leadership acumen.

Conclusions and Outlook

The CMIO profession has been rapidly changing over the past three decades. The author hesitates to use the word "maturing" because it is not clear that the job is going to stabilize anytime soon. These decades have been a source of constant change for the profession. Initially, the CMIO was a lesser professional and perhaps not even considered a healthcare executive. However, the role gained an external boost with execution of the HITECH Act, which, for better or worse, digitized the American healthcare industry. With this digitization, the CMIO's role changed yet again to focus on fully leveraging this digitization with twenty-first century data tools.

What will not change though is the central premise that the only way we will be able to fix our broken healthcare system is via the intelligent and strategic use of IT and data tools.

Useful Resources: Include Any Online Resources Via Landing Page Here
1. What is the HITECH Act? https://www.hipaa-journal.com/what-is-the-hitech-act/
2. American Medical Informatics Association (AMIA): https://www.amia.org/
3. What is computerized provider order entry (CPOE)? https://www.healthit.gov/faq/what-computerized-provider-order-entry

4. U.S. Office of the National Coordinator for Health Information Technology (ONC): https://www.healthit.gov/

Review Questions
1. How does the Institute of Medicine's "To Err is Human" propose to solve our mistake prone medical system?
2. How did the HITECH Act stimulate the growth of the CMIO profession in the U.S.?
3. How does a CMIO bridge the socio-technical gap?
4. How is a CMIO's role changing?
5. What is a CMIO's mission?

Appendix: Answers to Review Questions

1. How does the Institute of Medicine's "To Err is Human" propose to solve our mistake prone medical system?.

The solution is not to make healthcare providers better but to create a system better able to accommodate our human fallibility.

2. How did the HITECH Act stimulate the growth of the CMIO profession in the U.S.?

The HITECH Act effectively mandated electronic records in almost all U.S. healthcare environments. Most healthcare organizations needed a CMIO to facilitate compliance with this mandate.

3. How does a CMIO bridge the socio-technical gap?

The CMIO brings a clinician mindset to technologists and a technology mindset to clinicians.

4. How is a CMIO's role changing?

The CMIO is evolving into a key member of healthcare organizations' strategy and data teams. Ideally, they are their organizations' futurists.

5. What is a CMIO's mission?

CMIOs have a mission to facilitate delivery of the right information and data to the right person at the right time and in a way that it is immediately actionable.

References

1. Institute of Medicine. Best care at a lower cost: the path to continuously learning health care in America. Washington, DC: National Academies Press; 2013.
2. Institute of Medicine. To err is human: building a safer health system. Washington, DC: The National Academies Press; 2000.
3. Friedman CP, Frisse ME, Musen MA, Slack WV, Stead WW. How should we organize to do informatics? Report of the ACMI debate at the 1997 AMIA fall symposium. J Am Med Inform Assoc. 1998;5(3):293–304.
4. Lincoln TL. Medical informatics: the substantive discipline behind health care computer systems. Int J Biomed Comput. 1990;26:73–92.
5. Leape L, Berwick D. Five years after to err is human, what have we learned? J Am Med Assoc. 2005;293(19):2384–90.
6. Aller RD. Clinical informatics as a medical subspecialty. Healthc Inf Manage. 1993;7:11–6.
7. AMIA. Clinical informatics board review course-history. AMIA [Online]. 2014. http://www.amia.org/clinical-informatics-board-review-course/history. Accessed 1 May 2020.
8. Leviss J, Kremsdorf R, Mohaideen MF. The CMIO—a new leader for health systems. J Am Med Inform Assoc. 2006;13:573–8.
9. Burde H. The HITECH act: an overview. Virtual Mentor. 2011;13(3):172–5.
10. Detmer DE, Shortliffe EH. Clinical informatics [published online ahead of print May 13, 2014]. JAMA. 2014;311(20):2067–8.
11. Felmeth W. The new CMIO. [Lecture]. Ojai, CA: s.n.; June 2013.
12. Moreno L, Peikes D, Krilla A. Necessary but not sufficient: the HITECH act and health information technology's potential to build medical homes. (Prepared by Mathematica Policy Research under contract no. HHSA290200900019I TO2.). Rockville, MD: Agency for Healthcare Research and Quality; 2010.
13. Cram P, Anderson ML, Shaughnessy EE. All hands on deck: learning to "Un-specialize" in the COVID-19 pandemic. J Hosp Med. 2020;15(5):314–3115.
14. Kuhn KA, Guiuse DA. From hospital information systems to health information systems. Method Inform Med. 2001;40:275–87.
15. McNickle M. 5 keys to evolving role of the CMIO [Online]. 2012. https://www.healthcareitnews.com/news/5-keys-evolving-role-cmio. Accessed 25 Jul 2020.
16. Joseph C. The arch collaborative and physician builders [Online]. 2018. https://klasresearch.com/resources/blogs/2018/10/03/the-arch-collaborative-and-physician-builders. Accessed 2 Aug 2020.
17. Numerof & Associates. The state of population health: fifth annual numerof survey report. 2020.
18. Doolan DF, Bates DW, James BC. The use of computers for clinical care: a case series of advanced U.S. sites. J Am Med Inform Assoc. 10(1):94–107.
19. Ingebrigtsen T, et al. The impact of clinical leadership on health information technology adoption: systematic review. Int J Med Inform. 2014;83(6):393–405.
20. Metzger J, Fortin J. Computerized physician order entry in community hospitals: lessons from the field. California Health Care Foundation and First Consulting Group. s.l.: California Health Care Foundation and First Consulting Group; 2003.
21. Kannry J, et al. The Chief Clinical Informatics Officer (CCIO). AMIA task force report on CCIO knowledge, education, and skillset requirements. Applied Clin Inform. 2016;7:143–76.
22. Shaffer V. 13th annual AMDIS-Gartner CMIO survey. Ojai, CA: s.n.; 2017.
23. Bensema D. What are you going to do now, CMIO? [Online]. https://healthsystemcio.com/2018/04/30/what-are-you-going-to-do-now-cmio/. Accessed 25 Jul 2020.
24. Ross H. From liaison to leader: the emergence of the CHIO [Online]. 2016. https://healthsystemcio.com/2016/10/18/liaison-leader-emergence-chio/. Accessed 15 Nov 2016.
25. Ross H, Durst Z. Industry voices—the 2nd-generation CMIO/CHIO is evolving into a strategic role and team leader [Online]. 2019. https://www.fiercehealthcare.com/tech/industry-voices-second-generation-cmio-chio-evolving-into-a-strategic-role-and-team-leader. Accessed 30 Sep 2019.
26. Fairview Health Services' new CIO, Sameer Badlani, MD, shares insights about the changing role of IT leaders and the dynamics at play behind the scenes [Online]. https://www.healthleadersmedia.com/innovation/physician-cio-how-one-mans-journey-reflects-it-transformation. Accessed 26 Jul 2020.
27. From CMIO to CIO. Health Data Manag. 2007;15(11):43.
28. Halamka J. Chief Medical Information Officer's role becoming more important [Online]. 2012. https://medcitynews.com/2012/01/chief-medical-information-officers-role-becoming-more-important/. Accessed 16 Aug 2020.
29. Roth M. Physician CIO: "I Refuse to Fall in Love with Technology." [Online]. 2019. https://www.healthleadersmedia.com/innovation/physician-cio-i-refuse-fall-love-technology. Accessed 26 Jul 2020.
30. Jha AK, et al. A Crisis in Health Care: A Call to Action on Physician Burnout. Waltham, MA: Jha AK; Iliff AR; Chaoui AA; Defossez S; Bombaugh MC; Miller YA; Massachusetts Medical Society; Massachusetts Health and Hospital Association; Harvard T.H. Chan School of Public Health; Harvard Global Health Institute; 2018.

31. Schulte F, Fry E. *Death by 1,000 clicks: where electronic health records went wrong.* s.l.: Kaiser Health News; 2019.
32. Mostrous A. Electronic medical records not seen as a cure-all. Washington Post. 2009;10:25.
33. Versel N. UCLA uses 'Physician Informaticists' to win over medical staff X [Online]. 2014. http://health.usnews.com/health-news/hospital-of-tomorrow/articles/2014/12/29/ucla-uses-physician-informaticists-to-win-over-medical-staff. Accessed 24 Feb 2015.
34. Scott DJ, et al. The impact of electronic medical record implementation on labor cost and productivity at an outpatient orthopaedic clinic. J Bone Joint Surg Am. 2018;100(18):1549–56.
35. The CIO-CMIO partnership; execs now work together to get more value out of IT. Health Data Manag. 2016;24(7):42.
36. Moreno L, Peikes D, Krilla A. Necessary but not sufficient: the HITECH act and health information technology's potential to build medical homes. Rockville, MD: U.S. Department of Health and Human Services; 2010.
37. Committee on the Robert Wood Johnson Foundation Initiative on the Future of Nursing at the Institute of Medicine. The future of nursing: leading change, advancing health. Washington, DC: National Academies Press; 2011.
38. Harrington L. AONE creates new position paper: nursing informatics executive leader. Nurse Leader. 2012;10(3):17–8.
39. Sieja A, Markley K. SPRINT: an optimization strategy that increases satisfaction, improves teamwork and reduces burnout. Verona, WI: s.n.; 2019.
40. Collins SA, Alexander D, Moss J. Nursing domain of CI governance: recommendations for health IT adoption and optimization. J Am Med Inform Assoc. 2015;22(3):697–706.
41. Gale Health and Wellness. Health system CIOs, CMIOs develop industry standard information management capability road map for coordinating accountable care. s.l.: Gale Health and Wellness; 2011. p. 36.
42. Kearns M. Developing the role of CIO in healthcare management: from "the IT Guy" to CIO [Online]. https://healthmanagement.org/c/healthmanagement/issuearticle/developing-the-role-of-cio-in-healthcare-management-from-the-it-guy-to-cio. Accessed 16 Aug 2020.
43. Eastwood B. How to cultivate a strong healthcare CIO-CMIO relationship [Online]. 2014. https://www.cio.com/article/2848236/how-to-cultivate-a-strong-healthcare-cio-cmio-relationship.html. Accessed 16 Aug 2020.
44. Scott JT, et al. Kaiser Permanente's experience of implementing an electronic medical record: a qualitative study. BMJ. 2005;331:1313.
45. Grulke W, Silber G. 10 lessons from the future: tomorrow is a matter of choice, make it yours. London: Financial Times Prentice Hall; 2000.

The View of Health Information Managers (HIM): Strategic Insights Through Data Analytics

10

Mervat Abdelhak and Angelika Haendel

Learning Objectives
- Describe the roles and responsibilities of Health Information Management (HIM) Professionals.
- Identify educational and credentialing paths available for the HIM profession.
- Describe the emerging roles of Health Information Management professionals.
- Discuss the Health Informatics (HI) and patient—centered priorities from the perspective of HIM and in collaboration with other professions.

Key Terms
- Health information management
- Data and information governance
- Clinical documentation
- Electronic health records
- Clinical coding
- Data quality
- Interoperability
- Data analytics
- Actionable data

- Access to the data
- Privacy
- Patient engagement

Introduction

The Health Information Management Profession, founded back in the 1900's, continues to serve a critical role in healthcare across the globe.

Health Information Management professionals' knowledge and skill sets are needed more than ever in today's and for tomorrow's healthcare. HIM practitioners across the globe, bridge the clinical, financial, legal and quality health data for the improvement of the quality of patient care, clinical research and population health.

Today's Health care organizations are dependent on an enormous amount of data, data that are created and maintained at different sources and in varied formats. HIM professionals by validating the integrity and quality of data can identify the "source of truth" from among all the data sources thus improving health care decisions for providers and consumers alike.

M. Abdelhak (✉)
University of Pittsburgh, School of Health & Rehabilitation Sciences, Pittsburgh, PA, USA
e-mail: abdelhak@pitt.edu

A. Haendel
University Hospital Erlangen, Erlangen, Germany
e-mail: angelika.haendel@uk-erlangen.de

© Springer Nature Switzerland AG 2022
U. H. Hübner et al. (eds.), *Nursing Informatics*, Health Informatics,
https://doi.org/10.1007/978-3-030-91237-6_10

Definition and Role
of the Profession in Health Care

What Is Health Information Management?

Health Information Management Professionals work in many settings assuming a variety of roles and functions across the entire healthcare sector. HIM professionals work in hospitals, long-term care or mental healthcare agencies, university research institutions, pharmaceutical industry, consulting and IT firms, community care and government agencies, to name but a few.

Health Information Management professionals provide leadership in Data Management and Information Governance, Clinical Documentation, Clinical Coding, Electronic Health Records (EHR) design and management, Regulatory Compliance and Risk Management, Revenue Cycle Management, Data Privacy and Security, Data Analytics, Statistics, Patient Registries and Tracking, as well as the Reporting of health status and delivering actionable data.

Figure 10.1 displays the practice domains of Health Information Management professionals across the globe.

As healthcare delivery systems become much more complex, interdisciplinary and interprofessional, as well as data driven, consumer-centric and digital, the roles, responsibilities and the education of Health information management professionals will continue to evolve and change to meet the demands of this transformed workplace.

There will be the need for a higher educated, more qualified HIM professionals who can assume additional leadership and management tasks such as assisting in the planning, design implementation and maintenance of electronic

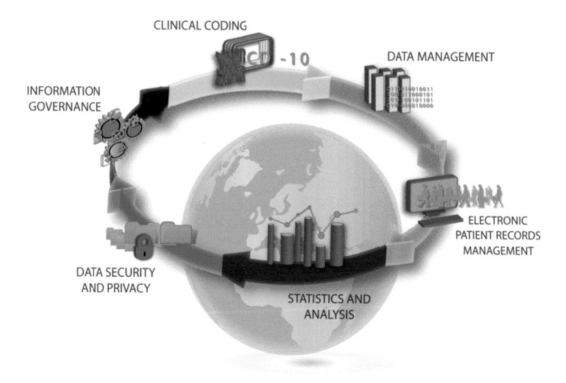

Fig. 10.1 Health information management practice across the globe

health records, telehealth systems, mobile health apps and technologies as well as patient portals. Furthermore, HIM professionals will continue to be responsible for clinical documentation improvement and clinical coding including the design and assessment of technology aided tools for the benefit of the user, provider and patient.

Many HIM professionals are already highly skilled in data analytics and data use. As health care organizations are faced with growing competition, the hospital management will need more statistical calculations and trend analysis. The related information for these statistics will probably come from a variety of sources. HIM professionals will be faced with merging and integrating complex data from these various sources. There will also be a growing need for comprehensive knowledge in the fields of data protection, confidentiality, especially with regard to the expanded patient rights, increased demand by patients, to access their health data and heightened consumer expectations. Classification systems including the International Classification of Diseases and

Related Health Problems (ICD-10, ICD-11) and the International Classification of Functioning, Disability and Health (ICF) as well as the implementation or the further development of reimbursement systems such as DRGs will also continue to add challenges for the HIM profession.

The roles and functions of Health Information Management Professionals will move beyond traditional task-oriented roles to leadership roles and responsibilities that include strategic planning, senior project management, data validation and integration as well as data and information governance oversight activities that govern access and use of data.

Figure 10.2 compares traditional and expanded tasks for HIM professionals.

Professional Associations

Advocacy and the advancement of the HIM profession are shepherded by HIM professional

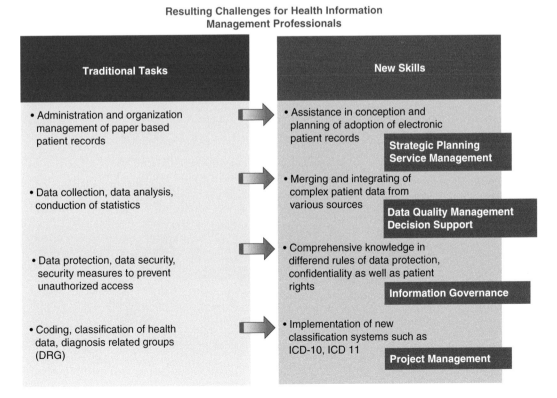

Fig. 10.2 Traditional and expanded tasks for Health Information Management Professionals

associations that have been established around the world. As the practice and education of HIM advances, countries recognize the need and value of organizing and connecting members who have similar goals and aspirations.

One association, the International Federation of Health Information Management Associations (IFHIMA) as described below, brings together many of the professional associations from around the globe.

IFHIMA was founded in 1968 as a forum for the exchange of Information regarding the profession. As an umbrella organization, IFHIMA acts as the "global voice" of Health Information Management for 23 member nations and hundreds of individual members. Moreover, IFHIMA is a non-profit, non-governmental and independent organization, with official relations with WHO.

IFHIMA member nations are grouped into the six WHO regions according to their geographical location: African Region, Region of The Americas, South-East Asia Region, European Region, Eastern Mediterranean Region and the Western Pacific Region (Fig. 10.3).

IFHIMA is dedicated to the professional growth and development of its members with particular emphasis on education and best-practices.

IFHIMA's goals are to:

- Promote the quality and use of patient records and health information globally.
- Provide best practices in health information management.
- Develop and implement international standards in health information management.
- Advise and assist developing countries with building and enhancing formalized training and education programs.
- Raise the profile of health information management professionals globally.

IFHIMA's mission is to strengthen the health information management profession globally. This includes sharing the latest news in the field of Health Information as well as sharing best practices. Moreover, IFHIMA's mission is to support its member nations and their members in advancing the need for well educated, trained HIM professionals who will ensure high quality documentation along the continuum of care as well as best practices in the field of clinical coding, analytics, research and planning in the field of healthcare. The mission includes assisting developing countries in the establishment of HIM associations, their workforce, as well as assisting nations that have mature health systems and care delivery organizations.

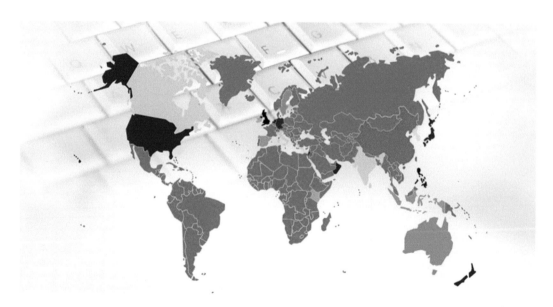

Fig. 10.3 IFHIMA member nations

Challenges of the Profession: Education and Certification

Overview

The educational pathways available and or required for HIM vary and differ across the globe. Some countries require an academic degree from an accredited institution of Higher education, while in other countries completing a certificate program is all that is required.

Academic degree preparation can be in HIM, or in Health Informatics encompassing HIM curricula, or in Medicine. The academic degree levels range from that of the Associate degree to Graduate degrees.

The educational preparation of Health Information Management professionals in the USA is offered at three academic degree levels: the Associate, Baccalaureate and master's level.

The Associate degree programs are housed at two -year colleges and are typically named "Health Information Technology" (HIT) programs. The Graduates of accredited Associate degree programs are eligible to sit for the Registered health Information Technician (RHIT) examination to obtain the Registered Health Information Technician (RHIT) credential.

HIM educational preparation is also offered at the baccalaureate level, at four -year colleges and Universities. Baccalaureate degree programs are typically named "Health Information Management" (HIM), or "Health Information Administration" (HIA), or more recently named "Health Informatics and Information Management (HIIM)". The Graduates from accredited HIM baccalaureate degree programs are eligible to sit for the Registered Health Information Administrator (RHIA) examination for the (RHIA) credential.

Master's degree level programs in HIM are also offered and are typically named "Health Information Management" (HIM), or "Health Informatics"(HI), or "Health Informatics and Information Management" (HIIM).Graduates of accredited HIM Master's degree programs are eligible to sit for the RHIA examination for the

(RHIA) credential as do Baccalaureate degree program graduates.

The accrediting organization, for all three degree level programs, is the Commission on Accreditation for Health Informatics and Information Management Education (CAHIIM). CAHIIM is an independent not-for profit organization that accredits HIM and HI degree programs.

In Europe Health Information Management Professionals are also known as Medical Documentalists, Professionals in Medical Documentation, or Medical Documentation Specialists. They work in hospitals, research institutes, pharmaceutical companies and other health care institutions. The career prospects are excellent, and the demand is expected to continue to increase in the future.

The education in the field of Medical Information Management is focused on the interface between medicine, information processing and health management. Essential contents of most of the study programs are documentation methods, computer science, medicine, statistics, information research as well as basics of business administration and management. Furthermore, students will also learn to communicate in a goal-oriented manner and to work scientifically. Most of the studies are practice-oriented through projects and practical phases as well as application-oriented courses.

In Europe, most of the Health Information Professionals or medical documentation professionals hold a bachelor's degree (B.Sc., or BA) or a three-year professional education in a technical college. Because of the increasing complexity of information management in the healthcare sector, there is a significant trend to complete a master's degree (M.Sc., or M.A.) for that profession.

Competencies

United States of America

The HIM profession across the globe, through professional associations, educators, researchers, practitioners and employers, authors competencies to ensure the successful practice in today's healthcare environment. These competencies provide the underpinnings for HIM curriculum development and for facilitating interprofessional collaborations.

Professional associations such as the American Health Information Management Association (AHIMA) in the USA has formed the Council for Excellence in Education (CEE) to set educational strategy and author competencies that are required in curricular design. The curriculum in the HIM Associate, baccalaureate and master's degree programs are built upon these competencies with a Bloom's level Taxonomy that is indicative of the depth at which each competency is addressed.

Table 10.1 provides a sample of the required competencies, and knowledge domains for HIM professionals in USA.

Global Academic Curricula Competencies for Health Information Professionals

In 2013, AHIMA in collaboration with IFHIMA established the Global Health Workforce Council (GHWC). This council consisted of 13 appointed members from 11 different nations with a cross section of expertise from around the globe. This international working group developed a global academic curricula standard to guide educational programming and workforce training in HIM, HI

Table 10.1 Selected competencies for HIM professionals in the USA

| Data content, structure & standards |
| Data governance |
| Information management strategic planning |
| Information integrity and data quality |
| Clinical coding |
| Clinical documentation |
| Regulatory compliance |
| Revenue cycle & reimbursement |
| Analytics, data use & decision support |
| Data protection, privacy and access |
| Health care statistics |
| Health information technologies |
| Project Management |
| Research methods |
| Leadership and organizational management |

and Health Information and Communication Technology (HICT). The curricula were completed in July 2015 and are available on the IFHIMA and AHIMA websites. https://ifhima.org/global-health-information-curricula-competencies/or http://www.ahima.org/about/global

Aims of this initiative was to develop recommendations for workforce strengthening through academic and workforce competencies for the health information professions including HIM, HI, and HICT—to ensure appropriate information governance throughout the healthcare ecosystem.

The curricula area has a practical guide to develop and implement academic programs in one or more of the health information professions (HIM/HI/HICT). Furthermore, the curricula serve as a roadmap that allows for customization of academic programs dependent on the specific needs of the country/region. The specific module selected (HIM, HI, HICT) and academic level (entry, intermediate, advanced) of the module chosen for implementation should be informed by the job roles needed in each specific country.

Table 10.2 shows the content of the curricula. Each of the 29 competencies is represented at an Entry, Intermediate and Advanced Level.

Health Informatics Priorities from the Perspective of This Profession

Emerging Roles Including Health Informatics and Patient-Centered Priorities

The Healthcare industry has for many years lagged behind in implementing modern e-technologies. However, the healthcare industry is now rapidly catching up especially with the adoption of electronic records, mobile health and the like. Health Informatics and patient-centered priorities (Table 10.3) have not only accelerated the adoption of electronic health records but also expanded the implementation of virtual

Table 10.2   Content of HIM curricula

1   Analytics and statistics:
2   Change management
3   Classification of disease, coding diagnoses and procedures
4   Clinical documentation improvement (CDI):
5   Data management and information governance
6   Data quality and information integrity:
7   Ethics
8   Financial management
9   Health information access, disclosure, and exchange
10 Health information systems and application design and planning:
11 Health information systems and application development and deployment:
12 Health information systems and application support:
13 Health law, regulation, accreditation, and/or certification:
14 Health record content & documentation:
15 Human resource management:
16 Information and information systems governance:
16 Information protection—data privacy, confidentiality and security:
18 Information security strategy and management:
19 Organisational management and leadership:
20 Project management:
21 Purchasing and contracting:
22 Quality management:
23 Research design and methods:
24 Risk management
25 Standards for data content, health information exchange, and interoperability:
26 Strategic planning:
27 Training and development
28 Work design and process improvement
29 Healthcare delivery systems:

Table 10.3   Health Informatics and patient-centered priorities and the challenges and opportunities for HIM

Health informatics and patient-centered priorities	HIM challenges and opportunities
Ongoing adoption of electronic health records (EHR) in health facilities	Increased volume of data and increased complexity and variability of data
Electronic health records depending on multiple data sources and different data formats	Challenges addressing data integration, interoperability, data security and data protection
Increasing use of mobile health and applications in health care	Challenges regarding privacy and confidentiality, quality of data and integrating mobile originated data into the EHR
Increased consumer engagement and assuming responsibility for their own health	Increased demand for patient education regarding their health condition and in the use of e-technologies
Cloud computing	Cybersecurity, data safety and data protection challenges
Demand for integrated care and cross-institutional sharing of electronic patient data	Increasing the complexity of data, interoperability issues, legal issues and heightened competition among health systems

Below is a list of but a few examples of how Health Informatics and patient-centered priorities are changing HIM.

- The ongoing shift from paper based to electronic health records (EHR) is a very important achievement as it enables a more widespread availability of patient data. Moreover, electronically accessible health data can be used in planning, managing and deploying resources, disease surveillance and research.
- The electronic health record contains data from different IT-Systems within a hospital, for example, data from the laboratory and pharmacy systems, which could differ in how these systems collect and maintain patient data. Therefore, health Informatics and HIM Professionals will have to collaborate in designing data validation and integration methods addressing interoperability challenges.

care, enhanced the application of Artificial Intelligence in the delivery of patient care as well as accelerated the implementation other technologies that improve engagement and access to care. It can be expected, that these technological and societal trends will add complexity to the management of health information. Furthermore, it can be expected that these challenges and opportunities cannot be addressed by HIM professionals in silo, but rather they can only be addressed successfully in collaboration with other professionals.

- Interoperability challenges also exist beyond the boundaries of one hospital or a multi-hospital system. Access to patient data whenever and wherever it is needed, has become an expectation by all.
- Consumer Engagement has expanded patients' rights and responsibilities. Patients are actively entering data into their EHR, for example by uploading self-collected data from their mobile health devices. The increasing use of mobile services will also bring challenges regarding privacy and confidentiality of data as well as challenges related to the quality and integrity of the data.
- The increasing participation of patients in their therapy and disease process imposes an increasing demand for training and education of patients regarding their health status and in the use of electronic health devices. Patients will be collecting and transferring data as well as deciding who can have access to their health data.
- Cloud computing and increased reliance on e-technologies creates additional challenges with cybersecurity and data protection.

Tasks

The following list provides an overview of high priority tasks.

- Comply with the Office of the National Coordinator (ONC) Interoperability and Information Blocking final regulations.
- Facilitating patient data access by ensuring that effective policies and procedures are in place for access, exchange and use of their electronic health information.
- Design and implement health IT systems that are secure in order to protect against cyber-attack and data breaches.
- Validate the quality and integrity of both structured and unstructured health data that are maintained thus providing actionable data for sound decisions.
- Redesign of EHRs to allow for the integration of external data such as social determinants of

health, mobile device and virtual visits data and the like.
- Advance and adopt a national patient identification strategy that would reduce the number of patients who are assigned duplicate or inaccurate medical record numbers thus enabling the exchange of health and interoperability.

Health Informatics Priorities in Collaboration with Other Professions

While the priorities of Health Information Management (HIM) are determined by the emerging roles of HIM professionals, there are Health Informatics priorities shared with other professions that arise from the increasing adoption of electronic health records and embrace the opportunities from analyzing EHR data. These priorities go beyond the management und use of data from the professionals' viewpoint and include the patients in their role as active users of health IT systems. The follow list provides an overview of these tasks.

- Enhance the development, availability and use of health IT tools and systems that allow patients to access their healthcare information via smartphones, mobile devices and portals, track and manage their health and wellness, and communicate with providers.
- Educate health professionals and vendors regarding their role in protecting patients' health information, the health care organization security incident response plans and their obligations to the consumer.
- Educate health care practitioners and facilitate clinical documentation improvements thus enhancing the quality of health data.
- Redesign of EHRs to reduce the burden on health care practitioners.
- Encourage and facilitate the use of health data and health IT for predictive analytics so that we can identify patients and communities at risk, marginalized groups and improve public health.

Summary

This chapter introduced the HIM profession as one that remains critical to the current and future healthcare industry. The roles and responsibilities of HIM professionals as well as the educational and certification pathways that exist for the profession were described. Promulgated competencies from the USA and globally were presented. These competencies are the guiding framework for education and practice. Health Informatics and patient-centered priorities have impacted the emerging roles in HIM. HIM professionals and other professionals collaborate and work together to ensure that tomorrow's healthcare is even more innovative, connected, transparent and accessible.

Conclusions and Outlook

Today's challenges of a greater volume and more complex data available in electronic format require traditional tasks of HIM to be re-designed. Consequently, privacy and confidentiality issues, data security, quality of data, interoperability and integrating mobile originated data into the electronic health records pose new challenges with which HIM is faced. These new obligations and tasks demand new competencies and skills to be developed and acquired. New competency areas embrace strategic planning, service management, data quality management, decision support, information governance and project management. Against this background, education of HIM students and upskilling the workforce is a major concern for HIM professionals.

Useful Resources

Links to HIM associations:
1. AHIMA—USA http://www.ahima.org/
2. CHIMA—Canada https://www.echima.ca/
3. DVMD—Germany https://dvmd.de/
4. HIMAA—Australia https://himaa.org.au/
5. IHRIM—United Kingdom https://www.ihrim.co.uk/
6. JHIM—Japan http://www.jhim-e.jp
7. KHIMA—Korea https://www.khima.or.kr/eng/1_main.php
8. SEDOM—Spain: http://www.sedom.es/

Review Questions
1. What is Health Information Management and what are classical subjects in study programs?
2. What are the fields HIM is moving into?
3. What are driving forces of HIM from the fields of health informatics and patient-centered care?

Appendix: Answers to Review Questions

1. What is Health Information Management and what are classical subjects in study programs?

HIM is a domain at the junction of medicine, information processing and health management. Typical study programs therefore include documentation methods, computer science, medicine, statistics, information research as well as basics of business administration and management.

2. What are the fields HIM is moving into?

HIMs is moving to leadership roles and responsibilities that include strategic planning, senior project management, data validation and integration as well as data and information governance oversight activities that govern access and use of data

3. What are driving forces of HIM from the fields of health informatics and patient-centered care?

The ongoing shift from paper based to electronic health records (EHR),

Interoperability of data originating from different systems that are compiled in electronic health records,

Interoperability challenges also exist beyond the boundaries of one hospital or a multi-hospital system,

Consumer Engagement has expanded patients' rights and responsibilities,

Patients are actively entering data into their EHR, for example by uploading self-collected data from their mobile health devices,

The increasing participation of patients in their therapy and disease process imposes an increasing demand for training and education of patients regarding their health status and in the use of electronic health devices,

Cloud computing and increased reliance on e-technologies creates additional challenges with cybersecurity and data protection.

Further Reading

1. Abdelhak M. Health information - management of a strategic resource. St. Louis and New York: Elsevier Health Science; 2015.
2. Ammenwerth E, Knaup P, Winter A, Bauer AW, Bott OJ, Gietzelt M, Haarbrandt B, Hackl WO, Hellrung N, Hübner-Bloder G, Jahn F, Jaspers MW, Kutscha U, Machan C, Oppermann B, Pilz J, Schwartze J, Seidel C, Slot JE, Smers S, Spitalewsky K, Steckel N, Strübing A, van der Haak M, Haux R, Ter Burg WJ. On teaching international courses on health information systems. Lessons learned during 16 years of Frank-van Swieten lectures on strategic information management in health information systems. Methods Inf Med. 2017;56(Open):e39–48. https://doi.org/10.3414/ME16-01-0124.
3. Dorsey AD, Clements K, Garrie RL, Houser SH, Berner ES. Bridging the GAP. A collaborative approach to health information management and informatics education. Appl Clin Inform. 2015;6:211–23.
4. Fenton SH, Low S, Abrams KJ, Butler-Henderson K. Health information management: changing with time. IMIA Yearb Med Inform. 2017;26:72–7.
5. Gibson CJ. Health information management workforce transformation: new roles, new skills and experiences in Canada. Perspectives in Health Information Management. 2015. http://perspectives.ahima.org/
6. Haendel A, MacDonald M, Skurka M, Nicholson L, Fernandes L. Strategic plan and accomplishments 2013-2016. www.ifhima.org.
7. IDC health insights: IDC FutureScape: worldwide healthcare 2015 predictions. 2015. http://www.idc.com
8. Marc D, Butler-Henderson K, Dua P, Lalani K, Fenton SH. Global workforce trends in health informatics & health information management. Stud Health Technol Inform. 2019;264:1273–7. https://doi.org/10.3233/SHTI190431.
9. Meidani Z, Meidani Z, Sadoughi F, Ahmadi M, Maleki MR, Zohoor A, Saddik B. National health information infrastructure model: a milestone for health information management education realignment. Telemed J E Health. 2012;18(6):475–83. https://doi.org/10.1089/tmj.2011.0189.
10. Stanfill MH, Marc DT. Health information management: implications of artificial intelligence on healthcare data and information management. Yearb Med Inform. 2019;28(1):56–64. https://doi.org/10.1055/s-0039-1677913.
11. World Health Organization (WHO) Western Pacific Region: Electronic Health Records. Manual for developing countries, 2006; WHO Library Cataloguing in Publication Data, ISBN 92 9061 2177 (NLM Classification WX 173).
12. Wissmann S. Addressing challenges to the health information management profession: an Australian perspective. Perspectives in Health Information Management. 2015. http://perspectives.ahima.org/
13. https://ifhima.org/global-health-information-curricula-competencies/.

The Educator's View: Global Needs for Health Informatics Education and Training

11

Toria Shaw Morawski, Johannes Thye, and Jessica Liston

Learning Objectives
- Discuss how increasing digitalization in health care affects health-related processes that impact the ability of informatics educators to create and continuously refine curricula and training materials.
- Introduce a few of the pain points and challenges experienced by educators in academic and clinical settings regarding curricula development aligned to competency attainment.
- Examine three case studies that bring to life challenges for educators to address and learn from when creating viable educational resources and training targeted at the informatics healthcare workforce.

Key Terms
- Electronic health (eHealth)
- The HIMSS TIGER Initiative
- Health information management
- Global workforce development
- Competency recommendations
- Curricula development

T. Shaw Morawski
Healthcare Information and Management Systems
Society (HIMSS), Chicago, IL, USA
e-mail: tori@torism44.com

J. Thye (✉)
University AS Osnabrück,
Osnabrück, Lower Saxony, Germany
e-mail: johannes.thye@hs-osnabrueck.de

J. Liston
Sutter Health, San Francisco, CA, USA

- Case studies
- Educate the informatics educators
- Competency attainment
- Lifelong learning
- TIGER International Competency Synthesis Project
- EU*US eHealth Work Project

Introduction

Increasing digitalization in health care affects health-related processes [1–4] and impacts the ability of informatics educators to create and continuously refine curricula and training that benefit their target audiences who comprise the future healthcare workforce. Information technology (IT) support is necessary to address progressively complex treatments/procedures, help integrate new treatment methods, speak to the growing demands on data and exchange, and finally, to make the processes more efficient and close service gaps [1, 2, 4–7]. Digitization thus has an impact on the activities of health professionals in direct patient care (DPC) such as physicians and nurses. This means that the use of IT is changing the tasks involved and, therefore, it must reflect in training and educational practices.

How does the digitization of healthcare systems connect to and help inform informatics focused teaching and training methods? How can

© Springer Nature Switzerland AG 2022
U. H. Hübner et al. (eds.), *Nursing Informatics*, Health Informatics,
https://doi.org/10.1007/978-3-030-91237-6_11

academic and clinical educators easily infuse new techniques and instruments into the design of educational materials? This chapter aims to address a few of the pain points that informatics educators are facing when it comes to curricula design aligned to competencies attainment to better support students and adult learners in the academic and clinical realms.

Advances in Nursing and Healthcare Drive Informatics Innovation and Evolution

In 2020, the Healthcare Information Management Systems Society's (HIMSS) Technology Informatics Guiding Education Reform (TIGER) Initiative released the fourth iteration of the "HIMSS TIGER Global Informatics Definitions" document. Since 2016, HIMSS TIGER has been highlighting established informatics terminology to shine a light on integrating informatics fluently into practice, education, research, and the development of resources on a global scale. For example, defining "nursing informatics" helped guide role delineation for nurses who specialize in informatics while helping those within and outside of nursing better understand the legitimacy of the practice and the competencies required to specialize in the role [8]. Global healthcare systems, medicine, nursing, and informatics are continuously evolving and expanding. This requires reflection on how the scope of disciplines themselves is changing rapidly enough to match their instruments [4, 9, 10].

Therefore, it is essential to universally define how informatics ties to each discipline, keeping in mind that informatics extends beyond geographic regions and borders; informatics concepts and their applications may vary locally, regionally and nationally. Discipline specific informatics definitions must frequently be revisited in scope. With definitions and scopes changing so rapidly, it makes sense that educators sometimes get lost in a sea of rapidly changing "informatics" terminology that can trigger comprehension challenges. It is important to point out that although concepts and definition of infor-

matics have been around for many years and evolved, the adoption of informatics has not followed suit. On the outside, the informatics field has changed rapidly due to the marketing of concepts; however, behind the scenes, it is clear that informatics has not yet become a fully organic part of delivering care, and this must change. Finally, educators must be encouraged and allowed time to acquire a firm grasp of the mental frameworks constructed to understand better and make sense of the swiftly changing terminology and concepts.

Educating the Informatics Educators

The first step in resolving educator pain points is to address them and then continuously "educate the educators" about the rapidly changing landscape of informatics in relation to their discipline specific learners. "Those responsible for educating or training the students or current providers, despite mandates to do so, themselves often lack in knowledge, skills, and attitudes so that there is not a transference of knowledge and skill that results in a demonstrable competency." [11].

Educators must first understand informatics in order to teach informatics better. Although healthcare continues to change rapidly in the digital age, informatics curricula development has not been prioritized, and many educators are not well-versed or equipped to teach informatics properly. "Health informatics programs should consider specialized tracks that include specific skills to meet the complex health care delivery and market demand, and specific training components should be defined for different specialties. There is a need to determine new competencies and skill sets that promote inductive and deductive reasoning from diverse and various data platforms and to develop a comprehensive curriculum framework for health informatics skills training." [12]. At the same time, educators in clinical settings should not simply focus on teaching software which may be replaced by new software in a few years' time anyway. They too must convey the overall picture of informatics in connection to digitization in order to make the principles understandable and thus, enable active participation in shaping and properly defining digital workplaces, for example, in software selection. They must also focus on the evaluation of enabling tools and resources to support those who are new to the workforce as they navigate digitized healthcare systems with the goal of bettering patient care. Regardless of setting, educators carry the weight of teaching students the full scope of digitalization while helping them understand informatics principles to play an active role in shaping the digital workplaces of the future. Historically, educators were not integrated into the development and design of technology systems, nor were the systems built in such a way that educators could seamlessly teach the tools leveraged in clinical settings.

Connecting Informatics Competency Attainment to Curricula and Skill Assessment Tools

Today, more than ever before, there is an emphasis on competency attainment connected to learning outcomes. While learning expectations and goals must be established early on by educators, they also need to be conscious of competency attainment focus and application as they develop curricula. "Competencies often serve as the basis for skill standards that specify the level of knowledge, skills, and abilities required for success in the workplace, as well as potential measurement criteria for assessing competency attainment." [13]. With this understanding in mind, future healthcare workers (HCWs) will need a firm grasp of their discipline's core competencies as they prepare to graduate and go out into the field. It is imperative that education must now encompass a conduit for competency attainment to assist students with the ability to use critical thinking in order to be competent while on the job.

Competency attainment can also be tied to the concept of lifelong learning, which "is a form of self-initiated education that is focused on personal development. While there is no standardized definition of lifelong learning, it

has generally been taken to refer to the learning that occurs outside of a formal educational institution, such as a school, university or corporate training." [14]. No longer are people expected to learn while in school only; HCWs are expected to continuously learn and refine their skills while on the job to succeed within digitized health care systems to impact care outcomes positively.

Definition and Role of the Educator in Health Care

Over the last two decades, healthcare systems have undergone enormous changes brought on by increasing pressures to improve quality, value, affordability, and, most importantly, safety. The burgeoning complexity of healthcare delivery systems, as well as regulatory forces, has resulted in demands to digitize the entire industry. These demands have forced educators to become more facile at managing and manipulating large amounts of data while requiring that health IT be incorporated into DPC at a rate that is faster than many educators and bedside clinicians can adapt to. Not only is speed a challenge with digitization but also the usability and usefulness of health IT. Not all IT is clinically meaningful, so educators must serve as the gateway to distinguish between relevant and non-relevant IT processes and also work to identify how they can guide measurement of the differences. Other issues to take into consideration is the standardization, validation, and implementation of informatics competencies to create an information-literate, highly skilled workforce that drives developing technology to enhance usability and ensure patient safety [15–17]. Educators have the additional burden of serving as the change agent that helps facilitate the adoption and integration of health IT into care in a useful manner. All of these outstanding needs further contribute to adverse side effects such as clinical burnout, alarm fatigue in clinical decision support systems (CDSS), the balance of mental health/wellness needs, and so on.

New Technologies Challenging Care Delivery and Education

Different health professions naturally have their own individual challenges. What they all have in common is the steadily increasing influence of digitalization and the need to work with technology efficiently. Digitalization can crystallize in different ways and different colors. For example, through new examination and treatment methods, for example, within the framework of telemedicine or new surgical methods, in addition to new methods and resource being developed in artificial intelligence (AI)/machine learning (ML) and augmented reality (AR) [2, 7, 10, 18]. ML is a statistical technique for data-driven learning by training models with data. Examples of data-driven health care are precision medicine (e.g. making predictions), within more complex cases, neural networks (e.g. determining whether a patient will acquire a particular disease) and deep learning (e.g. detecting potentially cancerous lesions in radiological images) [2]. In addition, there are already many well-known and long-established instruments such as reminder functions, alerting, and decision support by IT [6].

Furthermore, digitalization can also be reflected in communication support. It can simply start with emails between employees and can go all the way upto communication across sectors between service providers located around the world. Robotics is another area that supports these vital care processes [10]. These varied challenges must be considered in training and curricula development. Educators must be familiar with the new opportunities offered by digitization and be able to teach them. In other words, informatics competencies must be included in the curricula of training courses and degree programs. In addition, the digitization of teaching offers the opportunity to provide e-learning methods [19–22].

Health Informatics Priorities from the Perspective of Educators

The TIGER International Competency Synthesis Project (ICSP) and the resulting frameworks 1.0 and 2.0 were described in Chap. 2 of this book. Here, it is important to showcase the area of sci-

Table 11.1 Top 10 Core Competency Areas in Science and Education (Taken from the TIGER International Recommendation Framework 2.0 [23])

Science and education (S&E)		
	Core competency area	*REL ± SD*
1	*Communication* [n = 218]	91.6 ± 16.1
2	*Teaching, training & education in health care* [n = 220]	89.2 ± 17.9
3	*Leadership* [n = 218]	88.2 ± 17.3
4	Learning techniques [n = 218]	88.1 ± 18.8
5	Ethics in health IT [n = 219]	86.5 ± 21.3
6	Documentation [n = 222]	86.3 ± 21.2
7	Information & knowledge management in patient care [n = 221]	86.3 ± 20.2
8	Principles of health informatics [n = 218]	83.3 ± 23.2
9	Quality & safety management [n = 220]	83.1 ± 22.9
10	Data analytics [n = 218]	81.9 ± 23.6

ence and education as the teachers of health care personnel were specifically surveyed to garner their insights and input, resulting in the following Table 11.1, which demonstrates competencies that are particularly important for educators:

It becomes apparent that in addition to more classical skills such as learning techniques and teaching and training methods, communication, and the ability to lead are of great importance. Likewise, as an overarching skill, ethics plays a stronger role before classical IT knowledge about documentation or principles of health informatics emerge. Educators, therefore, do not need to possess complete knowledge of IT; however, they must have the ability to educate and communicate it to ultimately link this information back to competency attainment. "The aim is to integrate health informatics core competencies into the traditional training, curricula, and courseware (at all educational levels) and to prepare the teachers as gatekeepers and multipliers in education." [24].

The EU*US eHealth Work Project's survey identified 33 core health informatics competency areas targeted toward a broad range of interdisciplinary health professions. The relevance ratings of these competencies for various health care professions (including science and education) were assessed on a scale of 0 to 100. These core competencies areas comprised 718 experts from 51 countries, yielding 1571 relevance ratings [23, 25]. Building on the project's survey results, 22 global case studies were created to highlight and enrich the survey and gap analysis results. The studies bring forth current and future needs to life in practical ways, revealing real-world examples, insights, and remedies meant to be learned from and built upon to overcome challenges within healthcare systems and to further access to education [26].

Health Informatics Priorities in Collaboration with Other Professions

There are differences and overlaps among disciplines in the need for informatics/digital skills across various health professions. These differences and overlaps are especially important for professional fields directly linked to patient care such as nurses, physicians, and so on [25, 27, 28]. This link offers the opportunity to develop further collaborative education and training aligned to competency attainment. Concerning the successful collaboration of different professions, it is vital to find a common language and a basis of trust [27–30]. The following case studies enabled global authors to paint a picture as they took a deep dive into the root of issues and, thus, could illuminate a path to overcome pain points in education and training development.

Case Study #1

Austria: An Online-Based Master's Program in Health Information Management for Health Care Professionals

Case Study 1 describes the Health Information Management (HIM) master's degree program for health care professionals at the Private University of Health Sciences, Medical Informatics and Technology (UMIT TIROL) in Hall in Tirol, Austria. This program began in 2017 as an online-based program focused on management and organizational-oriented access to HI. HIM is defined as the management of health information systems, covering fields such as design, development, introduction, customizing, and application of IT-based innovations in healthcare. The mas-

ter's program targets physicians, nurses, quality managers, process managers, computer scientists working in healthcare, and other health care professionals interested in gaining in-depth knowledge of HIM. Among others, the following topics are covered and thus, reflect acquired competencies such as IT project management, applied computer sciences, process management, interoperability, health IT evaluation, clinical data analytics, as well as data protection and security.

The competencies outlined are entirely taught online using a modern and cooperative instructional design that enables learning together within interdisciplinary groups. The instructional design of the HIM master's degree program matches the needs of part-time students. In particular, all online courses follow the same basic structure: Each course first contains meta-information, including information on learning objectives, content, instructor, and literature. Then, each course consists of a set of weekly learning activities. Each week, a set of learning activities have to be completed by all participants. The learning activities are not meant to test competencies but to allow the students—alone and in interaction with the others—to accomplish the intended learning objectives. Examples for learning activities include reading literature on a given concept, preparing and presenting a case study, searching and presenting additional literature, contrasting different approaches, criticizing a given approach, conducting a statistical analysis, or designing a database schema for a given situation. All communication within the online courses is asynchronous. Students work on learning activities and post messages or reply to messages anytime they want (24/7). The instructor is present each day to answers questions and address problems while also providing tailored input and discussion summaries in response to student feedback and submissions.

Lessons Learned

There is a strong need for academic qualification related to health IT and HIM for healthcare professionals directed at every academic level. Overall, basic informatics modules should be included in medical and nursing programs. At the secondary level, short in-depth intensive courses must be offered to allow healthcare professionals to better understand the field of health IT and HIM. Finally, universities should offer full academic qualifications (such as professional master degrees) to allow healthcare professionals to become experts in health IT and HIM. These programs for health care professionals must be based on a management-oriented and organizational-oriented (and not purely technically oriented) approach to health IT and HIM. Only this allows physicians and nurses to obtain competencies in the field without the need to acquire in-depth technical skills. The program's evaluation showed that the instructional strategy successfully facilitates a trusting, interactive, and collaborative learning environment.

Case Study #2

China: Developing Informatics Competencies of ICU Novice Nurses Based on Miller's Pyramid Model

Case Study 2 describes the Sir Run Run Shaw Hospital (SRRSH), affiliated with the Zhejiang University School of Medicine, established in 1994. Over the last nearly 30 years, the hospital developed into a tertiary, research-oriented general with two campuses (Qingchun and Xiasha) totaling 190,333 square meters with 2400 beds, 32 specialty clinics, 77 nursing units, and 9 ancillary departments. SRRSH was the first Chinese public hospital to be accredited by the Joint Commission International (JCI). SRRSH has also pioneered the "Shaw Hospital Model," which combines Western and Chinese healthcare management methods. In 2017, SRRSH successfully achieved the HIMSS Electronic Medical Record Adoption Model (EMRAM) Stage 7 accreditation. This is an indicator that SRRSH is employing the best level of clinical IT and advanced safety features to provide the best patient care. SRRSH obtained Magnet Hospital in March 2019, the first in China at present.

Recently, the National Health and Family Planning Commission of the People's Republic of China (PRC) raised requirements for core nursing competencies as the growth of the profession has developed substantial evidence which links IT with improved patient safety, care quality, access, and efficiency. SRRSH's main concern was that nurses might not have the required proficiency, and nurse educators did not possess the skill or curriculum for clinical informatics instruction within traditional training methods. To address these potential deficits, nurse managers, educators, and five experienced instructors within the SRRSH intensive care unit (ICU) joined forces to create new activities designed to help new nurses acquire informatics competencies. Ten inexperienced nurses also engaged in the design to better understand how to fully support the new ICU nurses learning needs. They chose Miller's Pyramid as the framework model for this effort. The training was developed into levels inclusive of two components: (1) Teaching Methods and (2) Performance Evaluation:

- **Knows Level**: A self-learning package was delivered via email to all new nurses ahead of class; the online test was taken prior to class.
- **Knows How Level**: Managers, educators, and experienced instructors created a standardized tool based on practice rules and documentation standards. Mind-mapping methodology was employed to examine if new nurses have a clear understanding of workflows.
- **Shows How Level**: Collaboration with an IT vendor to develop a Clinical Information System (CIS) specifically designed for the lecture room; nurses, already using information system for seven months plus, were tested again via a simulated documentation scenario.
- **Do Level**: Development of a scoring scale based upon documentation standards to monitor the quality of electronic documentation; post three months of supervision, new nurses began working independently.

Results & Lessons Learned

The 30 new ICU nurses completed the program and successfully acquired specialized informatics skills. The participants confirmed that peer-led instruction and mind-mapping helped them better understand workflows. They preferred the lecturer to use peer-instruction and mind-mapping as opposed to conventional teaching and testing formats.

SRRSH's orientation model aimed to improve informatics competencies to enhance the performance and efficiency of clinical nursing. Their hospital also constructed an "Advanced Technology Learning Center" that could be leveraged to simulate the clinical practice environment via built-in patient cases and coordinate with realistic manikins (high and low-fidelity human patient simulators). To complement the simulations labs, new nurses were able to apply their recently acquired nursing knowledge to practice patient-care within a safe environment. The standardized high fidelity simulation approach, in compliment to the clinical informatics competency-based training, strived to better patient care and outcomes.

Case Study #3

United States—California: Sutter Health: Informatics Pioneers

Case Study 3 describes Sutter Health, a non-profit unified healthcare network providing comprehensive medical care in more than 100 Northern California cities with 24 acute care hospitals. Sutter has 53,000 employees and 12,000 physicians in their network, making them the eighth largest health system in the United States (U.S).

Status/Current Developments: Sutter Health is made up of 24 acute care hospitals throughout Northern California. Educational materials related to electronic health record (EHR) changes are developed at the system level by the information system (IS) Learning and Transformation team. Each facility takes responsibility for educating EHR users for all upcoming changes. Data from hospitals has shown that many EHR users do not read the system notices, which increases communica-

tion variation and continues to be problematic within hospitals.

A number of Sutter facilities have implemented a "super user" program that is supported financially by operations in order to facilitate education, training, and communication of staff throughout the hospital system. Some of these hospitals have a robust super user group comprised of members that attend monthly or quarterly meetings to obtain information regarding all upcoming EHR changes.

Currently, nurses on the system level informatics team also hold other positions while trying to carry out informatics duties. The deficiency of dedicated nursing informatics (NI) positions at all hospitals, along with missing infrastructure to support this, leads to a lack of preparation and miscommunication for EHR upgrades or enhancements, driving increased dissatisfaction among the staff.

Measures & Results Survey

In 2017, Sutter Health developed an online survey, yielding 76 respondents, consisting of five questions to better understand the current state of informatics for their 150 registered nurses (RNs) throughout the system. The survey questions were as follows:

1. Are you aware of the nursing informatics field/discipline?
2. How would you best define Nursing Informatics?
3. How have you engaged and interacted with Nursing Informaticists within Sutter Health?
4. How different are the roles between an Information Service Analyst and a Nursing Informaticist?
5. Describe how the NI program at Sutter Health could serve their needs.

Lessons Learned

The Sutter Health NI team learned many lessons based upon the survey results, which will be used to tackle the following key themes:

- Communication is critical, particularly in a large health system. Sutter has made numerous changes to enhance partnership and clinical representation across the integrated network to improve transparency and exchange ideas.
- Ongoing training and education is needed to improve informatics competencies and to better address the issues and pain points identified by staff via the survey. Sutter is in the process of developing a NI program that encompasses all aspects of the American Nursing Informatics Associations (ANIA) NI standards of assessment, diagnosis, planning, implementation and evaluation.
- Improve partnership with leaders to continue the development of formal governance structures for EHR changes, the inclusion of informatics in various IS and clinical groups. Senior leadership identified the importance and value of NI throughout the Sutter Health network to continue decreasing documentation burden to prevent clinician burnout.

As a result of these changes, implementations, optimizations, and EHR downtimes have occurred with less interruption to hospital operations. Patient safety has improved as Sutter continues to enhance technology tools that enhance value for patients and clinicians.

Summary

Stepping further into the digitalization of healthcare systems will demand that academic and clinical educators think outside of the box regarding education and training methods and models leveraged to teach the next generation of healthcare professionals. This chapter showcases three global case studies tied to informatics knowledge and competency attainment. We hope that the studies featured, pain points discussed, and resources highlighted, be leveraged to create supplemental resources, curricula, and training materials inspired by the development of competency-based education, tools, and resources from the TIGER ICSP and EU*US eHealth Work Project's publications and competency recommendation frameworks.

Conclusions and Outlook

In the future, global and local curricula must be developed, adapted, and tied to target competencies for each discipline. In the recent past, clinicians and academic educators focused more on computer science skills, while today, there is more of an emphasis on the development of communication, leadership, and ethics in IT skills. This new focus will need to be further explored and reviewed on local and global levels. The case study examples shared and the overarching global case study compilation represent a current section of time, requiring continuous review and refinement, against the backdrop of technical developments, social changes, and clinical practice advancement.

Useful Resources

1. HIMSS TIGER Global Informatics Definitions document: https://www.himss.org/resources/tiger-informatics-definitions
2. HIMSS TIGER International Competency Synthesis Project's Recommendation Frameworks: https://www.himss.org/tiger-initiative-international-competency-synthesis-project.
3. HIMSS Health Informatics Guide: https://www.himss.org/resources/health-informatics
4. EU*US eHealth Work Project page: http://ehealthwork.org/
5. EU*US eHealth Work Project Transatlantic Workforce Case Studies Report and link to each case study compiled under the project: https://www.himss.org/resources/developing-skilled-transatlantic-ehealth-workforce-case-studies-report
6. The HIMSS TIGER Initiative: https://www.himss.org/tiger
7. Sutter Health: https://www.sutterhealth.org/
8. TIGER International Competency Synthesis Project and Recommendation Frameworks for download: https://www.himss.org/tiger-initiative-international-competency-synthesis-project
9. Sir Run Run Shaw Hospital, Zhejiang University School of Medicine: http://www.srrsh-english.com/
10. Private University of Health Sciences, Medical Informatics and Technology

(UMIT) in Hall in Tirol, Austria: https://www.umit-tirol.at

11. Health Informatics Research Group, University of Applied Sciences Osnabrück, Germany: https://www.hs-osnabrueck.de/en/health-informatics-research-group/

Review Questions

1. How often should discipline specific informatics definitions be revisited in scope?
   (a) It is not necessary to revise definition scopes.
   (b) Scopes must be revisited frequently.
   (c) Each discipline should be revisited annually.
   (d) Every year.
   (e) Every five years.

2. True or False: Educators must first understand informatics in order to better teach informatics.
   (a) True
   (b) False

3. The three case studies showcased in this chapter come from the following countries:
   (a) Austria, China, and the U.S.
   (b) Austria, China, and Nigeria
   (c) China, Nigeria, and the U.S.
   (d) Australia, China, and the U.K.
   (e) Australia, Cambodia, and the U.S.

4. How many core health informatics competency areas were identified on the EU*US eHealth Work Project's survey that were woven into the TIGER ICSP's interdisciplinary Recommendation Framework 2.0?
   (a) 22
   (b) 33
   (c) 44
   (d) 55
   (e) 66

Appendix: Answers to Review Questions

1. How often should discipline specific informatics definitions be revisited in scope?

Discipline specific informatics definitions must frequently be revisited in scope. With definitions and scopes changing so rapidly, it makes sense that educators sometimes get lost in a sea of rapidly changing "informatics" terminology that can trigger comprehension challenges.

2. True or False: Educators must first understand informatics in order to better teach informatics

True: Educators must first understand informatics in order to better teach informatics. Although healthcare continues to change rapidly in the digital age, informatics curricula development has not been prioritized and many educators are not well-versed or equipped to properly teach informatics.

3. The three case studies showcased in this chapter come from the following countries:

The three case studies featured in this chapter hail from Austria, China, and the U.S.

4. How many core health informatics competency areas were identified on the EU*US eHealth Work Project's survey that were woven into the TIGER ICSP's interdisciplinary Recommendation Framework 2.0?

The EU*US eHealth Work Project's survey identified 33 core health informatics competences areas targeted toward a broad range of interdisciplinary health professions.

References

1. Arvanitis S, Euripidis NL. Investigating the effects of ICT on innovation and performance of European hospitals: an exploratory study. Eur J Health Econ. 2016;17:403–18. https://doi.org/10.1007/s10198-015-0686-9

2. Davenport T, Kalakota R. The potential for artificial intelligence in healthcare. Future Healthc J. 2019;6(2):94–8. https://doi.org/10.7861/futurehosp.6-2-94

3. Kuperman G. Reflections on AMIA—looking to the future. J Am Med Inform Assoc. 2013;20(e2):e367. https://doi.org/10.1136/amiajnl-2013-002435

4. Williams PAH, Lovelock B, Cabarrus T, Harvey M. Improving digital hospital transformation: development of an outcomes-based infrastructure maturity assessment framework. J Med Internet Res. 2019;7(1):e12465. https://doi.org/10.2196/12465

5. Jobst F. IT zur Prozessgestaltung im Krankenhaus - Wie bekommt man die optimale Kombination von IT-Anwendungen? In: Schlegel H, editor. Steuerung der IT im Klinikmanagement. Wiesbaden: Vieweg + Teubner Verlag; 2010. p. 225–51.

6. Jones SS, Rudin RS, Perry T, Shekelle PG. Health information technology: an updated systematic review with a focus on meaningful use. Ann Intern Med. 2014;160(1):48–54. https://doi.org/10.7326/M13-1531

7. Reddy S, Fox J, Purohit MP. Artificial intelligence-enabled healthcare delivery. J R Soc Med. 2019;112(1):22–8. https://doi.org/10.1177/0141076818815510

8. Shaw Morawski T, Fanberg H, Pitts J. Illuminating the specialty of health informatics. Nurs Manag (Springhouse). 2021;52(11):52–4.

9. HIMSS. HIMSS TIGER global informatics definitions. Chicago: HIMSS; 2020. https://www.himss.org/resources/tiger-informatics-definitions. Accessed 27 Oct 2020

10. Mesko B, Drobni Z, Bényei E, Gergely B, Györffy Z. Digital health is a cultural transformation of traditional healthcare. mHealth. 2017;3(9):38. https://doi.org/10.21037/mhealth.2017.08.07

11. Wilson ML. Health informatics. Aligning core health informatics competencies. Chicago: HIMSS; 2020. https://www.himss.org/resources/health-informatics. Accessed 27 Oct 2020

12. Sapci AH, Sapci HA. Teaching hands-on informatics skills to future health Informaticians: a competency framework proposal and analysis of health care informatics curricula. JMIR Med Inform. 2020;8(1):e15748. https://doi.org/10.2196/15748

13. Fanberg H. Health informatics. Workforce development. Chicago: HIMSS; 2020. https://www.himss.org/resources/health-informatics. Accessed 27 Oct 2020

14. Valamis lifelong learning. https://www.valamis.com/hub/lifelong-learning. Accessed 27 Oct 2020.

15. Hübner U, Shaw T, Thye J, Egbert N, Marin H, Ball M. Towards an international framework for recommendations of core competencies in nursing and inter-professional informatics: the tiger competency synthesis project. Stud Health Technol Inform 2016;228:655–659. https://doi.org/10.3233/978-1-61499-678-1-655

16. Egbert N, Thye J, Hackl W, Müller-Staub M, Ammenwerth E, Hübner U. Competencies for nursing in a digital world. Methodology, results, and use of the DACH recommendations for nursing informatics core competency areas in Austria, Germany, and Switzerland. Inform Health Soc Care. 2018;44(4):351–75. https://doi.org/10.1080/17538157.2018.1497635

17. Hübner U, Shaw T, Egbert N, Marin HF, Chang P, O'Conner S, et al. Technology informatics guiding education reform – TIGER*. An international recommendation framework of core competencies in health informatics for nurses. Methods Inf Med. 2018;57(S01):e30–42. https://doi.org/10.3414/ME17-01-0155

18. Alami H, Gagnon M-P, Fortin J-P. Digital health and the challenge of health systems transformation. mHealth. 2017;3(8):31. https://doi.org/10.21037/mhealth.2017.07.02

19. Breil B. Digitale transformation durch eLearning. In: Matusiewicz D, Pittelkau C, Elmer A, editors. Die Digitale transformation im Gesundheitswesen. Transformation, innovation, disruption. Berlin: MWV Medizinisch Wissenschaftliche Verlagsgesellschaft mbH & Co. KG; 2017. p. 234–8.

20. Tolks D. eLearning in der medizinischen Aus-, Weiter- und Fortbildung. In: Fischer F, Krämer A, editors. eHealth in Deutschland. Anforderungen und Potenziale innovativer Versorgungsstrukturen. Berlin: Springer-Verlag; 2016. p. 223–39.

21. Uprichard K. E-learning in a new era: enablers and barriers to its implementation in nursing. Br J Community Nurs. 2020;25(6):272–5. https://doi.org/10.12968/bjcn.2020.25.6.272

22. Walsh K. Strengthening primary care: the role of e-learning. Educ Prim Care. 2019;30(5):267–9. https://doi.org/10.1080/14739879.2019.1641751

23. Hübner U, Thye J, Shaw T, Elias B, Egbert N, Saranto K, et al. Towards the TIGER international framework for recommendations of core competencies in health informatics 2.0: extending the scope and the roles. Stud Health Technol Inform. 2019;264:1218–22. https://doi.org/10.3233/SHTI190420

24. Thye J. Health informatics. Understanding health informatics core competencies. Chicago: HIMSS; 2020. https://www.himss.org/resources/health-informatics. Accessed 27 Oct 2020

25. Thye J, Shaw T, Hüsers J, Esdar M, Ball MJ, Babitsch B, et al. What are inter-professional eHealth competencies? Stud Health Technol Inform. 2018;253:201–5. https://doi.org/10.3233/978-1-61499-896-9-201

26. Hübner U, Shaw Morawski T, Elias B, Bell S, Blake R. Developing a skilled transatlantic eHealth workforce case studies report. Chicago: HIMSS; 2020. https://www.himss.org/resources/developing-skilled-transatlantic-ehealth-workforce-case-studies-report. Accessed 28 Oct 2020

27. Foronda C, MacWilliams B, McArthure E. Interprofessional communication in healthcare: an integrative review. Nurse Educ Pract. 2016;19:36–40. https://doi.org/10.1016/j.nepr.2016.04.005

28. Gum LF, Sweet L, Greenhill J, Prideaux D. Exploring interprofessional education and collaborative practice in Australian rural health services. J Interprof Care. 2019;34(2):173–83. https://doi.org/10.1080/13561820.2019.1645648

29. Käppeli S. Interprofessional cooperation: why is partnership so difficult? Patient Educ Couns. 1995;26:251–6. https://doi.org/10.1016/0738-3991(95)00755-o

30. Thye J, Hübner U, Weiß JP, Teuteberg F, Hüsers J, Liebe JD, et al. Hospital CEOs need health IT knowledge and trust in CIOs: insights from a qualitative study. Stud Health Technol Inform. 2018;248:40–6. https://doi.org/10.3233/978-1-61499-858-7-40

Part III

Using Data and Information to Generate Knowledge

Learning Health Systems: Concepts, Principles and Practice for Data-Driven Health

12

Jens Rauch and Ursula H. Hübner

Learning Objectives
- To convey the concept of a learning health system (LHS) as a socio-technical system at the junction between care and research.
- To learn core values and drivers of an LHS and their role in governing an LHS.
- To recognize the cyclical nature of an LHS and give examples for each phase.
- To identify the difference between an operational and an analytical information system and the role of data warehouses for these purposes.
- To understand the role of observational data and the practice-based evidence approach.
- To provide examples of how longitudinal observational can be analyzed.

Key Terms
- Learning health system
- Continuous quality improvement
- Data-driven health.
- Data-to-knowledge
- Knowledge-to-performance
- Performance-to-data
- Hierarchical model

- Socio-technical system
- Practice-based evidence
- Evidence-based practice
- Data processing automation
- Forecasts
- Benchmarks
- Research support
- Real-time monitoring
- Lhs governance
- Culture
- Trust-building
- Lhs core values
- Data warehouse
- Operative information system
- Analytical information system
- Extract-transform-load processes
- Observational data
- Data analytics
- Survival time analysis
- Time series analysis
- Patient phenotyping

Introduction

A Learning Health System (LHS) is an overarching concept of a data-driven learning organization. Learning organizations follow the idea of continuous quality improvement through cycles of learning. These learning cycles are determined by input into the cycles, performance of the organization, and feedback based on the performance.

J. Rauch
University AS Osnabrück, Osnabrueck, Germany
e-mail: j.rauch@hs-osnabrueck.de

U. H. Hübner (✉)
University of Applied Sciences (UAS) Osnabrück,
Osnabrück, Niedersachsen, Germany
e-mail: U.Huebner@hs-osnabrueck.de

© Springer Nature Switzerland AG 2022
U. H. Hübner et al. (eds.), *Nursing Informatics*, Health Informatics,
https://doi.org/10.1007/978-3-030-91237-6_12

For example, an organization that strives at improving the patient handover and transfer processes needs to describe these processes (data input), analyze, and evaluate them with regard to key indicators such as access to up-to-date patient information (performance) and provide information to change these processes accordingly (feedback). These loops are governed by the concept of improving the organization in terms of

- resources (structural quality), for example qualified staff,
- adapting the patient care processes to the current needs (process quality), for example lean processes,
- and gaining new insights into health conditions and their treatment in general (outcome quality), for example fewer complications.

As a result of this, the entire learning cycle can be divided into three phases: *data-to-knowledge, knowledge-to-performance*, and *performance-to-data* [1]. For an integrated view on a patient or group of patients to be obtained, it is necessary to extract data from multiple heterogeneous individual systems and integrate them into a comprehensive IT infrastructure. Its purpose is to make the data available in a standardized form and to provide algorithms for knowledge acquisition. This step is called the *data-to-knowledge* phase [1] and it is typically implemented through *data warehouses* and subsequent data analysis via classical statistics or machine learning (ML). The translation of newly acquired knowledge is called the *knowledge-to-performance phase*. Data on patient care is mainly generated and captured internally at the point of care, that is, in the electronic health record (EHR) of health care institutions. Management of data capture and storage is called the *performance-to-data phase*. Relevant external data is located in further systems (e.g., scientific databases and information systems of federal offices for environmental data). The cycle can start anew analyzing data in the *data-to-knowledge* phase. Health informatics strives to answer questions of how information technology can support the prerequisites for an LH in all phases.

Thus, an LHS resides at the junction of patient care and health sciences research, for example, neurology and brain research, nursing practice and nursing science, process engineering, and health service research. It is a mechanism of weaving research findings from analyzing observational data from the practice, for example, from EHRs, immediately into the practice. This is why this approach is sometimes called *practice-based evidence* to contrast *evidence-based practice*, that is, utilizing medical guidelines based on randomized controlled trials (RCTs) to guide patient care. Although these two approaches reflect different methods, they can be used in a synergistic way so that RCT findings stimulate the analysis of observational data or vice versa. While *evidence-based practice* represented by RCT-based guidelines is criticized for its long dissemination process, the hope that goes along with *practice-based evidence* is to generate new knowledge from large amounts of observational data nearly in real-time (Fig. 12.1).

Speaking in practical terms, LHSs are socio-technical systems composed of care delivery organizations that employ information technology (IT) to continuously generate new knowledge from data of their patients and other sources to improve patient care [2]. Socio-technical means that such systems are constituted of the people of the organization and of the technology used for collecting, storing, communicating, analyzing, and visualizing the data. There are further terms, such as *learning systems for healthcare*. They are largely used synonymously and typically refer to individual organizations or networks of organizations. Sometimes *rapid* or *high-functioning* is added to emphasize that IT is intended to accelerate and comprehensively expand the transformation from data into knowledge. The notion of a health system does not necessarily refer to a national health system. An LHS may be implemented at the level of single institutions (e.g., hospitals), health systems (e.g., hospital groups) as well as at the level of regions, countries, or the supra-national level that is, involving several countries.

LHSs are inevitably connected with the ongoing digitization of society, especially in the health care sector with its increasing availability of accu-

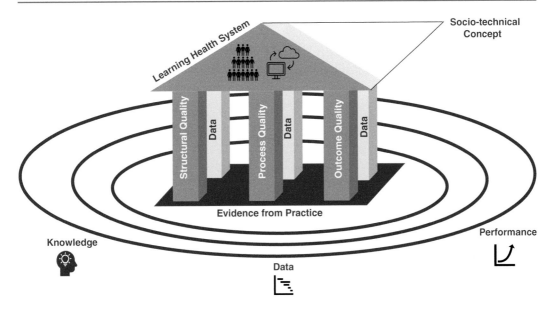

Fig. 12.1 Concept of a Learning Health System: the learning organization that rests on evidence in a rapid data-driven system to improve the quality of patient care

rate and comprehensive health-related data. This trend will enhance the benefits arising from LHSs since new knowledge can be continuously gained from the newly obtained data. This data may range from patient and process characteristics (e.g., multi-morbidities and sequences of treatment events) to factors impacting the state of health of individuals and public life (e.g., air quality, public activity, weather, and traffic recordings). One of the most significant challenges within health informatics is making these kinds of data accessible so that they can be used to better health care [3]. While new evidence and decision support on clinical and health care issues that arises from an LHS can be offered to health care professionals [4], patients can expect benefits from a more effective, more efficient, and safer care, for example, reduced waiting times through better use of resources, *precision medicine* through better capturing patient characteristics [5].

cal models, depending on their focus. While the hierarchical models describe how LHSs can be implemented by IT at the micro, meso and macro-level of a health system, the cyclical models focus on the learning and feedback cycle of continuous production of evidence. The cyclical models thus correspond to a process view of an LHS because they represent how data and knowledge must continuously flow between the individual phases or components of the learning system (e., g. health care professionals, systems for data capture, integration, and evaluation). In contrast, hierarchical models provide a static view by showing the purposes and context of an LHS at the levels of the hierarchy. Here, the focus is not on the process of learning or data flow but rather on the components, purpose, and context of LHS at the various levels of the health care system.

Models and Dimensions of a Learning Health System

There is a whole range of conceptual reference models for the use of IT for LHSs [1, 6–10]. These models can be divided into hierarchical and cycli-

Cyclical Models

Cyclical models describe the phases into which the IT-supported feedback cycle of an LHS can be divided. The most widely accepted model is that of Friedman et al. [1], which distinguishes between the three phases *performance-to-data* (P2D), *data-to-knowledge* (D2K), and

Fig. 12.2 Learning
health system—cyclical
model

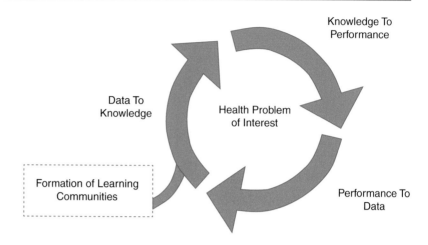

knowledge-to-performance (K2P) (Fig. 12.2). The model describes a process of iterative improvement of health services, in which knowledge is gained from data (D2K). This knowledge can then be used to improve the quality of care (K2P). Changing care practice will in turn, entail new and changed data traces so that the process can continue [6]. The external path in Fig. 12.1 indicates that groups of learning systems, that is, learning communities, can form collectives, supplying each other with data [11].

Hierarchical models

The Heimdall model by McLachlan et al. [10] and the model by Rouse et al. [9] belong to the hierarchical models (Fig. 12.3). Both models describe IT's role within an LHS at the levels of the individual, organization, and society. The Heimdall model starts at the level of the patient, for whom an LHS provides individual knowledge (e.g., for shared decision support in the choice of a therapy or the calculation of an individual risk). At the level of the organization, processes and resource provision can be optimized, e.g., the prediction of patient numbers and the minimization of waiting times. At the societal level, that is, regional, national, or transnational, the information infrastructure of an LHS serves to monitor health care for the population as a whole or for subgroups: this includes the promotion of research and benchmarking of care services. The model by Rouse

et al. [9] briefly presents the beneficial aspects of LHSs on four hierarchical levels and additionally lists IT components supporting the LHS [10]. It is shown that quality indicators can be derived from EHR data, from which knowledge can be gained for decision support in an organization. By exchanging data across organizations (health information exchange (HIE)) and analyzing them, it is possible to describe populations and derive health policy measures. At the national and international level, studies can be conducted with integrated data from many sources in order to develop improved guidelines for health care.

Dimensions of a Learning Health System

The overarching goal of an LHS is to improve the quality of healthcare. This can be achieved in a variety of ways using IT. A typology for the use of IT has been proposed by [12]. They identify six dimensions on which a given system can be classified (Table 12.1):

Automation describes the extent to which the system automatically performs routine procedures, for example, filling out forms, providing building blocks for patient summaries, thereby relieving the health care staff from routine tasks, intended to increase safety and to speed up the process. In an LHS, the automated provision of data ready for analysis is another excellent example.

Fig. 12.3 Learning
health system—
hierarchical model

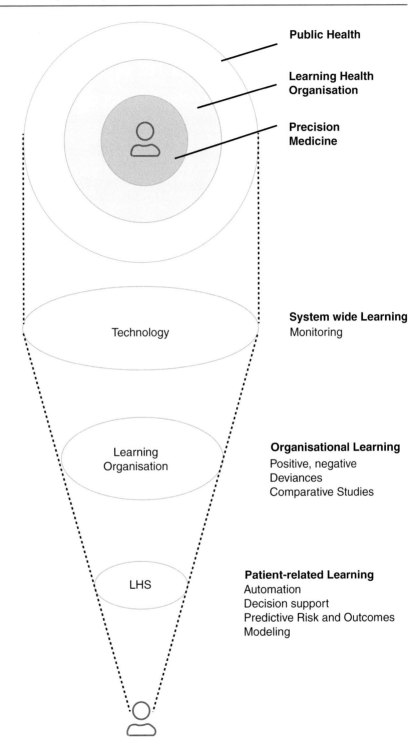

Public Health

Learning Health
Organisation

Precision
Medicine

System wide Learning
Monitoring

Organisational Learning
Positive, negative
Deviances
Comparative Studies

Patient-related Learning
Automation
Decision support
Predictive Risk and Outcomes
Modeling

Table 12.1 Dimensions of an LHS with examples

Dimensions	Examples
Automation	Pre-populated forms for ordering lab tests
Benchmarks	Comparison with the best in emergency department throughput
Forecasts	Consumption of medical products such as wound dressings, prescription of antibiotics
Decision support	Decision support in differential diagnosis of a chronic wound
Real-time monitoring	Infection rate of newborns
Research support	Identification of patient cohorts for heart failure and patients older than 65 years

Benchmarks allow health care providers or their organizational units, for example, departments or teams to compare themselves with one another over time based on predefined quality metrics. In this way, best practices can be identified in addition to success criteria and risk factors. These quality indicators can be computed from regularly captured data, hinting at potentials for improvements.

Forecasts are assertions about the likelihood of future events or developments. They may concern factors within the organization, for example, bed occupancy, resource consumption, or maybe patient-related topics, for example, occurrence of adverse events or the success rate of a treatment.

The system provides *decision support* when it gives data-driven recommendations to users in decision-making situations, for example, with respect to therapy or preventive measures.

Real-time monitoring refers to the capability of the system to display data resulting from care-related events with minimal time delay. In this way, situations requiring intervention, for example, supply bottlenecks, increased infection rates, or adverse events can be identified immediately, and appropriate measures may be taken.

Research support refers to the extent to which the system enables scientific studies to be conducted based on routine data, for example, for pragmatic clinical trials investigating the outcome of a treatment regime.

The dimensions, *automation, forecasting* and *decision support* are by design rather tied to the individual characteristics of a given health organization. This is because these aspects are strongly dependent on local conditions and idiosyncrasies, such as equipment available, range of therapies provided, facilities, and human resources. In contrast, the other three dimensions, *benchmarking, real-time monitoring and research support,* possess cross-organizational potential. The larger the circle of participating organizations, the more likely it is that different approaches with both positive and negative effects on the quality of care will be identified. Real-time monitoring of environmental events, on the other hand, would make it possible to mobilize the right resources at all health care facilities nearby promptly in the event of extreme situations, for example, disasters, epidemics [13]. Finally, *research support*, refers to the goal of analyzing data more quickly and on a broader scale to provide evidence for health care in a real-time manner [14].

The literature on LHSs mainly discusses approaches with cross-organizational goals, as these are expected to have a much broader impact on public health and the quality of care [6, 12]. However, the heterogeneous landscape of health care makes the use of health IT standards necessary. When regional, national, or even transnational initiatives are to be established, cooperation rules have to be implemented. These rules pertain to routine data initially generated at the point of care and are subject to the administration of the respective service provider [14, 15]. Previous project initiatives pursued this goal according to a top-down approach and thus, started with joint data integration for networks of health care organizations. This approach has proven to be very costly due to the large number of heterogeneous systems and organizational obstacles [16]. For this reason, Smoyer et al., [16] recommend a bottom-up approach, which first establishes local LHSs for individual health care facilities, and only then merges them into cross-organizational networks (Fig. 12.4).

This *bottom-up* approach intends to start with the individual institution to prepare and use their

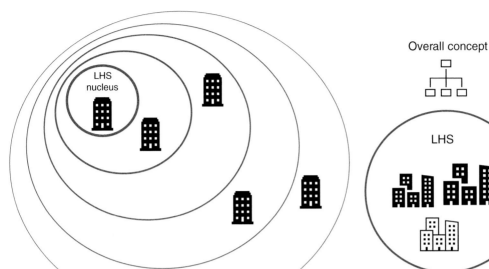
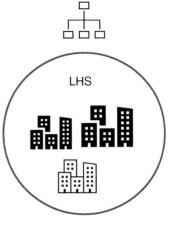

Fig. 12.4 Bottom-up development of an LHS (left), top-down development of an LHS (right)

data for knowledge acquisition. The resulting systems can then gradually be developed into a regional, national, and transnational LHS in order to anchor them on the macro level of the entire national health care system [10, 17]. These local LHSs not only serve as the starting point for larger LHS but also allow the health care providers to focus and analyze their own data, an approach that may go along with greater trust in the results.

Governance and Management of a Learning Health System

LHSs as socio-technical systems are inherently complex and require a systematic approach to governing and managing the structures, processes, and outcomes. Friedman and colleagues [1] name core values of an LHS as high-level guiding principles and mission statements: LHSs embrace values that relate to individuals, families, communities, and populations as the focus of an LHS that have to benefit from all its undertakings. These LHS essentials stipulate that an LHS has to provide added value in terms of health care quality and affordability. Outcomes should be accessible and transparent to all its partici-

pants to instill trust and demonstrate added value. The process to achieve these outcomes is underpinned by applying rigorous scientific methods to ensure data integrity, including all efforts to safeguard privacy. In terms of participants, it has to be inclusive, allowing for interested groups to join and participate. A cooperative leadership respects the diverse stakeholders. LHS leaders apply governance rules to enable trustful, stable, and sustainable cooperation while also allowing for flexibility and adaptability of goals and procedures.

As a new structure in a well-established environment, an LHS has to apply a governance model that meets the established core values and fits into the traditional settings of providing care. The model is dependent upon the type of LHS. As Lessard and colleagues summarized, within an organization, (e.g., a single hospital or group of hospitals), a matrix structure could be the solution of choice —where the lines represent the different domains, (e.g., medical and health sciences, informatics, and technology, data management, and ethics), and the columns stand for clinical departments and care units. Combining different organizations as communities of practice, network models that reflect the relationship between the organizations as the nodes in the network seem to be more appropriate. In any case, the involvement of patients and patient representatives is mandatory to ensure that the goals of the LHS meet the core values as outlined above and the use of the patient data complies with ethical understandings and public interests [18].

In order for an LHS to survive the project status, a reliable and stable funding scheme must be put into place. This can include federal and regional state funding either for research or for care delivery. However, other funding sources have to be considered that originate in the organizations involved. They are the ones who have to identify their interests and benefits in such an endeavor, as they are the ones who have to provide the resources such as staff, time, and equipment. Thus, one evaluation criterion is the programmatic return on investment [19].

Applications and Challenges of Learning Health Systems

Since the publication of the results from the initial Institute of Medicine (IOM) workshop on an LHS [2], a great number of LHS initiatives emerged on different themes, including different numbers of players and pursuing different goals. All of them share the vision of data-driven continuous quality improvements. Hereby, a cyclical approach constitutes the underlying understanding of an LHS, and an LHS culture serves as the main driver [20].

These findings were further substantiated regarding the vital contribution of an LHS culture, which embraces governance, vision, and leadership to ensure their success. The alliance of the various stakeholders, for example, clinicians, administrators, and industry, is forged and managed by LHS leaders and champions. Continuity and sustainability are achieved by ongoing learning and feedback loops that become "business as usual". For the clinical workforce to become active LHS users, they must have the right skills and competencies, including data literacy. LHSs are not free; they consume resources inclusive of a financial budget and time must be adequately allo-

cated. Finally, the data systems, as an LHS prerequisite, enable access, storage, linkage of datasets and platforms for retrieval and visualization [21].

Three examples of LHSs are presented to illustrate these guiding principles:

Example 1

The Veterans Health Administration belongs to the US Department of Veterans Affairs (VA), and is the largest integrated health care system in the country, which provides care at 1,255 health care facilities, including medical centers and outpatient sites of care [22]. It operates an extensive network of EHRs. A clinical data warehouse integrates patient data from local EHRs to make them available for application in a nationwide LHS. To improve the quality of care for veterans with a transient ischemic attack (TIA) and thus reduce the stroke risk, the VA started the PREVENT program as an LHS application [23]. The primary outcome is the provision of all types of care TIA patients are eligible for, such as anticoagulation therapy, brain imaging, carotid imaging, and statin therapy. A dashboard serves as a hub for the LHS that integrates and visualizes data on the performance of a hospital site which allows benchmarking. The dashboard serves as a source of clinical guidelines and other educational and scientific material. It is intended to be used as a meeting place for teams from different locations in the VA and professions. When evaluating this system, the users appreciated the access to data and their integration as well as the opportunity to monitor the progress in their own department. They found that it motivated teams to drill down to individual cases when overall rates got worse or did not meet the expectations. This contributed to active team learning and establishing a community of practice across the organization involving providers from different departments and reaching a multidisciplinary approach to achieve quality improvements. The hub turned out to be a catalyst for learning how to learn [23].

Example 2

The Michigan Surgical Quality Initiative [24] is a regional undertaking that comprises 70 hospitals in Michigan including those with major surgery. Organized as a regional LHS, it seeks to reduce opioid consumption of patients and fight the problem of opioid abuse. The LHS cycle is organized in three phases: The "performance to data" phase embraces the inclusion of new variables on pain killer prescription, consumption, and the perception of pain. The "data to knowledge" phase revealed that far less opioids were consumed than prescribed. This notion led to new prescription guidelines within the "knowledge to performance" phase. Continuous follow-up measures indicated that the prescription rate dropped steadily while the patients did not report more pain. The current data and their trend over time are displayed on a dashboard. The dissemination of these findings include, amongst others monitoring the refill requests and extending the LHS activities to all types of surgeries. To ensure the sustainability of these efforts and results, the hospitals offer incentives to the clinicians focused on reducing the administrative work and offering continuing medical education credit points for participating in meetings and calls of the LHS activities for reducing opioid prescription [24].

Example 3

The National Health Service (NHS) in England and Wales is the United Kingdom's national public health system. Clinical Commissioning Groups (CCGs) are bodies within the NHS consisting of general practitioners, clinical care providers, care consultants, and laymen responsible for planning and commissioning care in a local area. An LHS infrastructure was established within the NHS Health and Social Care Network to aid CCGs in monitoring antibiotic prescription in primary care and feedback these results to the health care providers at the patient and practice level. The antibiotics prescription dashboard displays longitudinal prescription rates for each practice and compares them to the national average, the type of antibiotic prescribed by infection, deviations from recommendations of the guidelines, and prescription behavior in relation to the risk to obtain a poor clinical outcome. The involvement of stakeholders, an active participatory design of the dashboard and the data provided were meant to increase the acceptance by care providers. Implemented in 70 primary care centers today, it is intended to be rolled out throughout the country to form a national learning health system. As a result of this, it is expected to reduce the number of unjustified antibiotic prescriptions [25].

While the concept and rationale of harnessing observational data in EHRs for generating actionable knowledge are straightforward, some challenges come along with it. First and foremost, access to the data in terms of technical, syntactic, and semantic access as well as legal access belong to the most significant problems to be solved. A centralized procedure, where data from different care delivery organizations are integrated into a single database, comes with the organizations' unwillingness to "give away" the data without really knowing what happens to it. Instead, federal solutions favoring local sovereignty and on-premises data analysis offer an alternative to the centralized approach. Pooled parameters of the local prediction models are then used to fine-tune and update the central prediction model. However, interoperability is an issue here as well. Using common data models (CDM) helps to overcome the problem of different data representations in electronic health records. The Observational Medical Outcomes

Partnership (OMOP) CDM is an example of such a model that has been developed, promoted, and extensively used by the Observational Health Data Sciences and Informatics (OHDSI) group to leverage big data worldwide for building clinical evidence. OMOP was developed to identify and characterize patient populations, predict the occurrence of a clinical phenomenon (e.g. condition, outcome) for individual patients and estimate the effect of interventions [26].

Also, unstructured data as found in clinical notes and reports can be exploited using natural language processing and mapping the relevant clinical entities to the CDM concepts. Semantic interoperability can be achieved by expressing clinical content in Systematized Nomenclature of Medicine Clinical Terms (SNOMED-CT) and Logical Observation Identifiers Names and Codes (LOINC), which is recommended by OHDSI. This procedure has been successfully applied to pathology reports as a data source for colon cancer patients, which were then merged with genomics data [27].

Evaluation of Learning Health Systems

The evaluation of an LHS is tied to the system's scope and requirements, both of which can be classified along the hierarchy, phase cycle, and dimensions that have been presented above. Overall measures of the performance of an LHS embrace the indicator cascade of:

- Knowledge-to-action latency, that is the time needed to put the data-driven knowledge into everyday practice,
- Systematic adoption of evidence, that is, performance of new practices, procedures, and processes based on evidence and
- Systematic elimination of harmful, inefficient and wasteful practices based on the evidence about good performance.

More indicators include patients' care experience, the work-life experience of the health workforce, and equity of care. Also, economic considerations such as utilization-cost measures and return on investment are relevant criteria for evaluating the outcome of an LHS. Finally, the impact on population health can be used as a high-level measure to evaluate an LHS [19].

Considering the phase cycle, the initial challenge is usually to integrate and make available data from clinical and administrative systems in the first place. This initial step can be seen as an outcome of the performance-to-data phase. Here, measures of success are the quality of the data and the ease of data access for health care professionals and data scientists. The data-to-knowledge phase requires appropriate algorithms to explore the data, test hypotheses, and visualize the findings. The outcome of this phase is to arrive at clinically meaningful findings that impact daily practice. Finally, the knowledge-to-performance phase is the stage in which interventions are designed and put in place, making use of the new knowledge. As a result of this, the outcome to be evaluated is the availability and implementation of such intervention. Only once the cycle has been run through entirely for the first time, the LHS as such can be evaluated in terms of clinical outcomes. In any case, all stakeholders, that is, patients and their relatives, health care and administrative professionals, researchers, as well as public health officials, should be considered to partake in such efforts.

The Technology of a Learning Health System

Since LHSs rely heavily on IT infrastructure, the concepts of information systems and data warehouses play an essential role. They must be understood as the technological backbone of an LHS. Information systems can be defined as software systems that "capture, transmit, store, retrieve, manipulate, or display information, thereby supporting people, organizations, or other software systems" [28]. There are two global types of information systems, which differ

Table 12.2 Operative versus analytical information systems

	Operative information systems	Analytical information systems
Purpose	Day-to-day information capture and retrieval, serves as legal document	Data analysis and visualization, research
Examples	Electronic health record systems, clinical information systems	Data warehouses with databases
Usage	documentation, retrieval	Forecasts, decision support, benchmarking, and others
Data types	Structured and unstructured data	Structured data
Architecture	Centralized and decentralized / distributed	Centralized and decentralized / distributed
Layers	vendor dependent	Data sources, staging layer, core integration layer, presentation layer, analytics software, frontend
Data quality	Heterogeneous	Transformed, cleaned and standardized data
Mode of operation	Manual input or data capture from medical devices	Extraction, transformation and loading (ETL) of data from operative into analytical information system
Role in LHS	Source of data	Integral part for data-driven learning

with respect to their aim, implementation, and data (Table. 12.2).

On the one hand, *operative information systems* focus on operative management, that is, supporting day-to-day operations in terms of information capture and retrieval. EHR systems and health information systems are typical examples. These systems are designed to provide fast and immediate data processing and access. For example, patient data being recorded at the regis-

tration desk of a hospital or medical prescriptions being updated during ward rounds are common tasks supported by these types of systems. In a health care organization, systems from different vendors may be in operation, resulting in a heterogeneous systems landscape. Within healthcare, it is reasonable to distinguish between administrative and clinical information systems. While the former are involved in administrative tasks such as registration, billing, scheduling, procurement, resource allocation, and alignment, the latter are used for all varieties of clinical tasks spanning documentation, diagnosis, and therapy [29]. Clinical information systems provide data and information to core processes of a health organization associated with patient care, that is, diagnostics, therapy, and rehabilitation. Administrative information systems provide supportive processes for the organization. While these systems used to be disjunctive in the past, more and more data from both system types are merged, for example, patient diagnoses from the EHR and materials data, such as endoprosthesis data from the materials management system.

Analytical information systems, on the other hand, predominantly serve analytical purposes, that is, enabling the extraction of knowledge from data and providing decision support [30]. Rather than capturing and providing small bits of data during the day-to-day health care provision, these systems are built upon the data stemming from the various operative information systems. As such, analytical information systems typically need to be tailored to extract and integrate data from heterogeneous systems landscape. Thus, a central requirement for these systems is a central integrated data storage, usually implemented as a data warehouse.

Analytical information systems must be an integral part of any LHS. Medical and health-related data usually have a high degree of complexity [31]. Most data also originate from a variety of heterogeneous operative source systems. This makes it necessary for LHSs to integrate the source data so that a uniform view and use of the data is possible, enabling analytical information systems.

Information systems are built upon databases. A database is, in its most conventional form, a collection of data tables, where each table holds data pertaining to a relevant concept (e.g., patient, medication, ward, lab results, etc.). The rows of a column represent individual instances of a concept (e.g., a patient, a lab result), while the columns represent attributes (e.g., date of birth, type of lab test). This type of data is called structured data. There are, of course, references between tables that allow data to be linked so that specific questions can be answered (e.g., "What test results have been obtained for a patient?"). In addition, databases provide a set of functions to filter and summarize data. Databases that use this conventional table representation of data are called *relational* databases, and the standard language to query these is SQL. Other types of databases, termed No-SQL databases, deviate from the relational data representation [12]. Other common approaches are document-based databases for unstructured data, which hold information objects (e.g., discharge letters, reports) as documents that do not need to pertain to a table-like format but follow other structures (e.g., XML, JSON).

The need for data integration and standardization stems from the possibility that the same kinds of information can be represented in databases in many ways. Data presented in a table or as a document is incompatible. But even within purely relational database tables, many possible data models arise. This is called *data heterogeneity.*

Both distributed and centralized approaches to data integration for LHS are being pursued [32]. The two approaches have their advantages and disadvantages [33]. Distributed solutions are particularly suitable when regulatory obstacles in organizational networks make central data integration difficult [1]. This is the case with cross-organizational LHSs that are developed according to the top-down principle. In this vein, a common global data schema is developed for all participating institutions, but without the data being kept centrally (Uniform Data Access). To ensure that data can still be accessed in all systems, interoperability must be established via standard-ization between the systems in such distributed solutions. This is achieved by standardized interfaces (e.g., HL7 FHIR) and data models (OpenEHR, OMOP), which provide a unified means to represent health-related data [34–36] and terminologies (e.g., SNOMED-CT).

On the other hand, central data warehouses are used as a central and high-performance integration solution (Common Data Storage) for analytical information systems [37–39]. For LHSs that are confined to a single organization, in which all data are available locally and integrated centrally, this is a more suitable approach. In this case, there is no strict need for standardization because the data models are predetermined by the source data and may be implemented ad hoc. However, the implementation of standardized interfaces and associated data models becomes necessary when several organizational LHSs are connected.

A data warehouse is implemented via a central database system, which in turn is divided into several layers. Usually, there are at least three layers (Fig. 12.5): an input layer (staging), which initially receives source data; a central layer (core integration layer), in which an integrated data schema unifies all data, places them in relation to each other and records temporal changes (historization); as well as a data presentation layer (consisting of specialized data marts), which is subdivided into specialized data stores (data marts) that arrange data for subsequent thematic analyses. The extended view on a data warehouse includes the data source layer and an analytical and frontend layer (Fig. 12.5).

For a data warehouse, the choice of a database depends on the type of data that is integrated and later analyzed. When we deal mainly with unstructured data, document databases are preferred (i.e., written texts and images that are possibly related and tagged by meta-information). Our interest here is to follow analytical routes like text mining or image analyses. Structured data, like patient demography data, lab results, diagnoses, treatment pathways, are usually in a table format and would be integrated within a relational database. Moreover, analysis of these types of data is done in the table format, too.

Fig. 12.5 Data
warehouse layers

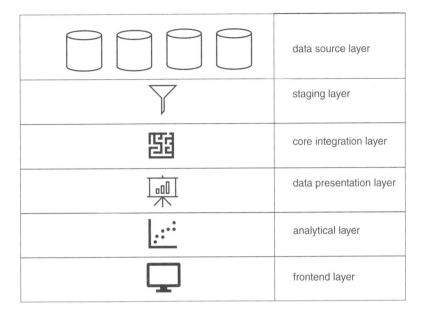

	data source layer
	staging layer
	core integration layer
	data presentation layer
	analytical layer
	frontend layer

Almost all statistics software tools work with data tables that are directly interoperable with relational databases.

While architectural layers and data schemas describe a structural view of a data warehouse, a dynamic view describes the data flow between the different layers of the data warehouse. Specifically, mappings between source and target data models need to be developed. The actual data streams are realized by Extract-Transform-Load (ETL) processes. Each of these specifies queries from a data source, transformations realizing the data integration, and a target for the transformed data. ETL processes are typically developed with specialized data integration software tools (e.g., Pentaho Data Integration).

Data Analytics in a Learning Health System

The analysis layer that builds on top of an integrated data store, such as the data warehouse, is less formalized than the data integration layer. This is because the procedure of data analysis is strongly oriented toward target groups evaluating the data and research questions that need to be answered. Depending on the end-users' methodological skills, simple reports, dashboards, reporting software, statistical programming, or data mining are used in the analysis layer [30]. To obtain new evidence from data, advanced methods must be employed that go beyond simple descriptive statistics, that is, means, distributions via histograms and trends via scatterplots. Moreover, assertions from descriptive analyses refer to the observed data only and may not be generalizable to future observations and other samples. Table 12.3 gives an overview of analytical methods. This overview is not exhaustive, and several methods have significant overlaps in particular data mining and machine learning.

Compared to classical conformational statistics, data mining algorithms are mainly used for exploratory analysis and pattern recognition in large data sets. In contrast, the more formal approach to inferential statistics involves verifying preconditions and proceeds strictly hypothesis-led [40], that is, clear assumptions leading the analysis. Methods from both areas are equally used for the acquisition of knowledge from databases in Learning Health Systems [41]. The central question for data mining, as well as for classical statistical analyses, is what data analytical methods are suitable for which questions. The diversity of possible questions that can arise from complex data in an LHS is reflected accordingly in the wealth of methods already in use [38].

Table 12.3 Overview of analytical methods

Analytical Method	Purpose	Examples
Descriptive statistics	Describe sample, obtain overview	Age distribution of patients in emergency department
Classical inferential statistics	Hypotheses testing	Do young physicians prescribe antibiotics more often than older physicians?
Data mining	Data exploration for new patterns, outliers (anomaly) detection, dependencies (associations, sequences)	Patient phenotyping, e.g., defining homogenous subgroups in obese patients
Time series analysis	Analysis of longitudinal data: detection of patterns and change, forecasting	Survival analysis of patients with full functional recovery from stroke, ARIMA time series models for forecasting the occupancy of ICU beds for COVID-19 patients
Machine Learning	Supervised learning, clustering, reduction of dimensions, structured prediction, anomaly detection, neural networks, reinforcement learning	Classification of chronic wounds from wound images, prediction of therapy outcomes

Some of the most appropriate methods in use with LHSs are survival analysis, time series analysis, and patient phenotyping, which will be introduced next. While the first and second approaches can be classified as statistical models, patient phenotyping tends to be more exploratory and belongs rather in the field of data mining. Finally, some issues of more advanced approaches relating to machine learning and artificial intelligence will be discussed.

The aim of *survival analysis* is to model the time course until the occurrence of certain events, such as hospital discharge, re-admission,

or death [42]. The time course is modeled via a survival function that gives the probability that the event will not occur before time t (Fig. 12.6). The complement of this function is the lifetime distribution function that is the probability of the event occurring before time t. The so-called hazard function is the momentary rate of event occurrence under the condition that the event has not happened before t. Predictor variables can be examined with respect to their effect on the hazard function for a given patient; for instance, a drug prescribed to prevent the occurrence of an infection might lower the infection risk by a certain percentage. Alternatives to classical survival analysis are Restricted Mean Survival Time [45].

While survival analysis can be seen as a special case, *time series analysis* generally deals with the prediction of trends and recurrent patterns in highly time-varying measures (Fig. 12.7). For instance, the number of patients arriving at an emergency department, the number of infections of a contagious disease or the prescribed dosages of a medication. A common approach is Autoregressive-Moving-Average (ARMA) models that aim to forecast a time series by decomposing its past course into portions of signal and noise [46]. In the moving average (MA) part of the model, forecasted value is composed of a fixed value and random noise. The autoregressive (AR) part of the model decomposition is given by a fixed value and a linear combination of the time series' prior values. Both parts are put into superposition to obtain an ARMA model. To account for a trend in the time series, the ARMA model may be applied to step-wise differences of the time series instead, which is called the integrated ARMA (ARIMA) model. When seasonal trends are present in the time series, additional seasonal AR and MA terms can be introduced (SARMA). External predictors might be added to the model, especially other time series that are thought to relate and precede the time series of interest. These are then called ARMAX models. Linear dependencies between several time series can be examined by cross-correlation [47]. The Granger causality test is suitable to determine the usefulness of a time series as an external predictor for a prediction [48].

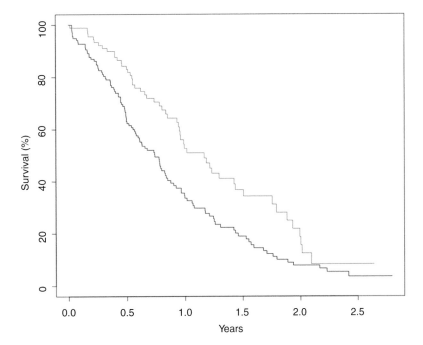

Fig. 12.6 Survival function—survival data for lung cancer patients (females in red, males in black) shown as a Kaplan-Meyer curve. Data from [43, 44]

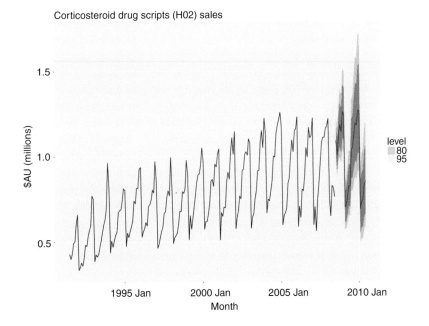

Fig. 12.7 Forecasts from an ARIMA model applied to monthly Australian corticosteroid (H02) prescription data (Australian $). The time series marked in blue denotes the predicted values and their range. Data stem from [46]

Phenotyping is a relatively new approach for identifying clusters of patients who resemble one another in terms of clinical appearance (phenotype). The aim is to find coherent and homogeneous groups of patients who behave similarly (Table 12.4). As such, methods used in this domain are primarily exploratory algorithms that are designed to find patterns of similarity. Similarity may be limited to specific process data [49] as well as biophysical signals (e.g., ECG, blood samples) [50] or might be extended over an entire array of patient EHR data making use of clinical notes [51]. The finding of coherent groups may be useful in predicting the future

Table 12.4 Diagnose clusters (triage) for frequent emergency department users obtained through non-negative matrix factorization [49]

Cluster	Summary	CCS codes	TOP ICD10	TOP ACSC (main diagnoses)
I	Nutritional deficiencies, infections, hypertension, gastritis & duodenitis; triage: 30 min	259, 3, 55, 159, 98,155, 52	Z74, B96.2, E87, N39.0, I10	Diseases of urinary system, intestinal infectious diseases
II	Device or implant complication, injuries, wounds, fractures; triage: 30–120 min; no admission	237, 239, 235, 205	T83, S30.0, S01, M54	Mental and behavioral disorders due to use of alcohol or opioids, back pain
III	Immobility, dementia, incontinence; triage: unspecific	95, 163, 68, 254	R26, F03, R39, Z50	Diseases of urinary system, metabolic disorders
IV	Heart failure, chronic renal failure, cardiac dysrhythmias; triage: 10 min	108, 259, 158, 106	I50.1, Z92.1, N18, I48	Heart failure, ischemic heart diseases, bronchitis & COPD

Legend: *CCS* Clinical Classification Software; *ACSC* Ambulatory Care Sensitive Conditions, *COPD* Chronic Obstructive Pulmonary Disease.

patient trajectories, assessing treatment risk, or estimating outcomes based on the other group members' data. Techniques used range from simple cluster algorithms (e.g., k-means) over factor analysis and principal component analysis to elaborate data mining (e.g., non-negative matrix factorization, Gaussian process regression) and machine learning algorithms (e.g., autoencoders, deep belief networks).

Apart from statistics and data mining, and due to its successes in the domain of artificial intelligence, machine learning plays an increasing role in the modeling of health-related data. Especially when it comes to classification and labeling tasks, sophisticated ML models (i.e., deep neural networks) prove superior compared to classical statistics and data mining approaches with regard to accuracy [52]. For example, there has been considerable progress in medical image analysis ranging from segmentation of lesions in the brain and breast cancer detection over diabetic retinopathy classification to leak detection in airway tree segmentation [53]. However, the emphasis of these models on accuracy typically comes at the cost of transparency. As a matter of fact, they may consist of hundreds of thousand individual numerical parameters that are being optimized during model training. Consequently, the model's reasoning, how it actually reaches its results or predictions, can hardly be understood due to the sheer number or model parameters and their interactions. This is why they are often called blackbox models. This poses a tremendous problem to patients and medical professionals, who seek intelligible information and rely on medical reasoning to make informed decisions. For example, a model that would propose a certain treatment based on disease patterns that were matched against a huge database of patients with similar complaints might yield obscure and medically unreasonable results. Such model output is unacceptable for patients and medical professions alike [54]. Therefore, the application of advanced machine learning in its current form has little to add to the body of knowledge in the health sciences because the knowledge gained is confined within the machine learning models themselves and cannot be revealed to users. Relating to the context of LHS, these models do not bring forth knowledge from data. Still, they are more likely to fulfill supportive functions, e.g., in raising a physician's awareness of case similarities or suspicious patches in a medical image.

Case Study

The Connected Health Cities (CHC) is a Learning Health System (LHS) in four regions in the North of England in the United Kingdom (UK). It has been established to address the inequalities in health between the North and the South of England, between social groups and men versus women, and overcome this health gap. The CHC consortium embraces partners from academia, the National Health Service (NHS), and industry in the regions of Greater Manchester, North West Coast,

Yorkshire, and the North East and North Cumbria. At the beginning of 2016, the three-year project with an extension of one year received 20 million pounds in funding from the Department of Health and Social Care (DHSC). The CHC initiative included different targets and applications depending on the region [55]:

1. **Yorkshire**: (a) collection and linkage of data on emergency and urgent care (EUC) provision and give a complete overview of the EUC demand in this region and (b) work with General Practitioners (GPs) on the aim of reducing inappropriate prescriptions of multiple drugs (polypharmacy) for the frail elderly,
2. **Greater Manchester:** (a) collection and analysis of antibiotics prescriptions by GPs to tackle antibiotics resistance through better decision making and optimization of the prescriptions, (b) linking data from ambulances and the hospital to improve the early recognition of stroke and the pursuant treatment in a stroke unit, (c) building an extensive database on patients with transient ischemic attacks and developing of predictive models for persons at risk, (d) management of timely referral of patients to neurosurgery after brain hemorrhage and (e) ensure that another stroke was prevented,
3. **North East/North Cumbria:** (a) development of predictive models for unplanned care, in particular for emergency and urgent care, and hereby support the demand management and service planning, (b) provision of special care for vulnerable groups through linkage of data from physical and mental health, social care, education, and housing,
4. **North West Coast:** (a) information sharing between agencies and services users and definition of best care paths through improved information collection and analysis, (b) improving care for people with chronic obstructive pulmonary disease (COPD) and epilepsy admitted to a hospital for emergency care through sharing information between health and social care.

All four regions set out to define and design a data sharing strategy and governance, develop an analytical platform, identify the requirements of the skill base, analyze a defined set of care pathways and look for improvements, plan the integration of research and development, and develop a business model for a sustainable LHS.

A systematic evaluation took place in 2018 using a survey that was cascaded to local staff and qualitative interviews. The aim was to identify the main challenges and emerging benefits. The findings were then triangulated, that is, combining the survey and the interview results. These findings were presented as major themes and they have been summarized below. Many participants remarked that such an ambitious project could run into time-related problems. For some, it took a year to clarify the ethical issues, obtaining the necessary approvals for data sharing. Many stated that the first two years were mainly used to lay the groundwork. Other challenges reported were:

1. missing access to high-quality electronic data and,
2. in some cases, the data was only available on paper,
3. and in other cases, the data quality was poor in terms of missing data, wrongly coded data, or duplicate data.

Many interviewees felt that obtaining a commitment at all levels for this project, was not easy, although it was of paramount importance for the executive level. Only with their support and direction could things be moved. Experts shared that due to the nature of a project with a limited timeline, it would be difficult to develop a culture of sustainability. Problems occurred because of short-term job contracts, and it also turned out that people in the different regions with different professions worked differently. Also, a common ground concerning the terminology and language used had to be achieved. Generally, communication was not as smooth and effective as necessary, leading to people not feeling connected [55].

Outside of the initial difficulties highlighted, experts agreed that an LHS project with multi-professional teams, opportunities for new collaboration and new research, embedding the results in a theoretical background looking out of the box, generated many positive effects that participants took advantage of. The data-driven approach was very much appreciated. Regarding the involvement of patients, the participants expressed that the voice of the patients was heard and it leveraged change. It was recognized that the research findings could be rolled out much faster than before, and could affect the clinical pathways directly. Alike, the research could be done must faster, and small pilots could be implemented [55].

Further studies followed this initial evaluation report. For example, the Hospital Frailty Risk Score calculation could be improved and proved to be a strong predictor for long length of stay and in-hospital mortality [56].

This report illustrates the LHS methodology employed, the initial challenges and the emerging benefits of a large regional LHS, and detailed practical insights reached due to the availability of the data.

Summary

A Learning Health System is a concept that can be put into practice in many different ways, in a single hospital or groups of hospitals at the local level. It can reach out to more participants at the regional, national, or supra-national level. Likewise, its scope can be broad and include different health problems as seen in the Connected Health Cities case study. However, it can also focus on only one urgent aspect, such as opioid abuse, antibiotics prescriptions, and the care of patients with transient ischemic attacks as seen in the application examples. Data-driven health within an LHS goes along with efforts of continuous and fast quality improvement realized by data, knowledge, and performance cycles. Evidence is built upon the observational data mostly found in electronic health records and supplemented by other external sources, for example, weather data, traffic data, and so on. Although the idea of an LHS is not new any lon-

ger, its realization was boosted by the increasing availability of large amounts of electronic data only recently. Its spread is further leveraged by interoperable information systems and common data models that allow data or findings to be shared and compared across different units and organizations. The use of informatics methods and an IT infrastructure are of paramount importance, as well as inter-professional cooperation and leadership that guides and governs the LHS based on core values. In this sense, an LHS is a true socio-technical system and a focal point of bringing added value through the broad spectrum of health informatics methods, such as health IT standards, terminologies, data models, data warehouses, ETL processes, data analytics methods, prediction and forecasting models, dashboards and decision support systems. Eventually, an LHS is meant to identify, implement, and evaluate these procedures and processes that are beneficial for the patient and eliminate the harmful and wasteful practice. Its advantage is the use of local and up-to-date data from the clinical field, ensuring a high validity. The better the informatics methods are implemented, the faster these data can be transformed into practical knowledge.

Conclusions and Outlook

Maximal use of observational data from EHRs is the key to the success of an LHS as a learning organization. Usage can be interpreted as applying informatics methods to data as well as the clinical use of the findings, for example, forecasts, predictions, alerts, and other types of advice given to the clinicians. Maximal use contrasts minimal use, that is, the situation when data that had been collected diligently and had so often resided in databases without utilization. Thus, LHS thinking requires a paradigm shift.

LHSs are complex systems composed of different stakeholders and technologies with many challenges lurking along the way. Although there are impressive LHS examples at the national and supra-national level, small local LHSs are equally important. They are robust with regard to feasibility and require a close connection between the users and data and this may help build trust in clinical decision support systems. Finally, establishing a local LHS does not preclude its participants from getting connected with other LHSs and constituting a regional or national LHS. It is the virtue of local LHSs to think big but act small.

Review Questions

1. Why is an LHS called a socio-technical system, and how do research and care interact?
2. What are the high-level governing principles of an LHS, and how can they be broken down?
3. How does the cyclical nature of an LHS contribute to continuous quality improvement, and how can these improvements be measured? Show some indicators.
4. Why can data from an Electronic Health Record not be immediately used for analytical purposes?
5. What are observational data? What are their strengths and weaknesses?
6. Give some examples of longitudinal data and their analysis.

Appendix: Answers to Review Questions

1. Why is an LHS called a socio-technical system, and how do research and care interact?

A Learning Health System is a complex undertaking that embraces people and technologies. People involved are first and foremost clinicians of all different types building the inter-professional team, furthermore administrators, scientists, informatics specialists, and patients. They can come from different units, departments, organizations, and countries depending on the goal, scope, and size of the LHS. Usually, the people represent some type of unit or organization that is part of the LHS. They work in patient care or in research; in the best case, they work in both areas or their work is highly integrated. They are the ones who set the agenda in terms of questions to be answered, data to be used and

indicators to be applied when measuring the success. The other components of an LHS are the technical systems and the data that reside in these systems. The technical side of the LHS includes the operational information systems, in particular the Electronic Health Record, as well as analytical information systems that have clean data ready for analyses. It is the technical layer where issues of interoperability between different data sources (operational information systems) are solved and where ETL processes are put into place to ensure that the data loaded are good, meaningful, and useful.

2. What are the high-level governing principles of an LHS, and how can they be broken down?

High-level principles or core values should help to govern an LHS. They embrace values of focusing on patients and their needs, values in terms of high quality and affordable care, and in terms of an additional value, accessibility and transparency of the findings, cooperative leadership and governance that builds trust, allows for sustainability and is guided by the inclusiveness of stakeholders and participants. Rigorous scientific methods, privacy measures at all levels and a flexible approach should be implemented to reach meaningful, valid, reliable, unbiased, legally and ethically compliant results. These principles have to be put into practice by appropriate governing and management structures and processes. They can follow different models, for example, the matrix structure model or the network model with well-defined responsibilities. In order for an LHS to become sustainable, a long-term financial structure has to be established.

3. How does the cyclical nature of an LHS contribute to continuous quality improvement and how can these improvements be measured? Show some indicators.

Continuous quality improvements build upon fast feedback and learning that is realized through the (many) iterations of the LHS cycle. This cycle embraces the phases "data to knowledge,"

"knowledge to performance" and finally "performance to data" that triggers the cycle to run once more. It is thus through continuity, incremental insights, and their application that improvement can happen. The outcome of an LHS can be measured at any level, that is, scrutinizing the success or failure after any of these phases. From an overall perspective, the indictor "knowledge-to-action latency" measures the speed of the LHS, the indicator "systematic adoption of evidence" reflects the degree of evidence of the adopted new procedures, while finally "systematic elimination of wasteful and ineffective practices" identifies and quantifies the inadequate procedures that have been stopped and discarded. More indicators include the "care experience of patients", the "work-life experience" of the health workforce, and "equity of care". Also, economic considerations such as "utilization-cost measures" and "return on investment" are relevant criteria for evaluating the outcome of an LHS. Finally, the "impact on population health" can be used as a high-level measure to evaluate an LHS.

4. Why can data from an Electronic Health Record not be immediately used for analytical purposes?

An Electronic Health Record belongs to the group of operational information systems employed for primary use, that is, for keeping the patient records, for documentation, as a legal document, and for supporting communication among the inter-professional team. These data are not intended for analysis that requires structured, comparable, clean, and consistent data representing similar types of information across organizational units and over time. They require that the same version of a classification system be used, for example. In the case of different versions, a transformation process has to be started. In case of different diagnoses of the same patient found in two different subsystems of the electronic health records, a rule, for example, the most recent data entry must be applied to determine which diagnosis will be used for further analysis.

5. What are observational data? What are their strengths and weaknesses?

Observational data are data that have been recorded at a single point of time or over an extended period of time and contrast with experimental data from RCTs. Typically, they originate from health records and represent routine data recorded for the purpose of patient care and not primarily for research. Their advantage is their availability to be used for real-time analysis. Data from the field have greater validity than those from the lab. Their disadvantage is that cause and effect are much more challenging to analyze and identify than from experimental data.

6. Give some examples of longitudinal data and their analysis.

Time series analyses are appropriate for studying longitudinal data, such as Auto-Regressive-Moving Average (ARMA) models and their derivatives ARIMA or SARMA models, for example, forecasting the rates of patients that arrive in the emergency department over two weeks. Survival analysis is another example of analyzing longitudinal data where the time is of interest until an event occurs, for example, time until a chronic wound has healed.

References

1. Friedman CP, Rubin JC, Sullivan KJ. Toward an Information infrastructure for global health improvement. Yearb Med Inform. 2017;26:16–23.
2. Olsen L, Aisner D, McGinnis JM. The learning healthcare system: workshop summary. 2007. https://doi.org/10.17226/11903.
3. Weng C, Kahn MG. Clinical research informatics for big data and precision medicine. Yearb Med Inform. 2016:211–8.
4. Devine EB, Capurro D, van Eaton E, Alfonso-Cristancho R, Devlin A, Yanez ND, Yetisgen-Yildiz M, Flum DR, Tarczy-Hornoch P. Preparing electronic clinical data for quality improvement and comparative effectiveness research: the SCOAP CERTAIN automation and validation project. EGEMS Wash DC. 2013;1:1025.

5. Nwaru BI, Friedman C, Halamka J, Sheikh A. Can learning health systems help organisations deliver personalised care? BMC Med. 2017;15:177.

6. Ethier J-F, McGilchrist M, Barton A, Cloutier A-M, Curcin V, Delaney BC, Burgun A. The TRANSFoRm project: experience and lessons learned regarding functional and interoperability requirements to support primary care. Learn Health Syst. 2018;2:e10037.

7. Abernethy AP, Ahmad A, Zafar SY, Wheeler JL, Reese JB, Lyerly HK. Electronic patient-reported data capture as a foundation of rapid learning cancer care. Med Care. 2010;48:S32–8.

8. Greene SM, Reid RJ, Larson EB. Implementing the learning health system: from concept to action. Ann Intern Med. 2012;157:207–10.

9. Rouse WB, Johns MME, Pepe KM. Learning in the health care enterprise. Learn Health Syst. 2017;1:e10024.

10. McLachlan S, Potts HW, Dube K, Buchanan D, Lean S, Gallagher T, Johnson O, Daley B, Marsh W, Fenton N. The Heimdall framework for supporting characterisation of learning health systems. J Innov Health Inf. 2018;

11. Rauch H, Hübner U, Denter M, Babitsch B. Improving the prediction of emergency department crowding: a time series analysis including road traffic flow. Stud Health Technol Inform. 2019;260:57–64.

12. Foley TJ, Vale L. What role for learning health systems in quality improvement within healthcare providers? Learn Health Syst. 2017;1:e10025.

13. Bengtsson L, Lu X, Thorson A, Garfield R, von Schreeb J. Improved response to disasters and outbreaks by tracking population movements with mobile phone network data: a post-earthquake geospatial study in Haiti. PLoS Med. 2011;8:e1001083.

14. Friedman C, Rubin J, Brown J, et al. Toward a science of learning systems: a research agenda for the high-functioning learning health system. J Am Med Inform Assoc JAMIA. 2015;22:43–50.

15. Owen J. General system theory and the use of process mining to improve care pathways. Stud Health Technol Inform. 2019:11–22.

16. Smoyer WE, Embi PJ, Moffatt-Bruce S. Creating local learning health systems: think globally, act locally. JAMA. 2016;316:2481–2.

17. Budrionis A, Bellika JG. The learning healthcare system: where are we now? A systematic review. J Biomed Inform. 2016;64:87–92.

18. Lessard L, Michalowski W, Fung-Kee-Fung M, Jones L, Grudniewicz A. Architectural frameworks: defining the structures for implementing learning health systems. Implement Sci. 2017 Jun 23;12(1):78. https://doi.org/10.1186/s13012-017-0607-7.

19. Allen C, Colemann K, Mettert K, Lewis C, Westbrook E, Lozano P. A roadmap to operationalize and evaluate impact in a learning health system. Learn Health Sys. 2021:e10258. https://doi.org/10.1002/lrh2.10258.

20. Hultman GM, Rajamani S, Wilcox A, Melton GB. Expert perspectives on definitions, drivers and informatics contributions to learning health systems. AMIA Jt Summits Transl Sci Proc. 2020 May 30;2020:251–8.

21. Enticott J, Braaf S, Johnson A, Jones A, Teede HJ. Leaders' perspectives on learning health systems: a qualitative study. BMC Health Serv Res. 2020 Nov 26;20(1):1087. https://doi.org/10.1186/s12913-020-05924-w.

22. Veterans Affairs. https://www.va.gov/health/

23. Rattray NA, Damush TM, Miech EJ, Homoya B, Myers LJ, Penney LS, Ferguson J, Giacherio B, Kumar M, Bravata DM. Empowering implementation teams with a learning health system approach: leveraging data to improve quality of care for transient ischemic attack. J Gen Intern Med. 2020 Nov;35(Suppl 2):823–31. https://doi.org/10.1007/s11606-020-06160-y.

24. Krapohl GL, Hemmila MR, Hendren S, Bishop K, Rogers R, Rocker C, Fasbinder L, Englesbe MJ, Vu JV, Campbell DA Jr. Building, scaling, and sustaining a learning health system for surgical quality improvement: a toolkit. Learn Health Syst. 2020 Jan 30;4(3):e10215. https://doi.org/10.1002/lrh2.10215.

25. Palin V, Tempest E, Mistry C, van Staa TP. Developing the infrastructure to support the optimisation of antibiotic prescribing using the learning healthcare system to improve healthcare services in the provision of primary care in England. BMJ Health Care Inform. 2020 Jun;27(1):e100147. https://doi.org/10.1136/bmjhci-2020-100147.

26. Observational Health Data Sciences and Informatics (OHDSI). Common data model. https://ohdsi.github.io/TheBookOfOhdsi/CommonDataModel.html

27. Ryu B, Yoon E, Kim S, Lee S, Baek H, Yi S, Na HY, Kim JW, Baek RM, Hwang H, Yoo S. Transformation of Pathology Reports Into the Common Data Model With Oncology Module: Use Case for Colon Cancer. J Med Internet Res. 2020 Dec 9;22(12):e18526. https://doi.org/10.2196/18526.

28. van der Aalst WM, Stahl C. Modeling business processes: a petri net-oriented approach. MIT press; 2011.

29. Wager KA, Lee FW, Glaser JP. Health care information systems: a practical approach for health care management. Wiley; 2017.

30. Gluchowski P, Chamoni P. Analytische Informationssysteme; 2016. https://doi.org/10.1007/978-3-662-47763-2.

31. Lenz R, Beyer M, Kuhn KA. Semantic integration in healthcare networks. Int J Med Inf. 2007;76:201–7.

32. Corbellini A, Mateos C, Zunino A, Godoy D, Schiaffino S. Persisting big-data: the NoSQL landscape. Inf Syst. 2017;63:1–23.

33. Ziegler P, Dittrich KR. Data integration–problems, approaches, and perspectives. In: Krogstie J, Opdahl AL, Brinkkemper S, editors. Concept. Model. Inf. Syst. Eng. Berlin, Heidelberg: Springer; 2007. p. 39–58.

34. Bender D, Sartipi K. HL7 FHIR: An Agile and RESTful approach to healthcare information

exchange. In: Proc. 26th IEEE Int. Symp. Comput.-Based Med. Syst. IEEE; 2013. p. 326–31.

35. Maier C, Lang L, Storf H, Vormstein P, Bieber R, Bernarding J, Herrmann T, Haverkamp C, Horki P, Laufer J. Towards implementation of OMOP in a German university hospital consortium. Appl Clin Inform. 2018;9:054–61.

36. Ulriksen G-H, Pedersen R, Ellingsen G. Infrastructuring in healthcare through the open EHR architecture. Comput Support Coop Work CSCW. 2017;26:33–69.

37. Khnaisser C, Lavoie L, Diab H, Ethier J-F. Data warehouse design methods review: trends, challenges and future directions for the healthcare domain. In: East Eur Conf Adv Databases Inf Syst Springer. 2015:76–87.

38. Meystre SM, Lovis C, Bürkle T, Tognola G, Budrionis A, Lehmann CU. Clinical data reuse or secondary use: current status and potential future progress. Yearb Med Inform. 2017;26:38–52.

39. Turley CB. Leveraging a statewide clinical data warehouse to expand boundaries of the learning health system. Methods Improve Patient Outcomes: EGEMs Gener. Evid; 2016. p. 4.

40. Zhao C-M, Luan J. Data mining: going beyond traditional statistics. New Dir Institutional Res. 2006; https://doi.org/10.1002/ir.184.

41. Cummins MR. Nonhypothesis-driven research: data mining and knowledge discovery. In: Richesson RL, Andrews JE, editors. Clin. Res. Inform. Cham: Springer International Publishing; 2019. p. 341–56.

42. Lawless JF. Statistical models and methods for lifetime data. John Wiley & Sons; 2011.

43. Therneau TM, Lumley T. Package 'survival'. R Top Doc. 2015;128(10):28–33.

44. Loprinzi CL, Laurie JA, Wieand HS, Krook JE, Novotny PJ, Kugler JW, Bartel J, Law M, Bateman M, Klatt NE, et al. Prospective evaluation of prognostic variables from patient-completed questionnaires. North central cancer treatment group. J Clin Oncol. 1994;12(3):601–7.

45. Royston P, Parmar MK. Restricted mean survival time: an alternative to the hazard ratio for the design and analysis of randomized trials with a time-to-event outcome. BMC Med Res Methodol. 2013;13:152.

46. Hyndman RJ, Athanasopoulos G (2018) Forecasting: principles and practice. OTexts.

47. Granger CW, Newbold P, Econom J. Spurious regressions in econometrics. Baltagi Badi H Companion Theor. Econom. 1974:557–61.

48. Schelter B, Winterhalder M, Timmer J. Handbook of time series analysis: recent theoretical developments and applications. John Wiley & Sons; 2006.

49. Rauch J, Hüsers J, Babitsch B, Hübner U. Understanding the characteristics of frequent users of emergency departments: what role do medical conditions play? Stud Health Technol Inform. 2018;253:175–9.

50. Lasko TA, Denny JC, Levy MA. Computational phenotype discovery using unsupervised feature learning over noisy, sparse, and irregular clinical data. PLoS One. 2013;8:e66341.

51. Wei W-Q, Teixeira PL, Mo H, Cronin RM, Warner JL, Denny JC. Combining billing codes, clinical notes, and medications from electronic health records provides superior phenotyping performance. J Am Med Inform Assoc. 2016;23:e20–7.

52. Ravì D, Wong C, Deligianni F, Berthelot M, Andreu-Perez J, Lo B, Yang G-Z. Deep learning for health informatics. IEEE J Biomed Health Inform. 2016;21:4–21.

53. Litjens G, Kooi T, Bejnordi BE, Setio AAA, Ciompi F, Ghafoorian M, van der Laak JAWM, van Ginneken B, Sánchez CI. A survey on deep learning in medical image analysis. Med Image Anal. 2017;42:60–88.

54. Strickland E. IBM Watson, heal thyself: how IBM overpromised and underdelivered on AI health care. IEEE Spectr. 2019;56:24–31.

55. Steels S, Ainsworth J, van Staa TP. Implementation of a "real-world" learning health system: Results from the evaluation of the Connected Health Cities programme. Learn Health Syst. 2020 Feb 26;5(2):e10224. https://doi.org/10.1002/lrh2.10224.

56. Street A, Maynou L, Gilbert T, Stone T, Mason S, Conroy S. The use of linked routine data to optimise calculation of the Hospital Frailty Risk Score on the basis of previous hospital admissions: a retrospective observational cohort study. Lancet Healthy Longev. 2021 Mar;2(3):e154–62. https://doi.org/10.1016/S2666-7568(21)00004-0.

Further Reading

Wager KA, Lee FW, Glaser JP. Health care information systems: a practical approach for health care management. Wiley; 2017.

EHR Data: Enabling Clinical Surveillance and Alerting

13

Vitaly Herasevich, Kirill Lipatov, and Brian W. Pickering

Learning Objectives
- To define barriers to implementation clinical surveillance and alerting platforms.
- To compare emerging technologies and strategies that may increase the clinical impact of surveillance and alerts.
- To recommend methodologies for evaluation of clinical surveillance technologies.

Key Terms
- Clinical Decision Support Systems (CDSS) or Decision Support System (DSS) or Clinical Decision Support (CDS)—Computer-based application provides reminders and best-practice guidance in the context of data specific to the patient that helps physicians make clinical decisions.
- Smart alerts or sniffers.
- Socio-technical systems.
- Rapid Response Team.

Introduction

Active or passive screening of patient populations for abnormalities is an integral part of the diagnostic and treatment process. The widespread adoption of the comprehensive electronic

health record (EHR) has opened up the potential for automated individual and mass clinical surveillance. Automation does not guarantee efficacy and may come with unintended consequence such as alert fatigue and information overload. This chapter will discuss how we can get the most out of automation and avoid some of the more harmful unintended consequences as we transition from our current situation to next generation solutions for clinical surveillance and alerting.

Historical Overview of Clinical Surveillance before Computerized Systems

The desire to monitor and track disease states and health outcomes has been with us for many centuries. The emergence of new communicable diseases or pandemics of established communicable diseases continues to be a key driver of discovery and innovation in health care. With the outbreak of the bubonic plague, for example, a system was put in place in docks around the world to quarantine passengers, crew, and the goods of those ships identified as carrying the disease. Improved understanding of the mechanism and risk factors promoting the spread of communicable diseases drove the development of monitoring and regulation programs. In the early eighteenth century, the economic and human cost of communicable

V. Herasevich (✉) · K. Lipatov · B. W. Pickering
Mayo Clinic, Rochester, MN, USA
e-mail: vitaly@mayo.edu; lipatov.kirill@mayo.edu;
pickering.brian@mayo.edu

© Springer Nature Switzerland AG 2022
U. H. Hübner et al. (eds.), *Nursing Informatics*, Health Informatics,
https://doi.org/10.1007/978-3-030-91237-6_13

disease became apparent, governing agencies directed resources toward rudimentary public health surveillance and on disease prevention through regulation of public water, sewage, and food supply. The need to monitor the efficacy of these measures through systematic analysis, led to the development of new public health surveillance tools such as births/deaths/marriages registries, point in time population census, analysis of living conditions, occupation, and socioeconomic status. In the United States (U.S.), the precursor of the public health service was formed in the nineteenth century with the purpose of compiling received physicians weekly contagious disease, morbidity, and mortality reports. In response to the devastating poliomyelitis pandemic, this initiative was expanded across all the states toward the beginning of the twentieth century as part of a federally funded public health initiative. The reporting practices continued to evolve in the U.S. and the responsibility for their compilation and dissemination was ultimately transferred to the Communicable Disease Center [1]. Toward the middle of the twentieth century, as the world became more connected, international cooperative organizations such as the World Health Organization (WHO) emerged to describe and monitoring the epidemiologic of disease in addition to develop policy and strategies that effectively contain, prevent and eradicate disease.

Public Health Surveillance

Public health agencies are responsible for ongoing, systemic collection, analysis, and interpretation of health-related data essential to the planning, implementation, and evaluation of public health practice. These agencies also manage the timely dissemination of data to those responsible for prevention control including appropriate public health agencies, government, healthcare administrators, and practitioners. Increasingly, as we have seen in the COVID-19 pandemic, those responsible include individual members of the public, private businesses and organizations. To carry out these activities, public health surveillance agencies must be able to reliably, investi-

gate the extent of public health problems, identify, and communicate with individual patients and their contacts, detect uncontrolled spread of a disease, characterizing disease trends, design prevention and treatment initiatives, monitor their effectiveness, and facilitate research [2]. All of this has to be done both as part of planning for potential threats and in response to emerging or present public health threats. A final consideration for public health agencies is how to manage the increasing burden of responsibility being placed on individuals and private businesses to take preventive actions and the loss of centralized control of the preventive strategy that accompanies this shift.

Several factors need to be considered prior to pronouncing a particular public surveillance program effective:

- The health condition in question must represent a large enough epidemiologic threat to prompt its surveillance. This requirement may be met if the disease specific mortality, prevalence, or rate of spread is sufficiently large.
- The data necessary for effective surveillance should be complete, relevant, and reliable.
- Collection and processing of this information has to be feasible and timely for the data to be actionable.
- Once acquired, the surveillance data must be useful in designing treatment and prevention strategies.
- Following implementation, surveillance tools should be constantly assessed for effectiveness and improvement opportunities.

The Deteriorating Patient and Emergence of Rapid Response Systems

Patients have a significant portion of their healthcare needs met in acute care hospital settings. Billions of dollars are spent on emergency visits and hospital admissions and this number continues to increase [3]. It is estimated that hospitalized patients in the U.S., Canada, Europe, and Australia experience adverse events at a rate of between 3% and 18% [4]. A considerable portion of these events is related to a failure to recognize deterioration. Over half of the patients admitted to intensive care units exhibit signs of worsening physiologic abnormalities hours before they transfer from hospital wards [5]. Those patients who are admitted late to the intensive care unit (ICU) have a worse outcome than those admitted earlier [6]. In an effort to reduce harm, rapid response systems (RRS), intended to bring critical care resources to the bedside of a patient who otherwise might suffer harm, have been proposed as a potential solution. The use of scoring systems as alerting triggers is considered important to reduce in-hospital mortality attributable to failures in recognition of severity of illness and inappropriate care of the deteriorating patients [7]. Despite the fact that, when formally studied, the evidence for their efficacy is inconsistent, the implementation of an RRS has been promoted as a key marker of quality and is strongly advocated for by organizations in the U.S. such as the Institute for Healthcare Improvement (IHI) and the Joint Commission [8]. The development of RRS illustrates some of the key challenges and lessons we need to learn if we are to move successfully into an era of highly effective clinical surveillance and alerting platforms.

The Adoption of Clinical Scoring Systems as Alerting and Surveillance Tools

Examples of validated scoring systems can be found in many areas of healthcare including, trauma, burns, sepsis, shock, and postoperative cardiac surgery. A variety of severity of illness scores exist in the ICU including the Therapeutic Intervention Scoring System (TISS), Simplified Acute Physiology Score (SAPS), and Sequential Organ Failure Assessment (SOFA) score [9]. The validation and refinement of these scores centers primarily on their ability to predict mortality. In general, scores developed for this purpose do not incorporate time series data and they are calculated at specific points in time. For example, the Acute Physiology and Chronic Health Evaluation

(APACHE) score used widely to predict the likelihood of mortality in critically ill patients, is calculated during the first 24 hours after the time of admission to the ICU. Importantly, the aforementioned scores have been primarily validated in the ICU settings and may not have similar predictive abilities when applied to other patient populations.

While primarily calibrated to predict mortality and allow patient population matching by severity of illness, these scores have been pressed into service as tools to indicate when individual patients may be at risk of clinical deterioration and require a higher level of care.

Multidisciplinary teams variably comprising nursing staff, respiratory therapists, and physicians have been formed in many health systems [7]. In order to function most effectively, these teams must be alerted to the presence of a distressed patient and be trained to immediately manage, appropriately triage, and transfer patients at risk for deterioration to a higher level of care, (or palliative care), if appropriate. Several initiatives have been designed to improve outcomes of deteriorating patients using scoring systems as triggers.

Designing Intelligent Surveillance and Alerting Systems

The reliability of the RRS is dependent on a number of factors. In contrast to scores, which are typically derived from a statistical analysis of a data base, alerting and surveillance platforms need to be designed with a deep understanding of the complex socio-technical health system [10], in which they will be deployed in order to be effective. Perhaps unsurprisingly, given the complexity of these systems, the evidence for the success of RRS has been conflicting. A summary of the key areas that need to be addressed, the suggested approach and expected impact are outlined in Table 13.1.

Table 13.1 Surveillance and alert systems are intended to be used in clinical environments. The optimal configuration of people, processes, incentives, and technology are essential if an alert

Table 13.1 Modified by permission from Springer Nature Critical Care journal: Clinical review: The hospital of the future—building intelligent environments to facilitate safe and effective acute care delivery, Brian W Pickering et al., 2012

Knowledge Domain	Approach	Impact
Health Care Stakeholders	Stakeholder engagement	Mechanistic understanding of disease Identification of meaningful problems to solve Stakeholder buy in to test and evaluate novel technology with significant potential risks Reduce likelihood of implementing high risk, low value technology
Human factors and cognitive science	SurveysField observation Interview Chart review Standard ontology of error	Identify the human factors that contribute to diagnostic, rescue, or care delivery failures that result in excess morbidity and mortality in the hospitalIdentify the modes of alert that are the most effective modifiers of behavior
Ergonomics and engineering	Field observation Process modeling Simulation	Understand processes of care deliveryIdentify and eliminate environmental factors that impede the delivery of careIdentify environmental artifacts that can be re-engineered to force best practiceTest the impact of changes in models of care delivery Test the impact on processes of care in high-fidelity simulation environments
Health care informatics, data analytics, and health information technology	Data warehousing Epidemiology Data mining Social networks Technology showcase Academic meetings and gatherings	Identify the best way to capture data from the environment (Electronic Medical Record (EMR), sensors, wearables, monitors) Reliably capture digital signatures of patient conditions and provider actionsBuild real time feedback to systems of health care delivery (provider and manager)Facilitate the reporting of errorsFacilitate secondary data use (e.g., the analysis of large data sets from multiple care delivery settings, research, learning health systems)Dissemination of knowledge
Culture	Represent the whole community Reporting error at a local level Lobbying Developing and enforcing standards Community consent	Knowledge of new or unanticipated errorsOrganized response re-enforces value of reportingFacilitate the implementation of recommendationsReform of incentivesPerpetuate the safety culture Facilitate research and development Reduce and eliminate disparities

or surveillance system is to successfully deliver the intended result. The knowledge deficits that must be addressed that facilitate reliable, safe, and compassionate delivery of appropriate interventions to hospitalized patients are summarized in the table below.

Clinical Informatics and the Development of Reliable Alerts

Identification of patients at risk of decompensation is the subject of ongoing research. Older severity-of-illness scores were not developed for use with electronic surveillance and alerting systems and so, they may be unreliable. Reporting of severity of illness scores can be cumbersome, particularly in the pre-EHR times. The validity of the calculated score can be compromised by variability or gaps in the record of individual parameters, such as heart rate or respiratory rate. These, if used in isolation from the overall trends, can suggest artificially higher severity of illness. Furthermore, some of the abnormal features may stem from pre-existing comorbidities and would not suggest a trajectory of imminent worsening condition [11]. Ultimately, the scores have been validated to predict overall mortality rather than deterioration during the hospital stay.

For accurate calculation, clinical scores require numerous pieces of information that are often unavailable at the time of urgent bedside assessment [12]. Vital signs are perhaps the most readily obtained, reliable, and easily reported clinical data. Currently, many early warning alert systems are based on these measurements. While isolated vital sign abnormalities have a poor ability to predict outcomes, such scores were utilized as triggers for first generation Medical Emergency Teams (METs) in Australia and were found to be associated with a significant reduction in cardiac arrests following implementation [13]. Because of their ease of use and the early success reported in Australia, single parameter triggers, have been adopted widely, and activated on wards in the U.S. Some studies in early adopter centers demonstrated a similar reduction in cardiac arrests and ICU admissions [14]. In contrast, a large cluster-randomized controlled trial, using similar criteria across a broader range of hospitals, failed to demonstrate a change in the rate of unplanned ICU admissions, cardiac arrests, or death despite substantially increasing the number of MET activations [15].

Many have concluded that the reliance on single parameter alerts is the source of the failure of MET and various combinations of vital sign derangements have been proposed. Aggregates of three or more vital signs above certain thresholds were found to have significantly higher association with in-hospital mortality [16]. These findings, combined with the widespread adoption of EMR digital systems and electronic medical records which make complex calculation less burdensome, sparked interest in multiparameter vital sign-based clinical alerts. One study analyzed the outcomes of MET activations triggered by more complex alerts and found that they were associated with increased survival [17]. These findings have highlighted the potential role of continuous vital sign monitoring as an alerting mechanism for MET to potential deterioration. While EMR's have enabled more complex score calculation [18], we should be cautious about a rush to adopt these as they have not been definitively associated with better outcomes [19].

EHR-Based Computerized Alerting Systems

Traditionally, health records were maintained using paper charts and documentation. Paper records present obvious challenges when it comes to collecting, preserving, and exchanging clinical information. The need for accessible, reliable, and efficient ways to exchange patient care information led to the development of EHR at the end of twentieth century [20]. A combination of a potential reduction in medical error, augmented billing and coding, and economic stimulus funding as part of the Health Information Technology for Economic and Clinical Health (HITECH) Act resulted in widespread adoption and implementation of EHR. However, despite the efforts to improve the user interfaces, bedside clinicians are increasingly overwhelmed by the amount of unprioritized information during chart review {Pickering, 2010 #76}.

In an effort to assist users in navigating the vast space of electronically stored patient data, an expanding set of software tools were introduced. Clinical Decision support (CDS) tools have been built on top of EHR data and are designed to make the user aware of unrecognized clinical events through alerts and predefined actions. The first implementation of CDS was through Computerized Physician Order Entry (CPOE) to alert for the presence of drug allergies, drug interactions, or unsafe abnormal clinical parameters [20]. Similar systems have subsequently been designed to notify healthcare professionals about critical laboratory values, deviations from standard of care, or to notify about a combination of findings that may suggest a condition needing immediate intervention. The latter have evolved into EHR-based alerting systems.

A modern surveillance algorithm would analyze the new data in patients record and upon meeting predefined parameters, would trigger an alert in various forms. These would include direct user notifications, interruptible and uninterruptible prompts, and pages sent out to care teams.

Rule Based Systems and Smart Alerts: Case STUDY of the Sepsis Sniffer

Some of the best examples of EMR-based alerts are surveillance systems utilized in the recognition and management of sepsis. Sepsis is a prevalent condition that may manifest in organ failure and shock. It continues to be prevalent in the hospital and ICU patients all across United States [21]. It is essential to recognize sepsis as early as possible. Delays in initiation of appropriate therapy have been repeatedly associated with increased mortality [22, 23]. Diagnosis of sepsis relies on recognition of or suspicion for infection in combination with specific vital sign and laboratory abnormalities [24–26]. EMR-based alert systems have been developed using these criteria in order to promptly advise care teams of suspected sepsis and facilitate timely treatment [27–29].

Sepsis recognition systems initially relied on similar parameters to their pre-EMR predecessors. Their validity largely was evaluated by comparing the data derived from the surveillance systems to a gold standard usually obtained from billing information such as International classification of Diseases (ICD) codes for sepsis and septic shock [30]. Other alerting systems used ICD codes for suspected or diagnosed infection in combination with a set of physiologic parameters consistent with sepsis [31]. When validated, those EMR-based sepsis sniffers achieved high sensitivity, specificity, and prediction values in several studies. However, initial implementation of sepsis sniffers was associated with alarm fatigue, disruption of workflow and poor acceptance [32, 33]. In addition to poor prospective clinical specificity, a major dissatisfactory feature was the "hard stop" interruptive nature of the alerts, forcing users to act before they could continue using the EMR [34]. Alternatively, non-interruptive alerts have been tested in various health care settings, including prescription and laboratory ordering, and they have been demonstrated to be ineffective with little impact on practice [35–37].

The implementation of EMR-based sepsis alerts has allowed us to learn much about their effectiveness as tools of early disease recognition and has enabled the development of more advanced clinical alerting surveillance systems that incorporate an afferent arm that is more nuanced that the hard stop alerts of the past. In more recent iterations, developers of sepsis alerting platforms have focused on using the alert as a trigger for a rapid review by a clinical expert or team of experts. This so-called afferent limb of surveillance is critical for success. Several hospitals have elected to form sepsis response teams variably comprising a combination of physicians, advanced practice providers, and nursing staff. Similar to the METs, introduction of these sepsis response teams leads to better outcomes in several before-and-after evaluation studies.

In a further effort to facilitate timely and appropriate action in response to clinical alerts is to augment the surveillance system with clinical decision support which prompts the user to either follow a predefined treatment algorithm or choose specific interventions that are considered the current standard of care. Several studies have found that this combination of surveillance and decision support is associated with improved outcomes [30].

Advantages and Disadvantages of EMR-based Surveillance

Early EMR-based surveillance systems, built on top of the original early warning scores are unlikely to perform better than traditional alert systems. Repeated triggering combined with automated notification can greatly increase alert fatigue, burden, and frustration resulting in poor system adoption by bedside clinicians.

However, EMR-based deterioration screening offers several advantages:

- With the amount of electronically available clinical data, it is substantially easier to add new features to the pre-existing sniffers and alert systems.

- With the automated alerts transmitted directly to the care team, there is less reliance on interdisciplinary communication and need for ongoing staff education.
- The data itself can be filtered and presented in the more prioritized fashion reducing the information overload associated with EMR implementation.

Machine Learning in Clinical Surveillance

With the widespread implementation of EMR and the integration of clinical analytics into healthcare teams, clinical data is increasingly accessible to healthcare stakeholders to guide practice, quality improvement initiatives, and research. An appetite to learn more from the vast amounts of data, derive new associations, and improve prediction capabilities has opened the door for machine learning (ML) in healthcare [38]. ML refers to the ability of computers to find relationships within large data that could be used to better understand diseases, estimate risks, tailor medical therapies, and much more.

At the core of ML is a technical process of identifying and weighing characteristics of variables that would defines relationships in a computational model. The process usually starts with selecting a large pool of data variables or features that could possibly contribute to a pattern. The selection of such features is often independent of an understanding of the process under study. Once the features are selected, a number of different ML techniques can be used to assign a value to each feature depending on its relationship to the outcome. Through a process of fitting the computer model is trained to estimate the known outcome as close as possible. Once the derived model is deemed successful on completing the task based on the training dataset, its performance is evaluated on a separate testing dataset. It is not unexpected that the accuracy of the outcome when the model is applied to the test example is significantly reduced compared to the accuracy from the training example. The differ-

ence should be evaluated and model changed to minimize discrepancy.

There are two classic subtypes of ML: supervised and unsupervised learning. In supervised learning, the task is to identify and fit parameters into a model that would best outline a path between selected input features and the desired outcome. In unsupervised learning, the outcome is not defined and the model instead tries to discover previously unseen patterns amongst large heterogeneous group of features.

Capabilities of ML go beyond analyzing numerical data. Much of the valuable clinical information is stored in the form of disorganized text narrative. Natural language processing (NLP) is a branch of ML dedicated to automation of text analysis in presenting the results in the structured way. Such technology has been utilized to process clinical notes, radiology, and pathology reports to obtain data on patient history, medications, characteristics of benign and malignant tumors, and clinical trials eligibility [39]. Such an approach may be of particular benefit in hospital surveillance as several studies demonstrate that subjective information in textual form such as nursing staff concerns being predictive of patient deterioration. A large retrospective study of over 100,000 patients reported performance of a mortality prediction model augmented by NLP. When compared to the predictive model based primarily on vitals and laboratory values, similar algorithm augmented by NLP demonstrated significantly better performance [40].

Using data available through the EMR, novel ML algorithms present us with an opportunity to develop faster and potentially more accurate hospital surveillance. The clinical use cases that have experimented with this approach include predicting; risk and prognosis of cancers; outcomes of neurosurgery [41] and radiation oncology [42]; complications from surgery [43, 44]; risk of heart attacks [45]; success of transplantation [46]; risk of hospital readmissions; and even the risk of violent behavior during a hospital stay [47]. An increasing number of studies are focusing on the application of ML to active patient monitoring. A recent review presented hundreds of new publications describing various approaches to combining routinely collected data from ICU patients with ML models to predict complications, mortality, and prognoses [48]. Most of those studies used models based on readily available ICU acquired data including vital signs.

Significant effort has been directed toward developing models that reliably predict patient deterioration. These studies have largely focused on creating intelligent early warning scores that are able to predict adverse outcomes such as mortality or unplanned ICU transfers. Advanced early warning scores, using multivariate regression or ML, were able to identify patients at risk with greater precision, when compared to conventional early warning scores [49].

Another ML surveillance focus is that of cardiac arrest prediction. Several of the highest performing models are based on vital signs while others included interpretation of electrocardiograms (ECGs) and heart rate variability measurements. Many of the most advanced models reach 100% sensitivity, specificity, and predictive values [50], at least in the laboratory. Whether ML based prediction performs better than conventional logistic regression in clinical practice remains a topic of debate. A recent systematic review shows no performance benefit of ML over logistic regression for clinical prediction models {Christodoulou, 2019 #77}.

What is clear is that ML has opened up different ways in which researchers, informaticians, and clinicians can examine data. One significant advantage of ML over traditional statistical methods is their ability to integrate different categories of static and dynamic data. This is particularly important in the hospital setting where the patient trajectory is often more important than their point in time clinical state. The recent increase of monitoring devices provides even more opportunities to obtain clinically relevant data close to real time with less intrusion than even the EMR currently provides. The new remote and wireless sensors are able to capture data continuously and the new ML tools can analyze trends and variations in vital signs, patient motion, and environmental noise to deliver new insights and alerts to a supervising clinician [51]. Sensors and cameras combined with appropriate networking capabilities are delivering advanced capabilities and driving down the cost of the growing field of telemedicine [52].

Information from live monitoring of vital signs, heart tracing, and laboratory values can be combined with chart data on demographics and comorbidities to enhance predictive performance. A novel hospital warning system combining EMR-derived early warning score with wireless sensors for continuous monitoring has been already developed [53]. Integration of such system with Rapid Response Team (RRT) activation was compared in a randomized controlled trial with usual care. The authors found modestly decreased hospital length of stay without significant change in mortality or need for post-hospitalization long-term care [54]. Nevertheless, this study demonstrates the safety and feasibility of combining modern monitoring techniques and EMR-based data into a novel hospital surveillance system.

Evaluation of Clinical Surveillance Technologies: Impact on Outcome and Diagnostic Performance, Satisfaction, and Usability

Clinical surveillance tools, as with any other health information technologies (IT), requires adequate evaluation before any implementation to practice [55]. Questions that matter most to patients and clinicians may be called "clinically oriented outcomes of interest" and are organized in the following four major domains:

1. Better health (clinical outcome measurements): Examples include rate of hospital acquired complications, discharge home, hospital mortality, hospital readmission, and so on.
2. Better care (clinical process measurements): Examples include adherence to and appropriateness of processes of care, provider satisfaction, technology adoption, and so on.

The following two domains would be secondary from the perspective of clinicians and patients but are primary for vendors and IT and purchase decision makers such as hospital administrators:

3. Lower cost (financial impact measurements): Examples include resource utilization, severity-adjusted length of hospital stay, cost, and so on.
4. Technical validity: Examples include technical stability and reliability, security, and so on.

Diagnostic accuracy studies are important tools for the evaluation of alerts. When new detection event (alerts) are developed, the creators need to compare it with the established best measurement—"the gold standard." This type of study is widely used in laboratory medicine, radiology, and diagnostic medicine. Sensitivity and specificity are basic performance measures of diagnostic testing and these metrics should always be presented together. They describe how well a test can detect if a condition is present or absent. Other important metrics of testing are positive and negative predictive values (PPV, NPV), likelihood ratios (LRs), and the area under the receiver operating characteristic (ROC) area under the ROC curve (AUC).

The standard way of summarizing the results of diagnostic performance studies is the 2-by-2 contingency table. The relationships between the diagnostic test (alert) and the occurrence of disease or event are shown in Fig. 13.1.

ROC curves show the ability of the diagnostic test to correctly classify subjects as different levels of threshold. The ROC curve is a plot of the sensitivity and specificity values for every individual point. The shape of an ROC curve and the calculated AUC, estimate the discriminative power of a test. The closer the curve is located to the upper left corner and the larger the AUC, the better the test for discriminating between diseased and non-diseased. A perfect diagnostic test has an AUC of 1.0. AUC 0.5 is an equal flip of the coin.

The Food and Drug Administration (FDA) has an excellent document called "Statistical Guidance on Reporting Results from Studies Evaluating Diagnostic Tests" that also describes the terminology and processes for estimation of agreement with a non-reference standard.

Case Study

Clinical Control Tower

EMRs contain large amounts of data with which we can assess a patient's status. Several approaches that were been combined with the EMR have been tried and tested to improve compliance with guidelines using checklists, educational initiatives, and protocoled bundles [56]. Although nurse-led remote screening and prompting using commercial EMR or e-ICU systems has been associated with modest improvements in adherence to selected evidence-based ICU processes, but the benefit was offset by poor communication with bedside teams and high additional staffing cost ($1–three million U.S. dollars annually) [57].

Fig. 13.1 2-by-2 diagnostic table

		Disease or Event (reference standard)	
		Present	Absent
Test or Alert (new test)	Positive	True Positive (TP)	False Positive (FP)
	Negative	False Negative (FN)	True Negative (TN)

However, important side effects of conventional EMR systems are indiscriminate data display and information overload posing a danger for timely decision-making in the ICU. This can be burdensome and time consuming, making the work of the clinician managing critically ill patients challenging. Facing these defects, our group (Clinical Informatics in Intensive Care Laboratory at Mayo Clinic) has developed novel visualization applications that have demonstrated decreased cognitive load and improved provider efficiency.

Control Tower for the hospital (or multi-facility healthcare systems) combines advanced analytics, visualizations, and alert-delivery mechanisms packaged as web-based application. A Control Tower was developed to assist the clinician in the identification of patients (or patient populations), who are at risk of diagnostic delay

and who may benefit from a diagnostic review with a specialist. It was developed with a multidisciplinary group of clinicians, informaticians, clinical researchers, data scientists, IT experts, and quality improvement experts (Fig. 13.2). The benefits of this approach include improvements in patient symptom control and satisfaction, reduced time to necessary specialist interventions, and a measurable impact on inpatient hospital mortality. Control Tower is a central alert-screening and response system developed at Mayo Clinic.

The concept behind Clinical Control Tower is to serve as a centralized alert and prediction "cockpit" for non-life-threatening conditions (Fig. 13.3). As we seek to understand people, processes and technology advances, the intention is to use this platform to manage conditions such as the detection of patients at risk of deterioration or of emerging critical illness.

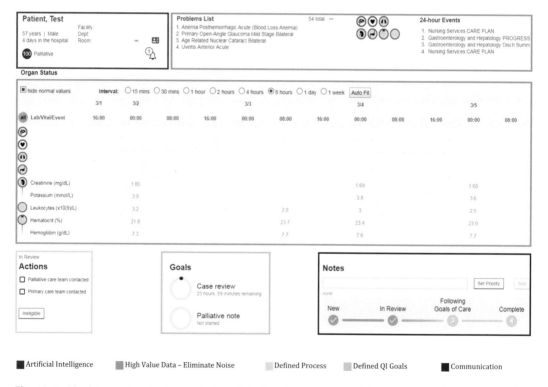

Fig. 13.2 Alerting interface for hospital wide clinical surveillance. The key elements that need to be considered in the design of a hospital wide clinical alerting and surveillance tool include an accurate and human readable alert; contextual high value data; a clear care pathway integrated into the workflow; real time status of key quality metrics or goals; and team communication tools. As can be seen here, the alert trigger or score is a small part of the integrated system. The development of control tower requires a deep understanding of the sociotechnical system into which it must be integrated

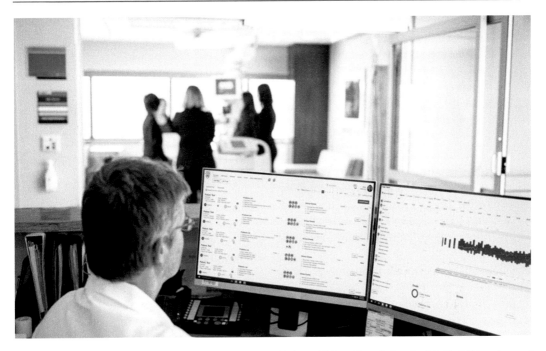

Fig. 13.3 Control tower in action. Photo used with permission of Mayo Foundation for Medical Education and Research; all rights reserved

This unified screening system is managed by a designated capsule communicator known as " `," analogous to the U.S. National Aeronautics and Space Administration ground-based astronaut, who maintains contact with astronauts during space missions. The CapCom in the healthcare context is the clinician responsible for screening incoming alerts and notifications (Fig. 13.3).

As no electronic alerts have 100% accuracy, it is essential to perform an initial validation of notifications by humans before activating specific workflows with bedside providers.

When the CapCom decides that an alert is valid, she/he communicates "down to the ground" to a bedside clinician and guides them through necessary and recommended tasks. Each step may be captured electronically in the control tower application. Workflow and actions are captured and they are analyzed using a feedback loop tool. Deviations from intended care processes may be identified.

Systems such as Control Tower represent a new generation of real time hospital or multi-hospitals clinical surveillance platform tools that complement and supplement existing EMR and telemedicine technologies.

Summary

Public health monitoring and surveillance has existed for centuries, however in-hospital surveillance progressed with the recent adoption of an EMR. The emergence of rapid response teams and adoption of scoring systems have become the standard of care for inpatient treatment. Clinical informatics methods allow for advance rule and ML based alerts. Nevertheless, optimal configuration of people, processes, incentives, and technology are essential to building successful alerts and/or surveillance systems.

Conclusions and Outlook

With the adoption of EMRs, more advanced and precise tools are needed to support bedside providers in real time. Clinical surveillance and advance alert systems are under development to serve needs of patients and clinicians. Platforms like Control Tower represent a new generation of hospital clinical surveillance systems.

Useful Resources

1. World Health Organization (WHO): https://www.who.int/
2. Mayo Clinic: https://www.mayoclinic.org/
3. FDA's Statistical Guidance on Reporting Results from Studies Evaluating Diagnostic Tests: https://www.fda.gov/regulatory-information/search-fda-guidance-documents/statistical-guidance-reporting-results-studies-evaluating-diagnostic-tests-guidance-industry-and-fda
4. Clinical In Intensive Care Laboratory at Mayo Clinic—https://www.mayo.edu/research/labs/clinical-informatics-intensive-care/

Review Questions

1. Rapid Response System in context of healthcare is:
   (a) Joint effort of City Mayor office, Sheriff, and public.
   (b) Extended Emergency Department.
   (c) Hospital activity to bring resources to deteriorated patient.
   (d) None of the above.
2. Reliable Clinical Alerts in clinical environment could be achieved by training ML tools on Big Data.
   (a) True.
   (b) False.
3. ICD codes are excellent sources of outcome diagnoses ("gold standard") for training computerized alerts.
   (a) True.
   (b) False.
4. Ideal clinical surveillance technologies should be carefully evaluated before implementation to practice in following domains (check all that apply):
   (a) Better health.
   (b) Profitability.
   (c) Better care.
   (d) Lower cost.

Appendix: Answers to Review Questions

1. Rapid Response System in context of healthcare is:
   (a) Joint effort of City Mayor office, Sheriff, and public.
   (b) Extended Emergency Department.
   (c) **Hospital activity to bring resources to deteriorated patient.**

Explanation: Rapid Response System (Team) is relatively now concept to healthcare. Those services established inside hospital and usually compound from Critical Care practitioners.

2. Reliable Clinical Alerts in clinical environment could be achieved by training Machine Learning tools on Big Data.
   (a) True.
   (b) **False.**

Explanation: Big data could be used to train Machine Learning tools. However, performance in clinical environment depends on other factors that not used during Big Data training.

3. ICD codes are excellent sources of outcome diagnoses ("gold standard") for training computerized alerts.
   (a) True.
   (b) **False.**

Explanation: ICD codes are used for billing and reporting purposes. That is documented in peer-review literature that ICD codes should not be used for using as "gold standard" for validation of clinical alerting and prediction models.

4. Ideal clinical surveillance technologies should be carefully evaluated before implementation to practice in following domains (check all what applies):
   (a) **Better health.**
   (b) Profitability.

(c) **Better care.**

(d) **Lower cost.**

Explanation: The Centers for Medicare & Medicaid Services (CMS) established those three goals as part of Affordable Care Act. Profitability of hospital/health care system is not part of that. Ideal technologies should address those three goals and not focus on increasing profitability.

References

1. Lee, L.M., Principles & practice of public health surveillance. 2010.
2. Smith PF, et al. "Blueprint version 2.0": updating public health surveillance for the 21st century. J Public Health Manag Pract. 2013;19(3):231–9.
3. Dieleman JL, et al. US Spending on personal health care and public health, 1996-2013. JAMA. 2016;316(24):2627–46.
4. Beitler JR, et al. Reduction in hospital-wide mortality after implementation of a rapid response team: a long-term cohort study. Crit Care. 2011;15(6):R269.
5. Hillman KM, et al. Duration of life-threatening antecedents prior to intensive care admission. Intensive Care Med. 2002;28(11):1629–34.
6. Barwise A, et al. Delayed rapid response team activation is associated with increased hospital mortality, morbidity, and length of stay in a tertiary care institution*. Crit Care Med. 2016;44(1):54–63.
7. Lyons PG, Edelson DP, Churpek MM. Rapid response systems. Resuscitation. 2018;128:191–7.
8. Berwick DM, et al. The 100 000 lives campaign setting a goal and a deadline for improving health care quality. JAMA. 2006;295(3):324–7.
9. Gunning K, Rowan K. ABC of intensive care: outcome data and scoring systems. BMJ. 1999;319(7204):241–4.
10. Carayon P. Sociotechnical systems approach to healthcare quality and patient safety. Work (Reading, Mass). 2012;41 Suppl 1(0 1):3850–4.
11. Smith ME, et al. Early warning system scores for clinical deterioration in hospitalized patients: a systematic review. Ann Am Thorac Soc. 2014;11(9):1454–65.
12. Downey CL, et al. Strengths and limitations of early warning scores: a systematic review and narrative synthesis. Int J Nurs Stud. 2017;76:106–19.
13. DeVita MA, et al. Use of medical emergency team responses to reduce hospital cardiopulmonary arrests. Qual Saf Health Care. 2004;13(4):251–4.
14. Moldenhauer K, et al. Clinical triggers: an alternative to a rapid response team. Jt Comm J Qual Patient Saf. 2009;35(3):164–74.
15. Hillman K, et al. Introduction of the medical emergency team (MET) system: a cluster-randomised controlled trial. Lancet. 2005;365(9477):2091–7.
16. Bleyer AJ, et al. Longitudinal analysis of one million vital signs in patients in an academic medical center. (1873–1570 (Electronic)).
17. Bellomo R, et al. A controlled trial of electronic automated advisory vital signs monitoring in general hospital wards. Crit Care Med. 2012;40(8):2349–61.
18. Downey CL, et al. The impact of continuous versus intermittent vital signs monitoring in hospitals: a systematic review and narrative synthesis. (1873-491X (Electronic)).
19. Cardona-Morrell M, et al. Effectiveness of continuous or intermittent vital signs monitoring in preventing adverse events on general wards: a systematic review and meta-analysis. (1742–1241 (Electronic)).
20. Evans RS. Electronic health records: then, now, and in the future. Yearb Med Inform. 2016;Suppl 1(Suppl 1):S48–61.
21. Rhee C, et al. Incidence and trends of sepsis in us hospitals using clinical vs claims data, 2009-2014. JAMA. 2017;318(13):1241–9.
22. Seymour CW, et al. Time to treatment and mortality during mandated emergency care for sepsis. N Engl J Med. 2017;376(23):2235–44.
23. Levy MM, et al. The surviving sepsis campaign: results of an international guideline-based performance improvement program targeting severe sepsis. Crit Care Med. 2010;38(2):367–74.
24. Seymour CW, et al. Derivation, validation, and potential treatment implications of novel clinical phenotypes for sepsis. JAMA. 2019;321(20):2003–17.
25. Seymour CW, et al. Assessment of clinical criteria for sepsis: for the third international consensus definitions for sepsis and septic shock (Sepsis-3). JAMA. 2016;315(8):762–74.
26. Singer M, et al. The third international consensus definitions for sepsis and septic shock (Sepsis-3). JAMA. 2016;315(8):801–10.
27. Alberto L, et al. Screening for sepsis in general hospitalized patients: a systematic review. J Hosp Infect. 2017;96(4):305–15.
28. Hooper MH, et al. Randomized trial of automated, electronic monitoring to facilitate early detection of sepsis in the intensive care unit*. Crit Care Med. 2012;40(7):2096–101.
29. Villegas N, Moore LJ. Sepsis screening: current evidence and available tools. Surg Infect. 2018;19(2):126–30.
30. Manaktala S, Claypool SR. Evaluating the impact of a computerized surveillance algorithm and decision support system on sepsis mortality. J Am Med Inform Assoc. 2017;24(1):88–95.
31. Thiel SW, et al. Early prediction of septic shock in hospitalized patients. J Hosp Med. 2010;5(1):19–25.
32. Ginestra JC, et al. Clinician perception of a machine learning-based early warning system designed to pre-

dict severe sepsis and septic shock. Crit Care Med. 2019;47(11):1477–84.

33. The Lancet Respiratory, M. Crying wolf: the growing fatigue around sepsis alerts. Lancet Respir Med. 2018;6(3):161.

34. Shah NR, et al. Improving acceptance of computerized prescribing alerts in ambulatory care. J Am Med Inform Assoc. 2006;13(1):5–11.

35. Amroze A, et al. Use of electronic health record access and audit logs to identify physician actions following noninterruptive alert opening: descriptive study. JMIR Med Inform. 2019;7(1):e12650.

36. Afshar M, et al. Patient outcomes and cost-effectiveness of a sepsis care quality improvement program in a health system. Crit Care Med. 2019;47(10):1371–9.

37. Lo HG, et al. Impact of non-interruptive medication laboratory monitoring alerts in ambulatory care. J Am Med Inform Assoc. 2009;16(1):66–71.

38. Deo RC. Machine learning in medicine. Circulation. 2015;132(20):1920–30.

39. Kreimeyer K, et al. Natural language processing systems for capturing and standardizing unstructured clinical information: a systematic review. J Biomed Inform. 2017;73:14–29.

40. Marafino BJ, et al. Validation of prediction models for critical care outcomes using natural language processing of electronic health record data. JAMA Netw Open. 2018;1(8):e185097.

41. Senders JT, et al. Machine learning and neurosurgical outcome prediction: a systematic review. World Neurosurg. 2018;109:476–486.e1.

42. Deist TM, et al. Machine learning algorithms for outcome prediction in (chemo)radiotherapy: An empirical comparison of classifiers. Med Phys. 2018;45(7):3449–59.

43. Hernandez-Suarez DF, et al. Machine-learning-based in-hospital mortality prediction for transcatheter mitral valve repair in the United States. Cardiovasc Revasc Med. 2020;

44. Hernandez-Suarez DF, et al. Machine learning prediction models for in-hospital mortality after transcatheter aortic valve replacement. JACC Cardiovasc Interv. 2019;12(14):1328–38.

45. Suzuki S, et al. Comparison of risk models for mortality and cardiovascular events between machine learning and conventional logistic regression analysis. PLoS One. 2019;14(9):e0221911.

46. Sousa FS, et al. Application of the intelligent techniques in transplantation databases: a review of articles published in 2009 and 2010. Transplant Proc. 2011;43(4):1340–2.

47. Menger V, et al. Machine learning approach to inpatient violence risk assessment using routinely collected clinical notes in electronic health records. JAMA Netw Open. 2019;2(7):e196709.

48. Shillan D, et al. Use of machine learning to analyse routinely collected intensive care unit data: a systematic review. Crit Care. 2019;23(1):284.

49. Linnen DT, et al. Statistical modeling and aggregate-weighted scoring systems in prediction of mortality and icu transfer: a systematic review. J Hosp Med. 2019;14(3):161–9.

50. Layeghian Javan S, Sepehri MM, Aghajani H. Toward analyzing and synthesizing previous research in early prediction of cardiac arrest using machine learning based on a multi-layered integrative framework. J Biomed Inform. 2018;88:70–89.

51. Joshi M, et al. Wearable sensors to improve detection of patient deterioration. Expert Rev Med Devices. 2019;16(2):145–54.

52. Albahri OS, et al. Systematic review of real-time remote health monitoring system in triage and priority-based sensor technology: taxonomy, open challenges, motivation and recommendations. J Med Syst. 2018;42(5):80.

53. Hackmann G, et al. Toward a two-tier clinical warning system for hospitalized patients. AMIA Annu Symp Proc. 2011;2011:511–9.

54. Kollef MH, et al. A randomized trial of real-time automated clinical deterioration alerts sent to a rapid response team. J Hosp Med. 2014;9(7):424–9.

55. Vitaly Herasevich MDPDMS, Brian MDMS, Pickering W. Health information technology evaluation handbook: from meaningful use to meaningful outcome. Taylor & Francis; 2017.

56. Weiss CH, et al. Prompting physicians to address a daily checklist and process of care and clinical outcomes: a single-site study. Am J Respir Crit Care Med. 2011;184(6):680–6.

57. Kahn JM, et al. Impact of nurse-led remote screening and prompting for evidence-based practices in the ICU*. Crit Care Med. 2014;42(4):896–904.

Interprofessional Structured Data: Supporting the Primary and Secondary Use of Patient Documentation

14

Kaija Saranto, Ulla-Mari Kinnunen, Pia Liljamo,
Minna Mykkänen, Anne Kuusisto, and Eija Kivekäs

Learning Objectives

This chapter aims to do the following:

- Describe important milestones in electronic records and interdisciplinary documentation.
- Illustrate the importance of structuring records.
- Discuss the opportunities and challenges of secondary use of data in clinical practice.
- Highlight the importance of continuity of care.
- Explain the changing roles of patients and professionals in a digital care environment.

Key Terms

- Coordination
- Continuity of care

- Digitalization
- Documentation
- Electronic health records
- Interdisciplinary
- Interprofessional
- Nursing discharge summary
- Standardized nursing terminology

Introduction

This chapter focuses on the electronic documentation of patient care, especially from an information processing and knowledge sharing point of view. In the early days of electronic patient records, the focus was on delivering information about symptoms and tests to be able to diagnose patients. It was also vital that the structure of screens followed the paper-based forms to have timely patient data [1]. Since those days, along with the development of health information technology (HIT), the importance is now on ways to easily find existing data on complex health problems of multimorbidity patients for decision-making. Further, electronic health records (EHR) are not designed for a single group of professionals, but more often, records are developed in interdisciplinary teams for interprofessional use in health care practice including financial administration [2, 3]. As EHRs, also health care service systems where they are operating are complex. Many changes are occurring due to limited resources in health care as well as

K. Saranto (✉) · U.-M. Kinnunen
Department of Health and Social Management,
University of Eastern Finland, Kuopio, Finland
e-mail: kaija.saranto@uef.fi;
ulla-mari.kinnunen@uef.fi

P. Liljamo
Oulu University Hospital, Oulu, Finland
e-mail: pia.liljamo@ppshp.fi

M. Mykkänen
Kuopio University Hospital, Kuopio, Finland
e-mail: minna.mykkanen@kuh.fi

A. Kuusisto · E. Kivekäs
Satakunta Hospital District, Pori, Finland
e-mail: anne.kuusisto@satasairaala.fi;
eija.kivekas@uef.fi

© Springer Nature Switzerland AG 2022
U. H. Hübner et al. (eds.), *Nursing Informatics*, Health Informatics,
https://doi.org/10.1007/978-3-030-91237-6_14

advances in science and medical practice. The role of patient participation in care processes is also changing since more care is provided virtually or online. This affects documentation as patients are also data providers, and patient-generated data is used in decision-making.

One important goal in present and future EHRs is to enable data integration and aggregation from various sources not only inside one service provider but also nationally—and even internationally. The need for timely health data is global as proved by the COVID-19 pandemic. Having a variety of secure standards to guarantee the interoperability of information systems globally is a huge challenge [3]. Interoperability has been considered a fundamental hindrance for nursing documentation although nurses and other health professionals have been active in developing tools to support continuity of care or data reuse. In practice, professionals need to agree on the codes and semantics of how to document patient care to ensure interdisciplinary communication based on interprofessional documentation [2]. This will support continuity of care, and most importantly, secondary use of patient data for quality control and administrative purposes. However, previous studies [3, 4] have highlighted the lack of functionalities of electronic records to be able support and follow the process of care due to poor system design. Most often, this follows multiple recording on various views by multiple professionals, which risks patient safety and continuity of care when timely data is not found and readily available.

Electronic Health Records for Interprofessional Use

Interprofessional health records comprise information that is especially needed in care transfer where timely data is crucial to guarantee continuity of care whether inside an organization or outside. Interprofessional data has also proved to be essential in emergency care, traumatology, nutrition, or cancer care, not to mention pediatrics or elderly care where patients may have multiple health problems. Thus, both structure and content of EHRs should assist clinical communication

and decision-making as well as have elements to summarize care episodes. One challenge for interdisciplinary documentation is both the differences and similarities of headings used in EHRs. In many records, or, more broadly, in information systems in health care, the views (meaning the various components) are designed based on specialties (e.g., surgical, internal medicine, psychiatric) for various professionals (e.g., physicians, nurses, physiotherapists, social workers, dietitians) or services (e.g., laboratory, radiology, rehabilitation) Further, health information systems may include components of administrative data such as visits and referrals, registers, or indicators (e.g., cancer, infections) as well as reports and certificates.

The model proposed by Donabedian (1992), which focuses on the structure, process, and outcome measures, has been used for quality assurance in health care for decades [5]. Broadly defined, structure measures refer to physical and organizational characteristics, whereas health care measures focus on the care delivered to patients (e.g., services, diagnostics, or treatments). Outcome measures refer to the effect of health care on the status of patients and populations [6]. In terms of data production in patient care, the model by Donabedian can be applied for structuring electronic records to classify the content into structure, process, and outcomes data. In many countries, data repositories have been created for patient data, achieving secured access based on the patient's consent for care providers or pharmacists at a regional or national level. These repositories are important for data sharing and secondary use of data (Fig. 14.1).

In many countries, like in Finland, patient records are continuous, starting from birth, and the key to personal data is a social security code unique to each citizen. Each professional should also have a smart card with an identifier to be able to use health information systems and national data archives in the national data repository named KANTA. Physicians use their cards to check previous notes and care episodes, to designate pharmacists to deliver medication, and to allow nurses to check orders and nursing discharge summaries. Patients use their own security codes to access the national data archives to

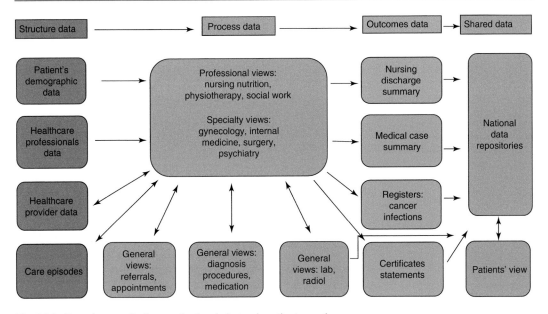

Fig. 14.1 Data elements for interprofessional electronic patient records

check their prescriptions, to read the summaries of care episodes, or to follow orders after a visit or hospital stay [7]. Many hospitals and health centers also provide online information through public or secured portals to provide digital health services. These have been especially useful in the COVID-19 pandemic.

Interdisciplinary health care demands unified documentation that follows this care process: assessment, diagnosis, goal setting, planning, intervention, and outcome assessment known by professionals and patients. This documentation requires defined data elements, classifications or terminologies, and standards to have high-quality data for multiple purposes. Most importantly, these should benefit patient participation in the care process.

Importance of Achieving Unified Documentation by Standardized Terminologies

Standardized nursing terminologies (SNT) have been under development and an object of interest for decades, beginning in the 1970s [e.g., 8, 9]. SNTs are content standards that include the terms or concepts that represent a focus on health concerning diagnoses, interventions, and outcomes consistent with the scope of practice for nursing. In literature, several terms such as "data set," "terminology," "language," "nomenclature," "classification," "vocabulary," and "taxonomy" have been used to describe the structures of nursing concepts in order to document and communicate practice [10]. According to Technology Informatics Guiding Education Reform (TIGER) recommendations [11] of nurses' health informatics competencies, nursing documentation including terminologies is one of the core competencies for clinical nursing, quality management, coordination of interprofessional care, nursing management, and information technology (IT) management in nursing. Thus, unified, uniform, and common language, SNT, is a prerequisite for interprofessional nursing practice and patient/disease-specific working groups.

The American Nurses Association (ANA) has worked since 1989 developing a process for recognizing nursing languages, vocabularies, and terminologies. The ANA has recognized two minimum data sets, two reference terminologies, and eight interface terminologies for facilitating standardized nursing documentation and interoperability of nursing data between different IT systems [9] (Table 14.1).

Unified documentation is a requirement for comprehensible content of nursing documenta-

Table 14.1 ANA recognized SNTs [9]

Interface Terminologies	Minimum Data Sets
Clinical Care Classification (CCC) System	Nursing Minimum Data Set (NMDS)
International Classification for Nursing Practice (ICNP)	Nursing Management Minimum Data Set (NMMDS)
North American Nursing Diagnosis Association International (NANDA-I)	
Nursing Interventions Classification System (NIC)	**Reference Terminologies**
Nursing Outcomes Classification (NOC)	Logical Observation Identifiers Names and Codes (LOINC)
Omaha System	SNOMED Clinical Terms (SNOMED CT)
Perioperative Nursing Data Set (PNDS)	
ABC Codes	

tion for all nurses and nursing administration. The need for developing a unified SNT in order to enhance comparability of nursing data is well recognized [8, 12]. Cross-mapping and coordination across classifications render it possible to evaluate the equivalence of the content and concepts used and to promote shared use of the various nursing classifications and data generated while avoiding redundancy in the information saved [13, 14].

The utility of the terminology in practice alongside the reliability and validity of the terminology must be evidenced through research [10]. In addition, patient care must be evidence-based, which refers to the best available evidence from scientific research. "Evidence based medicine is the conscientious, explicit, and judicious use of current best evidence in making decisions about the care of individual patients" [15]. A recent study [16] shows that terminologies in use must also be evidence-based. Vice versa, by using terminologies in nursing care documentation, we can make nursing visible and evidence the best possible patient care [10].

As an example from Finland, the national Finnish nursing documentation model is based on a defined nursing core data (nursing minimum data set, NMDS), a standardized nursing terminology: Finnish Care Classification (FinCC),

which is originally based on CCC terminology, and a nursing process model in decision-making. The nationally agreed key structured data elements, the core data in nursing includes nursing diagnoses, nursing interventions, nursing outcomes, nursing intensity, and nursing discharge summary. In the enhancement and updating of the FinCC, the aim was to ensure that the FinCC system is more thoroughly founded on evidence-based data. To achieve this, the expert group searched for evidence, including Current Care Guidelines and other guidelines for care; familiarized themselves with the legislation, relevant guidebooks by the Finnish Institute for Health and Welfare, instructions, and various models; and searched scientific publications. The new FinCC 4.0 was published in December 2019 [17] (Fig. 14.2).

The FinCC consists of the Finnish classification of nursing diagnoses (FiCND), the Finnish classification of nursing interventions (FiCNI), and the Finnish classification of nursing outcomes (FiCNO). Both the FiCND and the FiCNI include 17 components, which is the highest and the most abstract level of documentation (e.g., Skin Integrity, Nutrition, Coping and Fluid Balance). The main and subcategory levels are the concrete levels of documentation. Nursing outcomes can be evaluated by means of the three qualifiers of the FiCNO: improved, stabilized, and deteriorated. Besides the evidence-based data, end-users have had a big role in the development of the FinCC. The content of the FinCC is a result of a cultural validation in 2001, and it has been revised by utilizing the user feedback in 2004, 2007, 2010, and 2019. The Finnish nursing documentation model is widely used today in different health care settings [17, 18].

Secondary Use of Nursing Data

Patient care data from the EHR systems are increasingly in demand for reuse in administration and resource planning. Nursing documentation along with coded concepts is expected to produce more reliable data and fulfill requirements for reuse better. It has been proven that

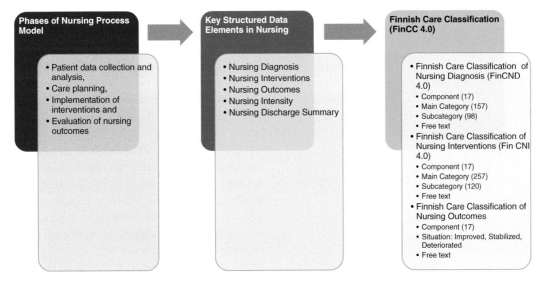

Phases of Nursing Process Model

- Patient data collection and analysis,
- Care planning,
- Implementation of interventions and
- Evaluation of nursing outcomes

Key Structured Data Elements in Nursing

- Nursing Diagnosis
- Nursing Interventions
- Nursing Outcomes
- Nursing Intensity
- Nursing Discharge Summary

Finnish Care Classification (FinCC 4.0)

- Finnish Care Classification of Nursing Diagnosis (FinCND 4.0)
  - Component (17)
  - Main Category (157)
  - Subcategory (98)
  - Free text
- Finnish Care Classification of Nursing Interventions (Fin CNI 4.0)
  - Component (17)
  - Main Category (257)
  - Subcategory (120)
  - Free text
- Finnish Care Classification of Nursing Outcomes
  - Component (17)
  - Situation: Improved, Stabilized, Deteriorated
  - Free text

Fig. 14.2 The national Finnish nursing documentation model including the FinCC 4.0. (see [17] for more information)

structured documentation can produce more complete and reliable patient records, better fulfilling the requirements of data quality for the purposes of secondary use. The different standards for representing, communicating, exchanging, managing, and reporting data, information, and knowledge in the EHRs have been developed in order to support nursing practice and to ensure the validity of the data. The most important standards for nursing are content, messaging, confidentiality, and security standards. Structured or coded concepts allow the performance of evaluation of the nursing process, the key structure for care plans and documentation, and the provision of valid electronically documented nursing clinical data shareable across HIT and EHR systems. The coded concepts also permit the measurement of nursing outcomes and effectiveness, providing evidence for decision-making [10].

Clinical documentation supports patient care, improves clinical outcomes, and enhances interprofessional communication. When nursing entries are made in the same consistent way everywhere using agreed-upon terminology, the documentation is comparable among different care units and organizations. The greatest benefit of structured data is that it enables the reuse of

recorded information because it can be identified [8, 10].

The rapidly changing environment of health care creates challenges for health care managers not only to have up-to-date information for daily management but also to have trends and scenarios of what is and will be happening in the future. Decision-making requires proper, accurate, and timely information that can be quickly and easily obtained. Reliable information on the reality of care is needed to support the monitoring of quality, safety, and costs of care as well as to plan development activities, to guarantee professionals' competences, and to benchmark research [19]. Clinical information systems contain large amounts of data on patient care, but little use is made of the accumulated data resources.

In health care, the primary use of patient data is to secure patient care. Structured data can be processed electronically, facilitating, for example, the access, retrieval, linking, and tracking of patient data. According to previous studies with nurses, using structured data enhanced the daily care processes, usability and quality of data, and secondary data use [6, 8, 19]. In health care organizations, managers and administrators are expected to benefit from structured patient data when already-stored data can be used in organizations for purposes other than patients' direct care. The secondary use of health care data means that data generated in health care activities is used for a purpose other than for which they were originally stored. The data is therefore used in non-therapeutic situations when the data is filtered and combined in different ways [20, 21], for example:

- Operational planning and information management.
- Development and innovation.
- Research, statistics, and teaching.
- Regulatory guidance and control.

In Finland, the secondary use of data is regulated by legislation, which harmonizes the use of health care customer data and other personal data related to health and well-being. The secondary use of EHR data imposes different requirements on the data stored and utilized in the patient record. Five dimensions have been defined for the quality of data entered into patient record systems: completeness, correctness, concordance, plausibility, and currency. Completeness of the data describes the reality of the patient's care. The data is accurate, high-quality, relevant, consistent, and reliable. The correctness of the data describes, for example, the accuracy of the data. Further, data correspondence describes the accuracy of data elements describing the same issue to each other. Plausibility where the data corresponds to the general medical and health scientific understanding is accuracy, validity, and believability. Currency means that the data has been stored up-to-date, meaning it has been updated [19, 22].

The reliability of the recorded data can be guaranteed by initially storing the data correctly. In order to use the accumulated data resources for secondary use, the information must be of consistent and comparable to draw reliable conclusions from it. The quality of the health care data must be good and easily accessible [21, 23]. Because of the usability of patient data, it is essential that the quality of the data is as high as possible because incomplete, inaccurate, or erroneous

recording makes the data unreliable. Clear, reliable, and accurate communication in health care between professionals is an essential part of patient safety and effective action [19, 23].

The structured nursing documentation makes it possible to easily assess the quality of recording. A nursing record audit is a prerequisite to having high-quality and valid data for secondary use [1, 19, 24]. Documentation in accordance with the nursing process has demonstrated the accuracy of documentation and the connection to legal requirements. In addition, patient orientation and the logical whole of documentation are key aspects of documentation evaluation [12]. Nursing documentation assessment models have primarily been developed for local or regional purposes, and a lack of international cooperation to assess the nursing record has been identified [25, 26]. The use of FinCC in nursing documentation can be assessed by an audit model developed for national use. In one university hospital in Finland, there is evidence from many years of systematic audits of nursing records, improving the quality and accuracy of records [27].

In many countries, where public health care is guaranteed for citizens, health care costs are referred with huge amounts of expenditure. From these figures/amounts, it is virtually impossible to find out nursing costs. One example of secondary use of nursing data is differentiating nursing care as part of a patient's billing. Everyday nurses document nursing diagnoses, nursing interventions, and nursing outcomes on each patient's EHR. By combining this data with other data required, one can determine the nursing input. Thus, in this way, we can understand the impact and effectiveness of nursing care.

The secondary use of data would not be possible without EHR functionalities. Most importantly, these should support nursing documentation during the caring process. An issue that should never be overlooked or underestimated is the alignment between the functionality of the new EHR system and users' requirements. In the case study at the end of our chapter, the use of structured nursing data for secondary purposes is described form nursing management point of view.

Securing the Continuity of Patient Care by Means of Electronic Nursing Discharge Summary

The nursing process model is a guiding structure of nursing discharge summary, which is a compact summary of the Nursing Minimum Data Set of the care period—in other words, a summary of nursing diagnoses, nursing interventions, nursing intensity, and nursing outcomes. Continuity of patient care (COC) often depends on the flow of information, preparation and sharing of patient records, and receiving of electronic nursing discharge summaries (ENDS). At the end of the patient's care period, a short, concise, and evaluative ENDS of the patient's care is prepared for the patient and for the follow-up care site. A medical case summary and ENDS include summary information about patient care and are separate documents. The ENDS is one part of an electronic patient record and is compiled from key issues in nursing records during the patient's care period (Fig. 14.4). The ENDS serves as care feedback and as referral in the patient transfer phase when a patient is transferred for follow-up care from one health care service to another and to the home. It should include all the necessary information required for patient care [28].

The purpose of the ENDS is to secure and improve the COC by excluding overlapping in documentation when each professional group documents their interventions and responsibilities. The ENDS should include the reason for hospital admission, how the patient has felt and how the condition has changed, what the patient's care consisted of, and whether the care will continue, and if so, how. The ENDS is a way to make nursing care visible [28]. It is essential that the information contained in the ENDS includes instructions for further care and allows the patient to continue self-care at home, in another place of care, or in subsequent care periods in the same unit if he or she re-enters care. In the patient's follow-up care setting, nurses can use the ENDS to develop a nursing care plan in addition to the medical case summary. For example, a specialist nurse in secondary care may provide instructions

to primary care nurses on appropriate stoma care aids after bowel surgery in the ENDS.

The ENDS should be recorded according to the nursing process, stored using a pre-agreed structure, and supplemented with patient-specific free-form text. Once the information is structured, it can be reused. Day-to-day nursing documentation, previously recorded with FinCC classification, can be compacted and reused in the compiling of ENDS. Standards for compiling the ENDS are rare [29], but they are often asked to support the ability to share comparable information with other health care organizations and settings [29–32]. The ENDS, adapted by standardized national definition work, have been used in Finland since 2005. It is compulsory to save the ENDS into the National Patient Data Repository in Finland.

The content of the ENDS consists of *personal data* (e.g., identification of the patient), *sociodemographic data* (e.g., information on the social life of patient), and *administrative* (e.g., identification of the care provider) and *clinical information* on a care period for purposes of follow-up care (e.g., functional ability, nutrition, digestion, medication, psychological regulation). Figure 14.3 shows that the process of compiling the content in ENDS consists of four nursing process model stages.

- *Patient admission* covers assessment for need of patient care, for example, the reason for hospital admission and background information such as the patient's housing conditions and functional ability.
- *Care planning* includes the most relevant nursing diagnosis defined according to the general health of the patient.
- *Implementation of intervention* covers the main interventions taken by the nurses. The responsibility of the nurse is to record in the ENDS medication administration-related matters, the effect of medication-related matters, medication taken on transfer day, as well as the medication to be given as needed, such as painkillers.
- *Evaluation of nursing outcomes* refers to major ratings at discharge and includes

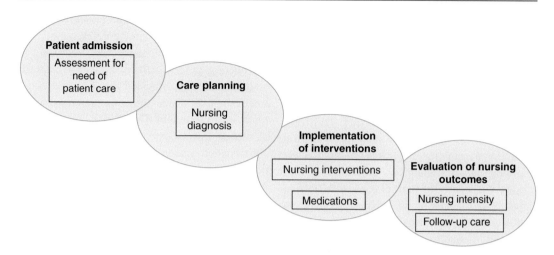

Fig. 14.3 National Electronic Nursing Discharge Summary titles in the Phases of Nursing Process Model in Finland

nursing intensity and issues related to follow-up care, for example, patient education, control visits, or suture removals, if not clear from the medical case summary.

In order to evaluate how continuity of care is achieved when using ENDS, the concept of COC needs to be defined. It is obvious that there is a need to determine explicitly what informational, management, and cross-border continuity of care mean. *Informational continuity of care* refers to data tool (e.g., paper or electronic nursing discharge summary), data content (e.g., medication), data structures (e.g., standards-compliant interoperability), or information quality (e.g., accuracy or adequacy of information) and related processes. *Management continuity of care* refers to information flow (e.g., timeliness or reliability), cooperation (e.g., understanding each other's work), coordination (e.g., care plan), and interprofessional (e.g., interprofessional documentation) or management (e.g., knowledge management) processes [33]. *Cross-border continuity of care* means that people receive the most appropriate treatment whenever they need it and wherever they are, and health care professionals have access to their patient data.

Based on the study findings, nursing staff in primary care evaluated the ENDS as a positive tool. Recipients assessed the flow of information to be more reliable and faster and collaboration to

be smoother and more responsive to the patient's situation than those who had not received them. The most important issue from the aspect of the receiving nurse is the patient's condition and well-being at discharge. There were some duplications and contradictions concerning the content of patient care in medical case summaries and in nursing summaries, especially concerning medication [34]. Further, a discharge checklist can be used to ensure that the information necessary for the safe COC generated during the patient's care period is recorded in the ENDS and is available for follow-up.

Recently, a structured electronic interdisciplinary discharge checklist was implemented into nursing documentation systems to support the safe discharge of the elderly from the beginning of care period. The content of the proposed document is based on FinCC and includes type of accommodation, toilet functions, dressing, and eating as well as aids and accessories. The checklist can be of practical use to health care professionals worldwide. For example, nurses responsible for the nursing discharge can utilize it to verify that all information relevant to follow-up is included when designing ENDS. Most importantly, timely information relevant to patient care is available where the care continues, and the checklist is interdisciplinary [35].

The ENDS deduce the patient's responsibility for data transmission because the patient can see the ENDS in My Kanta Pages, which is a citizens' online service used in Finland that displays information recorded by health care professionals about patients and their medications [7]. Studies have shown that patients have not always understood the follow-up instructions recorded in the medical case summaries or the medical terminology they contain and have not asked for clarification. In other words, they have lacked important information, and the need for a plain language medical case summary has been raised [32, 36]. The ENDS provide the patient with an individual follow-up plan and care instructions in an easy-to-read format. Interdisciplinary usage possibilities can be seen as a benefit of the ENDS. Written practically, the ENDS avoid medical terms not only by the patient but also by the staff of the home health service [37]. Currently, the ENDS are produced by nursing professionals. The aim is that in the future, the information produced by the patient such as well-being information or living wills could be integrated into the ENDS.

The Changing Role of Patients and Professionals in a Digital Care Environment

For decades, patients and citizens have been experienced in using the Internet to search for health-related information. Although patients trust their physicians, due to their expertise and experience, they prefer the Internet because it provides easy access to information [38]. In the beginning, patient portals were standalone websites with no connection to health care delivery contexts or providers. Currently, patient portals are promising instruments to improve patient-centered care, as they provide patients with information and tools that can help them better manage their health. The implementation of portals in both the inpatient and outpatient settings gives health care providers opportunities to support patients both during hospitalization and after discharge.

Patient portals for chronic disease management have shown some promising results regard-

ing patient outcomes [39]. A typical electronic patient portal allows patients to see their visit history, current medication list and allergies, recent laboratory results, and other medical data captured in their health care providers' electronic health records [40]. Self-Treatment and Digital Value Services and Virtual Hospital 2.0 projects have led to the development of digital services for citizens and health care professionals in Finland [41, 42]. These services have enabled service and treatment chains to merge in new ways in different specialized fields in both primary and specialized medical care service networks. Digital services allow better cooperation between those working in social welfare and health care service organizations. In addition, patients can store information about their well-being using different applications. A well-being application for example, may be an application on a mobile phone, an online service used via the browser on a computer, or a measuring device such as a blood sugar monitor or an activity tracker. In Finland, the My Kanta Personal Health Record stores citizens' health and well-being data conveniently and securely in one place [7]. It can store data collected by a patient's heart rate monitor or activity bracelet in the digital health service (Virtual Hospital/Health Village), allowing the patient to view the data in My Kanta Pages. The illustration of digital health services in the care process provides insight into the extent of the change when transforming traditional services to digital services.

Studies have been demonstrated in a review that socio-demographic characteristics and medical conditions of patients were predictors of portal use. Some patients wanted unlimited access to their electronic health records, personalized health education, and nonclinical information. In addition, patients were eager to use portals for communicating with their health care teams. Although some studies found that patient portals improved patient engagement, some patients perceived certain portal functions as inadequate. Patients and staff thought portals could improve patient care but could cause anxiety in some patients. However, portals improved patient safety, adherence to medications, and patient-provider communication but had no impact on objective health outcomes. Furthermore, preliminary results of a systematic review of patient portals did not reveal clear evidence of substantial and consistent positive effects of patient portals on patient empowerment and health-related outcomes.

Digital services have increased customer satisfaction and the impact of services offered to patients or customers while continually gathering data for service development. The projects achieved their goals. Digital services integrated with care paths enhance the efficiency of treatments and preventive health care, allow customers to access care at the right time, reduce the number of outpatient visits, and increase the efficiency of working time. Using a modern big data analytics methodology, the use and impact of digital services should be monitored. Service paths and structures should be continuously developed based on customers' behavior and the impact of services. Providing patients access to their health records has been linked to theorized benefits in four major domains of health care quality: patient-centeredness, effectiveness, safety, and efficiency. In addition, secure access to medical and nursing records improves patient satisfaction and enhances patient–provider communication.

Patient portals can be difficult to navigate, and patients may struggle to understand their medical information. According to studies, patients want their providers to encourage them and explain how to use the portal as well as provide multiple opportunities for training [43]. Low health literacy has been associated with a decreased use of preventive services, increased risk of developing a chronic disease, poorer treatment adherence, and poorer health outcomes [38]. In addition, health literacy also influences patient–provider communication. Individuals with low health literacy are less likely to engage in shared decision-making with their health care providers and are less likely to ask questions. McAlearney and colleagues' (2019) survey proved that patients identified viewing their health information, managing their schedules, and communicating with providers as notable activities [44]. Convenience, access

to information, and better engagement in care were indicated as benefits. Conversely, concerns were related to technology issues, privacy, and security risks.

Clinicians often cite inadequate visit time as a barrier to developing a relationship and communication with patients. Also, creating EHRs during patient interviews has diminished clinicians' ability to connect with patients, leading to clinicians' dissatisfaction with clinical practice [45]. When patients were able to input agendas into electronic health record notes before visiting a health care provider, both patients and clinicians felt that communication during the visit was improved and that time was optimized. They expressed interest in future patient-written agendas. The preliminary results of the Digital Health Village® patient portal [42] surveys revealed that patients were motivated to monitor their wellness with electronic health care services based on their experiences with such services, and the patients were confident about the effectiveness of such services. While the project manager, team, organizational structure, culture, and atmosphere are still regarded as key components in enabling a project's success, it was important to recognize all the factors influencing success. It has been proved that leadership was the most important project success factor. Finally, investing in the leadership and project management skills of project participants could improve the success of future projects.

Case Study

FinCC Supporting Nurse Managers in Decision-Making

Utilization of structured data for nursing care supports the development of nursing practices and the will to utilize nursing information in nursing management to ensure the best patient care. The produced data also helps to support decision-making for health care managers. The aim is to utilize statistics in nursing development founded on evidence-based care and day-to-day management. This case study aims to describe the possibilities structured documentation with a standardized terminology offers to daily nursing management. First, the process of data gathering is described, following the data analysis, and implications to practice.

The FinCC was implemented in 2007 into nursing records of a hospital district's wide EHR system. A systematic in-service training was created to support the daily use of the FinCC. Further, to guarantee the quality of the documentation a nursing audit system and a mentoring system were launched to support the maintenance of nursing documentation quality. The daily use in nursing documentation since the beginning has created a huge database to analyze trends, changes, and forecast challenges in patient care. Nurse managers can access this database through the EHR. The system includes a reporting tool based on the structured data, data retrieval, and its compilation according to the defined conditions, for example, component, main, and subcategory levels according to the FinCC. The IT department has created tools for data analytics, for example, for patient profiles by wards and

units, relations between nursing diagnosis and interventions, and further to nursing outcomes.

In the following figure (Fig. 14.4), the use of the 17 components of the Finnish classification of nursing diagnoses (FiCND) of two different wards, the gastrosurgical ward and the cardiac care unit, demonstrates the differences between patient needs. Nursing diagnoses in the gastrosurgical ward focus on sensory and neurological functions (including acute pain), coordination of care, elimination, coping, and nutrition. The cardiac care unit focuses on sensory and neurological functions (including chest pain), cardiac functions, respiration, skin integrity, and coping.

The use of the FinCC highlights how patients' care needs (diagnoses) and the content of nursing practice and interventions are different on various wards. The care unit profiles become more visible, which can help in the allocation of nursing resources, education, research, and teaching. By linking these statistics with other structured data, they can be used to describe the allocation of resources used as well as the quality and

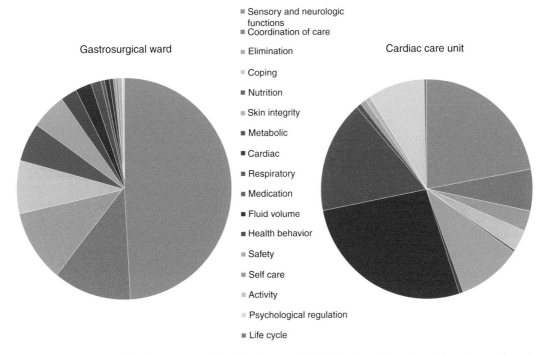

Fig. 14.4 Distribution of used components of nursing diagnoses (FiCND) on two different wards from January through May 2020

outcomes of treatment. We have to bear in mind that patients are individuals regardless of the same medical diagnosis and treatment processes. For example, patients may respond differently to anesthesia, or the patient may experience postoperative pain in very different ways. And thus, nursing needs and interventions in the patient treatment process can be very different despite the same medical diagnosis or procedure.

The use of the FinCC has many implications to both nursing and interprofessional practice. With the help of structured documentation, nursing care data can be retrieved from large amounts of patient data and, among other things, the above-mentioned differences in patient care processes can be found. By combining nursing diagnoses and interventions with, for example, medical diagnoses and procedures, it is possible to further develop interprofessional patient care from common care processes toward more and more individualized patient care. In addition, the data will influence the associated side diagnosis of the main medical diagnosis, for example, diabetes, changes in nursing diagnoses or interventions, extended care times, or increased costs. The use of the FinCC has also given a new language to discuss more in-depth about the nursing care and possibilities to share ideas for developments. The results produced by analytics and tools are discussed at ward level and at interdisciplinary meetings.

Summary

Although interdisciplinary documentation involves many challenges, it often has huge possibilities to improve data quality, data aggregation and transfer, and information flow. Interdisciplinary documentation is essential for professionals responsible for care, and it is meaningful for patients who often participate actively in decision-making in the care context. The role of technologies (e.g., patient records or health information systems) is evident, but the implementation and adoption processes still need continuous attention despite the past years of existence in practice.

The transition from a paper-based system to electronic and structured records has been more feasible than changing from an electronic to a new structured system. This indicates that health professionals have high expectations toward new systems. Still, it is not clear whether this is based on poor functionality in the system design or lack of training, which is an important feature in the implementation process. Incomplete functionality causes frustration among users when, for example, the same information must be recorded multiple times or search tools are totally lacking in the system. Additionally, this harms patient safety. Functionalities also concern patients since already in many health information systems, patients can have their own dashboard to record their information (e.g., social determinants, symptoms, or measures to be linked by professionals to the system).

Besides the system requirements, the structure of the record needs standards and common terminologies for successful use. Developing unified and evidence-based terminologies for recording patient care has been widely recognized and is of high importance. Several standardized nursing terminologies are in use globally. Further, the mapping of various terminologies has revealed that they have common elements to describe nursing care. Thus, whatever terminology is used, the content of patient care remains the same based on patients' signs and symptoms, and the visibility of evidence-based care is guaranteed. In many nursing faculties, curricula updates and developments are needed for nursing informatics competencies concerning documentation. The lack of skills and competencies as well as not understanding the value of standardized documentation is a risk for nursing practice, management, and patient safety.

In spite of great advancements, challenges still exist in interprofessional documentation and interdisciplinary data content if the EHR does not support standardized patient care documentation. Opportunities have been shown in informational, management, and cross-border continuity of care by means of shared data. However, the shared data is not useful unless the essential data content for patient care has not been recorded or if the recorded data is not unified, good quality, and up-to-date. As for continuity of care, there are challenges in duplication and diversity of data content between nursing discharge summaries and medical case summaries.

Patient portals have increased powerfully during the COVID-19 pandemic. A typical electronic patient portal allows patients to see their visit history, current medication list and allergies, recent laboratory results, and other medical data captured in their health care providers' electronic health records. The development of digital services for citizens and health care professionals has enabled service and treatment chains to merge in new ways in different specialized fields in both primary and specialized medical care service networks. In addition, digital health care services allow better cooperation among those working in health care service organizations. The illustration of digital health services in the care process provides insight into the extent of the change when transforming traditional services to digital services.

Conclusions and Outlook

A common understanding of the importance of accurate and timely documentation in interprofessional collaboration is important. Structured data recorded by nurses and other health professionals can be used many times for various purposes—first as the basis of patient care in many phases or settings, and then reused for summary and administrative purposes. Often, data is utilized for secondary purposes to evidence care quality, resource allocation, and the need for changes in treatment processes through research and development activities. In the future, patients will be more involved in and better responsible for data sharing in interdisciplinary teams in health care.

Useful Resources
1. Kanta Services in Finland. https://www.kanta. fi/en/
2. Digital Health Village in Finland. https:// www.digitalhealthvillage.com/en/home
3. Omaolo services https://www.omaolo.fi/

Review Questions
1. What opportunities does interdisciplinary documentation have?
   (a) Standardized EHR structure
   (b) Agreed headings
   (c) Improved information flow
2. Why must nursing terminologies be evidence-based?
   (a) In order to show evidence-based patient care
   (b) In order to develop terminologies based on evidence-based practices
   (c) So that the end users can refer to evidence-based research
3. FinCC is an acronym of:
   (a) Final Clinical Cooperation
   (b) Finnish Care Classification
   (c) Finnish Clinical Classification
4. Electronic Nursing Discharge Summary includes:
   (a) Nursing diagnosis
   (b) Nursing interventions
   (c) Nursing outcomes
   (d) Nursing intensity
5. What does secondary use of data mean?
   (a) Clinical data is used a second time.
   (b) Clinical data is copied to another location in the her.
   (c) Clinical data is used for a purpose other than that for which it was originally stored.
6. How does the digitalization of health care affect interprofessional collaboration or interdisciplinary documentation?
   (a) Because of digitalization, no interprofessional collaboration is needed in the future.
   (b) Only health professionals will continue to collaborate.
   (c) The role of the patient is strengthened, and patients participate, becoming increasingly involved in and responsible for data sharing.
   (d) Digitalization does not change anything.
7. What kind of services digitalization (digital transformation) allow?
   (a) Better cooperation among professionals in social welfare and healthcare service organizations.

(b) Patient can store information on his well-being using different applications.

(c) Digital services give instruments to improve patient-centered care.

(d) Digital services have enabled service and treatment chains to merge in new in different fields in medical care service networks.

Appendix: Answers to Review Questions

1. What opportunities do interdisciplinary documentation have?

   (a) Standardized EHR structure

   (b) Agreed headings

   (c) Improved information flow

Explanation: Interdisciplinary documentation is based on a standardized structure, which has agreed headings used in the EHR. When the multidisciplinary team is committed to use a structured EHR, information flow will improve between the team members.

2. Why must nursing terminologies be evidence-based?

   (a) In order to show evidence-based patient care

   (b) In order to develop terminologies based on evidence-based practices

   (c) So that the end users can refer to evidence-based research

Explanation: Terminologies in use must be evidence-based, and by using terminologies in nursing care documentation, we can make nursing visible and evidence the best possible patient care.

3. FinCC is an acronym of?

   (a) Final Clinical Cooperation

   (b) Finnish Care Classification

   (c) Finnish Clinical Classification

Explanation: FinCC is an acronym of Finnish Care Classification.

4. Electronic Nursing Discharge Summary includes:

   (a) Nursing diagnosis

   (b) Nursing interventions

   (c) Nursing outcomes

   (d) Nursing intensity

Explanation: ENDS is a compact summary of the Nursing Minimum Data Set of the care period, i.e., a summary of nursing diagnoses, nursing interventions, nursing intensity, and nursing outcomes.

5. What does secondary use of data mean?

   (a) Clinical data is used a second time.

   (b) Clinical data is copied to another location in the her.

   (c) Clinical data is used for a purpose other than that for which it was originally stored.

Explanation: Secondary use of health care data means that data generated in health care activities are used for a purpose other than that for which they were originally stored. The primary patient data in EHR is filtered and combined in different ways for secondary use purposes like operational planning and information management and health care development and innovation. Patient data can be utilized in research, statistics and teaching, and regulatory guidance and control.

6. How does the digitalization of health care affect interprofessional collaboration or interdisciplinary documentation?

   (a) Because of digitalization, no interprofessional collaboration is needed in the future.

   (b) Only health professionals will continue to collaborate.

   (c) The role of the patient is strengthened, and patients participate, becoming increasingly involved in and responsible for data sharing.

   (d) Digitalization does not change anything.

Explanation: The development of different kinds of digital services for citizens and health care professionals has enabled service and treatment chains to merge in new ways in different specialized fields in both primary and specialized medical care service networks. Digital health care services allow better cooperation among those working in health care service organizations. Patients will be able to view and produce their own health information as new digital tools and transactional portals are developed. Information systems and electronic identification enable secure patient participation.

7. What kind of services digitalization (digital transformation) allow?

   (a) Better cooperation among professionals in social welfare and healthcare service organizations.

   (b) Patient can store information on his well-being using different applications.

   (c) Digital services give instruments to improve patient-centered care.

   (d) Digital services have enabled service and treatment chains to merge in new in different fields in medical care service networks.

Explanation: Digital services have increased customer satisfaction and the impact of services offered to patients or customers while continually gathering data for service development. Digital services allow better cooperation between those working in social welfare and healthcare service organizations. In addition, patient can store information on his wellbeing using different applications. These services have enabled service and treatment chains to merge in new ways in different specialized fields in both primary and specialized medical care service networks.

References

1. Häyrinen K, Saranto K, Nykänen P. Definition, structure, content, use and impacts of electronic health records: A review of the research literature. Int J Med Inform. 2008;77:291–304.
2. Furlow B. Information overload and unsustainable workloads in the era of electronic health records. Lancet Respir Med. 2020;8(3):243–4.
3. Shull JG. Digital Health and the Sate of Interoperable Electronic Health records. JMIR Med Inform. 2019;7(4):e12712/1-8.
4. Joukes E, Kiezer N, de Bruijine MC, Abu-Hanna A, Cornet R. Impact of electronic versus paper-based recording before EHR Implementation on health care professionals' perceptions of EHR use, data quality, and date reuse. Appl Clin Inform. 2019;10(2):199–209. https://doi.org/10.1055/s-0039-1681054.
5. Donabedian A. The role of outcomes in quality assessment and assurance. Qual Rev Bull. 1992;11:356–60.
6. Pagulayan J, Eltair S, Faber K. Nurse documentation and the electronic health record. Use the nursing process to take advantage of EHRs' capabilities and optimize patient care. American Nurse Today. 2018;13(9):58–61.
7. Kanta Services. The Social Insurance Institution of Finland. 2020. https://www.kanta.fi/en/ Accessed 23 February 2020.
8. Saranto K, Kinnunen UM, Kivekäs E, Lappalainen AM, Liljamo P, Rajalahti E, Hyppönen H. Impacts of structuring nursing records: a systematic review. Scand J Caring Sci. 2014 Dec;28(4):629–47. https://doi.org/10.1111/scs.12094.
9. Office of the National Coordinator for Health IT. Standard nursing terminologies: a landscape analysis. Identifying Challenges and Opportunities within Standard Nursing Terminologies. 2017. Available at https://www.healthit.gov/sites/default/files/snt_final_05302017.pdf Accessed March 4, 2020.
10. Westra BI, Subramanian A, Hart CM, et al. "Achieving" meaningful use "of electronic health records through the integration of the nursing management minimum data set.". J Nurs Adm. 2010;40(7/8):336–43.
11. Hübner U, Shaw T, Thye J, Egbert N, de Fatima MH, Chang P, O'Connor S, Day K, Honey M, Blake R, Hovenga E, Skiba D, Ball MJ. Technology informatics guiding education Reform–TIGER. Methods Inf Med. 2018 Jun;57(S 01):e30–42. https://doi.org/10.3414/ME17-01-0155.
12. Muller-Staub M, de Graaf-Waar H, Paans W. An internationally consented standard for nursing process-clinical decision support systems in electronic health records. Comput Inform Nurs. 2016;34:493–502.
13. Wieteck P. Furthering the development of standardized nursing terminology through an ENP®-ICNP® cross-mapping. Int Nurs Rev. 2008;55:296–304.
14. Kim TY, Coenen A, Hardiker N. Semantic mappings and locality of nursing diagnostic concepts in UMLS. J Biomed Inform. 2012;45(1):93–100.
15. Sackett DL, Rosenberg WMC, Gray JAM, Haynes RB, Richardson WS. Evidence based medicine: what it is and what it isn't. BMJ. 1996;312:71.
16. Puhl RM. What words should we use to talk about weight? A systematic review of quantitative and qualitative studies examining preferences for weight-related terminology. Obes Rev. 2020 Feb 12. 2020; https://doi.org/10.1111/obr.13008.

17. Kinnunen U-M, Liljamo P, Härkönen M, Ukkola T, Kuusisto A, Hassinen Ti, Moilanen K. User guide, the Finnish care classification system, FinCC 4.0. Finnish Institute for Health and Welfare. 2020. Available: https://www.julkari.fi/handle/10024/140289

18. Liljamo P, Kinnunen U-M, Saranto K. Health care professionals' view on the mutual consistency of the Finnish Classification of Nursing Interventions and the Oulu Patient Classification. Scand J Caring Sci. 2016;30:477–88.

19. Macieira TGR, Chianca TCM, Smith MB, Yao Y, Bian J, Wilkie DJ, Lopez KD, Keenan GM. Secondary use of standardized nursing care data for advancing nursing science and practice: a systematic review. J Am Med Inform Assoc. 2019;26(11):1401–11.

20. White P, Roudsari A. Use of ontologies for monitoring electronic health records for compliance with clinical practice guidelines. Stud Health Technol Inform. 2011;164:103–9.

21. Goossen WTF, Epping PJMM, Dassen T. Criteria of nursing information systems as a component of the electronic patient record. an international Delphi study. Computer In Nursing. 1997;15(6):307–15.

22. Safran C, Bloomrosen M, Hammond WF, Labkoff S, Markel-Fox S, Tang PC. Toward a national framework for the secondary use of health data: an American Medical Informatics Association White Paper. J Am Med Inform Assoc. 2007 Jan;14(1):1–9.

23. Meystre SM, Lovis C, Bürkle G, Tognola A, Lehmann CU. Clinical data reuse or secondary use: current status and potential future progress. IMIA Yearbook of Medical Informatics. 2017:38–52.

24. Ackley J, Ladwig GB. Nursing diagnosis handbook: an evidence-based guide to planning care. 10th ed. St Louis, MO: Mosby/Elsevier; 2014.

25. Jefferies D, Johnson M, Griffiths RA. Metastudy of the essentials of quality nursing documentation. Int J Nurs Pract. 2010;16(2):112–24.

26. Saranto K, Kinnunen U-M. Evaluating nursing documentation–research designs and methods: systematic review. J Adv Nurs. 2009;65(3):464–76.

27. Mykkänen M, Saranto K, Miettinen M. Nursing Audit as a method for developing nursing care and ensuring patient safety. NI 2012.: 11th International Congress on Nursing Informatics, June 23–27. Montreal, Canada; 2012. https://pubmed.ncbi.nlm.nih.gov/24199107/

28. Kuusisto A, Asikainen P, Lukka H, Tanttu K. Experiences with the electronic nursing discharge summary. Stud Health Technol Inform. 2009;146:226–30.

29. Hübner U, Flemming D, Heitmann U, Oemig F, Thun S, Dickerson A, Veenstra M. The need for standardised documents in continuity of care: results of standardizing the eNursing Summary. Stud Health Technol Inform. 2010;160(Pt 2):1169–73.

30. Matney SA, Warren JJ, Evans JL, Kim TY, Coenen A, Auld VA. Development of the nursing problem list subset of SNOMED CT®. J Biomed Inform. 2012;45(4):683–8. https://doi.org/10.1016/j.jbi.2011.12.003.

31. Sockolow P, Hellesø R, Ekstedt M. Digitalization of patient information process from hospital to community (home) care nurses: international perspectives. In: Rotegård AK, et al., editors. International Medical Informatics Association (IMIA) and IOS Press; 2018.

32. Dionisi S, Di Simone E, Alicastro GM, Angelini S, Giannetta N, Iacorossi L, Di Muzio M. Nursing summary: designing a nursing section in the electronic health record. Acta Biomed. 2019;90(3):293–9.

33. Kuusisto A, Asikainen P, Saranto K. Contents of informational and management continuity of care. Stud Health Technol Inform. 2019 Aug;21(264):669–73. https://doi.org/10.3233/SHTI190307.

34. Kuusisto A, Asikainen P, Saranto K. Medication documentation in nursing discharge summaries at patient's discharge from special care to primary care. J Nursing Care. 2014; http://omicsgroup.org/journals/medication-documentation-in-nursing-discharge-summaries-at-patient-discharge-from-special-care-to-primary-care-2167-1168.1000147.pdf/

35. Kuusisto A, Joensuu A, Nevalainen M, Pakkanen T, Ranne P, Puustinen J. Standardizing key issues from hospital through an electronic multi-professional discharge checklist to ensure continuity of care. Stud Health Technol Inform. 2019 Aug;21(264):664–8. https://doi.org/10.3233/SHTI190306.

36. Romagnoli KM, Handler SM, Ligons FM, Hochheiser H. Home-care nurses' perceptions of unmet information needs and communication difficulties of geriatric patients in the immediate post-hospital discharge period. BMJ Quality & Safety. 2013;22(4):324–32.

37. DESI. The digital economy and society index. Human capital digital inclusion and skills. 2019. Available at: https://ec.europa.eu/newsroom/dae/document.cfm?doc_id=59976

38. Champlin S, Mackert M, Glowacki EM, Donovan EE. Toward a better understanding of patient health literacy: a focus on the skills patients need to find health information. Qual Health Res. 2017;27:1160–76.

39. Coughlin SS, Prochaska JJ, Williams LB, et al. Patient web portal, disease management, and primary prevention. Risk Manag Healthc Policy. 2017;10:33–40.

40. Kruse CS, Krowski N, Rodriquez B, Tran L, Vela J, Brooks M. Telehealth and patient satisfactions: a systematic review and narrative analysis. BMJ Open. 2017;7:e016242.

41. Omaolo services. 2020. https://www.omaolo.fi/ Accessed June 6th 2020.

42. Digital Health Village in Finland. 2020. https://www.digitalhealthvillage.com/en/home. Accessed June 6th, 2020.

43. Sarkar U, Bates DW. Care partners and online patient portals. JAMA. 2017;311(4):357–8.

44. McAlearney AS, Sieck CJ, Gaughan A, Fareed N, Volney J, Huerta TR. Patients' perceptions of portal use across care settings: qualitative study. J Med Internet Res. 2019;21(6):e13126.

45. Anderson MHO, Jackson SL, Oster NV, Peacock S, Walker JD, Chen GY, Elmore JG. Patient typing their own visit agendas into an electronic medical record: pilot in a safety-net clinic. Ann Fam Med. 2017;15(2):158–61.

Reusing Data from the Point-of-Care: Collect Once Use Many Times

15

Renate Ranegger and Dieter Baumberger

Learning Objectives

- Understand the possibilities of reusing data from the electronic medical record for multiple purposes.
- Understand the necessary prerequisites for reusing data from the electronic medical record.

Key Terms

- Workforce management (WFM)
- Sociotechnical systems (STS)
- Process interoperability
- Use of clinical data for multiple purposes
- COUMT paradigm (collect once, use many times)
- Motivated healthcare professionals
- Data accuracy
- Coding systems for the electronic medical record
- International standards

Introduction

The excessive burden caused by a "pointless bureaucracy"—as perceived by the healthcare professionals at the point of care—is not new and often remains an issue despite the move from paper-based documentation to an electronic medical record.[1] Due to terminological and methodological difficulties, few comparable results are available on this topic. It can be confirmed, however, that the implementation of a structured and standardized electronic medical record is likely to result in increased documentation time. The actual times mentioned in the literature are heterogeneous. The study by Joukes et al. [1], for example, examines the different baseline situations, revealing a significant increase of 8.3% in the time spent on documentation tasks when switching from paper-based documentation to an electronic medical record. The study by Baumann et al. [2], for example, reports that the implementation of an electronic medical record increases the documentation time from 16% to 28% for physicians, from 9% to 23% for healthcare professionals, and from 20% to 26% for interns.

R. Ranegger (✉)
LEP AG St. Gallen, St. Gallen, Switzerland

UMIT–Private University for Health Sciences, Medical Informatics and Technology, Hall in Tirol, Austria
e-mail: renate.ranegger@lep.ch

D. Baumberger
LEP AG St. Gallen, St. Gallen, Switzerland
e-mail: dieter.baumberger@lep.ch

[1] In our chapter, we use the term "electronic medical record" which is a digital version of a chart with patient information stored in a computer and contains the patient's medical history, diagnoses, and treatments by a particular physician, nurse practitioner, specialist, and so on. An EMR is a narrower view of a patient's history, while an EHR is a more comprehensive report of the patient's overall health, such as ELGA in Austria or EPD in Switzerland.

© Springer Nature Switzerland AG 2022
U. H. Hübner et al. (eds.), *Nursing Informatics*, Health Informatics,
https://doi.org/10.1007/978-3-030-91237-6_15

This perception by the healthcare professionals at the point of care—that repeated documentation merely feeds an excessive bureaucracy with redundant information—negatively impacts the cooperation between healthcare professionals and management. This consequently affects the quality of the data needed by management, such as the completeness of coded diagnoses or interventions.

One challenge on the way to preventing this situation is to structurally define and differentiate the data that is required to achieve a specific purpose. With respect to the data required for management purposes, this could mean identifying which data can already be obtained from the electronic medical record and which data may need to be collected separately. In a best-case scenario, it may be possible to avoid the previous need to collect additional data separately, for example by using state-of-the-art software solutions to exploit the existing data for management purposes.

The entries documented by the healthcare professional at the point of care refer to specific patients during a treatment and they are primarily used for communication among the healthcare professionals involved in the treatment process. The necessity for this type of documentation, in which the treatment-related content is decisive for patient safety and the quality of care, is undisputed among the healthcare professionals at the point of care. The consequences of a poor, delayed, or incomplete electronic medical record for patient safety and treatment efficiency are obvious, as is the importance of accurate documentation for legal certainty [3, 4].

This type of documentation entry is therefore not experienced as "pointless bureaucracy" by the healthcare professionals at the point of care. The documentation becomes a burden when the management specifies additional forms to be filled out. The demand for such data and the corresponding interest in additionally documenting this data usually do not originate with the healthcare professionals at the point of care, nor are they part of the primary processes of a healthcare organization, but come from the management itself in order to generate metrics for operationally relevant support processes. The additional data collected for this purpose can in turn be used for a variety of other purposes such as quality assurance, workforce health management, documentation of work activities for staffing purposes and job planning, the assignment of classification codes to diagnoses or procedures for billing in various pricing structures, for clinical or epidemiological registries such as tumor registries, in the context of clinical research, and much more [3, 4].

From a sociotechnical systems perspective, the healthcare professionals at the point of care should not experience documentation for management purposes as an unnecessary practical constraint that limits their ability to treat and care for patients. On the contrary, the healthcare professionals should find that software developments add value to their core tasks. The electronic medical record is a good way of reducing additional documentation time. In order to be able to base management decisions on data from the primary process, the healthcare professionals at the point of care should be actively involved and informed about the purpose of the data use. The aim should be to optimize the electronic medical record as a subsystem of a sociotechnical system. Connected optimization means more than simply adapting the technical subsystem to the social one or vice versa. The concept of sociotechnical system design explicitly postulates the necessity of joint optimization of the technology use and organization as well as the need to be oriented to both productive and social purposes.

The eight-dimensional model of Sittig and Singh [5], which was designed to address the sociotechnical challenges involved in development and implementation, is suitable for this purpose. The eight dimensions are not independent, sequential, or hierarchical, but rather are interdependent and interrelated concepts. (1) *Hardware and software*, that is, computing infrastructure, refers to equipment and software that is used to support and operate clinical applications. (2) *Clinical content* refers to textual or numeric data and images and represents the "language" of clinical applications. (3) The *human-computer interface* refers to all aspects of the computer that users can see, touch, or hear when interacting with the technology. (4) *People* refers to everyone who interacts with the system in any way, from the developer to the end user, including potential patients/ users. (5) *Workflow and communication* are the processes or steps required to ensure that patient care tasks are performed effectively. Two additional dimensions of the model are (6) *internal organizational features* (e.g. *policies, procedures, and culture*) and (7) *external rules and regulations*, both of which may facilitate or constrain many aspects of the previous dimensions. The last dimension is (8) *measurement and monitoring*, which refers to the process of measuring and assessing the intended and unintended consequences of implementing and using health information technology.

The most important secondary task which sociotechnical systems are confronted with externally is the handling of unpredictable and unforeseeable fluctuations and disturbances in workflows induced by turbulences in the environment, with their "control" being one of our human tasks. From a psychological point of view, intertwined with contingency theory, sociotechnical systems are understood as working environments in which, due to the limited controllability of the process dynamics as well as the fluctuations and disturbances, stress arises by definition and the workers must have an optimal level of resources (e.g. in the form of social support in semi-autonomous working groups, polyvalent qualification, and scope for self-regulation) in order to actively cope with and buffer this stress [6].

Especially in healthcare organizations with a high level of technology, agility must be understood as an ongoing capability to be developed and anchored in the corporate culture. When it comes to operational design and organization, however, healthcare organizations still tend to fall back on linear change and implementation frameworks that are often based on traditional, hierarchical, and structural models. Instead, change can be seen as an ongoing integrated transformation, with healthcare professionals at the point of care working together to fulfill primary tasks. The electronic medical record, with a work content associated with relevance, collabo-

ration, completeness, and opportunities for growth, is a motivating factor. It should be noted that the target group of users and adopters of electronic medical records increasingly comprises the so-called millennials, a cohort with a fundamental affinity for technology. Millennials are increasingly assuming leadership positions in the healthcare sector and are helping to shape the digital work environment in healthcare organizations with their changed expectations, values, and motivations. *"Placing a high value on autonomy, meaning, teamwork, personal development, self-expression, fun, and life balance, these workers decry bureaucracy and hierarchy"*. Millennials prefer choice and self-direction in their work environment. These aspects go hand in hand with the design possibilities from the sociotechnical system and represent current concepts that can be seen as the opposite of distinctly hierarchically structured work environments [7].

One of the eight dimensions in the sociotechnical model of Sittig and Singh [5] refers to the user interface, also called the *front end*, that is, what healthcare professionals see when recording or entering data, for example, "position patient in lateral position", in a computer or in an electronic medical record during the documentation of a standardized health intervention. For the purpose of supporting secondary processes, such data could be used in the back end for automated extraction, for example, of a pricing code, to secure revenue (Fig. 15.1, page 4) without the healthcare professional having to document "position patient in lateral position" a second time in any form. Of course, this also applies to unnecessary double documentation at higher aggregation levels such as "patient positioning" or "movement".

Collect Once, Use Many Times: A Guiding Principle

The COUMT Paradigm

Implementation is based on the "collect once, use many times" (COUMT) paradigm [8], a prerequisite being the use of modern information and

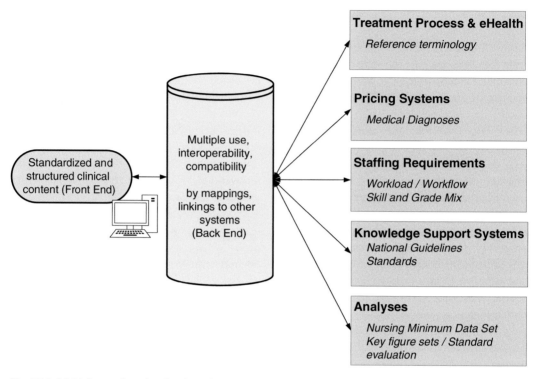

Fig. 15.1 Multiple use of nursing data from the electronic medical record

communications technologies (ICT). The basic idea is that structured data at the point of care is documented once in the electronic medical record to not only ensure cooperative patient care in the primary process, but also to be able to use the documented data for a variety of cross-patient issues for management and support processes. This reuse of documented data for purposes beyond the treatment and care process—for example for research, process optimization, risk management, financial controlling, or workforce management—is referred to as secondary use.

Guided by the COUMT paradigm, structured and standardized coding systems must be established in the front end for various uses in relation with other classifications, systems, instruments, or standards. The relations are created by so-called mappings or linkages and are basically implemented in the back end. This enables versatile data uses without additional documentation time. Such possible uses are illustrated in the model in Fig. 15.1.

Possible advantages include the automated data exchange between different healthcare organizations within the context of eHealth using reference terminologies (e.g. hospital and community care), the automated use of data for billing processes in healthcare pricing systems (e.g. national case-rate pricing plans, DRGs), or direct access at the point of care to practical knowledge within the context of knowledge management (guidelines, quality standards).

Added Value for Management and Support Processes

Data from the electronic medical record can be used for management and support processes as follows:

- to obtain information on the situation-appropriate use of staff and resources, which, among other things, enables the optimization of the grade mix and supports the needs-based deployment of staff, explains the importance of specializations, or identifies trends and developments in care requirements and nursing effort;

- to provide information to identify opportunities for improvement related to the possibility of streamlining interdisciplinary practices in order to optimize work, education, and patient processes;
- to enable analyses of efficiency and effectiveness in nursing and healthcare on the basis of condition- and intervention-related data;
- to provide support for health policy decisions on financing and cost calculation;
- to enable the benchmarking of organizations/regions (national and international); or,
- to contribute to quality assurance in healthcare through studies of misuse, overuse, underuse, and prevalence/incidence rates in connection with nursing interventions or patient safety indicators.

This illustrates the variety of possible uses of data from the electronic medical record—without additional documentation time at the point of care. Achieving this goal requires the solving of methodological challenges in the collection, processing, and validation of data as well as new approaches to data analysis [9].

Prerequisite for the Use of Data from the Electronic Medical Record

Introduction

Data can be used for secondary processes if various interlocking conditions are satisfied. These prerequisites can be roughly divided into the following categories: clinical content, documentation modality, and software-related prerequisites. This requires the availability of high-quality and, if possible, standardized primary data that can be transferred for analysis, using suitable software.

Coding Systems

To be able to exchange and reuse data from the primary process across sectors and with different communication standards, a suitable form of presentation of the documentation contents must be selected. The use of coding systems, among other things, is recommended for this purpose.

A coding system is a set of entities and their relations founded on certain principles. One coding principle, for example, is a classification involving the subdivision of entities into classes at different hierarchical levels. These classes, which can also be referred to as groups, categories, or chapters, are further subdivided. Each class has a title that serves as a heading to describe the contents of that class. In addition to this textual descriptor, each class usually also has a numeric notation.

The purpose of the classification determines its structure and content selection. This knowledge is key to achieving an understanding of classifications, as the selection process determines which information will ultimately remain in a classification. The selection is therefore based not only on the observed data but also on the purpose of the classification. Meanwhile, the context in which the issues are addressed is also relevant. Depending on the issues to be addressed, the perspectives change as well and, with it, the selection of the relevant information [10].

For an expert understanding of classifications, it is important to note that the contents, the division of classes, and their level of detail are determined by the intended application of the classification itself. Classifications are used for content structuring and statistical evaluation. When making classifications, details are deliberately omitted in favor of the statistical evaluability of coded data. The nursing intervention classification "oral administration of medication", for example, requires supplementary terminology, such as "metoclopramide drops", to describe the actions and to facilitate the communication between the healthcare professionals. Terminology (the set of all technical terms within a specialty) is therefore to be understood as a necessary complement to classifications [11].

Documentation Modality

Besides the mandatory framework conditions specific to each country (e.g. those relating to liability, regulatory issues, or social security and benefits), another decisive factor in determining documentation requirements are the data needed for analyses.

The documentation process is affected by (a) personal factors such as the experience, values, or motivation of the healthcare professional, (b) working conditions such as software process support in terms of practicability, or (c) situation-related factors such as time, that is, when there is only a limited amount of time for documentation because of the great number of tasks to be completed.

Generally, the time of documentation is extremely important for data quality. All further interpretations of the documentation entries, calculations, and analyses depend on the quality of the documentation. The systematic and timely management of the electronic medical record is essential for the benefit of the patient and of central importance for the quality of both the treatment and the data. The documentation times should therefore be optimally integrated into the workflow, with documentation entries made several times a day. When documentation entries are made in a timely manner, the intervention data can be expected to be more complete and more accurate.

Analyses, as mentioned in Sect. 4.1, page 9, can only be performed if the data is entered accordingly in the electronic medical record. For example, it is necessary that

- the time of the planned nursing intervention can be adjusted and that the plan and documentation time is saved,
- the person performing the intervention documents the intervention performed in a timely manner,
- more than one person performing the intervention documents the intervention performed,
- an intervention performed only once ("ad hoc") is documented in a structured and stan-

dardized manner and not noted as free text in the nursing report,
- the documented activities are reviewed for their correctness, and existing inaccuracies are recognized and corrected (securing of documentation/data quality), or,
- the entire care and treatment process is documented and saved on a storage device (i.e. there is no separation between electronic and paper-based documentation media, such as a separate paper-based positioning plan).

Software Requirements

The use of coding systems requires the development of a feasible and practical software system. Considering the purposes of evaluation and nursing documentation, the challenge is to implement the documentation contents in the software in such a way that the treatment process and the support and management processes are supported in a user-friendly manner in all phases and that the documentation time is kept to a minimum.

Important software-related prerequisites for the successful use of data from the electronic medical record include:

- data already available in other software applications are taken over and processed for analyses—for example, wage costs, data on treatment and care material, or data from a workforce management system (WMS) on absences or overtime in order to determine the case-related intervention perspective /staff-related working time;
- the plan, performance, and documentation time is documented and saved;
- the individual patient situation can be documented in a practical way;
- the documented data can be exported from the primary system to guarantee the possibility of evaluating the data documented.

To process data from coding systems, the following is useful:

- the filtering of data,
- the aggregation of data—for example, aggregating the health intervention "position patient in lateral position" to the next higher intervention group "positioning",
- the calculation of statistical measures, and,
- the drawing of diagrams.

Challenges in Using Data from the Electronic Medical Record

Key aspects associated with the use of nursing data from the electronic medical record relate to the documentation time and modality in the daily documentation as well as the complexity and usability of the data from the electronic medical record for supporting secondary processes [8, 12].

The use of data for secondary purposes therefore requires a clear picture of the quality and quantity of the data that is available in the information systems of the facilities. Another aspect is that care facilities often do not know whether they want to use their documented data and what they want to use it for. The use of data from the electronic medical record only functions well if clear purposes are pursued or specific questions need to be answered—from the point of view of management, quality assurance, patient safety, or research. Different data from the electronic medical record may be needed depending on the issue at hand. For patient care and treatment, it seems essential to have the individual, treatment-relevant information presented as completely and clearly as possible. In contrast, the comparability and reproducibility of data in the form of standardized information may be of particular interest for care-related examinations or scientific studies, although the questions posed and the data needed can diverge here as well.

If a health care organization wants to use the manifold possibilities of nursing data from the electronic medical record for data analysis purposes, this requires not only an appropriate methodical approach to data selection, preparation, and analysis but also the fulfillment of certain requirements regarding documentation

quality. In contrast to data from the financial domain (e.g. sales figures), nursing data is highly contingent on context. This means that individual nursing interventions cannot easily be combined for cross-patient analysis without more detailed information about their origin (for what purpose, when, by whom and how they were collected), and without information about influencing factors such as current diagnosis or health status. This is basically true for all clinical parameters and makes the handling of this data so complex [13].

The systematic planning of documentation projects (primary processes) and the use of nursing data (secondary processes) is necessary to make the best possible use of the possibilities of reusing data from the electronic medical record multiple times. The SPIRIT[2] framework, for example, describes how a platform for secondary data analysis can be created step by step, based on an analysis of the question to be answered and a survey of existing data sources while taking the context into account. The framework illustrates the complexity in connection with the use of data from the electronic medical record [14].

A problem, however, is the fact that documentation is often still paper-based and is therefore not analyzable at all, or the electronic documentation is incomplete and not very significant, making it of low quality [15].

Case Study on the Multiple Use of Data Collected Once for the Electronic Medical Record

LEP[3] Nursing 3 is a classification for nursing interventions [16] that is currently being used in the electronic medical records in over 700 healthcare organizations in Germany, Austria, and Switzerland. LEP enables the use of data from the electronic medical record for multiple pur-

---

[2] Systematic Planning of Intelligent Reuse of Integrated Clinical Routine Data

[3] *Leistungserfassung in der Pflege* ("documentation of nursing activities"; i.e. nursing workload measurement)

poses through mappings and linkages (cf. Figure 15.1, page 4).

The implementation of LEP involves more than 20 software applications in different information and hospital systems offering a wide range of implementation possibilities. The different purposes pursued by the respective healthcare organizations have a particular impact on the design of the electronic medical record and on data evaluation. This means that the application of LEP but also the use of the documented data from the electronic medical record varies.

At one Swiss university hospital, for example, LEP Nursing 3 is used as clinical content in the primary care and treatment process documentation. Guided by the COUMT paradigm, LEP Nursing interventions are documented once, automated, and used multiple times. The following three examples are intended to illustrate such applications at the university hospital:

(1) Multiple use of data from medical charts.

In order to avoid double documentation and data redundancy at the university hospital, the LEP nursing intervention "measure blood pressure" is automatically documented in the back end when a numerical blood pressure value, for example 120/90, is entered in the electronic medical record. Such an intervention can be used automatically for activity statistics or, with the additional entry of a time value, to calculate staff costs or workforce scheduling. Redundant data refers to already documented information that is available multiple times following repeated data collection. This would be the case at the university hospital if, in addition to the blood pressure value of "120/90" already documented in the medical chart, "measure vital signs" or "monitoring" were recorded additionally for cost accounting or intervention documentation purposes.

(2) Use of data for case-rate pricing.

Mapping LEP nursing interventions into the Swiss Surgery Classification (CHOP) 99.C1 Comprehensive Care automatically derives billing-relevant nursing data for the case-rate reimbursement of hospitals. The mapping algorithm, which was developed according to a specific set of rules, is implemented in the software application in such a way that the documented LEP interventions trigger the revenue-relevant pricing items directly, that is, automatically and without additional documentation.

(3) Use of data for working time productivity.

The LEP interventions documented in the electronic medical record are transferred via an interface into an analysis software program, where they are used for strategic management decisions. For example, the time spent by a ward carrying out interventions on a case is compared with the available staff time (net working time). The latter is transferred via an interface from the data of the workforce management system (WMS) into the analysis software. The comparison makes it possible to determine and interpret the working time productivity of the ward, for example, 75%, and use this information for possible decisions regarding staff deployment.

Besides the coding systems and the software, the documentation modalities (Sect. 2.2, page 6) are another essential prerequisite for the use of data for multiple purposes.

Global experience with Multiple Use of Data Collected Once

Grade Mix: Data for Resource Management

A common management purpose is the identification and calculation of an optimal grade mix in nursing. This requires concept-guided, comprehensible, and needs-based methods. Various workforce distribution and workforce calculation methods are used, such as nurse-to-patient ratio, nurse hours per patient day (NHPPD), activity and process analyses, or categorization methods of patient groups [17]. Ideally, the effectiveness of a grade mix is considered in connection with care-sensitive outcome measures, patient safety, and patient satisfaction [18], taking into consideration the work-life balance of nursing staff [19].

Despite numerous contributions on the topic, there are no widely accepted procedures for nursing managers on how to best integrate a new occupational group into nursing practice and how to optimally support the coordination of occupational groups in the daily ward routine.

In Germany, for example, there is ongoing debate about "minimum workforce requirement standards" in the nursing sector. The focus is on regulatory systems that stipulate binding minimum staffing levels. A metric such as the nurse-to-patient ratio is envisaged for this purpose. A minimum workforce requirement can also be understood as a maximum workforce requirement when viewed from another angle. For this reason, its determination depends on reliable and up-to-date data from practice in order to ensure that the nurse-to-patient ratio can meet changing patient and system needs [20, 21].

Numerous studies make recommendations for optimizing the nurse-to-patient ratio. The study by Aiken et al. [22], for example, examines correlations between the nurse-to-patient ratio and patient morbidity/mortality rates. The findings show that a lower workload of nursing staff is associated with better patient outcomes. However, the establishment of a nurse-to-patient ratio is expected to produce not only desired effects, such as greater safety for patients and nursing staff in the work environment or an incentive for nursing professionals to return to work at the point of care. Negative effects resulting from a rigid standardization of the nurse-to-patient ratio include, for example, the loss of nursing influence on or indifference for the expertise of different specialties of nursing professionals with or without work experience [21].

Next to the nurse-to-patient ratio as prescribed by law or regulation, the model of nursing hours per patient day is the most widespread method in Australia, for example. NHPPD presents the actual net working time of nursing staff on a ward in minutes per patient and day [20]. This method has been examined in numerous studies with regard to accompanying effects such as the impact on care quality, with results showing that a realistic NHPPD is associated with beneficial effects such as a reduction in complication rates or a shorter length of stay [23, 24].

Activity analyses based on the documented data additionally support the decision-making for a needs- and skills-based grade mix. The analysis of a needs-based allocation of the various occupational groups or the examination of shifts in actions within the occupational groups involved in the care and treatment process can further support the coordination in the daily ward routine [17]. Against the background of the possibility of reusing data from the electronic medical record, the study by Ranegger et al. [25] examined whether and to what extent activity analyses can cover a transparent and skills-based grade mix in nursing. Based on data automatically extracted from the electronic medical record, standardized and structured nursing interventions [16] were analyzed over a period of six months. The calculations were used to generate meaningful metadata on the nursing grade mix in a health care organization and its departments. On the basis of these study results, it could be shown that decision-makers can use data to determine an optimal grade mix in their healthcare and nursing facilities by determining which tasks should be performed by more highly qualified employees and which by less qualified employees. In addition, it was possible to calculate and depict the staffing and financial effects associated with shifts in nursing actions and skills. The calculation methods as applied in this study offer a suitable starting point for further questions regarding the calculation of case complexity, effects of changes in the grade mix on care and treatment costs [17], nursing outcomes [18, 22], or the work-life balance of nursing staff [19]. If the topic of action shifts is mentioned in connection with the grade mix in nursing, these must be examined regarding to the process logic. This is because not all action shifts that appear to make sense from an arithmetical perspective actually fit into the work processes.

During process-oriented analyses, activity offerings and actions are analyzed in terms of process organization. This method offers the opportunity to critically question and reflect on procedures and processes. This can help support decision-makers in deciding whether it makes sense to shift activities between occupational groups and whether the respective organizational unit becomes more efficient as a result. Within the framework of process-oriented analyses, incidents or actions are analyzed over time and used to depict the number of interfaces, process interruptions, and occupational groups involved. Using process-oriented analyses, the study by Ranegger et al. [25] showed that the occupational groups at the healthcare and nursing facilities are deployed in a needs-based manner and that therefore there is no need for optimization in this respect. With a focus on process optimization, the range of activities of the health care organization was also reviewed. The results show a broad variability of the range of activities over time, with a decline in activities on weekends. Such conspicuous occurrences can be assessed and reflected in detail at a later stage. It is possible, for example, to examine whether the reduction in activities on weekends involves optional or mandatory activities and whether this reduction in activities has an

impact on the quality of nursing care. Individual case analyses such as those carried out in this study made it possible to identify both optimal care processes as well as approaches to functional care—nursing tasks are divided into individual work steps and assigned to individual occupational groups. As an example of functional nursing, processes were identified in which a total of ten different persons from four different occupational groups were working on patients during day duty alone (Fig. 15.2).

Such process-oriented information on a meta-level is unbelievably for the management in healthcare and nursing facilities and can also provide an indication of qualitative aspects related to the grade mix. On the basis of detailed analyses (Fig. 15.3), processes can be analyzed at a micro level in order to break up work processes that may have become entrenched and to test them for efficiency and effectiveness.

Considerations with regard to process optimization (target process, Fig. 15.4) refer, on the one hand, to the reduction of the occupational groups involved. On the other hand, the aim is also to reduce and rearrange process steps in order to minimize interfaces and the susceptibility to errors [25]. It is also generally known that optimal work processes have a positive effect on employee and patient satisfaction.

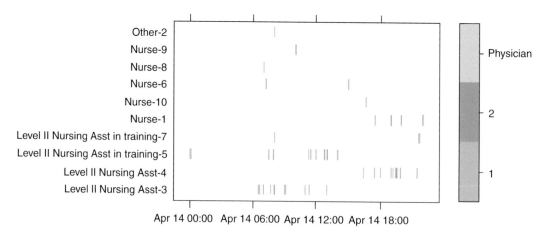

Fig. 15.2 Example of a single case analysis for process mapping based on a structured and standardized classification (1 = low qualified intervention, 2 = high qualified intervention)

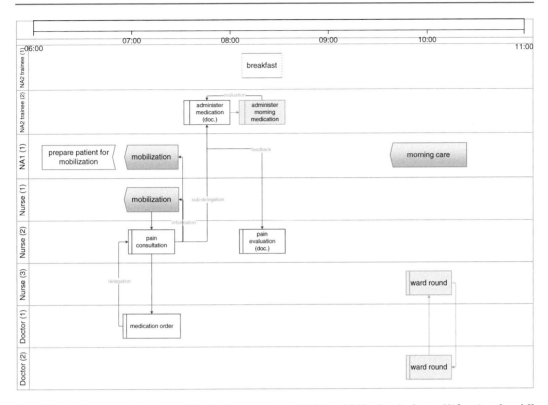

Fig. 15.3 As-is process based on an individual case analysis. *NA1* Level I Nursing Assistant; *NA2 trainee* Level II Nursing Assistant in training

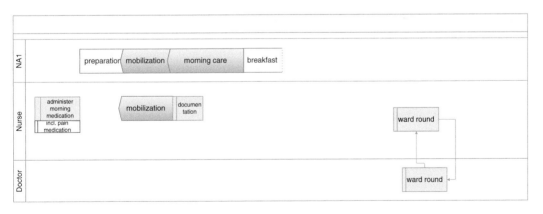

Fig. 15.4 Target process for the purpose of primary nursing. *NA1* Level I Nursing Assistant

In conclusion, it can be said that individual methods are not sufficient to answer the question of what constitutes an optimal grade mix in nursing. Instead, a combination of workforce distribution and workforce calculation methods should be used to coordinate the relevant aspects of an overall concept.

Knowledge Management: Retrieving Practical Knowledge While Working

One management objective is to have the best possible quality of treatment in the healthcare organization. For this purpose, knowledge management systems can be made available at the point of care to support the competence of the healthcare professionals in practice [26, 27]. By linking standardized and structured nursing interventions with knowledge management systems or internal standards or guidelines, the direct use of practical knowledge at the point of care is made available promptly and locally in the electronic medical record. The study by [28] shows that knowledge management (including knowledge acquisition, knowledge sharing, and knowledge utilization) positively impacts the "quality of healthcare and the social (e.g. employee and client satisfaction) and economic outcomes (e.g. productivity, financial performance) of a health organization".

Modern software technologies could be used to support healthcare professionals directly in their work with up-to-date specialist knowledge. If, for example, a wound is cared for and this is documented via the standardized healthcare intervention "wound care", the practical instructions for "care of infected surgical wounds" or "treatment of stage 1 pressure ulcers" can be called up directly from the electronic medical record and integrated into practice. Such knowledge describes how an intervention is carried out effectively and efficiently according to the current state of knowledge ("doing the right things right").

Using Data from the Electronic Medical Record for the Nursing Minimum Data Set

Another relevant management objective is process optimization. This can be based on data comparisons with a nursing minimum data set (NMDS). An NMDS is defined as "a minimum data set of items of information with uniform definitions and categories concerning the specific dimension of nursing, which meets the information needs of multiple data users in the health care system" [29].

Particularly in the 1990s, efforts were made to establish nursing minimum data sets as a way to answer national questions on nursing issues, for

healthcare reporting, and to support political decision-making. The purpose of an NMDS is to use aggregated nursing data for the description of nursing care, allocation of financial resources, benchmarking, workforce management, trend analyses, and quality assurance. To date, with the exception of Belgium, there is no binding data set that allows for national or international comparisons of nursing data [30].

The potential of an NMDS lies in the fact that, for the purpose of external comparability and opportunities for further development (thinking out of the box), operational comparisons can be carried out in order to question resources, costs, or processes, for example.

Data for NMDS analyses should also not be recorded additionally. In a current project [31], an automated mapping pipeline for nursing data documented in a structured and standardized manner from the electronic medical record were transformed into a nursing minimum data set (NMDS).

Data comparisons across different facilities or even countries can provide decision-makers with important information for a variety of purposes. As is the case with the use of routine data in general, however, successful data comparison is not without obstacles. Finding valid and accurate information for comparison is an enormous challenge in this context. Specifically, this pertains to documentation quality, which can be very heterogeneous depending on how the documentation is performed [15].

Summary

IT applications in a healthcare organization should be designed in such a way that the information documented by healthcare professionals can be interpreted and processed for a specific purpose. For the management purpose of staff planning, for example, a system should be able to find and process the corresponding intervention codes in the electronic medical record.

In this process, the electronic medical record is understood to be a central information hub in a sociotechnical system in which information technology is experienced not as a practical constraint but as a tool supporting all work processes. The electronic medical record supports the healthcare professionals in the care and treatment process, the core or primary process of any healthcare organization. At the same time, the data from the electronic medical record can be used "automatically" in the secondary processes of the healthcare organizations, for example for accounting or for staff planning purposes.

In this type of application, the healthcare professionals at the point of care need to collect the data only once, thus eliminating the need for additional documentation time, which is often perceived as pointlessly "administrative" or "bureaucratic". As healthcare professionals are involved, management decisions can be based on information that is more accurate and derived directly from the primary process. This simplifies the interaction between the healthcare professionals and the management for quick, documentation-based changes in response to new purposes.

In accordance with the guiding principle "collect once, use many times", the focus must be on fully exploiting, for management purposes, the current software options with regard to the electronic medical record, use suitable coding systems such as classification or nomenclatures for documentation entries, and comply with international standards for the use of clinical data for secondary purposes. The aim is to reduce additional documentation time at the point of care while making the best possible use of the data for secondary processes.

Conclusions and Outlook

The data in the electronic medical record can and should be used multiple times for management purposes without the healthcare professionals at the point of care having to collect data more than once.

The real-life case studies reveal individual applications within the COUMT framework. Data collected at the point of care and documented in the electronic medical record is used not only for treatment processes but is also automated and reused several times with the help of coding systems: for resource and knowledge management as well as for a nursing minimum data set. At the same time, there are extended application possibilities for management and support processes, for example methods of process mining. Further conceptual and content-related improvements will certainly be necessary with a focus on the COUMT paradigm; for now, we are still at the beginning of implementation in everyday practice with the first case studies. It is apparent that the applications have become increasingly plausible and therefore feasible.

As a guiding principle, methodological transformations and networking with regard to documentation and subsequent data processing should be implemented in a more target-oriented manner so that healthcare professionals at the point of care do not have to document data that would not be required under a COUMT paradigm.

The corresponding software applications are to be designed according to those sociotechnical perspectives that have a direct benefit for patients, healthcare professionals at the point of care, and management, so that the COUMT paradigm can be propagated in the healthcare organizations. It is important to know the attitude of healthcare professionals at the point of care regarding the use of data from electronic medical records, for example with respect to activity documentation or knowledge transfer, and to integrate this into the development of applications. The potential for the misuse of data from the electronic medical record must be made transparent and prevented. One of the challenges is to ensure that, when data and information are reused, the context of the transferred data and information is not lost and can be reproduced correctly. Unexpected or adverse effects of the use of clinical data for secondary purposes must be identified. Acceptance by the healthcare professionals at the point of care should be reviewed regularly: How do the healthcare professionals assess the information and reports derived from the analysis of the data from the electronic medical record? Do they find them helpful? [32, 33].

For management, it is essential to prevent "scope creep" and to critically and repeatedly review whether there is a shift in the originally intended purpose of using the data from the electronic medical record toward other or additional purposes. An evaluation should be able to answer the question of whether the selected data or key figures from the electronic medical record meet the needs and expectations of the interest groups while still fulfilling the purposes defined by the management and the healthcare professionals at the point of care [32].

Useful Resources

1. Ranegger R, Baumberger D, Bürgin R. Forschungsbericht. Bedarfs-und kompetenzorientierte Personaleinsatzplanung gemäss GuKG 2016—eine Tätigkeitsanalyse Teil A. St. Gallen, 2016. https://www.lep.ch/de/literatur.html. Accessed 31 August 2020.
2. Ranegger R, Baumberger D, Bürgin R. Forschungsbericht. Bedarfs-und kompetenzorientierte Personaleinsatzplanung gemäss GuKG 2016—eine prozessorientierte Analyse Teil B. St. Gallen, 2017. https://www.lep.ch/de/literatur.html. Accessed 31 August 2020.

Review Questions

1. What does the COUMT paradigm stand for? Can you give a practical example?
2. Why should healthcare professionals at the point of care only need to document data once?
3. What are the advantages of data that can be used directly from the electronic medical record?
4. What sorts of management and support processes can the data be used for?
5. What is the relationship between the data required by management for evaluation purposes and the necessary documentation of the data at the point of care?
6. According to Sittig and Singh [5], which eight dimensions can help address sociotechnical challenges involved in development and implementation?
7. From a sociotechnical perspective, what considerations must be observed in the system design for a successful implementation according to the COUMT paradigm?
8. What software requirements are necessary for implementation?
9. Looking to the future, can you outline an exemplary case study showing how data from the electronic medical record could be used for staff planning with regard to the skill/grade mix in an extended/better/additional way?

Appendix: Answers to Review Questions

1. What does the COUMT paradigm stand for? Can you give a practical example?

It means, "collect once, use many times". The basic idea is that structured data at the point of care is documented once in the electronic medical record to not only ensure cooperative patient care in the primary process, but also to be able to use the documented data for a variety of cross-patient issues for management and support processes.

2. Why should healthcare professionals at the point of care only need to document data once?

Eliminating the need for additional documentation time, which is often perceived as pointlessly "administrative" or "bureaucratic". This perception by the healthcare professionals at the point of care—that repeated documentation merely feeds an excessive bureaucracy with redundant information—negatively impacts the cooperation between healthcare professionals and management. This consequently affects the quality of the data needed by management, such as the completeness of coded diagnoses or interventions.

3. What are the advantages of data that can be used directly from the electronic medical record?

Possible advantages include the automated data exchange between different healthcare organizations within the context of eHealth using reference terminologies (e.g. hospital and community care), the automated use of data for billing processes in healthcare pricing systems (e.g. national case-rate pricing plans, DRGs), or direct access at the point of care to practical knowledge within the context of knowledge management (guidelines, quality standards).

4. What sorts of management and support processes can the data be used for?

- to obtain information on the situation-appropriate use of staff and resources, which, among other things, enables the optimization of the grade mix and supports the needs-based deployment of staff, explains the importance of specializations, or identifies trends and developments in care requirements and nursing effort;
- to provide information to identify opportunities for improvement related to the possibility of streamlining interdisciplinary practices in order to optimize work, education, and patient processes;
- to enable analyses of efficiency and effectiveness in nursing and healthcare on the basis of condition- and intervention-related data;
- to provide support for health policy decisions on financing and cost calculation;
- to enable the benchmarking of organizations/regions (national and international); or,
- to contribute to quality assurance in healthcare through studies of misuse, overuse, underuse, and prevalence/incidence rates in connection with nursing interventions or patient safety indicators.

5. What is the relationship between the data required by management for evaluation purposes and the necessary documentation of the data at the point of care?

As healthcare professionals are involved, management decisions can be based on information that is more accurate and derived directly from the primary process. This simplifies the interaction between the healthcare professionals and the management for quick, documentation-based changes in response to new purposes.

6. According to Sittig and Singh [5], which are the eight dimensions that can help address sociotechnical challenges involved in development and implementation?

(1) *Hardware and software*, that is, computing infrastructure, refers to equipment and software that is used to support and operate clinical applications. (2) *Clinical content* refers to textual or numeric data and images and represents the "language" of clinical applications. (3) The *human-computer interface* refers to all aspects of the computer that users can see, touch, or hear when interacting with the technology. (4) *People* refers to everyone who interacts with the system in any way, from the developer to the end user, including potential patient users. (5) *Workflow and communication* are the processes or steps required to ensure that patient care tasks are performed effectively. Two additional dimensions of the model are (6) *internal organizational features* (e.g. *policies, procedures, and culture*) and (7) *external rules and regulations*, both of which may facilitate or constrain many aspects of the previous dimensions. The last dimension is (8) *measurement and monitoring*, which refers to the process of measuring and assessing the intended and unintended consequences of implementing and using health information technology.

7. From a sociotechnical perspective, what considerations must be observed in the system design for successful implementation according to the COUMT paradigm?

From a sociotechnical systems perspective, the healthcare professionals at the point of care should not experience documentation for management purposes as an unnecessary practical constraint that limits their ability to treat and care for patients. On the contrary, the healthcare professionals should find that software developments add value to their core tasks. The electronic medical record is a good way of reducing additional documentation time. In order to be able to base management decisions on data from the primary process, the healthcare professionals at the point of care should be actively involved and informed about the purpose of the data use. The aim should be to optimize the electronic medical record as a subsystem of a sociotechnical system. Connected optimization means more than simply adapting the technical subsystem to the social one or vice versa. The concept of sociotechnical system design explicitly postulates the necessity of joint optimization of the technology use and organization as well as the need to be oriented to both productive and social purposes.

8. What software requirements are necessary for implementation?

The challenge is to implement the documentation content in the software in such a way that the treatment process and the support and management processes are supported in a user-friendly manner in all phases.

Important software-related prerequisites include:

- data already available in other software applications are taken over and processed for analyses;
- the plan, performance, and documentation time is documented and saved;
- the individual patient situation can be documented in a practical way;
- the documented data can be exported from the primary system to guarantee the possibility of evaluating the data documented.

To process data from coding systems, the following is useful:

- the filtering of data,
- the aggregation of data—for example, aggregating the health intervention "position patient in lateral position" to the next higher intervention group "positioning",
- the calculation of statistical measures, and,
- the drawing of diagrams.

9. Looking to the future, can you outline an exemplary case study showing how data from

the electronic medical record could be used for staff planning with regard to the skill/grade mix in an extended/better/additional way?

Open Answer.

References

1. Joukes E, Abu-Hanna A, Cornet R, de Keizer NF. Time spent on dedicated patient care and documentation tasks before and after the introduction of a structured and standardized electronic health record. Appl Clin Inform. 2018;9:46–53. https://doi.org/10.1055/s-0037-1615747.
2. Baumann LA, Baker J, Elshaug AG. The impact of electronic health record systems on clinical documentation times: a systematic review. Health Policy. 2018;122:827–36. https://doi.org/10.1016/j.healthpol.2018.05.014.
3. Schulz S. Kontroversen in der Medizinischen Informatik. Wozu benötigen wir standardisierte Terminologien wie SNOMED CT? Swiss Med Informatics. 2011;141:27–32. https://doi.org/10.4414/smi.141.73.272.
4. Padden J. Documentation burden and cognitive burden: how much is too much information? Comput Inform Nurs. 2019;37:60–1. https://doi.org/10.1097/CIN.0000000000000522.
5. Sittig DF, Singh H. A new sociotechnical model for studying health information technology in complex adaptive healthcare systems. Qual Saf Health Care. 2010;19(Suppl 3):i68–74. https://doi.org/10.1136/qshc.2010.042085.
6. Schüpbach H. Arbeitstätigkeit und Arbeitshandeln in soziotechnischen Systemen—ein Beitrag zur Diskussion. In: Rau R, Mühlpfordt S, editors. Arbeit und Gesundheit: Zum aktuellen Stand in einem Forschungs- und Praxisfeld: Festschrift anlässlich der Emeritierung von Prof. Dr. Peter Richter. Lengerich: Pabst Science Publishers; 2007. p. 28–41.
7. Pasmore W, Winby S, Mohrman SA, Vanasse R. Reflections: sociotechnical systems design and organization change. J Chang Manag. 2019;19:67–85. https://doi.org/10.1080/14697017.2018.1553761.
8. Joukes E, Cornet R, de Keizer N, de Bruijne M. Collect once, use many times: end-users don't practice what they preach. Stud Health Technol Inform. 2016;228:252–6.
9. Swart E, Gothe H, Hoffmann F, Ihle P, Schubert I, Stallmann C, March S. Sonderheft Methodische Aspekte der Sekundärdatenanalyse. Gesundheitswesen. 2020;82:S1–3. https://doi.org/10.1055/a-1083-5461.
10. Straub HR. Das interpretierende System: Wortverständnis und Begriffsrepräsentation in Mensch und Maschine mit einem Beispiel zur Diagnose-Codierung: ZIM; 2009.

11. Ingenerf J. Klassifikationen und Terminologien–Eine Übersicht. In: Rienhoff O, Semler SC, editors. Terminologien und Ordnungssysteme in der Medizin: Standortbestimmung und Handlungsbedarf in den deutschsprachigen Ländern. Berlin: MWV Medizinisch Wissenschaftliche Verlagsgesellschaft; 2015. p. 35–50.

12. Meystre SM, Lovis C, Burkle T, Tognola G, Budrionis A, Lehmann CU. Clinical data reuse or secondary use: current status and potential future progress. Yearb Med Inform. 2017;26:38–52. https://doi.org/10.15265/IY-2017-007.

13. Hackl W, Ammenwerth E. Percise data statt big date. EHEALTHCOM. 2017;4:32–5.

14. Hackl WO, Ammenwerth E. SPIRIT: systematic planning of intelligent reuse of integrated clinical routine data. A conceptual best-practice framework and procedure model. Methods Inf Med. 2016;55:114–24. https://doi.org/10.3414/ME15-01-0045.

15. Ranegger R, Hackl WO, Ammenwerth E. Implementation of the Austrian nursing minimum data set (NMDS-AT): a feasibility study. BMC Med Inform Decis Mak. 2015;15:75. https://doi.org/10.1186/s12911-015-0198-7.

16. Baumberger D, Hieber S, Raeburn S, Studer M, Bürgin R, Ranegger R, et al. LEP–structure and application. Gallen: St; 2016.

17. World Health Organization. Skill mix in the health workforce. Determining skill mix in the health workforce: guidelines for managers and health professionals/Jane Buchan, Jane Ball and Fiona O'May. 2000. https://apps.who.int/iris/handle/10665/66765. Accessed 31 August 2020.

18. Driscoll A, Grant MJ, Carroll D, Dalton S, Deaton C, Jones I, et al. The effect of nurse-to-patient ratios on nurse-sensitive patient outcomes in acute specialist units: a systematic review and meta-analysis. Eur J Cardiovasc Nurs. 2018;17:6–22. https://doi.org/10.1177/1474515117721561.

19. Mosadeghrad AM. Occupational stress and turnover intention: implications for nursing management. Int J Health Policy Manag. 2013;1:169–76. https://doi.org/10.15171/ijhpm.2013.30.

20. Simon M, Mehmecke S. Nurse-to-Patient Ratios. 2017. https://www.boeckler.de/pdf/p_fofoe_WP_027_2017.pdf. Accessed 6 May 2020.

21. International Council of Nurses. Nurse-to-Patient Ratios (NtPR). 2015. https://www.dbfk.de/media/docs/download/Internationales/ICN-Faktenblatt-Nurse-to-Patient-Ratios-2016.pdf. Accessed 6 May 2020.

22. Aiken LH, Sloane DM, Bruyneel L, van den Heede K, Griffiths P, Busse R, et al. Nurse staffing and education and hospital mortality in nine European countries: a retrospective observational study. Lancet. 2014;383:1824–30. https://doi.org/10.1016/S0140-6736(13)62631-8.

23. Min A, Scott LD. Evaluating nursing hours per patient day as a nurse staffing measure. J Nurs Manag. 2016;24:439–48. https://doi.org/10.1111/jonm.12347.

24. Twigg D, Duffield C, Bremner A, Rapley P, Finn J. Impact of skill mix variations on patient outcomes following implementation of nursing hours per patient day staffing: a retrospective study. J Adv Nurs. 2012;68:2710–8. https://doi.org/10.1111/j.1365-2648.2012.05971.x.

25. Ranegger R, Baumberger D, Bürgin R. Bedarfs- und kompetenzorientierter Grademix in der Pflege: Eine prozessorientierte Tätigkeitsanalyse auf Basis von LEP Nursing 3. Pflegewissenschaft. 2017;11(2):504–16.

26. Dogherty EJ, Harrison MB, Graham ID, Vandyk AD, Keeping-Burke L. Turning knowledge into action at the point-of-care: the collective experience of nurses facilitating the implementation of evidence-based practice. Worldviews Evid-Based Nurs. 2013;10:129–39. https://doi.org/10.1111/wvn.12009.

27. Bjørk IT, Lomborg K, Nielsen CM, Brynildsen G, Frederiksen A-MS, Larsen K, et al. From theoretical model to practical use: an example of knowledge translation. J Adv Nurs. 2013;69:2336–47. https://doi.org/10.1111/jan.12091.

28. Popa I, Ştefan SC. Modeling the pathways of knowledge management towards social and economic outcomes of health organizations. Int J Environ Res Public Health. 2019;16:1114. https://doi.org/10.3390/ijerph16071114.

29. Werley HH, Devine EC, Zorn CR, Ryan P, Westra BL. The nursing minimum data set: abstraction tool for standardized, comparable, essential data. Am J Public Health. 1991;81:421–6. https://doi.org/10.2105/ajph.81.4.421.

30. Ranegger R, Ammenwerth E. Nursing minimum data sets (NMDS)–eine Literaturübersicht bezüglich Zielsetzungen und Datenelementen. Pflege. 2014;27:405–25. https://doi.org/10.1024/1012-5302/a000393.

31. Ranegger R, Hackl WO, Eberl I, Baumberger D, Bürgin R, Ammenwerth E. Automated mapping of LEP nursing data to nursing minimum data sets. Stud Health Technol Inform. 2020;270:38–42. https://doi.org/10.3233/SHTI200118.

32. Scott PJ, Rigby M, Ammenwerth E, Brender McNair J, Georgiou A, Hypponen H, et al. Evaluation considerations for secondary uses of clinical data: principles for an evidence-based approach to policy and implementation of secondary analysis. A position paper from the IMIA technology assessment & quality development in health informatics working group. Yearb Med Inform. 2017; https://doi.org/10.15265/IY-2017-010.

33. Shaw T, Janssen A, Crampton R, O'Leary F, Hoyle P, Jones A, et al. Attitudes of health professionals to using routinely collected clinical data for performance feedback and personalised professional development. Med J Aust. 2019;210(Suppl 6):S17–21. https://doi.org/10.5694/mja2.50022.

Leveraging Health and Community Data: Insights into Social Determinants of Health

16

Ruth Metzger, Andrew F. Beck, and Adrienne W. Henize

Learning Objectives

Upon completion of this chapter, the learner will be able to:

- Explain the importance of informatics in identifying adverse social determinants that affect the health of individuals and populations.
- Describe the role of informatics in identifying connections between adverse social determinants and increased burden, both human and economic, to the health care system and patients.
- Describe the various types of informatics tools and systems that are used to gather, store, analyze, and share data of pertinence to addressing adverse social determinants of health.

Key Terms

- Informatics
- Electronic Health Records (EHR)
- Data
- Database
- Social determinants of health (SDOH)

- Emerging trends in Health Information Technology
- Disparities
- Indicators

Introduction

In the early 1960's, when computers came into common use for business purposes, there were visionaries who also recognized their potential to gather and share data in health care. Fast forward to the present day, and the first enormous mainframe computers have given way to networks of smaller, more powerful computers, to desktop computers, and to the light-weight and user-friendly mobile devices that are ubiquitous today. The average person now carries more computing power and visualization capabilities in the smartphone in their pocket than the first mainframe computers possessed. The tremendous computing ability that has been realized is now a tool that can be leveraged to improve individual and population health.

Informatics and Social Determinants of Health

Good health is a result of far more than good medical care alone. Every person's living circumstances greatly influence their ability to do the necessary things for good health—access medical care when

R. Metzger (✉)
University of Texas at Arlington, Arlington, USA

A. F. Beck
Cincinnati Children's Hospital Medical Center,
University of Cincinnati College of Medicine,
Cincinnati, USA
e-mail: andrew.beck1@cchmc.org

A. W. Henize
Cincinnati Children's Hospital Medical Center,
Cincinnati, USA

© Springer Nature Switzerland AG 2022
U. H. Hübner et al. (eds.), *Nursing Informatics*, Health Informatics,
https://doi.org/10.1007/978-3-030-91237-6_16

needed, live in a safe and stable home, obtain an education and employment, and be able to maintain a healthy diet and be physically active. The U.S. Centers for Disease Control and Prevention (CDC) defines these circumstances as "community-level conditions in the environments in which people live, learn, work, play, worship, and age that affect health and health outcomes" [1], commonly called social determinants of health (SDOH). These determinants are so influential to health that Dr. Melody Goodman, in her keynote address to the first annual symposium by the Harvard Department of Biostatistics, spoke those now oft-repeated words, "Your ZIP code is a better predictor of your health than your genetic code" [2].

Informatics can help us understand the connection between health conditions and people's SDOH by enabling the collection, storage, management, and analysis of pertinent data from multiple sources. In this way, informatics can help drive better health by bringing us information that helps us to act and resolve problems, improve the health of individuals and populations, and decrease the economic and human burden on health care systems and providers.

Until recently, most health care organizations did not systematically collect data on patients' SDOH. Several factors, such as the drive to value-based care and the realization of the affects the SDOH has on individual and population health, are rapidly changing that reality [3]. No longer is it sufficient for health care organizations to cure a disease; it is increasingly essential to also maintain patients' health by helping them to resolve circumstances that contributed to the disease or condition in the first place. Before the circumstances can be resolved, however, they must first be identified. One very effective place to identify these circumstances is the primary care setting, where patients come into contact with the health care system for routine checkups and episodic illnesses. Primary care offers a potentially ideal setting to screen those patients for risks and needs related to the SDOH.

There are multiple challenges to collecting SDOH data from patients. A recurring issue is that providers who are already handling a heavy workload have little time to do more. Some providers find it difficult to open a conversation with a patient about sensitive SDOH topics such as domestic violence or depression, or may feel reluctant to approach a topic if they lack knowledge or resources to help the patient [4]. Other challenges include patient concerns about privacy, the potential for abuse of data, and the need for providers to turn the information into actionable takeaways. At a population scale, the data collected across health care organizations can be limited and inconsistent. This becomes even more challenging moving outside of health care with even more limited coordination and even more inconsistency between sectors (e.g., health care, education, government).

As collection of SDOH data migrates into mainstream practice, however, providers are finding new and better ways to identify and respond to associated health-relevant social needs. These data, from the patient to the population level, can be matched and cross-referenced with external data from a magnitude of sources to connect health conditions with potential causes and exacerbating or mitigating factors, to inform interventions, and to influence public policies that affect health.

Drawing Connections: Vulnerable Populations

Informatics is a valuable tool for studying the health of any population or group of people. Certain populations, however, face far greater struggles to remain healthy than others because of factors that exist outside the health care system. In particular, many lower-income individuals struggle daily to obtain the bare necessities of food and shelter. Systemic segregation and discrimination often mean that these challenges are disproportionately experienced by racial and ethnic minorities. These struggles arise from long-standing inequities rooted in poverty and structural racism and are difficult to overcome.

Some of these inequities are visible to the eye and can be contextualized using already collected data. One example is poor-quality housing, for which data can be found in places such as housing code violation records, judicial records, and municipal records of property ownership. Despite civil resources responsible for maintaining safe and habitable dwellings, sometimes properties fall into such disrepair that tenants' health suffers. Sometimes landlords or building managers opt not to respond even in the face of potential litigation. A common health problem that is associated with moldy or vermin-infested housing is asthma. Mold and vermin feces are well-known triggers for asthma, and frequent asthma exacerbations can lead to preventable use of emergency rooms and hospitalizations. In a 2014 study, researchers discovered a significant association with "population-level rates of children's asthma-related emergency room visits and hospitalization" and the density of housing code violations. In this case, data from the health care system were analyzed in conjunction with data from the city's housing code violation records to pinpoint key links between context and health [5].

Other struggles may stay hidden inside families where they are not visible to the community or to health care providers—struggles such as hunger, depression, or stress from working multiple jobs or lacking reliable transportation to get to work. These struggles and stresses can and do manifest in people's physical and mental health, but there are often no meaningful data collected on these. One way these issues can be discovered is by screening patients during the course of providing health care. Once issues are identified, referrals can be made through the electronic health record (EHR) that connects patients directly to resources to help overcome them.

Data that are collected from patients can be combined and monitored for trends in health problems to pinpoint when and where they are occurring, and to whom they are occurring. The case study in this chapter illustrates such an example, where monitoring data from patient charts led to identification of recurrent health issues among pediatric patients and to a common denominator shared by most of them. The common denominator was a cluster of federally sub-sidized apartment buildings that were in a deplorable state of disrepair. In response, the health care organization partnered with the city's legal aid organization, which initiated legal action and eventually resolved the problem with the property's ownership in partnership with tenants. The patient population in those buildings is now being monitored to track potential improvements in the children's health that might have resulted from this action.

Data Sources

Data collected by health care providers are entered into each patient's EHR, which receives physician notes, medication orders, lab results, images and reports, nurses' and therapists' notes, vital signs, and more for the individual. Over the patient's life, the EHR creates a history of the progression of the individual's health. All the EHRs for a health care organization are combined into a collection of data called a database that becomes a valuable tool for studying the health of the population the organization serves.

Health data are collected, stored, and analyzed for many purposes by many different organizations. All of these sources offer potentially valuable information to those seeking SDOH-related factors to health conditions. Some examples of quality data sources are:

- *Disease registries* are a "tool for tracking the clinical care and outcomes of a defined patient population" [6]. These registries serve the research process and care management for groups of patients with chronic conditions such as diabetes, cancer, or coronary artery disease.
- *Vital statistics* are an important source of data on births, deaths, marriages, divorces, and so on. Birth certificates include key health indicators such as birth weight, gestation, birth defects, parents, race, and so on. Death certificates include key health indicators such as age and cause of death, as well as demographic information. Collected locally, these data are

submitted to government agencies, and eventually are included in the databases of the National Center for Vital Statistics where they serve to inform research.

- *Claims data from Medicaid, Medicare, and third-party insurers* are a rich resource for information related to patient diagnoses, procedures, and health care utilization [7]. The analysis of these data contributes to better decision-making and improvement of population health by enabling comparison of services provided and patient outcomes by provider, cost and quality of care, whether providers adhered to recommended treatment protocols for patients, and more.
- *U.S. Centers for Disease Control and Prevention (CDC)* systematically collects data from many sources through the National Notifiable Diseases Surveillance System (NNDSS), a "system of systems" they coordinate at the national level [8].
- *World Health Organization (WHO)* collects and analyzes data from its 194 member countries and "produces burden of disease and mortality health estimates, which are published in the 'World Health Statistics'" [9]. The estimates are like a "report card" for the world, and they enable countries to "target their health problems and prioritize the use of precious health resources."

The advent of the internet and social media have spawned new applications that can potentially track health conditions in real-time, a concept called *syndromic surveillance*. One example is FoodBorne Chicago, a Twitter-based surveillance system that tracks complaints of symptoms related to foodborne illness. Sponsored by the Chicago Department of Public Health, the app "tracks tweets using a machine-learning algorithm that identifies the keywords 'food poison'" [10]. As those words appear in tweets, the app tweets the user a link to a form to provide details, collecting data that might lead the food inspectors to the source of the illness.

Other types of data that are useful to health care are collected, stored, and analyzed by many organizations outside the health care system. This may or may not be done in partnership or cooperation with health care organizations. Some examples of these organizations include:

- Health Foundations such as Robert Wood Johnson Foundation, John A. Hartford Foundation, the Commonwealth Fund, and many others produce reports on population health outcomes, health care systems quality, and other health care-relevant issues.
- Academic institutions such as the University of Wisconsin Population Health Institute which track health and health environment data on their *"County Health Rankings"* web site [11].
- Municipal offices such as building commissions, assessors, township trustees, the court systems, and the local commissions which make an effort to address homelessness and food insecurity.
- Non-profit organizations and businesses that collect data on economic conditions and employment.

Role for Informatics

Informatics' basic function of systematically collecting, storing, analyzing, and sharing data supplies a platform for "bridging" the divide between clinical data in the health care system and data from other sources. While informatics is used to build the platform, meaningful action only occurs when astute providers ask critical SDOH-relevant questions or when they use contextual data to recognize potential connections between health issues and community-level characteristics. With informatics as a tool, health care providers and researchers are able to "proactively identify, monitor, and improve a range of medical, environmental, and social factors relevant to the health of communities" [12]. In this way, data can support individual and population health by identifying a basis for intervention and the identification of needed community partners who can help drive the resolution of the problems. At its very best, data can be used to establish or influence public policies that prevent the problems that adversely impact individual and population health.

Data Analytics Tools for SDOH

Technology has given researchers the ability to rapidly analyze data from different sources to pinpoint problems and trends. The concept is not new, but tasks that once took weeks or months to perform manually can now be done in a matter of hours.

Geospatial Mapping

One of the most useful tools for understanding the connections between people's circumstances and their health is the mapping of geospatial data. Geospatial data are any data that are related to a geographic location [13]. Geospatial data may originate from geographic positioning data, satellite imagery, geographic information systems (GIS), or other sources. These data can be manipulated, analyzed, mapped in 2D or 3D, layered, and used to "identify problems, monitor change, manage and respond to events, perform forecasting, set priorities, or understand trends" [14]. This tool allows researchers to overlay health data with mapped community-level data.

Geospatial data can be integrated with health data to pinpoint concentrations of health problems, or patients, in relationship to external factors. Figure 16.1, for example, illustrates how home addresses of low-income children with

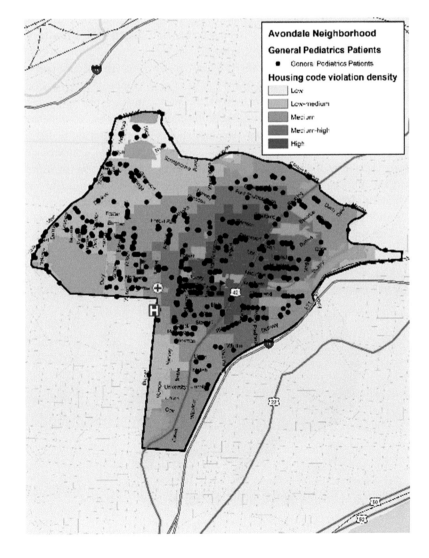

Fig. 16.1 Visualization of where Avondale Neighborhood General Pediatrics patients live overlaid with housing code violations. Source: Beck, Andrew F

chronic health problems who were patients of one clinic were overlaid with a map of housing code violations from the city's building code department records. The map illustrates how the children's homes were heavily concentrated in areas where the number of housing code violations was high. These circumstances can negatively affect people's health because of the unhealthy and unsafe condition of the housing. Even though states and localities have housing and building codes that require residences and commercial buildings to meet minimum health and safety standards, some property owners neglect to meet the standards. This leads properties to fall into serious states of disrepair and vermin infestation that negatively affect the occupants' health. When complaints are filed, municipalities may respond by issuing notices of violation, penalizing property owners, or by working with them to bring the property up to standards. Enforcing housing codes can be challenging for municipalities for several reasons. One reason is chronically negligent property owners who ignore notices of violation. Some property owners are difficult to locate and contact, especially if they are out-of-town; others engage attorneys to continuously challenge the violations in court. Again, data play a key role in identifying and responding to the issues.

The need for data from sources outside the health care system can stymie the process of finding negligent property owners, as delinquent or foreclosed mortgages cause the record of ownership to change frequently, as happens when banks buy and sell bundles of mortgages to each other. The actual owner of record can change faster than the municipal records can catch up. This creates difficulties for local code enforcement officials to deliver the notices of violation to the correct property owner [15]. These are a few of the reasons why the resolution of such problems can often take a great deal of time. Helping patients (and populations) find help to navigate such challenges falls within the purview of health care professionals, given the undeniable link between living circumstances and health outcomes.

Data Visualization

Another useful tool for informatics is data visualization. When massive amounts of data and information are involved in informing data-driven decisions, a graphical representation can help communicate findings more quickly than sifting through numbers, text, and tables. Data visualization provides a user-friendly way to observe trends and patterns in data.

Figure 16.2 provides a visualization of data representing hundreds of thousands of cases of reported COVID-19 across the U.S. in the spring of 2020. These data are routinely tracked by the CDC. At a

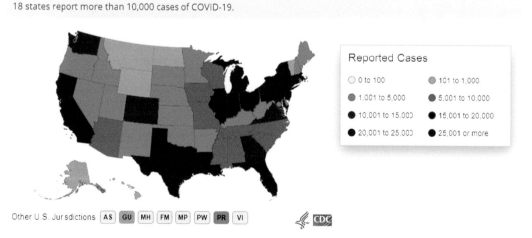

Fig. 16.2 Data visualization of the density of COVID-19 cases across the U.S., April 2020. Source U.S. Centers for Disease Control and Prevention https://www.cdc.gov/coronavirus/2019-ncov/cases-updates/cases-in-us.html

glance, it is easy to see the states with the highest number of reported cases, those with over 25,001 cases. It is also easy to see the states with the fewest reported cases. Information like this can help guide decisions on where to focus treatment, prevention, and testing efforts to fight the disease.

Cloud Computing

Cloud computing is a tool that gradually evolved from ever-developing technology and people's need to store, analyze, and share data and computing capabilities. In the early 1950's, users accessed information from mainframe computers through "dumb terminals" that had no computing capabilities but operated with the mainframe's capabilities instead. As computers grew smaller in size and more powerful on their own, different types of networking tools and data transmission protocols were developed to move and store data among them. With the advent of the internet in the late 1990's, far more complex and capable means of accessing and using data, such as cloud computing, have continually increased.

Cloud computing is "a model of computing where servers, networks, storage, development, and even applications (apps) are enabled through the internet" [16]. Cloud computing enables organizations to fulfill their data needs through a cloud service provider, without the need to invest in their own expensive equipment, hire and train staff, provide system security, and maintain equipment and technical support. This platform provides organizations with a cost-effective way to share resources and scale their usage to their changing needs. Figure 16.3 shows an example of how cloud computing may be configured.

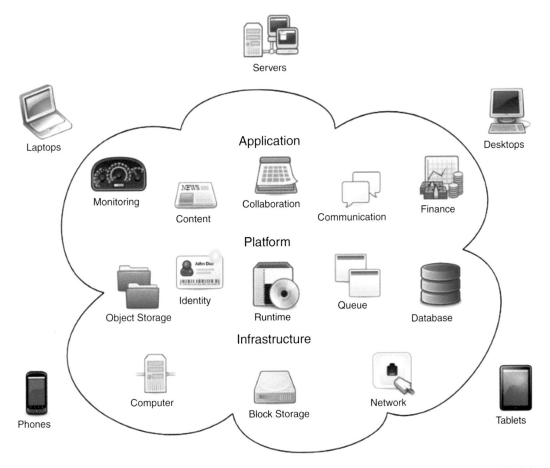

Fig. 16.3 Cloud computing structure, courtesy of Sam Johnston under Creative Commons Attribution-Share Alike 3.0 license

The data from electronic health records (EHRs) that are now the norm in health care are contributing to databases of health information that are growing exponentially. EHR data are one type of data that is called "big data," or data that businesses generate on a daily basis through the course of business. These databases are so large and growing so rapidly that they can be analyzed computationally to identify patterns, trends, and associations in population health and human behaviors. EHR data can be combined with data from other sources to add value and insight to research.

In the U.S., there are stark racial and ethnic disparities in health and health care. At the root of these disparities are socioeconomic determinants that are known to drive individual risk for certain chronic conditions, injuries, and failure to recover from health-related events. Big data is a valuable tool for analyzing these disparities among different demographic groups, understanding their health risks, recognizing and closing gaps in preventive care, and creating predictive alerts to inform decision making. These efforts constitute a holistic approach to care than in the past, and they are beginning to yield benefits in the form of improved health outcomes and cost savings to health care organizations.

Artificial Intelligence

Artificial, or augmented, intelligence (AI) is assuming an increasingly important role in health care by helping providers improve patient and population health outcomes while simultaneously reducing costs. AI is "the simulation of human intelligence processes by machines, especially computer systems" [17]. AI is based on specialized hardware and software that is used to write and train machine learning algorithms that utilize the human processes of learning, reasoning, and self-correcting. While AI is expensive to purchase, users can subscribe to services that suit their needs through cloud computing.

What can AI do for health care? Some organizations utilize AI to make better, more rapid diagnoses than humans are able to do. Some of the best-known technologies can understand natural language and respond to human commands or questions, which many people experience when they call a pharmacy for prescription refills or interact with a virtual chatbot or health assistant. AI can assist users to find medical information, inquire about bills, or schedule an appointment.

AI technologies are also being deployed in the battle against pandemics such as COVID-19 to understand the behavior of the disease and to predict its spread [18]. Avidon (2020) explains that.

"AI tools in analytics platforms pull data from disparate sources and use it in algorithms to almost instantaneously turn the data into the models used to comprehend potential scenarios" such as assessing and predicting the spread of disease.

During the 2020 COVID-19 pandemic, all the decision-making related to isolation, quarantine, and the economy were based on an analytical model, including analytics from China and other countries, that was employed to predict future global spread of the virus. The model included assumptions about infection and mortality rates that were utilized to create a predictive model. Researchers and economists used the model to simulate multiple possibilities based on the data and scenarios [18].

Data Analytics Tools

The market abounds with hundreds of different data and business analytics tools that are used in every industry. These tools are used for many purposes, including:

1. Retrieving data from one or more data systems and combining it into a larger repository, where they can be reviewed and analyzed.
2. Data mining, which examines large datasets in order to discover and analyze patterns in the data.
3. Combining data into reports and dashboards for easy visualization.
4. Predictive modeling which uses data and statistical methods to predict a range of potential outcomes.

5. Risk stratification, which uses data elements to differentiate the potential for risk and right-size the service that is then provided (e.g., in health care, this could mean distinguishing between patients based on their medical history, age, lifestyle, and other health indicators, etc.)

Though data analytics are used extensively in industry and health care, their use to target SDOH is just emerging and currently lacks "clearly defined strategies on how to use this information to inform patient care" [19]. One approach that is gaining favor is to integrate such data to promote improved, coordinated care, using such data to inform deployment of resources and connections. Kent also notes insights made by the eHealth Initiative (eHI) Foundation, that

> SDOH health data can lead to better care management and personalized care by providing a unique lens into the health and well-being of individuals…For instance, recognizing issues such as food insecurity, lack of transportation, and unsteady employment or housing, offers meaningful insights into circumstances that directly affect lives.

Ideally, caregivers, patients, and sometimes families will collaboratively identify which interventions and resources will work best. This includes caregivers educating patients on how certain SDOH play a role in their health. It also may include patients educating caregivers on which interventions are desired and effective.

Potential Partners and Collaborators

When health-harming SDOH situations are discovered during the course of health care, the partners and resources necessary for effective interventions to resolve the issues are often located outside the health care system. This means health care providers must collaborate with external partners to drive the actions that need to occur. The choice of partner(s) depends on the patients' needs.

In the example given in the case study, at the root of adverse health outcomes was unsafe, unhealthy housing. The responsible party was an out-of-town property owner who failed to properly maintain the property. The needed intervention was legal action to enforce health and safety standards for the apartments, so the health care organization partnered with the city's Legal Aid agency to resolve the issue. The provider had an existing, ongoing relationship with the local Legal Aid Society, a growing trend nationwide in the U.S. known as a medical-legal partnership MLP [20]. Other issues are similarly addressable, and health care providers may consider developing formal (or informal) partnerships with other social service agencies to support patients who need food and rental assistance, counseling services, senior resources, and safe places to stay if experiencing domestic abuse.

Neighborhood-Level Approach to Population Health

When Dr. Goodman pointed out the importance of our ZIP code for determining our health, it was because of factors such as "housing, education, job opportunities, child care, and transportation" that reflect our living conditions and our opportunities to experience health [21]. Even within a single community, there are tremendous differences in morbidity and mortality from one zip code to the next. The same is true in many parts of the developed world. For this reason, the goal of a "health in all policies" approach has emerged that incorporates an inter-sector approach to "embedding health considerations into decision-making processes" [22]. First voiced in Finland in 2006, the concept has been promoted by the World Health Organization and many countries. In the U.S., numerous states and cities have adopted the approach.

Improving the health of a neighborhood requires a focus on mitigating any underlying unhealthy condition that may exist there. The stories of those unhealthy conditions are told by data on the neighborhood—data on diseases and deaths, data on resources such as access to healthy food (full-service supermarkets vs. number of convenience stores and fast food joints), data on transportation, crime, income and employment, housing costs and conditions, home ownership vs. rentals, and so on. Inequities in health outcomes often parallel inequities in a range of SDOH, driven by generational poverty, structural racism, poor quality housing, and lack of socioeconomic opportunity [23]. Just as challenges may exist within such zip codes, or neighborhoods, so too do solutions.

An example of a neighborhood-level approach to population health improvement, and attention paid to the SDOH, occurred when a cross-sector team targeted a defined population of high-medical-need children in two low-income neighborhoods. These neighborhoods were identified as morbidity "hot spots," or areas of high concentration, through the use of geospatial methods that extracted data from the EHR and paired it with a range of community-level indicators. Together, these data told a powerful story, one where children experienced disproportionately high rates of hospitalization as well as housing and food insecurity, limited access to pharmacies to fill prescriptions, and greater barriers to participation in preventive services. Within these neighborhoods, the chronic disease that contributed to the most hospitalizations was asthma, so among the team's plan was a focus on interventions directed towards better control and prevention of asthma-related exacerbations. The focus later extended beyond asthma to other medical conditions and to a range of SDOH thought to be highly relevant root causes (Beck, Sandel, Ryan, & Kahn, 2016).

The health system data from July 2012 to July 2015 formed the baseline data. The improvement period began in July 2015 and continued through July 2018. During this improvement period, the research team adopted a patient/family-centered approach, engaged community partners from different disciplines to help families navigate the means to address their "complex, multidimensional problems" (Beck, et al., 2017), and engaged families to be part of designing their own interventions. By focusing on this specific population, and by using key data fields within the EHR and within additional datasets, the health care team and its partners were able to reduce children's hospitalization days by approximately 20%. These were more days that children spent at home and in school. Since then, the team has applied the same efforts to other "chronic conditions…pairing a data-driven approach with front-line knowledge of family and community needs" [23].

Case Study: Using Population Health Informatics to Address Health Inequities

Introduction

Health disparities are differences in overall health outcomes between populations of people. These disparities are often linked to socioeconomic status, with poorer people having poorer health status. Race and ethnicity also play an important role, with Hispanics, African Americans, and Native Americans more often living in poverty and having overall poorer health as compared to whites. These conditions that promote such disparities are defined as the social determinants of health (SDOH), or the circumstances in which people are "born, grow, live, work and age" [9].

Health disparities exist across the life course and are present among the youngest children, even those under the age of five [24]. Although data illustrating health disparities inform us about the differences in health outcomes among and between populations, they alone cannot explain the reasons why those disparities exist.

Primary care is one setting that has been found to be an effective place to screen for, identify, and address potentially health-harming circumstances experienced by patients and families. This case study takes a look at how one primary care system partnered with a legal aid organization to establish a medical-legal partnership, utilizing population health informatics to support the identification and mitigation of key risks related to the SDOH, risks known to adversely affect the health of low-income, minority families and to perpetuate disparities across populations.

Partners

Cincinnati Children's Hospital Medical Center (Cincinnati Children's) strives to be a force in improving children's health through excellence in clinical care and research. With their three pediatric primary care clinics, they serve approximately 37,000 patients per year, providing nearly 75,000 annual visits. The population they serve is primarily a low-income pediatric population, predominantly of minority race. More than 85% are insured through Ohio Medicaid [25]. Cincinnati Children's partner, the Legal Aid Society of Greater Cincinnati (Legal Aid), has approximately 40 attorneys on staff, many of whom work with clients referred from the Cincinnati Children's pediatric clinics. Together, the two organizations established a medical-legal partnership, the Cincinnati Child Health-Law Partnership (Child HeLP), in 2008.

The partnership strives to improve the health and well-being of children and families by identifying and mitigating certain risks known to be linked to health outcomes and that have potential legal solutions (e.g., adverse housing conditions, public benefit denials or delays). The identification and mitigation processes are enabled through a robust informatics infrastructure that enables social needs screening, sharing of relevant data, referral, and increasingly proactive data analytics and outcomes tracking.

Enabling Informatics Infrastructure

Data collection begins with the primary care visit, where screening for health-harming social risks had been integrated into the patient's health history within the EHR. The data collection tool has evolved with technology and currently is completed by the child's caregiver on a tablet at the time of intake. Responses are then delivered directly into Epic, the clinic's current electronic health record (EHR). Providers are then able to review those responses and integrate them into the clinic visit. Providers are encouraged to use responses as a "conversation starter," to dive more deeply into both positive and negative

responses in an effort to ensure that care delivery is appropriately targeted to need. If potentially actionable risks or problems are identified during the visit that could have a legal remedy, the provider can make a referral to Child HeLP and, by extension, a legal aid advocate (attorney or paralegal). This referral is made directly within the EHR, sending an electronic notice to Legal Aid personnel staffing the medical-legal partnership. Once the referral is received, the advocates initiate contact with the client, investigate the case, and intervene when legal action is warranted. Advocates are present within the largest clinic office multiple days a week and are often able to converse directly with the clinical team and the referred family. If they are not able to meet face-to-face at the time of the referral, they follow up by phone.

The Case

Poor quality housing, in particular, has been "shown to contribute to asthma, developmental and behavioral pathology, elevated [blood] lead levels, injury, and transmission of infectious diseases" [25]. In 2009, Child HeLP began to observe patterns in referral data that suggested a serious cluster of housing-related issues [25]. In a very hot spring, they began to see multiple children presenting for respiratory complaints including asthma exacerbations. They also began to see many housing complaints related to conditions and to the threat of eviction over the use of window air conditioning units. By examining the data, the medical-legal partners were able to pinpoint the origin of the problem, a set of apartment complexes that were owned and managed by an out-of-town developer. This owner consistently ignored code violations and orders from the city's health and building departments to resolve pest infestations and water damage. Clients complained of mold, cockroaches and rodents, peeling paint, and water leakages during their well-child checkups. They also frequently highlighted threats of evictions for mere complaints and for trying to maintain a healthy temperature within their units.

In July 2010, the owner of these complexes defaulted and a mortgage company took ownership. At that time, there were 19 building complexes which included 677 federally subsidized housing units. All of the buildings had code violations and outstanding orders to make repairs. The buildings were home to at least 45 children cared for at the Cincinnati Children's primary care centers, all African American, and all covered by Ohio Medicaid. Baseline data on the children revealed higher than normal rates of asthma and other airway diseases, developmental delays and behavior disorders, and elevated [blood] lead levels [25].

With the cluster, and pattern, recognized, Legal Aid advocates assisted both individual clients and a range of additional complex residents. One strategy was to facilitate the formation of a cross-complex tenants' association for which Legal Aid provided legal representation. Attorneys helped the tenant association work with the mortgage company to prioritize repairs. They also met with the city health and building departments, filed motions in court, and spoke out at city council meetings. Their efforts ultimately resulted in major repairs, including "new roofs, new ceilings and drywall, integrated pest management, replacement of sewage systems, refurbishment of air conditioning and ventilation systems, replacement of hallway lights, and repair of playground equipment" in the affected buildings [25].

Tracking and Follow-Up

The actions taken and SDOH-related successes of this case illustrate the positive impact such medical-legal partnerships can have on both patient and population health. Across the U.S., these partnerships are integrating the expertise of medical providers, attorneys, social workers, and case managers to attack problems at their root causes [20]. As of 2019, at least 333 health organizations in 46 states were actively engaged in these partnerships.

Data sharing is an essential ingredient for the effectiveness of the partnerships. In this case, the protected health information (PHI) remains within the health care system where sharing is governed by privacy and security laws such as HIPAA (Health Information Portability and Accountability Act), while clients agree to share the specific data the legal advocate needs to assist them. Legal outcomes are tracked on the Legal Aid database, while health outcomes are tracked in the EHR as they relate to clinic visits, hospital admissions, emergency room visits, and test results.

Future goals for Child HeLP, the Cincinnati medical-legal partnership, include being increasingly more proactive with data analysis and geospatial mapping to identify SDOH-related, contextual patterns amenable to both patient- and population-level action. At the same time, the team is actively pursuing research to better understand the linkage between the interventions and actions Child HeLP enables and a range of pediatric health outcomes.

Summary

The circumstances in which people live their day-to-day lives have a far greater influence on their health and longevity than the medical care they get. Those social determinants dictate where people can afford to live, how safe their neighborhoods are, how much they can earn, what type of food they can afford, where their children go to school, and much more. Sometimes those circumstances have a very negative impact on health. Health informatics is a valuable tool that can be used to collect, store, manage, and analyze data on social determinants to identify circumstances that are adversely affecting the health of individuals or populations. New technology tools enable health researchers and health care organizations to have information rapidly at their fingertips for faster and better diagnoses, recognizing patterns and trends in population health, and a deeper understanding of how to improve people's health and use limited health care resources more effectively.

Conclusions and Outlook

The future holds great promise for increased understanding of factors at the root of poor health. A move in this direction can be accelerated through the integration and analysis of data from health care systems combined with data from external sources. By leveraging patient and population-level data with community-level data, providers can gain insights into potential causative factors of adverse health conditions that can inform interventions to resolve them.

The focus on prevention of sickness by addressing "upstream" factors is a marriage of public health and health care, encompassing both prevention and treatment. In a recent interview with Dr. Joshua Vest of the Center for Health Policy at Indiana University [26], he elaborated on the importance of "prevention and addressing inequalities and supporting more effective, proactive use of resources and dealing with challenges and risks before they manifest as ill-health or unintended and undesirable consequences." His recommendations for the future include:

- Broader focus by health care organizations, pivoting from patient's illness to patient's health.
- Having common goals as health care organizations to address upstream factors.
- Development and building of an adequate informatics infrastructure.
- Development of the culture and values in health care organizations to support necessary infrastructure and capacity-building.

As the volume of data collected grows rapidly, the challenges of collecting, storing, and making meaningful use of those data grows, too. Some of those challenges include [27, 28]

- Integrating data from disparate sources in different formats.

- Protecting data that must be kept secure.
- Translating data into actionable knowledge.
- Data growth, including unstructured data such as documents, photographs, audio and video, free text, and so on.
- Gaining insights from data in a timely manner.
- Recruiting and retaining people with the necessary skills and expertise to manage and analyze the data.

The growing and evolving field of health informatics is transforming the delivery of patient-level health care and population-level health management. In doing so, there is a concomitant transformation in the education of health care professionals, development of newly needed skills, and modifications to the culture in which they will practice. There is the creation of new career paths, drives toward innovation in technology, and collective agreement that patients must be active participants in managing their own health as never before, using new technologies. Ultimately, health informatics is a vital tool for achieving the national Quadruple Aim [29] of improving population health, increasing patient satisfaction, reducing per-capita health care spending, and improving clinician and staff satisfaction.

Review Questions

1. As a health services researcher, you are interested in a pattern you observed in population health data that indicate a higher-than normal prevalence of pancreatic cancer in the lower Ohio River Valley in the U.S. You want to explore potential factors associated with this cancer, including the characteristics of the people who developed this cancer and any environmental exposures people with this cancer may have experienced. Identify at least two sources of data you might explore and the types of data you would need to find there. Then describe how you would compare the data to see if there might be an association

between the disease and certain environmental factors.

2. Discuss the importance of informatics in identifying health-harming SDOH by describing how relevant data are collected, who collects data, and how patterns in the data that reveal adverse SDOH are discovered.
3. Identify three challenges health care providers experience that are related to collecting relevant data on patients' SDOH. Suggest one potential solution to each challenge.
4. Describe the difference between geospatial mapping and data visualization.
5. You are a social worker helping a family that is struggling to obtain disability payments and health coverage for the husband, who was injured on his job as a construction worker. He has applied for disability and workmen's compensation and been denied. The family is very frustrated with the "run around" he has gotten from the Social Security and Workmen's Compensation offices and is suffering financially. Identify at least one external resource the health care provider could engage to help the family resolve this problem.

Useful Resources

1. Big Data Science: Opportunities and Challenges to Address Minority Health and Health Disparities in the 21st Century: https://www.ncbi.nlm.nih.gov/pmc/articles/PMC5398183/
2. Centers for Medicare & Medicaid Services Accountable Health Communities Model: https://innovation.cms.gov/innovation-models/ahcm
   Cleardata: Addressing the Social Determinants of Health with Cloud-Based Data Strategies: https://www.cleardata.com/research/social-determinants-health/
   https://www.ncbi.nlm.nih.gov/pmc/articles/PMC5398183/
3. County Health Rankings & Roadmaps: https://www.countyhealthrankings.org/

4. diversitydatakids.org (data for a diverse and equitable future): http://www.diversitydatakids.org/
5. Health Begins: https://healthbegins.org/
6. Health Leads: https://healthleadsusa.org/
7. National Center for Medical Legal Partnership: https://medical-legalpartnership.org/
8. Population health informatics—NYC Macroscope: look at EHRs and population health surveillance: https://soundcloud.com/phii-podcast/14-nyc-macroscope-a-look-at-ehrs-and-population-health-surveillance/
9. Social Interventions Research & Evaluation Network: https://sirenetwork.ucsf.edu/

Appendix: Answers to Review Questions

1. As a health services researcher, you are interested in a pattern you observed in population health data that indicate a higher-than normal prevalence of pancreatic cancer in the lower Ohio River Valley in the U.S. You want to explore potential factors associated with this cancer, including the characteristics of the people who developed this cancer and any environmental exposures people with this cancer may have experienced. Identify at least two sources of data you might find available in the cloud where you can explore data you need.

There are many resources for information; here are some examples.

Resource	Type of data
Cancer registries	Detailed information about cancer patients, distribution of cancer cases by gender, race/ethnicity, age, and other demographic factors, what prevention efforts work best, who is most likely to get cancer. Cancer registries analyze data and share with groups working to fight cancer.
National Vital Statistics database (CDC)	Captures all deaths from all causes across every state in the nation. These data help track the characteristics of those dying in the United States, help determine life expectancy, and allow comparisons of death trends with other countries

Resource	Type of data
Death certificates	Details vary from state to state, but often include: • Full name, • Address, • Birth date and birthplace, • father's name and birthplace, • mother's name and birthplace, • If a veteran, the discharge or claim number, • Education, • Marital status and name of surviving spouse, if any, • Date, place, and time of death, and, • Cause of death.
Labor statistics	Types and prevalence of employers and industries in the areas, products manufactured, services provided.
Environmental Protection Agency	Toxic discharges from industry, agriculture, or other sources in the area where the patient lived
Interviews with patients and families	Qualitative data regarding where the patient's place of employment, lifestyle, smoker or non-smoker, other relatives with cancer and what type of cancer, possible exposures to toxins

2. Identify three challenges health care providers experience that are related to collecting relevant data on patients' SDOH. Suggest one potential response to each challenge.

There are many challenges and these are a few examples:

Challenge	Response
Lack of standards for defining social determinants of health	Work within your organization and across organizations to be part of developing standards; be consistent within your own organization; provide input to national organizations working to define standards
Inadequate healthcare-based solutions for the core problems such as access to care, poverty and food insecurity	Develop partnerships with partners who can provide solutions, such as social work agencies and medical-legal partnerships
Reluctance of some providers to bring up sensitive topics such as abuse with patients	Educate providers—include opportunities to practice in with classmates before taking the skills to patients; allow clients to self-report via paper or electronic survey; ensure privacy during face-to-face conversations

3. You are a social worker helping a family that is struggling to obtain disability payments and health coverage for the husband, who was injured on his job as a construction worker. He has applied for disability and workmen's compensation and been denied. The family is very frustrated with the "run around" he has gotten from the Social Security and Workmen's Compensation offices and is suffering financially. Identify at least one external resource the health care provider could engage to help the family resolve this problem.

The most useful resource to address denial of benefits is legal assistance through a medical-legal partnership. If an MLP is not available, the local Legal Aid Society is another option.

References

1. National Quality Forum. National Quality Partners™ action brief. 2019. Retrieved from https://www.qualityforum.org/News_And_Resources/Press_Releases/2019/National_Quality_Forum_Leads_National_Call_to_Address_Social_Determinants_of_Health__through_Quality_and_Payment_Innovation.aspx.
2. Datz, T. ZIP code better predictor of health than genetic code. *The Harvard Gazette.* 2014, August 13. Retrieved from https://www.hsph.harvard.edu/news/features/zip-code-better-predictor-of-health-than-genetic-code/
3. Mullangi S, Pollak J, Ibrahim S. Harnessing digital information to improve population health. Harvard Business Review. 2019, May 14;
4. Metzger R, Hall M. A teaching strategy for social determinants of health screening in primary care. Annals of Nursing and Practice. 2018;5(3)
5. Beck A, Huang B, Chundur R, Kahn R. Housing code violation density associated with emergency department and hospital use. Health Aff. 2014;33(11):1993–2002.
6. Agency for Healthcare Research and Quality (AHRQ). Computerized disease registries. n.d.. Retrieved May 17, 2020 from https://digital.ahrq.gov/key-topics/computerized-disease-registries.
7. National Rural Health Resource Center. Using claims data. 2020. Retrieved May 17, 2020, from https://www.ruralcenter.org/population-health-toolkit/data/using-claims-data.
8. U.S. Centers for Disease Control and Prevention. National notifiable diseases surveillance system: data collection and reporting. 2018. Retrieved May 17, 2020 from https://wwwn.cdc.gov/nndss/data-collection.html.

9. World Health Organization. What are social determinants of health? 2019. Retrieved from https://www.who.int/social_determinants/en/.

10. Ellison K. Social media posts and online searches hold vital clues about pandemic spread. Sci Am. 2020; Retrieved from https://www.scientificamerican.com/article/social-media-posts-and-online-searches-hold-vital-clues-about-pandemic-spread/

11. University of Wisconsin Population Health Institute. County health rankings and roadmaps. 2020. Retrieved from https://www.countyhealthrankings.org/.

12. Gamache R, Kharrazi H, Weiner J. Public and population health informatics: the bridging of big data to benefit communities. In: IMIA yearbook of medical informatics; 2018. Retrieved May 17, 2020 from https://www.thieme-connect.com/products/ejournals/pdf/10.1055/s-0038-1667081.pdf.

13. Omnisci.com. Geospatial–a complete introduction. 2020. Retrieved from https://www.omnisci.com/learn/geospatial.

14. esri.com. What is GIS? 2020. Retrieved from https://www.esri.com/en-us/what-is-gis/overview#image.

15. Metzger R. Substandard rental housing in the promise zone of a mid-sized U.S. city. (doctoral dissertation). Minneapolis, MN: Walden University; 2018.

16. Accenture.com. Introduction to cloud computing. 2020. Retrieved from https://www.accenture.com/us-en/insights/cloud-computing-index?c=acn_glb_cloudgoogle_11261453&n=psgs_0620&gclid=CjwKCAjw34n5BRA9EiwA2u9k3-nJRhnT4OgIi19lhvHi-UrXHIWAqiSdaWjuJCU618v_d01BDxDxaxoC5SE-QAvD_BwE&gclsrc=aw.ds.

17. Rouse M. Artificial intelligence. Business Analytics. 2020; Retrieved from https://searchenterpriseai.techtarget.com/definition/AI-Artificial-Intelligence#:~:text=Artificial%20intelligence%20(AI)%20is%20the,speech%20recognition%20and%20machine%20vision

18. Avidon E. AI tools in analytics software key in fighting COVID-19. Business Analytics. 2020, April 3; Retrieved from https://searchbusinessanalytics.techtarget.com/feature/AI-tools-in-analytics-software-key-in-fighting-COVID-19?_ga=2.131220742.820365397.1596209138-1883762057.1596209138

19. Kent J. 5 ways to ethically use social determinants of health data. Health IT Analytics. 2019, June 27; Retrieved from https://healthitanalytics.com/news/5-ways-to-ethically-use-social-determinants-of-health-data

20. National Center for Medical-Legal Partnerships. We're helping to build an integrated health care system that better addresses health-harming social needs by leveraging legal services and expertise to advance individual and population health. 2019. Retrieved November 18, 2019 from https://medical-legalpartnership.org/.

21. Centers for Disparities in Health, Build Health Places Network, Robert Wood Johnson Foundation. How do neighborhood conditions shape health? An excerpt from making the case for linking community development health. 2015. Retrieved from https://www.buildhealthyplaces.org/content/uploads/2015/09/How-Do-Neighborhood-Conditions-Shape-Health.pdf.

22. American Public Health Association. Health in all policies. 2020. Retrieved from https://www.apha.org/topics-and-issues/health-in-all-policies.

23. Beck A, Sandel M, Ryan P, Kahn R. Mapping neighborhood health geomarkers to clinical care decisions to promote equity in child health. Health Aff. 2017;36(6):999–1005. https://doi.org/10.1377/hlthaff.2016.1425.

24. Colorado Department of Public Health and Environment. The connection between health disparities and the social determinants of health in early childhood. Health Watch. 2010. Retrieved from https://www.cohealthdata.dphe.state.co.us/chd/Resources/pubs/ECHealthDisparities2.pdf

25. Beck A, Klein M, Schaffzin J, Tallent V, Gillam M, Kahn R. Identifying and treating a substandard housing cluster using a medical-legal partnership. Pediatrics. 2012;130(5)

26. Shah G, Waterfield K. Promoting determinants of health services; informatics is the answer. J Public Health Manag Pract. 2019; Retrieved from https://jphmpdirect.com/2019/03/13/promoting-social-determinants-of-health-services-informatics-is-the-answer/

27. IBM Big Data & Analytics Hub. 3 top data challenges and how firms solved them. 2018. Retrieved from https://www.ibmbigdatahub.com/blog/3-top-data-challenges-and-how-firms-solved-them.

28. Datamation. Big data challenges. 2017. Retrieved from https://www.datamation.com/big-data/big-data-challenges.html

29. Agency for Healthcare Research and Quality. Quadruple aim proposed to address workforce burnout. 2019. Retrieved from https://integrationacademy.ahrq.gov/news-and-events/news/quadruple-aim-proposed-address-workforce-burnout

Citizen Generated Data: Opening New Doors in Health IT Research and Practice

Patricia Hinton Walker and John M. Walker

Objectives

- Explore the History and Future Relevance of Citizen Science.
- Compare and Contrast Citizen Science from Community/Individual Participatory Research.
- Differentiate Citizen Science Scientific Steps and Process Issues from other Scientific Studies in health care.
- Explore Journey from Biomarkers to Neural Networks.
- Application of Citizen Science for Improved Health and Personal Change.
- Examine Citizen Sciences Emerging Possibilities in Health Care.
- Explore, Ethics, Legal and Policy Aspects of Citizen Science.

- Technology and Implications for Underserved Populations and Social Determinants of Health
- Useful Resources
- Review Questions
- References

Key Terms

- Scientific citizenship
- Patient Engagement
- Community-based Participatory Research
- Health Information Technology Implications
- Use of mHealth technology for improving healthcare
- Wearable Technology Advances
- Biomarkers, Sensors, Apps and Neural Networks

Introduction to Citizen Science

In the book The Field Guide to Citizen Science: How You Can Contribute to Scientific Research and Make a Difference [1] by Darlene Cavalier, Catherine Hoffman and Caren Cooper, the authors introduce the readers to the history, process, and future opportunities of Citizen Science. Beginning with a bit of the history and exploration including the introduction of the Crowd Sourcing and Citizen Science Act as part of the American Innovation and Competitiveness Act in early 2017, 'Citizen Science outcomes are regularly included in peer-reviewed journals and in 2018 with the National Academy of Sciences published a report titled "Designing Citizen Science to Support Science Learning.' This movement is/was not only in the United States but also part of the European Union's Horizon and The Government of Canada's Citizen Science Portal lists citizen projects happening across Canada. More from Canadian contributions will be discussed later in this chapter. In this chapter,

P. H. Walker (✉) · J. M. Walker
Coaching Stepping Stones, Canton, GA, USA

© Springer Nature Switzerland AG 2022
U. H. Hübner et al. (eds.), *Nursing Informatics*, Health Informatics,
https://doi.org/10.1007/978-3-030-91237-6_17

we will discuss: The history, development and future relevance of citizen science; the variety of ways citizen science is designed, such as and including community-based, participatory research; the highlight the data process issues and interoperability issues from body sensors and biomarkers to artificial intelligence-driven decision making. Additionally, the authors will highlight the current and future possibilities in health care that are emerging through the implementation of citizen science and new technologies and finally provide a discussion of ethical, legal and policy related issues for the future. This chapter is purposefully designed to reflect global interest and advances in citizen science in the context of the international, interprofessional reach of the TIGER Initiative (Technology Informatics Guiding Education Reform).

Brief Background and History of Citizen Science

It is important to note that the idea of scientific work taken on by the general public is NOT NEW! There is a long history of citizens engaging in science, primarily focused on weather and the environment. According to 1890, the U.S. Government created the Cooperative Observer Program (COOP) to assist gathering meteorological data and the Audubon Society's Christmas Bird Survey is over one hundred years old. Citizens were monitoring the migration of butterflies in the 1960's and tracking observing lilacs and honey suckles in the early 1970's. Also, outside the USA, in Japan citizens were observing mutations of spiderworts for those living near nuclear reactors.

In 1972, citizens became involved in assessing the impact of laws on water supply and quality of water. Kimura and Kinchy [2]. In 2019, "2800 citizen scientists from 69 countries submitted nearly 9500 observations from nearly 3500 sites as part of the Mosquito Habitat Mapper community … predicting outbreaks of West Nil virus in U.S.A". Cavalier, et.al [3]. Under the Obama administration, the website *citizenscience.gov* was established which was "designed to acceler-

ate the use of crowdsourcing and citizen science across the U.S. government." (BOOK—Kinde). Subsequently, the Crowd Sourcing Citizen Science Act which aimed to 'encourage and increase the use of crowdsourcing and citizen science methods with the Federal Government' was passed in 2017 [2]. From a global perspective, the European Union's Horizon 2020 initiative is large responsible for the growth in the EU due to its substantial Funding, This project is aimed at elevating public engagement with science across Europe from passive engagement with the process of developing science to an active one. Citizen Science and Do It Yourself (DIY) scientific efforts demonstrate that this is possible, and our aim is to ensure that the European Research Area will become leader in 'deep' public engagement that is afforded by these advances.

As Environmental and health sensors like Fitbits and air-quality monitors become lower cost, people without science credentials are assessing the quality of their environment, providing a check on industries to make sure regulations are followed. In ports like Oakland, California—with significant truck traffic and in New Orleans—the communities have discovered excessive exposures to pollution where scientists and regulatory enforcers have potentially failed to look. "Citizen science has the power to transform science and society, recruiting volunteers or producing new tools. 'IT IS A Canvas—in many ways—with open space remaining to be filled'. And it's a movement that will undoubtedly shape your life, from finding a cure for Alzheimer's disease to gathering data in your own backyard." Cavalier, in Discover Magazine, Feb 27, 2020.

Citizen Science provides scientific observations and data, but it can do more. It can help make science more diverse and inclusive, provide a voice to the marginalized and challenge power inequalities. Examples over time that involved 'citizen science' were primarily focused on issues related to environment, economic and/or safety—including nutritional and air-related safety issues. Some examples include 2011 report by "Farming Concrete (in New York City) with a mission of protecting concluded that community gardeners were able to group some crops more efficiently than conventional farmers … with environmental, social, health and economic data." Kimura and Kinchy, [2] Feminist philosopher Iris Marion Young contends that 'the inclusion and participation of everyone … sometimes requires the articulation of special rights that attend to group differences in order to undermine oppression and disadvantage" Saroli, Brianna [4]. Later, the public became engaged in citizen science related to the AIDS crisis. Many people who were concerned about how clinical trials were being done (meaning that those who received placebos in randomized clinical trials were essentially getting a death sentence). In these citizen studies, they came to be known as 'patient activists', they became very engaged, and began to require 'a seat at the table'. Cavalier, and Kennedy [5]. This historic discussion helps us begin to understand some of the different approaches to citizen science, crowdsourcing, activism, and other forms of community-based participatory research.

Citizen science can be socially transformative when it responds to this problem and offers alternative knowledge and interpretations of bodies, environments, and social worlds. Environmental movements have been great examples of this potential … with positive impacts on scientific discovery, bringing new problems to light and 'alternative pathways' to research and development. (9.1). Examples of where difference has been made … Norco, Louisiana, residents of a predominantly African American neighborhood—bordering an oil company … concerned about health ailments that were thought to be related to toxic releases. One example of citizen science expanding the research data collection (beyond company researchers) was the Louisiana Bucket Brigade—trained local residents in 'air-sampling method' to send plastic bags of suspected air pollution. Kimura and Kinchy, [2] Citizen science can be 'produce knowledge from vantage points historically left out of science. Academic science as a social institution has been highly elitist, Western-centric and male dominated through most of its history.

"Academic institutions and research organizations have historically been populated by well-to-do men of Western European origin and people of color, the poor, and women have historically been underrepresented in positions of scientific authority. While science is diversifying, this history continues to have an effect on long-term research agendas and ideas about what kinds of questions are interesting and important.

Citizen Science, Community/Individual Participatory Research & Crowdsourcing

Citizen science has garnered strong interest in last several decades. Not only academic scientists, but policy makers and non-profit organizations are now embracing the concept. Supporters claim citizen science produces a wide range of virtues such as scientific literacy, engaged citizens, responsible research democratized science, and stronger environmental policing that is important to explore diverse ways that citizen scientists navigate common dilemmas. Participatory research efforts differed not only in terms of the issue areas and their contribution to scientific knowledge, but also in the style of participation and connections to policy. Citizen science projects are situated in different social contexts reflecting different histories of activism, state-science relations, and forms of civil society needs and progress toward health. THE TRANSFORMATIVE POTENTIAL: participatory environmental research, for example, does at least three things. It should bring diverse participants into the research process to produce knowledge from different vantage points. It should learn from and support efforts to create a more equitable society. And Finally—the collegiate practices of citizen science should construct a platform for broader political participation (Community-based participatory)! These are the hopes for citizen science.

Citizen science is a tool for groups to articulate their life experiences and counter sometimes dominant narratives. Citizens, through citizen science can (and have) provided resistance to assaults on environmental science ensuring that research on environmental topics that impact citizens continued. Including 'water monitoring,' participatory research does not necessarily or automatically lift up perspectives of marginalized people—but it can inspire volunteers to participate in data collection and contribute to change.

Key: 'Fostering trusting relationships between academic researchers and community groups takes time and significant commitments. While challenges are great—practitioners of citizen science have begun to address this issue more explicitly than before. There is growing recognition that gender, race, ethnicity, and socioeconomic backgrounds shape participation in citizen science. The U.S. Citizen Science Association (WHEN) was established on inclusion, diversity and justice recognizing that barriers for engagement exist.

Participatory environmental research can call attention to unfair distribution of pollution burdens and the ways that social inequality and power relationships shape environmental problems. In the case of fracking, grassroots air monitoring is revealing that people living in extractive communities (many of them economically marginalized and geographically isolated)—are exposed to toxic pollution.

Beyond this—there are models of participatory research that involve not only probing the biophysical aspects of a particular environmental issue but also asking questions about equity, power, and justice. Example in Marseille France … for years residents claimed excessive illnesses related to hundreds of gas, chemical and steel installations, yet official health data did not support the concerns. Barbara Allen—a social scientist collaborated on an environmental health study and worked with citizens to collect, interpret, and contextualize health data. Results indicated higher prevalence of asthma and cancer compared to the rest of the country. *Allen called it 'knowledge justice'; first observations as residents included as the basis of the questions asked in the health survey. Second, after the random sample is collected—worked with focus groups with the local* *populations and local doctors to interpret the data in context and got further analysis.* Finally, focus group participants were asked to think collectively about next steps and as a result of policy decisions, health clinics were able to be expanded.

This changes—so that research is not exploitative or purely extractive and only benefits paid researchers but it also provides opportunities for scientists and communities seeking environmental justice.

Giving Voice

The third virtue we see in participatory environmental research is capacity to give public voice to participants when scientific knowledge and technical expertise is important to decisions. Participative environmental research can grant access to regulatory decision making and provide an opportunity for those who have experienced social (AND HEALTH) injustice. *Greater participation of citizens brings increased scientific understanding to communities/citizens … and strengthens participation, dialogue and in the context of health (HEALTH BEHAVIOR CHANGE).*

FINALLY, science itself is/can be contentious with possibility of controversy. Research questions are shaped by disciplinary history and social contexts and interpretation of research results can have much broader impact. With suggestions for scientists, administrators, funding bodies, nonprofit organizations, activists, volunteers … SCIENCE ADVOCATES can best advance a transformative vision of citizen science. This addresses anti-scientific ideas (which may be on the rise). For instance, "the March for Science in 2019 attracted millions of people in more than six hundred cities around the world … to advocate and participate in scientific research, thinking and ultimately policy!" ([2] Science By the People).

IMPORTANT—Volunteers should not be considered merely as data collectors but considered as collaborators who bring necessary knowledge and perspectives. Instead of more efforts to make volunteers just participant-led, tit is important to make them truly collaborative (CBPR) and this is also an excellent means of science education where participants can also educate project leaders and each other. *Participants know more about the environmental history and other information that can assist with interpretation of data—which are issues that may be left out of traditional researcher-driven/funding driven research topics and processes. Quite often, it is good to have interdisciplinary research partners social scientists, historians, epidemiologists, and other groups.*

It remains to be seen how universities might successfully promote citizen science that is transformative. Public universities have a clear mandate to serve the public—but private universities are frequently not bound to certain community funders—making them sometimes easier to bring unique topics to the table. CITIZEN Scientists can insist on greater inclusion and diversity of volunteers. Are volunteers mostly all one gender, racial or ethnic group or social class. Is this by design or due to barriers to participation?

Scientific Steps and Process for Conducting Citizen Science

Steps to Take in a Citizen Science Project

As early as 2012 the now … **17**(2): 29. https://doi.org/10.5751/ES-04705-170229

To further the understanding of Citizen Science, this section will summarize the main steps in the process.

1. *What is the Problem?*
   Define and explore the problem. Is a solution needed or just knowledge of the problem's cause/effect? Why does it matter that the problem is solved or investigated? Who is interested in solving the problem? What can be accomplished by solving the problem? Has the problem been solved or partially solved by others?

2. *Project Design*
   Goals and Resources. Define the project goals and delineate the financial, human, and infor-

mation or other technology resources that will be required to gather the data that will prove or disprove those goals. Evaluate and/or define resources that will be used/required to accomplish the project goals. Resources may include skills, staff, students, sensors, surveys, or soil samples, for example. Software applications that may or may not exist may be needed; if the software does not exist, then plan to develop one. If one needs to be developed, then a data schema or structure that will support the project goals will need to be designed and tested.

3. Project Management
   Who should be included as participants and who should be project manager? Determine who is to be paid and who are the participant volunteers? Test and change elements of the project, if necessary, until the data, timing, software, hardware, and processes all support the goals. "Identify what tasks– including recruitment, training, data collection, quality assurance, analysis, and application of results– need to fit into your workflow. How long will each one take? Are there limits (for example, academic calendar or budget year) on when each can take place?" (1). Federal Crowdsourcing Webinar Series, Episode 1: Citizen Science. Retrieved from https://www.citizenscience.gov/toolkit/howto/step2/#. (April 2019).

4. *Community*
   It takes a community to do Citizen Science; some will be participants, and some will be professionals. "You will need to address the challenge of building and sustaining a trusting relationship with your community, which will include people with many different things to contribute and reasons for participating" (2). Federal Crowdsourcing Webinar Series, Episode 1: Citizen Science. Retrieved from https://www.citizenscience.gov/toolkit/howto/step3/#. (April 2019).

   The Citizen volunteers are particularly important members of the community. Without them there are no data and no knowledge gleaned. "Acknowledge their efforts early, often, and after a project. Recognize their contributions during regularly scheduled progress meetings during an ongoing project and champion their achievements when you formally document the results at the conclusion of an initiative" (2). Federal Crowdsourcing Webinar Series, Episode 1: Citizen Science. Retrieved from https://www.citizenscience.gov/toolkit/howto/step3/#. (April 2019).

5. *Data Management*

(a) Prepare a Data Management Plan. Primarily, the data gathered and the standard publicly accessible format within which it is stored must support the project goals. Decide how and from whom the data will be collected, stored for analysis, checked, certified, analyzed, safeguarded and, determine how and to whom the data will be distributed.

"To ensure the usefulness of your data, think of it as an asset with a "data lifecycle" of interlinked phases, including planning, acquisition, processing, analyzing, preserving and sharing. You will need to answer questions related to documentation, storage, quality assurance and ownership for each stage of the data lifecycle. At each stage, consider crosscutting elements, such as description (including metadata and documentation), quality management, backup and security" (3). Federal Crowdsourcing Webinar Series, Episode 1: Citizen Science. Retrieved from https://www.citizenscience.gov/toolkit/howto/step4/#. (April 2019).

(b) Analyze Data. Analyzing the data approaches the reason why the data were gathered. Your project is attempting to answer questions; the data contain those answers if the project's planning and data acquisition have been successful. In order to find those answers within those data, data analysis must be done.

"As in any scientific undertaking, analysis helps you document and describe facts, detect patterns, develop explanations, test hypotheses and check for error. Analysis of citizen science or crowdsourcing data isn't necessarily different from analysis of data collected by other methods and can vary widely depending on the nature of the study and type of data" (4). Federal Crowdsourcing Webinar Series, Episode 1: Citizen Science. Retrieved from https://www.citizenscience.gov/toolkit/howto/step4/#processhttps://www.citizenscience.gov/toolkit/howto/step4/#process. (April 2019).

(c) Share Data. Find out who will want to use your data and decide the best way to share it. Determine whether raw or analyzed data are appropriate for what groups of users. Are charts sufficient or are spreadsheets better? Ensure your organization has approved release and that the release is in accordance with federal requirements for open data and open access.

"For participants, being able to see (and use) the data generated by a project is an absolute must. Data that participants submit must not simply go into a black hole. Being able to see their data and see what others contribute keeps people engaged" Federal Crowdsourcing Webinar Series, Episode 1: Citizen Science. Retrieved from https://www.citizenscience.gov/assets/files/mping-weather-reports.pdf. (April 2019).

(d) Preserve Data. Make the data persistent and findable.

"Plan to preserve your data for the long term, meeting the data retention policies and practices of your agency as well as of the National Archives and Records Administration. You can preserve your data by archiving it or submitting it to an authorized data repository" (6). Federal Crowdsourcing Webinar Series, Episode 1: Citizen Science. Retrieved from https://www.citizenscience.gov/toolkit/howto/step4/#processhttps://www.citizenscience.gov/toolkit/howto/step4/#process. (April 2019).

6. *Sustain and Improve Project*

(a) Participation Adaptation: There are many reasons why people participate in Citizen Science projects; some are casual, some are serious super users who need little to no appreciation. Sometimes there are personal reasons why even super users need to quit participating, but those reasons should be analyzed so that appropriate changes within the project can be made. Appreciation and reward go a long way to foster continued participation but showing that the data that they helped gather have solved the problem is most appreciated. "… Galaxy Zoo collectively acknowledged its volunteers in a scientific paper. By validating the work of your volunteers, you encourage them to keep coming back" (19) (U.S. General Services Administration, 2019).

(b) Communicate effectively with participants and staff.
(c) Use formal documents to ensure clarity.
(d) Solicit feedback from participants to help evaluate the project.
(e) Sustain funding to ensure project efficacy.
(f) Evaluate data quality.
(g) Evaluate participant engagement throughout the project enhances data quality and quantity and success of the project.
(h) Evaluate project flexibility, especially within Project Management; this can ensure project success.
(i) End the project. There are several aspects to ending the project such as, when, why and how, data security, permissions to use data, awards, acknowledgements, press releases, articles, abstracts, presentations, and website results.

Technology and Body Sensor-Based Healthcare Data Flow

"A biomarker (short for biological marker) is an objective measure that captures what is happening in a cell or an organism at a given moment". (National Institute of Environmental Health Services. *Biomarkers*. Retrieved from https://www.niehs.nih.gov/health/topics/science/biomarkers/index.cfm. [March 2020]). Biomarkers include many measurements that are taken with a variety of chemical tests, genetic tests, measurements of the body such as blood pressure, heart rate, body weight, Body Mass Index and others. Biomarker sensors are increasingly influencing healthcare systems and individuals, [12–14, 15]. Some sensor packages to date can transmit their biomarker measurements via smartphone technologies such as Near Field Communication or BlueTooth and some rely on non-digital transmission of information such as a color change. Massachusetts Institute of Technology has even developed a wearable biosensor that continuously monitors biochemical biomarkers [16]. In the authors' opinions, soon we will need to integrate biomarker sensors into full or partial spectrum healthcare support systems. But, for the purposes of this chapter we will proceed to trace the flow of data from Citizen Science Data Donor biomarker sensor(s) through to the end "user" of that data.

In the past, biomarker data relied on transporting the person to a clinic, hospital, or doctor's office where a nurse, technician, or doctor used instruments to measure and then recorded in a paper chart the patient's biomarker data as BP, HR, heart and lung sounds and ordered lab tests to get chemical biomarker data. Then, after someone pulled the chart from the shelves, the doctor read the data on the paper chart and possibly diagnosed a health problem/issue. These data, compared to the information technology of the present, were slow to acquire, aperiodic, sparse, prone to the possibility of human errors, slow to retrieve, and to visualize. Compared to today's potential of integrating information technology and biomarker sensors, there were no advantages (see Fig. 1).

Current and possible citizen science health care data flow starts with the citizen's body:

1. Body: The body is the source of biomarker data. So, the Citizen Science Data Donor, interested in providing biomarker data to a data warehouse, causes sensor(s) to measure and record some of their biomarkers. So, at this point in the data flow, the body "contains" the data waiting to be sensed, measured, stored, and used.

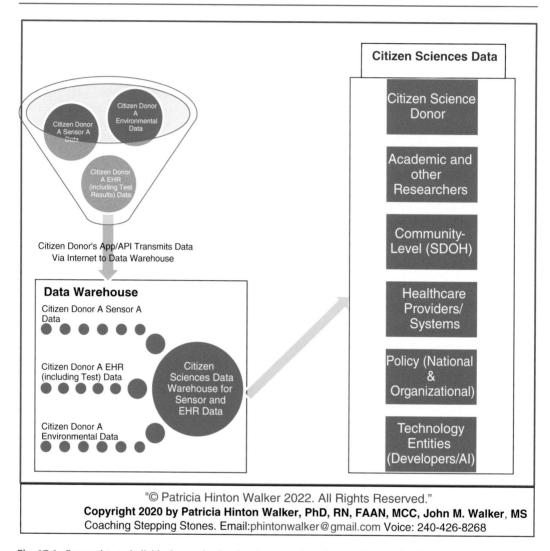

Fig. 17.1 Sensor data to individual, organizational and community science to improve health

2. Biomarker Sensor: "Noninvasive biomarker sensors that accurately measure changes in sweat and other biological fluids, can allow for a more personalized—also known as a "patient-centered"—approach to fitness goals and healthcare management" [17]. Today, many biomarker sensors are available such as those embedded in watches or, sensors that are external to SmartPhones but communicate via technologies such as BlueTooth or Near Field Communications. Heartrate, blood sugar, and blood oxygen sensors are examples. The sensor begins measuring the attribute of the Data Donor's body that it was designed to measure. Once the body attribute has been "sensed", a datum is created and stored. The datum might be a blood oxygen level of 94% and that value is then written to memory located either:

(a) on the sensor's memory for later transmission to a device such as a SmartPhone where it will await even later transmission to a Data Warehouse,

(b) another option is that the datum might instead be transmitted in near real-time from the sensor to the SmartPhone for storage and later transmission to the Data Warehouse.

So, sooner or later, the Citizen Science Data Donor's data will be located on her/his SmartPhone and will need to be transmitted to what we call (for the purposes of this publication) a 'Data Warehouse' which would essentially be a cloud-based database, a warehouse of data. A computer program (an App) located on the SmartPhone will be used to transmit the data to the warehouse.

3. App: "App" is a modern word that is short for "computer application" which is another word for "computer program," and finally, the words "computer program" are ways to describe "software". Then, there are Application Programming Interfaces; "An application programming interface (API) is a set of protocols, routines, functions and/or commands that programmers use to develop software or facilitate interaction between distinct systems" [18]. In this case, 'interaction between distinct systems' simply means that the app will be taking data that is resident on one system (Smart Phone) and transmitting it to another system (Data Warehouse). Think of an API as a small portion (a subroutine within a program or App) that does something that the programmer wants to occur at a scheduled time or when the user "clicks" on a button. For the purposes of this article, it is not necessary to focus on APIs, so the author will use the more commonly used word, "App" from this point onward. To continue the description of the current and possible Citizen Science data flow regarding Apps, we will describe one example where the Citizen Science Donor has decided it is time to Send out their Electronic Health Record (HER) data. The Citizen Science Donor starts the appropriate App and navigates to the screen where a Send button exists. The action of clicking on the Get & Send HER button causes a few lines of computer program code that is embedded in the Send button to request, receive, and store their EHR data on their smartphone and also to securely Send some or all of that EHR data and all of the recently acquired sensor data to the intended Citizen

Science Data Warehouse, a Cloud-based database. This App would use the Smart Phone's connection to the Internet to perform a secure data transmission. So, when the user clicks on the Get & Send HER button, an intended copy of the data is sent to the warehouse.

4. The Data Warehouse' would be comprised of computer server(s) and those servers would run database management software such as IBM DB2, Microsoft SQL Server, or Oracle, to perform four important functions:

   (a) to accept, store and organize donor data in a structured donor database and,

   (b) to possibly study the data via AI software and could, depending on its evolution and/or its commercial goals, create individual or population level health predictions and,

   (c) to provide (Send) selected and in most cases, anonymized, records *to customers/ users* (researchers, donors, Healthcare Delivery Organizations, Community Level SDOH, Policy Makers, and AI users) and,

   (d) to maintain database integrity and security.

At some point in a Citizen Science project, the Data Warehouse would make data available to the user(s) who would be able to run statistical software for research on the data or, to train Neural Networks to create individual or population health predictions. "The complexity and rise of data in healthcare means that artificial intelligence (AI) will increasingly be applied within the field" [19].

- Disadvantages: Cost of sensors/SmartPhone or Smart Phone-like device, possibility of errors caused by software bugs/errors.
- Advantages: Close to real-time data delivery rate and density largely determinable by the system, human errors (e.g., incorrect placement of sensors) would be minimized by reasonable effort, timely population-based healthcare risk assessment.

We have traced the flow of biomarker data from the body through sensors, apps, and communications to data warehouses and back to donors or users where personal and/or population level benefits can be realized. However, there are capital costs to this current data flow which could be reduced with systems integration processes. The complexity of healthcare data is growing rapidly, and the accuracy speed of some AI methods can alleviate some of that provider burden.

A common application of deep learning in healthcare is recognition of potentially cancerous lesions in radiology images" [20]. Deep learning is increasingly being applied to radiomics, or the detection of clinically relevant features in imaging data beyond what can be perceived by the human eye [21]). "Both radiomics and deep learning are commonly found in oncology-oriented image analysis. Their combination appears to promise greater accuracy in diagnosis than the previous generation of automated tools for image analysis, known as computer-aided detection or CAD [22].

The healthcare industry is rapidly approaching a point where integrating wearable sensor data, SmartPhone apps, existing communications, possibly Artificial Intelligence, and data security will be far less expensive and far more effective for far more people than ever.

The Citizen Scientist Donor flow of data is almost complete, but there are important possible and further uses for the donor's data regarding publicly available individual and population disease risk prediction and management. Citizen Scientists have a remarkable opportunity soon. Inexpensive AI software, for example, Neural Network desktop software, is currently available for download; this software is not difficult to use and does not require

knowledge of software programming. The problem is that the Citizen Scientist that would be using this AI software must have lots of data, some relevant to the project question(s) and some not, with which to train it and, unless the Citizen Scientist is a healthcare professional or a scientist who can find/detect many key heath biomarker records that have disease outcomes appropriate to the issue of interest, the Citizen Scientist cannot adequately train her/his AI neural network. Without successful training, the neural network is useless. So, another scenario is needed to make available to the public the benefits of professionally trained neural networks, or other AI software.

The Data Warehouse organization wishing to use neural network software create individual and/or population disease risk models.

A neural network typically takes a single set of data, partitions it into two non-overlapping subsets, and uses one subset to train the neural network such that the underlying behavior of the data are identified while not overly training it such that the 'noise' is treated as a component of the behavior." The other dataset is then inputted though the network to identify the actual patterns, outcomes, etc. based on the previously identified ideal behavior [23].

To do so, the organization would hire/retain experts knowledgeable in AI methods and software and healthcare professionals knowledgeable in the health issues of interest. In this example a simple neural network process, includes the following main steps after the data integrity standards are met (see Fig. 2).

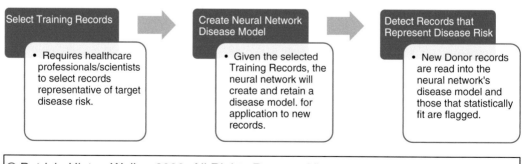

Fig. 17.2 Partial data flow for neural networks

1. Select Training Records: Teams of healthcare professionals/scientists will scour the Data Warehouse records to flag enough of those records that contain the biomarkers of interest and the outcomes of interest. The selected records are called *training records*. These training records will be used in the next step as human-selected examples of a problem/disease.
2. Create Neural Network Disease Model: All Training Records will then be read into the neural network software. Using only these training records, the neural network will create a disease model. The neural network's disease model will be retained within the neural network and will be ready to evaluate new records to determine whether those new records fit within the neural network's model of disease within a specified statistical significance.
3. Detect Records that Represent Disease Risk: The last major step is that new Donor records heretofore unseen by the AI model are read into the neural network's model of disease. The neural network, thanks to the training records, will then flag some new records that statistically fit its disease model and the organization should notify those donors of this finding. Similarly, the Citizen Science project will be able to contact relevant governments or local authorities regarding population disease risk details to inform policy.

Funding the Data Warehouse organization is probably the most problematic portion of the above AI scenario. It will need to support itself in some way; at some point in the project's lifespan it could sell access to its AI models, it could sell access to its anonymized data, or some other profit-oriented business model. However, assuming sufficient data are available to other organizations, price competition would soon reduce margins. On the other hand, a non-profit business model might work better and for longer; philanthropic donations could fund the training and ongoing maintenance of the AI models and other needs of the Citizen Science project organization and its data.

The healthcare industry is rapidly approaching a point where, among other data inputs, integrating wearable sensor data, SmartPhone apps, existing communications, artificial intelligence, and data security will probably form the basis for a significant increase in individual and population disease risk management. This will impact self-managed health/wellness and chronic care management, community level care, particularly in communities that have historically been underserved in health care, healthcare delivery organizations responsible for delivering healthcare, and future research for both community-based participatory research and academically-generated research grants from the National Institutes of Health and healthcare initiatives in private foundations.

Future Directions of Citizen Science

Emerging Future: It Is Becoming Difficult to Cast into the Future with it all around us

Where is Citizen Science taking us within the healthcare domain? Are we headed for a future where we will be monitored by biometric sensors in our refrigerators, embedded in our walls, floors, toilets and sinks and reported to insurance companies or authorities as some science fiction writers have portrayed that future? Or are we simply going to find ourselves in a future where our health and wellbeing are enriched by the knowledge gleaned by Citizen Science projects all over the world? Data can be immensely powerful; imagine millions of citizens providing their individual longitudinal biomarker data over their lifespans to a database. That database could be used to provide an overview of the overall human condition where *statistical measures* of each human biological system can easily be derived. But on the other hand, insurance companies could reasonably argue to legislators that given access to that database those companies could use it to decrease some individuals' policy cost, essentially precisely targeting people who would be healthier over their lifespan and those who would not be. As genetics becomes more detailed in its ability to identify problematic genes, that database would be immensely valuable to health insurance companies. All of the technology that is required to make, analyze, and distribute that corporate cost-saving knowledge is currently available. Genome research to identify problematic issues is active and has been for decades, database technology has been around for decades, artificial intelligence technology is currently worth billions of dollars and increasing in value, smartphone technology is significantly popular worldwide and powerful in its ability to detect, measure and report biomarker data to a cloud-based server with hardly any effort from the citizen, and citizens are willing to provide their biomarker data to a worthy cause.

Citizen Science and COVID-19. One example of a worthy cause is that the American Lung Association partnered with Northwestern University and University of California, San Francisco in a Citizen Science study of COVID-19. The project consists, in part, of a free and secure smartphone application. The project is estimated to last about 12 months and will require the user to attend to the application for 5 to 15 minutes per week. During that weekly time and while social distancing, the application will ask the user questions about potential COVID-19 exposures and symptoms.

> The COVID-19 Citizen Science study has the potential to be the largest-ever prospective epidemiological study of infectious disease. By collecting daily data from individuals around the world (with a goal of reaching 1 million users), researchers hope to gain insight into how the novel coronavirus spreads to help reduce future infections [24].

Precision Medicine

> Citizen Science seems to be poised to amplify the Precision Medicine area. Due to data donations that can be inherent in some Citizen Science projects, Precision Medicine can benefit greatly. The definition of Precision Medicine is the development of prevention and treatment strategies that take individual variability into account. Precision Medicine needs Citizen Science. The potential gains may be significant. "The active involvement of citizen scientists in setting research agendas, partnering with academic investigators to conduct

research, analyzing and disseminating results, and implementing learnings from research can improve both processes and outcomes" [25].

While not a Citizen Science project currently, one can just imagine the applications that a Smart Toilet could have in one. In Science News for Students, Smart Toilets are being envisioned by a lab in Stanford University in Palo Alto, California.

> The prototype can take pictures of your feces, track how often you go and measure how long each poop takes. Artificial intelligence then evaluates the consistency of the poop using a so-called Bristol scale. (Its seven categories range from 'rabbit droppings' through sausage-shaped to 'gravy.') The toilet also can measure the number of white blood cells and types of protein in urine. Such information could indicate an infection of the urinary tract or bladder [26].

The Smart Toilet project envisions that the data gathered will be analyzed by artificial intelligence and reported to the health care provider. Surely there should be user identification requirements and perhaps keyboard password entries or facial/voice/fingerprint recognition credentials. Or perhaps the smart toilet of the future will have DNA identification sensors thereby continuing the tension between privacy and better health care. A Citizen Science project using Smart Toilets would probably require significant funding due to the probable equipment costs but could feasibly uncover and/or confirm knowledge.

Analyzing and Interpreting Data. It is no secret that advances in Artificial Intelligence (AI) have made that technology useful in most situations. AI includes automated reasoning, machine learning, computer vision, computer hearing, knowledge representation and ontologies, natural language processing, and robotics. The most significant disadvantage of some AI is that it is sometimes impossible or difficult to determine how the software arrived at its conclusions; however, research and development is ongoing and will probably solve that issue. On the other hand and depending on the project, a correct answer is all that is required and knowledge of how the answer was derived/calculated is not needed. Given many records and subject matter experts who can select records with which to train an AI, a Citizen Science project can benefit from its application. There are AI applications in dermatology that are as accurate as humans in detecting disease.

> Members of the public are making substantial contributions to science as citizen scientists, and advances in technologies have enabled citizens to make even more substantial contributions. Technologies that allow computers and machines to function in an intelligent manner, often referred to as artificial intelligence (AI), are now being applied in citizen science [27]).

IBM Watson

IBM Watson is a huge enterprise within IBM. In 2011 Watson beat Jeopardy's best human contestants. It used natural language processing, hypothesis generation and evaluation and dynamic learning. It can quickly read millions of lines of free text information, such as academic articles. Citizen Science projects could provide IBM Watson Health with data that it would analyze to form conclusions and ongoing recommendations for those projects' goals.

> Companies are using IBM Watson to grow and transform their businesses in huge ways that are making a lot of professionals nervous. Instead of writing it off as "another new supercomputer," let's take a look at what actually makes Watson unique. Watson is a cognitive technology that processes information much more like a smart human than a smart computer. Rather than thinking humans will be replaced by a computer, you should realize that this is, in fact, a huge opportunity (Burrus).

AI & Dermatology

AI has been shown to be about as accurate as a human professional in diagnosing skin cancer. After training, the AI only requires an image of the skin lesion. "Research involving AI is making encouraging progress in the diagnosis of skin lesions. However, AI is not going to replace medical experts in the near future. In the first place, a human is needed to select the appropriate lesion for evaluation—often among hundreds of unimportant ones" [28].

MetaOptima Technology Inc. is using their DermEngine platform to provide teledermatology services. They developed a Deep learning visual search tool that "compares a user-submitted image in a database of thousands of pathology-labelled images gathered from expert dermatologists around the world" [28]. Citizen Science projects could provide more images to be added to that database.

Gaming

Eyewire is a game to map the brain from Sebastian Seung's Lab at Princeton University; it will support researchers who are modeling the information processing circuits of the brain. If you are interested in puzzles, you might be interested in Eyewire, a three-dimension game that challenges you to find all of the parts of a neuron within a thin slice of a brain. Join Eyewire, play the game and participate to help map a brain's neural connections. After analysis, researchers will hopefully "…discover how neurons connect and network to process information. You also help develop advanced artificial intelligence and computational technologies for mapping the connectome" [29]. Similarly, a new game named Neo is coming soon.

Eye Tracking

Some Citizen Science projects within psychology, neuroscience, infant and child research, human factors and engineering research, clinical and medical research, education, marketing, industry and human performance could benefit from application of eye tracking technology such as Tobii or Tobii Pro or Tobii Pro Fusion, "…*a fully portable, powerful eye tracker that enables researchers to run lab standard experiments in places not previously accessible*" [30].

Smart Phones

Future Citizen Science projects potentially have all the technology they will need in the smartphone that many of us have in our pocket or purse.

…the smartphone can be a powerful device to collect data—especially with the various sensors that the modern smartphone carries. The most common built-in sensors are the accelerometer, gyroscope, magnetometer, GPS receiver, microphone and camera. Other sensors that are seen in the higher-end models are for example gravity and rotational vector sensors, and environmental sensors such as barometers, photometers, thermometers and for example air humidity sensor. Some of the newer models even have a heart rate monitor built in, or a pedometer to track your steps, and there is even a Japanese model that can detect radiation levels [31].

An idea has been proposed to use smartphone camera technology to detect and report ultra-high energy cosmic rays. If enough people with smartphones participated in a Citizen Science project, that network of tiny smartphone camera sensors would have "significant observing power at the highest energies" [32]. The previous citations are only a small look at an enlarging scene; for example, another smartwatch has just recently been approved by the FDA to detect atrial fibrillation and to measure blood pressure from the wrist. The authors believe that Citizen Scientists will make many more contributions to science.

Ethics, Legal and Policy Aspects of Citizen Science

The first issue related to ethical, legal, and policy issues is to be clear about the language. For example, is the research Community-Based Participatory Research or is it crowdsourced data—that is generated about the environment, and so on but may or may not have donated physiological data? One example is 23andMe—which is a privately held testing company. They provide consumer data and have used genomic and voluntary phenotypic data for genomic research. Language that invites human participants to 'opt in' and share and/or 'donate data is different that when participants agree to allow data to become publicly available. Of course, how privacy is protected is critical as well as whether or not sometime in the future the data could be used related to 'pre-existing condition(s). Also, whether the data could be used sometime in the future for legal

purposes, for example, against companies that might be damaging some environmental aspects that could damage health (particularly impacting Social Determinants of Heath). The bottom line involves the nature of the public/private partnerships where data is involved and clarifying risks and opportunities for improvement of health and wellness for individuals, families, and communities.

From a policy perspective, it is important to clarify the terms of use, clarity the role of private companies whose products/devices are used to collect and store the data, as well as how the data is used both publicly and privately. Finally it is important to always address the question in a 'democratic society' is the citizen autonomy respected and what is the relationship to government or company authority, and how is both the autonomy and longer-term impact of the data collected protected. Beyond familiarity of the US Precision Medicine Initiative PMI and those partnerships with citizens, there are still ethics, policy and legal issues that will undoubtedly emerge in the future.

Use Citizen Science or Scientific Citizenship [33].and connection to EHR and PHR systems, and even a new direction called Local Health and Care Record Exemplars (LHCREs) have information regarding real-time data sharing and the question remains—what is identifiable and de-personalizeable—and what data do the 'citizen scientists' have access to, based on contributions? The big questions are: will individuals have to pay for results of the research that might be relevant to their health and will they 'know' the results related to industries that may have contaminated the environment(s) within which they live, work, eat, and sleep? https://www.nap.edu/catalog/25183/learning-through-citizen-science-enhancing-opportunities-by-design

Case Study: The Biomarker Toilets in a Senior Living Residence

A Senior Living home with several elderly residents was managed by a very tech-savvy administrator. Jay, the administrator, heard about a new product that he believed could save money for his organization and prevent health-related conditions from becoming serious for the senior residents. Jay reviewed the prototypes that were emerging from research at Stanford and at Duke.

Parker, S [26]. Waiting for a 'smart' toilet? It's nearly here. ScienceNewsforStudents. Retrieved from https://www.sciencenewsforstudents.org/article/smart-toilets-are-almost-here

Jay worked with an innovative toilet vendor to integrate these new prototype toilet's' data that use AI, to stream individual resident's data into his Wi-Fi-based local area network. This would track records of activity and data values for various biomarkers could be securely stored, retrieved, and reports and notifications generated quickly. Jay was careful to ensure that the system notified the Nurse Desk of important events and measurements. He knew that the toilets contained various sensors including, chemical analyses, presence of blood cells, temperature, seat force-measurements, and audio levels; so, he had worked with the vendor to ensure that certain events could be detected and notifications sent to the appropriate people in a timely way.

Jay consulted with the nurses to determine what events were important to know about and they told him that they wanted to know about the presence of blood in the stool or urine, a fall, and various chemical values such as prescribed drug levels. The latter was determined important because that would provide evidence that the resident was being administered the proper meds at the prescribed dosage and that the presence of any unprescribed medicine was a notifiable event. The vendor took the nurses' information and wrote the computer program that was stored in each of their BioMarker Toilets to ensure that the sensors and miniature chemical analysis lab inside each toilet was working properly and certified accurate and would notify the Nurse Desk of the nurse-defined important events reliably and in a timely manner.

A few days after installation of the toilets, residents paid little attention to the BioMarker Toilets. One night in the wee hours, the Nurse Desk received BioMarker Toilet notification that Mr. Red, one of the residents, had blood in his stool. The nurse read through his chart and scheduled him for an exam that next morning to determine whether it was hemorrhoidal or worse. The following week a resident's BioMarker Toilet notified the Nurse Desk that a fall had occurred in Mrs. Fellman's bathroom; the toilet's seat force-level sensor and audio sensor had supplied sufficient levels for the software to determine that a fall had probably occurred. The nurse responded with help and evaluated the fall as serious and took proper and early action preventing further issues. A few days later, nurses received a startling notification of the presence of a drug in Mr. Strangely's urine that had not been prescribed. BioMarker Toilet's neural network had benefit of the toilet's onboard mini chemical analysis lab results and had concluded that there had been an event and dutifully sent the notification. Upon seeing the notification, the nurse evaluated the resident's record and saw that the drug that had been detected in Mr. Strangely's urine could be serious and contacted the physician to discuss interventions. Those interventions were taken and the resident is safely back on the prescribed medicine. After investigation, Jay found that Mr. Strangely had, for some reason, willingly taken his neighbor's prescription and inappropriately self-medicated.

These events are just examples of many things that can occur without detection in today's Senior Living Residence's and with early detection and intervention proper application of appropriate, competent, and certified technology can prevent health issues from becoming serious.

Summary

With the arrival of COVID- 19, the focus on Citizen science has become even more important to scientists, citizens locally and globally. One project is engaging citizens, building on the National Academies of Sciences Engineering, and Medicine report [34], it is critical that community scientists assist health care leaders and agencies learn more about equity, diversity and including. This report highlights equity as a 'distribution of opportunities and resources that enables all participants to engage successfully … Diversity focuses on the differences among individuals, including demographic differences such as sex, race, ethnicity, sexual orientation, socioeconomic status, ability, languages and country of Origin, among others. Finally, the report stresses that how important it is to 'attend to inclusion with emphasis on intentional engagement with diversity [34]. And the 2019 Citizen Science study that has recently been launched by the American Lung Association [24] is a great example of how current health events can be initiated with intent to collect 'citizen data' from diverse populations in real time as we look to the future. With scientists still learning about this particularly deadly, communicable disease, scientists will increasingly need to rely on citizens across the globe to bring new scientific light to scientific understanding and even new treatment(s) for viral pandemics across the globe in the future,

Conclusions and Outlook

This chapter spans a significant period of time, beginning in 1890 and even going beyond 2020 with examples of the origins and growth and development over the year related to Citizen Science. Content in the chapter takes Citizen Scientists through the process of developing a citizen science project and highlights the detailed steps in the process that can be used currently and will inform researchers and health care provider systems of the value of this particular area of emerging research in the future.

Technological advances in many areas in addition to the increasing interest of populations such as the Boomers (with our growing aging population in the USA and globally; members of both Generation X and Generation Y who are very technology savvy are already engaged with use of advanced technology related to health and health monitoring. The outlook for Citizen Science projects which has been enhanced through social activism and will be even further enhanced in the future by these technology savvy populations and environmentally sensitive young people who are already engaged in making changes. This was highlighted earlier in the chapter related to AIDS research and with environmental issues such as the Louisiana project related to environmental monitoring of air quality.

There is increasing interest in use of sensors beyond wearables that are already in experimentation in different elderly care facilities with use of sensors in beds, measuring sleep, oxygen saturation during sleep, sensors in floors to identify individuals susceptible to falls. And although in the early stages of development, the toilet sensors mentioned in the case study highlight even more opportunities for citizens—and citizen scientist volunteers to participate in studies in the future. Finally, with the challenges globally with COVID-19, additional Citizen Science projects will be emerging beyond data collection using surveys locally and globally. Sensors that measure temperature and oxygen saturation and other health-related issues will certainly be emerging in the future as the research community better understands the impact of what is now called 'long-hauler's syndrome' and also the impact of participation (or not) in the use of vaccines (when they become available. In many ways, citizen science has 'only just begun' and will grow in the coming years. Increases in innovation and efficacy of technological sensors, combined with growing community interest and activism related to needs of under-served, diverse communities (globally) Citizen Science will be increasingly valued. It is critical that individual researchers, health care providers, health care systems, and policy makers who providing funding for research need to be prepared for the growing demands of individuals and communities in the future.

Review Questions
Questions Related to Developing a Citizen Science Project:

1. Questions related to defining and exploring the Problem.
2. Who is the population of Interest?
3. Why is it important to define and explore the problem?
4. Who is interested in solving the problem?

5. Who should be included as participants and who should be project manager?
6. "Identify what tasks—including recruitment, training, data collection, quality assurance, analysis, and application of results—need to fit into your workflow.
7. Who should be considered on the research team for effective Citizen Science research projects?
8. What are some of the important evaluation considerations for Citizen Science researchers when the project is completed?
9. Where is Citizen Science taking us within the healthcare domain?
10. Are we headed for a future where we will be monitored by biometric sensors in our refrigerators, embedded in our walls, floors, toilets and sinks and reported to insurance companies or authorities as some science fiction writers have portrayed that future?

Appendix: Answers to Review Questions

1. Questions related to defining and exploring the Problem?

Researchers and members of communities of interest would need to collaborate in identifying the problem for Citizen Science research projects sine engagement of the 'citizens' is critical for the success of citizens. This is based on whether the project involves wearable sensors or merely the process of assessing aspects of the environment that can have an impact on health but does not require wearable sensors that provide biometric data. It may be that the citizen science research project involves tracking of some aspect of the environment and a select number of bio-markers that can be tracked through use of 'wearable sensors'.

2. Who is the populations of interest?

Researchers/scientists and/or provider organizations can identify populations of interest based on challenges related to outcomes, re-hospitalizations, increased costs of health care for management of individuals with chronic conditions that may be related to some of the following examples:

(a) Chronic conditions of underserved populations that may have growing issues and costs related to diabetes, cardiac-related conditions, respiratory problems, and other conditions that are currently creating challenges in provider and self-management.

(b) Health care risks that may be related to environmental challenges that impact health including, but not limited to:
   • Contamination of the water (such as some of the damage to health even in children). An example was the negative impact of contaminated water in Flint Michigan.
   • Challenges with air quality which has been identified in several industrial areas that have created challenges with headaches such as the previously cited Louisiana Project and now may be related to cause of headaches related to fracking.
   • Future examples related to care of aging populations that are increasingly interested in all forms of sensors for self-monitoring to not only extend life but quality of life for a growing population of senior citizens.

3. Why is it important to define and explore the problem?

For the purposes of Citizen Science research projects, it is important that members of the scientific community identify data elements that can be captured reliably on wearable and/or environmental sensors. Then to identify interest from potential funding groups including federal, private organization and/or non-profit organizational funders. Finally, in order to engage communities in participating in data collection for citizen science, it is important that members of 'communities of interest' will help define participants and volunteer citizen scientists.

4. Who is interested in solving the problem?

For the individuals/groups establishing the Citizen Scientist, it is critical to identify funders of interest that are interested in or benefit from a Citizen Science research project. Funders may be interested because of 'mission/purpose' which is relevant to some not-for-profit groups; or health-care systems that have re-admission of certain populations and groups that are not responding to treatment and traditional health care approaches; and finally, to explore new knowledge that may be related to growing knowledge of the potential negative impact on health from the environment.

5. Who should be included as participants and who should be project manager?

For Citizen Science to be effective, community-based participatory research (CBPR) is one of the best options for a scientific approach to research. This approach involves a team which is made up of research science leader(s) and community members that become a form or a 'steering committee' and help ensure the success of the research. Historically, unfortunately much of community-based research involves predominately senior members of academic communities going into underserved communities for research projects 'about the citizens' and not with the citizens. Frequently, the research questions DO NOT address the community-member's concerns and leaders in the community are not engaged nor involved in the 'definition of the problem' instead of 'engaging communities' to ensure maximum participation in data collection (whether through use of sensors or collecting other information including demographics, etc.

6. "Identify what tasks– including recruitment, training, data collection, quality assurance, analysis, and application of results– need to fit into your workflow.

One of the first critical tasks is to recruit subjects. And, as mentioned previously the value of using a community-based participatory research process is that community engagement and creating a team with community leaders helps address this problem early. Next it is critical that data ele-

ments that are possible for subjects to obtain/track are identified. During this step it is critical to stake data collection steps to ensure that data if anonymized, records to customers identity and home location. This step also includes examining and ensuring the reliability of sensors designed to collect the data. Next it is critical to explore training of data contributors and identified leaders in the community that are part of the research coordination team.

A critical step is to attend to the collection, transfer of data to the data storage system (at the health care provider system or research data-base and work with IT leaders to ensure that data is stored in a structure donor database. Additionally, applying AI Software to this step is critical for options of community sensor reliability, organizing the data, analysis strategies for assessing groupings of the data including: individual level, group level for example - based on age and location within the community, and overall population-based data. This can ultimately also be correlated with data that may also be collected (again by same or other groups within the same community related to environmental sensor data,

Finally, it is important to create the data-warehouse which needs to be maintained for security and can be analyzed related to community level SDOH, connections to health care delivery systems for the purpose of exploring practice changes utilizing one of the evidence-based practice models that are relevant to the research and to the communities. And finally ensure long-term data integrity and security for secondary analysis and future research.

7. Who should be considered on the research team for effective Citizen Science Research projects?

Members of the research team include the primary scientists who design the research project, sometimes involves companies that have developed the instruments (watches and other sensor data collectors including smart beds, etc). Members include community leaders and representatives of the 'citizens that will be involved in the science" and IT professionals that can assist in development of the data-base management system and security measures that are critical to protect the citizen scientists. Finally, AI experts and systems are required for current and future data analysis related to potential SDOH content which can include environmental data but also other factors including resources such as housing, availability of healthy foods, transportation, etc.

8. What are some of the important evaluation considerations for Citizen Science researchers when the project is completed?

As researchers (whether part of a health sciences center, researchers in local educational institutions, or other scientific groups) design the Citizen Science projects, it is critical that evaluation methods are put in place. First, for CITIZEN SCIENCE it is critical to get input and evaluation data from the citizens and communities that have participated in data collection and use of sensors to determine challenges, reliability of data and value input for future potential projects. Additionally, of course it is critical that data collection, data analysis and relationship of data to location, to types/ages of citizen scientists and also impact of the AI systems that may or may not have been used.

9. Where is Citizen Science taking us within the healthcare domain?

Given the advancements in health-related sensors which are increasingly being approved by the FDA such as smart watches which can now measure oxygen saturation, blood pressure, regularity of cardiac function, temperature, and other date that has been available such as: number of steps and other activity, hours sitting, and with emerging gaming even eye movement which may highlight early signs of neurological functioning. The use of smart phones for surveys such as the current COVID-19 related survey by the American Lung Association is another example that relates to health behavior 'just-in-time' evidence related to health and health-behavior change.

10. Are we headed for a future where we will be monitored by biometric sensors in our refrigerators, embedded in our walls, floors, toilets and sinks and reported to insurance companies or authorities as some science fiction writers have portrayed that future?

There are articles that have identified opportunities to measure a variety of indicators that are increasingly related to health in terms of prevention and also to sometimes measure the effectiveness of treatment. Some examples that are already highlighted in the literature and mentioned earlier in this chapter include but are not limited to: the smart toilets which can identify early signs of diabetes (related to urine samples); gastro-intestinal related disorders (related to stool samples; sensors already in beds which have predicted respiratory distress related to early diagnosis of pneumonia (in some senior centers), floor sensors that identify unsteady gait that can potentially predict falls, etc. These are just some examples of the potential future use of sensors within home and housing. And there is an increasing focus on sensors (that are wearable and non-wearable that measure environmental elements including but not limited to quality of air and water in different communities, locations. It is important to note that these sensors are increasingly being implanted on a global level.

References

1. Cavalier D. The future of citizen science. Discover magazine. 2020. Retrieved from https://www.discovermagazine.com/planet-earth/when-the-people-investigate-how-citizen-science-has-transformed-research.
2. Kimura A, Kinchy A. Science by the people: participation, power, and the politics of environmental knowledge. New Brunswick, NJ: Rutgers University Press; 2019.
3. Cavalier D, Hoffman C, Cooper C. The Field guide to citizen science: how you can contribute to scientific research and make a difference. Portland, OR: Timber Press, Inc; 2020.
4. Saroli B. Indoctrination of young adults the college way: conservatives are cast out. From themorningwatchmsu. 2018. Retrieved from https://www.themorningwatchmsu.com/post/indoctrination-of-

young-adults-the-college-way-conservatives-are-cast-out.

5. Cavalier D, Kennedy E, editors. The rightful place of science: citizen science. Tempe, AZ: Consortium for Science, Policy & Outcomes; 2016.

6. U.S. General Services Administration. Federal Crowdsourcing Webinar Series, Episode 1: Citizen Science. 2019. Retrieved from https://www.citizen-science.gov/toolkit/howto/step2/#.

7. U.S. General Services Administration. Federal Crowdsourcing Webinar Series, Episode 1: Citizen Science. 2019. Retrieved from https://www.citizen-science.gov/toolkit/howto/step3/#.

8. U.S. General Services Administration. Federal Crowdsourcing Webinar Series, Episode 1: Citizen Science. 2019. Retrieved from https://www.citizen-science.gov/toolkit/howto/step4/#.

9. U.S. General Services Administration. Federal Crowdsourcing Webinar Series, Episode 1: Citizen Science. 2019. Retrieved from https://www.citizen-science.gov/toolkit/howto/step4/#process.

10. U.S. General Services Administration. Federal Crowdsourcing Webinar Series, Episode 1: Citizen Science. 2019. Retrieved from https://www.citizen-science.gov/assets/files/mping-weather-reports.pdf.

11. U.S. General Services Administration. Federal Crowdsourcing Webinar Series, Episode 1: Citizen Science. 2019. Retrieved from https://www.citizen-science.gov/toolkit/howto/step5/#adapt.

12. Ren C, Bayin Q, Feng S, et al. Biomarkers detection with magnetoresistance-based sensors. Biosens Bioelectron. 2020;165. Retrieved from https://www.sciencedirect.com/science/article/pii/S0956566320303353

13. The Optical Society. "Chip-based optical sensor detects cancer biomarker in urine". 2019. Retrieved from https://phys.org/news/2019-12-chip-based-optical-sensor-cancer-biomarker.html

14. Yirka B. Skin patch biomarker sensor that doesn't need batteries. TechXplore: Retrieved from; 2019. https://techxplore.com/news/2019-01-skin-patch-biomarker-sensor-doesnt.html

15. Cathcart N, Chen J. Sensing biomarkers with Plasmonics. Anal Chem. 2020;92(11):7373–81. Retrieved from. https://doi.org/10.1021/acs.analchem.0c00711.

16. Pataranutaporn P. "Wearable Lab on Body". MIT Media Lab. 2019. Retrieved from https://www.media.mit.edu/projects/wearable-lab-on-body/overview/.

17. Irwin R. "Sensors advance for biomarker monitoring". Medical design and outsourcing, Jan 2018. Retrieved from https://www.medicaldesignandoutsourcing.com/sensors-advance-for-biomarker-monitoring/.

18. Technopedia. "Application programming interface (API)". 2017. Retrieved from https://www.techopedia.com/definition/24407/application-programming-interface-api).

19. Davenport T, Kalakota R. The potential for artificial intelligence in healthcare. Future Healthcare Journal. 2019;6(2):94–8. https://doi.org/10.7861/futurehosp.6-2-94. Retrieved from https://www.ncbi.nlm.nih.gov/pmc/articles/PMC6616181/

20. Fakoor R, Ladhak F, Nazi A, Huber M. Using deep learning to enhance cancer diagnosis and classification. A conference presentation The 30th International Conference on Machine Learning, 2013. Retrieved from Google Scholar.

21. Vial A, Stirling D, Field M, et al. The role of deep learning and radiomic feature extraction in cancer-specific predictive modelling: a review. Transl Cancer Res. 2018;7:803–16. Retrieved from Google Scholar

22. Price L. Digital health hype cycle 2020. Healthcare. Digital. 2020. Retrieved from https://www.healthcare.digital/single-post/2020/01/29/Digital-Health-Hype-Cycle-2020.

23. Buscema P, Tastle W. Artificial neural network what-if theory. Int'l Journal of Information Systems and Social Change. 2015;6(4):52–81. Retrieved from https://www.researchgate.net/publication/280110097_Artificial_Neural_Network_What-If_Theory

24. The COVID-19 Citizen Science Study. 2020. Retrieved from https://www.lung.org/research/about-our-research/covid19-action-initiative/covid-citizen-science-study

25. Petersen C, Austin R, Backonja H, et al. JAMIA Open. 2020;3(1):2–8. https://doi.org/10.1093/jamiaopen/ooz060.

26. Parker S. Waiting for a 'smart' toilet? It's nearly here. ScienceNewsforStudents. 2020. Retrieved from https://www.sciencenewsforstudents.org/article/smart-toilets-are-almost-here

27. Ceccaroni L, Bibby J, Roger E, et al. Citizen science: theory and practice. Collection articles: ethical issues in citizen science. 2019. Retrieved from https://theoryandpractice.citizenscienceassociation.org/collections/special/ethical-issues-in-citizen-science/.

28. Goyal M, Yap M, Oakley A, et al. Artificial intelligence in dermatology: what is artificial intelligence. 2019. Retrieved from https://www.dermnetnz.org/topics/artificial-intelligence/.

29. Eyewire.org. About Eyewire, a game to map the brain. 2020. Retrieved from https://blog.eyewire.org/about/.

30. Tobii. Tobii Pro Introduces Tobii Pro Fusion–a portable and powerful eye tracker for scientific research. 2019. Retrieved from https://www.tobii.com/group/news-media/press-releases/2019/10/tobii-pro-introduces-tobii-pro-fusion%2D%2Da-portable-and-powerful-eye-tracker-for-scientific-research/.

31. Stoop J. New ways to use smartphones for science. Elsevier Connect. 2017. Retrieved from https://www.elsevier.com/connect/new-ways-to-use-smartphones-for-science.

32. Whiteson D, Mulhearn M, Smimmin K, Cranmer K, Brodie K, Burns D. Searching for ultra-high energy cosmic rays with smartphones. Astropart

Phys. 2016;79:1–9. https://doi.org/10.1016/j.astropartphys.2016.02.002.

33. Woolley P, McGowan M, Teare H, Coathup V, Fishman J, Settersten R, Sterckx S, Kaye J, Juengst E. 2016. BMC medical ethics.

34. National Academies of Sciences, Engineering, and Medicine. "Learning through citizen science. Enhancing opportunities by design" Consensus Study Report. 2018. Retrieved from https://www.nap.edu/catalog/25183/learning-through-citizen-science-enhancing-opportunities-by-design

Further Readings

1. 23andMe. Find out what your DNA says about you and your family. 2014. Retrieved from http://www.23andMe.com.

2. Bietz M, Patrick K, Bloss C. Data donation as a model for citizen science Health Research. Citizen Science: Theory and Practice. 2019;4(1) 6:1–11. https://doi.org/10.5334/cstp.178.

3. Bullard RD. Confronting environmental racism: voices from the grassroots. Boston: South End Press; 1983.

4. Burrus D. What can watson do for your company? Wired.com. 2015. Retrieved from https://www.wired.com/insights/2015/02/what-can-watson-do-for-your-company/.

5. Cooper C. Citizen science: how ordinary people are changing the face of discovery. New York, NY: The Overlook Press, Peter Mayer Publishers, Inc; 2016.

6. COSMOQUEST. What is Citizen Science? 2020. Retrieved from https://cosmoquest.org/x/about-cosmoquest/what-is-citizen-science/. Retrieved Sept. 2020.

7. Hinckson E, et al. Citizen science applied to building healthier community environments: advancing the field through shared construct and measurement development. The International Journal Of Behavioral Nutrition And Physical Activity. 2017;14(1):133. https://doi.org/10.1186/s12966-017-0588-6.

8. Katapally TR. The SMART framework: integration of citizen science, community-based participatory research, and systems science for population health science in the digital age. JMIR Mhealth Uhealth. 2019;7(8):e14056. https://doi.org/10.2196/14056.

9. King AC, et al. Maximizing the promise of citizen science to advance health and prevent disease. Preventive Med. 2019;119:44–7. https://doi.org/10.1016/j.ypmed.2018.12.016.

10. Merkel C, et al. Participatory design in community computing contexts: tales from the field. PDC 04: Proceedings of the eight conference on Participatory design: Artful integration: interweaving media, materials and practices–Volume 1, 2004, pages 1–10. https://doi.org/10.1145/1011870.1011872.

11. National Academies of Sciences Engineering and Medicine. 'New reports says: 'Citizen Science' can support both science and research goals'. 2018. Retrieved from https://www.nationalacademies.org/news/2018/11/new-report-says-citizen-science-can-support-both-science-learning-and-research-goals

12. National Institute of Environmental Health Services. Biomarkers. 2020. Retrieved from https://www.niehs.nih.gov/health/topics/science/biomarkers/index.cfm.

13. Newman G, et al. The future of citizen science: emerging technologies and shifting paradigms. Ecol Environ 2012. 2012;10(6):298–304. https://doi.org/10.1890/110294.

14. Penn Medicine News. Penn medicine study reveals promise of "Human Computing Power" via crowdsourcing to speed medical research. 2013. Retrieved from https://www.pennmedicine.org/news/news-releases/2013/july/penn-medicine-study-reveals-pr.

15. Smith E, Belisle-Pipon J, Resnik D. Patients as research partners: how to value their perceptions, contribution and labor? Citizen Science: Theory and Practice. 2019;4(1) 15:1–13. https://doi.org/10.5334/ctsp.184.

16. Stacey D, Legare F, Col NF, Bennett CL, Barry MJ, Eden KB, et al. Decision aids for people facing health treatment or screening decisions. Cochrane Database Syst Rev. 2014;1:CD001431. https://doi.org/10.1002/14651858.CD001431.pub4.

17. Staggers N, Gassert CA, Curran C. A Delphi study to determine informatics competencies for nurses at four levels of practice. Nurs Res. 2002;51(6):383–90. https://doi.org/10.1097/00006199-200211000-00006.

18. Symons JD, Ashrafian H, Dunscombe R, et al. From EHR to PHR: let's get the record straight. BMJ Open. 2019;9:e029582. https://doi.org/10.1136/bmjopen-2019-029582.

19. Torres T, Loehrer S. ACOs: a step in the right direction. Healthc Exec. 2014;29(4):62–5. Retrieved from http://www.ihi.org/resources/Pages/Publications/ACOsStepinRightDirection.aspx

20. U.S. Department of Health & Human Services. National strategy for quality improvement in health care (congressional report no. DHHS-2012). Rockville, MD: Agency for Healthcare Research and Quality; 2012.

21. World Health Organization. Framework for action on interprofessional education & collaborative practice. (No. WHO/HRH/HPN/10.3). Geneva, Switzerland: Author; 2010.

Data from Social Media: Harnessing Social Medial for Health Intelligence

18

Michael A. Gaspar, Janae Sharp, Geeta Nayyar, and Danielle Siarri

Learning Objectives
- Bolster your foundational understanding of how health, information, care delivery, policy, consumerism and social media coalesce in an increasingly digital society.
- Explore how health and consumerism work together to create healthier habits, improve literacy and impact health outcomes outside care encounters.
- Untangle the nuances of information privacy, security and integrity as it relates to public health and social discourse.
- Contextualize lessons learned from the COVID-19 pandemic and an increasingly divided political landscape for future social media use in health and wellness.
- Examine caregiver empowerment and wellness as it relates to delivering care amid social media misinformation and a 24/7/365 news cycle—while also using social media as a platform for structural change in our exam rooms, homes and communities.
- Familiarize yourself with applications of social media in public health surveillance and opportunities for future research and innovation.
- Define a realistic and healthy relationship between yourself and social media that allows you to thrive as a person and nursing informaticist.

Key Terms
- Effects social media has on consumer expectations for health and care delivery.
- Social media regulation impact on health and care delivery.
- Role of misinformation in consumer health literacy.
- Social media as a social determinant of health.
- Caregiver and clinician use of social media for advocacy and health equity.
- Social media applications for public health surveillance and population health management.

M. A. Gaspar (✉)
Savvy Cooperative, Chicago, USA
e-mail: michael@infointegrity.org

J. Sharp
Sharp Index, Salt Lake City, UT, USA
e-mail: janae@sharpindex.org

G. Nayyar
Salesforce, California, USA

D. Siarri
InnoNurse, North Las Vegas, USA
e-mail: dsiarri@innonurse.info

Introduction

When it comes to the intersection of social media, health and information, the truth is we currently have more questions than answers. It may be enticing to take aim at the COVID-19 pan-

© Springer Nature Switzerland AG 2022
U. H. Hübner et al. (eds.), *Nursing Informatics*, Health Informatics,
https://doi.org/10.1007/978-3-030-91237-6_18

demic—which persists even as these words are written—as the culprit for many of these challenges and uncertainties. However, systemic and cultural issues that existed before and will persist after the global health emergency ail much of what is still needed to scale thoughtful, health-related social media applications.

At the onset of 2020, global society was already struggling with the following issues—all of which have been prevalent discussion topics across social networks:

- Struggling to navigate divisive and dangerous political rhetoric
- Debating sustainable health, social justice, government and economic reform
- Combating clinician and caregiver burnout
- Bringing awareness to and making progress on racial and social injustice
- Escalating social and tech company regulatory concerns
- Acknowledging the need to repair global citizenship among nations
- Wavering trust in the scientific community
- Surges in cybercrime, election interference and social media mis- and disinformation

For reasons likely to be explored further by experts in the future, the COVID-19 pandemic seemingly managed to accelerate the discussion and global imagination surrounding these issues, respectively. One glaring example was mounting evidence that indigenous and communities of color were upward of 4.1 times more likely to be hospitalized and 2.8 times more likely to die of COVID-19 [1], bolstering already surging Black Lives Matter protests for racial justice and equity. What started as an already nascent behavioral and technological phenomenon leading into the pandemic, social media's scope of impact is proving to be an even more mysterious and challenging element of our digital lives than previously anticipated.

On one hand, health innovators are promisingly honing social media to extract valuable behavioral insights and establish predictive modeling that can have a meaningful impact on health outcomes. On the other, social media is marred with information integrity issues, vitriol and noise from malactors that prove to be detrimental to the health of patients and caregivers and public health research efforts. Given the interconnectedness of social media's impact on the public and healthcare alike, it's no longer tenable to contemplate these phenomena in silos—especially seeing how global social media adoption is expected to increase to 4.4 billion users, 23%, by 2025 [2].

The signals are clear: social media is here to stay, and healthcare needs to adapt to thoughtfully navigate what comes next.

If cogent and sustainable progress is to be made in responsibly wielding and understanding social media, we will likely need to accept that taking on such a task is a holistic and collaborative effort that requires diverse voices and expertise at the table—both inside and outside of healthcare. The 2019 research paper "A Call for a Public Health Agenda for Social Media Research" [3] provides a detailed analysis of what research, interdisciplinary collaboration and innovation are necessary to account for the evolving complexities of social media—in addition to noting the field's key challenges. In their analysis of the health and social media research field revealed opportunities for collaboration and academic cross-training in the following fields:

- Biomedical science
- Computer science
- Data science
- Economics
- Engineering
- General science/medicine
- Human computing interface
- Infections disease/vaccines
- Medical internet science
- Public health
- Public policy
- Social psychology/communication

Given the interdisciplinary challenges that lie ahead, the goal of this chapter is to lean on compelling research, examine case studies and reflect on evolving social media, societal and healthcare attitudes in hopes of establishing a holistic foundation of understanding for nursing informatics leaders to navigate an ever-evolving social media and health information landscape.

As noted, so much work is yet to be done, but a lot of insightful work exists to illuminate the path forward. Among this foundational work is the Social Media-Based Health Information Management (SMHIM) conceptual framework [4] outlined in the research article "Harnessing Social Media for Health Information Management" [4]. The framework draws from nine different disciplines and helpfully categorizes the landscape by the following:

- *Participants* within the intersection of social media and health information
- *Problems* in health that are being addressed or perpetuated by social media
- *Platforms* where social engagement takes place
- *Processes* by which social media data is generated, retrieved, integrated, analyzed and then applied within the context of health encounters
- *Opportunities* for researchers to expand on the study of social media and health information

This work proves exceptionally useful especially considering the complexity, intersectionality and shortage of research to date [3] on social media in healthcare. Table 18.1 draws upon the SMHIM framework to reflect new observations from the global COVID-19 pandemic, shifts in the social media and digital health landscapes, and more simply illustrate the relationship between stakeholders and factors within the ecosystem.

The aim is that this resource will serve as a starting point for meaningfully unpacking the following themes throughout this chapter to inform nursing informatics projects of the future:

- More fully understanding social media as a social determinant of health
- Maximizing advocacy efforts for consumers, patients and caregivers via public policy and regulation

Table 18.1 A quick reference guide to the social media and health information landscape

	Intersection of Social Media and Health Information	Description of Intersection	Research and Policy Opportunities
Benefits *Why?*	Care	Improve care quality and safety while optimizing care delivery	Digital health infrastructure Emerging health, consumer technology Health innovation Health reform Quality care delivery
	Communication	Improve communication between caregiver-caregiver, caregiver-patient and patient-patient	
	Convenience	Empower self-care and improve patient, caregiver access to information and care	
	Cost	Improve cost-effectiveness (value) of care delivery and public health surveillance	
Participants *Who?*	Caregivers[a]	Clinical and non-clinical care teams, including both healthcare-specific and consumer social media use	Caregiver burnout mitigation Consumer protection efforts Corporate responsibility initiatives Cultural difference exploration Health literacy advancement International collaboration and policy Social network regulation
	Companies[a]	Products and services within and outside health sector	
	Consumers/patients[a]	Health information consumers, social media users	
	Organizations[a]	Government agencies and mission-based organizations	
	Public figures[a]	Celebrities, influencers, community leaders and policymakers	

(continued)

Table 18.1 (continued)

	Intersection of Social Media and Health Information	Description of Intersection	Research and Policy Opportunities
Problem *What?*	Chronic disease	Chronic disease management, support (e.g., addiction, cancer, chronic pain, arthritis, diabetes and depression)	Critical health populations Disease management effectiveness
	Mental health	Adverse effects of social media use (e.g., caregivers, consumers, populations); mental health management, support	Health management effectiveness
	Public health surveillance	Population health analysis, forecasting and countermeasures (e.g., coronavirus, climate, influenza)	
	Public policy + regulation[a]	Caregiver and patient advocacy; health and social justice reform	
	Preventive health + wellness[a]	Health communication, engagement, behavior change and literacy improvement	
	Rare disease	Rare disease management, support and treatment	
Platform *Where?*	Publishers and curators	Blog, social curation and website discussion (e.g., Digg, Flipboard, medium, the *New York Times*, YouTube)	Multimedia and platform behaviorsplatform-specific privacy rulessocial and web anonymity
	Social networks[a]	Microblog and social media sites (e.g., Facebook, twitter, Instagram)	
	Thematic networks + forums[a]	Review platforms (e.g., Healthgrades, yelp); segmented discussion forums (e.g., Reddit, Quora)	
	Wikis	Community-curated bodies of knowledge (e.g., Wikipedia)	
	Professional networking[a]	General and healthcare-specific professional social networks and forums (e.g., LinkedIn, Sermo, Doximity)	
	Virtual reality and gaming	Gaming platforms for networking, therapeutics and medical training (e.g. Altspace, oculus, twitch)	
Processes *How?*	Data generation[a]	User-generated data from social media, including keywords, behavioral markers, geolocation and so on	Application programming interfacescausal assessment Data preparedness
	Data retrieval	Data extracted and organized from examining content analytics, social media datasets	Data privacy and confidentiality Data quality
	Data integration[a]	Data standardization, mobility, sharing for integration with/among care and business systems; interoperability	Disease intervention Health impact assessment Misinformation and
	Data analysis	Automation, streamlining of data analysis using machine learning, AI, natural language processing; information extraction for health intelligence applications	disinformation Multi-modal, −source, −role data fusion Patient education Personalized health
	Data application	Applied information extraction for care, business, public insights	management Public health data infrastructure

[a]Denotes updates to intersections originally outlined in the conceptual framework for SMHIM, "Harnessing Social Media for Health Information Management" 2017 [4].

- Shaping care practices using social media listening tools, analytics and engagement strategies
- Applying and scaling social media data capture for care, disease intervention and predictive modeling
- Co-designing a healthier and more sustainable health and social media ecosystem to enable all of the above

Examining Health Consumerization and Literacy

When you think of social engagement and intelligence, what comes to mind? For most people, the answer probably revolves around Facebook, Twitter and LinkedIn. While popular social media platforms play a critical role in this area, their potential ends neither with them nor the way typical users engage with their products. In fact, at a time when social media companies are under scrutiny for enabling the spread of misinformation and disinformation, social engagement and intelligence technologies used properly hold power to aid health consumerization and nurture health literacy.

Not convinced? We need only to examine successful use cases in, adjacent to and outside of healthcare to understand social engagement and intelligence strengths—including fostering impassioned engagement, community building, and fact-based content moderation. Access to the outdoors is a social equalizer [5] and has demonstrated physiologic and mental health benefits. Engaging in a successful social media campaign was part of the "Healthy Parks Healthy People" [6] initiative, which centers on national parks as a cornerstone for health improvement and fun.

This section will explore several examples/case studies of social media's role in consumer engagement opportunities with health and healthcare. Finally, we will close by attempting to understand how the application of consumer-focused social technology principles can grow and sustain health literacy.

Case Studies

The U.S. National Park Service

In his 2009 documentary series, the storied filmmaker Ken Burns elevated the belief that the national parks were "America's best idea." A historian devised the tagline, arguing that the parks deserved the honor because of their democratic nature and ability to "reflect us at our best rather than our worst." Put simply, these places offered beauty, adventure and fond memories to everyone, no matter who they were outside park boundaries.

In many ways, the U.S. National Park Service's use of social media has grown to reflect that optimistic view. Every day, from the agency's headquarters in Washington and dozens of parks across the country, staffers share photographs of towering mountains, stunning forests and vast deserts with their millions of social media followers on Facebook, Instagram, Twitter, Flickr and YouTube. Just as the parks themselves welcome all travelers, their social media accounts invite everyone to embark on an adventure. The National Park Service does this with high-quality content, educational information, community engagement—and a little bit of humor. "We use social media to reach new audiences," the organization notes [7], "and create a vibrant community of park advocates."

And the park service's use of mainstream social technologies is a rousing success.

As the agency's plethora of good press shows, its social media presence has earned praise from marketers [8], journalists [9] and advocates [10] alike. For instance, when a government shutdown in January 2019 forced National Park Services accounts to go dark, writers mourned their silence [10]. Audiences have taken to the main agency social media accounts and its 59 digital outposts for individual parks. More than 3 million people follow the National Park Service's Instagram account alone, while leading parks such as Yosemite and Yellowstone have 1.8 million and 1.1 million, respectively. From the launch of its first digital campaign, in 2015, the efforts have fueled an increase in visitors—so much so that some observers [11] believe the agency is doing *too good* of a job promoting its sites.

How has the National Park Serviced achieved this success? Its digital consultant, Accenture, attributed the growth [12] to extensive research into audience wants and needs and existing digital capabilities, a clear strategy and institutional support. But what consumers see less of a social engagement and intelligence play than information they want, delivered through appealing and personable accounts with a unique voice. The content, whether it be video rundowns about animals in Arizona or lessons on park history, is too compelling to not promote social engagement.

The lesson here is that social technology projects can win greater interest and develop a community built on shared values through a well-defined need and strategy, exceptional content and proper investment. Still, as in the case of overcrowded national parks, impassioned engagement brings unforeseen risks.

Reddit's /r/StopDrinking

Quitting drinking is hard. As many as 40%–60% of people who receive treatment for alcohol or drug addiction end up relapsing, researchers have found [13]. The more they drink, the more likely they are to face devastating consequences such as liver problems, heart issues, cancer and the condition's many social and emotional effects. One small corner of the internet, however, has cropped up to try to help its members accomplish lasting sobriety.

The community, /r/StopDrinking [14], operates on a popular and sometimes-controversial forum named Reddit. There, more than 260,000 participants describe their experiences with alcohol use disorder and recovery, cheering each other on and gathering tips along the way. Every day, for example, /r/StopDrinking posts a daily check-in in which users commit to avoiding alcohol for the next 24 hours. Some members display flair that tracks their time sober. Others do not subscribe to the forum but pop in to ask questions, while some regularly read the day's discussions but opt to stay silent.

Though anecdotal, the results can be astonishing. Scroll through /r/StopDrinking, and you will find many users who have been sober for months or even years, and many attribute their success to the community. "Your stories over the years showed me it was possible and slowly chipped away the defenses of addiction," one user, sober for 2 years, recently wrote [15]. "I can't be more grateful." The group's power has also earned glowing coverage [16] in the mainstream. Even in its early days, /r/StopDrinking caught the attention of researchers, helping some to lay the groundwork [17] for an early-warning system to proactively identify whether a social media user is abstinent.

So, what makes this forum effective?

At least in part, it appears to be the personal nature of its community-building efforts. On /r/StopDrinking, sharing one's story is simultaneously a selfless benefit to all onlookers and a self-serving act with the potential to reinforce or spark sobriety. Those who respond to user-submitted posts—which account for the sum of the community's content—typically do so without annoyance or negligence. Members of /r/StopDrinking seem to recognize that the very act of posting is an exercise in reckoning with one's own vulnerability. It is forgivable to think that this means that the forum has a high bar to entry, but it is untrue. Anyone can "lurk," allowing them to become comfortable with engaging the community at their own pace.

A strict set of guidelines [18] and committed content moderators make this environment possible. For example, the forum requires users to "speak from the 'I'" and contribute only when sober while prohibiting critiques, medical advice and nasty behavior. When someone breaks that contract, moderators often remove the offending comment quickly and sternly. As they note in their warnings, they do not hesitate to ban trolls. As a result of these efforts and participant buy-in, some users have labeled /r/StopDrinking [19] "the friendliest and best corner of the internet."

This example is important because it highlights real clinical benefits achieved with the aid of a non-clinical social support group. But what can healthcare learn from /r/StopDrinking? Clear goals, an internally incentivized audience and strong content moderation build a positive environment that is conducive to engagement and community building.

Opportunities to Boost Consumer Engagement with Health and Healthcare

The National Park Service's social media strategy and /r/StopDrinking's progress in helping people combat alcohol use disorder should inspire us to seek similar opportunities to increase and improve consumer engagement with health, wellness and the healthcare system. These case studies suggest that healthcare's approach to social technology must be neither one-size-fits-all nor lacking aspiration. Instead, healthcare leaders can use these examples as guidestones in crafting unique engagement and intelligence strategies to meet ambitious goals.

Community Building for Better Health Outcomes

Jumping off from /r/StopDrinking, many non-clinical social technologies have aided similar services around weight loss, grief, mental health, fitness, meditation and so on. In many cases, these non-clinical community-building initiatives have helped participants realize clinical benefits. Imagine if such a project were led by a healthcare provider organization, an insurer or a reputable vendor. How might they lend more credibility to the mission? Could they bake in a clinical component and measure its efficacy?

Some healthcare organizations are already doing this. In the United Kingdom, for example, more than 500 healthcare organizations use the platform Care Opinion [20] to better understand the needs of their patients and caregivers. Healthcare marketers like Jennings have created dozens of online communities [21] for healthcare providers, such as the UNC Lineberger Comprehensive Cancer Center, which launched a website for cancer patients to connect and share their stories. In one study [22], researchers built an online community for hospitalized patients and found that inpatient peer support could boost patient experiences, care quality and safety.

Applying Consumer-Focused Social Technology Principles to Growing and Sustaining Health Literacy

With the rise of digital misinformation and disinformation, health literacy is at risk. Although the phenomenon threatens consumers' lives, as we have seen in the COVID-19 pandemic, it offers healthcare stakeholders a chance to step in as arbiters of truth.

The Office of the National Coordinator (ONC) for Health Information Technology's (Health IT) *Patient Engagement Playbook* [23] sets forth a roadmap for how healthcare provider organizations and clinicians alike can help meet that need, focusing primarily on patient portals. The strategy calls for direct exchange between consumers and health systems. "By involving users in your content, you will motivate them to take action," a developer of the action plan notes.

Leading healthcare provider organizations like Mayo Clinic, meanwhile, have committed substantial resources to educate and engage patients. The health system's [24] website empowers users to search for information based on diseases, symptoms, tests and procedures, and drugs and supplements. Further, Mayo Clinic publishes a barrage of health-related content designed to bust myths and raise health literacy. The COVID-19 pandemic, for example, prompted staffers to publish an article debunking common misconceptions [25] about the outbreak. Twitter users have regularly shared and discussed [26] the page since its inception in May of 2020.

Still, for any healthcare organization to create an environment that grows and sustains health literacy, they need to strive for impassioned engagement, community building and robust content moderation.

The work starts with optimized and effective websites, for which the U.S. Department of

Health and Human Services (HHS) has written a comprehensive health literacy guide for building user-friendly health websites [27]. The gist, however, is simple:

- Deliver actionable and engaging content.
- Build an easy-to-navigate website.
- Reassess and improve the website as needed with users at the center of all developments.

Healthcare stakeholders may also look to forums like /r/StopDrinking, the industry-focused #HCLDR Twitter chat and Jennings' community-building projects for inspiration surrounding content moderation, curation and community building. Transparent and well-defined guidelines can support fact-based discussion while at the same time ensuring people of all levels of expertise feel comfortable. Consider how /r/StopDrinking's rule barring medical advice is complemented with a mandate to be kind. Even when someone crosses a line, the right community can keep attackers at bay.

But the balance is challenging to strike, according to a recent report [28] from Stanford, as enforcing rules designed to cull health misinformation could damage the personal and human qualities necessary for these tools to succeed in raising health literacy, disenchanting some users. "Where healthcare has a low tolerance of failure due to the consequences that can follow, online health communities thrive on stories of what went wrong and how people battled the system," the Stanford authors wrote. "The result is that the medical and the social, for all intents and purposes, operate in different realms."

The work might be messy, but it is worthwhile.

Meaningful Digital Engagement

Mayo Clinic's use of social technology has earned it about 3.5 million followers across Facebook, Instagram and Twitter. Its reach may well be due not just to its authority but also its ability to inform *and* excite. "One of the most effective kinds of content the clinic uses is narra-

tive," an industry observer wrote [29]. "Uplifting stories often drive patient engagement, and the Mayo Clinic takes full advantage of this."

The personable, smart and fact-based use of social technologies can engage patients in a way that simultaneously safeguards them from misinformation and promotes health and well-being. But that mission requires an understanding of an actual engagement with real, breathing people—and quite a few of them.

Unpacking Privacy, Regulation and Policy

Given the potential of consumer-focused social engagement and intelligence technologies, it is reasonable to wonder what is keeping healthcare from diving in headfirst. There is no simple answer, but it encompasses the perceived risk and the challenges inherent to most major social technology platforms. Most noteworthy are social media giants' suspect approach to data privacy and apparent inability to thwart misinformation and disinformation and police bad actors on their platforms.

Two striking examples of social media gone wrong occurred via Facebook's namesake platform. Each says a great deal about what is at stake, both for consumers and healthcare.

First, there is a major international scandal that came to light [30] in early 2018 when Facebook acknowledged that it had failed to protect more than 50 million users' personal data. Not long after, the company revised the total number affected to 87 million. A political data consulting firm named Cambridge Analytica had improperly accessed the personal data of these users several years earlier through a personality quiz hosted on Facebook. The quiz harvested data from 270,000 participants and their Facebook friends, which Cambridge Analytica then used to create psychological profiles for use in political campaigns. When Facebook uncovered the overreach, it eventually told Cambridge Analytica to delete the information, but the data remained available online years later.

The incident outraged Facebook users, privacy advocates and politicians who believed it spotlighted the social media platform's loose approach to data protection and consumers' ignorance of their exposure level. Cambridge Analytica ultimately shuttered, and Facebook faced billions in fines and incalculable damage to its reputation.

Then, in April 2018, a Health I.T. security expert and the founder of a breast cancer data blog filed a complaint against Facebook over the data breach and a glaring security flaw. The fault enabled third parties to enter a backdoor and steal membership information and personal data from Facebook groups—even if they were private or hidden.

The revelation was particularly troubling, considering the thousands of health-related groups on the platform. Andrea Downing, the blog owner and data privacy activist, said the security flaw put patients at risk [31] by threatening to unearth their most personal information, including their health data. "There are vulnerable groups out there where the stakes and the danger are much higher," she said in 2019. "… If you think about patient support groups, you realize that experts in patient engagement have not been talking about the implications of having closed groups on Facebook and what that means for patient privacy. Most users of these groups do not really know that such groups are not secure and that posting our health identity in a closed group in no way guarantees privacy."

Facebook claimed to have fixed the issue. By September 2020, the company also restricted the visibility [32] of health-related groups and encouraged more active moderation due to the rise of coronavirus misinformation. Still, observers have argued that Facebook's data-gathering tools, like the pixel—a behavior tracking social advertising and audience segmentation tool ubiquitously employed by social media and ecommerce giants—are not HIPAA compliant [33] and therefore should be viewed with caution by patients, clinicians and healthcare organizations alike.

In this section, we will further examine data privacy and misinformation, their effects on the healthcare ecosystem, and current and possible attempts to regulate social technologies for the benefit of their users and the global health information ecosystem.

Who Ensures Data Privacy on Social Media?

For the past several years, social media platforms have fallen under the microscope of politicians and government regulators around the world. Horror stories of large-scale data privacy violations recently surfaced details about how these platforms track users, and the prevalence of misinformation and perceived bias prompted the scrutiny. In the United States, for example, lawmakers have held a series of Congressional hearings during which Democrats grilled social media executives about how they combat misinformation and Republicans levied accusations of censorship of conservative content. In response to such concerns, some nations have enacted stauncher privacy laws, while others continue to debate how to move forward.

First, we will take a more in-depth look at how the United States regulates social media and what it means for users.

The country that unleashed social media into the world, for all its good and bad, has no designated authority [34] that regulates these platforms, according to an October 2020 TechCrunch review of social media regulation. Contrast that with companies in other industries, for example, pharmaceutical companies, whose activities are regulated by the U.S. Food and Drug Administration (FDA). That does not mean that Facebook and Twitter operate without any rules. On the contrary, the Federal Trade Commission (FTC) issued a $5 billion fine [35] in 2019 against Facebook for its privacy failures, establishing new structures inside the company to better safeguard user data. Meanwhile, Sect. 230 of the Communications Decency Act frees social media companies from liability over illegal content posted on their platforms, provided they remove the offending material. While these companies may face penalties from the federal government, they do not answer to any single entity within it.

For the past several years, members of Congress have attempted to push through [36] several pieces of legislation designed to tighten control over social media platforms. So far, none has become law, but there is bipartisan support for the broad idea of regulating social media. The devil is in the details, though, as Democrats tend to focus on misinformation, and Republicans often focus on contested claims of "censorship." In May 2020, the Trump administration signed an executive order to remove the protections provided under Sect. 230 and nudging government agencies to investigate and oversee social media companies. Later, in October 2020, the Federal Communications Commission (FCC) announced plans [37] to seek to regulate social media platforms in the name of fighting censorship.

However, the onus of regulating social technology companies appears to fall on individual states. So far, California has embarked on the most stringent attempt to rein in social media in the United States. In 2020, the California Consumer Privacy Act took effect [38] to limit how social media platforms can use the heaps of intensely personal data harvested from users. The law guarantees Californians the right to learn which data businesses earning more than $25 million per year gather, use, share or sell, and they may choose to delete or halt the sale of their personal information. Companies may not exclude users who opt to protect their data. Since the legislation began making headlines, other states have begun to advance similar privacy bills.

Still, any social media regulation in the United States can only follow in the footsteps of the European Union. In May 2018, the EU's General Data Protection Regulation (GDPR) took effect, placing unprecedented new data privacy mechanisms [39] in the hands of citizens and new controls on any business in possession of their data. For example, GDPR ensured EU residents the rights to delete their personal information, restrict its spread, object to its use and receive information notices from companies. The regulation also cemented the ability to withdraw consent previ-

ously given to companies using personal data—such as Facebook's pixel [40]. The EU labeled GDPR [41] the "toughest privacy and security law in the world," and other governments, including the United States, have reportedly drawn inspiration from its protections.

Why Social Technology Companies Need Our Data and Our Trust

Since most social media platforms are free to join, a good rule of thumb applies: If you are not *paying* for the product, you *are* the product. This is indeed how most social technology companies make their money, from Google and Twitter to Facebook and LinkedIn. They collect substantial amounts of data from their users on an ongoing basis, analyze the information, and then use their insights to sell billions of dollars in targeted advertising to companies small and large all over the world. Platforms like Facebook are so good at this practice that they often get accused of spying on users [42], but the truth is, they know everything they need from the data. Social technology expertise in this area [43] is why balding users get ads for hair-loss products, food writers see promotions for niche cheese products, and teenage Target customers receive coupons for pregnancy products before their parents know [44].

Targeted advertising is big business. In 2019, Facebook garnered nearly all of its revenues [45], $20.7 billion, from advertising. YouTube, owned by Google, earned $15 billion [46] for its targeted promotions. Twitter, meanwhile, surpassed $1 billion in revenues, much of it from ads [47], in the same year.

Without intimate personal data—and lots of it—social technology platforms simply have less to offer their clients. Advertising is less valuable when a company cannot target it to a precise demographic. If you have any doubt, just ask the newspaper industry.

That explains why social media giants have fiercely defended their business model, in some cases taking to the courts [48] to ward off stronger data privacy regulations, like in California. Social technology leaders have also tried to convince Congress that self-regulation is enough to enhance privacy and ease the public's concerns. Still, at the same time, even the most successful social media companies understand that their users are the product—and to keep them, they must rebuild their trust. That could be why some executives have appeared to welcome, with hesitance, the prospect of regulation—but only time will tell how that could unfold for users globally.

The Global Weaponization of Social Media

Information warfare is hammering the world, pitting nation against nation and citizen against citizen on every conceivable social media platform. The United States felt [49] the 2016 presidential election's effects when Russia directed an army of trolls to interfere by flooding the space with disinformation. In the years since, users took up the mantle themselves, knowingly and unknowingly sharing falsehoods and warping the national dialogue. The detrimental effects have not spared the health of the nation, particularly amid the uncertainty of the COVID-19 pandemic. But what precisely is happening, and what does it mean for healthcare?

Let us start with *disinformation*, or false information whose purpose is to deceive audiences, often to serve a political agenda, help its creators profit or simply sow chaos. Consider the famous film *Plandemic*, which went viral during the height of the global COVID-19 outbreak. A researcher who studies disinformation wrote that the film tied together several conspiracy theories and false narratives [50] to undermine the U.S. coronavirus response. It may well have been an example of disinformation, as the star subject had been on a campaign to elevate her profile in advance of a book release. However, it is all but impossible to distinguish disinformation from misinformation without knowing the creator's intent.

What, then, is *misinformation*? Much like its counterpart, it is false or inaccurate information, but its deceptive qualities need not be deliberate. So, if the director of *Plandemic* believed the film's untrue narratives, the piece would be misinformation, not disinformation. Misinformation has thrived across social media throughout the coronavirus outbreak, manifesting as unproven miracle cures, egregious claims of corruption and the bogus idea that the virus does not exist.

The effects of widespread inaccurate information can be deadly. Roughly 800 people have died because of pandemic conspiracies and rumors, according to one study, though others claim the report itself could be misinformation [51]. Still, one study found that regions of the United States that were exposed to coverage downplaying the pandemic suffered from more COVID-19 cases and deaths [52]. In another example, consider the anti-vaccination movement, which is proven to thrive [53] on social media. One survey in the United Kingdom found that half of all British parents of children under five saw anti-vaxxer messages [53] on social media. Meanwhile, preventable diseases like measles have seen a resurgence [54] thanks to the spread of misinformation. Between September 2018 and August 2019, New York City reported 649 confirmed cases [55] of the disease. Just as bad information has discouraged mask-wearing and promoted miracle cures during the COVID-19 pandemic, it may well fuel resistance to the vaccine, merging two groups of non-believers into one dangerous machine. This likely has profound effects on healthcare professionals and their organizations, though researchers are only beginning to study them. However, anecdotally, clinicians have attributed surges in their hospitals—and thus greater personal danger, more stress and longer hours—to people defying COVID-19 safety guidelines. Some healthcare workers said they felt "burned out" [56] and emotionally distraught. "We're here to take care of people, and we're even risking our own lives, only to then be completely undermined," a physician co-author of this chapter said. All the while, health systems and clinics battling the roaring pandemic have struggled to stock enough personal protective equipment, maintain hospital capacity and retain proper staffing levels.

Anti-vaccination groups, COVID-19 deniers and conspiracy theorists hawking dangerous or unproven "health supplements" have risen to prominence on social media platforms. Social media organizations have taken steps to stem the flow, such as banning conspiracy theorists like Alex Jones, labeling tweets from public figures as misleading or inaccurate, preventing the sharing of dubious articles and preemptively spotlighting reliable sources of information. But social media companies are under no obligation to rid their platforms of misinformation and disinformation—and they have shown little success in doing so.

A More Social Clinical Mindset?

Social networks have unfurled a myriad of inspiring and devastating outcomes from their growing ubiquity and sophistication since early iterations emerged in the mid-1990s. What healthcare and society are unearthing in 2020 is a foundation, decades in the making, calcified with some of the best and worst of us therein.

In short, the status of society's—and therefore healthcare's—relationship with social media is the most complicated it has ever been.

The evolution of the comprehensive issues with social media detailed previously in this chapter will inevitably be a backdrop on which nursing informatics leaders work to streamline and democratize care delivery—especially as its use

- proves to have a direct impact—both positive and negative—on patients' and caregivers' overall well-being;
- persists as a source of health information for populations globally;
- serves as an advocacy platform to influence health reform for health workers, organizations and the general public;
- creates a healthcare marketplace where people engage with, review and monitor their clinical care teams' performance and digital footprints; and
- helps clinical teams identify population health behaviors and potential localized health interventions.

While these challenges existed before and will persist after the COVID-19 pandemic, the global health crisis broadened social media's scope as a social determinant of health like never seen before.

Now more than ever, it is clear that social media and healthcare are inextricably connected.

In the section, we will discuss the paradoxical nature of social media and how social technologies affect health and care delivery in an ever-changing digital world. This means not only examining the data applications of social media in care delivery (applications that are explored in the following section) but also how it impacts caregivers' well-being and mission to build healthier communities.

Lessons Learned from COVID-19

Due to what some researchers are calling an "infodemic," content and information shared on social networks had started actively working against caregivers' and governments' efforts to curb the virus. Italian researchers applied epidemiological modeling to examine the behavior of social misinformation contagions [57] based on the networks on which they were distributed. While this research only scratches the surface in what it reveals about information integrity online, it did suggest that questionable information can garner up to three times more engagement than reliable information—especially when shared on less popular and less regulated social networks.

Compounding this misinformation phenomenon with an exhausted healthcare workforce, lacking in supplies, support and thinning emotional wherewithal pushed caregivers to a breaking point after months of global protest. At the forefront of demands for caregiver safety were 3400 nurses of the Massachusetts Nurses Association at Brigham and Women's Hospital in Boston who urged healthcare executives to provide safer work environments with universal N95 masking, shuttle safety, improved infection communication and quarantine protocols. The story was picked up by the *New York Times* [58],

Boston Globe [59] and other notable media outlets and became social media fodder thereafter.

As hospitals reached capacity and COVID-19 cases spiked both in the United States and globally, clinicians turned again to social media to plead with people to take the pandemic seriously by sharing harrowing accounts of their experiences caring for patients and themselves under such dire circumstances. These stories then got mainstream media attention, including coverage on *Good Morning America* [60], the leading U.S. morning show with 3.77 million viewers, and in locked stride with the news cycle, shared across social networks immediately thereafter coupled with action-oriented hashtags like #SocialDistance,   #WearAMask, #WashYourHands and #StayHome.

The first COVID-19 vaccine was administered in the United Kingdom on December 8, 2020. While a vaccine brought hope, it also stoked vaccine-related conspiracies and misinformation online. Sandra Lindsay, a New York–based critical care nurse, was the first to receive the vaccine in the United States. Her vaccination was nationally broadcast and came with the following remarks to the *New York Times* [61]:

> I trust science.
> That was the goal today. Not to be the first one to take the vaccine, but to inspire people who look like me, who are skeptical in general about taking vaccines.

Sandra Lindsay was the #19 global trending topic on Twitter on December 14, 2020 and started the social media world's vaccine journey by advocating for health information integrity and racial equity to a world aching for an end to the pandemic. Since then, vaccinations among healthcare workers and top political officials that followed have come with a similar message to their collectively massive social audiences hoping that the public will actively participate in vaccination programming.

This chain of events during the COVID-19 pandemic reveals the power of social media in helping close gaps in health literacy and amplifying healthcare workers' voices for structural change, safer working conditions and equitable patient care. However, the damage unreliable health information and divisive political rhetoric has done for the well-being of populations and caregivers alike is undeniable and far from fully understood.

Healthcare faces an evolving, complicated and likely tenuous relationship with social technologies. COVID-19 lessons learned aside, which will be significant, longitudinal studies [62] reveal increasing mental health concerns associated with social media use—especially among young people. That being said, social media, given its ubiquity in our lives, is now ubiquitous as a social determinant of health. That means health, technology and society will now need to evolve in concert if a positive structural change is going to take hold.

Refocusing the Mission of Medicine

As overwhelming as the unending nuances of social media might seem, there might be hope in normalizing the connection between health, information and social technology on the horizon as pathways for structural change.

Moved by what has unfolded in the media and online, the University of Pittsburgh School of Medicine Class of 2024 felt compelled to modernize their oath to "do no harm" during their White Coat Ceremony in August 2020. In a unique addendum [63] to their reciting of the Hippocratic Oath, the incoming class of physicians drafted their own commitment to "repairing the injustices against those historically ignored and abused in medicine." The first of its kind in Pitt Medicine history, the revised oath came in direct response to a world-shattering albeit revealing COVID-19 pandemic and a "national civil rights movement reinvigorated by the killings of Breonna Taylor, George Floyd, and Ahmaud Arbery."

While this new blueprint for, inclusive and empathetic care delivery does not outright mention social media, the following excerpts and the mounting evidence of its coding into our digital DNA provided in this chapter suggest that the intersection seems inevitable if not already inferred:

I will care for my patients' holistic well-being, not solely their pathology. With empathy, compassion and humility, I will prioritize understanding each patient's narrative, background and experiences while protecting privacy and autonomy.

I will educate myself on social determinants of health in order to use my voice as a physician to advocate for a more equitable healthcare system from the local to the global level.

I will restore trust between the healthcare community and the population in which I serve by holding myself and others accountable, and by combating misinformation in order to improve health literacy.

In making this oath, I embrace the ever-changing responsibilities of being a physician and pledge to uphold the integrity of the profession in the clinic and beyond.

Such a call for stronger roots in "social medicine' is one that exists, can be built upon, and has a long-lasting positive impact on access and community health to date. The intersectionality between policy and medicine is one that has been championed and nurtured by the late, lifelong health activist H. Jack Geiger, MD, MsciHyg [64]. Dr. Geiger, who pioneered the modern community health center model in the United States, spent his professional career dedicated to health, poverty and civil rights as an Institute of Medicine Lienhardt Award winner for "outstanding contributions to minority health," founding member and president of Nobel Peace Prize awardee organizations, Physicians for Human Rights (1986) and Physicians for Social Responsibility (1961).

In 2017, Dr. Geiger authored an article with the *Journal of the Association of American Medical Colleges* titled "The Political Future of Social Medicine: Reflections on Physicians as Activists" [65]. The invited commentary explores the notion that healers are inherently political as "most social determinants of health are politically determined." Like the incoming Pitt Medicine class of 2024, he contends that clinical programs can support structural change outside of the clinical setting and vice versa—with the help of interdisciplinary collaboration. For better or worse, in 2020, the venue for that public discourse is online and on social networks. As Dr. Geiger frames it,

the challenge is not letting the persistence of cynicism and bureaucracy "erode" the idealism of emerging healthcare leaders.

And from what we know now, social media very much is the place to elevate these clinical values—if they can cut through the noise.

Mining Social Media for Health Intelligence

As it relates to health intelligence, this chapter's predominant focus on the culture of social media and healthcare is an intentional one. Like with digital and health literacy among populations, nursing informaticists and healthcare at large stand to benefit from more robust social media literacy. With a stronger foundational knowledge of these platforms, the greater our ability to establish a more substantial public health infrastructure and thoughtfully apply health intelligence in large-scale and individualized care settings. Only time will tell what value a more harmonized social media and health information ecosystem will mean for society. Still, advancements in what has been observed to date look promising despite their very early stages of maturity.

A 2013 innovation scan reported that 66% of reviewed studies [66] showed that social media-based surveillance had comparable performance to traditional surveillance programs. However, the same report also noted that "with the potential to greatly improve disease surveillance and mitigation, there is a significant need to understand key chronological developments of the tools and methodologies in order to inform future endeavors and to assess this technology application for potential end-users." Fast forward to today, and the scientific research community is still seeking out a unified framework for social media's use in care delivery [3]. In addition to calls for more structured research, a 2015 landscape analysis [67] cited other challenges facing the validation of public health applications of social media data, including data biases, privacy concerns, data quality, social anonymity and methodology consistency, among others noted in the *Processes—*

Research and Policy Opportunities section of Table 18.1.

That same 2015 analysis [67] also summarized the uses of social media in public health surveillance, distinguishing them by the following three applications: [67].

1. *Epidemiological monitoring and surveillance*:
   (a) Monitoring official information
   (b) Disease detection—syndromic surveillance
   (c) Disease detection—event-based surveillance
   (d) Timely estimates and forecasting of disease incidence
2. *Situational awareness during natural disasters and humanitarian crises*:
   (a) Surveillance for situational awareness
3. *Communication surveillance to monitor perceptions, attitudes from public health events and messages*:
   (a) Global awareness
   (b) Specific reactions

In this section, we will summarize three case studies with key takeaways for each of these above applications—one from each category. Takeaways from these case studies should be examined in the context of the population in which the analysis was conducted and are not necessarily universally applicable. This varying sample of social media data applications will hopefully catalyze ideation around how nursing informaticists can creatively solve healthcare's most challenging problems with data-driven empathy and understanding in an ecosystem that is yet to be appropriately defined.

Application #1: Forecasting Flu Impact

There are 500,000 deaths worldwide attributed to influenza [68]. One study, "Forecasting Influenza-Like Illness Dynamics for Military Populations Using Neural Networks and Social Media" [69], aimed to mitigate flu mortality using deep-dive intelligence techniques to measure and predict flu and flu-like infection (ILI) rates using social media signals and machine learning. Overall, social media was validated as a viable supplemental data source to improve upon traditional forecasting methods provided by historical and CDC data—or even where no historical data was available at all.

Notable Takeaways

- Explicitly focused on military influenza sprawl across 26 U.S. and 6 international locations.
- Mined user-generated data via keyword mentions and hashtags—analyzing topics, embeddings, word n-grams, stylistic patterns and communication behavior.
- Sourced Twitter data from a social media vendor and through the public API—anonymized for usernames, user IDs and tweet IDs using an encryption algorithm.
- Examined social user data from the military population in particular geolocations using influenza as well as weather, personal welfare and travel keywords.
- Validated social media and search activity as supplemental in real-time data sources to enhance the predictive ability for health officials.
- Closed two-week gap in CDC's ILI data reporting, potentially shortening intervention timelines.
- Social media signals significantly outperformed models that relied solely on ILI historical data, but results did vary across locations.
- Social media data signals can potentially be used to forecast ILI trends where data is lacking or unavailable altogether.

Application #2: Predicting Health Impact of Climate and Natural Disasters

The European heatwave during the summer of 2003 could be attributed to between 22,000 and 70,000 deaths, while the Russian heatwave of 2010 claimed 56,000. In the research article

"Mining Social Media to Identify Heat Waves" [68], researchers took aim at what is one of humanity's deadliest natural threats, especially as climate change takes hold globally. Overall, behavioral signals from Twitter were found to be better at predicting heat-related mortality than traditional climate indicators.

Notable Takeaways

- Focused on two of the Indian states most impacted by heat-related mortality, Andhra Pradesh and Telangana.
- Collected tweet data containing India heat wave related keywords between January 1, 2010 and December 31, 2017, without geolocation.
- Leaned on "scraping" algorithm contained in the GetOldTweets-Python package to access Twitter keyword queries.
- Positively correlated increases in Twitter activity to India's news cycle while also revealing higher amplification rates among tweets containing links.
- Examined not only keyword-related tweets but also retweets of this content to better gauge totality of affected populations.
- Uncovered a possible exponential effect of heat waves on mortality given new social media analysis findings.
- Highlighted the value of socioeconomic and demographic context in social media data, previously lacking from traditional data sources.

Application #3: Understanding Behaviors Driving Misinformation During COVID-19

Much of the impact from misinformation that flowed through social channels amid the COVID-19 pandemic are yet to be known, granted, touched upon in this very chapter. Authors of the research article "The COVID-19 Social Media Infodemic" [57] leveraged Natural Language Processing techniques, various social media datasets, content credibility tools and epidemiological modeling to develop critical bench-

marks for pandemic-related misinformation mitigation strategies in the future. This research provided a robust analysis of content behaviors across five social networks and revealed compelling social dynamics among less regulated social networks and potentially ideologically homogenous user groups.

Notable Takeaways

- Leaned on Google Trends COVID-19-related search queries to identify social media data collection.
- Analyzed social media content behaviors related to COVID-19 across five social networks—Gab, Reddit, YouTube, Instagram and Twitter.
- Sourced social media data sets from respective platform APIs (Gab, YouTube, Twitter), third party (Reddit) and custom process (Instagram).
- Applied epidemiological modeling to simulate the exponential spread of information on social media.
- Classified information credibility using data from independent fact-checking organization Media Bias/Fact Check.
- Revealed higher propensity of misinformation sharing on fringe social networks like Gab, which happens to appeal to a politically far-right user base.
- Suggested that misinformation virality is potentially unique to the social network, its design and the engaged participants.

Summary

While flawed, social media has the potential to make significant positive impact on health and care delivery. The prevailing notions you will find in this chapter are as follows:

- From individuals to organizations, social media users have both an opportunity and an obligation to bridge gaps in social and health inequities.
- Regulation toward information integrity on social networks is critical to achieve equity,

maintaining healthy digital environments and innovation in public health surveillance.

- Access to and use of social media should be embraced as a social determinant of health and factored into health management, care delivery and health reform.
- Social media's promise will only be as resonant as the thoughtfulness that goes into wielding it.

Our findings show that significant work and resources need to be invested in digital and health literacy, research, application development, information integrity, regulation, public trust and policymaking to maximize the value of social networks for health and wellness. To that end, this chapter is a current state exploration of four core components of the health information and social media landscape that will collectively influence how we move forward as an industry and society:

- Social engagement for health and wellness.
- Information integrity, regulation and privacy of social media.
- Culture of medicine amid social media ubiquity.
- Applications of social media for public health surveillance and clinical intervention.

It is our sincere hope that this chapter stokes a discussion on how to create a more equitable, inclusive, safe and intelligent health information ecosystem that builds on the best of what social media has to offer.

Conclusions and Outlook

Looking to the Future of Social Engagement and Health Intelligence

While social engagement and intelligence represent a challenge for healthcare and nursing, in particular, they offer an opportunity of equal weight. Consider, for a second, the benefits at stake.

A healthcare-focused business may achieve data gathering and analysis to drive better decision-making and stronger, more relevant products and services. Community health organizations may use social technologies to improve patient engagement, expand care outside the clinic's walls and target information to at-risk populations. In the exam room, nurses and other clinicians can leverage these tools to bridge the divide between what patients say and what their symptoms suggest. They may use social innovation to engage patients further and personalize care delivery—two goals that nurses and their administrators alike are embracing more each day.

If social engagement and intelligence deliver on their promise, healthcare is standing on the precipice of an incredible change. But how might a mainstream digital health economy function? And which challenges must we overcome to make this vision a reality?

Envisioning a Mainstream Digital Health Economy

Social technologies are one part of the ever-growing digital health market, which is among the few spaces to have secured increased investment in 2020 [70], during the height of the COVID-19 pandemic. Broadly, the space contains everything [71], from electronic health records, artificial intelligence (AI) and machine learning and genomics for more personalized care to mobile computing, big data and wearable technologies that foster the collection and use of patient-generated data. Although each technology is unique, they are all linked.

For example, wearable devices allow consumers to capture health data, which they may soon choose to upload to their electronic health records. From there, the data can be used in extensive analyses designed to examine and enhance population health or run through AI systems that identify individual risks and aid, or perform, diagnoses. Should an algorithm flag an issue, a clinician on the floor could receive an alert directly through their mobile phone, suggesting they follow up. When a patient receives a diagnosis, the care team has the power to collaborate through virtual assistants and clinical apps that ensure coordinated care. That kind of unity stands to unearth opportunities to personalize care through genomics, clinical trials and other avenues that unconnected clinicians might have previously overlooked.

In the mainstream digital health economy, technologies that strengthen social engagement and intelligence play a vital role. The cycle described above, for instance, is unlikely to occur, at least at scale, without an informed and engaged base of patients. Consumers are unlikely to adopt, much less consistently use, wearable healthcare technology if they do not perceive its usefulness—a phenomenon that researchers have found [72] depends on health belief and health information accuracy. Social engagement and intelligence can push patients from health illiteracy to literacy, and then even ownership over their wellness and care. They do not need to initiate interest in these tools, but it is up to healthcare organizations and clinicians to ensure patients begin to understand their benefits. The same goes for clinicians and their adoption of clinical apps and other social technologies—researchers have also found [73] that their buy-in is associated not only with improved workflows but also noticeable results.

At their core, social technologies are the spark that could ignite digital health at scale.

Key Challenges to Overcome

Still, a dream does not become a reality only because it sounds good. Given the stigmatization and concrete barriers to the widespread adoption of social technologies noted in this chapter, there is no guarantee that they will enter daily administrative or clinical operations. Here are some of the challenges that social technology developers, healthcare organizations, clinicians and researchers must overcome if these innovations are to make a difference:

- **Destigmatization.** To avoid an uphill march, all stakeholders must agree to view social technologies for healthcare less as a new version of Facebook and more like another tool at the caregivers' disposal.

- **Data privacy concerns.** Derailing destigmatization requires purchasers and users to be confident that their chosen technology and use of it will not expose patients to unnecessary risk.
- **Misinformation and disinformation.** This is a plague that no one knows how to quell, but healthcare organizations will need to do precisely that if they plan to shift from a communications model built on broadcasting to one grounded in information exchange and relationship building.
- **Budgetary restrictions.** Can an enterprise buyer justify investing in a new social technology when other needs might be more pressing?
- **Evidence-based efficacy.** Proof is critical to overcoming that hurdle. Vendors and advocates cannot rely on glitzy marketing—they must produce and distribute data that supports a technology's benefits across the continuum of care.
- **Clinician adoption.** If clinicians on the ground are not excited about a social technology, why would their patients be?
- **Patient adherence.** When more patients begin to engage with social technologies, healthcare organizations will need to use insights assembled to keep them on board.
- **Current and future regulatory roadblocks.** It is unclear how HIPAA and other information-related rules might evolve to support or stifle this market, but everyone will need to match their innovation plans to the law.

Nurses and Health Professionals Can Change the World

The future can start with a single person. For example, many news organizations failed to quickly launch websites in the 1990s when the internet was catching on. Later, in the mid-2000s, some did not transition to social media until their competition had already built an effective presence there. But the news organizations that moved early and with intent—like the *New York Times*—now have millions of digital subscribers, while their competitors institute layoffs and sometimes close altogether.

Nurse and health informaticists can take simple steps now to ensure they and their organizations do not fall behind:

- Examine your clinical needs.
- Research how social engagement and intelligence technologies might fill those needs.
- Identify tools and applications that have evidence supporting their efficacy.
- Lobby for their adoption, inside the boardroom, the clinic and beyond.
- Lead by example, using social media to have the conversations you want your organization to initiate.
- Do not give up.

If each healthcare stakeholder follows this outline, it will only be a matter of time until healthcare decision-makers begin thinking about why they are falling behind the times and failing to develop cutting-edge solutions to their problems. And that could be just the catalyst to drive change.

Useful Resources

1. Zhou L, Zhang D, Yang C, Wang Y. HARNESSING SOCIAL MEDIA FOR HEALTH INFORMATION MANAGEMENT. Electron Commer Res Appl, 2018. https://doi.org/10.1016%2Fj.elerap.2017.12.003
2. Haldar S, Mishra SR, Kim Y, Hartzler A, Pollack AH, Pratt W, Use and impact of an online community for hospital patients, Journal of the American Medical Informatics Association, Volume 27, Issue 4. 2020; 549–557, https://doi.org/10.1093/jamia/ocz212.
3. Mayo Clinic: Patient Care and Health Information. https://www.mayoclinic.org/patient-care-and-health-information. (2020). Accessed Oct 2020.
4. Health.gov: Health Literacy Online: A guide to writing and designing easy-to-use health web sites. https://health.gov/healthliteracyonline/2010/Web_Guide_Health_Lit_Online.pdf. (2010). Accessed Oct 2020.
5. Grey D, Nigl A. The Impact of New Privacy Laws (GDPR) on Social Media Platforms. https://www.researchgate.net/publication/331821021_The_Impact_of_New_Privacy_Laws_GDPR_on_Social_Media_Platforms (2019). Accessed Oct 2020.
6. Bernardo TM, Rajic A, Young I, Robiadek K, Pham MT, Funk JA. Scoping review on search queries and social media for disease surveillance: a chronology of innovation. J Med Internet Res., 2013. https://doi.org/10.2196/jmir.2740.
7. Fung IC, Tse ZT, Fu KW. The use of social media in public health surveillance. Western Pac Surveill Response J., 2015. https://doi.org/10.5365%2FWPSAR.2015.6.1.019
8. Fung IC, Tse ZT, Fu KW. The use of social media in public health surveillance. Western Pac Surveill Response J., 2015. https://www.ncbi.nlm.nih.gov/pmc/articles/PMC4542478/table/T1/?report=objectonly
9. Volkova S, Ayton E, Porterfield K, Corley CD. Forecasting influenza-like illness dynamics for military populations using neural networks and social media. PLoS ONE 12(12): e0188941. https://doi.org/10.1371/journal.pone.0188941.
10. Cinelli M, Quattrociocchi W, Galeazzi A. et al. The COVID-19 social media infodemic. Sci Rep 10, 16,598, 2020. https://doi.org/10.1038/s41598-020-73510-5
11. Cory N, Stevens P. 2020. Information Technology and Innovation Foundation: Building a Global Framework for Digital Health Services in the Era of COVID-19. https://itif.org/publications/2020/05/26/building-global-framework-digital-health-services-era-covid-19. Accessed Oct 2020.
12. Cheung ML, Chau KY, Lam MHS, Tse G, Ho KY, Flint SW, Broom DR, Tso EKH, Lee KY. Examining Consumers' Adoption of Wearable Healthcare Technology: The Role of Health Attributes. Int J Environ Res Public Health, 2019. https://doi.org/10.3390%2Fijerph16132257
13. Jacob C, Sanchez-Vazquez A, Ivory C. Factors Impacting Clinicians' Adoption of a Clinical Photo Documentation App and its Implications for Clinical Workflows and Quality of Care: Qualitative Case Study, JMIR Mhealth Uhealth, 2020. https://doi.org/10.2196/20203.

Review Questions

1. What benefits does health consumerization have on the current state of healthcare delivery? What are its pitfalls?
2. How does an erosion of user trust in social media companies impact relationships between patients and their care teams?
3. What specific recommendations would you make to social network and other tech executives that would both promote a healthier space to exchange ideas and enable use of de-identified social network data for public health surveillance?
4. Where does public policy and advocacy intersect with healthcare for you? What intersectional issues should healthcare professionals consider in their treatment plans, health applications and community organizing? Who are potential collaborators for these activities?
5. How can social media data analysis practically impact day-to-day care right now? What applications need more work and why?
6. Where do you stand with social media? How do you use it personally? Professionally? What might you do differently after reading this chapter?

Appendix: Answers to Review Questions

1. What benefits do health consumerization have on the current state of healthcare delivery? What are its pitfalls?

Efforts to embrace health consumerization serve as a virtue signal to the public that caregivers are listening to needs, opportunities and attitudes that make care more accessible, frictionless— and hopefully affordable. Like so many sectors, social media has become a means of building relationships with care providers and the greater healthcare community. And with healthcare being a commodity in a private system, like many consumer brands, providers are competing for new patients seeking out the best care experience possible.

In many ways, this competition does incentivize organizations to rigorously pursue excellence in care delivery and digital operations to differentiate with experience. The Mayo and Cleveland Clinics of the world make social media a part of that core offering that not only builds trust in those brands but also meets a public need for trustworthy health information.

But, not every caregiving organization can be a Mayo or Cleveland Clinic nor is social media the only channel to create differentiating experiences for patients and consumers. Experiential touch points can be websites, emails, text, community programming, search engine marketing, or even word of mouth. The goal is to create a value proposition for users and honor it across channels that make sense to them and meets them where they are.

That said, the benefits for consumerization are inherent to the exercise of meticulously trying to delight end-users:

- You get to know them better.
- You get to understand how they behave.
- You get to hone in on their attitudes toward health and care.
- You get to learn how to deliver better care at scale.
- You get to explore how to make them partners in their own care.

As for pitfalls, there really aren't many. Consumerization for the sake of itself is obviously unhelpful. However, a thoughtful look at how to best serve patients and populations is never really a wasted endeavor. The areas where organizations might find this to be painful are as follows:

- Organizational change management to initiate and sustain change.
- Resourcing to ensure services and experiences are thoughtfully delivered.
- Market relevance, as information, technology and care environments are highly competitive.
- Information and digital tool security.

2. How does an erosion of user trust in social media companies impact relationships between patients and their care teams?

This chapter highlights how the impact of a lack in accountability among social tech companies can disrupt social and political discourse, lead to dangerous health decisions, strain mental health of patients and caregivers alike, and contaminate data retrieval and applications for public health use. These breakdowns serve as roadblocks for enhancing care delivery for all stakeholders:

Disrupt social and political discourse. As all social determinants of health are politically determined one way or another mis- and disinformation regarding critical health policy and reform that can close systemic gaps in health and wellness—affecting both patients and caregivers and the dynamics with which they interact.

Lead to dangerous health decisions. During the run up to the 2016 U.S. elections and the COVID-19 pandemic alone, poor information integrity and a lack of regulation has had a significant impact on global society. Most notably, weaponized political content and anti-science sentiments later diminished messaging around social distancing, masking up and vaccine credibility while also sowing political unrest. In other instances, people turned to dangerous, and sometimes fatal, self-care measures to avoid contracting the virus—much of which could be found on social networks. Finally, the ailing information environment paired with a failure to monitor social media user activity has harbored organization for political extremism that have led to death and injury for both people and democratic institutions.

Strain mental health of patients and caregivers. Even prior to the COVID-19 pandemic, excessive social media use had been linked to mental health decline. Serving as arbiters of highly coveted information, hosts to tenuous social discourse and connection points for friends, family and colleagues, there are many dimensions of daily life in the era of COVID-19 that were tied to social platforms. Paired with the volume of information, social networks, while critical, also can be seen as sources of additional stress and anxiety. This effect compounds even more powerfully for healthcare workers who were already pushed to their limits, not to mention at-home caregivers whose resources might have been inhibited or maxed out because of the pandemic. No matter where you sit in the healthcare ecosystem, no one is at their best when they are overwhelmed, burnt out, stressed or anxious.

Contaminate data retrieval and applications for public health. If the practice of mining social media data for health intelligence is going to evolve, it will need to do so with information integrity considerations in mind. As it stands, population health and health information professionals who are looking to social media data to identify interventions will need to filter out fake social accounts and be mindful of how information degradation impacts observed populations, not to mention how conflicting information might be working against their efforts altogether. Regulation and collaboration would likely be useful mechanisms in enabling social media health surveillance, but tech and social media companies' incentives to change are, at least currently, diametrically in conflict with how these companies have been accustomed to earning revenues. After considerable backlash from lawmakers, watchdogs and users alike, some companies are starting to show glimmers of effort toward user privacy and information integrity. Even so, some might argue that the damage has already been done, and meaningful reform is not imminent enough. On this issue, only time will tell.

3. What specific recommendations would you make to social network and other tech executives that would both promote a healthier space to exchange ideas and to enable use of de-identified social network data for public health surveillance?

Accountability matters—especially among tech company leadership given social media's ubiquity as a platform for connection, discourse and advocacy globally. Accountability, though, can come in multiple forms and from a multitude of channels. Those that come to mind in respect to social media regulation for health include:

- Regulation through policy and federal oversight.
- Mutual value proposition through creative partnership.
- Organized advocacy with intersectional stakeholders.
- Direct feedback to social media and tech companies.

This exercise will likely evolve as the landscape does, but some of the following can serve that allows for the context of current events to be factored in to a timely and productive discussion about healthy social media use in addition to its applications for health intelligence and literacy:

Public Health Collaboration
- How can public health agencies, researchers, providers and tech companies collaborate to improve purposeful and properly de-identified data collection for health surveillance and clinical interventions?

Information Integrity
- How can public health information be prioritized and appropriately integrated into the social media user experience?
- What safeguards will tech companies put in place to ensure misinformation, disinformation and hate speech are eradicated from social networks?

Data Privacy and Security
- Whether in a health context or not, what can be done to empower users to keep their data safe and their information private?
- Within a health context, how can users ensure that any data used for health intelligence is secure and de-identified?

Consumer Trust
- Social media has immense value. What must social/tech companies do to allow health professionals to wield these platforms as trusted tools for better health today and or years to come?

Health Citizenship
- Social media and tech companies arguably have a moral imperative to do no harm and to elevate inclusivity, equity, justice and health where possible.
- What do these companies' citizenship footprints look like? Are they meeting expectations?

4. Where does public policy and advocacy intersect with healthcare for you? What intersectional issues should healthcare professionals consider in their treatment plans, health applications and community organizing? Who are potential collaborators for these activities?

If we are asking for collective health citizenship, how can we advocate and work toward it? This is an essential question for the health sector, especially as social determinants of health become more widely used in our understanding of health and care delivery. However, health is also extremely personal as we all experience it differently. Intended objectives of this discussion could be:

- Personalize students' mission in health and nursing informatics.
- Explore diverse healthcare experiences in a classroom setting.
- Establish a connection between advocacy and attaining health equity.
- Contextualize informatics work through a health citizenship and equity lens.
- Identify intersectional stakeholder groups for readers to consider for future collaboration.

5. How can social media data analysis practically impact day-to-day care right now? What applications need more work and why?

Depending on the sophistication of the organization, social media data analysis is already likely having an impact on care delivery across settings. Although scaled health surveillance and intelligence is awaiting robust supportive research, academic cohesion and enhancements to regional and global public health data infrastructures, health and care organizations can still leverage social media data with reasonable accessibility to make a difference.

At the time in which this chapter is read and discussed, there very well may be advancements in these above areas. In the meantime, serviceable social media data analyses and applications can be used to inform and support innovation at the organizational level, if not spanning into surrounding physical and digital communities:

> Social media and broader digital operations analytics capabilities are swiftly maturing across public and healthcare ecosystems. Social analytics vendors in this space can offer an extreme amount of value to health organizations looking to leverage social listening capabilities for business and health surveillance purposes. These social analytics capabilities are also being added to out-of-the-box enterprise business data management and operational software tools making them even more commonplace in organizations' technology stacks. Health organizations with savvy wielders of data and technology, and the resources to invest in them, can begin to hone solutions of their own. However, how that contributes to a larger public health infrastructure remains to be seen.

> One particularly interesting application of social media listening is geofencing—essentially monitoring social media use for a particular geographic location. Currently, hospitals leverage the technology to engage and inform social media use on their campuses. Event organizers use the same technology for tracking chatter happening among their attendees. Tools like these have compelling applications in the public and population health space. The issues surrounding public health surveillance and health intelligence do not reside in technology, but more the cultural surrounding the application of these technologies.

6. Where do you stand with social media? How do you use it personally? Professionally? What might you do differently after reading this chapter?

As noted in this chapter and likely from personal experience of readers, social media can offer value both personally and professionally to those in the health and wellness sector. From professional development and networking to sophisticated data applications, it's now a developmental necessity from childhood through adulthood to understand and hone our unique relationships with social media—thoughtfully and with purpose.

References

1. CDC: COVID-19 Hospitalization and Death by Race/Ethnicity 2020. https://www.cdc.gov/coronavirus/2019-ncov/covid-data/investigations-discovery/hospitalization-death-by-race-ethnicity.html. Accessed Dec 2020.
2. Clement J. Number of social network users worldwide from 2017 to 2025. 2020. https://www.statista.com/statistics/278414/number-of-worldwide-social-network-users. Accessed Dec 2020.
3. Pagoto S, Waring ME, Xu R. A call for a public health agenda for social media research. J Med Internet Res. 2019;21(12):e16661. https://doi.org/10.2196/16661.
4. Zhou L, Zhang D, Yang C, Wang Y. Harnessing social media for health information management. Electron Commer Res Appl. 2018; https://doi.org/10.1016/j.elerap.2017.12.003.
5. Lachowycz K, Jones AP. Does walking explain associations between access to greenspace and lower mortality? Soc Sci Med. 2014;107:9–17. https://doi.org/10.2196/jmir.2740.
6. National Park Service. Healthy Parks Healthy People Resources 2020. https://www.nps.gov/subjects/healthandsafety/healthy-parks-healthy-people-resources.htm. Accessed Feb 2021.
7. National Park Service: Social Media. 2020. https://www.nps.gov/subjects/digital/social-media.htm Accessed Oct 2020.
8. Hurrdat Marketing: Five reasons the national park service is dominating social media. 2015. https://hurrdatmarketing.com/digital-marketing-news/five-reasons-the-national-park-service-is-dominating-social-media. Accessed Oct 2020.
9. Marotti A. Chicago tribute: five reasons the national park service is dominating social media. 2016. https://www.chicagotribune.com/business/blue-sky/ct-national-park-service-centennial-bsi-20160825-story.html. Accessed Oct 2020.
10. The Trust for Public Land: No joke: the national park service is hilarious on Instagram. 2020. https://www.tpl.org/blog/no-joke-national-park-service-hilarious-instagram. Accessed Oct 2020.
11. Hill A, Hollenhorst M. How social media hurts and helps the great outdoors. 2017. https://www.marketplace.org/2017/05/29/how-social-media-hurts-and-helps-great-outdoors/. Accessed Oct 2020.
12. Accenture Federal Services: National parks. 2016. https://www.accenture.com/us-en/case-studies/us-federal-government/national-parks. Accessed Oct 2020.

13. NIH: Drugs, Brains, And behavior: the science of addiction. 2020. https://www.drugabuse.gov/publications/drugs-brains-behavior-science-addiction/treatment-recovery. Accessed Oct 2020.

14. Reddit/Stop Drinking. 2020. https://www.reddit.com/r/stopdrinking/. Accessed Oct 2020.

15. Reddit/Stop Drinking. 2020. https://www.reddit.com/r/stopdrinking/comments/jse1lx/a_small_thank_you/. Accessed Oct 2020.

16. Dewey C. Washington Post: the surprising Internet forum some alcoholics are choosing over A.A. 2016. https://www.washingtonpost.com/news/the-intersect/wp/2016/01/05/the-surprising-internet-forum-some-alcoholics-are-choosing-over-aa/. Accessed Oct 2020.

17. Tamersoy A, De Choudhury M, Chau DH. Characterizing smoking and drinking abstinence from social media. HT ACM Conf Hypertext Soc Media. 2015; https://doi.org/10.1145/2700171.2791247.

18. Reddit/Stop Drinking. 2020. https://www.reddit.com/r/stopdrinking/wiki/index. Accessed Oct 2020.

19. Reddit/Stop Drinking. 2020. https://www.reddit.com/r/stopdrinking/comments/bxglfu/this_is_the_friendliest_and_best_corner_of_the/. Accessed Oct 2020.

20. Care Opinion. 2020. https://www.careopinion.org.uk/info/about Accessed Oct 2020.

21. Jennings Healthcare Marketing. 2020. http://www.jenningshealthcaremarketing.com/healthcare-marketing/online-communities/. Accessed Oct 2020.

22. Haldar S, Mishra SR, Kim Y, Hartzler A, Pollack AH, Pratt W. Use and impact of an online community for hospital patients. J Am Med Inform Assoc. 2020;27(4):549–57. https://doi.org/10.1093/jamia/ocz212.

23. Harris L. health.gov. Practicing what we preach: health literacy online and the ONC patient engagement playbook. 2016. https://health.gov/news-archive/blog/2016/10/practicing-what-we-preach-health-literacy-online-and-the-onc-patient-engagement-playbook/index.html Accessed Oct 2020.

24. Mayo Clinic: Patient Care and Health Information. 2020. https://www.mayoclinic.org/patient-care-and-health-information. Accessed Oct 2020.

25. Mayo Clinic: Debunking COVID-19 (coronavirus) myths. 2020. https://www.mayoclinic.org/diseases-conditions/coronavirus/in-depth/coronavirus-myths/art-20485720. Accessed Oct 2020.

26. Twitter: Mayo Clinic. 2020. https://twitter.com/search?q=https%3A%2F%2Fwww.mayoclinic.org%2Fdiseases-conditions%2Fcoronavirus%2Fin-depth%2Fcoronavirus-myths%2Fart-20485720&src=typed_query&f=live. Accessed Oct 2020.

27. Health.gov: Health Literacy Online: A guide to writing and designing easy-to-use health web sites. 2010. https://health.gov/healthliteracyonline/2010/Web_Guide_Health_Lit_Online.pdf. Accessed Oct 2020.

28. Hodgkin P, Horsley L, Metz B. Stanford social innovation review: the emerging world of online health communities. 2018. https://ssir.org/articles/entry/the_emerging_world_of_online_health_communities. Accessed Oct 2020.

29. Matthews K. HIT consultant: 4 hospitals leveraging social media to improve patient engagement. 2020. https://hitconsultant.net/2020/02/27/4-hospitals-leveraging-social-media-to-improve-patient-engagement. Accessed Oct 2020.

30. Ma A, Gilbert B. Business insider: Facebook understood how dangerous the trump-linked data firm Cambridge Analytica could be much earlier than it previously said. Here's everything that's happened up until now. 2019. https://www.businessinsider.com/cambridge-analytica-a-guide-to-the-trump-linked-data-firm-that-harvested-50-million-facebook-profiles-2018-3. Accessed Oct 2020.

31. Sharp J. Inside digital health: speaking with the woman behind the Facebook health data. Breach Complaint. 2019; https://www.idigitalhealth.com/news/speaking-with-the-woman-behind-the-facebook-health-data-breach-complaint. Accessed Oct 2020

32. Robertson A. The verge: Facebook will stop recommending health groups. 2020. https://www.theverge.com/2020/9/17/21443742/facebook-health-groups-recommendations-new-admin-rules. Accessed Oct 2020.

33. Larson A. Paubox: is Facebook pixel HIPAA compliant? 2020. https://www.paubox.com/blog/facebook-pixel-hipaa-compliant/. Accessed Oct 2020.

34. Coldewey D. TechCrunch: who regulates social media? 2020. https://techcrunch.com/2020/10/19/who-regulates-social-media. Accessed Oct 2020.

35. Coldewey D, Lomas N. TechCrunch: Facebook settles with FTC: $5 billion and new privacy guarantees. 2019. https://techcrunch.com/2019/07/24/facebook-settles-with-ftc-5-billion-and-new-privacy-guarantees. Accessed Oct 2020.

36. Newton C. The verge: new legislation is putting social networks in the crosshairs. 2019. https://www.theverge.com/2019/8/1/20749517/social-network-legislation-hawley-privacy-research. Accessed Oct 2020.

37. Kelly M. The verge: FCC will move to regulate social media after censorship outcry. 2020. https://www.theverge.com/2020/10/15/21518097/fcc-social-media-censorship-moderation-ajit-pai-section-230-nypost-biden. Accessed Oct 2020.

38. Wong Q. Cnet: CCPA: what California's new privacy law means for Facebook, twitter users. 2020. https://www.cnet.com/news/ccpa-what-californias-new-privacy-law-means-for-facebook-twitter-users. Accessed Oct 2020.

39. Grey D, Nigl A. The impact of new privacy Laws (GDPR) on social media platforms. 2019. https://www.researchgate.net/publication/331821021_The_Impact_of_New_Privacy_Laws_GDPR_on_Social_Media_Platforms Accessed Oct 2020.

40. Facebook: General Data Protection Regulation (GDPR). 2020. https://developers.facebook.com/docs/facebook-pixel/implementation/gdpr. Accessed Oct 2020.

41. GDPR.eu: What is GDPR, the E.U.'s new data protection law? 2020. https://gdpr.eu/what-is-gdpr/ Accessed Oct 2020.

42. Gebhart G, Williams J. EFF.org: Facebook Doesn't need to listen through your microphone to serve you. Creepy Ads. 2018; https://www.eff.org/deeplinks/2018/04/facebook-doesnt-need-listen-through-your-microphone-serve-you-creepy-ads. Accessed Oct 2020

43. Jennings R. Vox: why targeted ads are the most brutal owns. 2018. https://www.vox.com/the-goods/2018/9/25/17887796/facebook-ad-targeted-algorithm. Accessed Oct 2020.

44. Hill K. Forbes: how target figured out a teen girl was pregnant before her father did. 2012. https://www.forbes.com/sites/kashmirhill/2012/02/16/how-target-figured-out-a-teen-girl-was-pregnant-before-her-father-did/?sh=785a851f6668. Accessed Oct 2020.

45. Williams R. Marketing dive: Facebook's ad revenue rises 25% to record $20.7B. 2020. https://www.marketingdive.com/news/facebooks-ad-revenue-rises-25-to-record-207b/571404/. Accessed Oct 2020.

46. Sterling G. Marketing land: YouTube kicked in $15 billion as Google ad revenues topped $134 billion in 2019. 2020. https://marketingland.com/youtube-kicked-in-15-billion-as-google-ad-revenues-topped-134-billion-in-2019-275373. Accessed Oct 2020.

47. Williams R. Marketing dive: Twitter's ad revenue rises 12% as users reach 152M. 2020. https://www.marketingdive.com/news/twitters-ad-revenue-rises-12-as-users-reach-152m/571886/. Accessed Oct 2020.

48. Morrison S. Vox: Facebook is gearing up for a battle with California's new data privacy law. 2019. https://www.vox.com/recode/2019/12/17/21024366/facebook-ccpa-pixel-web-tracker. Accessed Oct 2020.

49. U.S. House of Representatives Permanent Selection Committee on Intelligence. Exposing Russia's Effort to Sow Discord Online: The Internet Research Agency and Advertisements. 2021. https://intelligence.house.gov/social-media-content/. Accessed Feb 2021.

50. Bangor Daily News: How the bogus 'Plandemic' video exploited false narratives to go viral. 2020. https://bangordailynews.com/2020/07/25/national-politics/disinformation-campaigns-are-murky-blends-of-truth-lies-and-sincere-beliefs-lessons-from-the-pandemic/. Accessed Oct 2020.

51. Islam MS, Sarkar T, Khan SH, Kamal AHM, Hasan SMM, Kabir A, Yeasmin D, Islam MA, Chowdhury KIA, Anwar KS, Chughtai AA, Seale H. COVID-19–related Infodemic and its impact on public health: a global social media analysis. Am J Trop Med Hyg. 2020;103(5):1621–9. https://doi.org/10.4269/ajtmh.20-0812.

52. Bursztyn L, Rao A, Roth CP, Yanagizawa-Drott DH. Misinformation during a pandemic. National Bureau of Economic Research Working Paper Series. 2020;27417 https://doi.org/10.3386/w27417.

53. Burki T. Vaccine misinformation and social media. The Lancet Digital Health. 2019;1(6) https://doi.org/10.1016/S2589-7500(19)30136-0.

54. Benecke O, DeYoung SE. Anti-vaccine decision-making and measles resurgence in the United States. Glob Pediatr Health. 2019:2333794X19862949. https://doi.org/10.1177/2333794X19862949.

55. NYC.gov: Measles. https://web.archive.org/web/20200510145035/https:/www1.nyc.gov/site/doh/health/health-topics/measles.page, 2019. Accessed Oct 2020.

56. Sharp Index: What does relentless misinformation mean for medicine? 2020. https://thesharpindex.com/blog1/what-does-relentless-misinformation-mean-for-medicine. Accessed Oct 2020.

57. Cinelli M, Quattrociocchi W, Galeazzi A, et al. The COVID-19 social media infodemic. Sci Rep. 2020;10:16598. https://doi.org/10.1038/s41598-020-73510-5.

58. The New York Times: Sept 30 COVID-19 Update. 2020. https://www.nytimes.com/live/2020/09/30/world/covid-19-coronavirus. Accessed Oct 2020.

59. Freyer FJ. Boston globe: at the Brigham, 'battle-weary' staff may have allowed virus to slip in. 2020. https://www.bostonglobe.com/2020/09/24/metro/brigham-womens-hospital-reports-cluster-10-covid-19-cases/. Accessed Nov 2020.

60. Kindelan K. Good morning America: nurses, doctors use social media to plead for public to take COVID-19 seriously as cases surge. 2020. https://www.goodmorningamerica.com/wellness/story/nurses-doctors-social-media-plead-public-covid-19-74320677. Accessed Dec 2020.

61. Otterman S. The New York Times: 'I Trust Science,' Says Nurse Who Is First to Get Vaccine in U.S. 2020. https://www.nytimes.com/2020/12/14/nyregion/us-covid-vaccine-first-sandra-lindsay.html. Accessed Dec 2020.

62. Riehm KE, Feder KA, Tormohlen KN, et al. Associations between time spent using social media and internalizing and externalizing problems among U.S. youth. JAMA Psychiatry. 2019; https://doi.org/10.1001/jamapsychiatry.2019.2325.

63. University of Pittsburgh: PittWire Modern-Day Hippocrates: Incoming School of Medicine Students Write Their Own Oath. 2020. https://www.pittwire.pitt.edu/news/modern-day-hippocrates-incoming-school-medicine-students-write-their-own-oath. Accessed Nov 2020.

64. Physicians for Human Rights: Dr. H. Jack Geiger, Founding Member and a Past President of PHR. 2020. https://phr.org/people/h-jack-geiger-md-m-sci-hyg/. Accessed Dec 2020.

65. Geiger JH. The political future of social medicine: reflections on physicians as activists. Acad Med. 2017;92(3):282–4. https://doi.org/10.1097/ACM.0000000000001538.

66. Bernardo TM, Rajic A, Young I, Robiadek K, Pham MT, Funk JA. Scoping review on search queries and social media for disease surveillance: a chronology

of innovation. J Med Internet Res. 2013; https://doi.org/10.2196/jmir.2740.

67. Fung IC, Tse ZT, Fu KW. The use of social media in public health surveillance. Western Pac Surveill Response J. 2015;6(2):3–6. https://doi.org/10.5365/WPSAR.2015.6.1.019.

68. World Health Organization: Influenza Fact Sheet. 2018. https://www.who.int/en/news-room/fact-sheets/detail/influenza-(seasonal). Accessed Oct 2020.

69. Volkova S, Ayton E, Porterfield K, Corley CD. Forecasting influenza-like illness dynamics for military populations using neural networks and social media. PLoS One. 12(12):e0188941. https://doi.org/10.1371/journal.pone.0188941.

70. Landi H. Fierce Healthcare: 2020 breaks record in digital health investment with $9.4B in funding. 2020. https://www.fiercehealthcare.com/tech/2020-breaks-record-digital-health-investment-9-4b-funding. Accessed Oct 2020.

71. Cory N, Stevens P. 2020. Information technology and innovation foundation: building a global framework for digital health services in the Era of COVID-19. https://itif.org/publications/2020/05/26/building-global-framework-digital-health-services-era-covid-19. Accessed Oct 2020.

72. Cheung ML, Chau KY, Lam MHS, Tse G, Ho KY, Flint SW, Broom DR, Tso EKH, Lee KY. Examining Consumers' adoption of wearable healthcare technology: the role of health attributes. Int J Environ Res Public Health. 2019;16(13):2257. https://doi.org/10.3390/ijerph16132257.

73. Jacob C, Sanchez-Vazquez A, Ivory C. Factors impacting clinicians' adoption of a clinical photo documentation app and its implications for clinical workflows and quality of care: qualitative case study. JMIR Mhealth Uhealth. 2020;8(9):e20203. https://doi.org/10.2196/20203.

Data Analytics, Artificial Intelligence and Data Visualization

19

Mustafa Ozkaynak and Diane Skiba

Learning Objectives
- Identify the significance of data analytics, artificial intelligence and data visualization in health informatics.
- Examine the relationships of data analytics, artificial intelligence and data visualization to solve complex health problems.
- Determine the challenges and risks associated with data analytics, artificial intelligence and data visualization.

Key Terms
- Decision-making
- Data science
- Prediction
- Artificial intelligence
- Deep learning
- Machine learning
- Algorithms
- Visualization

Introduction

The first chapter of this textbook discussed learning health systems (LHS) in detail. The ability to retrieve and use data from and about the clinical practice is important to LHS. This chapter first dis-

cusses data analytics in general and then the correlation of data analytics in relationship to artificial intelligence (AI) and data visualization. The chapter will also describe how these approaches can be an essential tool for informatics and health care.

Finally, the chapter will provide a high-level survey of data analytics, AI and visualization while highlighting some controversial issues, risks and challenges of these techniques within the healthcare arena.

Data Analytics

Definition

Data analytics is the process of extracting meaning from raw data to gain insights into an issue. It exists at the intersection of information technology (IT), statistics and operation management. Data analytics may examine historical data over time. The size of data used, however, may vary among projects. In general, there are four types of data analytics: descriptive (answers the question of what happened), diagnostic (i.e., why things happened), predictive (i.e., what will happen in the future under given conditions) and prescriptive analytics (i.e., what decision-makers should do). Data analytics can inform nursing decision-making (at the bed side [e.g., pain management] and administrative levels) and the design, implementation and evaluation of nursing informatics interventions (e.g., symptom-tracking apps).

M. Ozkaynak (✉) · D. Skiba
College of Nursing, University of Colorado,
Aurora, CO, USA
e-mail: mustafa.ozkaynak@cuanschutz.edu;
diane.skiba@cuanschutz.edu

© Springer Nature Switzerland AG 2022
U. H. Hübner et al. (eds.), *Nursing Informatics*, Health Informatics,
https://doi.org/10.1007/978-3-030-91237-6_19

Why Do We Use Data Analytics in Health Care?

Various user groups can benefit from data analytics as summarized in Table 19.1 (adapted from Matheny et al. [1]).

Data availability offers support to empower all of the actors in health care to engage in ways that promote collaboration with each other. Data analytics tools and approaches can be used to help put health information into context in the decision-making process of health management.

The wide variety of uses of data analytics in health care can be accomplished by multidisciplinary teams. Such a team should include clinicians, patients, informal caregivers, informaticians, health IT (HIT) designers, public health specialists, business administrators, statisticians and data scientists.

Data Sources for Data Analytics

Current healthcare systems can utilize various data sources for data analytics such as: electronic health record (EHR) [2–4], images [5], sensors [6, 7], genomics, clinical notes, patient observations, patient narratives, biomedical literature and social media [8, 9] and other daily living activities such as media consumption, restaurant selection, transportation use and illicit drugs. These diverse data sources can be used individually; however, even more powerfully multiple data sources can be used together. For example, social media postings combined with the biomedical literature to identify potential flu pandemic provide more meaningful/ robust information. Clinical notes, patient observations and EHR can help with identifying specific individuals who have the flu. Additionally, sensor data can be used to trace the patient's contacts. A good example is provided by Lorgelly et al., who linked cancer data with commonwealth reimbursement data to infer which patient, disease, genomic and treatment characteristics explain variations in health expenditure [10]. However, aggregating diverse data sources is a technical and semantic interoperability challenge [11].

In current practice, the dominant data source for data analytics is EHR in clinical environments. The potential for patient-generated data has been well acknowledged; however, using patient-data in clinical practice is still limited.

Table 19.1 User groups of data analytics in health care

User Group	Category	Examples of Applications/Data Resources
Patients and families	Health/symptom tracking, self-management	Mobile devices, wearables, sensors, smart homes
	Rehabilitation	Cardiac rehabilitation using apps and robots
	Social support	Identifying social isolation, chatbot applications, social robots
Clinician care teams	Early detection, prediction and diagnostic tools	Early cancer detection (e.g., melanoma), individual opioid addition risk prediction based on health records
	Symptom management	Evaluation of pain management practices in various units and identifying the root causes of poor practice
	Patient safety	Early detection of fall
Public health program managers	Identification of individuals at risk	Identifying suicide risk using social media
	Pandemic	Contact tracing of COVID19
	Population health	Eldercare monitoring (ambient sensors) Epidemiology of air pollution Restaurant selection
Business administrators	Cybersecurity	Protection of personal health information
	Nurse scheduling	Developing nurse scheduling algorithms that optimize cost while maintaining patient safety
Payers	Fraud detection	Healthcare billing fraud

For example, the type of data patients can enter is restricted, reducing the use of data in decision-making.

Data Analytics and Precision Medicine

Precision medicine (or precision health) has been fueled by the rising availability/affordability of mobile, ubiquitous sensing and documenting technologies, and data analytics tools and approaches. Precision health focuses on the uniqueness of the individual's characteristics and uniqueness of the (social, organizational, cultural etc.) context associated with them. However, we are facing an increasing gap between our ability to generate large biomedical data ("big data") and our ability to analyze and interpret them.

Data Quality in Health Care

EHRs and other information routinely collected during or about healthcare delivery and management can help address the critical need for evidence about the real-world effectiveness, safety and quality of healthcare delivery. However, individual data resources can be insufficient to develop comprehensive solutions. Therefore, combining multiple data sources (sites, environments, etc.) is often necessary [11].

Data quality is an important determinant of the value of a data source, and it is even more important when data are needed to be aggregated from multiple data sources. For example, EHR databases contain data collected during routine clinical care by practitioners focused on patient care, or by patients focused on capturing their healthcare experiences, rather than the more rigorous data collection associated with research. Differences in clinical workflows, practice standards, patient populations, available technologies and referral resources impact what data are collected and how they are documented.

The viability of a LHS is dependent on a robust understanding of the quality, validity and optimal secondary uses of routinely collected electronic health data within distributed health data networks. Robust data checking can strengthen confidence in the findings based on a distributed data network.

Data quality is a complex, multidimensional concept that defies a one-size-fits-all description [12]. Data quality is particularly important when data coming from different resources is aggregated [12]. A key data quality concept is "fitness for use." Data are considered fit for use "if they are free of defects and possess desired features … for their intended uses in operations, decision making, and planning" [13]. Data quality is context dependent, which means the same data elements or data sources may be deemed high quality for one use and poor quality for a another use. The purpose of use determines which variables are relevant or have a high Impact in a specific context.

Weiskopf defined five high-level dimensions of data quality for EHRs (Table 19.2) [14].

Kahn et al. proposed a health-care-specific "Harmonized Data Quality Assessment Terminology and Framework for the Secondary Use of Electronic Health Record Data" [15]. They described three data quality categories (Table 19.3).

Although both of the frameworks were developed for EHRs, they can be applied to other data sources as well. Data quality is a multidimensional process that can require trade-offs between dimensions because of organizational and data-use priorities and resource constraints. Data quality characterization is itself a data collection and analytic activity with costs inherent in the pro-

Table 19.2 Five dimensions of data quality for EHR [14]

Dimension	Synonyms
Completeness	Accessibility, accuracy, availability, missingness, omission, presence, rate of recording, sensitivity, validity
Concordance	Agreement, consistency, reliability, variation
Correctness	Accuracy, corrections made, errors, misleading, positive predictive value, quality, validity
Currency	Recency, timeliness
Plausibility	Accuracy, believability, trustworthiness, validity

Table 19.3 Data quality categories of Kahn et al.'s framework [15]

Category	Subcategories	Definition
Conformance	Value conformance Relational conformance Computational conformance	"Features that describe the compliance of the representation of data against internal or external formatting, relational, or computational definitions"
Completeness	Not available	"Features that describe the frequencies of data attributes present in a data set without reference to data values"
Plausibility	Uniqueness plausibility Atemporal plausibility Temporal plausibility	"Features that describe the believability or truthfulness of data values"

cess of data quality assessment, monitoring and governance. Developing a comprehensive cost-benefit analysis of a better administrative and clinical data quality is still an open area to study.

Data Analytics and Human Factors

Several aspects of human cognition should be considered in attempting to reap the benefits of big data. Limitations of human beings in processing such large data repositories require new ways of interacting with large data sets (e.g., new ways of visualizing complex health data; for more detail please see Sect. 6 of this chapter). Human information processing is limited by cognitive capacity; for example, humans tend to remember a very limited number of elements (seven plus or minus two) in their working memory, limiting the amount or complexity of information that can be effectively presented to them. In addition, humans are susceptible to a range of cognitive biases when using data to make decisions or reason [16, 17].

State-of-the-art data analytics applications in clinical settings will not reach their full potential unless they are integrated into clinical workflow [18], but there are multiple barriers, including: data privacy concerns, algorithm transparency, data standardization, interoperability and patient safety concerns. Workflow studies that consider the fragility of data analytics models in real-world heterogeneous and noisy clinical environments are critical to the integration of data analytics systems into clinical decision-making.

Artificial Intelligence

Introduction to Artificial Intelligence

Healthcare professionals are using a variety of tools to maximize the value of their clinical data. One such tool is the use of artificial intelligence (AI). From a historical perspective, Alan Turing first introduced the idea of a "thinking machine," in his classic 1950 article "Computing Machinery and Intelligence." In this article [19] he asked the question "Can machines think?" He proposed an imitation game which has translated into/resulted in the Turning Test. "The Turing Test is a method of inquiry in artificial intelligence (AI) for determining whether or not a computer is capable of thinking like a human being. Turing proposed that a computer can be said to possess AI if it can mimic human responses under specific conditions" [20].

John McCarthy, a cognitive scientist, first coined the term AI in 1955 for a presentation at the 1956 Dartmouth Conference. He presented a proposal for a summer research project on AI. "The study is to proceed the basis of the conjecture that every aspect of learning or any other feature of intelligence can in principle be so precisely described that a machine can be made to simulate it" [21]—thus, the beginning of the field of AI.

For many years, there were very few advances in AI. Bengio [22] stated that even the term "AI seemed to leave the domain of serious science." Scientists and writers described the dashed hopes of the period from the 1970s until the mid-2000s as a series of "AI winters." During these AI winters, Kulikowski [23] noted there was some work related to clinical AI. Kulikowski [23] highlighted a visionary article by Schwartz, in which Schwartz made the following statement, "Computing science will probably exert its major effects by augmenting and, in some cases, largely replacing the intellectual functions of the physician" [24]. His message was that we need to harness the power of the computer to work for physicians in an effective and efficient manner. Here are a few early examples of clinical AI: In the 1970s, a system called MYCIN, developed by Stanford University, identified bacterial infections and recommended treatment options [25]. "MYCIN contained three components: a knowledge base created by experts, an inference engine with rule-based algorithms, and a user interface. Although there were other instances of expert system designed in that era, there was never a critical mass of users to adopt them for clinical practice" [26]. Kulikowski also described the development of the CASNET (for CAusal Associational Network) consultation program for glaucoma. "The program showed how causal explanations of disease could be combined with empirical knowledge of presumptive diagnoses, prognoses, and treatments to provide advice on glaucoma patient management" [23]. In nursing, one of the early applications of AI was the development of an expert system for nursing practice [27]. This expert system, COMMES (Creighton Online Multiple Modular Expert Systems), was "a group of artificial-intelligence based expert systems designed to provide decisions support nursing practice" [28].

The acceptance and use of AI in the clinical setting was dormant for many years. In the mid-2000s there was a resurgence in the field and the definition of AI was evolving. Here are some of the more recent definitions. The first two definitions are simple and represent a layman's perspective:

The English Oxford Living Dictionary (https://www.lexico.com/definition/artificial_intelligence) defined AI as "The theory and development of computer systems able to perform tasks normally requiring human intelligence, such as visual perception, speech recognition, decision-making, and translation between languages."

Merriam-Webster (https://www.merriam-webster.com/dictionary/artificial%20intelligence) dictionary defined artificial intelligence as "A branch of computer science dealing with the simulation of intelligent behavior in computers and the capability of a machine to imitate intelligent human behavior."

West [29] offered the following theoretical definition: AI generally is thought to refer to "machines that respond to stimulation consistent with traditional responses from humans, given the human capacity for contemplation, judgment, and intention." McGrow [30] builds upon Pan's [31] computer science perspective of AI as "the theory and development of computer systems able to complete tasks that typically require human intelligence, such as visual perception, speech recognition, decision-making, and/or language translation."

To summarize, AI is a field within computer science in which a machine is able to mimic human intelligence. It has evolved into an umbrella term [30] that encompasses such areas as cognitive computing (CC), machine learning (ML) and deep learning. To follow is an examination of these areas with AI.

To understand cognitive computing, it is important to note that computer science as a discipline has transitioned from a tabulation era to a programming era and now to a cognitive era. Advances in brain science and the understanding of how the brain learns provide a foundation for the cognitive era of computing. According to Marr [32], cognitive computing (CC) is a "mashup of cognitive science—the study of the human brain and how it functions—and computer science." Kelly [33] further defined CC as "systems that learn at scale, reason with purpose and interacts with humans naturally." An interesting component that CC adds is the ability to handle unstructured data. In the past, most AI applications were based on structured or numeric data.

Many consider ML as a subset of AI, and deep learning as a subset of ML. "Machine learning is a family of statistical and mathematical modeling techniques that uses a variety of approaches to automatically learn and improve the prediction of a target state, without explicit programming" [1]. ML learns inductively. Various techniques (such as random forests and Bayesian networks) are used to parse the data and to permit learning within an algorithm. Three techniques commonly used are: supervised, unsupervised and enforced learning. The supervised technique trains the computer with explicitly labeled data, which means data that are tagged and represent certain characteristics. A common example would be email spam filtering. An example in health care of a supervised technique would be interpretation of radiological images. An unsupervised technique uses non-labeled data in which the algorithm seeks to find the patterns or relationships in the data. An example in health would be identifying a subgroup of cancer patients with a particular gene expression. Lim, Tucker, and Kumara [34] used unsupervised ML to identify latent infectious diseases from Twitter data. Reinforced learning technique does not "indicate the correct output for a given input, the training data in reinforcement learning are assumed to provide only an indication as to whether an action is correct or not; if an action is incorrect, there remains the problem of finding the correct action" [35]. An example of a reinforced technique is a study that used personalized messages to encourage diabetic patients to continue their physical activity [36].

Deep learning is a subset of ML. It is a different model that uses artificial neural networks. These neural networks are "based on general mathematical principles that allow them to learn from examples" [22]. Common examples of deep learning include: speech recognition, natural language processing (NLP), image analysis and driverless cars. The next section will describe the various AI uses in health care and nursing.

Uses of AI in Nursing and Health Care

In the last few years, AI has exploded in the world of health care. Several factors served as driving forces. According to the Executive Office of the President, National Science and Technology Council Committee on Technology [37], AI is "driven by three mutually reinforcing factors: the availability of big data … dramatically improved machine learning approaches and algorithms … and the capabilities of more powerful computers."

Over the last decade this explosion of AI in health care has led to numerous articles on this topic. In 2019, the National Academy of Medicine (NAM) convened a meeting to examine the hope, the hype, the promise and the peril of AI in health care [1]. AI examples were classified by stakeholder groups. This classification provided a framework to examine the various uses of AI in health care according to the following stakeholders: patients and families; clinical care team; public health program managers and business administrators; and researchers. In nursing, McGrow [30] promoted the use of AI in nursing by classifying how AI was being used based on three types of analytics. For clinical analytics, AI examples included: "clinical pathway prediction, disease progression prediction, health risk protection, predictive risk scoring, and virtual assistants embedded in clinical systems for workflow improvements" [30]. McGrow also notes, "AI may also be used in disease management, assisting with the differential diagnosis on medical images and combining patient data with academic evidence and regulatory guidelines to personalize treatment plans" [30]. In terms of operational analytics, AI examples were: monitoring operations such as safety metrics, equipment and supplies; identification of fraud and improvements in documenting coding. The last category, behavioral analysis, is consumer-centric and uses AI to facilitate and support patient engagement related to health and wellness as well as to deter hospital readmissions. Given these frameworks, what follows is a sampling of AI uses in nursing and health care.

One example that has emerged within the last decade is IBM's Watson. Skiba [26] described IBM Watson Health "as a cognitive computing system that can ingest, combine, and understand massive volumes of structured and unstructured data. It can reason and learn from its interactions with the data." It is probably best known for its work in oncology. In particular, Watson can help

facilitate evidence-based practice treatment decisions for oncology patients. This is based on
work with Memorial Sloan Kettering Cancer
Center (MSKCC). This collaborative project
allows for the AI to learn from an MSKCC dataset and "interpret cancer patients' clinical information and identify individualized,
evidence-based treatment options that leverage
our specialists' decades of experience and
research" (https://www.mskcc.org/videos/
mskcc-and-ibm-collaborate-applying-watson-
technology-help-oncologists). Another example
of using Watson in population health is to identify
care gaps for patients. For example, the Iowa
clinic used the system to automatically search
patient records to identify care gaps, such as
women who need mammograms (https://www.
ibm.com/blogs/watson-health/catching-cancer-
time/?mhsrc=ibmsearch_a&mhq=mammog
ram%20reminders).

With the rapid growth of consumerism and
access to smart devices and wearables, there are
many AI applications within this category. AI is
being used for health monitoring, health assessments, disease prevention, chronic disease management, medication management and
rehabilitation.

Conversational agents, virtual agents or chatbots use AI as a basis for their applications. The
most common conversational agents are Apple's
Siri, Amazon's Alexa or Microsoft's Cortana. In
health care, conversational agents are more than
voice-only agents and make use of human (nurse)
and non-human (animal or robot) images. These
images, along with the voice, gestures and facial
expressions, "provide a richer interactive experience. These are called embodied conversational
agents (ECAs)" [38]:

> Meet Molly, a chatbot that can assess a patient's
> problem and determine if self-care therapies are
> sufficient or is there a need for intervention by a
> health care professional. Molly uses AI algorithms
> based on clinical content related to chronic dis-
> eases and medical protocols. The patient can use a
> smartphone and when asked about their symptoms,
> they can respond using speech, text, images and/or
> video. Molly can also be used to monitor patients
> at home with chronic diseases such as chronic
> heart failure. Here is a link to a demonstration of
> Molly: https://youtu.be/AU1nGpOmZpQ

> Meet Florence who can help you with medication
> management, track your health, educate you about
> a disease and find you a provider or pharmacy.
> Florence is your personal health assistant on your
> cellphone. To learn more, visit: https://youtu.be/
> BtqJaHv53g0

In terms of chronic disease management, here are
a few examples of how AI can be used with
patients. In the "self-management" domain, conversational agents already exist to address depression, smoking cessation, asthma and diabetes:

> A conversational agent mobile app, WoeBot, that is
> used to deliver cognitive behavior therapy (CBT)
> to young adults with depression and anxiety issues.
> In their study, the researchers found that a conver-
> sational agent was feasible and effective CBT
> modality. Participants in this study had lower
> depression scores and less anxiety [39].

> Another example is the use of a chatbot to imple-
> ment smartphone CBT interventions for self-
> management of pain. The text-based chatbot,
> SELMA (Self Management), was found to be fea-
> sible and the intervention group appreciated the
> empathic and responsible interaction of the chatbot
> [40].

> AI and facial recognition were used for assessment
> of pain in patients who may not be able to com-
> municate pain, such as an Alzheimer's patient.
> Using a smartphone, one can use an app PainChek®
> (https://painchek.com/), that analyzes facial mus-
> cle movements to determine pain. The patient's
> data are stored to enable coordinated care
> management.

In a review of AI use in diabetes [41], there were
four different categories: "improved screening
and detection of diabetic retinopathy (DR) and
macular edema; individualized predictive risk
stratification and treatment; decision-support
tools for clinicians; and patient self-management
aids." To follow are some examples of uses in
patient self-management:

> Zhang, Yu, Siffiquie, Divakaran & Sawhney [42]
> described the development of a patient tool, "Snap-
> n-Eat" that allows patients to assess the nutritional
> assessment of their food by taking pictures with
> their smartphone. The AI system recognizes the
> food and can estimate the caloric and nutritional
> value of the specific item of food. To accomplish
> this task, they used a dataset of 2000 images clas-
> sified into 15 different food groups to train the AI
> system. The dataset allowed the AI recognition
> system to have an accuracy rate of 85% within
> these 15 different categories of food.

Another example was the use of an AI recognition system to measure the activity of diabetic patients using their smartphones [43]. Using ML and symbolic reasoning, the system could quantify high level daily activities and provide advice to adjust their activity choices.

A final example was the use of a wound assessment tool for diabetic patients. This smartphone app allows patients to take pictures of their wounds which are then analyzed using a machine learning algorithm. The picture and the analysis can then be shared with their wound nurse on a daily basis. This particular study found the "system can be efficiently used to analyze the wound healing status with promising accuracy." [44]

In terms of clinicians use of AI in a hospital setting, Cedar Sinai Hospital used a hands-free (HF) voice-activated device (Amazon Echo) to facilitate communication between patients and nurses. Avia (https://aivahealth.com/) provided a system that allowed patients to control their patient experience and communicate with the nurses. Nurses could then better manage their workflow with this communication device.

Another example is the use of unsupervised ML algorithm on home health data. This was used to identify three subgroups of patients with HF using telehealth. The ML algorithm identified that had distinct levels of healthcare utilization outcomes of home health length of stay and the number of hospitalizations. Various clustering techniques were used to examine "intercluster differences for patient characteristics related to medical history, symptoms, medications, psychosocial assessments, and healthcare utilization" [45].

In terms of the primary care arena, Babylon Health has implemented two components of AI: a symptom checker and a conversational agent. This is a consumer-facing product where patients using their smartphone can connect to the conversational agent. Patients interact with the conversational agent and ask questions about their symptoms, to identify a likely diagnosis. The system is based upon clinical data from multiple sources, which include billions of symptom combinations to provide a presumptive diagnosis and course of action [46]. The product has many other features such as a virtual visit with your general practitioner, digital assistance with medication adherence, and clinical record and pharmacy services. The National Health Service (NHS), in various health districts in the United Kingdom (UK), used this system (https://www.abdn.ac.uk/staffnet/documents/BabylonDigital-HealthcareLeaflet.pdf). It is also being used in Rwanda (http://www.babyl.rw/), where it has over two million users, who have done over one million consultations.

Another area where AI is growing is the use of robotics in health care. For many years, surgeons have been using robotic surgery. In the last decade, robotics has expanded to include robots for consumers and for healthcare providers. These robots can perform operational functions while also serving as emotional companions. Robert [47] provided some examples of robots for use in health care or as personal companions:

- Pepper (https://www.softbankrobotics.com/emea/en/industries/healthcare} is a humanoid robot that can express empathy and serve in many capacities within hospitals.
- ROBOBEAR (https://www.youtube.com/watch?v=J3edDaPSdY4) is a strong helper for both patients and clinicians but has a gentle touch.
- Pillio (https://pillohealth.com/devices) is an AI health companion for your home.
- Aflac Duck (https://aflacchildhoodcancer.org/) is an interactive supportive tool to help distract children while getting their cancer treatments. The duck can express the children's feelings and also has a port so the clinician can demonstrate how the duck gets an injection.
- TRINA (Tele Robotic Intelligent Nursing Assistant) (https://youtu.be/Ms0iTdDAL20) is a project to train a robot to perform common nursing tasks, especially under hazardous circumstances.

There is a tremendous potential to use AI in health care. AI has the potential to transform health care and allow healthcare delivery systems to be more efficient and effective, while maintaining safety. Topol stated: "he expects to see AI help healthcare organizations give physicians and patients 'the gift of time'—to get back to where medicine was decades ago, when the relationship was characterized by a deep bond with trust and empathy" (https://www.beckershospitalreview.com/artificial-intelligence/dr-eric-topol-how-ai-will-restore-humanity-of-medicine-this-decade.html). It is important for all clinicians to be knowledgeable about AI and embrace its power to provide quality care that is safe and patient-centric.

Challenges

The adoption and implementation of AI in health care is not without its challenges and issues. One such challenge is that "much of healthcare data are siloed and unstructured" [30] and do not include consumer driven data. The lack of Interoperability across systems is also a hindrance. "This fragmentation increases the risk or error, decreasing the comprehensiveness of datasets and increases the expense of gathering data" [48].

Like all digital tools, privacy and security is always a challenge. It is important to ensure that patients' data are protected. As massive amounts of data are collected, the security of these datasets is important. Patients and healthcare institutions want to ensure security provisions have been established for all datasets that may be used in AI. In addition, since data are gathered from multiple sources, there needs to be assurance and protection that the patient's permission to access their data is obtained. If permissions are not obtained, there is a risk that there could be a violation of privacy laws. AI techniques could also make conclusions without explicit data. For example, "AI system might be able to identify that a person has Parkinson's disease based on the trembling of a computer mouse, even if the person had never revealed that information to anyone else (or did not know). Patients might consider this a violation of their privacy, especially if the AI system's inference were available to third parties, such as banks or life insurance companies" [48]. "Machine learning techniques can instead be used to infer new meaning within and across contexts and is generally unencumbered by privacy rules in the United States (U.S.)" [49]. An example is using Twitter postings to identify new mothers, who may be at risk for postpartum depression (PPD). The analysis of unstructured data could be used to train algorithms to predict risk. Accordingly, "using publicly available Twitter posts to infer risk of PPD, for example, does not run afoul of existing privacy law" (49). It is extremely important that "both privacy and security of data is critical to comply with the law and act ethically" [50].

Informed consent is a potential ethical issue in using various AI technologies. One such example would be the growing application of AI techniques associated with the use of facial recognition technology (FRT) for a variety of healthcare issues. This technology has been used in health care for "diagnosing genetic disorders, monitoring patients, and providing health indicator information (related to behavior, aging, longevity, or pain experience, for example)" [51]. If FRT is to be used in a healthcare setting, informed consent needs to be obtained from the person. The informed consent must be obtained from the patient regarding data collection and storage and the specific purpose for the use of these FRT images [52].

A major ethical concern is the potential for a biased dataset. If biased data are used to train your algorithm, then your AI will be biased. It is important for healthcare professionals to think about the impact of social determinants on health care, and how are they are accounted in datasets. It is also important that biases are examined in terms of algorithm transparency [47]. It is the healthcare provider's responsibility to determine what data was used to train the system, and what controls were placed on the system to avoid bias [47].

With the growth of AI, another challenge is the liability when mistakes are made and patients are injured or die. "The implementation of AI raises complex legal questions regarding the health care professionals' and technology manufacturers liability" [53]. This is of particular importance, if AI techniques are used that fail to explain the reasoning behind the AI conclusion. This is sometimes called the "black box" phenomena [53]. For example, "consider a situation in which a black box AI system assists in detection of breast cancer using mammography data and suggests an erroneous diagnosis, resulting in injury to a patient. Are our legal doctrines of tort liability sufficient to handle medical malpractice?" [53].

A longer-term risk is how AI will impact the relationship between providers and patients. As more AI tools become available, will patients still trust their healthcare providers? In an editorial, Nundy, Montgomery and Wachter [54] raise the following question: Does AI have the "potential to enable and disable the 3 components of trust: competency, motive, and transparency?" In terms of competency, AI can augment the provider's level of expertise and enable trust. If the AI "lacks explainability and inappropriately conflicts with physician judgement and patient autonomy" [54], it can be a disabler of trust. In terms of motive, AI could enhance the workflow of providers and thus allow more time with the patient which in turn promotes trust. But if more AI tools are used for screening and addressing certain health issues, there may be less trust with the AI or the provider. Transparency refers to acknowledging how clinical decision-making is using data based on evidence. This would facilitate trust. If patient data are being used for a variety of purposes, patients may be more distrustful.

In order to achieve some of the benefits of AI in health care, healthcare professionals must be involved to ensure challenges and issues are addressed. This will allow maximum benefit to providers, patients and their families, caregivers and healthcare institutions.

Data Visualization

Definition

Visualization can be defined as the communication of information using graphical representations. Data visualization is the visual representation of otherwise abstract data.

Although qualitative data can also be visualized (e.g., word clouds), the big majority of the visualization efforts focus on quantitative data. Visualization is mainly about mapping variables to visual properties (space, color, line, etc.). Two main reasons for data visualization are exploration and informing and persuading. Visualization allows for containing a large amount of data and information in a relatively small space.

In health care, there is an increasing amount of data to be dealt with on a daily basis. Many care-related activities performed by nurses and other clinicians involve either collecting data (e.g., physical assessment), recording data (e.g., charting), retrieving data (e.g., history review) or using data (e.g., decision-making). However, in many applications, raw data have not much value in themselves; instead, information should be extracted from a group of data—additionally, the information overload problem [55], which "refers to the danger of getting lost in data which may be:

- irrelevant to the current task at hand,
- processed in an inappropriate way,
- presented in an inappropriate way" [56].

High-quality care and patient safety depend on the right information being available at the right time to the right person. Additionally, the information should not only inform the user but also make the user able to take an action toward better care delivery.

Visual representations and interaction techniques take advantage of the human eye's broad-bandwidth pathway to the mind and allow users to see, explore and understand large amounts of information. Visualizations can provide cognitive support by (1) exploiting advantages of human perception (such as parallel visual processing) and (2) compensating for cognitive deficiencies, such as limited working memory. When visualizing data we need to pay attention to two level of processes: (1) perception (the low-level activity of sensing the visual aspects of a display); (2) cognition (the higher-level process of interpreting the display and translating it into meaning).

Visual analytics is a similar term to visualization and can be defined as the science of analytical reasoning facilitated by advanced interactive visual interfaces [57].

Florence Nightingale as the First Data Visualizer

Florence Nightingale (1820–1910; lady with the lamp, medical reformer and campaigner for soldiers' health) is considered the founder of the modern nursing profession. However, she is one of the first people who realized that visualization was the most effective way of bringing data into life.

When Florence Nightingale arrived at the British military hospital in Turkey in 1856 during the Crimean War, the scene was severe. The mortality rate was high, and the hospital was chaotic—even the number of deaths was not recorded accurately. Florence Nightingale established much needed order and method within the hospital's statistical records. She also collected a lot of new data. In doing so, Nightingale learned that poor sanitary practices were the main perpetrator of high mortality in hospitals. She was determined to reduce such avoidable deaths. By using visualization, she made a case for eliminating the practices that contributed to the unsafe and unhealthy environment.

The specific organization of Nightingale's chart allowed her to represent more complex information layered in a single space. Her coxcomb chart was divided evenly into 12 slices representing months of the year, with the shaded area of each month's slice proportional to the death rate that month. Her color-coding shading indicated the cause of death in each area of the diagram. Her drawings can be accessed at http://www.archive.org/details/mortalityofbriti00lond.

Selected Principles of Visualization

The general principle when developing visualization is to use the design which minimizes cognitive burden for the task at hand. There are many principles about how to achieve this. Although discussing each of these principles is beyond the scope of this section, we would like to provide some selected principles.

In his book *Beautiful Evidence* [58], Edward Tufte illustrates the following principles for the analysis and display of data:

1. Show comparisons, contrasts and differences.
2. Show causality, mechanism, explanation and systematic structure.
3. Show multivariate data; that is, show more than one or two variables.
4. Completely integrate words, numbers, images and diagrams.
5. Thoroughly describe the evidence. Provide a detailed title, indicate the authors and sponsors, document the data sources, show complete measurement scales and point out relevant issues.
6. Analytical presentations ultimately stand or fall depending on the quality, relevance and integrity of their content.

Zhu [59] defined the effectiveness of data visualization in terms of three principles: accuracy, utility and efficiency. Accuracy refers to what extent the attributes of visual elements match the attributes of data items, and the structure of the visualization shall match the structure of the data set. Utility refers to what extent the visualization help users achieve the goal of specific tasks. Efficiency refers to what extent the visualization reduces the cognitive load for a specific task over non-visual representations.

Case Study

Primary Care Provider Using AI as Part of Their Practice?

You are a healthcare professional working in a primary health clinic. Your Chief Information Officer (CIO) is exploring new technologies to expand healthcare access. One such mechanism is to use an AI-based product that patients can use to get accessible care on their schedule rather than on clinic availability. The company is going to demonstrate the product and you are being asked to attend so you can ask questions and provide feedback from a clinician's perspective.

The demonstration highlights a patient, Alexandra, who has been experiencing some dizziness. She is a 30-year-old marketing executive at a small firm. Since her days are consumed in meetings for a special project, she decides to try the virtual assistant platform on her smartphone that is connected to her primary care clinic.

After work, she logged into her patient portal to access Maria, the virtual assistant. Maria greets her as the platform scans her face and determines if the patient on the screen is associated with that patient portal account. Using facial recognition, it verifies Alexandra and brings up her electronic health record (EHR).

Maria, then, proceeds to engage Alexandra in a conversation about her specific reason for contacting the virtual assistant platform. Maria determined that her primary complaint is dizziness that she experienced twice in the last few days. Once it was when she was home and the second episode happened when she was driving home from work. She was able to pull over and call a friend to take her home. Maria listens carefully and then begins to ask Alexandra some questions. Based on Alexandra's answers, Maria moves from one knowledge domain to another domain to ascertain the potential diagnosis.

Once the potential diagnoses are determined, Maria presents the top three diagnoses and their corresponding probabilities. Alexandra listens carefully and her voice starts to crack as she asks Maria a question out the primary potential diagnosis. Maria recognizes that Alexandra's voice is noticeably different and she appears more emotional. Given this recognition, Maria asks Alexandra if she is worried. Alexandra states she is very nervous. Maria asks her if she wants to either schedule an appointment with her primary care provider or immediately talk with a telehealth clinician. She opts to talk with a telehealth clinician. She is connected to this clinician, who had access to her records and a summary of her interactions with Maria.

Given this scenario, please address the following questions:

- What is your first reaction to this demonstration?

- What are the benefits to patients using this platform?
- What are some issues that you would raise about the patient's use of this platform?
- What issues do you think providers would raise about this platform use?
- Are there any legal or ethical issues you would ask?
- List three to five other questions you would ask about this product.

Summary

This chapter provides a high-level introduction to world of data analytics, artificial intelligence (AI) and data visualization. This chapter also defines the concepts associated with these three emerging areas and provides examples of applications to nursing and health care. As with any new innovation, there are both benefits and challenges associated with data analytics, AI and data visualization.

Conclusions and Outlook

There is no doubt that health care has begun to embrace data analytics, AI and data visualization as an important component of healthcare delivery. It is projected that "the next 20 years are likely to see further acceleration in the capabilities of computers to analyze complex data and mimic human cognition" [60]. This is particularly true as we have moved from an information-driven system to a knowledge management system. As healthcare providers use these tools to augment their knowledge and to harness the power to guide patient care, it will become more apparent that healthcare professionals will need to remember the art of caring for patients [60].

Given this outlook, it is important for healthcare professionals education to gain a better understanding of how data are being collected, aggregated, manipulated and analyzed to provide AI tools with the capacity to deliver personalized care for patients [61].

If you are a healthcare professional, you need to be acutely aware of data analytics, AI and data visualization techniques. If your healthcare organization is using or developing AI tools, Robert [47] recommends that as an expert or an end-user, a healthcare professional should work with the data science team to ensure the validity of the data and be the quality check for data inputs and outputs. As part of a clinician's role, one should ask the following questions: Do the results make sense or are they surprising; any missing data; do you have confidence that you understand what the data represent and how to best use the results; and mostly importantly, do you trust the results to use in the care of your patient? [47].

Useful Resources

Resources on Data Analytics:

1. Website and Videos:
   - Clinical & Business Intelligence: Data Management—A Foundation for Analytics. https://www.himss.org/data-management-resources-and-tools
   - Office of the National Coordinator for Health Information Technology, Patient Demographic Data Quality Framework. https://www.healthit.gov/playbook/pddq-framework/introduction/
   - Highlights of PCORI-Funded Research Results. https://www.pcori.org/research-results-home

Resources on Artificial Intelligence:

2. Books:
   - Eric Topol- *Deep Medicine: How Artificial Intelligence Can Make Healthcare Human Again* first Edition Basic Books 2019.
   - Arjun Panesar. *Machine Learning and AI for Healthcare: Big Data for Improved Health Outcomes* Apress Books. February 5, 2019.
3. Website and Videos:
   - AI: Healthcare's new nervous system. https://www.accenture.com/us-en/insight-artificial-intelligence-healthcare%C2%A0
   - A Reality Check On Artificial Intelligence: Are Health Care Claims Overblown? Kaiser Health Organization. https://khn.org/news/a-reality-check-on-artificial-intelligence-are-health-care-claims-overblown/
   - Wired *Magazine's COVID-19 will accelerate AI in the Health Care Revolution.* https://www.wired.com/story/covid-19-will-accelerate-ai-health-care-revolution/
   - *National Academy of Medicine AI and Health Care.* https://nam.edu/event/webinar-artificial-intelligence-and-health-care/
   - *Healthcare IT News: The Vast promise (and very real hurdles) of healthcare AI.* https://www.healthcareitnews.com/video/vast-promise-and-major-challenges-healthcare-ai
   - *Initial Wins of AI.* https://youtu.be/j5ASmVnATc0
   - *The advent of AI in health care (Cleveland Clinic).* https://youtu.be/H0etieBDxeY
   - *Artificial Intelligence can change the future of medical diagnosis.* https://youtu.be/HrKzXLgGohA
   - *MD* vs Machine: Artificial Intelligence in Health Care. https://youtu.be/xSDf-ma4VEx8
   - Better *Medicine through machine learning.* https://youtu.be/Nj2YSLPn6OY
   - Artificial *Intelligence in Healthcare—It's about time.* https://youtu.be/3LkbUxqGTfo
   - The *state of artificial intelligence in medicine—Stanford Medicine.* https://youtu.be/PZQMyj-9z-w
   - Pratik *Shah: How AI is making it easier to diagnose disease.* https://www.ted.com/talks/pratik_shah_how_ai_is_making_it_easier_to_diagnose_disease
   - Rosalind *Picard: An AI smartwatch that detects seizures.* https://www.ted.com/talks/rosalind_picard_an_ai_smartwatch_that_detects_seizures
   - Sylvain *Duranton: How humans and AI can work together to create better businesses.* https://www.ted.com/talks/sylvain_duranton_how_humans_and_ai_can_work_together_to_create_better_businesses
   - *Anab Jain: Why we need to imagine different futures.* https://www.ted.com/talks/

anab_jain_why_we_need_to_imagine_different_futures

- *Cynthia Breazeal: The rise of personal robots.* https://www.ted.com/talks/cynthia_breazeal_the_rise_of_personal_robots

Resources on Data Visualization:

4. Books:
   - *Tufte* ER. The Visual Display of Quantitative Information: Graphics Press; 2001.
5. Website and Videos:
   - Andrew Abela's Chart Chooser (https://datavizblog.com/2013/04/29/andrew-abelas-chart-chooser/).
   - Visualizing Health. http://www.vizhealth.org
   - David McCandless: The beauty of data visualization. https://www.ted.com/talks/david_mccandless_the_beauty_of_data_visualization?language=en#t-732781
   - Agency for Healthcare Research and Quality. Data Visualizations. https://www.ahrq.gov/data/visualizations/index.html
   - Agency for Healthcare Research and Quality Research Data Infographics. https://www.ahrq.gov/data/infographics/index.html
   - University of Toledo. Locating Health Statistics. https://libguides.utoledo.edu/health_stats/data_visualization
   - National Center for Health Statistics. Data Visualization Gallery. https://www.cdc.gov/nchs/data-visualization/index.htm

Review Questions

1. Which one of the following option is an appropriate use of data analytics in health care?
   (a) Studying medical errors in clinical settings without notifying anyone know in the clinic.
   (b) Selling some individuals' complete health history to third parties for profit purposes.
   (c) Picking the embryo with the gender of preference by families in an embryo transplantation.
   (d) Pain tracking of a patient to recommend indivitdualized therapy.

2. Which of the following option is synonym for correctness dimension of EHR data quality according to Weiskpf et al. 2013?
   (a) Accessibility
   (b) Variation
   (c) Accuracy
   (d) Timeliness
3. Which of the below product is not considered an example of AI?
   (a) Chatbot that interacts with patients
   (b) Database that predicts mortality rates
   (c) Conversational agent that facilitates cognitive behavioral therapy
   (d) Facial recognition to assess pain
4. Which one of the following is an appropriate visualization option for qualitative data?
   (a) Bar charts
   (b) Word clouds
   (c) Scatter plots
   (d) Pie charts

Appendix: Answers to Review Questions

1. Which one of the following option is an appropriate use of data analytics in health care?
   (a) Studying medical errors in clinical settings without notifying anyone know in the clinic.
   (b) Selling some individuals' complete health history to third parties for profit purposes.
   (c) Picking the embryo with the gender of preference by families in an embryo transplantation.
   (d) Pain tracking of a patient to recommend indivitdualized therapy.

2. Which of the following option is synonym for correctness dimension of EHR data quality according to Weiskpf et al. 2013?
   (a) Accessibility
   (b) Variation
   (c) Accuracy
   (d) Timeliness

3. Which of the below product is not considered an example of AI?

(a) Chatbot that interacts with patients

(b) Database that predicts mortality rates

(c) Conversational agent that facilitates cognitive behavioral therapy

(d) Facial recognition to assess pain

4. Which one of the following is an appropriate visualization option for qualitative data?

(a) Bar charts

(b) Word clouds

(c) Scatter plots

(d) Pie charts

References

1. Matheny M, Thadaney Israni S, Ahmed M, Whicher D. Artificial intelligence in health care: the Hope, the hype, the promise, the peril. Washington, DC: National Academy of Medicine; 2019.
2. Ozkaynak M, Dziadkowiec O, Mistry R, Callahan T, He Z, Deakyne S, et al. Characterizing workflow for pediatric asthma patients in emergency departments using electronic health records. J Biomed Inform. 2015;57:386–98.
3. Jang H, Ozkaynak M, Amura CR, Ayer T, Sills MR. Analysis of medication patterns for pediatric asthma patients in emergency department: does the sequence placement of glucocorticoids administration matter? J Asthma. 2019;1-10
4. Jang H, Ozkaynak M, Ayer T, Sills M. Factors associated with first medication time for children treated in the emergency Department for Asthma. Pediatric Emergency Care Accepted.
5. Gillies RJ, Kinahan PE, Hricak H. Radiomics: images are more than pictures. They Are Data Radiology. 2016;278(2):563–77.
6. Demiris G, Thompson H. Smart homes and ambient assisted living applications: from data to knowledge-empowering or overwhelming older adults? Contribution of the IMIA smart homes and Ambiant assisted living working group. Yearb Med Inform. 2011;6:51–7.
7. Le T, Reeder B, Chung J, Thompson H, Demiris G. Design of smart home sensor visualizations for older adults. Technol Health Care. 2014;22:657–66.
8. Gittelman S, Lange V, Gotway Crawford CA, Okoro CA, Lieb E, Dhingra SS, et al. A new source of data for public health surveillance: Facebook likes. J Med Internet Res. 2015;17(4):e98.
9. Kuehn BM. Twitter streams fuel big data approaches to health forecasting. JAMA. 2015;314(19):2010–2.
10. Lorgelly PK, Doble B, Knott RJ. Realising the value of linked data to health economic analy-

ses of cancer care: a case study of cancer 2015. PharmacoEconomics. 2016;34(2):139–54.
11. Weng C, Kahn MG. Clinical research informatics for big data and precision medicine. Yearb Med Inform. 2016;1:211–8.
12. Kahn MG, Brown JS, Chun AT, Davidson BN, Meeker D, Ryan PB, et al. Transparent reporting of data quality in distributed data networks. EGEMS (Wash DC). 2015;3(1):1052.
13. Wang RY, Strong DM. Beyond accuracy: what data quality means to data consumers. J Manag Inf Syst. 1996;12(4):5–33.
14. Weiskopf NG, Weng C. Methods and dimensions of electronic health record data quality assessment: enabling reuse for clinical research. J Am Med Inform Assoc. 2013;20(1):144–51.
15. Kahn MG, Callahan TJ, Barnard J, Bauck AE, Brown J, Davidson BN, et al. A harmonized data quality assessment terminology and framework for the secondary use of electronic health record data. EGEMS (Wash DC). 2016;4(1):1244.
16. Kushniruk AW. Analysis of complex decision-making processes in health care: cognitive approaches to health informatics. J Biomed Inform. 2001;34(5):365–76.
17. Patel VL, Arocha JF, Kaufman DR. A primer on aspects of cognition for medical informatics. J Am Med Inform Assoc. 2001;8(4):324–43.
18. Naylor CD. On the prospects for a (deep) learning health care system. JAMA. 2018;320(11):1099–100.
19. Turing AM. Computing machinery and intelligence. Mind. 1950;LIX(236):433–60. https://doi.org/10.1093/mind/LIX.236.433.
20. Rouse M. Turing Test 2019. Available from: https://searchenterpriseai.techtarget.com/definition/Turing-test
21. McCarthy J, Minsky ML, Rochester N, Shannon CE. A proposal for the Dartmouth summer research project on artificial intelligence. 1955.
22. Bengio Y, Shladover SE, Russel S. The rise of AI. Sci Am. 2016:44–5.
23. Kulikowski CA. Beginnings of artificial intelligence in medicine (AIM): computational artifice assisting scientific inquiry and clinical art–with reflections on present AIM challenges. Yearb Med Inform. 2019;28(1):249–56.
24. Schwartz WB. Medicine and the computer. The promise and problems of change. N Engl J Med. 1970;283(23):1257–64.
25. Shortliffe E. Computer-based medical consultations: MYCIN. New York, NY: Elsevier; 1976.
26. Skiba DJ. Augmented intelligence and nursing. Nurs Educ Perspect. 2017;38(2):108–9.
27. Ryan SA. An expert system for nursing practice: clinical decision support. In: Saba VK, Rieder KA, Pocklington DB, editors. Nursing and computers: an anthology. New York, NY: Springer; 1989. p. 270–83.
28. Cuddigan JE, Norris J, Ryan SA, Evans S. Validating the knowledge in a computer-based consultant for nursing care. Proc Annu Symp Comput Appl Med Care. 1987;74-8

29. West D. What is artificial intelligence 2018. Available from: https://www.brookings.edu/research/what-is-artificial-intelligence/

30. McGrow K. Artificial intelligence: essentials for nursing. Nursing. 2019;49(9):46–9.

31. Pan Y. Heading toward artificial intelligence 2.0. Engineering. 2016;2(4):409–13.

32. Marr B. What everyone should know about cognitive computing 2016. Available from: https://www.forbes.com/sites/bernardmarr/2016/03/23/what-every-one-should-know-about-cognitive-computing/#e4068bf5d6e7

33. Kelly JE. Computing, cognition and the future of knowing: how humans and machines are forging a new age of understanding [IBM Research White Paper] 2016. Available from: https://www.research.ibm.com/software/IBMResearch/multimedia/Computing_Cognition_WhitePaper.pdf

34. Lim S, Tucker CS, Kumara S. An unsupervised machine learning model for discovering latent infectious diseases using social media data. J Biomed Inform. 2017;66:82–94.

35. Jordan MI, Mitchell TM. Machine learning: trends, perspectives, and prospects. Science. 2015;349(6245):255–60.

36. Yom-Tov E, Feraru G, Kozdoba M, Mannor S, Tennenholtz M, Hochberg I. Encouraging physical activity in patients with diabetes: intervention using a reinforcement learning system. J Med Internet Res. 2017;19(10):e338.

37. Executive Office of the President. Artificial intelligence, automation, and the economy 2016. Available from: https://obamawww.whitehouse.archives.gov/sites/whitehouse.gov/files/documents/Artificial-Intelligence-Automation-Economy.pdf

38. Roski J, Chapman W, Heffner J, Trivedi R, Del Fiol G, Kukafka R, et al. How artificial intelligence is changing health and healthcare. In: Matheny M, Israni ST, Ahmed M, editors. Artificial intelligence in health care: the Hope, the hype, the promise, the peril. Washington, DC: National Academy of Medicine; 2019.

39. Fitzpatrick KK, Darcy A, Vierhile M. Delivering cognitive behavior therapy to young adults with symptoms of depression and anxiety using a fully automated conversational agent (WoeBot): a randomized controlled trial. JMIR Ment Health. 2017;4(2):e19.

40. Hauser-Ulrich S, Künzli H, Meier-Peterhans D, Kowatsch T. A smartphone-based health care Chatbot to promote self-Management of Chronic Pain (SELMA): pilot randomized controlled trial. JMIR Mhealth Uhealth. 2020;8(4):e15806.

41. Dankwa-Mullan I, Rivo M, Sepulveda M, Park Y, Snowdon J, Rhee K. Transforming diabetes care through artificial intelligence: the future is here. Popul Health Manag. 2019;22(3):229–42.

42. Zhang W, Yu Q, Siddiquie B, Divakaran A, Sawhney H. "Snap-n-eat": food recognition and nutrition estimation on a smartphone. J Diabetes Sci Technol. 2015;9(3):525–33.

43. Cvetković B, Janko V, Romero AE, Kafalı Ö, Stathis K, Luštrek M. Activity recognition for diabetic patients using a smartphone. J Med Syst. 2016;40(12):256.

44. Wang L, Pedersen PC, Strong DM, Tulu B, Agu E, Ignotz R. Smartphone-based wound assessment system for patients with diabetes. IEEE Trans Biomed Eng. 2015;62(2):477–88.

45. Bose E, Radhakrishnan K. Using unsupervised machine learning to identify subgroups among home health patients with heart failure using telehealth. Comput Inform Nurs. 2018;36(5):242–8.

46. Middleton K, Butt M, Hammerla N, Hamblin S, Mehta K, Parsa A. Sorting out symptoms: design and evaluation of the "Babylon check" automated triage system. arXiv. 2016;

47. Robert N. How artificial intelligence is changing nursing. Nurs Manag. 2019;50(9)

48. Price WM. Risks and remedies for artificial intelligence in health care 2019. Available from: https://www.brookings.edu/research/risk-and-remedies-for-artificial-intelligence-in-health-care

49. Horvitz E, Mulligan D. Data, privacy, and the greater good. Science. 2015;349(6245):253–5.

50. McCarthy MK. Artificial intelligence in health: ethical considerations for research and practice 2019.

51. Martinez-Martin N. What are important ethical implications of using facial recognition technology in health care? AMA J Ethics. 2019;21(2):E180–7.

52. Balthazar P, Harri P, Prater A, Safdar NM. Protecting your Patients' interests in the era of big data, artificial intelligence, and predictive analytics. J Am Coll Radiol. 2018;15(3 Pt B):580–6.

53. Sullivan HR, Schweikart SJ. Are current tort liability doctrines adequate for addressing injury caused by AI? AMA J Ethics. 2019;21(2):E160–6.

54. Nundy S, Montgomery T, Wachter RM. Promoting trust between patients and physicians in the era of artificial intelligence. JAMA. 2019;322(6):497–8.

55. Eppler MJ, Mengis J. The concept of information overload–a review of literature from organization science, accounting, marketing, MIS, and related disciplines (2004). In: Meckel M, Schmid BF, editors. Kommunikationsmanagement im Wandel: Beiträge aus 10 Jahren =mcminstitute. Wiesbaden: Gabler; 2008. p. 271–305.

56. Keim D, Andrienko G, Fekete J-D, Görg C, Kohlhammer J, Melançon G. Visual analytics: definition, process and challenges. In: Kerren A, Stasko JT, Fekete J-D, North C, editors. Information visualization–human-centered issues and perspectives. Springer; 2008. p. 154–75.

57. Thomas J, Cook K. Illuminating the path: the research and development agenda for visual analytics. IEEE Comput Soc Press; 2005.

58. Tufte ER. Beautiful evidence: graphis Pr; 2006.

59. Zhu Y. Measuring effective data visualization. Advances in visual computing. Berlin, Heidelberg: Springer Berlin Heidelberg; 2007.

60. Johnston SC. Anticipating and training the physician of the future: the importance of caring in an age of artificial intelligence. Acad Med. 2018;93(8):1105–6.

61. Wartman SA, Combs CD. Medical education must move from the information age to the age of artificial intelligence. Acad Med. 2018;93(8):1107–9.

Part IV
Interoperable Systems

Interoperability: There is no Digital Health without Health IT Standards

20

Joyce Sensmeier

Learning Objectives
- Define interoperability in the context of a digital health ecosystem.
- Describe the role of data standards in achieving interoperability.
- Delineate data standards categories and initiatives.
- Identify the key approaches for achieving health information exchange.
- Explore the drivers of standards implementation and adoption.

Key Terms
- Application Programming Interface
- Data Standards
- Digital Health
- Health Information Exchange
- Interoperability
- Terminology

Introduction

Today's healthcare environment expects interoperability and information exchange across the continuum of care to ensure patient safety, inform decision-making and improve health outcomes. For decades, the healthcare industry has expressed the need and vision for the exchange of electronic health information, and a multitude of well-intentioned efforts have been launched to address the interoperability challenge. Across the globe, numerous entities have developed methods for sharing data among providers, patients and other authorized parties to revolutionize the delivery of care. However, to truly achieve this goal, stakeholders must embrace, widely adopt and implement standards-based, interoperable health information technology (IT) systems.

Interoperability (or the lack of) continues to be a high-profile topic today. Yet, in spite of our best collective efforts, we are still unable to ensure that individuals and their healthcare providers have ready access to health information whenever and wherever it is needed, governed by the appropriate privacy and security requirements. One roadblock to widespread interoperability is that healthcare stakeholders are used to working in silos, with information tailored primarily to individual requirements, or those of their organization. For decades, hospitals and other provider organizations have cobbled together systems using proprietary interfaces, focusing on their specific integration needs.

Bridging the information gap between individuals and their health systems to advance health and wellness is dependent on the transformation of today's healthcare environment toward a digitally enabled health ecosystem. According to the Healthcare Information and Management

J. Sensmeier (✉)
HIMSS, Chicago, USA

© Springer Nature Switzerland AG 2022
U. H. Hübner et al. (eds.), *Nursing Informatics*, Health Informatics,
https://doi.org/10.1007/978-3-030-91237-6_20

285

Systems Society (HIMSS), "digital health connects and empowers people and populations to manage their health and wellness, augmented by accessible and supportive provider teams working within flexible, integrated, interoperable and digitally-enabled care environments that strategically leverage digital tools, technologies and services to transform care delivery" [1].

Aligning individuals, populations and health teams to optimize health and wellness is a key outcome of the interoperability component of digital health systems. Interoperability is a critical foundation of health systems to enable data that are seamlessly available across multiple sources [2]. Realizing the vision of a digital health ecosystem will make it possible for an individual to share health information with formalized health system teams when and where connectivity is needed.

Defining the Role of Interoperability in the Digital Health Ecosystem

In the digital health ecosystem, interoperability advances the goal of optimizing health by providing seamless access to the right information needed to more comprehensively understand and address the health of individuals and populations. According to HIMSS [3], interoperability is "the ability of different information systems, devices and applications ('systems') to access, exchange, integrate and cooperatively use data in a coordinated manner, within and across organizational, regional and national boundaries, to provide timely and seamless portability of information and optimize the health of individuals and populations globally. Health data exchange architectures, application interfaces and standards enable data to be accessed and shared appropriately and securely across the complete spectrum of care, within all applicable settings and with relevant stakeholders, including by the individual." This comprehensive definition was updated in 2019 to better reflect the evolving healthcare environment.

Health IT systems, or applications, participating in information exchange do so with variable degrees of interoperability. As described in Fig. 20.1, each level of interoperability defines the type of information exchange that entities may simultaneously engage in [3].

Countries and territories across the globe sit at varying stages of adoption and implementation of standards-based, interoperable health IT sys-

Four Levels of Interoperability

Foundational- establishes the inter-connectivity requirements needed for one system or application to securely communicate data to and receive data from another

Structural- defines the format, syntax, and organization of data exchange including at the data field level for interpretation

Semantic- provide for common underlying models and condification of the data including the use of data elements with standardized definitions from publicly available value sets and coding vocabularies, providing shared understanding and meaning to the user

Organizational- includes governance, policy, social, legal and organizational considerations to facilitate the secure, seamless and timely communication and use of data both within and between organizations, entities and individuals. These components enable shared consent, trust and integrated end-user processes and workflows.

Fig. 20.1 Four levels of interoperability. Source: Healthcare information and management system society

tems. Thus, harmonization is necessary in promoting the interoperability of health information and empowering patients with their own data. Some of the key barriers to interoperability include the following elements as described by the Global Digital Health Partnership [4]:

- Lack of electronic health record (EHR) capability to take action based on exchanged data
- Poor usability of EHRs and negative impact on provider workflows
- Lack of universal adoption of standards-based EHRs
- Increasing cost due to interoperability infrastructure that is unaffordable
- Challenges managing coordinated action among and across multiple organizations
- Economic incentives that do not encourage data exchange

Overcoming these barriers will require advancing both near- and long-term strategies [5]. In the near term, aligning on a clear definition of interoperability, and widely adopting and implementing standards-based, interoperable health IT systems will bear fruit. Long-term strategies rely on embracing a culture shift wherein interoperability is driven by transparency, value and innovation.

Overview of Current Data Standards, Categories and Initiatives

The global standards landscape consists of multiple entities, systems, regulations, protocols and processes. Governments and the private sector participate in international standards activities in a variety of ways: through global treaty organizations where governments are members; through private, voluntary organizations where each country is represented by a single "national body" organization; through professional and technical organizations with individual or organizational members; and through industry consortia [6].

Global standardization is best achieved through domain-specific activities and through alliances and processes supported by associations, companies, standards development organizations (SDOs), consortia and collaborative projects. Organizations such as consortia that enable worldwide participation of stakeholders are creating an innovative environment that evolves with the changing needs of the global marketplace. Users of standards are increasingly aware of their importance and expect an ecosystem that can produce and deliver standards with maximum efficiency and minimum cost, eliminate duplication and optimize ease of adoption. SDOs work to create consensus within a community of practitioners before releasing a standard. Governments rely on voluntary consensus standards in regulation and procurement to minimize additional regulatory requirements. Voluntary consensus standards are the foundation of global commerce, providing the "essential infrastructure," or recipe that enables interoperability to achieve widespread health information exchange (HIE).

Data Standards Categories

A wide range of SDOs operate in the arena of healthcare interoperability, sharing the field with as few overlaps as possible, such as Health Level Seven (HL7) for health data communication, SNOMED CT and LOINC for terminologies, and DICOM for medical image processing [7]. Data standards can also reference implementation specifications, or profiles which provide a more detailed description of the method or approach for implementing a standard or multiple standards for a particular use. Standards from non-healthcare-specific standards organizations are also used within healthcare, such as W3C, OASIS and IETF for Internet standards, and IEEE for device communications.

This complex picture also includes international, regional and national standards bodies (ISO, CEN, NIST, etc.) which publish standards while ensuring collaboration with other SDOs through liaison roles in order to avoid duplication. However, having a host of standards to pick from can be confusing, especially as the various available standards have been developed for different purposes and designed to accomplish entirely different objectives [8].

For the purposes of describing the health data standards landscape, we suggest four broad categories [9]. Services/exchange standards are used to establish a common, predictable, secure communication protocol between systems (i.e., infrastructure). Vocabulary/code sets/terminology standards consist of nomenclatures and code sets used to describe clinical problems and procedures, medications and allergies (i.e., semantics). Content/structure standards are used for sharing clinical information such as clinical summaries, prescriptions and structured electronic documents (i.e., syntax). Administrative standards are used for payment, operations and other non-clinical interoperability needs.

Services/Exchange Standards

Services/exchange standards primarily address the format of messages that are exchanged between information systems, document architecture, clinical templates, the user interface and patient data linkage. To achieve compatibility between systems, it is necessary to have prior agreement on the infrastructure of the messages to be exchanged. The receiving system must be able to divide the incoming message into discrete data elements that reflect what the sending system wishes to communicate.

The following section describes some of the major entities involved in publishing services/exchange standards.

Personal Connected Health Alliance The Personal Connected Health Alliance (PCHAlliance) publishes and promotes the Continua Design Guidelines. These guidelines provide an open implementation framework for authentic, end-to-end interoperability of personal connected health devices and health IT systems. They are built upon common international standards defined by recognized SDOs. The guidelines further clarify the underlying standards or specifications by reducing options or by adding missing features to improve interoperability, with

a specific focus on personal health devices. Continua also develops commercial ready source code that simplifies and accelerates implementation of the capabilities described within the framework [10].

Health Level Seven Health Level Seven (HL7) develops standards in multiple categories, including services/exchange and content that are widely adopted in healthcare. Numerous HL7 standards focus on facilitating the exchange of data to support clinical practice within and across organizations. HL7 standards cover a broad spectrum of information exchange vehicles, including medical orders, clinical observations, test results, admission/transfer/discharge data, document architecture, clinical templates, user interface, EHR data and billing information. Consolidated CDA (C-CDA) is an HL7 standard that defines the structure of specific medical records, such as discharge summaries and progress notes, serving as a structured way to exchange this information between providers and patients while preserving its meaning.

HL7 FHIR (Fast Healthcare Interoperability Resources) is an emerging standard describing data formats and elements (known as "resources") and a web-based Application Programming Interface (API) for exchanging health information. An API is a set of routines, protocols and tools for building software applications, and specifying how the software components, or building blocks, should interact [11]. APIs are used when building graphical user interfaces. The FHIR specification is rapidly being adopted as a next-generation standards framework for the exchange of EHR data due to the ease of implementation.

Institute of Electrical and Electronic Engineers The Institute of Electrical and Electronic Engineers (IEEE) has developed a series of standards known collectively as P1073 Medical Information Bus (MIB), which support real-time, continuous and comprehensive capture and communication of data from bedside medical devices such as those found in intensive care units, operating rooms and emergency departments. These data include physiological parameter measurements and device settings. IEEE 11073 standards are designed to help healthcare product vendors and integrators create interoperable devices and systems for disease management, health and fitness.

Integrating the Healthcare Enterprise Integrating the Healthcare Enterprise (IHE) is an international standards-profiling organization that publishes a detailed framework for constraining multiple standards to address specific use cases, filling the gaps between standards and their implementation. Through its profiling process, IHE enables the coordinated use of standards such as DICOM and HL7 to address specific clinical needs in support of optimal patient care. IHE has published a large body of specifications made up of domain-specific integration profiles that are being implemented globally by healthcare providers and regional entities to enable standards-based safe, secure and efficient health information exchange.

World Wide Web Consortium The World Wide Web Consortium (W3C) is the primary international standards organization for development of World Wide Web infrastructure. W3C publishes transport protocols, including the Representational State Transfer (REST) architectural style, which was developed in parallel with the Hypertext Transfer Protocol (HTTP), used in web browsers. The largest known implementation of a system conforming to the REST architectural style is the World Wide Web.

Content/Structure Standards

Content/structure standards define the structure and content organization of the electronic message or document's information content. They also define a "package" of content standards (messages or documents) which, when grouped together, make up the syntax of a message. Content is typically structured by data elements, including data collected on people, events or encounters. Unstructured data are not organized in a pre-defined manner, and are typically docu-

mented as text, but may also contain dates, numbers or facts.

The following section describes some of the major entities involved in publishing content/structure standards.

Clinical Data Interchange Standards Consortium The Clinical Data Interchange Standards Consortium (CDISC) is a global, multidisciplinary consortium that has established standards to support the acquisition, exchange, submission and archive of clinical research data and metadata. CDISC foundational standards are the basis of the complete suite of standards, supporting clinical and non-clinical research processes from end to end. Foundational standards focus on the core principles for defining data standards and include models, domains and specifications for data representation. CDISC develops and supports global, platform-independent data standards that enable information system interoperability to improve medical research and related areas of healthcare.

National Council for Prescription Drug Programs The National Council for Prescription Drug Programs (NCPDP) develops both content and transport standards for information processing in the pharmacy services sector of the healthcare industry. Electronic prescription transactions consist of messages flowing between healthcare providers (i.e., pharmacy software systems and prescriber software systems) that represent prescription orders. NCPDP's Telecommunication Standard Version 5.1 was named the official standard for pharmacy claims within the Health Insurance Portability and Accountability Act (HIPAA). Other NCPDP standards include the NCPDP SCRIPT standard for electronic prescribing.

National Electrical Manufacturers Association The National Electrical Manufacturers Association (NEMA), in collaboration with the American College of Radiologists (ACR) and others, formed DICOM (Digital Imaging and Communications in Medicine) to develop a generic digital format and a transfer protocol for biomedical images and image-related information. DICOM enables the transfer of medical images in a multi-vendor environment and facilitates the development and expansion of picture archiving and communication systems (PACS). The DICOM standard is the dominant international data interchange message format for biomedical imaging.

Vocabulary/Code Sets/Terminology

A fundamental requirement for effective communication is the ability to clearly and accurately interpret concepts shared between the sender and the receiver of the message. Natural human languages are complex in their ability to communicate subtle differences in the semantic meaning of messages. Most communication between health IT systems relies on the use of structured vocabularies, terminologies, code sets and classification systems to represent health information. Standardized terminologies enable data collection at the point of care and retrieval of data, information and knowledge in support of optimal clinical practice.

The following section describes some of the major entities involved in publishing vocabulary/code sets/terminology standards.

Current Procedural Terminology The Current Procedural Terminology (CPT) code set, maintained by the American Medical Association (AMA), describes medical, surgical and diagnostic services. It is designed to communicate uniform information about medical services and procedures among physicians, nurses, coders, patients, accreditation organizations and payers for administrative, financial and analytical purposes. In addition to descriptive terms and codes, it contains modifiers, notes and guidelines to facilitate correct usage.

International Statistical Classification of Diseases and Related Health Problems: Tenth Revision International Statistical Classification of Diseases and Related Health Problems (ICD) is a medical classification list published by the World Health Organization (WHO). It contains codes for diseases, signs and symptoms, abnormal findings, complaints, social circumstances and external causes of injury or diseases. For disease reporting, the United States utilizes its own national variant of ICD-10 called the ICD-10 Clinical Modification (ICD-10-CM). A procedural classification called ICD-10 Procedure Coding System (ICD-10-PCS) has also been developed for capturing inpatient procedures.

LOINC Logical Observation Identifiers Names and Codes (LOINC) is the international standard developed and maintained by the Regenstrief Institute for identifying health measurements, observations and documents. LOINC enables the exchange and aggregation of clinical results for care delivery, outcomes management and research by providing a set of universal codes and structured names to unambiguously identify things you can measure or observe. Since its inception, the LOINC database has expanded to include not just medical and laboratory code names but also nursing diagnosis, nursing interventions, outcomes classification and a patient care data set.

NEMSIS The National Emergency Medical Services Information System (NEMSIS), administered by the National Highway Traffic Safety Administration's Office of Emergency Medical Services, provides a universal standard for the collection and transmission of emergency medical services (EMS) operations and patient care data. NEMSIS provides the framework for collecting, storing and sharing standardized EMS data from states nationwide. Data from NEMSIS is also used to benchmark performance, determine the effectiveness of clinical interventions and facilitate cost-benefit analyses.

Nursing Terminologies The American Nurses Association (ANA) has recognized the following nursing terminologies that support nursing practice: ABC Codes, Clinical Care Classification, International Classification of Nursing Practice, LOINC, North American Nursing Diagnosis Association, Nursing Interventions Classification (NIC), Nursing Outcomes Classification (NOC), Nursing Management Minimum Data Set, Nursing Minimum Data Set, Omaha System,

Patient Care Data Set (retired), Perioperative Nursing Data Set and SNOMED-CT. These standard terminologies enable knowledge representation of nursing content. Nurses use assessment data and nursing judgment to determine nursing diagnoses, interventions and outcomes. These nursing terminologies have become a significant vehicle for facilitating interoperability between different concepts, nomenclatures and information systems [12].

RxNorm RxNorm is used as a tool for supporting semantic interoperability between drug terminologies and pharmacy knowledge base systems, serving as a normalized naming system for generic and branded drugs. The National Library of Medicine (NLM) produces RxNorm, which is used by hospitals, pharmacies and other organizations to record and process drug information. RxNorm provides normalized names and unique identifiers for medications and over the counter drugs in the United States.

SNOMED International SNOMED International owns and maintains SNOMED CT, the global common language for health terms. SNOMED CT is a resource with comprehensive, scientifically validated clinical content that enables consistent representation of clinical content in EHRs. The NLM distributes SNOMED CT-related files to licensed individuals in the United States via the Unified Medical Language System terminology services.

Unified Medical Language System The Unified Medical Language System (UMLS) is a set of files and software that brings together many health and biomedical vocabularies and standards to enable interoperability between information systems. The UMLS integrates and distributes key terminology, classification and coding standards, and associated resources to promote creation of more effective and interoperable biomedical information systems and services, including EHRs. The NLM licenses and distributes the UMLS in its role as the central coordinating body for clinical terminology standards within the U.S. Department of Health and Human Services (HHS).

Administrative Standards

Administrative standards and implementation specifications are used in healthcare for payment, operations and other non-clinical interoperability needs. These standards outline the requirements for electronic business transactions, operating rules, privacy, security protocols and authentication.

The following section describes some of the major entities involved in publishing administrative standards.

Accredited Standards Committee X12N Accredited Standards Committee (ASC) X12N has developed a broad range of electronic data interchange standards to facilitate electronic business transactions. In healthcare, X12N standards have been adopted as national standards for such administrative transactions as claims, enrollment and eligibility in health plans, and first report of injury under the requirements of the Health Insurance Portability and Accountability Act (HIPAA) of 1996. HIPAA directed the Secretary of HHS to adopt standards for transactions to enable health information to be exchanged electronically, and the Administrative Simplification Act (ASA), one of the HIPAA provisions, requires standard formats to be used for electronically submitted healthcare transactions.

CAQH CORE Operating Rules CAQH CORE is a multi-stakeholder collaboration of more than 110 organizations, including providers, health plans, vendors, government agencies and standard-setting bodies that work together to publish operating rules to simplify healthcare administrative transactions. These operating rules leverage a range of existing standards to make electronic data transactions more predictable and consistent, regardless of the technology. CAQH CORE has been designated by the Secretary of HHS as the author for federally mandated operating rules per Sect. 1104 of the Patient Protection and Affordable Care Act (ACA).

Health Insurance Portability and Accountability Act To reduce paperwork, streamline business processes and protect the privacy and security of certain health information across the healthcare system, the Health Insurance Portability and Accountability Act (HIPAA) of 1996 and the Patient Protection and Affordable Care Act (ACA) set national standards for electronic transactions, code sets and unique identifiers. The Administrative Simplification provisions of HIPAA apply to the adoption of electronic transaction standards and operating rules for use in the healthcare industry.

HIPAA Security Standards for the Protection of Electronic Health Information were developed to protect electronic health information and implement reasonable and appropriate administrative safeguards that establish the foundation for a covered entity's security program. Prior to HIPAA, no generally accepted set of security standards or general requirements for protecting health information existed.

Internet Engineering Task Force The Internet Engineering Task Force (IETF) is an open international community of network designers, operators, vendors and researchers focused on the evolution of Internet architecture and the smooth operation of the Internet. IETF has published and maintains OAuth which is the industry-standard protocol for authentication. OAuth is an open standard for access delegation, commonly used as a way for Internet users to grant websites or applications access to their information on other websites but without giving them the passwords.

Multiple standards development efforts, some collaborative, some competing, have long been underway to advance the goal of interoperability, but those efforts have not, until now, provided us with clear guidance on what are the "best available" standards and implementation specifications to use. The Interoperability Standards Advisory (ISA) [13] process represents the model by which the Office of the National Coordinator for Health Information Technology (ONC) coordinates the identification, assessment and public awareness of data standards and implementation specifications, or profiles, that can be used by the healthcare industry to address specific interoperability needs. These needs include, but are not limited to, interoperability for clinical, public health, research and administrative purposes.

ONC encourages all stakeholders to implement and use the standards and implementation specifications identified in the ISA as applicable to the specific interoperability needs they seek to address. Each standard or specification included in the ISA is characterized by the level of maturity and adoption, whether it is federally required, cost and the availability of test tools. With this publication, ONC has taken a non-regulatory, practical approach, including an interactive, predictable process for annual updates. The ISA provides a single, public list of the best-available standards and implementation specifications reflecting on-going dialogue, debate and consensus. The ISA also enables a 'first pass' viewpoint for standards selection by government programs, procurements, testing or certification programs, and standards-profiling efforts.

Interoperability Initiatives

As a result of the expanding health data standards landscape, new interoperability opportunities, initiatives and industry consortia are continually being formed. This evolving ecosystem creates the need for an interactive resource that is current, factual and curated. To this end, HIMSS has published the *Interoperability Initiatives Environmental Scan* [14], which provides a review of the current landscape of networks, initiatives and frameworks which support interoperable, nationwide health information exchange. The Environmental Scan is a dynamic resource which incorporates relevant information about key interoperability initiatives within the United States, including an overview of types of exchange services, data being exchanged, covered, onboarding requirements and business models.

The United States Nationwide Interoperability Roadmap [15] is a timely resource that defines a Learning Health System. The Learning Health System describes a future state where

- individuals are at the center of their care;
- all stakeholders are able to securely, effectively and efficiently contribute, share and analyze data;
- providers and patients have a seamless ability to securely access and use health information from different sources and technologies;
- an individual's health information is not limited to what is stored in EHRs, but includes information from many different sources and care-settings;
- technologies that individuals use are featured, and this future state portrays a longitudinal picture of their health, not just episodes of care;
- diagnostic tests are only repeated when necessary, because the information is readily available; and
- public health agencies and researchers can rapidly learn, develop, test and deploy the very best in clinical, evidence-based guidelines.

The Learning Health System, once realized, should lower healthcare costs, improve population health, empower individuals and drive innovation.

ONC has also outlined a set of Guiding Principles [16] to help the United States achieve its ten-year vision of the future interoperable health IT ecosystem:

- *Build upon the existing health IT infrastructure.* Significant investments have been made in health IT across the ecosystem. To the extent possible, we must encourage stakeholders to build from existing health IT infrastructure, increasing interoperability and functionality as needed.
- *One size does not fit all.* We will strive for baseline interoperability across health IT infrastructure, while allowing innovators and technologists to vary the user experience in order to best meet the user's needs based on the scenario at hand, technology available, workflow design, personal preferences and other factors.
- *Empower individuals.* Health information from the care delivery system should be easily accessible to individuals and empower them to become more active partners in their health just as other kinds of data are empowering them in other aspects of their lives.
- *Leverage the market.* Demand for interoperability from health IT users is a powerful driver to advance our vision. As payment and care delivery reform increase the demand for interoperability, we will work with and support these efforts.
- *Simplify.* Where possible, simpler solutions should be implemented first, with allowance for more complex methods in the future.
- *Maintain modularity.* Complex systems are more resilient to change when they are divided into independent components that can be connected together. Modularity creates flexibility that allows innovation and adoption of new, more efficient approaches over time without overhauling entire systems.
- *Consider the current environment and support multiple levels of advancement.* We must account for a range of capabilities among information sources and information users, including EHR and non-EHR users. Individuals and caregivers need to find, send, receive and use their own health information both within and outside the care delivery system and the interoperable infrastructure should enable this.
- *Focus on value.* We will strive to make sure our interoperability efforts yield the greatest value to individuals and care providers; improved health, healthcare and lower costs should be measurable over time and at a minimum, offset the resource investment.
- *Protect privacy and security in all aspects of interoperability.* To better establish and maintain trust, we will strive to ensure that appropriate, strong and effective safeguards for health information are in place as interoperability advances across the industry. We will also support greater transparency for individuals regarding the business practices of entities that use their data.

These Guiding Principles are intended to inform our work as we improve the interoperability of health information systems, devices and networks, and scale existing approaches for fluidly exchanging health information across the health ecosystem to optimally support the continuum of care and inform population health.

Each of these interoperability initiatives outlines best practices and highlights current successes taking place within the digital health ecosystem. They also emphasize the importance of embracing an environment that will empower and engage individuals in their own health management.

Leveraging Data Standards to Achieve Health Information Exchange

The goal of health information exchange is to facilitate access and retrieval of clinical data to provide safe, timely, efficient, effective, equitable, patient-centered care. Health Information Exchanges (HIE)s are entities that provide the capability to electronically move clinical information among disparate health information systems and maintain the meaning of the information being exchanged [17]. The term "HIE" is generally used as either a verb or a noun. HIE as a verb means the act of exchanging electronic information to deliver better patient-centered care. HIE as a noun refers to an entity that has agreed upon the governance, policies, trust and/or the collaboration necessary to provide a successful HIE framework.

There are several types of HIE entities currently operating across the United States and its territories. State-wide HIEs are run by the governments of their respective states. Some statewide, or regional, HIEs use an umbrella approach, serving as the aggregator for multiple disparate private health information exchanges. Regional or community HIEs are interorganizational and depend on a variety of funding sources. Most are non-profit. Private or proprietary HIEs are made up of a single community or network, often based within a single organization, which executes overall management, finance and governance. Examples of private HIE's include hospital/integrated delivery networks (IDN), payer-based, or

disease-specific HIEs. Hybrid HIE's may consist of collaborations between organizations, such as an accountable care organization, or a vendor network of clients, operating within a state or region.

Health information exchange entities can provide many important benefits for providers, patients and health systems, such as

- enhanced care coordination through shared communication of essential information for optimal patient care. Due to this shared communication, HIEs can reduce, or even eliminate, redundant and unnecessary testing;
- timely access to the right information for providers, patients and all other stakeholders;
- improved efficiency and reliability through the elimination of unnecessary paperwork and access to clinical decision support tools; and
- improved quality and safety by reducing medication and medical errors.

There are three primary HIE architectures. In a centralized architecture, patient data are collected and stored in a central repository, data warehouse or other databases. This HIE architecture allows full control over the data, including the ability to authenticate, authorize and record transactions among participants. In a federated or decentralized architecture, interconnected but independent databases allow for data sharing and exchange, granting users access to the information only when needed. The third type of HIE architecture is the hybrid architecture which incorporates variations of federated and centralized architectures to leverage the advantages of each. Hybrid HIEs are becoming increasingly common as various combinations of available services are implemented.

Today there are many successful HIEs exchanging and sharing data across the United States. The eHealth Exchange is the largest health data-sharing network in the United States, with connectivity spanning across all 50 states [18]. The eHealth Exchange network includes exchange partners who securely share clinical information over the Internet using a standardized approach. By leveraging a common set of standards, legal agreement and governance, eHealth Exchange participants are able to securely share health information with each other, without additional customization and individual legal agreements.

Carequality is an interoperability framework, or network of networks, that leverages common rules, well-defined standards-based technical specifications and a participant directory to enable its participants, HIE networks, vendors, payers and others, to establish connectivity across the U.S. health ecosystem [19]. The Carequality Framework consists of multiple elements, including legal terms, policy requirements, technical specifications and governance processes, which operationalize data sharing under principles of trust. The participants benefit from accelerated, less costly health-data-sharing agreements, because they no longer need to develop individual legal agreements between each data-sharing partner.

San Diego Health Connect [20] is an example of a community-wide HIE that securely connects hospitals, health systems, patients, private HIEs and other healthcare stakeholders. As a not-for-profit organization, San Diego Health Connect serves the San Diego health ecosystem. The EMS Hub is one type of service they provide to close the gap that exists between the transporting EMS service and the receiving hospital. Using wireless technology, the Hub transmits pre-hospital data from EMS vehicles in route to the hospital. Because emergency departments (ED) receive this health information—such as electrocardiograms—from EMS before the patient arrives, ED staff are able to appropriately prepare resources and reduce time to treatment.

The Strategic Health Information Exchange Collaborative (SHIEC) [21] is a member organization that serves as a forum for HIEs to work collaboratively together, sharing best practices and identifying joint solutions to address individual and collective needs. SHIEC has the capacity to influence legislation relevant to the common business interests of its members. It also provides education regarding the benefits, functions and roles of HIEs. SHIEC promotes the improvement of business conditions for sustainability of HIEs, acting on behalf of its members to achieve economies of scale without compromising the ability of each member to serve local interests.

Influencers and Accelerators of Standards Implementation and Adoption

The Twenty-first-century Cures Act, published by HHS in 2020, holds public and private entities in the United States accountable for enabling easy, appropriate access to electronic health information. The ONC Final Rule establishes new regulations to prevent information-blocking practices and anti-competitive behaviors by healthcare providers, developers of certified health IT products, HIEs and other information networks. The rule updates certification requirements for health IT developers and establishes new provisions to ensure that providers using certified technologies have the ability to communicate about usability, user experience, interoperability and security [22].

The United States Core Data for Interoperability (USCDI), as outlined by the Final Rule, consists of a standard set of health data classes and constituent data elements representing essential clinical data to be included in EHRs to enable nationwide, interoperable health information exchange [23]. Within this core data set, each data element is linked with applicable standards to guide implementation. ONC has established a predictable, transparent and collaborative process to expand the USCDI, providing stakeholders with the opportunity to offer comments. The Final Rule also defines requirements for standards-based APIs to support an individual's access and control of their own electronic health information. The overall goal is for patients to be empowered to more securely and easily have access to their health information from their provider's medical record, using the smartphone application of their choice.

The National Academy of Medicine released a publication in 2018 titled "Procuring Interoperability: Achieving High-Quality, Connected, and Person-Centered Care" [24] to offer guidance for acquiring interoperable health

IT solutions and devices. As illustrated in Fig. 20.2, health systems are encouraged to establish a comprehensive, ongoing procurement strategy focused on functional system-wide interoperability, rather than purchasing individual software and hardware which require proprietary interfaces. This publication advocates for the acquisition of standards-based, industry-driven and modular interoperable products to enable health delivery systems to achieve optimal care quality, safety and efficiency. By implementing better procurement practices health systems can more rapidly achieve the interoperability that is implicit in the digital health ecosystem of the future.

In order to more rapidly advance global, standards-based health data interoperability, the HL7 FHIR Accelerator Program [25] was established to assist communities with the creation and adoption of high-quality FHIR implementa-

tion guides and other standard artifacts. HL7 FHIR has gained rapid acceptance as an innovative interoperability platform standard. As an increasing number of use cases emerge, end users and implementers can apply the capabilities of FHIR to address discrete business needs. HL7's Accelerator Program helps communities more efficiently navigate through the standards development process. Example projects cover a variety of use cases, including the Argonaut Project, CARIN Alliance, CodeX, Da Vinci Project, Gravity Project and Vulcan. The program also offers infrastructure and collaboration tools, support services, including self-service guidelines, project and/or financial management and other infrastructure services.

Collectively, these efforts will accelerate the global adoption of innovative, standards-based, health IT systems to help realize the vision of a digital health ecosystem.

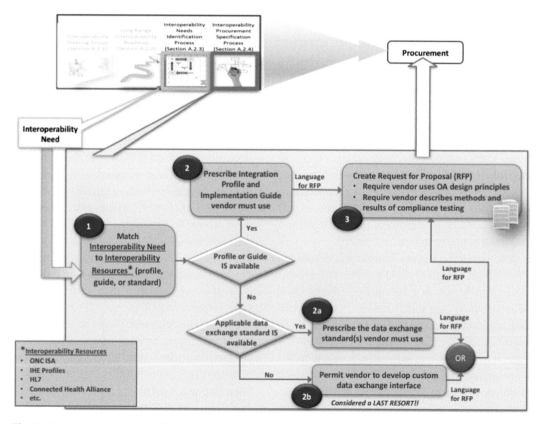

Fig. 20.2 Procuring interoperability: Achieving high-quality connected, and person-centered care. Source: National Academy of Sciences, Courtesy of The National Academies Press, Washington, D.C

Interoperability Case Study

The Oregon Clinic (the Clinic) is an independent specialty physician organization based in the Pacific Northwest, which coordinates with local hospital systems to deliver patient care [26]. The practice consists of about 260 providers, 160 physician shareholders and 20 specialty practices. The physicians at the Clinic are affiliated with multiple hospitals across the region where they use different EHR systems, as well as their own EHR system at their respective private practices, which presented them with unique interoperability challenges. The Clinic decided to look into alternate solutions to exchange information with local hospitals. The goal was to find a cost effective solution that would get the information they needed into their patients' charts in a timely, legible, accurate and relevant manner while using multiple systems across the continuum of care.

Technical Approach

Prior to beginning on their path to interoperability, the Clinic shared information with hospitals by faxing referrals and other patient information between facilities. This was time-consuming and often failed to produce patient information in a timely manner. Their two local partners, Providence and Legacy Health Systems, were already exchanging health information with other systems, which proved instrumental in helping the Clinic address their interoperability needs. The Clinic began the process by learning more about IHE profiles, HL7 standards and HL7 C-CDA, which prepared them for the launch of the interoperability pilot.

Their first project involved using C-CDA referrals via Direct Messaging with Providence and Legacy Health Systems. Since the Clinic represents specialty providers and receives many external referrals, they wanted to use standards-based interoperable exchange to create a type of closed referral loop. This referral processing involved use of the C-CDA standard and Direct Messaging, along with a service called Automated Clinical Messaging (ACM) which sends a secure message via a portal with structured information attached.

Overview of Clinical Workflow

1. An external primary care physician (PCP) sends a C-CDA referral to a specialty provider at the Clinic.
2. Once the Clinic receives the referral, a receipt message is sent back to the PCP. This not only alerts the PCP that the referral has been received, but also confirms the communication pathway between the PCP and the specialist to confirm that Direct Messaging is working.
3. After the patient visits the specialist and the encounter is documented and signed, the consult note is then sent back to the PCP via Direct Messaging. The ACM service queries data in the EHR for an appointment type that matches the referral. If it finds a match, it will initiate sending the consult note back to the referring provider.

Thus far, there has been a positive response from specialists and referring providers as this process eliminates extra steps for collecting data and verifying that the patient visited the specialist.

The second project was to implement bi-directional, real-time C-CDA exchange with the local hospital systems. In September 2016, the Clinic began to collaborate on a pilot program to publish clinical documents to a shared registry through which clinicians could query and retrieve documents from their respective repositories. The last essential piece of this project was joining Carequality, which allows its members access to a vast, trusted network of clinical documents wherever they reside. This bi-directional sharing of clinical documents is made possible through Carequality by the implementation of the IHE cross-gateway-sharing infrastructure Cross Community Access (XCA) profile.

Lessons Learned

- Listen carefully to physicians and clinical staff and incorporate their feedback. Work to build trust and do not implement a technical solution that they do not perceive as an improvement.

- Do not underestimate the power of physician champions to break through the status quo. People often become "stuck in a groove" and will do things the way they have always done them unless they can see a clear reason to change.
- Develop close relationships with important community partners and determine who is ready and motivated to take on an interoperability project. It does not work to implement change before a partner is ready and willing to collaborate.

The Clinic went from little to no interoperability to sharing information bi-directionally, previewing records and proactively surfacing pertinent information from inbound C-CDA documents. They process over 90% of referrals electronically via the automated referral management system outlined above. The referring physicians are happy to get their referrals handled quickly and to get detailed, consistent information back from the Clinic's specialists. They have reached a tipping point with thousands of C-CDA documents now exchanged every month; the other clinics are clamoring to be included and physicians are seeing improvements in how their charts are prepared.

Summary

This chapter lays the foundation for understanding the ability of interoperability and standards-based systems to empower digital health by defining key terms and initiatives. Interoperability is a critical foundation of health systems to enable data that are seamlessly available across multiple sources. Four levels of interoperability are described, including foundational, structural, semantic and organizational. Barriers to interoperability are discussed as well as short- and long-term strategies for overcoming such barriers. For the purposes of outlining the health data standards landscape, four broad areas are used to categorize health data standards, including services/exchange, content/structure, vocabulary/code sets/terminology and administrative standards. Major entities involved in publishing each of these health data standards are described. The Interoperability Standards Advisory process, which coordinates the identification, assessment and public awareness of the best-available data standards that can be used by the healthcare industry to address specific interoperability needs, is also described.

The evolving digital health ecosystem creates a need for initiatives that inform and advance the interoperability landscape. Such initiatives include the HIMSS Interoperability Initiatives Environmental Scan, the United States Nationwide Interoperability Roadmap and the Learning Health System. Guiding principles for achieving an interoperable health IT ecosystem are outlined. Active health information exchange entities are described, including common types of HIE architecture and potential benefits. Efforts to accelerate the global adoption of innovative, standards-based health IT systems are needed to realize the promise of digital health. Such efforts described in this chapter include the Twenty-first-century Cures Act, the USCDI and the HL7 FHIR Accelerator Program. The chapter concludes with a case study describing one organization's successful interoperability journey, including lessons learned.

Conclusions and Outlook

Many of us share the same goal. That all individuals, our families and our healthcare providers are able to send, receive, find and use electronic health information in a manner that is appropriate, secure, timely and reliable. The digital health ecosystem will leverage clinical integration to achieve a wider sharing of health information and facilitate use of standards-based systems by individuals and members of the care team. Providing secure, timely and reliable information exchange will improve the health and wellness of individuals through comprehensive data that inform shared decision-making. Once realized, the digital health ecosystem will enable individuals, their families and care providers to access, send, receive and use electronic health information to achieve optimal health outcomes.

Useful Resources
1. Accredited Standards Committee (ASC) X12. www.wpc-edi.com

2. American Medical Association (AMA). www.ama-assn.org
3. American National Standards Institute (ANSI). www.ansi.org
4. American Nurses Association (ANA). www.nursingworld.org
5. Carequality. https://carequality.org
6. Clinical Data Interchange Standards Consortium (CDISC). www.cdisc.org
7. Digital Imaging Communication in Medicine Standards Committee (DICOM). www.nema.org
7. eHealth Exchange. www.ehealthexchange.org
8. Health Level Seven (HL7). www.hl7.org
9. HIMSS. www.himss.org
10. Institute of Electrical and Electronic Engineers (IEEE). www.ieee.org
11. Integrating the Healthcare Enterprise (IHE). www.ihe.net
12. International Organization for Standardization (ISO). www.iso.org
13. International Statistical Classification of Diseases and Related Health Problems (ICD-10). www.cdc.gov/nchs
14. Internet Engineering Task Force (IETF). https://www.ietf.org
15. Logical Observation Identifiers Names and Codes (LOINC). www.loinc.org
16. National Council for Prescription Drug Programs (NCPDP). www.ncpdp.org
17. National Electrical Manufacturers Association (NEMA). www.nema.org
18. National Emergency Medical Services Information System (NEMSIS). https://nemsis.org/
19. National Library of Medicine (NLM). www.nlm.nih.gov/.
20. Office of the National Coordinator for Health Information Technology (ONC). www.healthit.gov
21. Personal Connected Health Alliance (PCHAlliance). www.pchalliance.org/continua-design-guidelines
22. RxNorm. www.nlm.nih.gov/research/umls/rxnorm
23. Strategic Health Information Exchange Collaborative (SHIEC). www.strategichie.com
24. Unified Medical Language System (UMLS). www.nlm.nih.gov/research/umls
25. World Wide Web Consortium (W3C). www.w3.org

Review Questions

1. HIMSS has published a definition of interoperability. According to HIMSS, which of the following is NOT included in the four levels of interoperability?
   (a) Functional
   (b) Semantic
   (c) Structural
   (d) Organizational
2. For the purposes of describing the health data standards landscape, four broad areas are used to categorize heath data standards. Which of the following are included in the health data standards categories?
   (a) Internet protocols
   (b) Imaging standards
   (c) Clinical summaries
   (d) Services/exchange standards
   (e) None of the above
3. Which standard is viewed as an emerging standard describing data formats and elements and a web-based API for exchanging health information?
   (a) Consolidated CDA
   (b) HL7 FHIR
   (c) DICOM
   (d) NCPDP
4. Which of the following resources provides clear guidance on what are the "best available" standards and implementation specifications to use to meet an interoperability need?
   (a) ONC Interoperability Standards Advisory
   (b) HIMSS Interoperability Initiatives Environmental Scan
   (c) U.S. Nationwide Interoperability Roadmap
   (d) Learning Health System
5. ONC has outlined a set of Guiding Principles to help achieve their 10 year vision of the future interoperable health IT ecosystem. Which of the following items are NOT included in the Guiding Principles?
   (a) Maintain modularity
   (b) Protect privacy and security
   (c) Focus on value
   (d) One size fits all

6. Health information exchange entities provide all of the following benefits for providers, patients and hospitals EXCEPT:
   (a) Enhanced care coordination through shared communication of essential information
   (b) Timely access to the right information for providers, patients and all other stakeholders
   (c) Discounts on purchasing software for proprietary interfaces
   (d) Improved efficiency and reliability through the elimination of unnecessary paperwork
7. The United States Core Data for Interoperability consists of a standard set of health data classes and constituent data elements representing essential clinical data to be included in EHRs to enable nationwide, interoperable health information exchange. Which of the following describes capabilities of the USCDI?
   (a) Each data element is linked with applicable standards to guide implementation.
   (b) Expansion of the USCDI will require financial investment by key stakeholders.
   (c) Standard APIs are excluded from the USCDI requirements in order to enable individual access.
   (d) The USCDI is subject to annual updates via a closed process as mandated by ONC.

Appendix: Answers to Review Questions

1. HIMSS has published a definition of interoperability. According to HIMSS, which of the following is NOT included in the four levels of interoperability?
   (a) Functional
   (b) Semantic
   (c) Structural
   (d) Organizational

Explanation: According to HIMSS, the four levels of interoperability that differentiate the types of information exchange are as follows:
• Foundational—establishes the interconnectivity requirements needed for one system or application to securely communicate data to and receive data from another.
• Structural—defines the format, syntax and organization of data exchange, including at the data field level for interpretation.
• Semantic—provides for common underlying models and codification of the data, including the use of data elements with standardized definitions from publicly available value sets and coding vocabularies, providing a shared understanding and meaning to the user.
• Organizational—includes governance, policy, social, legal and organizational considerations to facilitate secure, seamless and timely communication and use of data both within and between organizations, entities and individuals. These components enable shared consent, trust and integrated end-user processes and workflows.

2. For the purposes of describing the health data standards landscape, four broad areas are used to categorize heath data standards. Which of the following are included in the health data standards categories?
   (a) Internet protocols
   (b) Imaging standards
   (c) Clinical summaries
   (d) Services/exchange standards
   (e) None of the above

Explanation: For the purposes of describing the health data standards landscape, we suggest four broad areas to categorize health data standards. Services/exchange standards are used to establish a common, predictable, secure communication protocol between systems (i.e., infrastructure). Vocabulary/code sets/terminology standards consist of nomenclatures and code sets used to describe clinical problems and procedures, medications and allergies (i.e., semantics). Content/structure standards are used to share clinical information such as clinical summaries, prescriptions and structured electronic documents (i.e., syntax). Administrative standards are used for payment, operations and other non-clinical interoperability needs.

3. Which standard is viewed as an emerging standard describing data formats and elements

and a web-based API for exchanging health information?

(a) Consolidated CDA
(b) HL7 FHIR
(c) DICOM
(d) NCPDP

Explanation: HL7 FHIR is an emerging standard describing data formats and elements and a web-based API for exchanging health information. The FHIR specification is rapidly being adopted as a next-generation standards framework for the exchange of EHR data due to the ease of implementation.

4. Which of the following resources provides clear guidance on what are the "best available" standards and implementation specifications to use to meet an interoperability need?
(a) ONC Interoperability Standards Advisory
(b) HIMSS Interoperability Initiatives Environmental Scan
(c) U.S. Nationwide Interoperability Roadmap
(d) Learning Health System

Explanation: The ONC Interoperability Standards Advisory provides a single, public list of the best-available standards and implementation specifications reflecting the ongoing dialogue, debate and consensus. The ISA also enables a 'first pass' viewpoint for standards selection by government programs, procurements, testing or certification programs, and standards-profiling efforts.

5. ONC has outlined a set of Guiding Principles to help achieve their ten-year vision of the future interoperable health IT ecosystem. Which of the following items are NOT included in the Principles?
(a) Maintain modularity
(b) Protect privacy and security
(c) Focus on value
(d) One size fits all

Explanation: According to the guiding principles, one size does NOT fit all. We should strive for baseline interoperability across the health IT infrastructure, while allowing innovators and technologists to vary the user experience in order to best meet the user's needs based on the scenario at hand, technology available, workflow design, personal preferences and other factors.

6. Health information exchange entities provide all of the following benefits for providers, patients and hospitals EXCEPT:
(a) Enhanced care coordination through shared communication of essential information
(b) Timely access to the right information for providers, patients and all other stakeholders
(c) Discounts on purchasing software for proprietary interfaces
(d) Improved efficiency and reliability through the elimination of unnecessary paperwork

Explanation: Health information exchange entities can provide many important benefits for providers, patients and hospitals, such as:
• Enhanced care coordination through shared communication of essential information for optimal patient care
• Timely access to the right information for providers, patients and all other stakeholders
• Improved efficiency and reliability through the elimination of unnecessary paperwork and access to clinical decision support tools
• Improved quality and safety by reducing medication and medical errors

7. The United States Core Data for Interoperability consists of a standard set of health data classes and constituent data elements representing essential clinical data to be included in EHRs to enable nationwide, interoperable health information exchange. Which of the following describes capabilities of the USCDI?
(a) Each data element is linked with applicable standards to guide implementation.
(b) Expansion of the USCDI will require financial investment by key stakeholders.
(c) Standard APIs are excluded from the USCDI requirements in order to enable individual access.
(d) The USCDI is subject to annual updates via a closed process as mandated by ONC.

Explanation: Within this core data set, each data element is linked with applicable standards to guide implementation. ONC has established a predictable, transparent and collaborative process to expand the USCDI, providing stakeholders with the opportunity to offer comments. The Final Rule also defines requirements for standards-based APIs to support an individual's access and control of their own electronic health information.

References

1. Snowden A. HIMSS defines digital health for the global healthcare industry. HIMSS. 2020; https://www.himss.org/news/himss-defines-digital-health-global-healthcare-industry. Accessed 15 May 2020
2. Snowden A. Digital health: a framework for healthcare transformation. HIMSS. 2020; https://go.himss.org/digital-health-a-framework-for-healthcare-transformation.html. Accessed 27 May 2020
3. HIMSS. What is interoperability in healthcare? HIMSS. 2019; https://www.himss.org/what-interoperability. Accessed 16 May 2020
4. Global Digital Health Partnership. Connected health: empowering health through interoperability. Global Digital Health Partnership. 2019; https://s3-ap-southeast-2.amazonaws.com/ehq-production-australia/57f9a51462d5e3f07569d55232fcc11290b99cd6/documents/attachments/000/102/278/original/GDHP_Interop_2.05.pdf. Accessed 15 May 2020
5. Powell K, Alexander G. Mitigating barriers to interoperability in healthcare. Online J Nurs Inform. 2019;23:2.
6. ANSI. United States standards strategy. ANSI 2015. https://share.ansi.org/shared%20documents/Standards%20Activities/NSSC/USSS_Third_edition/ANSI_USSS_2015.pdf. Accessed 17 May 2020
7. Brandstätter J. Overview of IHE/HL7/FHIR. eHealth Suisse. 2019; https://www.e-health-suisse.ch/fileadmin/user_upload/Dokumente/E/overview-ihe-hl7-fhir.pdf. Accessed 17 May 2020
8. Busch L. Standards: recipes for reality. Cambridge, MA: MIT Press; 2011.
9. Office of the National Coordinator for Health IT. Interoperability standards advisory. ONC. 2019; https://www.healthit.gov/isa. Accessed 20 May 2020
10. Continua. Fundamentals of medical grade data exchange. Personal Connected Health Alliance. 2018; https://www.pchalliance.org/sites/pchalliance/files/Fundamentals_Medical-Grade_Data_Exchange_Sep2018.pdf Accessed 28 May 2020
11. Webopedia. API - application program Interface. Webopedia. 2020; https://www.webopedia.com/TERM/A/API.html. Accessed 27 May 2020
12. Sensmeier J. Health data standards: development, harmonization, and interoperability. In: Saba VK, McCormick KA, editors. Essentials of nursing informatics. 6th ed. USA: McGraw-Hill Education; 2015. p. 101–13.
13. Office of the National Coordinator for Health IT. Interoperability standards advisory: reference edition. ONC. 2020;2020. https://www.healthit.gov/isa/sites/isa/files/inline-files/2020-ISA-Reference-Edition.pdf. Accessed 15 May 2020
14. HIMSS. Interoperability initiatives environmental scan. HIMSS. 2019; https://www.himss.org/environmental-scan. Accessed 15 May 2020
15. Office of the National Coordinator for Health IT. Connecting health and care for the nation: a shared nationwide interoperability roadmap. ONC. 2017; https://www.healthit.gov/sites/default/files/hie-interoperability/nationwide-interoperability-roadmap-final-version-1.0.pdf. Accessed 15 May 2020
16. Office of the National Coordinator for Health IT. Connecting health and care for the nation: a 10-year vision to achieve an interoperable health IT infrastructure. ONC. 2014; https://www.healthit.gov/sites/default/files/ONC10yearInteroperabilityConceptPaper.pdf. Accessed 15 May 2020
17. HIMSS. FAQ: What is health information exchange? HIMSS. 2014. https://www.himss.org/resources/faq-what-health-information-exchange-hie. Accessed 24 May 2020.
18. EHealth Exchange. 2020. https://ehealthexchange.org. Accessed 24 May 2020.
19. Carequality. 2020. https://carequality.org. Accessed 27 May 2020.
20. San Diego Health Connect. 2020. https://www.sdhealthconnect.org. Accessed 24 May 2020.
21. Strategic Health Information Exchange Collaborative. 2020. https://strategichie.com. Accessed 24 May 2020.
22. Miliard M. HHS publishes final regs on info blocking, interoperability. Healthcare IT News. 2020; https://www.healthcareitnews.com/news/hhs-publishes-final-regs-info-blocking-interoperability. Accessed 24 May 2020
23. Office of the National Coordinator for Health IT. United States Core data for interoperability. ONC. 2020; https://www.healthit.gov/isa/united-states-core-data-interoperability-uscdi. Accessed 25 May 2020
24. Pronovost P, et al. Procuring interoperability: achieving high-quality, connected, and person-centered care. National Academy of Medicine. 2018; https://nam.edu/procuring-interoperability-achieving-high-quality-connected-and-person-centered-care. Accessed 25 May 2020
25. HL7. HL7 FHIR accelerator program. 2020. https://www.hl7.org/about/fhir-accelerator. Accessed 25 May 2020.
26. HIMSS. HIMSS Interoperability Case Study: The Oregon Clinic. HIMSS. 2018. https://www.himss.org/resources/developing-health-information-exchange-case-study. Accessed 26 May 2020.

Clinical Decision Support: The Technology and Art of Providing Support Where the Clinicians Need it

21

Ann Kristin Rotegård and Bente Christensen

Learning Objectives
- Understand what clinical decision support (CDS) means.
- Understand the Five Rights and barriers within for nurses.
- Understand the meaning and importance of clinical data models.
- Understand what interoperability means in clinical decision support.
- Understand the interaction between an electronic health record (EHR) system and the decision support tool.
- Understand the deficiencies in CDS within nursing.
- Understand the connection between evidence-based practice and clinical decision support.
- Understand the methodological foundations of the CDS VAR Healthcare.

Key Terms
- Closed loop between clinical practice
- Research and education
- Provision of knowledge and person-specific information

- Five rights model,
- Identification of content
- Evidence-based healthcare

Introduction

In this chapter, we describe clinical decision support systems (CDSS), challenges and success criteria as well as the development of a knowledge and decision support tool for nurses with a case study: VAR Healthcare.

Some of the first concepts relating to health informatics were mentioned in a paper presented at the New Jersey Industrial Health Conference, Somerville, in 1966. It stated: "Obviously a computer is not and cannot be a replacement for the flesh and blood physician or nurse, but it represents a powerful tool to help them both. But the use of this instrument extends far beyond just the physician or nurse in medicine. For example, hospitals are considering using computers to support virtually every phase of patient care, from admission through diagnosis and treatment to follow-up" (p. 10, [1]).

Electronic patient records (EPRs) have gradually become an essential tool for planning, providing and improving clinical care. So far, the data generated from the different systems and devices have been combined, interpreted and applied manually when decisions in clinical practice have been made. However, the emerging

A. K. Rotegård (✉)
Cappelen Damm AS, Oslo, Norway
e-mail: ann.kristin.rotegard@cappelendamm.no

B. Christensen
Nord University, Bodø, Norge
e-mail: bente.christensen@nsf.no

© Springer Nature Switzerland AG 2022
U. H. Hübner et al. (eds.), *Nursing Informatics*, Health Informatics,
https://doi.org/10.1007/978-3-030-91237-6_21

complexity of clinical care calls for more advanced information and communications technology (ICT) support to assist healthcare personnel in keeping track of patients. The situation may be compared with the evolution of traffic: there was a time when there were few cars on the road, roads were not conducive to driving at high speeds and road safety was not particularly an issue. Today, this picture is very different, and cars can assist drivers in reading and coping with traffic. Caring for patients has evolved along similar lines. Multiple professions are involved; there are numerous handovers of patients and information, much parallel treatment and assessments, and a higher turnover of patients. Nurses are at the centre of these processes. Additionally, medicine, and consequently nursing care, has become extremely advanced, and healthcare personnel deal with large amounts of knowledge that must be processed and applied. Thus, there is a need for, and an expectation, that ICT would assist healthcare personnel in maintaining an overview of their patients and provide updated treatment and care.

There has been an increasing recognition of the benefits of EPRs in health care. If clinical decision support (CDS) is provided within EPRs based on practice guidelines, care can be provided based on evidence and best practice in order to achieve better quality and efficiency [2–5]. Healthcare procedures or guidelines are central to nursing care and treatment, and their quality may be highly significant to patient outcomes by ensuring patient safety and reducing errors [6, 7].

Still, perhaps the most promising potential is the ability to close the loop between clinical practice, research and education [8].

Traditionally, guidelines or procedures have been developed locally and with little or no coordination within or across hospitals, healthcare institutions and other healthcare delivery systems. There are examples of hospitals that have several variations of the same procedure (up to 50 in our experience). Lack of consistency and quality of procedures/guidelines are a threat to patient outcomes and patient safety. Standardised digital tools that are anchored in best evidence

are needed to support nurses and other healthcare professionals to improve efficiency, save money and improve communication and treatment. There is also a need for support systems across healthcare systems and education to bridge practices strengthen the perspective and need for continuous learning and keeping up to date with the latest research and development.

What Is Clinical Decision Support (CDS)?

Clinical decision support system (CDSS) was introduced as a MeSH (Medical Subject Headings) term in the US National Library of Medicine in 1998. CDSS was defined as "Computer-based information systems used to integrate clinical and patient information and provide support for decision-making in patient care" (https://www.ncbi.nlm.nih.gov/mesh/?term =decision+support+systems%2C+clinical).

Along with development and research within clinical decision support, there are a variety of definitions of the term. The following is a more recent one:

"Clinical decision support (CDS) provides clinicians, staff, patients or other individuals with knowledge and person-specific information, intelligently filtered or presented at appropriate times, to enhance health and health care. CDS encompasses a variety of tools to enhance decision-making in the clinical workflow. These tools include computerised alerts and reminders to care providers and patients; clinical guidelines; condition-specific order sets; focused patient data reports and summaries; documentation templates; diagnostic support, and contextually relevant reference information, among other tools" (https://www.healthit.gov/topic/safety/clinical-decision-support).

Clinical decision support (CDS) systems are computer-based systems that combine medical, health professional and other knowledge with individual patient information to support decision-making, and the assessment, care and treatment of patients. Accordingly, clinical decision support depends on good-quality clinical data repositories, and reinforces the need for standardised data representation and storage. Lack of a good clinical data warehouse will have a significant impact on the quality of advice emanating from the CDS systems. Data mining algorithms require good-quality clinical data repositories to be able to extract knowledge to support clinical decision-making [9–11]; therefore, there is a heavy reliance on large volumes of readily accessible, existing clinical data sets that are usually extracted from the repository content of EPRs. Lack of standardised data in the repository may lead to data sets that are not representative of the patient population [9]. It is therefore essential that standardised data representations are used for leveraging the knowledge base repositories so as to facilitate the generation of patient-specific care recommendations [9, 10, 12]. Therefore, besides standardised and structured data, decision support presupposes a knowledge base that can be combined with the data [13].

Decision support comprises a variety of tools and interventions such as computerised alerts and reminders, clinical guidelines, order sets, patient data reports and dashboards, documentation templates, diagnostic support and clinical workflow tools, and may be categorised according to their level of complexity [14].

Related Work on Clinical Decision Support

Several reviews conclude that there is little evidence to support the cost-effectiveness of CDS within medicine [15, 16] and nursing. Nevertheless, Lobach [17] found that CDS has the greatest impact on process outcomes, for example, providing knowledge related to specific medical conditions and ordering clinical treatment. Research on CDS utilisation has mostly targeted physicians, with little mention of nurse practitioners [18].

At the core of decision support for nurses is evidence-based interventions with associated nursing diagnosis and patient outcomes. Specifically, nurses need support to define and document nursing diagnosis, and these should be predefined and anchored in research and provided automatically [19].

A recent integrative review of clinical decision support in acute care settings for nurses reveals that CDS is used in nursing practice for various purposes: supporting nursing diagnostics, medication management, improving situational awareness, supporting guideline adherence, triage and non-medication based nursing interventions [20]. This review found that CDS statistically improved outcomes, but there was no statistic significant improvement of nursing diagnosis support. However, none of the studies reported negative outcomes. Most of these publications had text-based recommendations, and half of these studies had integrations in the EHR (electronic health record) [20]. Automatic extraction of patient data from the patient record occurred in 7 out of 28 studies, and 50% were based on input from nurses.

Most of the studies of CDS in nursing are within acute care settings and relate to single clinical conditions. Examples are pressure ulcers [20], prediction of haemodynamic instability, respiratory distress and infection detection [11]. Bennett and Hardiker [21] also looked at studies within acute care settings.

According to Dunn Lopez [20], a general CDS that can support nurses across patient conditions and systems that are fully integrated with the EHR systems are lacking. There is also a lack of studies that include CDS development as well as a lack of usability studies (ibid.). Hence, more research and development is needed in CDS for nursing care, more broadly, and with more automation for optimal support [18].

The case study in this chapter will address these gaps in previous research.

Challenges and Success Criteria for CDS

Despite great expectations of achieving quality, it has been difficult to introduce the adoption of clinical decision support systems [22]. A systematic review of randomised controlled trials of

CDS identified four characteristics that significantly contributed to improving clinical practice: CDS is automatically available in the clinical workflow, support is provided through the system at the time and place (site) of the decision, and practical advice/references are provided and are computer-based [3]. CDS systems that were an integrated component of the patient record or order entry systems were also significantly more likely to improve clinical practice than stand-alone systems [3]. The latter is also supported by Goossen-Baremans, Collins and Park [13].

Based on the amount of development and research on CDS in the last two decades, the CDS Five Rights model was developed in 2006 and pursued [14]. This model is considered a best-practice approach for quality improvement and healthcare outcomes, when the interventions in the CDS transfer the right information, to the right person, in the right format, through the right channel at the right time in the workflow (ibid.).

The right information means evidence-based information that provides guidance or advice on relevant best practices. Examples include clinical guidelines, procedures or pathways.

The right person refers to the person who needs support for best-possible processes and outcomes. This includes healthcare professionals (doctors, nurses, pharmacists etc.), patients and/or their next of kin/caretakers.

The right format refers to how the support is given, that is, data displays, documentation tools, care plans and registry reports.

The right channels might be a clinical information system like the electronic health record system or more general channels like the Internet, mobile technology systems, smart home devices and patient portals.

The right time refers to the timing of the support or guidance in the clinical workflow or process.

The CDS Five Rights framework is used to analyse and document the development and use of CDS and also uncover barriers and optimise the CDS utilisation and care processes in practice. The framework is recommended when implementing new CDSS in clinical practice [11].

Borum [18] found that research uncovers barriers in the CDS Five Rights areas. The most common barrier for nurse practitioners utilising hospital CDS systems is within the area of *right information*. Relevant clinical knowledge, up-to-date, evidence-based practice guidelines, accurate clinical pathways and current clinical algorithms are key elements that encourage nurse practitioners to accept and use CDS in the hospital setting. Healthcare procedures or guidelines are at the core of nursing care and treatment, and their quality and evidence may be highly significant to patient outcomes by ensuring patient safety and reducing errors [6, 7].

Barriers have also been found due to the requirement of *the right people*. Automatic provision of decision support as part of workflow and support at the time and location of decision-making presupposes that the person targeted for the support must be the person entering the data. In the multidisciplinary nature of heath care, this is often not the case, as, for instance, nurses and secretaries make data entries on behalf of the doctor. Hence, changing work procedures is often necessary to achieve CDS, and this is one of the reasons why CDS has been shown to be difficult to implement [23]. Studies reveal that nurses are likely to accept and use CDS systems [24]. Many frameworks/models for evaluating of technologies are based on a medical perspective. A framework for outcomes based on digital technologies for nurses has recently been developed. This framework comprises four outcome target groups; persons in need of care, formal caregivers, informal caregivers and healthcare organisations (Krick et al., 2020).

Barriers and possibilities have also been described within *the right format* perspective. Medic et al. [11] stress the importance of the Five Rights when implementing CDS in acute care settings, and they point to user interface (participatory design), sufficient training, continuous feedback to clinicians as well as presenting underlying data and rationale for decisions as factors for success.

Several studies look at the importance of the *right channels*. We have already mentioned Kawamoto [3] and Goossen-Baremans, Collins and Park [13], who recommend integrations between the patient record, knowledge bases and decision support bases and/or standardised procedures/guidelines. Hyruk [25] also claims that clinical support systems produce best results when integrated into other systems and work processes, such as in electronic patient records.

Alarms have been a focus of many CDS systems to ensure *the right time*; however, several studies report "alarm fatigue," as a clinician may be exposed to many types of alarms during their work [11, 18]. Thus, the care providers may neglect or overlook the alarms, and the aim of the CDS fails.

A recent study has found that the design of the CDSS should provide adequate support for clinical tasks, the workflow and cognitive activities, and should be followed up by organisational policies and procedures to ensure correct implementation and use. Methods like lean process improvement and business process management (BPM) are recommended for identifying and eliminating barriers and a poor fit between human, technological and organisational factors [26].

CDS in EPR Systems

Legislation in many countries imposes strict requirements for professional reliability and relevant documentation. Decisions that healthcare providers make are planned and documented in the patient's record/health record system, and decision support is therefore a central feature of the EHR system. There is currently some decision support integrated into the EPR systems; however, it is still in the early stages.

The aim of health information systems and EPR systems is to ensure continuous, clinical care of good quality and to ensure patient safety and best-possible health outcomes. To achieve these aims and so that it can be used for statistical purposes and as a foundation for financing, data has to be structured, of good quality and followed up using quality indicators and quality improvements, research and decision support [27].

Structure, standards and detailed clinical data models (CDM) are needed. CDM is used to "analyse, sort, formalise, structure, and standardise data elements for clinical use" ([28], p. 212; [29], p. 428), and the core of clinical data models are described as expressions of data elements with their relationships, structures and codes. Terminologies or conceptual representations and standards are needed in relation to the content. This may include scientific evidence as well as clinical practical knowledge [13, 28, 29]. One standard, ISO TS 13972, describes requirements and a logical model of clinical concepts to define structured clinical information. This chapter will not go into details about this standard, but the core of this standard is to ensure semantic interoperability, that is, "ensuring that the precise meaning of exchanged information is understandable by any other system or application not initially developed for this purpose" [30].

The flow of information between a decision support system and the EHR system can go either way: from the CDS to the EHR or from the EHR to the CDS. The clinical information that is being transferred has to be understood accurately and consistently by both systems (ibid.).

Also, as part of a detailed clinical management system, the ISO 9001 Quality Management System can be used for the development, application and governance of the system.

Reference terminologies or models are also needed in terms of standardised term sets and units of measure (ibid.). SNOMED CT is a globally defined terminology for such representation in healthcare systems. The International Classification for Nursing Practice (ICNP) is regarded as a global and formal terminology system for standardised documentation of nursing care, representing the core of nursing documentation, nursing diagnosis, nursing goals and nursing interventions. ICNP complies with ISO 18104, which "specifies the characteristics of two categorical structures, with the overall aim of supporting interoperability in the exchange of meaningful information between information systems in respect of nursing diagnoses and nursing actions" [30]. Thus, ICNP is regarded as a reference terminology system that provides statistics based on descriptions and comparisons of nursing at all levels of health care, within and across countries (https://www.icn.ch/what-we-do/projects/ehealth-icnp; [13]). ICNP has been mapped to SNOMED-CT and ensures alignment between the systems and also ensures connections to and representation of nurse-sensitive concepts in SNOMED-CT (https://www.twna.org.tw/frontend/un07_international/file/2015/3%20Benefits_of_ICNP_-_SNOMED_CT.pdf). Furthermore, ICNP represents nursing terminologies in the WHO family of classifications along with ICD (International Classification of Diseases) and ICF (International Classification of Functioning, Disability and Health) (https://unstats.un.org/unsd/classifications/Family/Detail/1024).

When the CDMs and semantic interoperability are defined and data elements understood, the next step is to put these elements "into proper actions" [29]. VAR Healthcare is an example of a clinical digital support system for nurses that has developed from being a knowledge support system to providing more decision support.

Case Study

VAR Healthcare-From Reference Book to Decision Support

This work started as a public research and development project from 2001 to 2003. The idea was to digitalise the pocket manual for procedures that the nurses used, based on the political strategies on digitalisation of health and the new quality reforms in health care. The project involved two hospitals and one nursing college.

The aim of this project was to

- develop and evaluate a practical, digital tool for updated and quality-controlled procedures, as well as a knowledge base for nursing care to replace the paper-based and "home-made" procedures employed at that time; and
- provide a solid foundation for education and lifelong learning at all levels, and ensure consistent, continuous care and patient safety.

The Norwegian Nurses Organisation assumed ownership of the project in 2002, partly to ensure further development and operation and to process the results, but also to make nursing care visible; show its complexity, professionality and impor-tance for patient safety and positive outcomes. A second project that involved two large municipalities and a nursing home/elderly institution was completed during the early maintaining phase, 2004–2005. This part of the project was funded by and completed in collaboration with a national, political trade organisation for competence enhancement in order to test, adapt and implement the tool in the municipalities. VAR Healthcare started out with installations of local compact discs (CDs), but also offered simple links/integrations with the original EHR/EPR vendors.

Evaluation and experience of using the tool are summarised as follows:

(a) Reduced resources in the development and maintenance of procedures, resulting in more time with the patient and more time to implement the tool/evidence-based practice.
(b) Increased quality of treatment and care—consequently reduced malpractice claims along with increased patient safety.
(c) Consistent treatment of the patient within and across units/healthcare settings.
(d) More efficient and better quality of nursing documentation.
(e) Efficient education of new employees and students—fewer resources spent on teaching and seminars.
(f) An important element of a national strategy for quality insurance in nursing care—building professionalism.

Today, VAR Healthcare is a web-based decision support system with more than 400 evidence-based procedures and guidelines for nursing practice, with associated knowledge summaries, knowledge tests and medical calculators (Fig. 21.1).

The procedures are richly illustrated and animated (Figs. 21.2 and 21.3). Furthermore, VAR Healthcare is brand-neutral and contains procedures that are used by nurses in situations across healthcare settings. VAR covers many needs: easy and ready access to procedures that are continuously updated and evidence-based, contributing to improved nursing documentation and care planning; continuous care and patient

Fig. 21.1 VAR Healthcare—making evidence usable, available on various devices

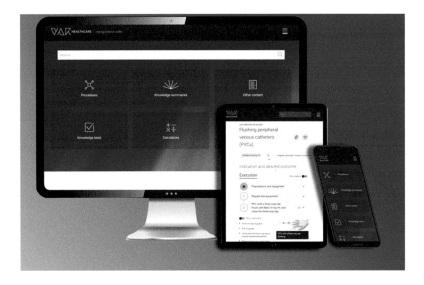

safety; education and lifelong learning as well as quality improvement and management in clinical practice. VAR is designed to facilitate various needs for and levels of information (Fig. 21.3).

The development and maintenance of VAR Healthcare have followed a rigid system, focusing on structure, language and consistency across the system. Based on technology development and new possibilities, there have been several platform changes and a continuous further development of technological solutions. The latest version (version 15) of VAR Healthcare goes beyond knowledge support for nursing by including initial support for decision-making. It was conceived as a digital reference book and developed into a digital decision support tool. VAR Healthcare supports the nursing process and documentation. The template includes indications for the procedure (nursing diagnosis), goals/expected outcomes for the procedure and descriptions of increasing efficacy of nursing documentation (Fig. 21.2). The procedure is in itself an intervention that can be linked to or integrated into the electronic patient record system or the health information system, and thus contribute to an improved overview, less documentation and evidence-based documentation and practice.

Evidence-based procedures are an important element of nursing documentation, as the quality of the planned and documented care affects patient safety and outcomes [19]. The International Classification for Nursing Practice (ICNP) terminology is used in the VAR application, providing more advanced search and decision support, for example, suggestions for current procedures due to a specific problem or risk situation.

Also, based on continuous updates, it is possible to give alerts when new research, legislation or development has contributed to new knowledge that affects and changes the performance of the procedure. In standardised care plans, as well as in quality management systems, automatically updated procedures are ensured without having to do this update manually in clinical practice.

In this way, we can reduce the number of years it currently takes to implement new research into practice. Also, experienced nurses are better prepared and alerted to actually perform evidence-based and best practice. The original EPR vendors have started an adaptation process for such integrated decision support.

Principles for Developing a General Evidence-Based Support Tool

Based on our experiences and in line with the CDS Five Rights model [14], we will describe some important elements involved in developing a CDSS.

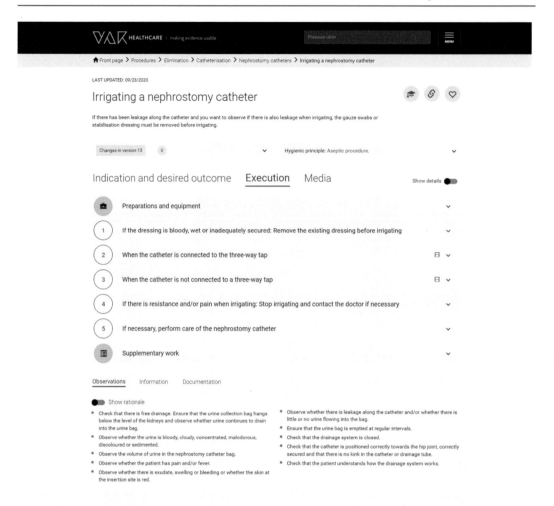

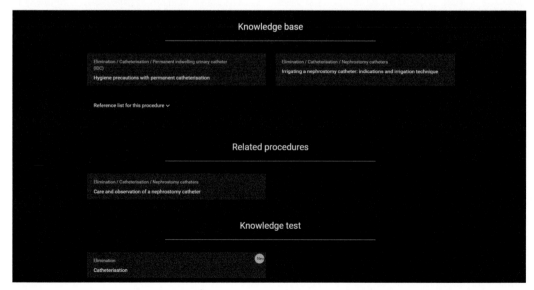

Fig. 21.2 A procedure in VAR Healthcare

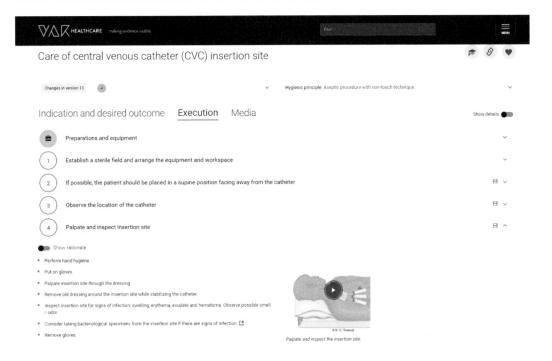

Fig. 21.3 Various levels of text can be shown

The foundation of a successful development is to have an innovative idea, not just based on research gaps or needs, but also anchored in society's or patients' needs. The idea should be described and operationalised as a project, with a project manager and a working group. The project should be performed stepwise and divided into phases, for example:

- Phase 1: Identifying content
- Phase 2: Prototype development
- Phase 3: System development
- Phase 4: Testing, evaluating and adjusting the tool
- Phase 5: Operation and maintenance

Figure 21.4 visualises the phases and process of such a CDSS development.

Phase 1: Identifying Content

To ensure the right information and content, a resource group with development experts should be established. It is a good idea to incorporate skills and competencies from practical as well as theoretical fields to ensure quality and anchoring in a broad understanding of knowledge, for example, experts from universities/colleges along with experts from hospitals/clinical practice.

To identify content for your CDSS, systematic literature searches and reviews should be performed, as well as using universally accepted methods, for example, PICO (Patient Problem/Population, Intervention, Comparison/Control, Outcome), AGREE II (The Appraisal of Guidelines for Research & Evaluation Instrument), and the EBHC (evidence-based healthcare) pyramid 5.0 for accessing pre-appraised evidence and guidance [31].

Seeking the best-possible knowledge is important, and with regard to the nature of nursing care and practice, several types of knowledge are important for the quality of its performance and outcomes. Therefore, the content should be based on the best-available knowledge, including legal, ethical, theoretical, practical and aesthetic knowledge. The knowledge base is, therefore, rooted in research and science, as well as personal and collective experience and professional traditions.

Fig. 21.4 Phases and process of CDSS development

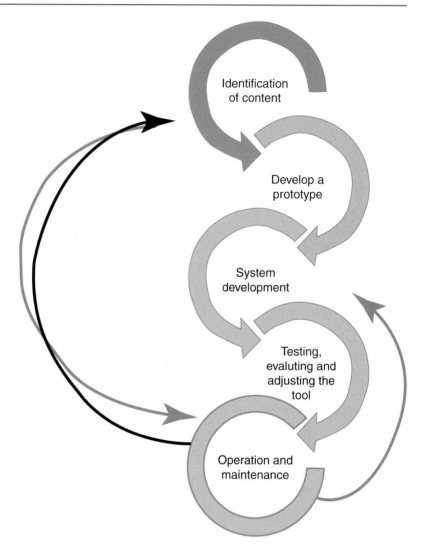

Also, transforming this knowledge for practical understanding and use, and making evidence usable are key factors that have significantly contributed to the success of the VAR Healthcare CDSS.

Furthermore, working in a structured, systematic manner is crucial. The content should be based on theories, models and/or standards that are in line with the aims of the project.

In the VAR Healthcare case study, we used Virginia Henderson's model of basic needs and the VIPS model [32, 33], as foundation for the categorisations of the procedures. The VIPS model was developed in 1991 to provide a common structure and keywords for representation of nursing care in patient records and was the prominent

model chosen for EPR infrastructure in Norway at that time. Henderson's basic needs were the core of nursing education in Norway. At VAR we also used the Model of Practical Skills Performance in Nursing [34] to address the complexity of a nursing procedure and as a fundamental principle that practical skills should be emphasised as being more than merely technical expertise.

Other standards and structures that should be considered are ISO standards, for example, ISO 9000 Quality Management Systems—Fundamentals and Vocabulary [35]. Such standards would cause one to consider and build systems for release management and control of the changes. The use of reference terminologies, like ICNP, contributes to a systematic use of nursing terms and consistency as well as the possibility of semantic interoperability between systems.

The content should be further validated by medical and/or nurse specialists from other hospitals and university colleges than just those involved in the working group. Involving the right persons, based on the Five Rights model, means involving professionals who will use the CDSS and ensures that they have the right information that they need.

Phases 2 and 3: Prototype and System Development

Our experience is that the technology and design should be developed in collaboration with IT vendors/experts to ensure a solid, enduring foundation. Working iteratively by first developing a prototype is a better use of resources and gives the end-user an idea and example for testing and providing feedback. In this collaboration between the different professions and experts, it may be a good idea to use a mediator with expertise or experience within both professions to "translate" the messages, ideas and possibilities as well as the consequences of decisions that are made. This is also part of finding the right person (the Five Rights model) and being able to develop the right technology/solution. It is important to avoid trying to "reinvent the wheel" and to get help to describe the intended use cases/needs, and translate them into technological possibilities. In this collaboration, you may discover that your mental map may be challenged and changed for an innovative and essential solution. Due to the Five Rights model, this collaboration between professions and expertise would increase the quality of the right format, right channel and right time.

Phase 4: Testing, Evaluating and Adjusting the Tool

All elements of the Five Rights should be tested and evaluated and the solution should be adjusted.

Qualitative and quantitative methods can be used. Tests and evaluations should be made on (a) the content—for example, quality and usefulness in performance, patient documentation, education, and (b) the technology—for example, user sequence and utility value, usability, implementation experiences. Methods that could be used include questionnaires, interviews and focus groups (e.g. dialogues to exchange experience based on the use of the system [qualitative]). Blind-testing of the technology can also be performed.

Adjustments and improvements based on the tests and evaluation should be performed between the phases, as well as prior to the release of the final version.

Phase 5: Operation and Maintenance

This is the most important phase and should be regarded as an ongoing phase. This step involves the dissemination of use of the tool and involves a plan and roll-out or an introduction of the tool for best-possible implementation.

The HOT-fit framework might be a good foundation for the preparation implementation of the CDSS [36]. This framework takes into account the fit and connection between humans using the system (system use and user satisfaction), the organisation they work in/where the system will be used in (environment and structure) and the technology (system, information and service quality). These factors may include barriers and success factors that can provide guidance or strategies for correct implementation.

A recent systematic review and gap analysis found that there are gaps in the research on organisational factors in evaluation studies of guideline-based CDSS systems [37].

Another recently developed framework is the Technology, People, Organisations and Macro-environmental factors (TPOM) framework that supports formative evaluations of implementation and digitally enabled transformation efforts [38]. This framework includes the same categories as the HOT-fit framework, but adds a macro-environmental factor and also provides more detailed dimensions. A recent study has found that the design of the CDSS should provide adequate support for clinical tasks, the workflow and cognitive activities, and should be followed up by organisational policies and routines to ensure correct implementation and use. Methods like lean process improvement and business process management (BPM) are recommended for identifying and eliminating barriers and a poor fit between human, technological and organisational factors [26].

By incorporating education and/or clinical practice in the development, it is likely that the intended end users will utilize the technology and can be ambassadors for the system and potentially other users.

One should consider again the use cases of the CDSS and potential collaboration with academia, other system developers, like the EHR vendors, QMS vendors and so on.

This phase also launches the project as a business and ensures that the CDSS is continuously up to date and can be used over time in education and/or clinical practice. Further technological changes, and possibly platform changes, will definitely be included, and funding will be required for these. You would need to involve someone who is willing to invest in your CDSS to ensure funding is available for further development, actualisation and use. Research funds are also an important source in supporting further research into your CDSS.

The underlying concept and core of maintenance and operations is to involve the users and bridge the academic and practical aspects of the tool. Establishing a user forum for key users (superusers) is preferable for networking, discussions, ideas, feedback and further development.

Summary

This chapter describes CDS in general, CDS in electronic patient record systems and the possible success of CDS and the VAR Healthcare case study, which is a general decision support system for nurses. Such a system has never been reported before. Most studies describe CDS for doctors much more than for nurses. Reports of CDS within nursing studies have mainly been conducted within acute care, and the support relates to a single clinical condition in a patient. There is a lack of the following: general CDS for nurses across patient conditions, systems that are fully integrated with the EHR systems, studies that include CDS development and usability testing. Hence, more and broader research and development is needed in CDS for nursing care and with more automation for optimal support.

The success of CDS development can be optimised when interventions in the CDS transfer the right information, to the right person, in the right format, through the right channel at the right time in the workflow. Also, to ensure continuous, clinical care of good quality that facilitates patient safety and best-possible health outcomes, data should be structured and of good quality. Clinical data models (CDM) and reference terminologies/models are needed to ensure semantic interoperability between systems.

The case study describes the development of VAR Healthcare, a general knowledge and decision support tool for nurses to be used across healthcare settings and that responds to many of the previous uncovered deficiencies of CDS for nursing care. VAR builds on nursing theories and learning theories, and uses standards and systematic processes in the development and maintenance of the tool. For many years, VAR has had links from various information systems like EPR systems, but it now also uses ICNP as a reference terminology system to ensure interoperability and the possibility of further development of sustainable integrations. Such integrations would bring CDS to the next step that could further optimise clinical practice and documentation—the next level of decision support for nurses.

Conclusions and Outlook

What important points can be summarised based on the case study in this chapter, VAR Healthcare? We would like to sum up our experiences and lessons learned based on the Five Rights.

The right information. VAR Healthcare is centred on procedures for nurses that are anchored in research and best evidence/practice and, furthermore, that can be used across settings in health care. Best evidence involves not just research, but also ethical, theoretical, practical and aesthetic knowledge. The knowledge base in VAR is therefore rooted in science, personal and collective experience, and professional traditions.

Systematic and structured use of nursing theories and models as part of the foundation of a CDSS has also played an important role. This is line with the findings of an integrative review of CDS in nursing, where the authors suggest the use of theories to improve the realisation of CDS in nursing practice [20]. Because VAR has been used across healthcare settings and education for over 20 years, practical and experience-based knowledge has developed cumulatively based on input from experts across settings, regions and countries. Thus, practical and experience-based knowledge is described at a collective level, in contrast to the individual experiences of the individual nurse. High-quality CDSS is dependent on high-quality content and technology, and thus a high level of competence in the professionals involved in the development of the content as well as the technology.

The right person. VAR Healthcare is developed for nurses, by nurses. Increasing and strengthening the competence of nurses is an important prerequisite for improving patient safety, continuity of care and positive patient outcomes. The aim of supporting nurses to provide and understand the rationale for their actions—why they perform care/procedures the way they do—involves not just providing the right content to the right person, but also providing the pedagogical perspective and evidence. This promotes increased reflection on practice and professionality.

The right format. VAR has provided evidence in a practical manner and language, where illustration updates concur with the text. Technology has also been used to provide various levels of information based on the user's needs; for example, a nursing student or a nurse who needs more in-depth information can access a complete view of the main steps of the procedure. Experienced nurses might only need the main steps of the procedure or just a glance at a detailed animation or illustration. A graduated system of changes and knowledge tests, where the user is guided to find the right answer, ensures lifelong learning and helps nurses keep up to date as a natural part of their work.

The right channels. VAR is available when nurses need it, wherever the nurse (or patient) is: on the Internet, on the computer, mobile phones and tablets. It can be integrated with EPR systems and into QMS for managers.

The right time. Furthermore, integrations with EPR systems by using ICNP will be of importance for building further support, including providing nurses with information at the right time. Certain information about the individual patient might trigger certain procedures, nursing diagnoses or goals (expected outcomes), and be made available to the nurses automatically. Although alarm fatigue has been reported [11, 18], alerting nurses when new research means changing how a procedure should be carried out is necessary for keeping even experienced nurses up to date.

Our experience of success with CDS is the following:

(A) An important part of quality assurance is achieved through sound technical expertise at each stage. It is important to verify the quality of the sources, knowledge and professionals who are responsible for development, evaluation and improvement throughout the process, from ideas to finished content and functionality. CDS connects knowledge between IT/informatics, technologies, and nursing professions and work processes. That means learning from and understanding each other and building bridges between the various competencies.

Long-term focus and follow-up. Maintenance of the system, including continuous further development of existing as well as new content and technology development—new possibilities, new platforms. Integration between a knowledge base, electronic patient record system and a reference terminology system may improve the foundation for research and statistics in nursing practice and patient outcome. The knowledge summaries in VAR also uncover gaps in research and show the potential for new knowledge and development within nursing care.

(B) Point A above also requires resource, investment, and business adaptation and knowledge. This is necessary for the success and longevity of a system.

(C) The innovative perspective of this project might slowly impact how CDS might change the mental image of "the reality." CDS should not only be an analogous system. However, we are challenged to think beyond what we currently know. In this VAR Healthcare project, we are transforming evidence into practice/daily work processes by utilising opportunities within technology (making evidence usable).

(D) With the solution and support described in the VAR Healthcare case study, evidence-based procedures form a natural part of nursing documentation/care planning, which in turn is essential for evidence-based practice and patient safety. This decision support system may turn the image of the care plan concept on its head and change the traditional view of care planning. In many ways, VAR is a standard "care plan" that is continuously anchored in best-practice knowledge and research and that keeps nursing process/documentation at the core of its template. That means saving resources that are currently being used to develop, update and control local work. These resources could instead be applied to ensure proper implementation and use, which the research has shown to be necessary and that currently poses a challenge.

Useful Resources

1. www.varportal.co.uk
2. www.varportal.de
3. www.varportal.dk

4. www.varnett.no
5. www.varhealthcare.com
6. ICNP: https://www.icn.ch/what-we-doprojects/ehealth-icnptm
7. SNOMED CT: http://www.snomed.org/
8. HL7: https://wiki.hl7.org/index.php?title=Detailed_Clinical_Models#Definition
9. ISO/TS 13972; 2015 (en). Health informatics—detailed clinical models, characteristics and processes.
10. ISO 18104, 2014.
11. WHO family of classifications: https://unstats.un.org/unsd/classifications/Family/Detail/1024

Review Questions

1. What is CDS?
2. Can you name the Five Rights?
3. In what settings has the use of CDS within nursing care been reported?
4. What is the most commonly reported barrier within the Five Rights for nurses?
5. What is CDM?
6. What is semantic interoperability?
7. In what direction should information be exchanged between the EHR system and the decision support tool?
8. What are the deficiencies in CDS within nursing?
9. For how long would the maintenance phase of a CDSS last?
10. Can you mention any standards that could be used in a CDSS, exemplified by the VAR case study?

Appendix: Answers to Review Questions

1. What is CDS?

CDS are computer-based systems that combine medical, health professional and other knowledge with individual patient information to support decisions, assessment, care and treatment of patients.

2. Can you name the Five Rights?

- The right information
- The right person
- The right format
- The right channels
- The right time

3. In what settings has the use of CDS within nursing care been reported?

Most of the studies of CDS in nursing are within acute care settings and relate to single clinical conditions.

4. What are the deficiencies in CDS within nursing?

According to Dunn Lopez [20], there is a lack of a general CDS that can support nurses across patient conditions, and of systems that are fully integrated with the EHR systems. There is also a lack of studies that include CDS development and a lack of usability studies.

5. What is the most commonly reported barrier within the Five Rights for CDS in hospitals for nurses?

The most common barrier for nurse practitioners using hospital CDS systems is within the area of *right information*

6. What is CDM (clinical data model)?

A detailed clinical model, that is, information model, of a discrete set of precise clinical knowledge which can be used in a variety of contexts.

7. What is semantic interoperability?

It means ensuring that the precise meaning of exchanged information is understandable by any other system or application not initially developed for this purpose.

8. In what direction should information be exchanged between the EHR/EPR system and the decision support tool?

The flow of information between a decision support system and the EHR system can either way: from the CDS to the EHR or from the EHR to the CDS.

9. For how long would the maintenance phase of a CDSS last?

This phase should be an ongoing phase and include implementation as well as continuous updating of the content and technology in line with new research, development and best practice.

10. Can you mention any standards that could be used in a CDSS, exemplified by the VAR case study?

Conceptual models like ICNP and SNOMED CT. ISO standards, for example, ISO 9000 Quality Management Systems—Fundamentals and Vocabulary [35] and ISO 18104:2014 Health Informatics—Categorical Structures for Representation of Nursing Diagnoses and Nursing Actions in Terminological Systems. Information models and theories like VIPS model [32, 33] and Virginia Henderson's basic needs. Learning models like the Model of Practical Skills Performance in Nursing [34].

Key words:

Clinical decision support, knowledge support, information standards, electronic patient record systems, documentation of nursing, documentation of health care, evidence-based procedures, evidence-based guidelines.

Clinical Decision Support: "Clinical decision support (CDS) provides clinicians, staff, patients or other individuals with knowledge and person-specific information, intelligently filtered or presented at appropriate times, to enhance health and health care. CDS encompasses a variety of tools to enhance decision-making in the clinical workflow. These tools include computerised alerts and reminders to care providers and patients; clinical guidelines; condition-specific order sets; focused patient data reports and summaries; documentation templates; diagnostic support, and contextually relevant reference information, among other tools."

CDM (Clinical Data Model): "Information model of a discrete set of precise clinical knowledge which can be used in a variety of contexts" (https://wiki.hl7.org/index.php?title=Detailed_Clinical_Models#Definition).

Interoperability: Ensuring that the precise meaning of exchanged information is understandable by any other system or application not initially developed for this purpose [30].

Reference Terminology: A reference terminology is defined as "a set of concepts and relationships that provide a common reference point for comparisons and aggregation of data about the entire health care process, recorded by multiple different individuals, systems or institutions" [39]. A clinical reference terminology is an ontology of concepts and the relationships linking them. A clinical reference terminology defines the concepts in a formal and computer-processable way [40].

References

1. Cassuto, J. Medical electronics in our future. Presentation at the New Jersey Industrial Health Conference, Somerville, November 5, 1966. https://journals.sagepub.com/doi/pdf/10.1177/216507996701500601. Accessed 13 April 2020.
2. Barretto S, Warren J, Goodchild A, Bird L, Heard S, Stumptner M. Linking guidelines to electronic health record design for improved chronic disease management. AMIA Symposium. 2003;66–70.
3. Kawamoto K., Houlihan CA., Balas. EA., Lobach DF. Improving clinical practice using clinical decision support systems: a systematic review of trials to identify features critical to success. MBJ 2005; 330: 765.
4. Sim I, Gorman P, Greenes RA, Haynes RB, Kaplan B, Lehmann H, Tang PC. Clinical decision support Systems for the Practice of evidence-based medicine. J Am Med Inform Assoc. 2001;8:527–34.
5. Wang P, Zhang H, Baohua L, Lin K. In: Sermeus W, et al., editors. Making patient risk visible: implementation of a nursing document information system to improve patient safety. IMIA and IOS Press; 2016. https://doi.org/10.3233/978-1-61499-658-3-8.
6. Murad M. Clinical Practice Guidelines. Mayo Clin Proc. 2017;92(3):423–33.
7. Trowbridge R, Weingarten S. Clinical decision support systems. In: Shojania KG, Duncan BW, KM MD, et al., editors. Making health care safer: a critical analysis of patient safety practices. Evidence Report/Technology Assessment No. 43 (Prepared by the University of California at San Francisco–Stanford Evidence-based Practice Center under Contract No. 290-97-0013), AHRQ Publication No. 01- E058. Rockville, MD: Agency for Healthcare Research and Quality; 2001.
8. van der Lei J. Closing the loop between clinical practice, research, and education: the potential of electronic patient records. Methods Inf Med. 2002;41:51–4.
9. Bonney W. Impacts and risks of adopting clinical decision support systems. In: Jao C, editor. Efficient decision support systems–practice and challenges in biomedical related domain; 2011. https://www.intechopen.com/books/efficient-decision-support-systems-practice-and-challenges-in-biomedical-related-domain/impacts-and-risks-of-adopting-clinical-decision-support-systems. https://doi.org/10.5772/16265.
10. Kwon APA, et al. Nurses seeing Forest for the trees in the age of machine learning. Comput Inform Nurs. 2019;37(4):203–12.
11. Medic G, Kosaner Kließ M, Atallah L, et al. Evidence-based clinical decision support systems for the prediction and detection of three disease states in critical care: a systematic literature review. F1000Research. 2019;8:1728. https://doi.org/10.12688/f1000research.20498.1.
12. Quama, R. Semantic mapping of clinical model data to biomedical terminologies to facilitate interoperability. PhD thesis submitted to University of Manchester. 2008. http://www.cs.man.ac.uk/~qamarr/papers/HealthcareComputing2007_Qamar.pdf. Accessed 29 July 2020.
13. Goossen-Baremans A, Collins S, Park HA. Semanticification in connected health. Stud Health Technol Inform. 2017;232:133–51.
14. Osheroff JA, Teich JA, Levick D, et al. Improving outcomes with clinical decision support: an Implementer's guide. 2nd Edition. Chicago, IL: HIMSS, 2012. American Medical Informatics Association. 2017;24(3):669–76.
15. Bright TJ, Wong A, Dhurjati R, et al. Effect of clinical decision-support systems: a systematic review. Ann Intern Med. 2012;157:29–43.
16. Verhugese J, Anilkrishna BT, Sajal KC, et al. Cost and economic benefit of clinical decision support systems for cardiovascular disease prevention: a community guide systematic review. J Am Med Inform Assoc. 2017;24(3):669–76.
17. Lobach, D. et al. Enabling health care decision making through clinical decision support and knowl-

edge management. Evidence Report/Technology Assessment No. 203. Rockville (MD); Agency for Healthcare Research and Quality. 2012. Report No.: 12-E001-EF. http://www.ncbi.nlm.nih.gov/books/NBK97318/. Accessed 29 July 2020.

18. Borum C. Barriers to hospital-based nurse practitioners utilizing clinical decision support systems. CIN Computers Informatics Nursing. 2018;36(4):1.

19. Muller-Staub M, de Graaf-Waar H, Paans W. An internationally consented standard for nursing process-clinical decision support Systems in Electronic Health Records. Computers, Informatics, Nursing: CIN. 2016;34(11):493–502.

20. Lopez K, Febretti A, Stifter J, Johnson A, Wilkie D, Keenan G. Toward a more robust and efficient usability testing method of clinical decision support for nurses derived from nursing electronic health record data. Int J Nurs Knowl. 2017;28(4):211–8.

21. Bennett P, Hardiker N. The use of computerized clinical decision support systems in emergency care: a substantive review of the literature. J Am Med Inform Assoc. 2017;24(3):655–68.

22. Wendt T, Knaup-Gregori P, Winter A. Decision support in medicine: a survey of problems of user acceptance. Stud Health Technol Inform. 2000;77:852–6.

23. Silsand L, Ellingsen G. Complex decision-making in clinical practice. In: Proceedings of the 19th ACM conference on Computer-Supported Cooperative Work & Social Computing, CSCW. 16. New York, NY, USA: ACM; 2016. p. 993–1004.

24. Staggers N, Weir C, Phansalkar S. Advances in patient safety and health information technology: role of the electronic health record. In: Hughes RG, editor. Patient safety and quality: an evidence-based handbook for nurses. Rockville (MD): Agency for Healthcare Research and Quality (US); 2008. Chapter 47.

25. Hyruk LA. Information systems and decision support systems: what are they and how are they used in nursing? AJN. 2012;112(1):62–5.

26. Olakotan O, Yusof MM, Puteh SEW. A systematic review on CDSS alert appropriateness. Studies of Health Technology Informatics. 2020;16(270):906–10. https://doi.org/10.3233/SHTI200293.

27. Goossen W. Representing knowledge, data and concepts for EHRS using DCM. Stud Health Technol Inform. 2011;169:774–8.

28. Goossen WTF. Detailed clinical models: representing knowledge, data and semantics in healthcare information technology. Healthc Inform Res. 2014;20(3):163–72.

29. Goossen WTF. Strategic deployment of clinical models. Nursing informatics 2016. In: Seremeus W, et al., editors. . IMIA and IOS Press; 2016.

30. ISO/TS 13972; 2015 (en). Health informatics–Detailed clinical models, characteristics and processes.

31. Alper BS, Hayenes RB. EBHC pyramid 5.0. For accessing preappraised evidence and guidance. Evidence Based Medicine. 2016;21(4):123–5.

32. Ehrenberg A, Ehnfors M, Thorell-Ekstrand I. Nursing documentation in patient records: experience of the use of the VIPS model. J Adv Nurs. 1996;24(4):853–67.

33. Ehnfors M, Ehrenberg A, Thorell-Ekstrand I. Nya VIPS-boken. Välbefinnande, integritet, prevention, säkerhet. 2. utg. Lund: Studentlitteratur; 2013.

34. Bjørk IT. Hands-on nursing: new graduate's practical skill development in the clinical setting [PhD]. Oslo: Institutt for Sykepleievitenskap, Universitetet i Oslo; 1999.

35. International Organization for Standardization. ISO 9000: 2015. Quality Management Systems — Fundamentals and Vocabulary (confirmed in 2021). https://www.iso.org/standard/45481.html.

36. Yusof MM, Kuljis J, Papazafeiropouloub A, Stergioulasb LK. An evaluation framework for health information systems: human, organization and technology-fit factors (HOT-fit). Int J Med Inform. 2008;77:386–98.

37. Kilsdonk E, Peute LW, Jaspers MWM. Factors influencing implementation success of guideline-based clinical decision support systems: a systematic review and gaps analysis. Int J Med Inform. 2017;98:56–64.

38. Cresswell K, Williams R, Sheikh A. Developing and applying a formative evaluation framework for health information technology implementations: qualitative investigation. J Med Internet Res. 2020;22(6):e15068.

39. Imel M, Campbell JR. Mapping from a clinical terminology to a classification. In: AHIMA's 75th anniversary National Convention and exhibit proceedings; 2003. http://bok.ahima.org/doc?oid=61537. Accessed 29 July 2020.

40. Campbell JR, Imel M. Function of rule-based mapping within integrated terminology management. In: AHIMA's 77th National Convention and exhibit proceedings; 2005. https://library.ahima.org/doc?oid=61602#.XyF5A54zY2w. Accessed 29 July, 2020.

Telehealth: Reaching Out to Patients and Providers

22

Ragan DuBose-Morris, Katherine E. Chike-Harris, Kelli Garber, Aric M. Shimek, and Kelli Stroud

Learning Objectives
- Describe telehealth modalities and applications.
- Identify the appropriate application of telehealth to support care teams.
- Extend best practices to professional roles.
- Place telehealth within the context of present and future state health informatics.
- Locate resources to inform current and future practice guidelines, legislation and policy.
- Analyze the use of systems to provide high-quality, secure telehealth encounters.

R. DuBose-Morris (✉)
The Center for Telehealth, Academic Affairs Faculty, Medical University of South Carolina, Charleston, SC, USA
e-mail: duboser@musc.edu

K. E. Chike-Harris
DNP Program, Medical University of South Carolina, College of Nursing, Charleston, USA
e-mail: chikehar@musc.edu

K. Garber
The Center for Telehealth, The Medical University of South Carolina, Charleston, USA
e-mail: garberk@musc.edu

A. M. Shimek
Ann & Robert H. Lurie Children's Hospital of Chicago, Chicago, USA
e-mail: ashimek@luriechildrens.org

K. Stroud
Atrium Health University City, Charlotte, USA
e-mail: Kkstroud@me.com

Key Terms
- Telehealth Technologies
- Remote Patient Monitoring
- Direct-to-Consumer
- Cross-state Licensure Requirements
- Reimbursement Parity
- Information and Communication Technology

Introduction

Telehealth is defined by the Health Resources and Services Administration (HRSA) as "the use of electronic information and telecommunications technologies to support and promote long-distance clinical health care, patient and professional health-related education, public health, and health administration. Technologies include videoconferencing, the internet, store-and-forward imaging, streaming media, and terrestrial and wireless communications" [1]. Though the terms are often used interchangeably, telemedicine usually involves clinical care while telehealth may or may not [2]. Telehealth can be used to deliver tele-education, teleconsultation, telepractice and teleresearch [3]. Tele-education refers to the delivery of live or stored educational content to health professions students, practicing providers and secondary education students, among others. Teleconsultation generally involves connecting a

© Springer Nature Switzerland AG 2022
U. H. Hübner et al. (eds.), *Nursing Informatics*, Health Informatics, https://doi.org/10.1007/978-3-030-91237-6_22

healthcare provider or patient under their care to a specialist or expert at a distant medical center. Telepractice refers to connecting healthcare providers in one location to patients in other locations such as a daycare, school, jail, skilled nursing facility or home. Teleresearch may include expanding a population base under study virtually or disseminating research findings from an academic institution to a local provider [3]. Furthermore, telementoring enhances the care provided by local clinicians. Project ECHO, the Extension for Community Healthcare Outcomes, is a model of medical education and care management that empowers clinicians to manage patients in their local community. It connects frontline providers with experts at distant institutions to gain the knowledge and support needed to care for patients with complex conditions within the local medical home [4]. Telehealth allows healthcare providers of all professions to work collaboratively and interprofessionally.

Overview

The concept of telehealth is not new. In fact, in the 1925 edition of *Science and Invention* magazine Hugo Gernsback described an instrument of the future called the "teledactyl." This instrument, predicted for the year 1975, would allow the clinician to "feel at a distance" [5]. The first true reference to telemedicine in medical literature appeared in 1950 and described the transmission of radiologic images by telephone a distance of 24 miles in Philadelphia [6]. The first medical use of video communications in the U.S. is believed to be in 1959 when clinicians at the University of Nebraska used two-way interactive television to transmit neurological examinations (Fig. 22.1). In 1963, Massachusetts General Hospital established telecommunications with a nurse staffed medical station at Boston's Logan Airport [7]. During the 1960s and 1970s, additional telemedicine applications evolved.

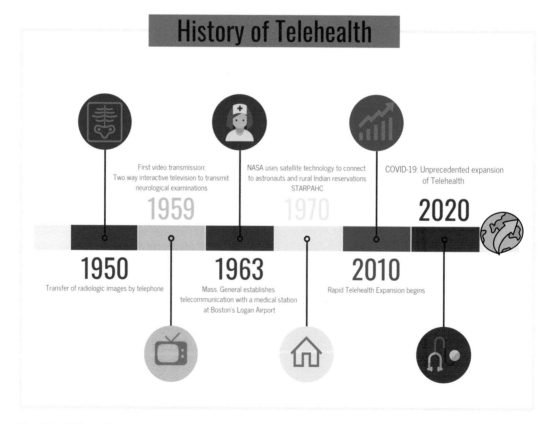

Fig. 22.1 Major milestones in the history of telemedicine. Image: Kelli Garber, created in Venngage

Interestingly, the U.S. Indian Health Service, the National Aeronautics and Space Administration (NASA), and the Lockheed company developed the Space Technology Applied to Rural Papago Advanced Health Care (STARPAHC) program. This program used satellite communications to provide medical services to both astronauts and a population living on an isolated Indian reservation [6]. In years since, technology has advanced along with the evolution of the voice over internet protocol and web 2.0, allowing for the transmission of dynamic content and improved sound and video quality. While telemedicine was gaining momentum in the 2000s, the arrival of the COVID-19 pandemic in 2020 thrust telehealth to the forefront of health care as a means to provide care and reduce transmission of the novel coronavirus (2019-nCoV). Many prior barriers to utilization, such as restrictions on originating sites and reimbursement, were removed during the pandemic, giving way to widespread adoption of telehealth. Whether this momentum will continue remains to be seen at the time this chapter is being written. However, it is likely the COVID-19 pandemic will mark the turning point in the widespread integration of telehealth into health care.

Technologies and Interoperability

The delivery of health care via telehealth can be performed through several modalities, which consist of four main categories: synchronous, asynchronous, remote patient monitoring (RPM) and mobile health (mHealth) [2, 8]. Synchronous televisits are what most people envision when thinking about telehealth and the use of real time, two-way audio-visual communication between the distant and originating sites. Typically, this communication utilizes a U.S. Health Insurance Portability and Accountability Act (HIPAA)-compliant, secured videoconferencing platform in conjunction with high-quality video and audio equipment, and peripherals (e.g., electronic stethoscope, otoscope, ultrasound equipment) if needed, in order to perform a comprehensive exam. Synchronous visits can occur patient-to-provider or provider-to-provider or can be medi-

ated by a telepresenter in alternate types of originating sites, such as school-based clinics. Some vendors offer telehealth devices that can be purchased for home use in order for a parent or other family member to facilitate a more detailed telehealth exam with the use of peripherals. This expands the scope of care that can be provided when the patient connects with a provider to be assessed, diagnosed and then treated for common acute conditions such as upper respiratory infections, strep throat or acute otits media. However, peripherals are not needed for all types of visits, especially those related to mental health, where a HIPAA-compliant and secured videoconferencing platform will suffice.

Asynchronous telehealth, also known as "store-and-forward," is based on capturing an item, either video, image or document, which is then electronically transmitted to another site for evaluation [2, 8]. A common asynchronous televisit is the evaluation of radiographic (X-ray) images within an urgent care or emergency room setting. The X-ray is obtained at the urgent care site and is then transmitted electronically to an offsite orthopedic provider who reads the image and then sends a report back with a diagnosis. Another example would be the ongoing assessment of a wound. In this case, the patient or caregiver takes daily pictures of a wound and emails the images to their provider, who assesses the status of the wound's healing and determines whether to modify the patient's treatment or if the patient needs an in-person visit.

RPM is the collection or real-time monitoring of patient health data that is evaluated via electronic means by a remote provider [2, 8]. Health data collected in a patient's home can consist of daily weights for the assessment of congestive heart failure, blood glucose measurements for the evaluation of diabetes, or blood pressure measurements. These measurements are transmitted to a provider who determines an appropriate intervention, if needed. RPM is also used in the hospital setting. Virtual sitters provide remote monitoring of patients to prevent falls and to monitor patients at risk for suicide. Tele-intensive Care Unit involves the remote monitoring of critically ill patients by intensivists and critical care nurses at a distant medical center thereby extending their expertise to patients in areas that lack sufficient specialized staff to care for critically ill patients.

Mobile health (mHealth), is similar to RPM in that data is collected using an electronic device [2, 8]. The difference between mHealth and RPM is that the data collected, for example, through a wearable sensor, is not necessarily sent to a provider for evaluation, but provides the wearer information about their own health, such as quality of sleep, number of steps, amount of activity and heart rate. mHealth often involves the use of health applications (apps) on mobile devices (smartphones, tablets) to collect information and provides health-related education to the consumer. These apps can also be used by healthcare providers as well in the form of medical dictionaries, medication prescription guides and review of patient records remotely. In addition to apps, several technologies that can be plugged into a mobile device can be employed to monitor patient data much like RPM. These adaptive devices can be added onto the mobile devices and collect health information such as blood pressure, blood glucose and EKGs that can be sent to the provider for evaluation. It is important to critically appraise health apps prior to using them to determine the developer, how often the content is updated, the expertise of the content experts, and the privacy and security of the app. Patients and providers should always be advised to read the privacy and security policies thoroughly before downloading and using any app.

Connectivity and Accessibility

The technologies that help to support all of the daily functions of health care are highly dependent upon the infrastructure on which they are built [9]. In the case of telehealth, combinations of wired and wireless networks are required to support connectivity between providers to hospitals, community facilities and their patients homes. These connections are generally supported through private vendors often in partnership with non-profit or governmental agencies

[10]. Accessibility is a key concern due to the lack of equitable and reliable broadband services. The same services that support daily commerce, education and entertainment are vital for the stable deployment of healthcare services. Prioritizing the development of broadband networks to support telehealth has taken national and international commitment [11, 12].

Within hospital and higher-level healthcare facility settings, the required broadband services are often available. Communicating with more rural or socially economically disadvantaged areas changes the options for connectivity at the local site [13]. The level of complexity increases when dealing with higher acuity services or with technology that requires more broadband capacity. Using lower bandwidth devices, such as those found in the remote patient monitoring realm, often allows providers to have direct-to-consumer access within a patient's home or at a central community location. Much as the evolution of modern economic systems, including electricity, telephones and running water, internet connectivity is equally important as a universal service in today's healthcare economy. Healthcare providers are essential to informing the development of these networks and the maintenance of their status as open for a variety of communication needs.

Security and Privacy

Telehealth offers the benefit of connecting with providers and specialists from around the world ,thus improving patient outcomes by matching the right patient to the right provider. However, utilizing technology to receive care is not without its challenges and risks. From the organization to the patient end user, everyone should take steps to ensure that their personal and private information remains just that.

The recent surge in users, types of applications and enabled devices has created unique challenges in data security and privacy. Recently, a wide variety of different platforms have emerged for use in the medical space—many of which were never designed for this kind of use— each with varying levels of security and privacy

[12]. In addition, the "bring your own device" (BYOD) trend is opening the door for additional security risks as patients and providers use personal technologies like smartphones, computers and tablets to access each other. This ultimately opens the door to more security and privacy risk when compared to consultations that occur on company-provided and maintained devices, which typically provide additional security features not found on most personal devices.

In addition, recent changes in response to the global COVID-19 pandemic have seen the rules and restrictions over U.S. HIPAA compliance relaxed slightly [14]. This is demonstrated by the Office for Civil Rights announcing in March 2020 that they would use discretion with regard to imposing penalties for HIPAA non-compliance against those using telehealth platforms which do not comply with current privacy regulations. This modification was intended to assist with rapid expansion of telehealth among providers who had previously not employed telehealth technology in their offices. It does not override state laws pertaining to privacy and security. While expanding telehealth has allowed for safer care of patients during the crisis, it does raise several privacy concerns. For example, researchers have found hackers targeting telehealth consultations for malicious activity in light of the recent surge in use and popularity.

Despite these recent changes, the onus to maintain security and privacy still lies heavily with the organization offering telehealth to its patients and with the providers conducting virtual visits. This is particularly important when providers are working remotely. What this looks like can vary across organizations but several key components have emerged. They include the organization's responsibility to conduct the steps in Fig. 22.2.

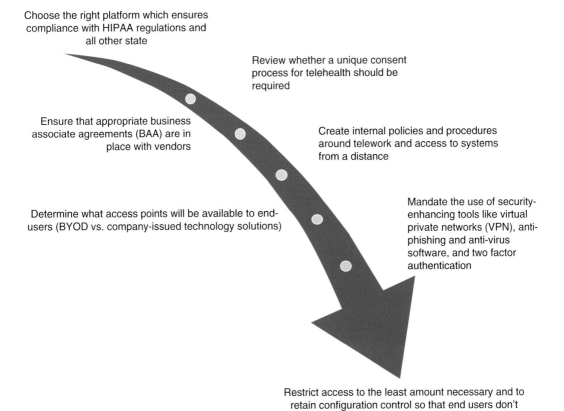

Fig. 22.2 Security planning, implementation and review steps (see Davis, 2020 for more details)

Some organizations have begun to seek an accreditation of their telehealth program and many of these components are important in that process. Going through the accreditation process typically includes the validation of privacy, security and safety technology requirements during the survey. Achieving accreditation can be used as a differentiator in the marketplace and also as evidence of achieving industry safety and security standards.

U.S. Regulatory Overview

Many who consider integrating telehealth into healthcare focus on the technology. While selecting the most appropriate technology is important, it is equally important for clinicians to review national and state legislation and regulations pertaining to telehealth and their practice prior to providing virtual care. In addition to telehealth specific legislation, one must consider a variety of legislation pertaining to health. Federal legislation and regulations, including the Ryan Haight Act and that of the Centers for Medicare and Medicaid Services (CMS) affect care provided via telehealth. The Ryan Haight Online Pharmacy Consumer Protection Act amended the Controlled Substances Act (CSA) with the purpose to prevent illegal distribution and dispensing of controlled substances over the internet [15]. Among other stipulations, CSA requires a clinician to have conducted at least one in-person medical evaluation with the patient prior to prescribing controlled substances (CS) via telehealth. If the patient has not been evaluated in person by the clinician, they may prescribe CS via telemedicine if real-time audio-visual communications are used while the patient is being treated by and physically located in a Drug Enforcement Administration (DEA)-registered hospital or clinic, or while the patient is being treated by and in the physical presence of a DEA-registered practitioner [16]. During the COVID-19 pandemic, the DEA adopted policies to allow DEA-registered clinicians to prescribe CS via telemedicine without an in-person visit with the patient. These policies were enacted only during the public health emergency and include specific requirements [17].

CMS legislation and regulation guides telehealth reimbursement for Medicare and Medicaid and often influences that of private payers. Medicare telehealth coverage was originally established in the Social Security Act 1834(m) of 1997. Because it was established in law, modifications to telehealth policy have been limited by the need to pass legislation. Restrictions on Medicare telehealth reimbursement include those pertaining to the specific services provided (based on the Current Procedural Terminology code), connecting provider type and geographic location of the patient at the time the services are rendered [18]. In 2019, CMS began reimbursing for certain services conducted remotely using communications technology that were not specifically defined as "Medicare telehealth services." These services include brief communication technology-based services or "virtual check-ins," remote evaluation of pre-recorded patient information and interprofessional internet consultation. An in-depth review of reimbursement for telehealth services is beyond the scope of this chapter, however it is important to recognize the complex nature of the telehealth reimbursement landscape. The Center for Connected Health Policy is an excellent resource for both national and state legislation and regulation pertaining to telehealth care and reimbursement [19].

In addition to Federal legislation, clinicians must be well-versed in state legislation and regulation pertaining to telehealth as well as their specific scope of practice. Some states integrate telehealth policies into law while others establish them through Medicaid program policies [20]. State telehealth laws may include a definition of telehealth or telemedicine, professional practice standards, consent requirements specific to telehealth, establishment of the provider-patient relationship via telehealth, prescribing requirements, telehealth specific licensure or certification requirements, cross-state licensure requirements and reimbursement parity.

No two states are alike in defining or regulating telehealth [21]. Furthermore, it is imperative that the clinician consider whether telehealth legislation applies to their specific healthcare profession by identifying what type of legislation it modifies (physician practice act, nurse practice act, stand-alone law, etc.) and whether the definitions of telemedicine or telehealth are inclusive of that profession. It is also important to look beyond telehealth legislation to that of the clinician's practice act and any advisory opinions or position statements put forth by governing boards such as the Board of Nursing. Following a 50-state review of Advanced Practice Registered Nurse (APRN) telehealth related legislation, advisory opinions and position statements, Garber and Chike-Harris found that most states have some telehealth guidelines, but that there is wide variation among states with regard to APRN practice and telehealth care [22]. Lack of uniformity in telehealth laws across jurisdictions can present a challenge for APRN practice as noted by the National Council of State Boards of Nursing (NCSBN) [23]. This illustrates the importance of carefully reviewing state laws in all of the states where care is being provided. A review of both the distant and originating site state laws is warranted.

Currently all states require that providers be licensed in the state where the patient is located. During the COVID-19 pandemic, CMS waived this requirement with regard to reimbursement, however this did not override requirements within state law. While this is an area of focused attention for telehealth advocates, all healthcare professions do not have options for cross state licensure or existing licensure compacts; a provider must apply for a license in each originating site state.

International Regulatory Overview

Despite its demonstrated benefits, global progress in telehealth has been varied, often non-linear, and predominantly confined to the national level. True international bodies for governing and regulating do not yet exist, but the past decades have seen the emergence of several large organi-

zations with both a global reach and an international focus. Of these, notable mentions include the eHealth arm of the World Health Organization (WHO), the Healthcare Information and Management Systems Society (HIMSS), the American Telemedicine Association (ATA) and the International Society for Telehealth and E-Health (ISFTeH). These organizations have been involved in telehealth for varying lengths of time but all aim to promote, advance and expand the use of telehealth globally.

As expected, the ways in which technologies are used vary in health care internationally. Researchers have noted that in high-income countries and regions with good information and communication technology (ICT) infrastructure, telehealth applications are used within a broad spectrum of services focused on diagnosis and clinical management [24]. RPM is increasingly used to monitor and manage patients with acute and chronic illnesses. Conversely, in low-income countries and areas with nascent or limited infrastructure, telehealth applications are primarily used to link providers with specialists, referral hospitals and tertiary care centers. The rapid development and release of new ICT, advancements in telecommunications infrastructure and new revenue opportunities for telehealth projects all signal a growing trend around the world. Of these, we highlight two here: the use of telehealth in public health/global health and in disaster response.

Expanding the International Reach of Medicine and Health Promotion

The WHO is a leader in global health and advocates for universal health coverage. Their 2018 Resolution on Digital Health explicitly included a call to action for countries to increase use of technology to strengthen health systems [25]. The challenges facing health systems across all nations range from the rise of non-communicable diseases, a growing shortage of the health workforce, manmade and natural disasters, and infectious disease outbreaks. The use of digital technologies continues to be explored as a means to address some of these challenges by a number of countries [26].

Technology is also changing how we care for others in public health settings, both locally and globally. Community health workers (CHWs) play an important role in reaching underserved populations and their utilization of telehealth technologies can assist in providing that care; these not only monitor patients and support the provision of care but they also aid with on the job training. One example showing promising outcomes is the e-Mamta program in Gujarat, India, which resulted in significant reduction in neonatal and maternal mortality [24]. This is just one example of how the uptake of technology can help expand the knowledge and reach of CHWs and help to promote health equity and address many of the social determinants of health (SDoH).

Emergency Care and Disaster Response

When time is of the essence, telehealth can be especially useful. Understanding that the main contributions of ICT to health care are through increasing the reach and speed of access, the role of telehealth in disasters becomes apparent [24]. The natural disasters in Puerto Rico are prime examples, from the 2016 Zika virus outbreak to *Hurricane Maria* in 2017 to the massive 2018 earthquake, many Puerto Ricans have been intermittently left without access to quality medical care [27]. These tragedies have helped to underscore both the value of, and the challenges in, using technology to provide care when demand overwhelms local capacity.

Despite these examples, the idea of using technology to assist in disaster response is not necessarily a new one. In 1995, the Global Emergency Telemedicine Services was launched by the Ministries of Health in France and Italy to provide an immediate telemedicine-based response to any emergency situation globally [24].

Looking at the four phases of disaster management, the potential uses of telehealth are

Table 22.1 Four phases of disaster management

Phase	Potential Uses of Telehealth
Mitigation	Vulnerability analyses, public education through the internet
Preparedness	Virtual simulations, scenario creations, support for evacuations, tele-training
Response	Teleconsults, telementoring, assisted evacuations
Recovery	Disease prevention, tele-support for long-term effects like PTSD

many (Table 22.1) [24]. Incorporating telehealth into common practice for disaster response has many benefits [27]. Tele-responders can help manage the influx of injured patients by remotely assisting with stabilization and rapid triage. They can also support local providers during complex cases which often require local practitioners to practice outside of their normal comfort zones. The peer-to-peer support offered through telehealth can help a patient receive the care they need but may not have otherwise been able to find. Another benefit lies with the volunteers and those who are charged with organizing them. Being able to volunteer virtually on a part-time basis may increase the number of volunteers willing to participate, while simultaneously allowing them to do so without the need to be transported, fed and housed at a disaster scene.

Emerging Trends

Health care is changing from a fee-for-service model to a value-based care model which bases insurance reimbursement more on the quality of care delivered to the patient rather than the specific services provided. Value-based care has three aims, including better health care for the patient, better health for the population, and lower overall costs [28]. Population health shares similar values since its focus is on the health outcomes of a group of individuals (i.e., population) and how these outcomes are provided to each individual, combining the concepts of health care and public health [29]. Telehealth technologies are transforming population health through meeting the three aims of value-based care.

With the increased integration of telehealth services into primary care practices, specialty practices, hospitals, skilled nursing facilities, prisons and schools, barriers to healthcare access are being minimized, especially for populations located in rural areas. These services are increasing patient compliance and engagement, reducing overall healthcare costs, and providing more effective and efficient care [30, 31]. Traditionally, rural populations have had barriers and challenges in accessing quality health care, either through lack of transportation, lack of services available in the area or the inconvenience of finding and securing a local primary care provider. With the increased adoption and utilization of telehealth, these barriers are being addressed and minimized. The benefits of telehealth are being recognized nationally and measures have been adopted to decrease the digital divide and increase broadband availability.

Telehealth has increased patient engagement and compliance by providing care to them in an environment where they feel the most safe and comfortable—their home. Instead of long waits in a medical facility's waiting room, patients are able to connect with their providers and specialists through on-demand consumer platforms, e-visits or virtual visits (synchronous and asynchronous). This is especially convenient for those who have transportation barriers, such as lack of a personal vehicle or the need for specialized transportation (e.g., people with physical disabilities). The use of eHealth or RPM is also increasing patient engagement and compliance by improving chronic disease management [32]. Patients can be monitored remotely, preventing escalation of negative trends (e.g., increased weight for a newly discharge congestive heart failure patient) which increases patient healthcare outcomes and reduces emergency visits or rehospitalizations [32]. This directly aligns with the aims of value-based care by increasing the health of the patient while decreasing overall healthcare costs.

Telehealth benefits the healthcare providers by reducing overhead costs, and no-show and cancellation rates [33]. Telehealth is changing the models of delivery of care, but not changing the standard of care. Literature has shown that telehealth can be effective in its delivery of care by allowing the identification and management of strokes at a faster rate, increasing the efficiency of ICU nurses and providers, increasing patient compliance and contributing to greater positive healthcare outcomes while making effective care easier and more efficient [30, 31]. Another benefit for providers, especially primary care providers in rural areas, is increased access to specialty care and consultation, as well as education. Rural primary care providers use telehealth to improve care of patients with chronic conditions by participating in such programs as Project ECHO [4]. In addition to reducing practice costs and increasing provider education, telehealth can also contribute to the reduction of provider burnout and improved patient care (Fig. 22.3). Telehealth offers a more controllable schedule for the provider without the pressure of rushing to see each patient within a set timeframe; this reduces stress for the provider and affords them the ability to concentrate more on the patient [34, 35].

Who Uses Telehealth?

Millennials, defined as those born between 1981 and 1996 [36], are the first generation to grow up with easily accessible electronics and therefore they are comfortable using technology to manage their everyday lives. Statistics from 2017 illustrate that 74% of millennials would choose a virtual visit over an in-person visit and 60% would like to see telehealth replace in-person office visits [37]. Even though millennials are tech savvy, approximately 81% of Americans own smartphones and three-quarters of American adults own either a laptop or desktop computer [38]. Contrary to widespread beliefs, 88% of adults >40 years old expressed interest in using telehealth according to the Associated Press-NORC Center for Public Affairs Research poll [37]. Moreover, telehealth has consistently shown that care provided via telehealth is equivalent to in-person care and that patient-provider communication using telehealth technologies has shown to be equal to in-person visits as well [39]. These

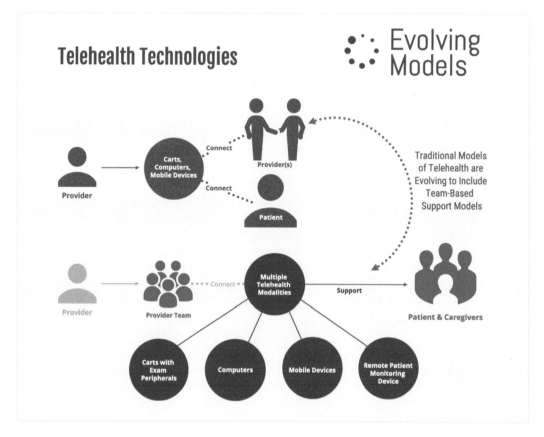

Fig. 22.3 Evolving models of team-based care supported by telehealth. Image: Ragan DuBose-Morris, created in Venngage

trends and facts suggest that telehealth is open for adoption by those who would benefit the most from it—the healthcare consumers. With increased adoption and utilization, healthcare delivery via telehealth will be a common modality in the near future.

Continuing Education and Evidence-Based Practice

Today's technology differs from the technology for tomorrow as telehealth will continue to evolve. Healthcare professionals must stay current with the latest education, competencies, certifications and evidence-based practice as it pertains to telehealth. Health professions training programs are rapidly seeing the need to train future healthcare providers in preparation for

practice and to demonstrate competencies as part of their formal training process [40]. In addition, accrediting bodies and professional associations are beginning to examine what it means to be a telehealth provider and how best to document knowledge, comfort and skills. The result will be a more formal assessment and possible inclusion of questions on board certifying exams.

Continuing education is another area of defined need as well as opportunity [41]. Many of the best ideas for the development of telehealth applications have flowed from the experiences of seasoned providers who understand the needs of their patients and want to better connect. Still, the training required for foundational telehealth knowledge was not typically included in most providers formative training and in the case of evolving systems of care, providers often rely on ongoing education to establish and enhance their skills. There are opportunities as well for students and residents to assist in the establishment of collaborative learning spaces where providers learn the technology skills needed and trainees acquire the medical skills required [42, 43] Performing a quick internet search will provide the general telehealth continuing education that may be beneficial. However, there are specific certifications that can be earned by healthcare professionals in telemental and telebehavorial health.

Next Generation Practice

Disruptive technologies like blockchain, artificial intelligence (AI), machine learning (ML) and virtual reality (VR) offer exciting potential for the delivery of health care. However, with new products, platforms and buzz words emerging almost daily, a simple cataloguing here of recent releases would be remiss.

The scope of nursing is evolving and through these changes, nurses now have a more interconnected role within the teams to which they belong. This has the potential to lead to new leadership opportunities within increasingly interprofessional teams and organizations. While this is an emerging trend in and of itself, today's nurse must also be prepared to tackle another emerging trend: playing a larger leading role in technology programs. Because of this, the nurse of tomorrow must focus on the skills needed to understand and incorporate healthcare technologies into their practice while simultaneously developing a critical eye on how to protect the very patients using them.

A nurse's unique clinical viewpoint is especially important in the integration of clinical patient-facing technologies. To meet this new edict, it will become increasingly important to ensure all current and future nursing professionals are equipped with the skills they will need to be a leader in technology. These range from how to assess technology products and the patient populations they're intended to serve to understanding the evidence-base around these technologies.

It will also become increasingly important to equip current and future nurses on the operational areas of project management such as planning, budgeting and change management in order to ensure a seamless implementation. This is a key role a nurse can play at all levels given the nurse's central role in communication and coordination.

Key components needed to build a new telehealth program include:

1. Performing a needs assessment can assist in finding the right partner, product or platform. This analysis will help clearly understand the program's need and its driver(s), the users, the key stakeholders and the kinds of data to be collected.
2. Begin by evaluating potential vendors across the six critical factors listed in Table 22.2 [44].

This trend in rapid technology proliferation is predicted to continue. "In the midst of a global pandemic and a U.S. recession, U.S. digital health companies raised $5.4B in venture funding across the first six months of 2020. The sector is on track to have its largest funding year ever" [45]. This continues the upward trend seen when comparing the increase from a then record $4.6B in 2014 to $8.2B in 2018, the last year where figures are available [45]. This surge in investment under-

Table 22.2 Developing a telehealth program

Factors to Compare	Key Elements
Business	Who are they as a business? Do they align with your mission and values?
Information technology	Can the technology integrate with your current system(s)? Is it customizable?
Security	Do they support compliance with HIPAA and local regulations? Is there transparency surrounding the collection of data and how it will be used?
Usability	How easy is it for the end user to operate? Can it be used by multiple types of specialties?
Customer service	How will they support your team through the process and your patients afterwards?
Clinical validation	Will this document outcomes in a way that can be used for published research?

scores the known trend: the use of technology in the provision of health care is increasing. The time is now to empower nurses to lead the way.

Case Study

John is a seven-year-old male student in the second grade. He has a history of severe asthma for which he has been hospitalized several times. He lives with his grandmother and two younger cousins in a small house in a very rural area. He sleeps in a sleeping bag on the floor in the living room along with his cousins because there is only one bed in the home. The family's main mode of transportation is walking since the grandmother doesn't drive and there is no public transportation in their county. John does not have a primary care provider; the closest pediatric office is over 30 miles away. He receives most of his care at the local emergency department (ED) which is approximately four miles from his home. Every time he is admitted to the hospital, he is referred to a primary care provider for follow-up but the family is never able to keep the appointments due to the aforementioned barriers. The literacy level of the family is low and therefore they have difficulty understanding the printed ED discharge instructions. However, John's school recently integrated a School-Based Telehealth (tSBH) program and he is now able to be evaluated and treated in the school nurse's office through synchronous telehealth visits with a pediatric-focused provider. Through the use of telehealth peripheral devices, a complete exam is completed at each visit with the assistance of the school nurse. Necessary asthma medications are prescribed and delivered to the school nurse by a local pharmacy in order for them to be administered at school. An asthma action plan was given to the school nurse, John, and his grandmother at an appropriate literacy level. Asthma education is reviewed with both John and his grandmother on a regular basis. John's asthma has been well controlled since the introduction of the tSBH program, enabling him to be seen by a pediatric provider on a regular basis and reducing the number of asthma-related ED visits.

Recently, the town was impacted by a category four hurricane causing significant damage to John's community and school. Due to the severity of the damage, recovery would take months for the town. With the school and its tSBH clinic closed, John again faced barriers in accessing consistent primary health care. However, the pediatric tSBH provider was able to connect with John and his grandmother at home through synchronous telehealth using their smartphone. While there are no telehealth peripherals, the provider is able to conduct enough of an assessment to ensure that John's care continues. During the visit, the provider is also able to assess the living conditions and potential triggers for John's asthma, as well as ensure that John is using his medications and inhalers correctly. She is able to advise the grandmother on ways to prevent triggers to better control John's asthma. To ensure that John receives his daily controller medications while at home and to monitor use of his rescue inhaler, he is provided with a Bluetooth-enabled inhaler. This inhaler uploads data about his medication administration to an app and its information is sent to his provider. This form of RPM is successful in assessing his compliance with his medication regimen, influencing the provider's decisions about modifying his medication management plan.

During the asthma visit, the grandmother tells the provider that John has been crying a lot and appears to be anxious since the hurricane. She notices that he appears the most upset whenever it rains. The provider conducts a thorough assessment, using the Trauma Symptom Checklist for Young Children, and suspects that he is suffering from post-traumatic stress disorder related to the hurricane. She then initiates a referral to the telemental health team who specializes in Trauma Focused Cognitive Behavioral Therapy. The team provides and uses a locked mobile device to provide this specialized therapy to John at home.

Review Questions

1. In managing asthma in the patient's home using telehealth technologies, how would you ensure that John and his low literacy grandmother understand the difference between the

maintenance and the rescue medication, as well as the prescribed asthma action plan?

2. What is needed to coordinate care between the local provider and the tSBH program to meet John's primary healthcare needs, such as regular well-child visits and immunizations?

3. What are some other options for providing health care to a community that has been struck by a natural disaster where existing healthcare facilities have been closed?

Conclusion: What's Next

Roles for Providers

With the adoption and expansion of telehealth, providers will need to become knowledgeable with this healthcare modality, not only in delivering it, but also in leading its implementation within their practice and participating in the development of protocols that benefit the entire population. Adopting telehealth will require the APRN to have basic knowledge of informatics in order to understand the technological requirements and keep abreast with its fast-paced change and evolution; research and adapt new telehealth technologies; participate in nursing research to enhance the use of informatics and telemedicine within their nursing practice; and continue to be advocates for patients who would benefit most from telehealth technologies. The future role of APRNs will be heavily influenced by advancing technology, particularly telehealth, and it is therefore essential that they be proactive and lead its integration.

As it relates to nursing, the roles and responsibilities within healthcare technology are growing. Nurses must develop the skills needed to assess patients for their level of digital literacy and their access to health information and communication technologies. Patients will also look to nurses for help in navigating these new systems and applications (e.g., electronic health records, patient access portals, wearable devices, etc.). Nurses will also play a key role in educating patients on when using telehealth is appropriate

and how to maintain privacy in the home during a telehealth visit.

In the long term, all providers must be prepared to address the risks created by patients seeking healthcare services from either on-demand, direct-to-consumer remote providers or from subspecialists outside of their normal network. As we have witnessed, the transition of the patient from a receiver to consumer of health care continues and this will have lasting effects on how, when and where a patient uses telehealth. Not only is the medical home at risk when patients seek care outside of their normal network, they may also be exposing themselves to increased risk as they attempt to connect using platforms and applications they are unfamiliar with. In these areas, the nurse's role of educator and advocate will become increasingly more important as technology plays a larger role in our patient's lives.

Evolution of Technologies

Current telehealth technologies were only a dream in the early 1920's when the cover of Radio News magazine showed the possibility of a future "The Radio Doctor" [5]. Now this "Radio Doctor" is a reality. How will telehealth evolve within the next decade? Will we be able to perform non-invasive medical diagnostics without even touching a patient as portrayed in today's sci-fi movies? Telehealth technologies will continue to become more advanced and encourage corresponding changes in healthcare delivery. One such advancement is AI, which is already being researched and utilized to develop remote healthcare models in such areas as tele-radiology, tele-pathology, tele-dermatology and tele-psychiatry [46]. AI is currently being utilized to assist the elderly to extend their independence and increase their quality of life through the use of eldercare-assistive robots [46]. AI may transform synchronous telehealth visits by employing AI and robotics to assess a patient in lieu of a medical person, which can assist in the evaluation and diagnosis of a patient before the patient is even seen by a provider [47]. With the rapid evolution of healthcare technologies, the most important characteristic that the healthcare professional needs to possess is an openness to learning and utilizing these technologies with the knowledge that this care is increasing the healthcare outcomes of a population and its individuals.

Changing Regulatory and Legal Space

Telehealth is a modality that is gaining greater popularity and usability within the current healthcare arena. Healthcare professionals should know that telehealth is affected by specific legal and regulatory issues. Currently, telehealth use outpaces policy and most likely always will. In an effort to ensure telehealth remains at the forefront, legislation must embrace and acknowledge telehealth as an extension of or additional option of current health care. Active healthcare policies should encompass telehealth. However, healthcare providers must be knowledgeable of federal and state laws that govern the privacy and security of medical information and ensure the technology they are using complies with applicable laws [48]. Each state has individual, if any, guidelines that offer guidance and suggestions for the management of telehealth services for differing levels of healthcare professionals [21]. In order to successfully expand telehealth, a mechanism for cross state practice must be implemented for all healthcare providers.

Your Challenge

The future of healthcare practice will indeed involve new technologies and ways in which provider teams can communicate across time, space and profession. For those interested in helping to advance the provision of service to achieve population health goals, much has been put in place that can be replicated in new settings or for new patient populations. We challenge you to be creative and equitable in the approach you take with the provision of telehealth services so that patients, providers and communities are all better served.

Summary

To summarize the evolution of telehealth at this point on the current trajectory of adoption is to note that there are significant opportunities and challenges remaining to bring telehealth into maturation. Beyond the different types of telehealth services and modalities supported, there advancements remain needed in how patients connect with providers, ways in which privacy and security can be assured throughout the transfer of highly sensitive private health information and the need for improved regulatory and legal environments in which telehealth can be expanded as well as regulated appropriately. Ideally, these advancements occur in a way that serves the greatest number of patients while also supporting a robust team of healthcare professionals that will ultimately be responsible for the care of patients through the efficacy of telehealth practice. Additional research and implementation science is needed within the scope of health informatics for telehealth to be a truly ubiquitous tool.

Useful Resources

1. Telehealth Implementation Playbook. 2020. Available from: https://www.ama-assn.org/system/files/2020-04/ama-telehealth-playbook.pdf
2. Center for Connected Health Policy. Available from: https://www.cchpca.org/
3. National Consor tium of Telehealth Resource Centers. Available from: https://www.tele-healthresourcecenter.org/
4. American Telehealth Association. Available from: https://www.americantelemed.org/

Review Questions

1. What is the definition of telemedicine?
   (a) Health care provided at a distance
   (b) Health care and provider education at a distance

(c) Health care that utilizes informatics and telecommunication

(d) Healthcare laws, regulations and applications

2. What telehealth modality involves the use of electronic devices to monitor patients at a distance?

(a) Asynchronous telemedicine

(b) Synchronous telemedicine

(c) Remote patient monitoring

(d) mHealth

3. Which statement is true regarding the use of telehealth across state lines?

(a) A provider must be licensed only in the state where they are located.

(b) A provider must be licensed only in the state where the patient is located.

(c) A provider must be licensed both in the state where they are located and in the state where the patient is located.

(d) A provider cannot provide telemedical services across state lines.

4. What are the four phases of disaster management?

(a) Notification, collaboration, preparation and response

(b) Mitigation, preparation, response and recovery

(c) Organization, preparation, response and recovery

(d) Mitigation, organization, preparation and response

Appendix: Answers to Review Questions

1. What is the definition of telemedicine?

While the terms *telehealth* and *telemedicine* have been used interchangeably, the definition of telemedicine is related to providing health care at a distance whereas telehealth may not may not include actual health care.

2. What telehealth modality involves the use of electronic devices to monitor patients at a distance?

Remote patient monitoring is the use of electronic collection devices which are used to assess a patient's information, such as weight, heart rate, blood pressure or blood glucose, by a distant provider.

3. Which statement is true regarding the use of telehealth across state lines?

In order to provide care across state lines using telemedicine, a provider must be licensed both in the state where he is located and in the state where the patient is located.

4. What are the four phases of disaster management?

Mitigation, preparation, response and recovery are the four phases or disaster management that should be used.

References

1. What is telehealth? | HHS.gov [Internet]. Health Resources and Services Administration (HRSA). 2020 [cited 2020 Jul 17]. Available from: https://www.hhs.gov/hipaa/for-professionals/faq/3015/what-is-telehealth/index.html

2. Telehealth Basics–ATA [Internet]. American Telemedicine Association. 2020 [cited 2020 Jul 17]. Available from: https://www.americantelemed.org/resource/why-telemedicine/

3. Burke BL, Hall RW. Telemedicine: Pediatric Applications. 2015; Available from: www.pediatrics.org/cgi/doi/10.1542/peds.2015-1517

4. Our Story | Project ECHO [Internet]. The University of New Mexico School of Medicine. 2020 [cited 2020 Jul 17]. Available from: https://echo.unm.edu/about-echo/#:~:text=Project ECHO (Extension for Community,people%2C right where they live.

5. Novak M. Telemedicine Predicted in 1925. Smithsonian.com [Internet]. 2012 [cited 2020 Jul 17];1905. Available from: https://www.smithsonianmag.com/history/telemedicine-predicted-in-1925-124140942/

6. Field M. Evolution and current applications of telemedicine. In: Telemedicine: a guide to assessing telecommunications for health care [Internet]. National Academies Press (US); 1996 [cited 2020 Jul 17]. p. 34–54. Available from: https://www.ncbi.nlm.nih.gov/books/NBK45445/

7. Bird KT. Cardiopulmonary frontiers: quality health care via interactive television [Internet]. Vol. 61,

Chest. Elsevier; 1972 [cited 2020 Jul 17]. p. 204–5. Available from: http://journal.chestnet.org/article/S001236921535892X/fulltext

8. Center for Connected Health Policy. Home Page | CCHP Website [Internet] [cited 2020 Jul 17]. Available from: https://www.cchpca.org/

9. Bauerly BC, McCord RF, Hulkower R, Pepin D. Broadband access as a public health issue: the role of law in expanding broadband access and connecting underserved communities for better health outcomes. J Law Med Ethics [Internet]. 2019 Jun 1;47(2_suppl):39–42. https://doi.org/10.1177/1073110519857314.

10. King K, Ford D, Haschker M, Harvey J, Kruis R, McElligott J. Clinical and technical considerations of an open access telehealth network in South Carolina: definition and deployment. J Med Internet Res. 2020;22(5):e17348. Available from: https://www.jmir.org/2020/5/e17348/

11. Drake C, Zhang Y, Chaiyachati KH, Polsky D. The limitations of poor broadband internet access for telemedicine use in rural america: An observational study. Ann Intern Med. American College of Physicians. 2019;171:382–4.

12. Koumpouros Y, Georgoulas A. A systematic review of mHealth funded R&D activities in EU: trends, technologies and obstacles. Informatics Heal Soc Care. 2020;45(2):168–87. Available from: https://www.tandfonline.com/doi/full/10.1080/17538157.2019.1656208

13. Struminger BB, Arora S. Leveraging telehealth to improve health care access in rural america: it takes more than bandwidth. Ann Intern Med. American College of Physicians. 2019;171:376–7.

14. Davis J. Must-have telehealth, remote work privacy and security for COVID-19. Helath IT Security Cloud News [Internet]. 2020; [cited 2020 Jul 17]; Available from: https://healthitsecurity.com/news/must-have-telehealth-remote-work-privacy-and-security-for-covid-19

15. Ryan Haight Online Pharmacy Consumer Protection Act of 2008 (2008; 110th Congress H.R. 6353) [Internet]. GovTrack.us. 2008 [cited 2020 Jul 17]. Available from: https://www.govtrack.us/congress/bills/110/hr6353/text

16. Congressional Research. The special registration for telemedicine: in brief. Washington, D.C; 2018.

17. U.S. Department of Justice Drug Enforcement Agency. COVID-19 Information Page [Internet]. usdoj.gov. 2020 [cited 2020 Jul 17]. Available from: https://www.deadiversion.usdoj.gov/coronavirus.html

18. Center for Connected Health Policy. Telehealth and Medicare [Internet] [cited 2020 Jul 17]. Available from: https://www.cchpca.org/telehealth-policy/telehealth-and-medicare

19. Health Information Technoloy [Internet]. Center for Connected Health Policy. 2020 [cited 2019 Mar 4]. Available from: https://www.cchpca.org/telehealth-policy/health-information-technology

20. Center for Connected Health Policy. Telehealth Medicaid and State Policy [Internet]. 2020 [cited 2020 Jul 17]. Available from: https://www.cchpca.org/telehealth-policy/telehealth-medicaid-and-state-policy

21. Center for Connected Health Policy. State Laws and Reimbursement Policies [Internet]. Public Health Institute. 2016 [cited 2020 Jul 17]. Available from: https://www.cchpca.org/telehealth-policy/current-state-laws-and-reimbursement-policies

22. Garber KM, Chike-Harris KE. Nurse practitioners and virtual care: a 50-state review of APRN telehealth law and policy. Telehealth Med Today. 2019 Jun;28:4.

23. Council of State Boards of Nursing N. NCSBN's environmental scan a portrait of nursing and healthcare in 2020 and beyond. J Nurs Regul. 2020;10(4):S1–35. Available from: www.journalofnursingregulation.com

24. Gogia S. Fundamentals of telemedicine and telehealth. Fundamentals of Telemedicine and Telehealth Elsevier. 2019:1–412.

25. Edelman PM and JK. Global Digital Health Index [Internet]. 2019. Available from: https://www.digitalhealthindex.org/stateofdigitalhealth19

26. WHO. Global diffusion of eHealth: Making universal health coverage achievable [Internet]. Report of the third global survey on eHealth Global Observatory for eHealth. 2016. Available from: http://apps.who.int/bookorders.

27. Lurie N, Carr BG. The role of telehealth in the medical response to disasters. JAMA Intern Med. 2018;178(6):745. Available from: http://archinte.jamanetwork.com/article.aspx?doi=10.1001/jamainternmed.2018.1314

28. Centers for Medicare and Medicaid Services. Telehealth General Inforamtion [Internet] [cited 2020 Jul 17]. Available from: https://www.cms.gov/Medicare/Medicare-General-Information/Telehealth

29. American Academy of Family Physicians. Population Health [Internet] [cited 2020 Jul 17]. Available from: https://www.aafp.org/about/policies/all/population-health.html

30. Morris S. How telemedicine is transforming healthcare [Internet]. HealthTechZone. 2019 [cited 2020 Jul 17]. Available from: https://www.healthtechzone.com/topics/healthcare/articles/2019/06/28/442557-how-telemedicine-changing-healthcare.htm

31. Hah H, Goldin D. Exploring care providers' perceptions and current use of telehealth technology at work, in daily life, and in education: qualitative and quantitative study. J Med Internet Res. 2019;21(4):e13350. Available from: https://mededu.jmir.org/2019/1/e13350/

32. Noah B, Keller MS, Mosadeghi S, Stein L, Johl S, Delshad S, et al. Impact of remote patient monitoring on clinical outcomes: An updated meta-analysis of randomized controlled trials. npj Digit Med. 2018 Dec 15;1(1):1–12. https://doi.org/10.1038/s41746-018-0027-3.

33. Ellimoottil C, An L, Moyer M, Sossong S, Hollander JE. Challenges and opportunities faced by large health systems implementing telehealth. Health Aff. 2018;37(12):1955–9. https://doi.org/10.1377/hlthaff.2018.05099.

34. Von Feldt K. Physician burnout: is telehealth the cure? iSalus Healthcare. 2019; Available from: https://isalushealthcare.com/blog/physician-burnout-is-telehealth-the-cure/

35. National Academies of sciences, engineering and MNA of MC on SA to IPC by SCW-B. taking action against clinician burnout: a systems approach to professional Well-being. Taking Action Against Clinician Burnout National Academies Press; 2019. 334 p.

36. Michael D. Where millennials end and generation Z begins | pew research center. Pew Res Cent. 2019;17:1–7. Available from: https://www.pewresearch.org/fact-tank/2019/01/17/where-millennials-end-and-generation-z-begins/

37. 6 Key Statistics About Millennials and Telemedicine [Internet]. Media Logic 2017 [cited 2020 Jul 17]. Available from: https://www.medialogic.com/blog/healthcare-marketing/6-key-statistics-millennials-telemedicine/

38. Pew Research Center. Demographics of Mobile Device Ownership and Adoption in the United States [Internet]. Pew Research Center 2019. [cited 2020 Jul 17]. Available from: https://www.pewresearch.org/internet/fact-sheet/mobile/

39. Shigekawa E, Fix M, Corbett G, Roby DH, Coffman J. The current state of telehealth evidence: a rapid review. Health Aff. 2018 Dec 3;37(12):1975–82. https://doi.org/10.1377/hlthaff.2018.05132.

40. Chike-Harris KE, Durham C, Logan A, Smith G, DuBose-Morris R. Integration of telehealth education into the health care provider curriculum: a review. Telemed e-Health. 2020 Apr 3;27(2):137–49. https://doi.org/10.1089/tmj.2019.0261.

41. van Galen LS, Wang CJ, Nanayakkara PWB, Paranjape K, Kramer MHH, Car J. Telehealth requires expansion of physicians' communication competencies training. Med Teach. 2019 Jun 3;41(6):714–5. https://doi.org/10.1080/0142159X.2018.1481284.

42. Pourmand A, Ghassemi M, Sumon K, Amini SB, Hood C, Sikka N. Lack of telemedicine training in academic medicine: are we preparing the next generation? Telemed e-Health. 2020; Apr 15

43. Kirkland EB, DuBose-Morris R, Duckett A. Telehealth for the internal medicine resident: a 3-year longitudinal curriculum. J Telemed Telecare. 2019;27(9):599–605. https://doi.org/10.1177/1357633X19896683.

44. Telehealth Implementation Playbook [Internet] 2020. Available from: https://www.ama-assn.org/system/files/2020-04/ama-telehealth-playbook.pdf

45. 2020 Midyear Digital Health Market Update: Unprecedented funding in an unprecedented time [Internet]. Rock Health. 2020 [cited 2020 Jul 17]. Available from: https://rockhealth.com/reports/2020-midyear-digital-health-market-update-unprecedented-funding-in-an-unprecedented-time/

46. AiT Staff Writer. AI In Telemedicine: Augmenting Healthcare Services in 2020 [Internet]. AiThority. 2020 [cited 2020 Jul 26]. Available from: https://aithority.com/ait-featured-posts/ai-in-telemedicine/#:~:text=AI in telemedicine is disrupting, develop new remote healthcare models.

47. Borole D. The Future of Telemedicine with the Rise of Artificial Intelligence [Internet]. DataFloq. 2019 [cited 2020 Jul 26]. Available from: https://datafloq.com/read/future-telemedicine-rise-artificial-intelligence/6744

48. Garber KM, Chike-Harris KE. Nurse practitioners and virtual care: a 50-state review of APRN telehealth law and policy. Telehealth Med Today. 2019 Jun 28;4. Available from: https://telehealthandmedicinetoday.com/index.php/journal/article/view/136/177

Public Health: Interoperability Applications to Support Population Health

Brian E. Dixon

Learning Objectives

- Define and distinguish between the terms public health and population health.
- Describe nursing roles in the use of information technologies to facilitate public health and population health.
- Explain the role of public health organizations in facilitating and participating in interoperability and health information exchange.
- List and describe common scenarios in which interoperability and health information exchange could facilitate improvements to population health outcomes.
- Describe the current adoption and use of interoperability and health information exchange by public health organizations.
- Define and describe existing as well as emerging standards for interoperability in the context of population health.
- Discuss the challenges to broader adoption of interoperability and health information exchange for population health use cases.

Key Terms

- Health information exchange
- Interoperability
- Public health
- Population health
- Electronic case reporting
- Care coordination
- Population health management
- Social determinants of health
- Learning health system

Introduction

The field of *public health* can be defined as "the science and art of preventing disease, prolonging life and promoting health through the organized efforts of society, organizations, public and private communities, and individuals" [1]. Public health as a science and practice focuses on the health and well-being of populations—collections of individuals who reside in communities. The ethos of public health is quite similar to that of nursing. Specifically, public health concerns itself not only with the care of patients but the prevention of illness and health promotion.

The commonalities between public health and nursing manifest themselves in multiple ways, including in the many roles that nurses play in governmental public health agencies across the globe. For example, most local health departments employ one or more nurses who deliver

B. E. Dixon (✉)
Department of Epidemiology, Indiana University (IU) Richard M. Fairbanks School of Public Health, Indianapolis, IN, USA

Center for Biomedical Informatics, Regenstrief Institute, Inc., Indianapolis, USA
e-mail: bedixon@regenstrief.org

© Springer Nature Switzerland AG 2022
U. H. Hübner et al. (eds.), *Nursing Informatics*, Health Informatics,
https://doi.org/10.1007/978-3-030-91237-6_23

care to individuals without (or without enough) insurance and/or coordinate the critical role of disease investigation. Public health nurses also lead vaccination campaigns to protect infants, children, and other populations from disease. Nurses further play critical roles in health systems with respect to infection control and prevention, a role nowadays titled "infection preventionist" (formerly "infection control practitioner").

Governmental public health organizations exist at federal, state, and local levels of modern society. Whereas federal agencies often coordinate responses to disease outbreaks like the COVID-19 pandemic, state and local agencies are often on the front lines of addressing everyday health challenges such as diabetes, obesity, influenza, and dementia. All public health agencies focus on ten essential services to support the health and well-being of populations in their jurisdiction.

The ten essential services of public health [2] include:

1. Monitor health status to identify and solve community health problems.
2. Diagnose and investigate health problems and health hazards in the community.
3. Inform, educate, and empower people about health issues.
4. Mobilize community partnerships and action to identify and solve health problems.
5. Develop policies and plans that support individual and community health efforts.
6. Enforce laws and regulations that protect health and ensure safety.
7. Link people to needed personal health services and assure the provision of health care when otherwise unavailable.
8. Assure competent public and personal healthcare workforce.
9. Evaluate effectiveness, accessibility, and quality of personal and population-based health services.
10. Research for new insights and innovative solutions to health problems.

The Commissioned Corps of the U.S. Public Health Service seeks to prevent disease, conduct research, and care for patients in underserved communities across the nation and throughout the world [3]. The Corps is one of the seven uniformed services serving the U.S. government, and its members staff numerous agencies across the federal government. The Corps includes a number of Registered Nurse and Nurse Practitioner professionals serving across dozens of federal agencies. These men and women serve on the front lines of health care, especially during disease outbreaks and public health emergencies.

Facilitating Population Health Through Interoperability

Interoperability refers to "the ability of two or more [EHR] systems or [health information technology] components to exchange information and to use the information that has been exchanged" [4]. When caring for patients, most interoperability scenarios will involve the exchange of information between two or more clinical information systems like electronic health record (EHR) systems, laboratory information systems, and electronic prescribing systems. For example, retrieving a patient's past medical history might involve using a health information exchange (HIE) application to access information on a patient's visits to other hospitals in the region.

Yet there exists a broader set of circumstances where clinical information systems need to exchange data with public health information systems. For example, in the recent COVID-19 pandemic, hospitals were required to report data on inpatients who tested positive for the disease to state health authorities as well as the federal government. The data were necessary to inform public health about hospital capacity as well as current supply levels of personal protective equipment (PPE). In Indiana, members of the state's national guard units would deliver PPE to health facilities running low to ensure they could care for patients arriving with COVID-19-like illness. Similarly, laboratory test results for patients with COVID-like illnesses were required to be reported electronically to state health departments, and detailed clinical case reports were submitted to public health by nurses and physicians treating infected patients. These scenarios would benefit from electronic exchange of information from inventory management, EHR, and laboratory information systems rather than requiring clinical staff to manually enter data into public health databases.

Public health agencies seek to facilitate information exchange in communities to enable multiple components of the health system to collaborate in addressing population health needs. Agencies host community-wide immunization registries, which are available to clinics and pharmacies where vaccines are delivered. Public health organizations also play a critical role in facilitating discussions among healthcare stakeholders to ensure that together these stakeholders can share data and information to identify and resolve the needs of those living in a community. Public health agencies bring a population health perspective to data and information exchange.

The Population Health Perspective

Whereas clinicians tend to conceive of health from the perspective of the patient, public health focuses on populations with an emphasis on prevention of disease, injury, disability, or environmental impact [5]. Populations can be thought of as a group of patients, such as all the patients for which I'm responsible as a clinician. Yet most often, populations are groups of individuals who have at least one common thread, such as the neighborhood in which they live, a disease or condition (e.g., diabetes mellitus, traumatic brain injury), or a personal trait (e.g., eye color, ethnicity).

The term *population health* (sometimes referred to as PopHealth) has several meanings. Governmental public health agencies conceive their role as advocating, providing support, and caring (many local public health agencies operate free or low-cost clinics) for the health and well-being of populations in their jurisdiction. Clinical organizations tend to focus on the health outcomes of defined populations as measured by targeted health status indicators. A more recently proposed definition is "a domain focusing on health outcomes of a group of individuals, including the distribution of such outcomes within the group" [6]. However, it is important to note that a consensus-based definition of population health does not exist.

Researchers at the Johns Hopkins Bloomberg School of Public Health developed a conceptual framework for population health that integrates the milieu of ideas on PopHealth [7]. An adapted version of this framework (Fig. 23.1) depicts the

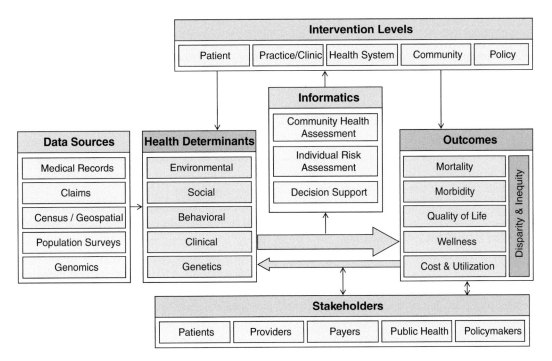

Fig. 23.1 A conceptual model for population-level data exchange and use to influence outcomes, adapted from [7]

exchange of clinical as well as non-clinical data for use in informatics applications to influence population health outcomes. Data on the determinants of health (e.g., genetic, behavioral, clinical, social, environmental) are derived from numerous sources, including EHR systems and insurance claims. Population-level data from the U.S. Census Bureau as well as population surveys (e.g., Behavioral Risk Factor Surveillance System) can be integrated with clinical and administrative data to derive information about health determinants. Informatics applications, including decision support engines and measurement of community health metrics, are used to derive knowledge about outcomes from the data and information. Knowledge informs the various stakeholders, including public health agencies, about the health and well-being of the populations. These stakeholders can implement various interventions into clinical practice as well as health systems and communities to influence change in outcomes.

The ultimate goal of a population health intervention, including informatics interventions, is to improve population-level health outcomes by modifying the underlying determinants of health. Population health interventions can target specific patient populations (e.g., African-American men with HIV, Veterans), a health system (e.g., payment adjustment in value-based contracts), or a community (e.g., neighborhoods with a high proportion of Hispanic residents). Interventions can also target one or multiple health determinants. For example, a health system may offer cancer screenings for high-risk patients in low-income neighborhoods. Community-level approaches might involve policies that expand access to expensive Hepatitis C treatment for Medicaid patients or homeless populations.

Current Use of Interoperability for Population Health

Many public health organizations have implemented processes that necessitate healthcare providers to report information for certain diseases. While providers may manually type this information into a website hosted by the health department, they nonetheless electronically report data to public health. Reciprocal sharing of data and information with healthcare organizations also exists, such as when clinics retrieve immunization records from a public health registry. But how much interoperability exists in the modern informatics landscape?

The current adoption and use of HIE by public health organizations, especially governmental local and state public health agencies, is difficult to ascertain. There exist few studies of HIE adoption, and virtually none of them focus on public health organizations. This may be due, in part, to the fact that the definition of adoption for public health organizations is unclear. While the U.S. Office of the National Coordinator for Health Information Technology (ONC) has defined four types of HIE functions for hospitals, similar measures for health departments do not exist. If a local health department exchanges data with the U.S. Centers for Disease Control and Prevention (CDC), does that count as HIE? While challenging to define and measure, there is some evidence that HIE adoption exists among public health organizations.

As of 2014, the CDC reported that two-thirds (67%) of health departments had implemented some form of HIE involving the electronic exchange of laboratory data [8]. While promising, this statistic pertains to the proportion of overall laboratory results received by public health departments. It does not provide insight into how those messages were received or whether the exchange involved a regional HIE organization or simply point-to-point transmission of the message. It is assumed that many exchanges of laboratory results involve point-to-point communication between the lab and the health department.

The most recent data on HIE adoption among local health departments, published in 2019 by Yeung [9], suggests that 13.4% of local health departments have adopted HIE as opposed to 24.7% adoption of EHR systems. These data are based on a survey of local health departments conducted in 2013 by the National Association of City and County Health Officials. A survey of hospital-based infection preventionists, who are often responsible for population surveillance in healthcare systems, reported that just 10% of respondents indicated their hospital was engaged in HIE activities [10]. Both of these surveys were conducted more than 5 years ago, making it challenging to understand current HIE adoption levels. Furthermore, there are no comparable surveys of state health departments or a census of HIE use by the CDC. Therefore, our best guess is that less than one in five or 20% of public health organizations is engaged in sustained interoperability with clinical organizations. This would suggest that many forms of public health HIE, such as disease case reporting and vaccine record history, involve manual information retrieval or reporting by a nurse or other clinician. These exchanges are most likely to involve a fax machine.

Population Health Use Cases for Interoperability

In this section of the chapter, we examine several scenarios in which interoperability and HIE are increasingly being adopted and used to enhance population health.

Reporting Notifiable Conditions to Public Health Agencies

One of the most common forms of interoperability and HIE is used to report notifiable conditions (also referred to as communicable or infectious diseases) to governmental public health agencies. Nearly all states have laws that require healthcare providers and/or laboratories to report new cases of diseases such as tuberculosis, malaria, chlamydia, and HIV. While these state laws vary with respect to which diseases should be reported, most necessitate reporting by both the laboratory and physician who ordered the confirmatory laboratory test. Agencies use these data to monitor the prevalence of disease as well as reduce the potential for disease spread through investigation and follow-up with the individuals who are diagnosed with the disease.

Historically data were either mailed or faxed into the health department. However, most states now have the capacity to receive data on notifiable diseases via electronic messages from laboratories [11]. The process of reporting data from laboratories to public health agencies for notifiable diseases is referred to as electronic laboratory reporting (ELR). Less common is the electronic reporting of notifiable disease case information from providers to public health agencies. This process is referred to as electronic case reporting (eCR).

Electronic Laboratory Reporting

Given variable adoption rates of ELR before 2011, ELR was incorporated into the regulations for both Stage 2 and Stage 3 of the Meaningful Use Program, as well as the 2018 Promoting Interoperability Program, managed by the U.S. Centers for Medicare and Medicaid Services (CMS). Laboratory information systems are required to electronically submit laboratory results to EHR systems for delivery to clinicians, and hospitals are encouraged to electronically report laboratory results for notifiable disease cases to public health departments using their EHR system.

Nearly all ELR implementations across the U.S. utilize HL7® Version 2.5.1 messages to report positive laboratory results for a notifiable disease. The tests performed by the laboratory are identified using Logical Observation Identifiers Names and Codes (LOINC®) codes. The outcome of the test (e.g., positive, detected) is identified using the Systematized Nomenclature of Medicine-Clinical Terms (SNOMED CT®) codes. Health departments typically parse the incoming HL7 messages into a case reporting system, such as the NEDSS Base System, which is used by 23 health departments representing 19 states plus Washington, DC; Guam; Puerto Rico; and the U.S. Virgin Islands [12].

Public health agencies that use ELR report a number of benefits. First, notifiable disease reports that arrive electronically arrive faster than the previously used paper-based reports [13–15]. Second, ELR has been shown to increase completeness or the proportion of reportable disease reports that are transmitted to public health [11, 13–15]. Thus, ELR can address the problem of underreporting of reportable disease cases [16, 17].

Electronic Case Reporting

Whereas ELR messages are sent from the laboratory, eCR messages are sent from physician practices or hospitals. These messages include details beyond what can be sent in an ELR message, such as the patient's disposition at the time of clinical diagnosis. An eCR message might also contain details about the patient's vaccination history, social determinants, and symptoms. These details can be used by disease investigation officers at the health department to identify suspected or probable cases.

In Stage 3 of the CMS Meaningful Use Program as well as the 2019 Promoting Interoperability Program, CMS promoted eCR as a valid public measure for hospitals. The requirement nudges hospitals to move "toward sending 'production data'" to public health authorities in their jurisdiction.

There are two available technical specifications for achieving interoperability and HIE with respect to eCR. The first method involves using the HL7 Clinical Document Architecture (CDA) standard to deliver a case report from an EHR system to a public health organization. The Electronic Initial Case Report (eICR) technical standard, published by HL7®, [18] enables providers to publish a standardized clinical document that contains details about the notifiable disease case. For example, a provider would use his or her EHR to manually initiate the creation of an eICR document and then hit a "submit to public health" button. The document would be electronically transmitted to public health.

The current version of the eICR standard (published in January 2018) is being pilot-tested in several communities across the U.S. as a part of the "Digital Bridge" [19]. The initiative plans to update the technical standard after the pilot testing using feedback from pilot sites.

An alternative to the eICR is the newer HL7® standard, referred to as Fast Healthcare Interoperability Resources (FHIR). Whereas the eICR involves clinical health organizations (or individuals) manually "pushing" a document to public health, a FHIR-based approach would involve public health organizations electronically querying specific information from clinical data sources (e.g., EHR system).

In partnership with the Georgia Tech Research Institute, the Regenstrief Institute piloted [20] a FHIR-based application within the INPC (Indiana Network for Patient Care), a community-based HIE network [21]. During the pilot, Regenstrief received an HL7® 2.5.1 compliant ELR message from a laboratory. The ELR message served as an electronic trigger for the application to query the INPC for additional details since the INPC contains data from multiple EHR systems. The query from the health department asked for FHIR-based resources, which are discrete health data exposed through web services [22], on the patient such as demographics, medications, and clinical diagnosis codes. The data requested from the INPC were then transmitted to the state health department case management system for use by disease investigators and epidemiologists.

While the pilot was considered a success, the testing of the FHIR-based approach identified several challenges. For example, the FHIR-based application required that providers had recorded an International Classification of Disease (ICD) code for a disease that matched the initial positive laboratory report. However, physicians did not record an ICD diagnosis in 25% of cases. Informatics applications need to be more lenient as humans do not always behave in an expected manner. More intelligent approaches that can examine structured as well as non-structured data (e.g., clinical notes, nursing documentation) are likely necessary to better automate disease reporting processes.

Health Indicators

Another application area for HIE in public health involves querying EHR systems and other electronic data sources to enhance the measurement and monitoring of population health indicators. Public health agencies rely upon a number of risk factor information systems to collect, manage, and share data for surveillance purposes [23]. These data typically identify the prevalence of disease (e.g., proportion of individuals who have been told by a healthcare provider they have diabetes) or risk factors for disease (e.g., proportion of individuals who report being a smoker).

While current methods produce reliable estimations of population health, many risk factor information systems publish data with wide confidence intervals and small sample sizes at the local level. For example, the 2015 BRFSS estimated hypertension prevalence in Marion County, Indiana, to be 28.4% (CI: 24.6%–32.2%) based on a sample size of 934 individuals [24]. The confidence intervals become more significant for sub-populations, such as the proportion of African Americans with hypertension. Moreover, many indicators are available only at state and national levels, which also complicates their application to county and sub-county public health jurisdictions.

Given these challenges, some health departments have attempted to leverage interoperability to gather EHR data that can be applied at the local level. For example, the New York City Department of Health and Mental Hygiene deployed its MACROSCOPE system in which the city electronically queries EHR systems representing more than 700 primary care practices in the metropolitan area [25]. Aggregate data on the prevalence of obesity, smoking, diabetes, hypertension, immunization, and depression are returned from the EHRs and synthesized into indicators for review by epidemiologists. In Indiana, the Marion County Public Health Department partnered with the Regenstrief Institute to similarly gather county-level data from EHR systems using the INPC. This project calculated prevalence rates for depression, diabetes, asthma, and other conditions of public health interest [26].

In both the New York City and Indianapolis cases, the EHR-based population health indicators possessed much tighter confidence intervals than BRFSS. For example, in New York, the prevalence of diabetes was measured at 13.9% (CI: 13.8%–14.0%) [27]. These cities also found that EHR-based measures are similar to risk factor information system estimates for most (but not all) indicators. Depression and asthma did not match BRFSS or NHANES estimates, while indicators for hypertension and diabetes were nearly equivalent.

Specialized Disease Registries

Another application area for HIE in public health is specialized disease registries. Given the ability of HIE networks to facilitate the collection, management, and sharing of data on health indicators as described above, public health organizations could routinely capture information on specific high-priority conditions of local interest. For example, many public health agencies are interested in establishing community-wide diabetes registries for primary or secondary prevention.

A registry is an organized system that uses observational study methods to collect uniform data to evaluate specified outcomes for a population defined by a particular disease, condition, or exposure, and that serves one or more predetermined scientific, clinical, or policy purposes [28]. It is common for public health agencies to maintain immunization registries [29]. The current CMS program Promoting Interoperability encourages providers to use EHR systems to support the development of specialized disease registries.

One example is a comprehensive registry for sexually transmitted infections (STIs) [30]. While public health agencies typically receive information from providers and laboratories when an individual tests positive for an STI, usually public health does not receive negative tests results. Using an STI registry developed by the Regenstrief Institute, the Marion County Public Health Department examined where patients received STI testing using positive and negative test results [31]. The researchers found that STI clinics were more likely to test men and outpatient practices more likely to test women. Yet they also discovered the emergency departments increasingly tested a larger proportion of the population and documented greater morbidity. This suggested that public health agencies might wish to partner with emergency settings to address rising rates of STIs in the community. Researchers further leveraged the STI registry to examine the validity of using ICD-10 codes to document STI cases [32] and syphilis testing rates among women with a stillbirth delivery [33].

Care Coordination Informed by Interoperability

Healthcare delivery is fragmented. Patients seek care from a variety of providers, whether or not those providers are part of the same organized network [34]. Moreover, many patients manage their health using devices as well as the Internet [35]. Given the mobility of individuals and populations, delivering high-quality, coordinated care requires that clinicians can access, manage, and share information.

Event notification is one form of interoperability involving the electronic reporting (or pushing) of information pertaining to a clinical event from one provider to another facilitated by a messaging standard [36]. Notification usually pertains to acute care events (e.g., hospitalization, emergency care), and the notifications are typically sent to primary care providers responsible for coordination of care [37]. Increasingly, nurses are asked to perform care coordinator roles in clinics and health systems. Therefore, future applications of event notifications may center around nursing roles rather than physician roles as nursing scopes of practice expand.

Currently we are studying the use of interoperable messages sent using HIE networks to inform care coordination processes. A randomized trial implemented in the Veterans Health Administration (VHA) system in New York and Indiana [36] recently completed. Final results are pending. However, preliminary analysis shows that providers were aware of the electronic notifications integrated into the EHR and supported their continued use. Moreover, physicians and nurses alike suggested that nursing roles take more ownership of the electronic alerts [38]. The alerts make nurses more aware of the outside hospitalization events, which normally only come to light when the patient informs the care team of the event. Some patients do not remember to report these events, and delays in primary care can occur if the patient forgets to follow up following discharge from an inpatient encounter. While more research is necessary to demonstrate effectiveness, many health systems are interested in using event notification to reduce rehospitalization rates while improving coordination and follow-up for patients. Informatics and interoperability are critical to the success of such interventions.

Challenges to HIE and Interoperability for Population Health

While HIE has much promise for population health and there exist several drivers toward HIE adoption in the U.S. and internationally, there remain a number of challenges to widespread adoption and use of HIE among public health organizations. The following challenges need to be addressed through future research as well as policy:

- *Workflow*: A significant barrier to better use of HIE and interoperability is clinical workflow. In a recent study of an HIE-based intervention to improve eCR [39], researchers found that while the intervention was initially targeted to physicians most clinics expect nurses to report notifiable diseases to public health agencies [40]. If EHR vendors build tools for physicians but these tools are not available to nurses, how can the interventions be successful in changing population health? Vendors as well as HIE organizations need to examine workflow patterns and design (or redesign) processes to achieve intended population health outcomes in a way to minimize burden on all healthcare professionals. Better workflow will result in higher adoption and use of HIE interventions, leading to maximal impact on populations.
- *Incentives*: Current policy in the U.S. encourages the use of interoperability to improve public health functions such as notifiable disease surveillance. Yet hospitals and clinics can meet the CMS Promoting Interoperability requirements by implementing just one "choice" in the menu of available public health use cases. This will boost utilization of public health HIE, but adoption will not be uniform or at levels on par with EHR functionality achieved under the earlier Meaningful Use program. Policymakers and public health authorities should consider additional policies

to incentivize the development and use of the public health HIE infrastructure.

- *Funding*: While many people wish it did not cost money to exchange information, the reality is the infrastructure necessary for HIE is expensive. Organizations that develop the infrastructure to facilitate HIE often establish business models that require organizations to pay for HIE services. Costs can create roadblocks for some health departments to engage in meaningful HIE with partners. Continued efforts are necessary to invest in the creation of interoperable highways in which all members of the healthcare system can participate, including federally qualified health centers and public health departments. Federal funds are necessary to further develop the public health infrastructure that could then be leveraged by healthcare systems to improve population health.

- *Complex Legal and Regulatory Environment*: Health information exchange is plagued by a complex legal and regulatory environment regarding electronic patient information sharing, security and privacy concerns, and governance rules that vary across states. States and the federal government need to work together to harmonize laws the same way informaticians work to harmonize data standards. Removing complexity will facilitate better exchange of data and information in health care. Recently, the Veterans Administration (VA) removed the requirement for patients to opt-in to HIE with non-VA providers, a policy that heretofore resulted in only a fraction of Veterans signing up for HIE services [41]. Policymakers need to consider the implications of policies designed to protect health information while encouraging organizations to protect data and intelligently share information when in the best interest of population health.

Case Study

A good example of public health interoperability is the Regenstrief Notifiable Condition Detector (NCD), which implements an interoperable approach to ELR [42]. The NCD is a technology developed by the Regenstrief Institute, which is now licensed to the Indiana Health Information Exchange (IHIE) for their use with Indiana-based healthcare systems. The NCD is distinct from the core HIE infrastructure, but it is integrated with the core systems that receive a variety of data from multiple health information systems. It is one of the few non-EHR technologies to be certified for meaningful use in support of the public health ELR criteria.

The NCD examines all incoming laboratory results that are reported from laboratories to IHIE. This includes white blood cell counts, glycosylated hemoglobin results, and stool cultures, among other routine lab tests. The NCD inspects both the lab test performed and the lab results for evidence of a notifiable disease. With respect to the lab test performed, the NCD examines the LOINC code that indicates the specific test ordered by the provider. The NCD specifically looks for the presence of certain LOINC codes known to be associated with notifiable diseases. The list of applicable LOINC codes is maintained by IHIE, but it is largely informed by the CDC Reportable Conditions Mapping Table [43], a nationally published list of notifiable diseases. IHIE customizes the list, based on those diseases required under state public health laws, and it can adapt the list to meet local needs. For example, in early 2020, IHIE added LOINC codes associated with laboratory tests for the detection of the SARS-CoV-2 virus that causes COVID-19 as they were created by LOINC before they could be added to the CDC's list. This allowed IHIE to nimbly respond to the emerging pandemic as hospital and commercial laboratories began running various tests for detecting the presence of the SARS-CoV-2 virus in populations.

With respect to the lab test result, the NCD examines SNOMED CT codes that identify the outcome of the lab test. There are specific SNOMED CT codes to indicate the presence of a given virus (e.g., 165,816,005 or HIV-positive) or organism (e.g., 112,283,007 or *Escherichia coli*), which are reportable in most jurisdictions. When these codes are provided in the results section of an ELR message, the NCD will flag the result as positive for the given virus or organism. There are also SNOMED CT codes that simply indicate the organism tested by the lab is simply "DETECTED" or "PRESENT," which is equivalent to the more specific organism codes.

Once detected, the NCD forwards the ELR message to the Indiana State Department of Health. Using an interface to the state's NEDSS Base System, IHIE delivers an appropriate technical message using the HL7 standard [44]. Sometimes, IHIE must reformat or enhance the original HL7 message to ensure it complies with the requirements of the meaningful use (now called Promoting Interoperability) program. The state agency can then integrate the information from the message into its case management system and assign the result to a county health department for follow-up. Contact tracing is likely a household topic these days due to the COVID-19 pandemic. That is one set of activities that local health departments often conduct for diseases, such as HIV as well as syphilis. Case management might also involve reaching out to clinics for confirmation a patient received treatment for a given notifiable disease, such as *salmonellosis* or tuberculosis.

In addition to sexually transmitted infections that are required under state law to be reported to public health, the NCD also detects multi-drug resistant organisms (MDROs). These organisms are particularly challenging for public health authorities as they can lead to greater disease burden and downstream health impacts for populations. The NCD reports MDRO cases to public health authorities as well as infection control practitioners in health systems [45]. These health professionals often track the presence of organisms internally to isolate such patients to prevent further spread of MDROs to other patients in a healthcare facility. Alerts to infection control nurses and physicians are sent by IHIE when a laboratory reports a new MDRO result. The system can further produce reports that count the various conditions and MDROs detected during the past day, week, or month.

A challenge faced by the NCD system is the usage of available standard terminologies in the lab messages received by the IHIE. Although most labs utilize LOINC codes to identify the test performed, some laboratories include only a local or proprietary code [46]. Similarly, not all laboratories identify the test results with the use of an available SNOMED CT code [46]. Instead, the results are either a proprietary code, perhaps one used by a major EHR vendor, or a block of text that is interpretable by a human but not a computer. For example, stool cultures often list a number of bacteria that were examined by the lab and found to either be "DETECTED" or "NOT DETECTED." When grouped into a long list of bacteria and their detection (or lack of detected), computers are challenged in making an accurate interpretation. Therefore, the NCD employs a range of critics (e.g., computer functions) that attempt to infer the result from non-standard results included in the lab message. These critics employ natural language processing (NLP) techniques to interpret the text [47]. Informatics applications must be designed to handle not only expected results (e.g., standardized LOINC and SNOMED CT codes) but also results that do not conform to standards. The applications cannot break or fail to work. The NCD flags results it cannot interpret as exceptions for humans to review and adjudicate when possible. Once adjudicated, the system can learn from the humans and next time infer a similar result. Adaptability and learning are important features for health informatics applications given the complexity of health data.

The NCD, originally developed in the early 2000s, has been shown to dramatically increase the volume of notifiable diseases detected when compared to manual, human processes [14]. In the most recent evaluation, the NCD performed well with respect to sensitivity, specificity, and positive predictive value [42]. Yet a challenge for the NCD remains the free text results in which laboratories list multiple answers or in which the result is buried in a large block of seemingly related text. This is particularly true when detecting organisms via cultures for MDROs as well as enteric diseases. Therefore, researchers are exploring the potential of advanced language rules-based approaches as well as machine learning to enhance the capability of the NCD. To date the performance of machine learning approaches is impressive, boosting positive predictive value for sexually transmitted disease results [48]. Yet there remains much work to study the use of advanced NLP as well as machine learning techniques and operationalize them in the context of a complex HIE environment.

Summary

The disciplines of public health and nursing complement one another. Nurses are often at the center of population health efforts, whether they are addressing a patient's social determinants of health or coordinating specialty care for individuals with a chronic condition. As illustrated in Fig. 23.2, nurse interactions with informatics applications facilitate bidirectional, interoperable exchange of information in support of population health. Data from the patient as well as measurements taken about the patient are entered into the EHR system. Documentation is shared with a regional or community HIE, which deposits the information into a database that contains records on populations (e.g., all patients with uncontrolled diabetes, all individuals <40 diagnosed with hypertension). The nurse can further use the HIE via her EHR system to retrieve information on populations to inform her care of the patient. Information from the HIE can be shared with the care team to discuss alternative diagnoses or treatment plans. Notifiable diseases diagnosed by the care team can be reported to public health agencies. Patients ready for discharge but who have social determinant challenges (e.g., lack of social support, lack transportation) can be connected to community-level resources. All of these workflows involve a nurse interacting with an informatics application to mediate care processes.

Conclusions and Outlook

While this chapter has described much of what is known today about the intersection of interoperability and population health, the story has only just begun. Many of the informatics interventions that exist are less than a decade in the making. More research and application of these technologies will be necessary to refine their

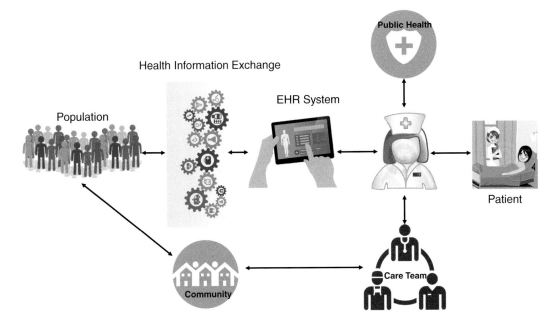

Fig. 23.2 A conceptual model for nurse interactions with informatics applications in support of population health

design and implementations to maximally improve population health. Furthermore, additional research and development of population health informatics interventions are necessary to fully cover the broad spectrum of processes involved in public as well as clinical health. Below are two specific examples of exciting areas on the horizon for public health interoperability. Readers likely can think of two or three additional examples or ideas.

An exciting but understudied area is the intersection of public health and personal health devices, such as the FitBit or Apple Watch©. Increasingly patients are adopting personal devices to record their health information, including data on their well-being. These devices are not yet fully utilized in clinical health processes, let alone public health processes. Yet many public health agencies would love to receive and analyze well-being data available at the population or community level. Applications that can make these data interoperable and accessible to public health are welcome. Nutrition, physical activity, and other experts in public health would be excellent partners with nursing to examine the use of such data for driving primary and secondary prevention efforts.

Another exciting area is population health analytics [49]. This area combines the massive computing power in health care with the non-clinical data assets available from public health organizations. It further presents the opportunity to develop algorithms that can drive detection of social determinant risk factors and/or prevention of disease. Nascent work is underway in population health analytics. More research and development will be necessary in the coming decade to apply emerging technologies while developing specific methods for this sub-discipline within the broader field of biomedical informatics.

Useful Resources

There exist a number of helpful resources to explore in the area of public health interoperability, including:

1. The Strategic Health Information Exchange Collaborative (SHIEC) is a national collabora-

tive representing HIE organizations and their strategic business and technology partners. The organization is currently sponsoring an initiative called the Patient-Centered Data Home project. This project ensures that patient information can follow them no matter where they go in the U.S., enabling cross-border exchange. Information can be found at https://strategichie.com/.

2. The Public Health Informatics Institute (PHII) is a non-governmental organization dedicated to promoting the appropriate use of informatics to support public health practice. The organization provides a number of free resources on its website relevant to HIE and public health. These resources can be accessed at https://phii.org/resources.

3. The Healthcare Information Management System Society (HIMSS) released a toolkit for public health departments to better understand HIE services and their role in public health [50]. The toolkit and the individual tools are available from the HIMSS website.

4. The Global Burden of Disease (GBD) project is hosted by the Institute for Health Metrics and Evaluation (IHME). GBD data are freely available for use in education and research as well as policymaking. All global, regional, national, and in some cases sub-national estimates of the burden of diseases, injuries, and risk factors can be downloaded from http://www.healthdata.org/gbd/data.

5. The book *Public Health Informatics and Information Systems* (third Edition, 2020) is a comprehensive text on the intersection of informatics and public health [51]. Individuals interested in learning more about public health informatics would benefit from this text on the subject.

6. The book *Health Information Exchange: Navigating and Managing a Network of Health Information Systems* (second Edition, 2022) is a comprehensive text on HIE, including its intersection with population health. Individuals interested in learning more about HIE and their design, development, and implementation would benefit from this text.

Review Questions

1. How does "public health" differ from "population health"?
2. Describe how interoperability can support population health in the context of a clinical encounter.
3. Describe how interoperability can support public health in the context of disease surveillance.
4. List and describe three informatics interventions which support population health that benefit from interoperability.
5. If you were to implement one of the public health information systems described in this chapter, which one would it be? Which stakeholders would be important to involve in the design of the intervention?

Appendix: Answers to Review Questions

1. How does "public health" differ from "population health"?

It is important to recognize that a consensus-based definition of population health does not exist. However, the distinction between these two concepts generally falls on the definition of population. In public health, the population is defined by geography or the jurisdiction of the governmental public health agency; whereas in population health, the population can be any group of individuals.

2. Describe how interoperability can support population health in the context of a clinical encounter.

There are multiple ways in which interoperability can support population health in the context of a clinical encounter. First, information about the population of individuals similar to the patient in front of the clinician could be queried to inform the patient's care plan. Next, information on multiple patients in the same area as the patient could be integrated to inform the likely prognosis or potential care plan for the patient. Sharing data with the next care provider could enhance care coordination.

3. Describe how interoperability can support public health in the context of disease surveillance.

Interoperability can connect clinical information systems with those used in public health to support disease surveillance. Medical systems can be used to identify individuals with a given condition of interest to public health authorities (e.g., syphilis) in a given geographic area. This allows public health officials to examine the prevalence of the disease in that population. Through case reporting, clinicians can report not only the prevalence of disease but also treatment and outcomes for patients with a given condition to public health authorities. Public health can use those data to examine outcomes as well as disease burden.

4. List and describe up to three informatics interventions which support population health that benefit from interoperability.

- Electronic laboratory reporting (ELR), the process of reporting data from laboratories to public health agencies for notifiable diseases.
- Electronic case reporting (eCR), the process of reporting details of a given disease case to public health agencies by providers.
- Health indicators, a system that can query electronic health records and other clinical information systems to derive the population-level prevalence of a given disease or risk factor.

Specialized disease registries, an information system that uses observational study methods to collect uniform data to evaluate specified outcomes for a population defined by a particular disease, condition, or exposure.

5. If you were to implement one of the public health information described in this chapter, which one would it be? What stakeholders would be important to involve in the design of the intervention?

Open-ended question—up to the instructor to interpret and/or grade.

References

1. Centers for Disease Control and Prevention US. Introduction to Public Health. CDC, Atlanta, GA. 2018. https://www.cdc.gov/publichealth101/public-health.html. Accessed May 1 2020.
2. Centers for Disease Control and Prevention US. The Public Health System & the 10 Essential Public Health Services. CDC, Atlanta, GA. 1994. https://www.cdc.gov/publichealthgateway/publichealthser-vices/essentialhealthservices.html. Accessed May 1 2020.
3. Commissioned Corps of the U.S. Public Health Service. America's Health Responders. U.S. Department of Health and Human Services, Washington, DC. 2020. https://www.usphs.gov/default.aspx. Accessed Aug 11 2020.
4. Bates DW, Samal L. Interoperability: What Is It, How Can We Make It Work for Clinicians, and How Should We Measure It in the Future? Health Serv Res. 2018;53(5):3270–7. https://doi.org/10.1111/1475-6773.12852.
5. Magnuson JA, Dixon BE. Public health informatics: an introduction. In: Magnuson JA, Dixon BE, editors. Public health informatics and information systems. Cham: Springer International Publishing; 2020. p. 3–16.
6. Kindig D, Stoddart G. What is population health? Am J Public Health. 2003;93(3):380–3. https://doi.org/10.2105/ajph.93.3.380.
7. Kharrazi H, Gamache R, Weiner J. Role of informatics in bridging public and population health. In: Magnuson JA, Dixon BE, editors. Public health informatics and information systems. Cham: Springer International Publishing; 2020. p. 59–79.
8. Lamb E, Satre J, Hurd-Kundeti G, Liscek B, Hall CJ, Pinner RW, et al. Update on progress in electronic reporting of laboratory results to public health agencies–United States, 2014. MMWR Morb Mortal Wkly Rep. 2015;64(12):328–30.
9. Yeung T. Local health department adoption of electronic health records and health information exchanges and its impact on population health. Int J Med Inform. 2019;128:1–6. https://doi.org/10.1016/j.ijmedinf.2019.04.011.
10. Dixon BE, Jones JF, Grannis SJ. Infection prevention-ists' awareness of and engagement in health informa-tion exchange to improve public health surveillance. Am J Infect Control. 2013;41(9):787–92. https://doi.org/10.1016/j.ajic.2012.10.022.
11. Nguyen TQ, Thorpe L, Makki HA, Mostashari F. Benefits and barriers to electronic laboratory results reporting for notifiable diseases: the New York City Department of Health and Mental Hygiene experi-ence. Am J Public Health. 2007;97(Suppl 1):S142–5. https://doi.org/10.2105/AJPH.2006.098996.
12. Centers for Disease Control and Prevention. NBS Overview. In: National Electronic Disease Surveillance System (NEDSS) Base System. U.S. Department of Health & Human Services, Atlanta, GA. 2019. https://www.cdc.gov/nbs/over-view/index.html. Accessed Jul 21 2019.
13. Effler P, Ching-Lee M, Bogard A, Ieong MC, Nekomoto T, Jernigan D. Statewide system of electronic notifiable disease reporting from clinical laboratories: comparing automated reporting with conventional methods. JAMA. 1999;282(19):1845–50.
14. Overhage JM, Grannis S, McDonald CJ. A com-parison of the completeness and timeliness of automated electronic laboratory reporting and sponta-neous reporting of notifiable conditions. Am J Public Health. 2008;98(2):344–50. https://doi.org/10.2105/AJPH.2006.092700.
15. Panackal AA, M'Ikanatha NM, Tsui FC, McMahon J, Wagner MM, Dixon BW, et al. Automatic electronic laboratory-based reporting of notifiable infectious diseases at a large health system. Emerg Infect Dis. 2002;8(7):685–91.
16. Lombardo JS, Buckeridge DL, editors. Disease sur-veillance: a public health informatics approach. Hoboken: Wiley; 2007.
17. Doyle TJ, Glynn MK, Groseclose SL. Completeness of notifiable infectious disease reporting in the United States: an analytical literature review. Am J Epidemiol. 2002;155(9):866–74.
18. Health Level Seven International. HL7 CDA® R2 Implementation Guide: public Health Case Report, Release 2–US Realm–the Electronic Initial Case Report (eICR). 2018. http://www.hl7.org/imple-ment/standards/product_brief.cfm?product_id=436. Accessed Jul 21 2019.
19. Digital Bridge. Implementation overview. 2019. https://digitalbridge.us/infoex/implementation/. Accessed Jul 1 2019.
20. Dixon BE, Taylor DE, Choi M, Riley M, Schneider T, Duke J. Integration of FHIR to facilitate elec-tronic case reporting: results from a pilot study. Stud Health Technol Inform. 2019;264:940–4. https://doi.org/10.3233/SHTI190362.
21. Overhage JM. The indiana health information exchange. In: Dixon BE, editor. Health information exchange: navigating and managing a network of

health information systems. 1st ed. Waltham, MA: Academic Press; 2016. p. 267–79.

22. Health Level 7. FHIR Overview. HL7.org. 2017. https://www.hl7.org/fhir/overview.html. Accessed Oct 25 2018.

23. Mokdad AH. The behavioral risk factors surveillance system: past, present, and future. Annu Rev Public Health. 2009;30:43–54. https://doi.org/10.1146/annurev.publhealth.031308.100226.

24. McFarlane TD, Dixon BE, Gibson PJ. Using electronic health records for public health hypertension surveillance. Online J Public Health Inform. 2018;10(1) https://doi.org/10.5210/ojphi.v10i1.8992.

25. Newton-Dame R, McVeigh KH, Schreibstein L, Perlman S, Lurie-Moroni E, Jacobson L, et al. Design of the New York City Macroscope: innovations in population health surveillance using electronic health records. EGEMS (Washington, DC). 2016;4(1):1265. https://doi.org/10.13063/2327-9214.1265.

26. Dixon BE, Zou J, Comer KF, Rosenman M, Craig JL, Gibson PJ. Using electronic health record data to improve community health assessment. Front Public Health Serv Sys Res. 2016;5(5):50–6. https://doi.org/10.13023/FPHSSR.0505.08.

27. Perlman SE, McVeigh KH, Thorpe LE, Jacobson L, Greene CM, Gwynn RC. Innovations in population health surveillance: using electronic health records for chronic disease surveillance. Am J Public Health. 2017;107(6):853–7. https://doi.org/10.2105/ajph.2017.303813.

28. Registries for evaluating patient outcomes: a user's guide. Agency for healthcare research and quality (US). Rockville (MD); 2014. https://www.ncbi.nlm.nih.gov/books/NBK208643/

29. Ekhaguere OA, Kareiva C, Werner L, Dixon BE. Improving immunization through informatics: perspectives from the BID initiative partnership with Tanzania and Zambia. In: Magnuson JA, Dixon BE, editors. Public health informatics and information systems. Cham: Springer International Publishing; 2020. p. 481–96.

30. Dixon BE, Tao G, Wang J, Tu W, Hoover S, Zhang Z, et al. An integrated surveillance system to examine testing, services, and outcomes for sexually transmitted diseases. Stud Health Technol Inform. 2017;245:361–5.

31. Batteiger TA, Dixon BE, Wang J, Zhang Z, Tao G, Tong Y, et al. Where do people go for gonorrhea and chlamydia tests: a cross-sectional view of the central Indiana population, 2003-2014. Sex Transm Dis. 2019;46(2):132–6. https://doi.org/10.1097/OLQ.0000000000000928.

32. Ho YA, Rahurkar S, Tao G, Patel CG, Arno JN, Wang J, et al. Validation of ICD-10-CM Codes for identifying cases of Chlamydia and Gonorrhea. Sex Transm Dis. 2021;48(5):335–40; https://doi.org/10.1097/olq.0000000000001257.

33. Ho YA, Allen K, Tao G, Patel CG, Arno JN, Broyles AA et al. Provider adherence to syphilis testing guidelines among stillbirth cases. Sex Transm

Dis. 2020;47(10):686–90. https://doi.org/10.1097/olq.0000000000001230.

34. Finnell JT, Overhage JM, Grannis S. All health care is not local: an evaluation of the distribution of emergency department care delivered in Indiana. AMIA Annu Symp Proc. 2011;2011:409–16.

35. Nazi KM, Hogan TP, Woods SS, Simon SR, Ralston JD. Consumer health informatics: engaging and empowering patients and families. In: Finnell JT, Dixon BE, editors. Clinical informatics study guide: text and review. Zurich: Springer International Publishing; 2016.

36. Dixon BE, Schwartzkopf AL, Guerrero VM, May J, Koufacos NS, Bean AM, et al. Regional data exchange to improve care for veterans after non-VA hospitalization: a randomized controlled trial. BMC Med Inform Decis Mak. 2019;19(1):125. https://doi.org/10.1186/s12911-019-0849-1.

37. Moore T, Shapiro JS, Doles L, Calman N, Camhi E, Check T, et al. Event detection: a clinical notification service on a health information exchange platform. AMIA Annu Symp Proc. 2012;2012:635–42.

38. Franzosa E, Traylor M, Judon KM, Guerrero Aquino V, Schwartzkopf AL, Boockvar KS, et al. Perceptions of event notification following discharge to improve geriatric care: qualitative interviews of care team members from a 2-site cluster randomized trial. J Am Med Inform Assoc. 2021;28(8):1728–35.

39. Dixon BE, Zhang Z, Arno JN, Revere D, Joseph Gibson P, Grannis SJ. Improving notifiable disease case reporting through electronic information exchange-facilitated decision support: a controlled before-and-after trial. Public Health Rep. 2020;135(3):401–10. https://doi.org/10.1177/0033354920914318.

40. Revere D, Hills RH, Dixon BE, Gibson PJ, Grannis SJ. Notifiable condition reporting practices: implications for public health agency participation in a health information exchange. BMC Public Health. 2017;17(1):247. https://doi.org/10.1186/s12889-017-4156-4.

41. Dixon BE, Ofner S, Perkins SM, Myers LJ, Rosenman MB, Zillich AJ, et al. Which veterans enroll in a VA health information exchange program? J Am Med Inform Assoc. 2017;24(1):96–105. https://doi.org/10.1093/jamia/ocw058.

42. Fidahussein M, Friedlin J, Grannis S. Practical challenges in the secondary use of real-world data: the notifiable condition detector. AMIA Annu Symp Proc. 2011:402–8.

43. CDC. Reportable Condition Mapping Table (RCMT). Centers for Disease Control and Prevention, Atlanta, GA. 2012. http://www.cdc.gov/EHRmeaningfuluse/rcmt.html. Accessed Jun 2 2016.

44. Grannis SJ, Stevens KC, Merriwether R. Leveraging health information exchange to support public health situational awareness: the Indiana experience. Online J Public Health Inform. 2010;2(2) https://doi.org/10.5210/ojphi.v2i2.3213.

45. Kho AN, Doebbeling BN, Cashy JP, Rosenman MB, Dexter PR, Shepherd DC, et al. A regional informat-

ics platform for coordinated antibiotic-resistant infection tracking, alerting, and prevention. Clin Infect Dis. 2013;57(2):254–62. https://doi.org/10.1093/cid/cit229.

46. Dixon BE, Siegel JA, Oemig TV, Grannis SJ. Electronic health information quality challenges and interventions to improve public health surveillance data and practice. Public Health Rep. 2013;128(6):546–53.

47. Friedlin J, Grannis S, Overhage JM. Using natural language processing to improve accuracy of automated notifiable disease reporting. AMIA Annu Symp Proc. 2008;207-11

48. Dexter GP, Grannis SJ, Dixon BE, Kasthurirathne SN. Generalization of machine learning approaches to identify notifiable conditions from a state-wide health information exchange. AMIA Joint Summits on Translational Science proceedings AMIA Joint Summits on Translational Science. 2020;2020:152–61.

49. Kasthurirathne SN, Ho YA, Dixon BE. Public health analytics and big data. In: Magnuson JA, Dixon BE, editors. Public health informatics and information systems. Cham: Springer International Publishing; 2020. p. 203–19.

50. Healthcare Information and Management Systems Society. Public Health & HIE Toolkit. 2015. https://www.himss.org/resources/public-health-hie-toolkit. Accessed Aug 11 2020.

51. Magnuson JA, Dixon BE. Public health informatics and information systems. 3rd ed. Cham: Springer International Publishing; 2020.

Part V

Safe Systems and Patient Safety

Patient Safety: Opportunities and Risks of Health IT Applications, Methods and Devices

24

Sayonara de Fatima F. Barbosa
and Grace T. M. Dal Sasso

Learning Objectives
- Understand patient safety from a health informatics perspective.
- Recognize the benefits and limitations of informatics to improve patient safety.
- Define applications that health professionals can use to improve patient safety.
- Provide an overview of the potential that major information technologies (ITs) have to impact the safety of care.

- Smart pumps
- Automated medication dispensing machine
- Wearables
- Internet of things
- Unsafe health IT

Key Terms
- Health informatics
- Patient safety
- Errors
- Unintended consequences
- Electronic health record
- Clinical decision support system
- Computerized practitioner order entry system
- Predictive analysis
- Big data
- Machine learning
- Deep learning
- Artificial intelligence
- Barcoding
- Radio frequency identification

S. de F. F. Barbosa (✉) · G. T. M. Dal Sasso
Federal University Santa Catarina,
Florianópolis, Brazil
e-mail: sayonara.barbosa@ufsc.br;
grace.sasso@ufsc.br

Introduction

Patient safety is a topic of worldwide importance and concern. However, this was already a concern of Florence Nightingale in 1863, when stating: "It may seem a strange principle to enunciate as the very first requirement in a hospital that it should do the sick no harm." This alert occurred 136 years before the report "To Err Is Human: Building a Safer Health System" from the United States Institute of Medicine (IOM) in 1999, which concluded that skilled care activity was not infallible and was likely to cause adverse events. The same study reviewed the obstacles to safe care in complex environments and made a series of recommendations for technology adoption by healthcare providers. The next report, "Crossing the Quality Chasm," also published by IOM, reviewed some of the challenges to effective use of information technology (IT) to improve care quality, like underinvestment by provider organizations, safety for patient health information, provision of adequate technical infrastructure to ensure connectivity in diverse settings, reimbursement for technology services and others [1].

© Springer Nature Switzerland AG 2022
U. H. Hübner et al. (eds.), *Nursing Informatics*, Health Informatics,
https://doi.org/10.1007/978-3-030-91237-6_24

In 2008, WHO World Alliance for Patient Safety reviewed global activities on the state of technology and patient safety, and the Patient Safety Technology program was established with the aims to identify areas where technology can be used to enhance the safety of patient care by "designing out" potential risks or by improving communication and the reliable transmission of information.

Nursing works intensively with information. The clinical condition of patients demands a lot of information, which needs to be communicated between the different healthcare professionals. The transfer of essential information and the responsibility for the care of the patient from one healthcare provider to another is an integral component of communication in health care, and information technology may facilitate access to information and communication among members of the healthcare team with different applications.

Internationally, improving nursing informatics is seen as the best way to improve hospital system performance, collaboration and the satisfaction of hospital personnel and patients as well [2, 3].

Every healthcare organization is concerned with patient safety, and although the adoption of Health information technology (HIT) has the potential to improve it, is necessary to consider the unanticipated and undesirable consequences of implementing HIT which could lead to new and more complex hazards, especially in developing countries, where regulations, policies and implementations are few, less standardized and, in some cases, almost non-existing [4]. Failed HIT implementation can become a new source of risk for the patient, due to poor designs, changes in workflow and lack of training are so important and frequent that they have been defined as "technological iatrogenic 'or' e-iatrogenesis" [5, 6].

There are many approaches to improve patient safety, and there is an agreement that the applications of information technology (IT) have the potential to support the healthcare environment through the reorganization process, making the procedures more accurate and efficient, and reducing the risk of human error. Health information technology can improve healthcare quality and patient safety in different categories, like [7]:

- Prevention: to prevent an adverse event before happening. It includes alerts, clinical decision support, implementation, interface design and customized health IT solutions.
- Identification: to identify a quality and safety event when it is about to occur. Electronic tracking tools, alerts, clinical decision support, implementation and customized health IT solutions.
- Action: action on a quality and safety event once it has already occurred. Documentation, implementation and culture relative to the use of health IT.
- Outcomes: includes protocol compliance, error reduction, length of stay, clinical outcomes and medical error reduction.

Health informatics to improve patient safety not only considers the technologic aspects but is also embedded in a sociotechnical work system, with people and workflows. The successful implementation and adoption of health information systems also depends on a better fit between human, contextual and technological factors. For this task, a framework can be useful. As an example, Singh and Sittig [8] proposed a conceptual framework that identifies health IT safety domains, related safety principles and measurement cycles. The proposed model identifies a network of different actors interconnected to each other, and also illustrates that a central issue with the evaluation of IT-based health care is influenced by the complexity of the evaluation objects and includes both social and technical considerations (Fig. 24.1).

Health IT Applications to Improve Patient Safety

Electronic Health Record

An electronic health record (EHR) is a longitudinal electronic record of patient health information generated by one or more encounters in any care delivery setting. Included in this information are patient demographics, progress notes, problems, medications, vital signs, past medical history, immunizations, laboratory data, and

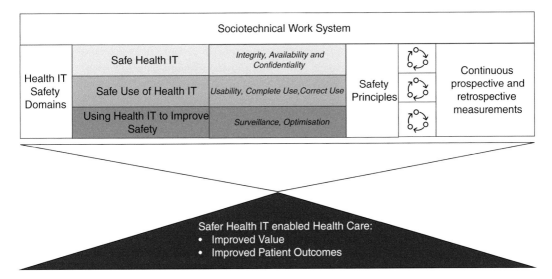

Fig. 24.1 Health Information Technology Safety Measurement Framework based on Singh and Sitting, 2016

radiology reports and images. The EHR automates and streamlines the clinician's workflow and can generate a complete record of a clinical patient encounter, as well as supporting other care-related activities directly or indirectly via the interface including evidence-based decision support, quality management and outcomes reporting [9]. The EHR has health-related information on an individual that conforms to nationally recognized interoperability standards and that can be created, managed and consulted by authorized clinicians and staff across more than one healthcare organization. Its role to ensure patient safety is to provide consistent, up-to-date data and information that is available for all providers involved in the care of a patient. It serves as an engine for information logistics; that is, it provides the right information, in the right amount and quality, at the right time to the right recipient. It, hereby, supports information continuity across all patient care processes.

Computerized Practitioner Order Entry (CPOE)

An order entry application is specifically designed to assist practitioners in creating and managing medical orders for patient services and medications. This application has a special electronic signature, workflow and rules engine functions that reduce or eliminate medical errors associated with practitioner ordering processes [9]. It is also defined as a computer application that accepts the provider's orders for diagnostic and treatment services electronically, instead of the clinician recording them on an order sheet or prescription pad. CPOE systems make use of pre-populated forms specific to the workflows and the patient condition. They are also known as computerized physician order entry, computerized patient order entry and computerized provider order entry.

CPOE development, advancement of EHR technology, has increased efficiency and safety, particularly when coupled with clinical decision support (CDS) tools. CPOE targets medication-prescribing errors, which are believed to be the most prevalent adverse events (ADE) in hospitals [9, 10]. Utilizing CPOE can detect medication errors more efficiently and automatically by checking that the right medication is prescribed at the appropriate dose for a patient. Likewise, adding CDS to CPOE improves adherence to the medication formulary and reduces ADEs by checking prescribed medications against a patient's listed allergies or adverse reactions as well as automatically checking for drug-drug interactions [10]. CDS may also use warnings or hard stops, which limit medication doses to an appropriate range based on a patient's age or size or may require high-risk medications (e.g., anticoagulants or insulin) to be ordered with appropriate monitoring.

Lastly, in the outpatient setting, CPOE can increase medication pick-up, particularly when linked to an automatic notification to primary care providers regarding non-compliance [10]. CPOE employment has been associated with reduced hospital mortality for pediatric patients [11].

A CPOE system can reduce the potential for error in increasingly complex environments by ensuring that orders are more legible, complete and appropriate. However, when CPOE is combined with clinical decision support to identify serious potential complications, including drug-drug interactions, potentially life-threatening allergies and conditions that require different treatment options, only then the true benefit of a CPOE system can be realized [12].

CPOE can help to decrease errors in the initial prescription order which typically carries the greatest risk of a serious harm, but also in each stage of the prescribing process [12], which embraces the following type of errors:

- decision errors: failure to account for relevant comorbidities, polypharmacy, previous reactions and incorrect decision;
- calculation errors: failure to calculate the appropriate dosage;
- communication errors: dosage written incorrectly, illegible handwriting, wrong patient, ambiguous information on prescription and medication not given in a timely fashion;
- monitoring error or incorrect length of treatment: failure to track drugs with a risk of accumulation of toxicity or where time-limited treatment is desirable; and
- slips: incorrect drugs or doses packaged at dispensation and drugs given to the wrong patient.

All these errors reflect potential sources jeopardizing patient safety.

Clinical Decision Support System (CDSS)

A clinical decision support system (CDSS) is an application that uses pre-established rules and guidelines that can be created and edited by the healthcare organization and integrates clinical data from several sources to generate alerts and treatment suggestions [13]. A CDSS can contribute to patient safety, as it can ensure the consistency of decision-making, the mitigation of risks of rule violation or omission and the control of specific risks and errors associated with cognitive lapses or biases [12]. Alerting systems are a type of clinical decision support. By notifying physicians and nurses about likely adverse events at the time those events occur, online alerts can improve the timeliness of the response. The results are fewer errors, improved quality of care and better patient outcomes. The challenge has been to deliver the message in real time to the healthcare professionals responsible for the patient so that they can take timely and appropriate action. The design and implementation of a CDSS are complex and involve many variables, including function, user, setting and desired outcome.

Clinical Decision Support Systems and Big Data

By adding innovative big data technologies, clinical decision support will become more accurate, more predictive and more meaningful for many outcomes, including early identification of clinical deterioration, pressure injury, delirium and healthcare-associated infections (urinary catheters, central venous access or surgical sites) [13].

Big data can be defined as digital data that is generated in large volume and wide variety and that is stored at high speed, resulting in very large data sets for traditional data processing systems, and requires the use of technology and analytical methods specific for its processing and transformation into knowledge or value [14].

Big data technology involves the so-called Four Vs: volume (processing large amounts of data); variety (from an integrated group of various databases and in different formats); velocity (perform analytical calculations at high speed, in real time); veracity (with high precision) [15]. In healthcare, other "Vs" can be added [16]: validity (accurate and correct data), viability, volatility (how fast the data is transformed), vulnerability (access permissions), visualization (data must be presented unambiguously, and attractive to the user) and value (data must provide better health services, such as better governance, better analysis and smarter decision-making).

Health professionals generate a large amount of free text, coded information about diagnoses or procedures, in addition to registration of interventions and medication administration. Large amounts of data are generated by medical devices, such as laboratory results, vital signs, images, sounds, videos and more. Today it is possible to store and process this information automatically and extract new knowledge and guidance to improve patient care [16], providing more personalized care.

The current state of technology makes it possible to process, in real time, this large amount of physiological data from the patient, early identifying clinical changes, executing validated and designed algorithms. In this type of system, different predictive algorithms to detect sepsis or apnea can be implemented. This system may be able to identify patterns in physiological data and quickly alert the health team to risk signs for patients, extracting knowledge from historical physiological data that ultimately help to early detect critical conditions. This type of system is known as real-time big data analytics.

Predictive Analysis and Artificial Intelligence

Outcome prediction, broadly, involves the forecasting of a patient event to assess interventions that would improve their treatment. Undoubtedly, early prediction of specific patient events among critical patients has the potential for faster and more precise steering of care and resources. Prognostic models leveraging large volumes of data and recent machine learning techniques are a promising approach to achieving data-driven medicine through artificial intelligence [17].

Artificial intelligence (AI) is defined as the theory and development of computer systems capable of performing tasks that normally require human intelligence, such as perception, speech recognition, decision-making and language translation languages [18]. It is also defined as a multidisciplinary science that seeks to develop and apply computational techniques that simulate human behavior in specific activities. These techniques can also serve as a toolset for ensuring patient safety through predictive analysis.

Machine learning is a subtype of AI that allows computers to learn from large amounts of data (big data) without being explicitly programmed [19]. It uses algorithms that can learn from the data to gain knowledge from experience and to make decisions and predictions automatically [20]. This "learning" refers to the self-tuning of the software that adjusts the algorithm over time to increase accuracy [21]. Some examples of machine learning are syntactic pattern recognition, natural language processing, search engines and computer vision [22].

Deep learning is a subfield of machine learning. A deep learning model is designed to reach the same conclusions as a traditional machine learning algorithm, but with much less human information. For this, deep learning algorithms use a layered structure, called an artificial neural network [21]. It is deep learning because the structure of artificial neural networks consists of several layers of input, output and hidden. Each layer contains units that transform the input data into information that the next layer can use to perform a particular predictive task. Due to this structure, a computer can learn through its own data processing.

The different artificial intelligence techniques associated with the use of data mining techniques and statistical algorithms allow the application of predictive analysis, to identify the probability of future results based on historical or current data. Different studies have been carried out with the application of artificial intelligence techniques. In the intensive care area, for example: application of deep learning methods to predict severe complications in the intensive care unit in real time after cardiothoracic surgery [23]; the use of a machine learning model to predict the onset of hypotension in patients in the ICU with an alert system for bedside implementation [24]; prediction of sepsis mortality in the ICU with machine learning methods [25].

Clinical databases are a fundamental tool for medical research, including for the application of machine learning. However, most of the patient data has access limited to small groups of researchers within the vendor, hospital or institution owning the systems where the data is collected. As such, confirming the validity of studies has been a challenge for the research community. Apart from the lack of established guidelines on the evaluation of algorithms, the use of proprietary data sets and the creation of proprietary models results in a lack of essential detail which is fundamental to the scientific process. This unfortunate medical norm results in algorithms that are incognito not only to other researchers but also to the care providers who may ultimately use them, and to the patients that may be affected by them [26].

Health IT Devices and Their Interconnection to Improve Patient Safety

Barcoding Medication Technology

A barcode is an optical machine-readable representation of data that relates to the object displaying the barcode. It records text information in an encoded format and serves as an index key in clinical databases. The system is supported by software that references expert databases to comply with the "Five Rights" of patient medication administration. Hospital pharmacies scan unit-dose packaging to improve security, build an audit trail and automate inventory record keeping. In a medication administration application, barcode architectures often include a barcoded wristband issued to the patient at the time of admission. Nurses' ID badges and medications also carry barcodes. At the time of administering medication, all three barcodes are scanned at the bedside, which links to an order in the EHR. This assures an identical match between patient and medication, identifies the nurse administering the medication and also protects patients from prescription, transcription and dispensing errors [18]. The nurse is warned not to proceed if the patient does not have an order for the specific medication, including dose and route, due at that time. Using barcode scanning has reduced wrong medication, wrong patient, wrong time, wrong route and wrong-dose errors. Though checking the five rights of medication administration will never be replaced by a digital system, barcode scanning, when used appropriately, can act as a safeguard to those administering medications [27].

Another example is if there is a physician order for a look-alike medication misinterpreted during its transcription. The system would alert the nurse with a warning, that the nurse needs to check, enabling the nurse to verify the prescription with the pharmacist or physician in the event an error has been made [28].

Scanning technologies like barcode can be used in a range of healthcare areas, including [18, 29] the following:

• Patient identification and profiling	• Dietary management
• Patient movement and handover	• Supply chain management
• Diagnosis, including pathology and radiology	• Storage and unit labeling
• Medication management	• Cycle counts
• Blood transfusion	• Annual equipment inventories
• Surgical procedures	• Preventative maintenance
• devices and implants	• Linen inventory and distribution
• Medical record tracking	• Sterile reprocessing
• Sterile services	• Security
• Asset management	• Employee identification

Barcodes can be matched with RFID tags (see Sec. 3.2) to create two-tiered identification and more robust point-of-care, patient-specific medical media. Pharmaceutical companies can locate and track each dose of medication produced in vast batches, equipment can be monitored and utilized with greater efficiency, and healthcare staff can more efficiently create and maintain healthcare records [18].

Barcode technology can be used as a stand-alone application or linked to CPOE and EHR systems, as well as to pharmaceutical and supply systems. This allows institutions to access financial information and to drill down to the patient level to report on the cost of providing care, as shown in Fig. 24.2.

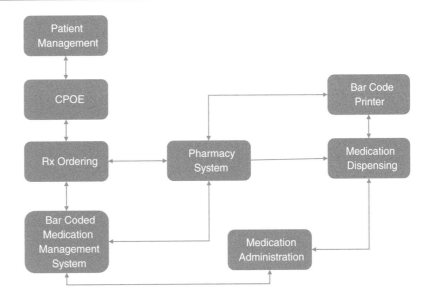

Fig. 24.2 Example of an integrated medication management system based on Zebra Technologies [28]

Radio Frequency Identification

The term RFID (radio frequency identification) describes a wireless identification technology that communicates data by radio waves. Data is encoded in a chip, which is integrated with an antenna and packaged into a finished "tag." [18]. The tag can be attached to a pallet of goods, high-value items or a patient wristband, or even inserted under the skin. The tag transmits a signal and an antenna and transceiver read the signal and transmit it to a server. RFID tags may be passive—requiring close proximity to a reader and are usually applied to track supplies—or may be active, in which case the RFID tag contains a small battery to allow continuous monitoring—mostly used to track equipment. RFID technologies offer different rewritable options, memory sizes and tag forms, and can be read from anywhere within range of the RFID reader. RFID labels can hold more data than bar codes and can be read automatically without any user intervention [18].

Radio frequency identification is believed to be the next-generation technology for tracking and data collection and has successfully been applied in several industries such as manufacturing, retail and logistics. RFID technology is also seen as the next disruptive innovation in healthcare and represents several opportunities for increased safety, operational efficiency and cost savings, by tagging inventory, assets, patients and personnel [30].

RFID for patient safety has basically four applications, with some examples [31]:

- Patient identification: smart wristband with a passive RFID tag, can be scanned to identify patients and reveal information such as date of birth, name, insurance information, allergies, blood type and medication requirements, and also be used for surgical patients to ensure that the surgical procedure is performed on the right patient.
- Patient tracking: as a technology for improving patient care and safety by tracking vulnerable patients, like the movements of elderly in long-term care.
- Patient monitoring: RFID in combination with other Internet-of-Things-based sensors like mobile networks or wireless sensor networks (WSN) can also be used for patient monitoring and collection of sensor-derived data, and can help in incidents such as patient falls or heartbeat irregularities.
- Patient drug compliance: used in the home after leaving the hospital by attaching an RFID tag to the medicine container that records each time it is opened. Through a connected information system, physicians can access this RFID data and thus monitor patient drug compliance.

However, RFID adoption in healthcare also has different challenges, as the following issues demonstrate [31]:

- Technological challenges: RFID wireless transmissions may cause electromagnetic interference with biomedical devices and electronic medical equipment, which pose a threat to patient safety in medical environments and medical equipment such as external pacemakers or syringe pumps, which could cause the equipment to switch off in the proximity of an RFID tag. Another technological challenge relates to the accuracy and reliability of RFID systems, which depends on factors like tag placement, read distance, the object tagged and angle of rotation, in addition to the presence of items containing liquid, metal objects and local magnetic interference.
- Security, privacy and data management challenges: mainly originate from counterfeiting unencrypted sensitive data within RFID tags, intercepting data during transmission or the unauthorized access of sensitive data. There are also some challenges when it comes to the privacy and security of patient information stored in RFID tags; for example, an unauthorized person might access a patient's electronic medical record or the patient could be exposed to physical tracking, because RFID tags automatically respond to queries from RFID readers without alerting the tagged person.
- Organizational and financial challenges: Although the cost of RFID tags has decreased significantly they are still considered substantial. In addition to the RFID tags and readers, the RFID infrastructure also requires middleware, databases, servers and applications. Also, training, business process redesign, organizational change and RFID infrastructure maintenance are costs that need to be accounted for.

Smart Pumps

Infusion pumps with dose calculation software, sometimes referred to as "smart pumps," offer the opportunity to identify and correct pump programming errors. The smart pump has a customized software that contains a drug library. This software essentially transforms a conventional IV pump into a computer that alerts you if a programmed infusion is outside of the medication's recommended parameters, such as dose, dosing unit (mcg/kg/min, units/h, etc.), rate or concentration [32]. Smart pumps log data about all such alerts, including the time, date, drug, concentration, programmed rate and volume infused, thus providing valuable continuous quality improvement (CQI) information [33]. Besides, smart pumps have free-flow protection—safety features that are designed to prevent unintentional overdoses of medication or fluid.

Advances in health IT are just beginning to address pump programming errors. While smart pumps using dosing error reduction software can mitigate some programming errors, many medication-infusion administration errors are still possible, including wrong rate, wrong concentration, wrong medication and wrong dose. Smart pump integration links smart pumps to the EHR, such that medication administration requires barcode scanning the patient's wristband, the medication and the pump channel. The pump is then automatically programmed using the available order from the linked EHR. Also, the pump automatically administers the medication volume documented in the EHR at the appropriate time, allowing for improved documentation. While relatively new, smart pumps have the opportunity to decrease ADEs by decreasing the keystrokes by approximately 86% [34] and improving pharmacy workflow by automatically notifying the pharmacy when a bag or syringe is at a pre-specified level and needs to be replaced.

Automated Medication Dispensing Machine

Automated dispensing cabinets (ADCs), also known as automated distribution devices or automated dispensing machines, function as an electronic point-of-care storage device for medication distribution [35]. ADCs, like all information technology systems, are not designed to replace human activity or to prevent all errors but instead to support humans in clinical decision-making [36].

An over-reliance on technology and trust in its proper functioning can develop among its users. However, the technology is not infallible and thus the risks associated with ADCs must be identified and safeguards must be employed to promote safe practice instead of contributing to new medication errors [35].

While improved technology is seen intuitively as a driver for increased patient safety, the presence of new technology may lead to new problems, particularly without a clear understanding of contributing factors at the time of implementation [37].

The process of automating the services of a pharmacy department using automated dispensing systems technology increases the efficiency at which medications are controlled, improves the accuracy of patient drug profiling, minimizes inappropriate dispensing and distribution and provides better utilization of human resources at the ever-busy pharmacy department. However, the process of switching into an automated system may have multiple challenges, such as [38]:

- inability to integrate lot numbering from the previous manual system to the new automated system;
- slight discrepancy between actual counts of medications versus the documented figures;
- human resource challenges in terms of administration during the phasing out and concurrent implementation of the automated system; and
- standard cabinets may not be appropriate for all units. They should be customized to suit the variety of medications common in the respective units.

Wearable Technology

Technology, worn in clothing or accessories, that records and reports information about behaviors such as physical activity or sleep patterns is known as wearables [39]. This technology aims to educate and motivate individuals toward better habits and better health. Wearable biosensors are non-invasive devices that capture, transmit and process health-related data [40]. Ideal sensors should be low cost, reliable, lightweight, easy to wear, easy to use, have long battery life and allow the wearer to ambulate normally [41].

Wearables as medical technologies are becoming an integral part of personal analytics, measuring physical status, recording physiological parameters or informing schedule for medication. These continuously evolving technology platforms do not only promise to help people pursue a healthier lifestyle, but also provide continuous medical data for actively tracking metabolic status, diagnosis and treatment. Advances in the miniaturization of flexible electronics, electrochemical biosensors, microfluidics and artificial intelligence algorithms have led to wearable devices that can generate real-time medical data within the Internet of Things. These flexible devices can be configured to make conformal contact with epidermal, ocular, intracochlear and dental interfaces to collect biochemical or electrophysiological signals [42] (Fig. 24.3).

Wearable sensors and digital technologies have the potential to improve patient safety for both hospital patients and those at home. Several sensor designs are available. Acute deterioration in patient's condition is accompanied by changes in their physiological parameters first. The vital signs can help detect several problems such as cardiac, respiratory, shock and sepsis [41].

A range of options is used to transmit the data from the sensor wirelessly, including Bluetooth, radiofrequency and WiFi signal. The wearable sensor technology can transmit data back to the clinicians via alerting through a centralized monitoring system, integrating into electronic health records and alerting to mobile applications for portable handheld devices such as smartphones and Personal Digital Assistant (PDA) [41].

The continuous monitoring of heart rate and respiratory rate can predict and reduce the occurrence of potential adverse events such as cardiac arrest and respiratory failure through measuring blood pressure, oxygen saturation, heart rate,

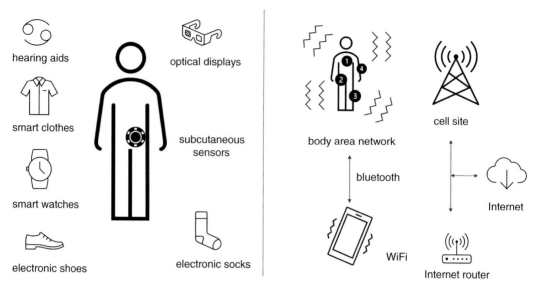

Fig. 24.3 Wearables devices for medical applications based on [44]

temperature, respiratory rate and level of cognition [41].

The wearable sensors can do even more and different measures, such as bed motion, body posture, fall detection and activity, and accelerometry data. The sensors can be placed for example under the patient's mattress or in different areas of the patient's body, for example, adhesive sensor that is placed on the patient's chest, sensors that are worn around the wrist, thumb sensor for oxygenation saturation [41] and three-axis accelerometers to detect motion.

Internet of Things

The Internet of Things (IoT) is an advanced network of objects (i.e., things) with unique identities, each of which interconnects or connects to a remote server to provide more efficient services [44]. The amalgamation of various fields such as data acquisition, communication and data analysis offer continuous connectivity for the objects to collect, exchange and combine data. Consequently, it is possible to achieve inclusive knowledge about the entire system. According to the specification and functionality of an Internet-of-Things-based system to collect, transmit and process healthcare-related data, the architecture

of the system can be specified in three layers, the perception layer, the gateway layer and the cloud layer [43, 45]. The perception layer is defined to capture comprehensive health and environmental data using heterogeneous sensors. This layer is the lowest and has the most contact with the studied or monitored entities, including persons such as patients, nurses and physicians, and objects. Medical devices (e.g., heart rate monitor, pulse oximeter and electrocardiography device), activity and localization devices (e.g., accelerometer and bed presence) and emergency buttons are items that stand in this layer to collect related data. The gateway layer is allocated to connect the sensors to a remote server. The captured data are transmitted via wireless protocols such as Bluetooth and WiFi to a local gateway. The gateway provides continuous connectivity for the sensors or other perception layer inputs and manages interruptions. Then, it transfers the gathered data to a remote or local server called a cloud for further analysis.

The cloud layer is the third and most remote section of the Internet-of-Things system. All the acquired data are transferred to the cloud via the gateway. The cloud can be obtained either via Internet-connected remote servers provided by third parties or by local servers connected to the local hospital information

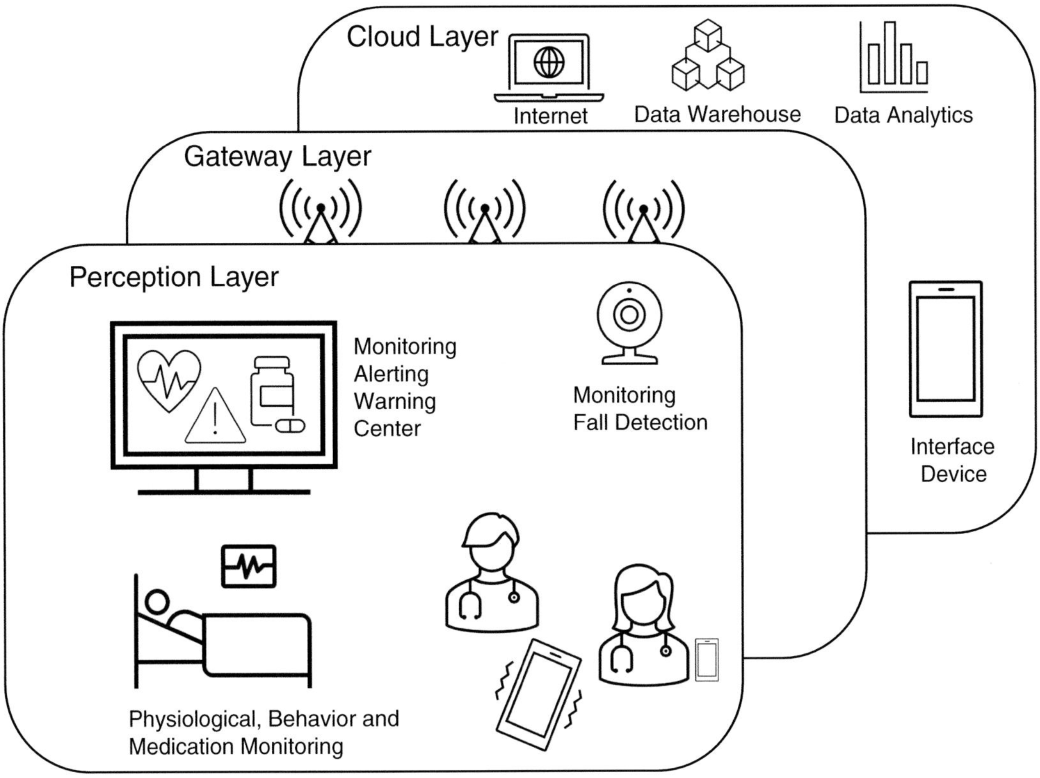

Fig. 24.4 Internet-of-Things solutions for nursing in hospital environment based on [46]

system (HIS) to provide more protective privacy and security.

Some examples of utilization of IOT for basic patient care can be presented in different categories:

- Periodical clinical reassessment: vital signs, neonatal monitoring, pain, medication.
- Activities of daily living: sleep detection, secretion monitoring (sense diaper wetness sends notifications in case of detecting soiled diapers; disposable wet sensors placed inside of diapers), fall detection, activity monitoring.
- Care management: decision-making support system, tracking (personnel, patients, devices), nursing calling system.
- Comprehensive assessment: real-time hand hygiene monitoring to monitor healthcare professionals in hospital rooms and provide a reminder whether hand hygiene is missed; hand hygiene monitoring using installed

sensors in hospital rooms and user-tags for clinical staff (Fig. 24.4).

Challenges in Health Information Technology–Related Patient Safety

Health system is complex and adaptative [47], and although the introduction of health information technology can improve care and patient safety, it also has the potential to cause unintended consequences, becoming necessary to understand the challenges it may impose.

Ensuring the safety of health IT and its use in the clinical setting has emerged as a key challenge, which may be present in any stage of the health IT lifecycle and can help healthcare organizations, health information technology (IT) developers, researchers, policymakers and funders focus their efforts on health IT-related patient safety.

According to Sittig and colleagues [48], some challenges in health information technology-related patent safety, according to the stage of the health IT lifecycle where they appear, are presented as follows:

- Design and development challenges
  - Developing proactive models, methods and tools to enable risk assessment.
  - Developing standard user interface design features and functions.
  - Ensuring the safety of software in an interfaced, network-enabled clinical environment.
  - Implementing a method for unambiguous patient identification.
- Implementation and use challenges
  - Developing and implementing decision support that improves safety.
  - Identifying and implementing practices to safely manage information technology system transitions.
- Monitoring, evaluation and optimization challenges
  - Developing real-time methods to enable automated surveillance and monitoring of system performance and safety.
  - Establishing the cultural and legal framework/safe harbor to allow sharing information about hazards and adverse events.
  - Developing models and methods for consumers and patients to improve health information technology safety. These challenges represent key "to-do's" that must be completed before we can expect to have safe, reliable and efficient health information technology-based systems required to care for patients.

Case Study

Brazilian Initiatives to Improve Patient Safety Related to Health Informatics

The potential to improve patient safety and quality through nursing informatics is a critical component and one of Brazil's goals. Among the Brazilian initiatives, we can highlight three pillars in particular.

The first pillar refers to the initiative to develop *a system of Electronic Patient Records called eRUE®*: Electronic registration and (tele) monitoring in health for the Urgency and Emergency Attention Network in the Santa Catarina State. The main objective of this system was to integrate the different services that make up health care in the urgency and emergency network, from primary health care to the hospital environment.

So, the eRUE® system integrated the system of Manchester® screening (risk rating), ICD® 10/11 (International Statistical Classification of Diseases and Health-Related Problems) and the ICNP® 2.0 (International Classification of Nursing Practices). ICNP and ICD have been integrated into SNOMED-CT® (Systematized Nomenclature of Medicine-Clinical Terms), which is the standard for the exchange of clinical health information and interoperability.

To improve the quality of health care and patient safety, the eRUE® system allows the user to classify the patient's risk with alerts that are issued since the initial patient care by the Manchester® protocol, categorizing the patient's clinical situation by priority and color. It also allows establishing the type of disease by region, that is, what is the highest frequency of the patient's problem in that geographic location; the total waiting time for the care process in different scenarios of the urgent and emergency healthcare network; the time for the first appointment; the type of transport used (land or air or sea); time for transportation; location of patient care; hypothesis medical diagnosis; nursing diagnosis—ICNP; final situation/destination of patient care Hospitalization and mortality rate.

The second pillar is *predictive analytics using machine learning and artificial intelligence to strengthen patient safety and improve the quality of care*. Technology that enables predictive analytics has data-retrieval capabilities. It can extract data from sources such as electronic health records, medical equipment and devices, and wearable technologies.

A practical example that was developed in Brazil is a predictive analysis model that makes it possible to verify the probability of a citizen to develop cerebrovascular diseases from their health conditions. In addition to the risk factors for cerebrovascular diseases, new factors related to eating habits and education level were included in the model as well. The prediction used the technique of logistic regression and was optimized by an algorithm of predictive analysis, stochastic descending gradient. Thus, it allowed estimating the probability associated with the occurrence of a cerebrovascular disease through a set of independent variables. The inclusion of the new risk improved the predictive analysis algorithm, increasing the average probability of a citizen develop a cerebrovascular disease by 45.3%, going from 47.6% to 69.2%. The variables related to eating habits showed the highest average probabilities, both for the minimum index and for the maximum. The education variable demonstrated that the higher the level of education the less likely is the development of cerebrovascular disease.

The model presented provides a tool for municipal managers and health professionals about the health condition of the population concerning cerebrovascular diseases. It can assist professionals in planning, as well as in making safer decisions related to the area and assisting citizens in providing adequate information. Furthermore, this model is planned to be applied to other needs, especially maternal morbidity and mortality.

The third pillar is the development of mobile apps. For example, we developed an app called mSmartAVC®: a mobile learning application for the detection and caring of individuals with cerebrovascular accidents. The results evidenced that the mSmartAVC® has a significant difference ($p < 0.001$) in the learning of nurses and students in decision-making when confronted with detection and care of stroke of patients after using the application. Also, the application showed internationally certified quality criteria and improves decision-making and clinical evaluation performed by nurses and students in the detection and care of stroke patients.

Digital Health Strategy for Brazil
The Brazilian Ministry of Health created the Digital Health Strategy for Brazil from 2020 to 2028 (ESD28). This Health Strategy systematized and consolidated the work carried out over the last decade, in particular, that of the National Policy for Health Information and Informatics— PNIIS (BRASIL, 2015), and the Digital Health Action, Monitoring and Evaluation Plan for Brazil (PAM & A 2019–2023). Thus, this document from Brazil, has aligned itself with previous initiatives and, together with a PNISS, performs the essential task of updating, expanding and complementing them.

ESD28, is structured around three axes of action:

1. *Strategic Vision of Digital Health*: Reaffirms, updates and expands the content of the e-Health Strategy document for Brazil, bringing a clear and concise vision of what we want to achieve by 2028.
2. *Digital Health Action Plan*: Describes the set of activities to be performed and the necessary resources for the implementation of the Digital Health Vision, associated with evolutionary stages.
3. *Digital Health Monitoring and Evaluation Plan:* Describes the activities necessary for the Action Plan to remain consistent and systematically adherent to the Digital Health Vision, making it possible to periodically review the Action Plan for readjustment, adapting it to new needs, and also take advantage of new opportunities to capture value.

Thus, in Brazil due to the various examples of Electronic Health Records both from public and private institutions, which are still not integrated and therefore compromise information and patient safety, there is a need to quickly test, validate and put them into practice. These activities should make use of innovation, knowledge and best practices developed in any of the sectors linked to health.

There is still a great lack of knowledge and enormous distrust among the actors (individuals and companies) in the public and private sectors, both in healthcare and in other industries related to health equipment, services and products. Therefore, digital health in Brazil is an extremely complex field, due to the diversity of actors and interests, the lack of maturity of health organizations, the scarcity of human resources and trained leaders and, above all, the complexity inherent to healthcare processes.

Therefore, the coordinated development of the three axes should provide that

- the computerization objectives of the Brazilian Unified Health System (SUS) be strengthened by innovation initiatives, models of services, applications and knowledge, fruits of collaborative and citizen participation;
- the results of the collaboration, such as service delivery models, knowledge extraction mechanisms, digital health applications and alerts in epidemiological or health surveillance, for example, are naturally integrated into the SUS, supplementary to private health platforms;
- the training of human resources resulting from collaborative efforts has a positive impact on the development of the Digital Health Strategy;
- health organizations, service companies, developers, and software and solution providers that participate in the Collaboration Space are better prepared for digital health;
- the Collaboration Space is an instrument for economic and social development, as it trains psycho-social,

organizational, and methodological topics necessary for digital health, an area of great specialization, promoting the emergence of innovative activities of great socio-economic value;
- ESD28 is born and remains in line with the best practices of Public Management, among which the Federal Government's Digital Transformation objectives stand out;
- ESD28 is aligned and remains inspired by the United Nations Sustainable Development Goals, particularly, "Goal 3: Ensure a healthy life and promote well-being for all, at all ages"; and
- ESD28 focuses on the needs identified in the National Health Plan in force and those that will succeed them.

Summary

As presented in this chapter there is a manifold of health IT applications, methods and devices to improve patient safety. Among them are electronic health records, computerized provider order entry systems and clinical decision support systems, and also those making use of big data and predictive analytics through machine learning algorithms and other AI methods. Furthermore, these systems can be supported and enriched by implementing sensors and devices such as barcoding and radio frequency identification use, smart pumps, automated medication dispensing machine and wearables, which all could become interconnected in an Internet-of-Things approach. Although these health IT applications, methods and devices already demonstrated their contribution to safe care, they can also pose a threat to patient safety. Ensuring the safety of health IT and its use in the clinical setting has emerged as a key challenge at any stage of the health IT lifecycle. In order for health informaticians and clinicians to understand what they are, their development process, utilization and evaluation, they must be well prepared, especially with the growing use of wireless technologies, big data and data analytics. The Brazilian case study shows the three pillars of the National Digital Health Strategy: electronic health records, predictive analysis and health apps.

Conclusions and Outlook

Health care is becoming increasingly data-driven, and technological advances are changing the way health professionals can provide patient care. The use of wireless devices and the storage and processing of large volumes of data, with artificial intelligence techniques, has created the possibility of continuous analysis of patient data, converting them into information and identifying trends and patterns. Predictive analysis of these data can forecast the occurrence of an adverse event or a change in the patient's clinical condition, promoting greater safety for the patient and allowing a better assessment of the quality of care provided. Physicians and nurses must understand the implications of these developments and implementations and the need for the evaluation of different information technologies in care and management. Also, they have to be aware of the skills necessary to improve patient care, based on a greater amount of data, and follow ethical and legal principles, respecting the legal and privacy issues.

Review Questions

1. In your clinical practice, how might you/a healthcare team use electronic patient records to improve patient safety?
2. You are developing your activities in a strategic sector of your clinical practice that has several predictive models of care integrated with the system used in the institution. What is its main use?
3. What are the opportunities and risks for RFID technology in health care?
4. Give examples of design and development challenges for the following aspect:
   (a) Developing proactive models, methods and tools to enable risk assessment.
   (b) Developing standard user interface design features and functions.
   (c) Ensuring the safety of software in an interfaced, network-enabled clinical environment.
   (d) Implementing a method for unambiguous patient identification.
5. How can smart pumps be integrated with electronic health records?

Appendix: Answers to Review Questions

1. In your clinical practice, how might you/a healthcare team use electronic patient records to improve patient safety?

Here are some examples of how your healthcare team might improve patient safety from electronic patient records: in workflow through reducing the time required to get charts, improving access to comprehensive patient data, helping to manage prescriptions, improving the scheduling of patient appointments and providing remote access to patients' charts. Also, through the electronic patient record alert systems, it is possible to quickly identify the problem that the patient is reformulating and intervene to reduce complications.

2. You are developing your activities in a strategic sector of your clinical practice that has several predictive models of care integrated with the system used in the institution. What is its main use?

Clinical analyses based on predictive models in health care can help, among so many examples, to detect early signs of patient deterioration in the ICU and general ward, identify at-risk patients in their homes to prevent hospital readmissions and prevent avoidable downtime of medical equipment. They can also support managers and health professionals in making safer decisions regarding the best health practices to be developed in a given situation or case.

3. What are the opportunities and risks for RFID technology in health care?

Opportunities of RFID: for example, patient identification, patient tracking, patient tracking and patient tracking. Risks of RFID: electromagnetic interference with biomedical devices and electronic medical equipment, counterfeiting unencrypted sensitive data within RFID tags, intercepting data during transmission, unauthorized access of sensitive data and high costs.

4. Give examples of design and development challenges for the following aspect:

Examples:
(a) Developing proactive models, methods and tools to enable risk assessment: *defining potential sources of risks and risk linkages, the definition of indicators how to measure the risks, classification of harm and probability of occurrence, mitigation strategy including risk management plan.*
(b) Developing standard user interface design features and functions: *icons are consistent throughout the user interface and placed at the same position on each screen.*
(c) Ensuring the safety of software in an interfaced, network-enabled clinical environment: *implementing technical and organizational measures to counteract potential tampering, hacking and other unauthorized manipulations, for example, firewalls, physically separated networks (internal and external), back-up schedules and anti-malware software.*
(d) Implementing a method for unambiguous patient identification: *using a master-patient index.*

5. How can smart pumps be integrated with electronic health records?

Smart pump integration links smart pumps to the EHR such that medication administration requires barcode scanning the patient's wristband, the medication and the pump channel. The pump is then automatically programmed using the available order from the linked EHR. Also, the pump automatically administers the medication volume documented in the EHR at the appropriate time, allowing for improved documentation.

Useful Resources and References
1. How Interoperability & Data Sharing Can Improve Patient Safety—https://www.youtube.com/watch?v=L5Hhok4_tcY
2. How Tech Secures & Enhances the Patient Experience in Hospitals—https://www.youtube.com/watch?v=bpaph88UYHY
3. SOPS Health IT Patient Safety Supplemental Items for Hospitals—https://www.youtube.com/watch?v=pRYSNj5otrA

References

1. Institute of Medicine. Crossing the Quality Chasm: A New Health System for the 21st Century. Washington, DC: National Academies Press; 2002.
2. Peltonen LM, Topaz M, Ronquillo C, Pruinelli L, Sarmiento RF, Badger MK, et al. Nursing informatics research priorities for the future: Recommendations from an international survey. Stud Health Technol Inform. 2016;225:222–6.
3. Peltonen LM, Alhuwail D, Ali S, Badger MK, Eler GJ, Georgsson M, et al. Current trends in nursing informatics: Results from an international survey. Stud Health Technol Inform. 2016;225: 938–9.
4. Park HA. Health informatics in developing countries: a review of unintended consequences of it implementations, as they affect patient safety and recommendations on how to address them. Yearb Med Inform. 2016;1:1–2. https://doi.org/10.15265/IY-2016-028.
5. Palmieri PA, Peterson LT, Corazzo LB. Technological iatrogenesis: the manifestation of inadequate organizational planning and the integration of health information technology. Adv Health Care Manag. 2011;10:287–312.
6. Weiner JP, Kfuri T, Chan K, Fowles JB. "e-Iatrogenesis": the most critical unintended consequence of CPOE and other HIT. J Am Med Inform Assoc. 2007;14:387–8.
7. Feldman SS, Buchalter S, Hayes LW. Health information technology in healthcare quality and patient safety: literature review. JMIR Med Inform. 2018;6:e10264. https://doi.org/10.2196/10264.
8. Singh H, Sittig DF. Measuring and improving patient safety through health information technol-

ogy: the health it safety framework. BMJ Quality & Safety. 2016;25(4):226–32. https://doi.org/10.1136/bmjqs-2015-004486.

9. Healthcare Information and Management Systems Society. HIMSS dictionary of health information and technology terms, acronyms and organizations. 5th ed. Boca Raton: Taylor & Francis Group; 2019.

10. Salmon JW, Jiang R. E-prescribing: history, issues, and potentials. Online J Public Health Inform. 2012;4(3):ojphi.v4i3.4304. https://doi.org/10.5210/ojphi.v4i3.4304.

11. Wang JK, Herzog NS, Kaushal R, Park C, Mochizuki C, Weingarten SR. Prevention of pediatric medication errors by hospital pharmacists and the potential benefit of computerized physician order entry. Pediatrics. 2007;119(1):e77–85. https://doi.org/10.1542/peds.2006-0034.

12. Bates DW, Teich JM, Lee J, Seger D, Kuperman GJ, Ma'Luf N, Boyle D, Leape L. The impact of computerized physician order entry on medication error prevention. J Am Med Inform Assoc. 2019;6(4):313–21. https://doi.org/10.1136/jamia.1999.00660313.

13. Huckvale C, Car J, Akiyama M, Jaafar S, Khoja T, Bin Khalid A, Sheikh A, Majeed A. Information technology for patient safety. Qual Saf Health Care. 2019;19(Suppl 2):i25–33. https://doi.org/10.1136/qshc.2009.038497.

14. Fiks AG. Designing computerized decision support that works for clinicians and families. Curr Probl Pediatr Adolesc Health Care. 2011;41(3):60–88. https://doi.org/10.1016/j.cppeds.2010.10.006.

15. Linnen DMS. The promise of big data: Improving patient safety and nursing practice. Nursing. 2016;46(5):28–34. quiz 34-5. https://doi.org/10.1097/01.NURSE.0000482256.71143.09.

16. McCormick K, Sensmeier J, Dykes P, et al. Exemplars for advancing standardized terminology in nursing to achieve sharable, comparable quality data based upon evidence. OJIN: Online J Nurs Informatics. 2015;19(2).

17. Pramanik PKD, Pal S, Mukhopadhyay M. Healthcare big data: a comprehensive overview. In: Bouchemal N, editor. Intelligent systems for healthcare management and delivery. IGI Global; 2019. p. 72–100. http://doi:10.4018/978-1-5225-7071-4.ch004.

18. Bulgarelli L, Deliberato RO, Johnson A. Prediction on critically ill patients: The role of big data. J Crit Care. 2020;60:64–8. https://doi.org/10.1016/j.jcrc.2020.07.017.

19. Pan Y. Heading toward Artificial Intelligence 2.0. Engineering. 2016;2(4):409–13.

20. Samuel AL. Some studies in machine learning using the game of checkers. IBM J Res Dev. 1959;3(3):210–29. https://doi.org/10.1147/rd.33.0210.

21. Holzinger A. Machine learning for health informatics. In: Holzinger A. (ed.) Machine learning for health informatics: state-of-the-art and future challenges. Springer; 2016;p.1–24.

22. Douthit BJ, Hu X, Richesson RL, Kim H, Cary Jr MP. How artificial intelligence is transforming the future of nursing. American Nurse. 2020 September 6. Available at https://www.myamericannurse.com/how-artificial-intelligence-is-transforming-the-future-of-nursing

23. Obermeyer Z, Emanuel EJ. Predicting the future–big data, machine learning, and clinical medicine. N Engl J Med. 2016;375(13):1216–9.

24. Meyer A, Zverinski D, Pfahringer B, Kempfert J, Kuehne T, Sündermann SH, Stamm C, Hofmann T, Falk V, Eickhoff C. Machine learning for real-time prediction of complications in critical care: a retrospective study. Lancet Respir Med. 2018;6(12):905–14.

25. Yoon JH, Jeanselme V, Dubrawski A, Hravnak M, Pinsky MR, Clermont G. Prediction of hypotension events with physiologic vital sign signatures in the intensive care unit. Crit Care. 2020;24(1):661–9.

26. Kong G, Lin K, Hu Y. Using machine learning methods to predict in-hospital mortality of sepsis patients in the ICU. BMC Med Inform Decis Mak. 2020;20(1):251.

27. A Zebra Technologies White Paper. Patient safety applications of bar code and rfid technologies. Lincolnshire. Zebra Technologies Corporation; 2010. Available at https://rmsomega.com/healthcare/wp-content/uploads/sites/2/2014/10/Zebra-PatientSafety-White-Paper.pdf

28. Morriss FH, Abramowitz PW, Nelson SP, Milavetz G, Michael SL, Gordon SN, et al. Effectiveness of a Barcode medication administration system in reducing preventable adverse drug events in a neonatal intensive care unit: a prospective cohort study. J Pediatr. 2009;154:363–8.

29. Eskew JA, Jacobi J, Buss WF, Warhurst HM, Debord CL. Using innovative technologies to set new safety standards for the infusion of intravenous medications. Hosp Pharm. 2002;37(11):1179–89. https://doi.org/10.1177/001857870203701112.

30. Bainbridge M, Askew D. Barcoding and other scanning technologies to improve medication safety in hospitals. Sydney: ACSQHC. Australian Commission for Safety and quality in Healthcare; 2017. Available at: https://www.safetyandquality.gov.au/sites/default/files/migrated/Barcoding-and-other-scanning-technologies-to-improve-medication-safety-in-hospitals.pdf

31. Haddara M, Staaby A. RFID applications and adoptions in healthcare: a review on patient safety. Procedia Computer Science. 2018;138:80–8. https://doi.org/10.1016/j.procs.2018.10.012.

32. Haddara M, Staaby A. Enhancing patient safety: a focus on RFID applications in healthcare. Int J Reliable and Quality E-Healthcare. 2020;9:1–17. https://doi.org/10.4018/IJRQEH.2020040101.

33. Wilson K, Sullivan M. Preventing medication errors with smart infusion technology. Am J Health Syst Pharm. 2004;61(2):177–83. https://doi.org/10.1093/ajhp/61.2.177.

34. Ritter T. Perspectives From ECRI. J Clin Eng. 2005;30(2):81–2.
35. Biltoft J, Finneman L. Clinical and financial effects of smart pump-electronic medical record interoperability at a hospital in a regional health system. Am J Health Syst Pharm. 2018;75(14):1064–8. https://doi.org/10.2146/ajhp161058.
36. Burton SJ. Automated dispensing cabinets can help or hinder patient safety based on the implementation of safeguard strategies. J Emerg Nurs. 2019;45(4):444–9. https://doi.org/10.1016/j.jen.2019.05.001.
37. Institute for Safe Medication Practices. Understanding human over-reliance on technology. ISMP Medication Saf Alert. 2016;21(18):1–4.
38. Boyd A, Chaffee B. Critical evaluation of pharmacy automation and robotic systems: a call to action. Hosp Pharm. 2018;54(1):4–11. https://doi.org/10.1177/0018578718786942.
39. Darwesh BM, Machudo SY, John S. The experience of using an automated dispensing system to improve medication safety and management at King Abdul Aziz University Hospital. J Pharm Practice Comm Med. 2017;3:114–9. https://doi.org/10.5530/jppcm.2017.3.26.
40. Patel MS, Asch DA, Volpp KG. Wearable devices as facilitators, not drivers, of health behavior change. JAMA. 2015;313(5):459–60.
41. Andreu-Perez J, Leff DR, Ip HM, Yang GZ. From wearable sensors to smart implants–towards pervasive and personalised healthcare. IEEE Trans Biomed Eng. 2015;62(12):2750–62. https://doi.org/10.1109/TBME.2015.2422751.
42. Joshi M, Ashrafian H, Aufegger L, Khan S, Arora S, Cooke G, Darzi A. Wearable sensors to improve detection of patient deterioration. Expert Rev Med Devices. 2019;16(2):145–54. https://doi.org/10.1080/17434440.2019.1563480.
43. Al-Fuqaha M, Guizani M, Mohammadi M, Aledhari and M. Ayyash. Internet of things: a survey on enabling technologies, protocols, and applications. IEEE Communications Surveys & Tutorials. 2015;17(4):2347–76. https://doi.org/10.1109/COMST.2015.2444095.
44. Yetisen AK, Martinez-Hurtado JL, Ünal B, Khademhosseini A, Butt H. Wearables in medicine. Adv Mater. 2018;11.:30(33):e1706910. https://doi.org/10.1002/adma.201706910.
45. Atzori L, Iera A, Morabito G. The internet of things: a survey. Comput Netw. 2010;54:2787–805. https://doi.org/10.1016/j.comnet.2010.05.010.
46. Mieronkoski R, Azimi I, Rahmani AM, Aantaa R, Terävä V, Liljeberg P, Salanterä S. The internet of things for basic nursing care-a scoping review. Int J Nurs Stud. 2017;69:78–90. https://doi.org/10.1016/j.ijnurstu.2017.01.009.
47. Sturmberg JP, O'an DM, Martin CM. Understanding health system reform–a complex adaptive systems perspective. J Eval Clin Pract. 2012;18(1):202–8.
48. Sittig DF, Wright A, Coiera E, Magrabi F, Ratwani R, Bates DW, Singh H. Current challenges in health information technology-related patient safety. Health Informatics J. 2020;26(1):181–9. https://doi.org/10.1177/1460458218814893.

Patient Safety: Managing the Risks

25

Andrea Diana Klausen, Rainer Röhrig, and Myriam Lipprandt

Learning Objectives

At the end of this chapter, the reader should

- know and be able to explain the terms Patient Safety, (Critical) Incident, Near-Misses, Adverse Event, Hazard and Risk;
- know and be able to explain the term Socio-technical System;
- be able to apply methods of Systematic Failure Analysis;
- be able to give examples of error causes in the interaction of humans and machines (computers) and the resulting hazards;
- be able to explain the two-stage training concept;
- be able to apply the training concept to their own use cases.

Key Terms

- Abnormal use
- Adverse event
- Correct use
- Harm
- Hazard
- Hazardous situation
- (Critical) incident
- Near-misses
- Normal use

- Patient safety
- Risk
- Risk analysis
- Safety
- Security
- Socio-technical system
- Use error

Introduction

For a long time, the significance of treatment errors was underestimated. This changed at the turn of the millennium in 2000. In its report "To Err Is Human: Building a Safer Health System," the Institute of Medicine (US) Committee on Quality of Health Care in America estimated that 98,000 hospital patients die each year in the United States due to treatment errors [1]. More recent studies also estimate that treatment errors are the third leading cause of death in the United States [2]. In Germany adverse events are estimated to be 900,000–1,800,000 per year or 5%–10% of hospital treatments, preventable adverse events are estimated to be 360,000–720,000 cases per year (2%–4%), adverse events caused by medical malpractice are estimated to be 188,000 cases per year (1%) and deaths caused by medical errors are estimated to be 18,800 cases per year (0.1% of hospital treatments) [3].

These data highlight the need to understand the causes and contributing factors of adverse

A. D. Klausen · R. Röhrig · M. Lipprandt (✉)
Institute of Medical Informatics, Medical Faculty of RWTH Aachen University, Aachen, Germany
e-mail: mlipprandt@ukaachen.de

© Springer Nature Switzerland AG 2022
U. H. Hübner et al. (eds.), *Nursing Informatics*, Health Informatics,
https://doi.org/10.1007/978-3-030-91237-6_25

events in patient care, and to develop and establish preventive interventions. This is summarized under the term *patient safety*. The World Health Organization (WHO) defines patient safety as follows:

> Patient safety is the reduction of risk of unnecessary harm associated with healthcare to an acceptable minimum. An acceptable minimum refers to the collective notions of given current knowledge, resources available and the context in which care was delivered weighed against the risk of nontreatment or other treatment. [18]

The patient safety perspective also found its way into nursing. There, the effects of nursing staffing, working environment, nursing workload and education, among others, have been studied [4–9]. Ultimately, single "cause-and-effect" relationships can rarely be demonstrated in complex systems as various compensatory mechanisms take place. Finally, patient safety is an interdisciplinary and interprofessional issue that must include all individuals, processes, devices, technologies and materials directly or indirectly involved in the treatment process.

A special significance is given to patient safety in the use of information technology, in particular the use and operation of medical software and digital devices. In this context, it is important to consider not only the technology, but also the socio-technical system: in addition to the entire technology, this also includes all persons involved in a process, their actions and interactions (human-human, human-machine and machine-machine).

Patient safety depends to a large extent on the "human factors". The term "human factors" refers to the cognitive, psychological and social factors of influence in socio-technical systems. Therefore, it is important to address the topic of patient safety in education and training as well as in equipment and system briefings in order to raise employee awareness of the topic and to build up the necessary competence.

For example, the topic of patient safety has been included in several curricula for nursing students [10], medical students [11] and healthcare informatics students [12]. The learning objectives in the curricula are to provide students with an overview of the motivation, methods and their own role in patient safety culture and management. Further education is then required depend-

ing on the role inside an organization. For example, post-incident failure analysis should only be performed by specially trained teams [13, 14]. Similarly, risk managers who manage the risk of medical software and digital devices should have special training. In the area of IT operations in hospitals, there are now specially trained incident response teams that are deployed in the event of IT blackouts [15].

An important aspect of patient safety is the user perspective, that is, strengthening the "human factors" through education and training. The need for user training on product-specific safety aspects is regulated by law in most countries. In contrast, education and training of other safety-relevant competencies, in particular the training of safety-relevant behaviors, are the responsibility of the company (nursing service, clinic) in certain areas.

In the following, a method is presented for identifying the weaknesses in the human factors from reported critical incidents with the help of systematic error analysis or the results of risk assessment, which can be improved through targeted training of knowledge, process skills and practiced behavior, including communication. Then, a training concept is developed for the educational needs identified in this way (prevention concept), and incorporated and implemented in a systematic training program (prevention application). Criteria should be established against which the success of the training program can be measured (evaluation). The above mentioned key terms will be defined as follows.

Abnormal Use	"Conscious, intentional act or intentional omission of an act that is counter to or violates normal use and is also beyond any further reasonable means of user interface-related risk control by the manufacturer" [16]
Adverse Event	Event that leads to a (patient) harm or damage.
	In context of medical devices, including medical software: "event associated with a medical device that led to death or serious injury of a patient, user or other person, or that might lead to death or serious injury of a patient, user or other person if the event recurs, Including the discrimination between preventable and non-preventable" [16]

Correct Use	*"Normal use without use error"* [16]
Harm	*"Injury or damage to the health of people, or damage to property or the environment"* [17]
Hazard	*"Potential source of harm"* [17]
Hazardous Situation	*"Circumstance in which people, property or the environment is/are exposed to one or more hazards"* [17]
(Critical) Incident	Event which may result in patient harm (adverse event)
Near-Misses	(Critical) Incident that doesn't lead to patient harm
Normal Use	*"Operation, including routine inspection and adjustments by any user, and stand-by, according to the instructions for use or in accordance with generally accepted practice for those medical devices provided without instructions for use"* [16]
Patient Safety	*"Patient safety is the reduction of risk of unnecessary harm associated with healthcare to an acceptable minimum. An acceptable minimum refers to the collective notions of given current knowledge, resources available and the context in which care was delivered weighed against the risk of non-treatment or other treatment"* [18]
Risk	*"Combination of the probability of occurrence of harm and the severity of that harm"* [17]
Risk Analysis	*"Systematic use of available information to identify hazards and to estimate the risk"* [17]
Safety	*"Freedom from unacceptable risk"* [17]
Security	Security is the degree of protection against danger, damage, loss and crime

Socio-technical System	Socio-technical System (STS) is an approach to describe a complex organizational work design that describes the organization and interaction between people and technology
Use Error	*"User action or lack of user action while using the medical device that leads to a different result than that intended by the manufacturer or expected by the user"* [16]

Developing of Teaching and Learning Concepts

The education concept consists of a five-step approach (see Fig. 25.1):

- *Reporting:* In this step of the concept, adverse events are reported.
- *Risk Management*: In risk management, a systematic error analysis is applied to a reported adverse event.
- *Prevention Concept:* The results of the systematic error analysis are reviewed and used to develop action strategies for risk minimization and are didactically developed.
- *Prevention Application:* The prevention concept is transferred into practice.
- *Evaluation*: In this stage, different evaluation methods are used to check the learning objectives. If the desired learning objectives are not achieved, a new risk analysis is started.

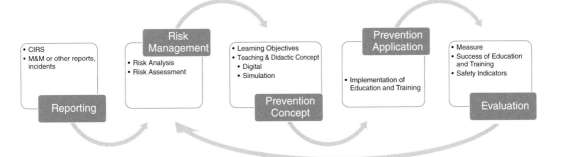

Fig. 25.1 Development of teaching concepts in response to safety-critical events

Reporting

The requirement for systematic error analysis includes the willingness of employees to report errors. If employees who report their own errors have to face a loss of reputation or other personal consequences, they won't report errors (shame-and-blame culture). Likewise, a one-sided focus on the nurse as the sole source of error is counterproductive. In order to learn from errors, an open error culture must be created in which errors are seen as an opportunity to learn from them and thus prevent damage. Instead of a mono-causal focus on individual errors, solution-oriented approaches become possible, which include the facilitating factors of an event [18, 19]. The leading question must not be "WHO is to blame?"; the leading question must be "HOW to prevent this error in the future?"

The concept of Critical Incident Report Systems (CIRS) was therefore adopted from the aviation industry. In a CIRS employees can report near-misses. In order to protect employees, anonymity must be guaranteed. However, if necessary, there should be a consultation option via a trusted party so that further questions can be answered for the systematic error analysis.

All reported errors are systematically analyzed. The results of the error analysis provide the basis for corrective measures and recommendations to avoid or minimize the extent of damage. In addition, these measures serve the

educational training concept to enable needs-based competencies in dealing with errors and emergencies. Systematic error analysis requires a team with appropriate competencies and resources, but in particular a culture of appreciation of reported errors and those reporting them.

Risk Management

A systematic analysis of critical events, hazards and risks that can occur in nursing is conducted. The results are the basis for the development of recommendations for action to acquire competence in emergency situations.

Risk Analysis

Patient harm due to adverse events is usually the end of a longer chain of errors. The error chain is usually triggered by an event that is causal for a possible patient harm. For patient harm to occur after a causal, or triggering, event, other contributory factors must be added. For example, a dosage error by a physician can be detected by a nurse and patient harm averted. The British psychologist and risk researcher James Reason developed the "Swiss cheese model": Each slice of cheese represents a level of safety (see Fig. 25.2). None of these safety levels is 100% safe; there are holes in every layer like in Emmental cheese. Although the Emmental

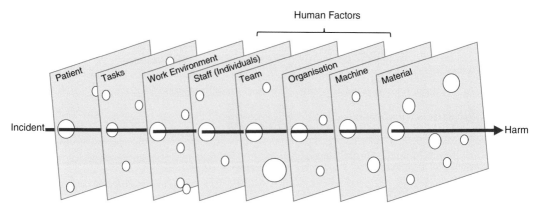

Fig. 25.2 Swiss cheese model according to Reason [20], with the various safety levels that prevent an incident from becoming a harm. The levels of the individual capabilities of employees, the team and the organization, and human interaction are summarized as follows

cheese is full of holes, it is usually not possible to see through the cheese from back to front. Figuratively transferred errors in the Swiss cheese system are normally intercepted by a safety layer. Only when several necessary and favorable factors come together does patient harm occur. The different safety levels can be assigned to different characteristics. The cognitive, psychological and social influencing factors, represented here by "staff" and "team," are summarized as human factors.

In risk management, a somewhat more formal approach is used. Here, too, a causal chain is assumed. After a causal event, a hazard arises in a sequence of further events. A hazard is a potential source of harm [17]. Further actions and events lead to a hazardous situation, that is, a state in which the patient is exposed to a hazard. The hazardous situation can then give rise to the harm. The risk is defined as the product of the severity of the harm and the probability of the harm occurring (see Fig. 25.3). The probability that harm will occur is the product of the probabilities that a sequence of events will create a hazardous situation (P1) and that this will lead to an incident (P2).

Safety Aspects of Human-Machine Interaction

A relevant source of error in the use of medical devices or software is the human-machine interface [21–24]. Incorrect handling can also lead to patient harm.

Normal Versus Abnormal Use

In usability standards, a distinction is made between intended actions and unintended actions. An intended action can be a correct use as well as an intended abnormal use (see Fig. 25.4). An abnormal use is defined as "conscious, intentional act or intentional omission of an act that is counter to or violates normal use and is also beyond any further reasonable means of user interface-related risk control by the manufacturer" [16]. Since to err is human, an unintentional erroneous condition must be assumed. Therefore, normal use includes both intended use and unintended use.

Use Error Versus User Error

In case of a communication error, it is always difficult to decide on which side the error occurred. The same applies to human-machine

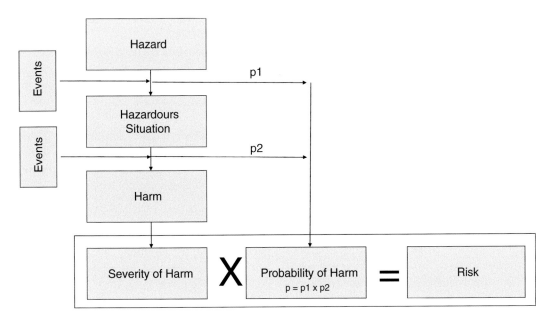

Fig. 25.3 Depiction of hazard, hazard situation and risk according to ISO 14971 [17]

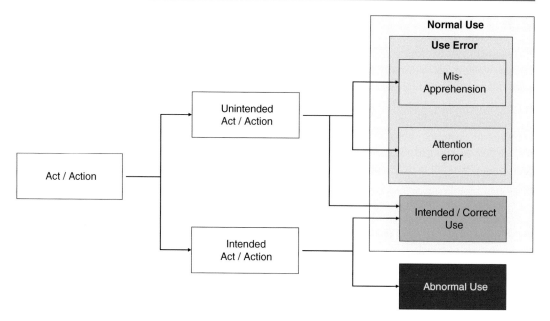

Fig. 25.4 Normal use and use error based on DIN EN 62366

communication. We always speak of a user error when the user is solely responsible for the error. In most cases, however, it is a combination of a usability weakness in the system and an error on the part of the user. In this case, we speak of a use error [25].

Example: A user reads a possible value from a blood glucose meter. However, the value is the batch code of the test strip and not the measured value. This results in incorrect treatment [26]. The device differentiates which value it displays according to the stage of the process. In the measured value display, the unit is also displayed small next to the digits. In this case, there is an error on the part of the user, but this error is to be expected. Thus, the error is a usability error and therefore also a device error. In this case we speak of a use error.

Risk Assessment

Classical error research deals with the analysis, classification and cause of errors [27]. Various qualitative methods from engineering and social research are available for this purpose. The different methods also have different strengths and weaknesses depending on the use case. Common to all methods is that they require a high level of methodological, technical and social competence from the investigators [13], which can often only be provided by an interdisciplinary and interprofessional team. Through structured questions, interviews and the reconstruction of the error event as well as the systematic outline of possible cause-and-effect relationships, undesired events, incidents, application errors with different effects can be analyzed and processed.

To minimize risks the hazards and their causes must first be discovered. Several methods are available for this purpose that systematically identify hazards and their causes and triggering events.

The *Preliminary Hazard Analysis* (PHA) is an experience-based and not very systematic listing of possible, known hazards. It is a brainstorming method that identifies the obvious hazards based on the medical device. It is based on experience and feedback.

In the *5-Why method* [28] starting from the possible harm, the question "Why does it happen?" is asked. By asking repeatedly, hidden faults and facilitating factors are found. In this method, you keep searching by asking "why" questions until you reach an end.

The *Ishikawa diagram* (fishbone diagram) is a graphical representation for a bottom-up approach that lists the influencing causes structured by categories that are considered to be causal for the effect (error, event). Originally, the categories included human, material, environment (milieu), machine or resource, measurement and method. In the London Protocol [13], the branches of the Ishikawa diagram were expanded to include categories that may have an influence on a patient from a medical perspective.

A forward analysis from causes to effects by creating a fishbone diagram, Ishikawa diagram (Fig. 25.5), serves to complete and categorize the causes and facilitating factors. Additionally, this diagram provides a deeper understanding of the situation.

The *Bow-Tie diagram* (Fig. 25.6) is used to analyze and document risks. It is a method that combines other methods such as the fault tree analysis and the cause-and-effect diagram. The adverse event (damage event) to be avoided is represented as a node in the center of the diagram. This can be hazards, incidents or adverse events. For each event a Bow-Tie diagram is created.

The causes are listed on the left side of the Bow-Tie diagram. Fault tree analysis or the cause-and-effect diagram can be applied here. On the right side, the effects resulting from the undesired event are entered.

On both sides, safeguards or barriers are incorporated that are either preventive or curative (green boxes). On the left side, hazard warnings can be specified as preventive. On the right side,

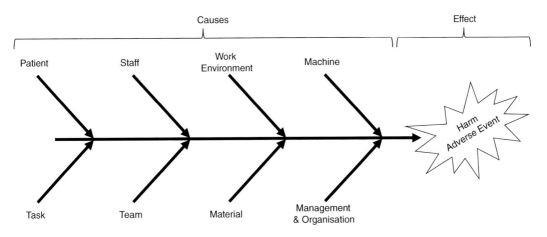

Fig. 25.5 Ishikawa diagram (fishbone diagram, invented by Kaoru Ishikawa, a Japanese analyst)

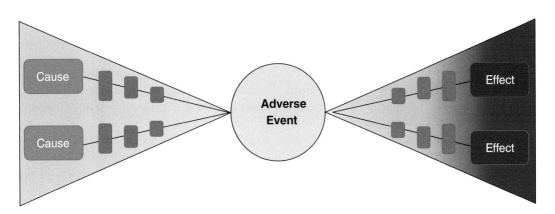

Fig. 25.6 Bow-Tie diagram

the measures to deal with the adverse event can be documented.

Prevention Concept

For the development of a preventive teaching concept in outpatient care, a methodical-didactical two-stage teaching concept is shown below. The structure is composed of a digital learning format and a simulation training. This concept is intended to make the goals of the training clear to learners. Through the structure, they experience the opportunity to acquire and consolidate new competencies both theoretically and practically. It offers opportunities to practice nursing procedures and medical emergency situations both in a digitally supported self-learning phase and in authentic problem situations under realistic conditions (simulation). The teaching concept for home ventilation is presented as an example in the case study.

Learning Objectives

The structure of a teaching concept includes learning objectives. They show the pedagogical-didactical planned goals of the teachers. Learning objectives describe the requirements for the learner's performance. They form criteria that enable learners to evaluate their own learning progress.

For the development of learning objectives, it is useful to choose a formulation that is easy to understand and clarifies what the learner should know and understand. The wording should be precise enough to list observable behavior (if possible). Learning objectives are action-oriented and should indicate what learning outcomes the learner will be able to apply after the unit. Precise learning objective wording allows both learners and instructors to better review learning outcomes. Precisely formulated learning objectives show what an (observable) learning outcome is based on. For the description of learning objectives, different levels of competence must be taken into account in the formulation.

Examples
1. *After working through this chapter, you should be able to explain the subject of patient safety.*
2. *After working through this chapter, you will be able to explain the terms risk and hazard.*
3. *You will be able to apply the methods of systematic failure analysis to your individual case.*

Teaching Concept

The development of the teaching concept takes into account the integration of new topics. For example, results of a risk analysis can be incorporated into a teaching concept. Digital learning materials and tools (e.g., in the form of online seminars, virtual reality, films, textbooks, internet resources: websites, portals, video/audio sequences) are provided. Learners should use the digital learning format in a self-learning phase. These tools allow learners to interact with instructors. They can get support from the teachers in their learning progress. The teachers are the learning guides and contact persons. They actively support the learning development of the learners.

Digital Learning Format

The digital learning format is divided into two areas. One area offers basic elements of medical and technical topics. Another area focuses on practical skills in different care contexts.

To enable learners to repeat familiar topics, medical topics such as anatomy, physiology and ventilation, but also in-depth topics such as anesthesia [29] are offered in the digital self-learning phase. Digital literacy is a central theme [30]. Learners should expand their technical knowledge through the use of tools. They should deal with the socio-technical system in a differentiated way through learning opportunities. Through the processing of learning tasks, all persons, actions and interactions involved in the process are considered and questioned.

In order to raise learners' awareness of the topic of patient safety, they are offered learning tasks in various tools for the acquisition of safety-relevant competencies/safety-relevant behavior in emergency care. In the following concept, elements of Crew Resource Management (CRM) [31, 32] are integrated into the teaching concept to strengthen the area of the "human factors". CRM, like Critical Incident Reporting Systems (CIRS), has its origins in aerospace. Originally, the concept was developed as Cockpit Resource Management and focused on the interpersonal aspects of the cockpit crew. The CRM concept has evolved over time and now represents comprehensive training on human factors [33]. Learners should learn about risk minimization activities through the application of the tools and apply recommendations for action in learning tasks.

Simulation Training
In order to achieve a successful theory/practice transfer of the self-learning phase, a collaborative simulation training is useful. The unifying structure of both formats is learning tasks and use cases, in different methodological/didactic formats. The simulation is structured in several practice phases that build on each other. It depicts care situations that have been processed as adverse events in a risk management process.

The simulation is designed as a face-to-face event in a realistic simulation laboratory. In the simulation situation, the theoretical content from the digital self-learning phase is deepened and transferred to practical application. This structure ensures reflection on the results of the digital self-learning phase. The joint processing of complex problems and the reflection on the applied measure expand the repertoire of actions. The risk minimization methods complete the learning offer and increase the learners' ability to act.

The demonstrated concept creates a practical connection and integration of existing competencies into a new field of nursing action (e.g., emergency situation) [34]. Technology acceptance is increased through the practical use of medical devices and software. The reflection of applied actions and an exemplary handling of an adverse event show the learners, a new way of dealing with errors. An open error culture creates sustainability in the learners' ability to act.

The simulation is conducted with a group of at least four to a maximum of six people. It begins with a reflection on the regular use of innovative care technologies. The learners thus deal with a socio-technical system right at the beginning of the simulation.

The nurses are divided into two teams. Each team has a different task. One team takes over the nursing actions on a simulation manikin. The other team takes the position of observing. The observing team is given a scoring grid with set criteria (to implement the CRM communication rules) to fill in during the observation. This method is intended to make it easier for the observing team to provide structured feedback to the care team.

Prevention Application

Based on the work of the previous section (Learning Objectives) is transferred into concrete training content. For this purpose, the risk control actions must be integrated with the nursing actions and mapped onto the digital and simulation concepts. For the digital learning unit, this includes dealing with diverse e-learning concepts such as web applications, collaborative, interactive tools, movies, podcasts, quizzes, mind maps and online lectures. For the simulation, the concepts have to be adapted to the real environment with a full-scale patient simulator. For this, the medical equipment technology of the patient simulator must be programmed for actual emergencies [35, 36]. Furthermore, simulation rooms must be prepared for the simulation at each appointment. The simulators are programmed, materials are provided (nursing supplies, assessment grids for observation, etc.) and all medical equipment is tested for function.

Evaluation

The evaluation of the training concept takes place in several steps. In the digital self-learning phase, learning progress is evaluated by the instructors and learners themselves. Learning progress is evaluated by completing learning tasks in different tools. The evaluation of the simulation takes place directly after the simulation in the form of a questionnaire. The questionnaire asks whether defined learning objectives of the training concept were achieved. After a defined period of time, this survey is conducted again and compared with the results of the first survey. The comparison enables a subjective assessment of the sustainability of the learning objectives achieved. In a final step, an indirect evaluation is carried out by applying the safety indicators [37] in professional practice.

Case Study

Care and emergency situation:

Mrs. K. (78 years old) lives in an apartment with her husband. She suffered a traumatic brain injury in a traffic accident in 2018. Since that time, she has required ongoing respiratory support. Mrs. K has a tracheostoma* and is supported in her breathing by a home ventilator via a tracheal tube. Mrs. K. is provided with a speaking valve daily for the time of personal hygiene.

At 04:00 p.m. Mrs. K reconnected to the ventilator. An acoustic and visual alarm sounds from the ventilator. The nurse deactivates the alarm as she is positioning the patient in bed. The audible and visual alarm beep at 04:01 p.m. again. The nurse deactivates the alarm again. Two minutes later the alarm sounds again and the oxygen saturation is too low. The nurse looks at the ventilator and sees the following alarms:

- Set ventilation pressure cannot be applied.
- Respiratory volume too low.
- Respiratory minute volume too low.

The nurse checks the ventilator settings without finding an error; meanwhile, the oxygen saturation drops to 85%. At 4:11 p.m. the nurse calls the ambulance. After ambulance arrives, a paramedic notices that the cuff of the tracheal cannula is not blocked. The paramedic blocks the tracheal cannula.

Risk Management

Using the example of an error message on the ventilator, the causes and effects as well as the risk-controlling measures are presented.

In the first step (1), an initial Preliminary Hazard Analysis (PHA) can be performed by repeatedly asking questions (5-Why method) to reveal the hazards. In the second step (2), the damage and impact can be determined. In the third step (3), actions for risk minimization and recommendations for action are given and the last step transfers it into the training concept.

| Step (1)—Identification of occurring errors or hazards and causes (risk analysis with 5-Why method). ||
Question	Answer
(a) Why did insufficiency ventilation occur?	Cuff was not blocked.
(b) Why was the cuff not blocked?	After changing from the speaking cannula to the "normal" tracheal cannula, the blocking was forgotten.
(c) Why was the ventilator connected to the unblocked tracheostomy tube?	Unblocked tracheal cannula was not detected.
(d) Why was the unblocked tracheostomy tube not detected?	Leakage was not detected.
(e) Why was the leak not detected?	• Breath sounds were not correctly interpreted. • The alarms of the ventilator (lack of pressure build-up + respiratory volume decreased indication of leakage) were not adequately interpreted. • Ventilator gives no indication of leakage volume. • No cuff pressure measurement was performed.
(f) Why was no cuff pressure measurement performed?	• Normally, a cuff pressure measurement is only performed once per shift. • It was not considered as a cause of error.
Step (2)—Potentially fatal outcome for the patient and traumatized caregiver	

Step (1)—Identification of occurring errors or hazards and causes (risk analysis with 5-Why method).	
Question	Answer
Step (3)—Risk minimization actions and recommendations for action	
User-centered view	
(a) Development of checklists for dealing with speaking valves	Material checklists (material for speech training, application of the speech valve)
(b) Standard Operating Procedures (SOP)/ recommendations for action	• Preparation for application of the speaking valve (material assembly, provision of emergency utensils such as resuscitation bag) • Application of the speaking valve (suctioning the patient at the tracheal cannula and in the pharynx to remove possible secretion before application—aspiration prophylaxis, removing the ventilator, unblocking the cuff, putting on the speaking valve, regular measurement of the oxygen saturation by a finger meter) • Follow-up on use of the speaking tube (check ventilator settings, check ventilator system, remove speaking valve, unblock cuff, connect ventilator)

After you get to step (3), you can apply the Bow-Tie diagram (see Fig. 25.7).

Prevention Concept and Application

The risk analysis shows lack of competence and behavioral patterns as necessary and facilitating factors. Preventive measures, processes, behaviors and competencies define what nurses need in this situation. Subsequently, the findings on the prevention of adverse events are incorporated into a training concept. The training needs identified in the systematic error analysis take up risk minimization measures and recommendations for action in the digital and simulated learning phase in various tools. To this end, topics in different training areas are offered on the learning platform. Exemplary training fields are shown in Table 25.1.

Evaluation

The evaluation consists of a direct feedback and a query of the learned contents after some time, as well as a check on the basis of fixed indicators from the routine care. In an assessment grid with fixed criteria to be carried out in the care, the care situation is observed and evaluated according to the fixed criteria.

After the simulation, the "observing team" discusses the emergency situations in an appreciative manner. It analyzes the nursing situation

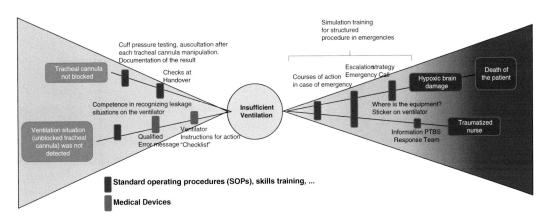

Fig. 25.7 Bow-Tie diagram. The "causes" (cuff was not blocked) and the "effect" (insufficient ventilation) are identified. The risk-controlling measures can be listed

Table 25.1 Based on the risk management, defining the learning objectives (didactics) and the methodology, divided into theoretical and practical skills and evaluation in everyday life

Didactics			Methodology		Risk Monitoring
Identified Possible Causes or Contributing Factors	Risk Control Measures	Learning Objectives "The caregiver …"	Knowledge Transfer (Digital Learning World)	Practice (Simulator Training)	Evaluation
Cuff was not blocked after change from speaking valve to ventilator and the situation was not detected	Instruction of action and training of the procedure	… knows the procedures and can apply them independently	Educational film, online seminar, learning tasks on a digital pin board	Practical training of the nursing process	Supervision/review on the patient at longer intervals
	Checking of cuff pressure, auscultation, ventilation parameters	… knows the procedure and can apply the interventions	Educational film, quiz	Training of the procedure with different clinical constellations.	Documentation check Repeat training on the simulator
Leakage on the ventilator is not detected	Qualified, self-explanatory alarm-message CDSS with notes and options for action (checklist)	Technical aspects. Nurses must be trained on the medical devices (ventilator, CDSS) Digital: online presentation, working on a case study in small groups			
	Skill development in ventilation physiology	Recognize possible sources of ventilator	Educational film, quiz	Simulator training with different clinical situations and errors	Repeat training on the simulator
Ambulance is called too late	Instructions for escalation scheme in emergencies.	… knows the criteria and can apply them even under stress.	Educational film, Materials, quizzes, online assignments	Training of emergency situations on the simulator	Debriefing of critical events
Location of resuscitation bag/emergency case not known or not found	Standard that in each facility/premises on the ventilator the most important information is on a sticker	… knows that the location of the emergency materials is always stuck on the side of the ventilator	Digital simulators of the facility—virtual tour followed by assignment tasks. Short film and online assignments on a digital pin board	On-site training during familiarization at home	Regular consultation by team leader/supervisor as part of the function check

based on the criteria of the assessment grid. Due to the different knowledge of the participants (skill mix, skill grade mix, interdisciplinary team), the participants' ability to act is sustainably expanded. Each profession brings its expertise to the analyses. The team composition allows to include different levels of multi-causal development of hazards or errors from the different professions.

Summary

Risks in nursing are omnipresent and often go undetected. Being on their own, nurses in home care must remain capable of acting as well as initiating the correct measures. This is true, for example, in cases of emergency in intensive home care where life-sustaining medical devices such as ventilators are often used. However, instruction in medical devices does not include specific handling in stressful situations, which can often lead to incorrect decisions. Equipment failure or emergencies are usually not part of the instruction in medical devices. This is where the methods of systematic risk analysis and risk management play a crucial role. Methodological competence about systematic failure analysis and measures of action are necessary to understand how failures and risks occur, and who is responsible for them. Systematic failure analysis can be used to identify causes of failures or, as in our approach, to look into the future with the question: "What if?" The selection and use of methods for failure analysis is one of the most difficult tasks. Time and personnel resources are needed, which, depending on the concrete topic, have both domain competence in care and methodological competence in the application of risk management and transfer to the training concepts to avoid critical incidence in future. The case study in intensive home care where life-sustaining medical devices such as ventilators are often used underpins the need for systematic risk analysis and management. It shows how the steps from *identified possible causes or contributing factors* and *risk control measures* lead to appropriate *learning objectives*. Knowledge transfer in a digital learning world and practical simulation training are proven methodological approaches to reach the learning objectives and are illustrated in the case study.

Conclusions and Outlook

In this chapter, methods of systematic risk management were discussed and demonstrated. The case study shows the fundamental role of the methodological competence of risk management in preventing future adverse events in the context of intensive home care. Integrating the results of the systematic risk analysis into a training concept enables nurses to apply action competencies in case of future adverse events. Here, the segmenta-

tion of the training concept into a digital and a simulated part is crucial. Particularly in view of the future digitalization and further development of medical technology, the human-machine interaction is becoming increasingly important. These interactions influence the entire socio-technical system and have the potential to improve patient safety on the one hand, but also bear new types of risks. Therefore, enhanced competencies are needed to identify new potential risks in the use with these technologies. The didactic implementation of the training gives nurses the opportunity to understand causes of errors and to identify them in order to avoid patient harm. In addition, the challenge of dealing with new digital devices is learned and further deepened.

Review Questions

1. What are the five steps in the teaching concept in response to safety-critical events?
2. How is risk defined according to ISO 14971?
3. What is the Bow-Tie diagram and what do the green boxes denote?
4. Please explain the teaching concept "Digital Learning Format."
5. Please explain the teaching concept "Simulation Training."

Appendix: Answers to Review Questions

1. What are the five steps in the teaching concept in response to safety-critical events?

   - Reporting: In this step of the concept, adverse events are reported.
   - Risk Management: In risk management, a systematic error analysis is applied to a reported adverse event.
   - Prevention Concept: The results of the systematic error analysis are reviewed and used to develop action strategies for risk minimization and are didactically developed.

- Prevention Application: The prevention concept is transferred into practice.
- Evaluation: In this stage, different evaluation methods are used to check the learning objectives. If the desired learning objectives are not achieved, a new risk analysis is started.

2. How is risk defined according to ISO 14971?

Severity of harm × probability of harm = risk.

3. What is the Bow-Tie diagram and what do the green boxes denote?

The Bow-Tie diagram is a method that is used to analyze and document risks. The adverse event (damage event) to be avoided is represented as a node in the center of the diagram. This can be hazards, incidents or adverse events. On both sides, safeguards or barriers are incorporated that are either preventive or curative (green boxes). On the left side, hazard warnings can be specified as preventive. On the right side, the measures to deal with the adverse event can be documented.

4. Please explain the teaching concept "Digital Learning Format."

To enable learners to repeat familiar topics, medical topics such as anatomy, physiology, and ventilation, but also in-depth topics such as anesthesia are offered in the digital self-learning phase. Digital literacy is a central theme [30]. Learners should expand their technical knowledge through the use of tools. They should deal with the socio-technical system in a differentiated way through learning opportunities. Through the processing of learning tasks, all persons, actions and interactions involved in the process are considered and questioned. Elements of Crew Resource Management (CRM) can be integrated into the teaching concept to strengthen the area of the "human factor."

5. Please explain the teaching concept "Simulation Training."

In order to achieve a successful theory/practice transfer of the self-learning phase, a collaborative simulation training is useful. The simulation is structured in several practice phases that build on each other. It depicts care situations that have been processed as adverse events in a risk management process. The simulation is designed as a face-to-face event in a realistic simulation laboratory. The reflection of applied actions and an exemplary handling of an adverse event show the learners a new way of dealing with errors. The simulation is conducted with a group of at least four to a maximum of six people. The nurses are divided into two teams. One team takes over the nursing actions on a simulation manikin. The other team takes the position of observing. The observing team is given a scoring grid with set criteria to provide structured feedback to the care team.

References

1. Kohn LT, Corrigan JM, Donaldson MS (eds). To Err is Human: Building a Safer Health System. Washington (DC); 2000.
2. Makary MA, Daniel M. Medical error-the third leading cause of death in the US. BMJ. 2016;353:i2139. https://doi.org/10.1136/bmj.i2139.
3. Klauber J, Geraedts M, Friedrich J et al. (2014) Krankenhaus-Report 2014. Schwerpunkt: Patientensicherheit. Schattauer
4. Aiken LH, Clarke SP, Sloane DM, et al. Hospital nurse staffing and patient mortality, nurse burnout, and job dissatisfaction. JAMA. 2002;288:1987–93. https://doi.org/10.1001/jama.288.16.1987.
5. Aiken LH, Cimiotti JP, Sloane DM, et al. Effects of nurse staffing and nurse education on patient deaths in hospitals with different nurse work environments. Med Care. 2011;49:1047–53. https://doi.org/10.1097/MLR.0b013e3182330b6e.
6. Clay AS, Chudgar SM, Turner KM, et al. How prepared are medical and nursing students to identify common hazards in the intensive care unit? Ann Am Thorac Soc. 2017;14:543–9. https://doi.org/10.1513/AnnalsATS.201610-773OC.
7. Fagerström L, Kinnunen M, Saarela J. Nursing workload, patient safety incidents and mortality: an observational study from Finland. BMJ

Open. 2018;8:e016367. https://doi.org/10.1136/bmjopen-2017-016367.

8. Schnall R, Larson E, Stone PW, et al. Advanced practice nursing students' identification of patient safety issues in ambulatory care. J Nurs Care Qual. 2013;28:169–75. https://doi.org/10.1097/NCQ.0b013e31827c6a22.

9. Wakefield A, Attree M, Braidman I, et al. Patient safety: do nursing and medical curricula address this theme? Nurse Educ Today. 2005;25:333–40. https://doi.org/10.1016/j.nedt.2005.02.004.

10. Kinnunen U-M, Rajalahti E, Cummings E, et al. Curricula Challenges and Informatics Competencies for Nurse Educators. Stud Health Technol Inform. 2017;232:41–8.

11. Varghese J, Röhrig R, Dugas M et al. Welche Kompetenzen in Medizininformatik benötigen Ärztinnen und Ärzte? Update des Lernzielkatalogs für Studierende der Humanmedizin. GMS Medizinische Informatik, Biometrie und Epidemiologie; 16(1):Doc02 / GMS Medizinische Informatik, Biometrie und Epidemiologie; 2020;16(1):Doc02. https://doi.org/10.3205/MIBE000205.

12. Borycki EM, Cummings E, Kushniruk AW, et al. Integrating Health Information Technology Safety into Nursing Informatics Competencies. Stud Health Technol Inform. 2017;232:222–8.

13. Taylor-Adams S, Vincent C. Systems analysis of clinical incidents. The London protocol. Clin Risk. 2004;10:211–20. https://doi.org/10.1258/1356262042368255.

14. Vincent C. How to investigate and analyse clinical incidents. Clinical Risk Unit and Association of Litigation and Risk Management protocol. BMJ. 2000;320:777–81. https://doi.org/10.1136/bmj.320.7237.777.

15. Sax U, Lipprandt M, Röhrig R. The Rising Frequency of IT Blackouts Indicates the Increasing Relevance of IT Emergency Concepts to Ensure Patient Safety. Yearb Med Inform. 2016;130–137. https://doi.org/10.15265/IY-2016-038.

16. IEC 62366-1:2015–02 Medical devices–Part 1: Application of usability engineering to medical devices.

17. ISO 14971:2019 Medical devices–Application of risk management to medical devices.

18. World Health Organization (2005) World alliance for patient safety: WHO draft guidelines for adverse event reporting and learning systems: from information to action. http://apps.who.int/iris/bitstream/handle/10665/69797/WHO-EIP-SPO-QPS-05.3-eng.pdf?sequence=1&isAllowed=y

19. Maas M, Güß T. Patient safety – mission for the future: The importance of Critical Incident Reporting Systems (CIRS) in clinical practice. Anasthesiol Intensivmed Notfallmed Schmerzther. 2014;49:466–72; quiz 473. https://doi.org/10.1055/s-0034-1386709.

20. Reason J. Human error: models and management. BMJ. 2000;320:768–70.

21. Lipprandt M, Klausen A, Alvarez-Castillo C, et al. Erweiterte systematische Fehleranalyse zweier CIRS-AINS Alert-Fälle: Vom Anwender- zum Anwendungsfehler. Anästhesiologie & Intensivmedizin. 2020;76–84. https://doi.org/10.19224/ai2020.076.

22. Magrabi F, Ong M-S, Runciman W, et al. An analysis of computer-related patient safety incidents to inform the development of a classification. J Am Med Inform Assoc. 2010;17:663–70. https://doi.org/10.1136/jamia.2009.002444.

23. Ong M-S, Magrabi F, Coiera E. Syndromic surveillance for health information system failures: a feasibility study. J Am Med Inform Assoc. 2013;20:506–12. https://doi.org/10.1136/amiajnl-2012-001144.

24. Wilken M, Hüske-Kraus D, Klausen A, et al. Alarm Fatigue: Causes and Effects. Stud Health Technol Inform. 2017;243:107–11.

25. Hölscher UM, Rimbach-Schurig M, Bohnet-Joschko S et al. Patientensicherheit durch Prävention medizinprodukt-assoziierter Risiken. Teil 1: aktive Medizinprodukte, insbesondere medizintechnische Geräte in Krankenhäusern. 2014. https://www.aps-ev.de/wp-content/uploads/2016/08/APS_Handlungsempfehlungen_2014_WEB_lang.pdf. Accessed 10 Oct 2018.

26. Berufsverband Deutscher Anästhesisten A supposedly too high blood glucose value turns out to be a code number of the test strip. CIRSmedical CASE-Report: 106016. https://www.cirsmedical.ch/AINS/

27. Badke-Schaub P, Hofinger G, Lauche K. Human factors. Springer; 2008.

28. von Eiff W. Risikomanagement: Kosten-Nutzen-basierte Entscheidungen im Krankenhaus. Wegscheid: Wikom-Verlag; 2007.

29. Shih Y-CD, Liu C-C, Chang C-C, et al. Effects of digital learning in anaesthesiology: a systematic review and meta-analysis. Eur J Anaesthesiol. 2021;38:171–82. https://doi.org/10.1097/EJA.0000000000001262.

30. Lall P, Rees R, Law GCY, et al. Influences on the implementation of mobile learning for medical and nursing education: qualitative systematic review by the digital health education collaboration. J Med Internet Res. 2019;21:e12895. https://doi.org/10.2196/12895.

31. Ashcroft J, Wilkinson A, Khan M. A systematic review of trauma crew resource management training: what can the United States and the United Kingdom learn from each other? J Surg Educ. 2021;78:245–64. https://doi.org/10.1016/j.jsurg.2020.07.001.

32. Buljac-Samardzic M, Doekhie KD, van Wijngaarden JDH. Interventions to improve team effectiveness within health care: a systematic review of the past decade. Hum Resour Health. 2020;18:2. https://doi.org/10.1186/s12960-019-0411-3.

33. Neuhaus C, Röhrig R, Hofmann G, et al. Patientensicherheit in der Anästhesie. Multimodale Strategien für die perioperative Versorgung (Patient

safety in anesthesiology: Multimodal strategies for perioperative care). Anaesthesist. 2015;64:911–26. https://doi.org/10.1007/s00101-015-0115-6.

34. Pacheco Granda FA, Salik I. StatPearls. Simulation Training and Skill Assessment in Critical Care, Treasure Island (FL); 2021.

35. Lei C, Palm K. StatPearls. crisis resource management training in medical simulation. Treasure Island (FL); 2020.

36. Moss H, Weil J, Mukherji P. StatPearls. Set up and execution of an effective standardized patient program in medical simulation. Treasure Island (FL); 2020.

37. Marquardt N, Hoebel M, Lud D. Safety culture transformation-The impact of training on explicit and implicit safety attitudes. Hum Factors Ergon Manuf. 2020; https://doi.org/10.1002/hfm.20879.

Cybersecurity: Ensuring Confidentiality, Integrity, and Availability of Information

26

Lee Kim

Learning Objectives
1. Understand the basics about cybersecurity.
2. Learn about the cybersecurity threat landscape in the healthcare sector.
3. Hear about what you can do to enhance your organization's cybersecurity posture.

Cybersecurity: The Basics

What Is Information Security?

Information security involves the protecting of information and assets from unauthorized access, use, and disclosure. The information can be in any medium or form—i.e., electronic or physical (such as paper records).

What Is Cybersecurity?

The National Institute of Standards (NIST) defines cybersecurity as the "ability to protect or defend the use of cyberspace from cyberattacks."[1] Cybersecurity falls under the umbrella category of information security. Information security relates to the protection of information in whatever medium it may exist. Cybersecurity is a subset of information security and deals with information in electronic form (e.g., mobile devices, computer networks, servers, laptops, etc.).[2]

Cybersecurity involves the protecting of **electronic** information and assets from unauthorized access, use, and disclosure.[3] As shown in Fig. 26.1, the three main objectives of cybersecurity are the confidentiality, integrity, and availability of information. This is also known as the "CIA triad."

Key Terms

- Administrative safeguard
- Anti-virus
- Asset
- Authentication
- Availability
- Breach
- Business associate
- Business associate agreement

---

[1] NIST. Computer security resource center: glossary. Available from: https://csrc.nist.gov/glossary/term/cybersecurity

[2] Bitsight. Cybersecurity Vs. Information Security: Is There A Difference? Available from: https://www.bitsight.com/blog/cybersecurity-vs-information-security

[3] Critical & Infrastructure Security Agency CISA. Available from: https://www.us-cert.gov/ncas/tips/ST04-001

L. Kim (✉)
HIMSS, Chicago, USA
e-mail: Lee.Kim@himss.org

© Springer Nature Switzerland AG 2022
U. H. Hübner et al. (eds.), *Nursing Informatics*, Health Informatics,
https://doi.org/10.1007/978-3-030-91237-6_26

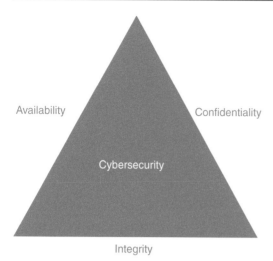

- Ransomworm
- Risk
- Safeguards
- Security awareness
- Security incident
- Shadow IT
- Spear-phishing
- Supply chain
- Technical controls
- Technical safeguard
- Threat
- Trojan horse
- Vulnerability
- Whaling

Fig. 26.1 CIA triad of cybersecurity (Confidentiality, Integrity, and Availability). The Key Terms and their definitions can be found in "Appendix: Definition of Key Terms" at the end of this chapter

- Compensating controls
- Confidentiality
- Countermeasures
- Covered entity
- Critical infrastructure
- Cyberattack
- Decryption
- Defense-in-depth
- Denial of service (DoS)
- Encryption
- Firewall
- General phishing
- HIPAA Privacy Rule
- Incident response
- Integrity
- Internet of Things (IoT)
- Legacy systems
- Malicious insider
- Malware
- Multi-factor authentication
- Nation-state actors
- Negligent insider
- Password spraying
- Patch
- Phishing
- Physical safeguard
- Protected health information (PHI)
- Ransomware

Introduction

Traditionally, the focus of healthcare information security was on avoiding data breaches. At the time, many healthcare providers relied on paper records and film. However, the digital transformation of healthcare has only occurred in the last ten to twenty years. Radiologists led the wave of digital transformation in the late 1990s by implementing picture archiving and communication systems (PACS) to replace film and light boxes. Additionally, electronic health records (EHRs) were adopted by many healthcare organizations starting in 2011 (namely, incentivized by the meaningful use program).[4] This led the way for healthcare information being processed and stored primarily in electronic form. Paper records and film became relics of the past for many healthcare providers.

Prior to 2013, the largest reported breaches in the healthcare industry were largely the result of lost or stolen devices, such as backup tapes, servers, or laptops. Physical theft and loss of assets (e.g., devices, laptops, workstations, etc.) while avoiding data breaches were the primary focus.

In 2013, a major retailer was breached as a result of a large-scale cyberattack on its heating, cooling, and air conditioning (HVAC) vendor. Stolen credentials from the HVAC vendor were

---

[4]HealthIT.gov. 2011 Edition. Available from: https://www.healthit.gov/topic/certification-ehrs/2011-edition

used to break into the retailer's systems. In essence, this was a **supply chain** attack since the cyberattackers had compromised the retailer's vendor to ultimately target the retailer. Subsequent to 2013, cyber supply chain attacks continue to compromise healthcare information systems (HIS) through stolen vendor credentials.

Additionally, ransomware has also evolved into a significant threat[5]. Ransomware, a type of malicious software (**malware**) that purports to deny access to a machine or device and demands that ransom be paid, has evolved since 1989, and ransomware was not a very significant threat up until about 2012, as most ransomware was scareware. However, since 2012, with the introduction of the Reveton ransomware[6] and, subsequently, many other ransomware variants such as CryptoLocker, CryptoWall, TeslaCrypt, Locky, Samsam, Petya, and Maktub,[7] ransomware has been a challenge to deal with. Ransomware is a significant threat to the **confidentiality, integrity, and availability** of information. Now, ransomware holds the computer system and data hostage, allegedly in exchange for the payment of ransom to the cybercriminals. However, as the United States (U.S.) Federal Bureau of Investigation (FBI) notes, there is no guarantee that a user will get his or her data back—even if the ransom is paid.[8] Due to these **risks**, it is important to regularly back up computer systems and devices so that data may be restored back to a good "clean "state, in case a machine or device has been compromised by ransomware.

But, ransomware is just one type of **malware**.[9] Other types include credential stealers whereby usernames, passwords, and other tokens are stolen by cybercriminals and **wipers** in which entire disk drives may be erased, and the data may be unrecoverable.

In summary, with the digital transformation of healthcare, cybersecurity is necessary to protect the **confidentiality**, **integrity**, and **availability** of electronic information. Robust cybersecurity programs in healthcare organizations are quintessential for normal operations and good quality patient care.

What Is the Role of Physical Security in Protecting Data?

Physical security is essential in order to ensure that data will be secure.[10] In essence, physical security measures help to prevent, detect, and correct unauthorized physical access. Ideally, **defense-in-depth** is deployed such that multiple layers of safeguards are put into place. If case one measure fails, another measure may help to detect, deter, correct, or otherwise prevent unauthorized physical access. Examples of physical security measures (also called **safeguards**) include locks, doors, cameras, etc.

If physical safeguards that are meant to protect computers and/or devices are compromised, then these **assets** may be in jeopardy. In other words, the data may be stolen or otherwise compromised by an unauthorized individual. There are many ways in which physical security may be compromised, such as by way of theft or loss. Examples include stolen, unencrypted backup tapes whereby cybercriminals can easily access data stored on the tapes. Another example is unauthorized access to a machine or device with an easy to guess password.[11]

[5] HIMSS. 2021 Healthcare Cybersecurity Survey. Available from: www.himss.org/cybersurvey

[6] FBI. FBI, This Week: Reveton Ransomware. Available from: https://www.fbi.gov/audio-repository/news-podcasts-thisweek-reveton-ransomware/view

[7] NJCCIC. NJCCIC Ransomware Variants. Available from: https://www.cyber.nj.gov/threat-center/threatprofiles/ransomware-variants/

[8] FBI. Ransomware. Available from: https://www.fbi.gov/scams-and-safety/common-scams-and-crimes/ransomware

[9] Roger A. Grimes. CSO. 9 types of malware and how to recognize them. Available from: https://www.csoonline. com/article/2615925/security-your-quick-guide-to-malware-types.html

[10] SANS. Physical Security and Why It is Important. Available from: https://www.sans.org/reading-room/whitepapers/physical/physical-security-important-37120

[11] Sucuri Blog. Password Attacks 101. Available from: https://blog.sucuri.net/2020/01/password-attacks-101.html

Yet another example is an unauthorized individual gaining physical access to an **asset** (e.g., computers, laptops, devices, etc.). For instance, the individual may "tailgate" his or her way into a restricted area at a healthcare provider and gain unauthorized access to a server containing sensitive information. In another example, an individual may carry his or her work laptop into a coffee shop and ask a stranger to watch the laptop while ordering a coffee or using the restroom. Such a careless action may lead to the laptop being stolen or an unauthorized individual getting access to the laptop (especially if the session has not been locked).

Another **risk** in terms of unauthorized access to a computer or a device includes tampering with the data, configuration, or functional/technical operation. For example, an unauthorized individual could potentially reconfigure a wireless infusion pump so that it delivers a fatal bolus of insulin to a patient. Alternatively, a smart elevator may be compromised, resulting in the interference with normal operations of a hospital's elevator. Accordingly, **physical safeguards** are very important to have. **Patient safety**, **physical security**, and **cybersecurity** depend upon each other.[12]

What Is a Cyberattack?

A **cyberattack** generally occurs via cyberspace and targets an organization's networks, computers, and/or information for the purpose of disrupting, disabling, destroying, or maliciously controlling a computing environment/infrastructure; or destroying the integrity of the data or stealing controlled information. A cyberattack may lead to a compromise regarding the **confidentiality**, **integrity**, and/or **availability** of networks, computers, devices, and/or data.

An attack against **confidentiality** generally means that a network, system, device, and/or information may have been disclosed to an unauthorized individual or entity. An attack against **integrity** generally means that a network, system, device, and/or information may have been altered or otherwise corrupted by an unauthorized individual or entity. An attack against **availability** generally means that a network, system, device, and/or information may have been rendered unavailable or otherwise inaccessible (e.g., disruption or otherwise). A **cyberattack** may compromise one of these three components of the triad (see Fig. 26.1 above), two components, or all three (i.e., confidentiality, integrity, and availability).

Additionally, an attack on integrity can lead to tampered or otherwise incorrect or inaccessible patient information. As an example, a patient's medication list may be tampered with and a clinician may rely upon the incorrect medication list, potentially risking the patient's life. In another example, a patient's allergies may be inadvertently mixed up with another patient's, thereby potentially leading to adverse consequences if the patient is given a medication which he or she is allergic to.

Further, an attack on **availability** may lead to an asset, such as a computer system, device, network, and/or information being unavailable at a particular moment in time. This may have dire consequences, especially in the case of an emergent situation, such as in the emergency room or intensive care unit.

In general, the likelihood of a **cyberattack** to succeed depends upon the **cybersecurity** defenses in place at the healthcare provider organization and the **cybersecurity** team's ability to block and tackle **security incidents** (also known as **incident response**). The more sophisticated the **cybersecurity** defenses with basic and advanced security controls, the more agile a healthcare provider's **cybersecurity** team is in terms of blocking and tackling incidents. This means that **cyberattacks** are either less likely to succeed or, if a **cyberattack** does happen, then that harm caused by the **cyberattack** may be less (compared with a healthcare provider organiza-

---

[12]United States Department of Homeland Security. A Lifeline: Patient Safety and Cybersecurity. Available from: https://www.dhs.gov/sites/default/files/publications/ia/ia_vulnerabilities-healthcare-it-systems.pdf

tion with virtually no cybersecurity defenses and a lack of a skilled cybersecurity team within the organization).

Why Are Good Passwords Important?

Passwords are often used to help protect networks, computer systems, devices, and/or information. Accordingly, password security is very important. If a cyberattacker were to obtain or otherwise correctly guess a password for a user account, this opens up the possibility to the cyberattacker to perform unauthorized functions and/or to gain unauthorized access to networks, computer systems, devices, and/or information. Thus, when a system is **breached**, there is a possibility that the information compromised may include usernames and passwords belonging to workforce members at the healthcare provider organization and others with trusted access.

In one example, systems and devices may have no password, a simple (easy to guess) password, or a default password (which one may be able to easily find in a manual). Ideally, passwords should be unique and easy to remember but difficult for others to guess. Complex passwords typically include a combination of upper and lower case letters, symbols (e.g., punctuation marks and otherwise), numbers, and are of a sufficient length.[13] Additionally, password complexity and password aging should be enforced so that passwords must be changed at regular intervals (e.g., 30, 60, or 90 days).

Passwords should never be reused. Passwords should not be shared between personal and work accounts. If a password is required to be changed, the substantially same or identical password should not be reused. A very common way to compromise password is by way of a password reuse attack. Cybercriminals know that individuals *typically* reuse passwords, and this attack tends to be fairly successful.[14] Data leaks and breaches are common ways in which cybercriminals gain stolen credentials, and these credentials may be used in a brute force attack to gain unauthorized access to systems and devices.[15]

What Is a Phishing Attack?

Phishing attacks are highly effective in terms of gaining access to protected computer resources and networks. While **phishing** may occur in many ways (e.g., e-mail, website, social media, telephone calls, etc.), phishing typically occurs by way of e-mail.

What Role Do Countermeasures Play in Thwarting Cyberattacks?

In the realm of cybersecurity, countermeasures (also referred to as **controls** and **safeguards**) are necessary in order to reduce vulnerabilities in networks, computer systems, and devices. The key to robust cybersecurity is to implement multiple layers of controls and safeguards (also referred to as a **defense-in-depth**). Accordingly, if one control or safeguard fails, then another may help to prevent or otherwise mitigate potential incidents.

As an example, **firewalls**, when properly configured, work to filter both incoming and outgoing network traffic. Depending upon the **firewall** configuration and rules, certain traffic that is incoming and/or outgoing may be blocked. However, not all malicious traffic is blocked by the firewall. Accordingly, there are other countermeasures that typically exist on computer systems, such as but not limited to **anti-virus software**.

---

[13] National Initiative for Cybersecurity Careers and Studies. Creating a Password. Available from: https://niccs.us-cert.gov/sites/default/files/documents/pdf/ncsam_creatingapassword_508.pdf

[14] Help Net Security. The password reuse problem is a ticking time bomb. https://www.helpnetsecurity.com/2019/11/12/password-reuse-problem/

[15] Kaspersky. Brute Force Attack: What you need to know to keep your passwords safe. Available from: https://www.kaspersky.com/resource-center/definitions/brute-force-attack

Patch management programs also should be deployed so that **vulnerabilities** may be mitigated. Virtually every type of technology, including hardware, software, and other devices, may have vulnerabilities. A manufacturer may develop a patch to address such vulnerabilities. It is then up to the organization to apply the patch to address these vulnerabilities. Please note: In terms of **legacy** systems **and software**, patches are not typically developed by the manufacturer since, by definition, such legacy systems and software are not **supported** by the manufacturer. Examples of legacy operating systems include Windows XP, Windows 7, and others. In the case of **legacy systems and software**, it may be necessary to use **compensating controls** to protect the machine or device.

While no countermeasure is foolproof, it is essential to ensure that basic and advanced security controls are in place to provide for as robust cybersecurity of the network, systems, and devices as much as possible.

Healthcare as a Critical Infrastructure Sector

The healthcare and public health sector is a critical infrastructure sector. Critical infrastructure is designated as such since the sector provides essential services and related assets that underpin society and serve as the backbone of the nation's economy, security, and health. The healthcare and public health sector constitute approximately fifteen percent of the gross national product, and roughly eighty-five percent of the sector's assets are privately owned and operated.[16] The healthcare and public health sector are designated as a critical infrastructure sector since everyone needs healthcare, and healthcare touches virtually everything. Accordingly, healthcare is intertwined with the nation's economy, national security, and health.

The healthcare and public health sector cannot function without the resources and services provided by many other critical infrastructure sectors, including transportation, communications, energy, water, and emergency services.[17] These sectors provide the necessary goods and services that support nearly every home and business across the country and are critical to disaster response and community resilience.[18]

Information sharing about threats is critical for the healthcare and public health sector to stay ahead of threats (which include cyber threats). Information sharing among healthcare and public health sector stakeholders helps to build situational awareness and also helps to enable risk-informed decision-making. Accordingly, information sharing may occur specifically within the healthcare and public health sector (called intra-sector information sharing).

Information sharing may also occur between the healthcare and public health sector and other critical infrastructure sectors (called **inter-sector information sharing**). As an example, inter-sector information sharing may occur between stakeholders in the financial services sector and the healthcare and public health sector. Information sharing may occur by way of word of mouth and/or automated, threat intelligence sharing.[19]

A History of Cybersecurity in Healthcare and Present Landscape

It used to be that healthcare providers were primarily concerned about breaches. Hacking of systems, devices, and networks did occur, but this was not a consideration until relatively recently.

---

[16] United States Department of Homeland Security. National Infrastructure Protection Plan: Healthcare and Public Health Sector. Available from: https://www.dhs.gov/xlibrary/assets/nipp_snapshot_health.pdf

[17] United States Department of Homeland Security Cybersecurity & Infrastructure Security Agency. Available from: https://www.cisa.gov/critical-infrastructure-sectors

[18] United States Department of Health and Human Services. Healthcare and Public Health Sector-Specific Plan. https://www.phe.gov/Preparedness/planning/cip/Documents/2016-hph-ssp.pdf (Figure 8, page 12).

[19] MITRE. Cybersecurity standards. Available from: https://www.mitre.org/capabilities/cybersecurity/overview/cybersecurity-resources/standards

In the United States, priorities traditionally were about avoiding breaches and complying with the **Health Insurance Portability and Accountability Act of 1996** (HIPAA) and, specifically, the **HIPAA Privacy Rule** and the **HIPAA Security Rule**. Thus, the approach to healthcare cybersecurity was namely a "checklist" type of approach in light of complying with the HIPAA regulations.

However, since at least 2013, the healthcare sector was also dealing with new, aggressive forms of **ransomware**. Essentially, any storage media that is connected, either physically or logically, to a computer system, device, or network may be vulnerable to a ransomware attack. Additionally, in August 2014, a major cyberattack on a health system was announced. Specifically, hackers had infiltrated the computer network and had stolen the **protected health information** of 4.5 million patients, and **nation-state actors** were allegedly to blame. The breached data allegedly included names, social security numbers, and contact telephone numbers.[20]

From this point forwards, organizations knew that hackers were intentionally targeting their networks, systems, devices, and information.

In addition to ransomware, **ransomworms** appeared on the scene. An example of a ransomworm was WannaCry,[21] which was the world's first reported international cyberattack as of May 12, 2017, and quickly spread to more than 200,000 Windows systems in 150 countries around the globe.[22] **Patches** were made available by various software manufacturers for their products to ensure that this **vulnerability** was addressed.[23] As a result, organizations that applied these patches resolved this vulnerability. Unfortunately, though, WannaCry has persisted as a problem due to the lack of patching at certain organizations.

NotPetya was discovered in Ukraine on June 27, 2017. **Nation-state actors** are said to be the originators of NotPetya, which was characterized as **wiper** malware that behaved like **ransomware**.[24] This was reportedly the second international cyberattack (the first being WannaCry) and affected countries around the world, including western European countries and the United States. In the United States, operations at pharmaceutical companies, couriers, and medical transcription companies were affected by the NotPetya malware.[25]

Further, **negligent insider threat** and the **malicious insider threat** are always concerns at healthcare provider organizations (and, generally, any organization). Any employee or other workforce member may become disgruntled and intentionally cause harm to an organization by way of abusing or misusing trusted access to a system or network. This is an example of a **malicious insider threat actor**.

Generally, though, negligent insider threat is much more common. Workforce members may ignore their cybersecurity training and negligently click on a link that they do not recognize or respond to an unusual e-mail asking for sensitive information, such as usernames and passwords, patient information, financial information,

[20] Steve Alder. HIPAA Journal. Community Health Systems Cyber Attack Puts 4.5 M Patients at Risk. Available from: https://www.hipaajournal.com/community-health-systems-cyber-attack-puts-4-5m-patients-risk/

[21] NCCIC. National Cybersecurity and Communications Integration Center. What is WannaCry/WannaCrypt0r? Available from: https://www.us-cert.gov/sites/default/files/FactSheets/NCCIC%20ICS_FactSheet_WannaCry_Ransomware_S508C.pdf

[22] Robert Lemos. Three Years After WannaCry, Ransomware Accelerating While Patching Still Problematic. DARKReading. Available from: https://www.darkreading.com/attacks-breaches/three-years-after-wannacry-ransomware-accelerating-while-patching-still-problematic/d/d-id/1337794

[23] Microsoft. Microsoft Security Bulletin MS17–017 Important. Security Update for Windows Kernel (4013081). Available from: https://docs.microsoft.com/en-us/security-updates/securitybulletins/2017/ms17-017

[24] Washington Post. Russian military was behind "NotPetya" cyberattack in Ukraine, CIA concludes. Available from: https://www.washingtonpost.com/world/national-security/russian-military-was-behind-notpetya-cyberattack-in-ukraine-cia-concludes/2018/01/12/048d8506-f7ca-11e7-b34a-b85626af34ef_story.html

[25] Wired. The Untold Story of NotPetya, the Most Devastating Cyberattack in History. Available from: https://www.wired.com/story/notpetya-cyberattack-ukraine-russia-code-crashed-the-world/

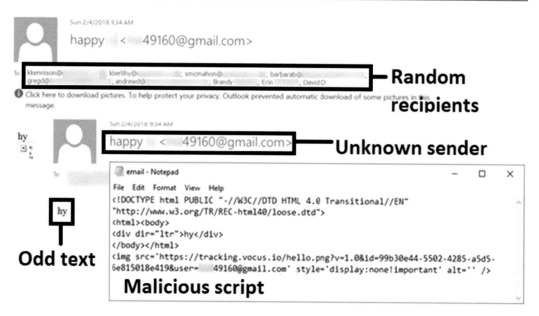

Fig. 26.2 Example of general phishing e-mail [United States Department of Homeland Security. 2018 Public-Private Analytic Exchange Program. Phishing: Don't be Phooled! Available from: https://www.dhs.gov/sites/ default/files/publications/2018_AEP_Vulnerabilities_of_ Healthcare_IT_Systems.pdf (p. 14). (Annotations are from the author)]

or otherwise.[26] A common example within healthcare provider organizations is an employee snooping on patient records without authorization or justification to do so.[27]

Phishing is a significant threat to healthcare providers.[28] For example, an online scam artist may send a **general phishing** e-mail to an employee at a healthcare provider organization with the intent of either eliciting sensitive information and/or infecting a computer system or device with **malware** (such as **ransomware** or a **credential stealer** which steals user credentials).

With **general phishing** e-mails, these e-mails do not target specific individuals but, rather, these e-mails are sent in such large numbers with the hope that some people will either respond and/or click on the malicious link and/or malicious attachment. Typical hallmarks of **general phishing** e-mails are too good to be true claims, misspellings and grammatical errors, and the like, as shown in Fig. 26.2.[29]

Alternatively, an online scam artist may send a **spear-phishing** e-mail to a specific employee within an organization or to a specific department or unit within an organization. Unlike general phishing e-mails, spear-phishing e-mails are tailored to the targeted recipients. The tailoring of e-mails may be possible due to information gathered by the online scam artist about the healthcare provider organization's website and/or the

[26]Carnegie Mellon Software Engineering Institute. Insider Threat. Available from: https://www.sei. cmu.edu/research-capabilities/all-work/display. cfm?customel_datapageid_4050=21232

[27]Imprivata. 5 Types of Insider Threats in Healthcare—and How to Mitigate Them. Available from: https://www. imprivata.com/blog/5-types-of-insider-threats-in-health-care-and-how-to-mitigate-them

[28]Phishing.org. History of Phishing. Available from: https://www.phishing.org/history-of-phishing

[29]United States Department of Homeland Security. 2018 Public-Private Analytic Exchange Program. Phishing: Don't be Phooled! Available from: https:// www.dhs.gov/sites/default/files/publications/2018_AEP_ Vulnerabilities_of_Healthcare_IT_Systems.pdf (pp. 2–3).

individual's social media profile, among other things. As a result of the specific tailoring of the e-mails, the spear-phishing e-mail may look authenticate and/or otherwise entice the intended recipient into responding to the e-mail and/or clicking on the malicious link and/or malicious attachment. Clicking on a malicious link may lead to a phishing website designed to steal a user's credentials. Opening a malicious attachment may cause a computer system to be infected with malware, such as a ransomware (which may result in being locked out of a computer/resource) or a credential stealer (in which case, sensitive information may be stolen, such as a username and password, patient information, etc.). An example of a spear-phishing e-mail is shown in Fig. 26.3.

Whaling occurs when an online scam artist targets a "big fish" such as a C-suite executive at a healthcare provider organization (e.g., CEO, CFO, Chief Informatics Officer (CIO), etc.). Like spear-phishing, whaling e-mails are also tailored to the recipient. As an example, a whaling e-mail may be sent from an online scam artist to a CFO in order to convince him or her to wire funds to an account that is controlled by the online scam artist. Like other kinds of phishing, the objective is to deceive the target, but not to arouse suspicion about the ruse. An example of a whaling e-mail is shown in Fig. 26.4.

Other forms of phishing exist, such as but not limited to SMS phishing (also called **SMiShing**). This is when the online scam artist crafts a deceptive message to the target via a text message to a mobile phone.

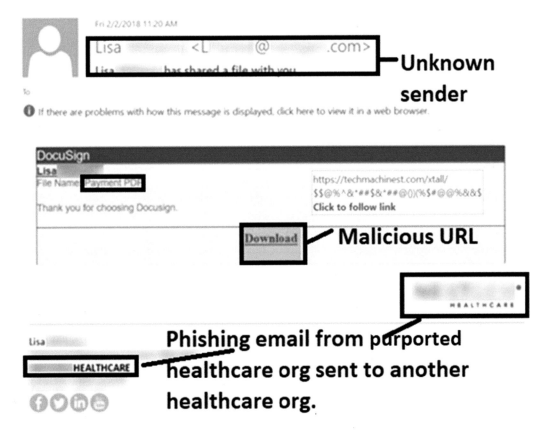

Fig. 26.3 Example of spear-phishing e-mail [United States Department of Homeland Security. 2018 Public-Private Analytic Exchange Program. Phishing: Don't be Phooled! Available from: https://www.dhs.gov/sites/ default/files/publications/2018_AEP_Vulnerabilities_of_ Healthcare_IT_Systems.pdf (p. 19). (Annotations are from the author)]

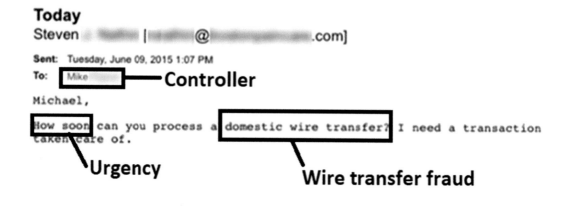

Fig. 26.4 Example of whaling e-mail [United States Department of Homeland Security. 2018 Public-Private Analytic Exchange Program. Phishing: Don't be Phooled! Available from: https://www.dhs.gov/sites/default/files/ publications/2018_AEP_Vulnerabilities_of_Healthcare_IT_Systems.pdf (p. 24). (Annotations are from the author)]

Generally speaking, **phishing** has been a primary means by which cyber threat actors gain a foothold into an organization's network, systems, devices, and information. In terms of cyber threats, **phishing** tends to be one of the major threats facing healthcare provider organizations of all types and sizes, regardless of geographic location.[30] The reason why **phishing** is so effective is because it bypasses the cybersecurity perimeter of an organization (which is often difficult to break into, due to robust security controls) and, instead, (when successful) tricks the human recipient into taking the desired action, as intended by the online scam artist (e.g., divulging of sensitive login credentials, clicking on a malicious link or attachment, etc.). In the wake of the COVID-19 pandemic, **phishing** attacks have been crafted based upon this special theme.

Security Awareness

Every organization can benefit from **security awareness** training. Through such efforts, individuals will learn about basic cyber hygiene (i.e., good security practices). Examples of topics for **security awareness** training include **phishing**, **anti-virus software**, maintaining good security practices while working from home or when traveling for work, and the like.[31] **HIPAA** also mandates security awareness training for healthcare-**covered entities** and **business associates**.[32] Many healthcare providers conduct security awareness training once a year, but more frequent intervals are recommended. In other words, workforce members need to be reminded of basic cyber hygiene on a regular basis (e.g., phishing, etc.).

---

[30]HIMSS. 2018 HIMSS Cybersecurity Survey. Available from: https://www.himss.org/sites/hde/files/d7/u132196/2018_HIMSS_Cybersecurity_Survey_Final_Report.pdf. HIMSS. 2019 HIMSS Cybersecurity Survey. Available from: https://www.himss.org/sites/hde/files/d7/u132196/2019_HIMSS_Cybersecurity_Survey_Final_Report.pdf

[31]NIST. Building an Information Technology Security Awareness and Training Program. Available from: https://nvlpubs.nist.gov/nistpubs/Legacy/SP/nistspecialpublication800-50.pdf (pp. 8–9).

[32]Code of Federal Regulations. Administrative Safeguards. 45 CFR 164.308.

Security Awareness Tips at Work

In terms of basic cybersecurity hygiene, there are certain principles that are evergreen. In regard to **phishing**, if a workforce member receives an e-mail that you are not expecting or that seems suspicious in some way, disregard the e-mail instead of responding or clicking on any links or attachments. However, if the healthcare provider has a policy to report such e-mails to the information technology (IT) team or the cybersecurity team, workforce members should follow the appropriate reporting protocol.

Security awareness on **phishing** is also essential for all workforce members. Workforce members need to carefully scrutinize e-mails and other messages that they do receive, making sure that the messages are authentic and not suspicious or unusual in any way. Clicking on a link[33] or opening up an attachment in an odd or unusual e-mail is never recommended. When in doubt, ask the IT helpdesk, cybersecurity team, and/or appropriate point of contact at the organization or business for assistance and/or report the **phishing** message to them. If the unusual or odd e-mail is from a recipient whom you recognize and you wish to verify the authenticity, place a phone call or physically talk to that person and ask about the message.

Additionally, in light of the COVID-19 pandemic, other future pandemics, and disasters, it is essential for good cyber hygiene and compliance in regard to the organization's policies, procedures, and applicable laws and regulations (including HIPAA) be adhered to. There will be situations like these that may call for individuals to work remotely, such as from home or other settings other than the traditional workplace setting. Some individuals may be provisioned with issued laptops and mobile devices. But, others may have to use their own laptops, mobile devices, and/or computers in order to do their work. Even though an individual may be using his or her device, it is still essential to practice good cyber hygiene and to be aware of any potential or suspected security incidents. In case a laptop, mobile device, and/or computer is exhibiting odd or unusual behavior or activity and/or if odd or unusual behavior or activity is found while using an organization's resource (such as e-mail, portals, or otherwise), it is important to report this information to the information technology helpdesk, cybersecurity team, and/or appropriate point of contact right away so that they are aware and can address any potential issues quickly.[34]

Cybersecurity Laws and Regulations

In the United States, **HIPAA** is a federal requirement that generally applies to **covered entities** and **business associates**. Covered entities include (1) health plans, (2) healthcare clearinghouses, and (3) healthcare providers who electronically transmit any health information in connection with transactions for which the United States Department of Health and Human Services has adopted standards. Examples of covered entities may include physician practices, ambulatory surgical centers, hospitals, long-term care facilities, health plans, healthcare clearinghouses, and others.

Business associates perform functions or services on behalf of **covered entities**. Business associates create, receive, transmit, or maintain protected health information on behalf of the covered entity. Examples of business associates are far and wide and include such entities and individuals as accountants, attorneys, cloud service providers, document storage companies, third-party billing services, and others.

As of this writing, the most current version of HIPAA is the HIPAA Omnibus Rule.[35] The

---

[33]The employer's or organization's policies and procedures should be adhered to and any questions should be directed to the information technology helpdesk, cybersecurity team, or the appropriate point of contact. Use caution when clicking on any links, opening any attachments, or responding to e-mails, social media messages, etc.

[34]Georgia Professional Tech Education. Staying Cyber-Safe While Teleworking. Available from: https://pe.gatech.edu/blog/industry-trends/staying-cyber-safe-while-teleworking

[35]Omnibus HIPAA Rulemaking. United States Department of Health and Human Services. Available from: https://www.hhs.gov/hipaa/for-professionals/privacy/laws-regulations/combined-regulation-text/omnibus-hipaa-rulemaking/index.html

HIPAA Omnibus Rule has three main components: Privacy Rule, Security Rule, and Breach
Notification Rule. Both covered entities and business associates must comply with HIPAA. Similar
to a covered entity, a business associate is directly
liable under the HIPAA Rules and subject to civil
and, in some cases, criminal penalties for making
uses and disclosures of protected health information that are not authorized by its contract or
required by law. A business associate also is
directly liable and subject to civil penalties for
failing to safeguard electronic protected health
information in accordance with the HIPAA
Security Rule. The HIPAA Rules generally
require that covered entities and business associates enter into contracts (also referred to as a
business associate agreement) with their business associates to ensure that the business associates will appropriately safeguard protected health
information.[36]

Additionally, the HIPAA Privacy Rule, 45
CFR Part 160 and Subparts A and E of Part 164,
sets forth permitted and required uses and disclosures of PHI. The PHI may exist in any form,
including on paper, film, and in electronic form.
Protected health information is a form of individually identifiable health information.

The **HIPAA Security Rule**, 45 CFR Part 160
and Part 164, Subparts A and C, sets forth requirements for ePHI. In other words, the confidentiality,
integrity, and availability of electronic protected
health information must be maintained by **covered
entities** and their **business associates**.[37]

The **HIPAA Breach Notification Rule**, 45
CFR §§ 164.400–414, requires HIPAA covered
entities and their business associates to provide
notification following a breach of unsecured protected health information.[38]

A breach is, generally, an impermissible use
or disclosure under the Privacy Rule that compromises the security or privacy of the PHI. An
impermissible use or disclosure of PHI is pre-
sumed to be a breach unless the covered entity or
business associate, as applicable, demonstrates
that there is a low probability that the protected
health information has been compromised based
on a risk assessment of at least the following
factors:

- The nature and extent of the PHI involved,
  including the types of identifiers and the likelihood of re-identification.
- The unauthorized person who used the PHI or
  to whom the disclosure was made.
- Whether the PHI was actually acquired or
  viewed; and.
- The extent to which the risk to the PHI has
  been mitigated.

Covered entities and business associates,
where applicable, have discretion to provide the
required breach notifications following an impermissible use or disclosure without performing a
risk assessment to determine the probability that
the protected health information has been
compromised.

There are three exceptions to the definition
of "breach." The first exception applies to the
unintentional acquisition, access, or use of PHI
by a workforce member or person acting under
the authority of a covered entity or business
associate, if such acquisition, access, or use
was made in good faith and within the scope of
authority. The second exception applies to the
inadvertent disclosure of PHI by a person
authorized to access PHI at a covered entity or
business associate to another person authorized
to access PHI at the covered entity or business
associate, or organized healthcare arrangement
in which the covered entity participates. In both
cases, the information cannot be further used or
disclosed in a manner not permitted by the
Privacy Rule. The final exception applies if the

[36]Business Associate Contracts. United States Department of Health and Human Services. Available from: https://www.hhs.gov/hipaa/for-professionals/covered-entities/sample-business-associate-agreement-provisions/index.html

[37]The Security Rule. United States Department of Health and Human Services. Available from: https://www.hhs.gov/hipaa/for-professionals/security/index.html

[38]Breach Notification Rule. United States Department of Health and Human Services. Available from: https://www.hhs.gov/hipaa/for-professionals/breach-notification/index.html

covered entity or business associate has a good faith belief that the unauthorized person to whom the impermissible disclosure was made, would not have been able to retain the information.[39]

Yet another United States federal privacy law is 42 CFR Part 2, which protects patient records created by federally funded programs for the treatment of substance use disorder.[40]

At the state level in the United States, healthcare provider organizations must also be aware of other applicable privacy and security laws.[41] Certain states make certain types of healthcare information as super PHI. Examples include records related to drug and alcohol abuse, HIV-related information, and the like.[42]

Case Study

Hypothetical Scenario

A **phishing** e-mail was sent to the chief nursing officer (CNO) in the late afternoon on a Wednesday. The CNO is juggling a wide variety of tasks and demands near the end of the shift. The sender appeared to be a vendor with whom the hospital regularly does business with. The phishing e-mail contained very convincing language, directing the CNO to immediately open the attachment. The CNO does so and, within minutes, an alarming message is displayed on the screen demanding that ransom is paid in exchange for the data, which is now purportedly locked up by the cybercriminals.

Because the CNO is involved in shift change, the problem is ignored. Ultimately, the CNO leaves work for that day. The IT department is not notified of the problem. Within a matter of a few hours, the **ransomworm** spreads across the entire hospital network. This results in millions of records—the entire patient database of the hospital—being breached.

As we can see in this scenario, the CNO failed to realize that the e-mail which was sent was actually from an online scam artist. The CNO also failed to notify the IT helpdesk of the problem. The appropriate steps would have been to not open up the malicious content sent via e-mail and called or otherwise notified the IT helpdesk of the problem. That way, any problem(s) would have been more quickly mitigated, and the egress of patient information may have been prevented, or at least significantly mitigated.

Summary

Healthcare cybersecurity is of the utmost importance in today's electronic world. Healthcare providers rely upon robust cybersecurity to ensure both normal operations in terms of business and clinical operations, as well as patient safety.[43] Everyone at a healthcare provider (and any other business) should take the time to understand at least the basics of cybersecurity so that they are literate. Anyone can potentially invite trouble into his or her organization by, for example, opening up a phishing e-mail or responding to a phony request (sent by e-mail or otherwise).

Threats will continue to multiply, and cybersecurity is a fast moving target. However, the basics relevant to cybersecurity are generally the

[39] Breach Notification Rule. United States Department of Health and Human Services. Available from: https://www.hhs.gov/hipaa/for-professionals/breach-notification/index.html

[40] SAMHSA. United States Department of Health and Human Services. Available from: https://www.samhsa.gov/about-us/who-we-are/laws-regulations/confidentiality-regulations-faqs

[41] State Health IT Privacy and Consent Laws and Policies. United States Department of Health and Human Services. Available from: https://www.healthit.gov/data/apps/state-health-it-privacy-and-consent-laws-and-policies

[42] Jill Arent. Comparison of Pennsylvania Confidentiality of HIV-Related Information Act (Act 148) and Federal Health Insurance Portability and Accountability Act. AIDS Law Project of Pennsylvania. Available from: http://www.aidslawpa.org/wp-content/uploads/2011/04/comparativechart.pdf

[43] Patrick Howell O'Neill. A patient has died after ransomware hackers hit a German hospital: This is the first ever case of a fatality being linked to a cyberattack. MIT Technology Review. Available from: https://www.technologyreview.com/2020/09/18/1008582/a-patient-has-died-after-ransomware-hackers-hit-a-german-hospital/

same. As a result, regular reminders about cybersecurity hygiene should be given to all workforce members. Additionally, in the case of workforce members who may be negligent insiders, additional time and effort should be spent to re-educate these individuals to prevent or mitigate future potential harm to the organization.

Conclusions and Outlook

Healthcare cybersecurity is an essential area for nurses, doctors, and other administrators and clinicians to understand. Good cyber hygiene is everyone's responsibility. Anyone who interacts with electronic patient data must first understand the basics of healthcare cybersecurity and the historical evolution. It is also essential for individuals to continuously learn about developments, such as new threats and mitigations.

nurses and others are frequently targeted by phishing e-mails, social phishing messages, and vishing calls. this is because cybercriminals know that people are the weakest link in any organization's cybersecurity program. whether it is patient information, financial information, or employee information, cybercriminals are eager to gain access. the end goal is often identity theft and fraud, but it also can be espionage and blackmail. the latter is especially true in the case of gaining access to information related to high-profile patients, such as celebrities, politicians, executives, and others.

Other threats include ransomware and the stealing of credentials by cybercriminals. Ransomware and credential stealing malware are frequently distributed by way of phishing attacks. To help mitigate these threats, it is best to adhere to the organization's policies and best practices. This includes not using unauthorized applications and services (also known as shadow IT). Additionally, strong passwords and other strong authentication methods should always be used. Passwords and other credentials should never be reused.

Looking to the future, phishing attacks will continue to increase in volume and sophistication. Individuals need to continue learning about new tactics, including examples of what to look for. While the technical security controls in place can block some phishing attempts, such controls are not one-hundred percent foolproof. As a result, security awareness and good cyber hygiene are also important to maintain a good security posture. Information sharing, though, is equally important.

Accordingly, individuals should share information, as appropriate, with the designated points of contact at their organization in regard to phishing attempts, malware attacks, and any other unusual or odd behavior or activity of a computer system, device, and/or IT asset (such as e-mail, portals, or otherwise). This will only help the organization bolster its security posture. In the end, good security is an essential part of patient safety.

Review Questions
1. What is cybersecurity?
2. What does patient safety have to do with cybersecurity?
3. What is the CIA triad and why is it important?
4. What is ransomware?
5. What is phishing?
6. What is HIPAA?
7. Why is security awareness important?

Resources
Further Reading

- NIST Glossary—https://csrc.nist.gov/glossary
- DHS AEP—Phishing: Don't be Phooled!—https://www.dhs.gov/sites/default/files/publications/2018_AEP_Vulnerabilities_of_Healthcare_IT_Systems.pdf
- DHS AEP—A Lifeline: Patient Safety & Cybersecurity—https://www.dhs.gov/sites/default/files/publications/ia/ia_vulnerabilities-healthcare-it-systems.pdf
- HHS—Health Information Privacy—https://www.hhs.gov/hipaa/index.html
- HHS—Cybersecurity Guidance Material—https://www.hhs.gov/hipaa/for-professionals/security/guidance/cybersecurity/index.html
- Health Care Industry Cybersecurity Task Force—Report on Improving Cybersecurity

in the Health Care Industry—https://www. phe.gov/Preparedness/planning/CyberTF/ Documents/report2017.pdf
- IMDRF—Principles and Practices for Medical Device Cybersecurity—http://www.imdrf. org/docs/imdrf/final/technical/imdrf-tech-200318-pp-mdc-n60.pdf
- National Cyber Security Alliance—https:// staysafeonline.org/

Organizations

- HIMSS—https://www.himss.org
- Cyber Health Working Group—https://www. intelligence.healthcare/
- InfraGard—https://www.infragard.org/
- US-CERT—https://www.us-cert.gov/
- ICS-CERT—https://www.us-cert.gov/ics

Appendices

Appendix 1: Answers to Review Questions

1. What is cybersecurity?
   The National Institute of Standards (NIST) defines cybersecurity as the "ability to protect or defend the use of cyberspace from cyberattacks." Cybersecurity falls under the umbrella category of information security. Information security relates to the protection of information in whatever medium it may exist. Cybersecurity is a subset of information security and deals with information in electronic form (e.g., mobile devices, computer networks, servers, laptops, etc.). Cybersecurity involves the protecting of electronic information and assets from unauthorized access, use, and disclosure.

2. What does patient safety have to do with cybersecurity?
   Within a cyberattack scenario, an attack on integrity can lead to tampered or otherwise incorrect or inaccessible patient information. This, in turn, can pose a potentially significant risk to patient safety. This is especially true in an instance where the clinician may rely on the tampered/altered information and/or if the tampered/altered information relates to the delivery of critical medication (such as insulin in an infusion pump) for the patient, and/or a life-saving or life-sustaining medical device (whose operation and/or configuration may have been altered). Thus, cybersecurity (and especially integrity) and patient safety are intertwined.
   Further, an attack on availability may lead to an asset, such as a computer system, device, network, and/or information being unavailable at a particular moment in time. Depending upon the timing and criticality of what needs to be accessed, this may pose a potentially significant patient safety problem for the patient, especially if the patient is in a critical situation (such as in the intensive care unit, in the operating room, or otherwise in need of emergency treatment).
   For more information, please see DHS AEP—A Lifeline: Patient Safety & Cybersecurity—https://www.dhs.gov/sites/ default/files/publications/ia/ia_vulnerabilities-healthcare-it-systems.pdf.

3. What is the CIA triad and why is it important?
   Cybersecurity involves the protecting of electronic information and assets from unauthorized access, use, and disclosure. There are three goals of cybersecurity, namely protecting the confidentiality, integrity, and availability of information. The three main objectives of cybersecurity are the confidentiality, integrity, and availability of information. All three are required in order for robust cybersecurity to be achieved. The failure of one or more of these components may mean that the business operations, clinical operations, and/or patient safety may be potentially placed in jeopardy.

4. What is ransomware?
   Ransomware is a type of malicious software, or malware, designed to deny access to a computer system or data until a ransom is paid.

5. What is phishing?
   Phishing means a social engineering tactic that is used to persuade individuals to provide sensitive information and/or take action through seemingly trustworthy communica-

tions. Phishing may take various forms, such as e-mail (e-mail phishing), social media (social phishing), phishing websites, voice calls (voice phishing), text messages (SMiShing), and the like.

6. What is HIPAA?

HIPAA is the Health Insurance Portability and Accountability Act of 1996. As of this writing, the most current version of HIPAA is the HIPAA Omnibus Rule. There are three components to the HIPAA Omnibus Rule: HIPAA Privacy Rule, HIPAA Security Rule, and the Breach Notification Rule.

The HIPAA Privacy Rule sets forth permitted and required uses and disclosures of protected health information. The protected health information may exist in any form, including on paper, film, and in electronic form. Protected health information is a form of individually identifiable health information.

The HIPAA Security Rule sets forth requirements for electronic protected health information. In other words, the confidentiality, integrity, and availability of electronic protected health information must be maintained by covered entities and their business associates.

The HIPAA Breach Notification Rule, 45 CFR §§ 164.400–414, requires HIPAA covered entities and their business associates to provide notification following a breach of unsecured protected health information.

7. Why is security awareness important?

Every organization can benefit from security awareness presentations and training. Through such efforts, individuals will learn about basic cyber hygiene (i.e., good security practices). Example topics for security awareness presentations and training include phishing, anti-virus software, maintaining good security practices while working from home or when traveling for work, and the like. (The difference between a security awareness presentation vs. training concerns depth. A more in-depth discussion of security awareness is usually provided during training, as opposed to listening to a mere presentation on the topic.) HIPAA also mandates security training

for healthcare-covered entities and business associates.

Appendix 2: Definition of Key Terms[44]

Administrative safeguard means a safeguard that is intended to protect the administrative aspects of securing an asset. For example, policies and procedures may be implemented to prevent, detect, contain, and correct security violations.

Anti-virus means a program specifically designed to detect many forms of malware and prevent them from infecting computers, as well as cleaning computers that have already been infected.

Asset means a resource that is valuable to an organization that must be protected.

Authentication means verifying the identity of a user, process, or device, often as a prerequisite to allowing access to resources in an information system.

Availability means that information is made available as needed. When availability is compromised, this means that information is not available when it is needed.

Breach generally means an impermissible use or disclosure that compromises the security or privacy of the information.[45] While not all security incidents are breaches, some security incidents may rise to the level of a breach. Breach notification laws exist at the federal and state levels.

Business associate means a person or entity, who is not a member of the workforce and performs or assists in performing, for or on behalf of a covered entity, a function or activity regulated by HIPAA, including the Privacy Rule, involving the use or disclosure of individually identifiable health information, or that provides certain ser-

---

[44]NIST. Computer security resource center: glossary. Available from: https://csrc.nist.gov/glossary. Definitions are generally from this source, unless otherwise noted.

[45]United States Department of Health and Human Services. Breach Notification Rule. Available from: https://www.hhs.gov/hipaa/for-professionals/breach-notification/index.html

vices to a covered entity that involve the use or disclosure of individually identifiable health information.[46]

Business associate agreement means contracts that the **covered entity** is required to enter into with their **business associates** to ensure that the business associates will appropriately safeguard protected health information.[47] (Please note: a contract has the same meaning as an agreement.)

Compensating controls means the security and privacy controls implemented that provide equivalent or comparable protection for a system or organization.

Confidentiality means that information is protected by preventing the unauthorized disclosure of information. When confidentiality is compromised, this means that there has been an unauthorized disclosure of information.

Countermeasures means the protective measures prescribed to meet the security requirements (i.e., confidentiality, integrity, and availability) specified for an information system. Safeguards may include security features, management constraints, personnel security, and security of physical structures, areas, and devices. Countermeasures are synonymous with **security controls**.

Covered entity means (1) health plans, (2) healthcare clearinghouses, and (3) healthcare providers who electronically transmit any health information in connection with transactions for which the United States Department of Health and Human Services has adopted standards.[48]

Critical infrastructure means essential services and related assets that underpin American society and serve as the backbone of the nation's economy, security, and health.

Cyberattack means an attack, via cyberspace, targeting an enterprise's use of cyberspace for the purpose of disrupting, disabling, destroying, or maliciously controlling a computing environment/infrastructure; or destroying the integrity of the data or stealing controlled information.

Decryption means the process of changing ciphertext into plaintext using a cryptographic algorithm and key.

Defense-in-depth means that multiple safeguards are layered to protect an asset.

Denial of service (DoS) means an attack that occurs when legitimate users are unable to access information systems, devices, or other network resources due to the actions of a malicious cyber threat actor. DoS attacks can cost an organization both time and money while their resources and services are inaccessible.[49]

Encryption means the process of changing plaintext into ciphertext using a cryptographic algorithm and key.

Firewall means a part of a computer system or network that is designed to block unauthorized access while permitting outward communication.

General phishing means a phishing attack that does not target specific individuals.[50]

HIPAA Privacy Rule, 45 CFR Part 160 and Subparts A and E of Part 164, means national standards that have been established to protect individuals' medical records and other personal health information (PHI) and applies to health plans, healthcare clearinghouses, and those healthcare providers that conduct certain healthcare transactions electronically. It is a **HIPAA** regulation. HIPAA Security Rule means security standards for the protection of electronic protected health Information that establish a national set of security standards for protecting certain

---

[46]National Institutes of Health. HIPAA Privacy Rule: Information for Researchers. Available from: https://privacyruleandresearch.nih.gov/pr_06.asp

[47]United States Department of Health and Human Services. Business Associate Contracts. Available from: https://www.hhs.gov/hipaa/for-professionals/covered-entities/sample-business-associate-agreement-provisions/index.html

[48]National Institutes of Health. HIPAA Privacy Rule: Information for Researchers. Available from: https://privacyruleandresearch.nih.gov/pr_06.asp

[49]Cybersecurity & Infrastructure Security Agency. Security Tip (ST04–015): Understanding Denial-of-Service Attacks. Available from: https://www.us-cert.gov/ncas/tips/ST04-015

[50]United States Department of Homeland Security. 2018 Public-Private Analytic Exchange Program. Phishing: Don't be Phooled! Available from: https://www.dhs.gov/sites/default/files/publications/2018_AEP_Vulnerabilities_of_Healthcare_IT_Systems.pdf (p.2).

health information that is held or transferred in electronic form (also known as **electronic protected health information or ePHI**).

Incident response means incident handling. Generally speaking, incident handling includes detection and analysis of an incident (e.g., whether an incident occurred and prioritizing the handling of the incident), containing, eradicating, recovering from an incident, and post-incident activity (such as gathering lessons learned).[51]

Integrity means that information is protected by keeping it intact. When the integrity of information is compromised, this means that the information has been modified without authorization from its original form.

Internet of Things (IoT) means devices, sensors, and the like (but other than computers, smartphones, or tablets) that connect, communicate, or otherwise transmit information with or between each other via the Internet.

Legacy systems mean systems which may not have any ongoing support from the hardware and software vendor(s) that provided these solutions.[52]

Malicious insider means individuals, such as employees, former employees, contractors, business associates, or business partners who has or had authorized access to an organization's network, system, or information and who has intentionally exceeded or misused that access so as to negatively affect the confidentiality, integrity, or availability of the organization's information or information systems.[53]

Malware means a computer program that is covertly placed onto a computer or electronic device with the intent to compromise the confi-

dentiality, integrity, or availability of data, applications, or operating systems. Common types of malware include viruses, worms, malicious mobile code, Trojan horses, rootkits, spyware, and some forms of adware.

Multi-factor authentication means authentication using two or more factors to achieve authentication. Factors include: (i) something you know (e.g., password/personal identification number (PIN)); (ii) something you have (e.g., cryptographic identification device, token); or (iii) something you are (e.g., biometric).

Nation-state actors are cyber threat actors who are typically motivated by political, economic, technical, or military agendas and who may engage in industrial espionage. Nation-state actors are typically highly sophisticated cyber threat actors.[54]

Negligent insider (also called an **unintentional** insider) means an individual, such as employees, former employees, contractors, business associates, or business partners who has or had authorized access to an organization's network, system, or information and who, through action or inaction and without malicious intent, causes harm or substantially increases the likelihood of future serious harm to the confidentiality, integrity, or availability of the organization's network, system, or information.[55]

Password spraying means an attack that tries a few commonly used passwords on a large number of accounts.[56]

Patch means a software component that, when installed, directly modifies files or device settings related to a different software component

[51]NIST. Computer Security Incident Handling Guide (Special Publication No. 800–61 Rev. 2). Available from: https://nvlpubs.nist.gov/nistpubs/SpecialPublications/NIST.SP.800-61r2.pdf

[52]Health Care Industry Cybersecurity Task Force. Available from: https://www.phe.gov/Preparedness/planning/CyberTF/Documents/report2017.pdf

[53]Daniel Costa. Carnegie Mellon University Software Engineering Institute. CERT Definition of "Insider Threat"—Updated. Available from: https://insights.sei.cmu.edu/insider-threat/2017/03/cert-definition-of-insider-threat---updated.html

[54]Chapter 7: Fighting Cyber Threats to the Growing Economy. https://www.govinfo.gov/content/pkg/ERP-2018/pdf/ERP-2018-chapter7.pdf (p. 329).

[55]Daniel Costa. Carnegie Mellon University Software Engineering Institute. CERT Definition of "Insider Threat"—Updated. Available from: https://insights.sei.cmu.edu/insider-threat/2017/03/cert-definition-of-insider-threat---updated.html

[56]Double Octopus. The Secret Security Wiki. Password Spraying (Low and Spray). Available from: https://doubleoctopus.com/security-wiki/threats-and-tools/password-spraying/

without changing the version number or release details for the related software component.

Phishing means a social engineering tactic that is used to persuade individuals to provide sensitive information and/or take action through seemingly trustworthy communications.[57] Phishing may take various forms, such as e-mail (e-mail phishing), social media (social phishing), phishing websites, voice calls (voice phishing), text messages (SMiShing), and the like.

Physical safeguard means a safeguard that is intended to protect physical security of an asset.

Protected health information (PHI) generally means information that is created, transmitted, received, or maintained by a covered entity or a business associate, including demographic information, related to the past, present, or future physical or mental health or condition of an individual, provision of healthcare to an individual, or past, present, or future payment for the provision of healthcare to an individual, together with certain identifiers (which may serve to identify the individual patient).

Ransomware is a type of malicious software or malware that denies access to a computer system and data and demands the payment of ransom.

Ransomworm means a type of computer worm that, upon infecting a new system, encrypts a victim's data and holds it for ransom until payment is received.[58]

Risk means a measure of the extent to which an entity is threatened by a potential circumstance or event, and typically is a function of: (i) the adverse impacts that would arise if the circumstance or event occurs; and (ii) the likelihood of occurrence.

Safeguards (also referred to as countermeasures and controls) means actions, devices, procedures, techniques, or other measures that reduce the **vulnerability** of a system. Safeguards may be physical, technical, or administrative in nature.

Security awareness means initiatives that are designed to change behavior or otherwise reinforce good security practices of individual users.

Security incident means an occurrence that actually or potentially jeopardizes the confidentiality, integrity, or availability of an information system or the information the system processes, stores, or transmits or that constitutes a violation or imminent threat of violation of security policies, security procedures, or acceptable use policies.

Shadow IT means the use of systems, devices, applications, software, and services that are not authorized for use by the organization's information technology department.[59]

Spear-phishing means a targeted phishing attack.[60]

Supply chain means the physical and informational resources required to deliver a good or service to the final consumer.

Technical controls (also referred to as security controls or technical security controls) means the security controls (i.e., safeguards or countermeasures) for an information system that are primarily implemented and executed by the information system through mechanisms contained in the hardware, software, or firmware components of the system.

Technical safeguard means a safeguard that is intended to protect the cybersecurity of an asset.

Threat means any circumstance or event with the potential to adversely impact organizational operations (including mission, functions, image, or reputation), organizational assets, or

---

[57] United States Department of Homeland Security. 2018 Public-Private Analytic Exchange Program. Phishing: Don't be Phooled! Available from: https://www.dhs.gov/sites/default/files/publications/2018_AEP_Vulnerabilities_of_Healthcare_IT_Systems.pdf (p.2).

[58] Peter Tsai. Spiceworks. What is a ransomworm? History, concerns, and implications: Word of the Week. Available from: https://community.spiceworks.com/topic/1995594-what-is-a-ransomworm-history-concerns-and-implications-word-of-the-week

[59] Forcepoint. Shadow IT defined. Available from: https://www.forcepoint.com/cyber-edu/shadow-it

[60] United States Department of Homeland Security. 2018 Public-Private Analytic Exchange Program. Phishing: Don't be Phooled! Available from: https://www.dhs.gov/sites/default/files/publications/2018_AEP_Vulnerabilities_of_Healthcare_IT_Systems.pdf (p.2).

individuals through an information system via unauthorized access, destruction, disclosure, modification of information, and/or denial of service.

Trojan horse means a computer program that appears to have a useful function, but that also has a hidden and potentially malicious function that evades security mechanisms, sometimes by piggybacking on a legitimate process.

Vulnerability means a weakness in information systems, system security procedures, internal controls, or implementation/configuration of the same that may be exploited by a threat actor.

Whaling means a targeted phishing attack that is aimed at wealthy, powerful, or prominent individuals (e.g., C-suite executives such as chief financial officers (CFO) and chief executive officers (CEO), politicians, and celebrities).[61]

---

[61] United States Department of Homeland Security. 2018 Public-Private Analytic Exchange Program. Phishing: Don't be Phooled! Available from: https://www.dhs.gov/sites/default/files/publications/2018_AEP_Vulnerabilities_of_Healthcare_IT_Systems.pdf (p.2).

Quality and Safety of Health Mobile Applications: Are They an Issue?

27

Célia Boyer

Learning Objectives

- Owning a smartphone is now almost a given, and with smartphone use comes the benefit of access to a large pool of apps on every topic conceivable, including health. So, it is not surprising that mHealth apps development is on the rise, as is the use of mHealth apps. However, unlike apps intended for other purposes, the use of mHealth apps carries, not only the advantage of improved health but also the burdens of potential misuse, misleading content and possible security breach of personal data. In this chapter, we present different initiatives involved in finding solutions to limit the issue of variability of the quality of health apps. We introduce how the mHONcode can be used to evaluate the possible hazards that you can find in some of the most popular mHealth apps in app stores. The mHONcode criteria will help you to identify and assess the trustworthiness of health apps, thus providing the end-user with trustworthy and quality tools to help in the management and maintenance of their healthcare.

Key Terms

- Mobile applications
- mHealth
- Trustworthiness

- Certification
- Quality
- Code of Conduct

Introduction

On the Web today, it is difficult to determine what information is valuable and what is useless. One of the concerns is the growing number of health websites of doubtful quality brought about by the popularity of the Internet. However, between 2012 and 2020, the number of existing websites increased by 180%, to nearly 1.8 billion in 2020, according to Internet Live Stats.[1] Health websites compete with health applications for smartphones and pose multiple dangers in the form of the quality of health content as well as the issues of confidentiality and security of private data.

It is estimated that over 200 health apps worldwide are being added each day to the top app stores, with over 325,000 health apps available in 2017 alone and downloaded 3.6 billion times and designed by 84,000 developers [1, 2]. Despite the short period of time, there is already evidence of health apps playing a positive role in both patient outcomes and the costs of care.

According to a survey conducted in 2018 (Day S. Zweig M.), both patients and physicians

C. Boyer (✉)
Health on the Net Foundation, Geneva, Switzerland

[1] Internet Live Stats (2020). Total number of websites. URL: http://www.internetlivestats.com/total-number-of-websites/#trend [Accessed 05 June 2020].

© Springer Nature Switzerland AG 2022
U. H. Hübner et al. (eds.), *Nursing Informatics*, Health Informatics,
https://doi.org/10.1007/978-3-030-91237-6_27

are ready for increased digital engagement. Approximately 85% of health apps in the market today are for wellness, designed to be used primarily by the consumer, and the remaining 15% are medical, designed to be used by physicians [3].

e-Health connects the companies that develop applications and the healthcare consumers who use them. Two major problems arise in this "digital care:" the reliability of the application and data security [4].

In the midst of this huge e-health market, how can we distinguish reliable, high-quality, and secure applications from those that may represent a danger to users and thus to public health?

Healthcare consumers continue to show strong use of digital technology, with numbers rising each year. In fact, the adoption of digital health technology is at its highest rate ever—with 89% of respondents using at least one digital health tool in 2018 [5]. Thus, it is very important that the quality of this technology be optimum, which is unfortunately not always the case. For example, some applications allow people to measure their blood pressure by placing the pulp of their finger on the camera of their smartphone. Unfortunately, the figures displayed are not reliable, and users are misled by the results of the apps. The need for an evaluation of the reliability and veracity of health applications is real, and many opinions agree on this matter.

The other point identified is that of the security of the application and of the data that the user transmits, sometimes without being aware of it, via the application, and which is sometimes shared with third parties without his consent [6]. The most blatant example is the one that appeared in the Wall Street Journal in February 2019 [7], revealing that several applications had sent the data collected to Facebook without authorization. Thus, a second, non-negligible need emerges— that of the user to be able to ensure that their data is not shared without their consent and that they are able to use the app safely without doubt of breach of privacy.

The former European Commissioner for Health Tonio Borg said in 2014 "mHealth has a great potential to empower citizens to manage their health and stay healthy longer, to trigger greater quality of care and comfort for patients, and to assist health professionals in their work. As such, exploring mHealth solutions can contribute to modern, efficient and sustainable health systems."[2] Mr. Borg's visionary comment was indeed true. However, as is the case with most things, there are always pros and cons. The pros are immense, with mHealth having the potential to greatly impact population health, but the cons are that there are no indicators to allow the public to discern trustworthy apps from the crowd. A systematic review conducted by McKay [8] has shown the lack of a uniform best practice approach to evaluate mobile health apps amongst the scientific community. In this huge market, how would the general public, without any medical knowledge or a health care provider recommending a health app, be able to gauge the trustworthiness, accuracy, and security of an app to use or recommend?

Carroll et al. [9] have shown that younger persons (18–44 years) with a higher education (college graduate or higher) have a higher likelihood of adopting health apps than the ones aged 45–65+ years. Furthermore, they highlighted the role of mobile phone health apps as a health promotion tool to change lifestyle behaviors (perform physical activity, change diet and lose weight). mHealth apps are in full expansion in the healthcare domain (Wellness. Education, Prevention, and Care), including in their use by the general public. However, the regulation measures for these apps have not kept up at the same pace.

The numbers are worrying: a study shows that 66% of the health apps certified as clinically safe by the UK NHS apps Library were, in fact, sending identifying information over the internet without encryption and disclosure [10]. Huckvale et al. [11], in another paper, demonstrate that 67% of the insulin dose calculator apps assessed provided inappropriate dosage recommendations. Plante in 2016 [12] showed that a blood pressure measuring app produced false measure-

---

[2] http://europa.eu/rapid/press-release_IP-14-394_en.htm

ments, and this app had been downloaded 150,000 times. These are only a few examples. Wisniewski et al. [13] highlight that apps based on six diseases (depression, schizophrenia, addiction, hypertension, diabetes, and anxiety) provide questionable content or unsupported claims. Scientific publications have shown that sharing of user data is routine and yet far from transparent despite the introduction of the European Union General Data Protection Regulation (GDPR) in 2018, preventing the user from making an informed choice regarding the transmission of their data to third parties [14, 15]. So, the ubiquity of smartphones, tablets, sensors, and similar smart devices means that huge volumes of data concerning health and personal data are being harvested and processed without even the users' knowledge.

Amid the massive choice available to the public along with the accompanying risks, no real, sustainable solution currently exists to help differentiate the trustworthy from the non-trustworthy. Additionally, knowing that 23% of the digital health marketers are non-healthcare professionals [2], how can users identify reliable applications? What are the criteria a mHealth app should fulfill to be available for download in the app stores? Are the security of health and personal data and the transparency of information considered a major issue to be considered in the mHealth arena? Are these issues taken seriously by mHealth developers and stakeholders commissioning the developments on their behalf?

Approaches to Assess Health Apps

The rapid development of the mHealth sector raises concerns about the potential risk of health functions apps providing transmission of health data, capture of health data via sensors, self-diagnoses, disease management or diagnosis and appropriate processing of the data collected through apps or solutions since mHealth solutions and devices can collect large quantities of personal information, including personal health information (e.g., data stored by the user on the device and data from different sensors, including

location) and processes them. Apps pose a new challenge that cannot be solved as we did for health content websites, mainly because of several reasons: (a) all the data is visible in health websites as it is part of the content and so it is easy to check the production process of the content; whereas in an app, the algorithms used to analyze the data are kept secret and not disclosed (industrial secrets); the privacy and security of transmission and storage is very difficult to test and assess (b) apps play the role of a "medical device" even if theoretically they are not which is unlike health websites which do not play a diagnostic role but only an informational role. So, the intrinsic risks posed by apps are totally different from health websites.

Health apps supporting citizen's empowerment through self-management, health promotion and disease prevention, providing personalized health advice and care has become a challenge worldwide [16].

The "annual study on mHealth" suggests that the ubiquity of smartphones, tablets, sensors, wearables, personal trackers, and similar wireless smart devices means that huge volumes of data concerning health, fitness, lifestyle, stress, and sleep are being harvested and processed [16]. This report foresees that in 2020, 551 Million users will by then actively (at least once a month) make use of a mHealth app.

The main issue then becomes how to identify the most appropriate, adapted, and trustworthy health app out of hundreds of thousands of similar health apps.

Another major risk of apps is that they work according to a set formula or standardized algorithms, which are relatively unchanged from patient to patient. This then does not allow the capture of the other aspects of clinical diagnosis such as clinical observation or personal medical history of the patient and his/her various signs.

Health apps have to undergo specific accreditation in the USA by the FDA to be categorized as medical devices [17]. So far in Europe, there is no such specific directive for apps except the Code of Conduct on privacy for mobile health apps submitted for approval to the Art 29 Data Protection Working Party [18]. So in Europe, health apps to be labeled as medical devices should respect the Council Directive 93/42/ECC concerning medical devices. This chapter does not address the health apps as medical devices as it is governed by clear regulation.

However, the majority of health apps labeled as non-medical device also provide medical functionalities such as auto-diagnosis and auto-medication. Mobile apps span a wide range of health functions, with potential benefits and risks to public health compounded by the fact that these apps are potentially available to billions of people worldwide. Depending on the type of the app and its intended use, the potential risk will vary and thus, the level of scrutiny given should be proportionate to the risk.

Different initiatives propose solutions to solve the problem of the quality and security of mobile apps. Below in Table 27.1 is a non-exhaustive list of some initiatives, guidelines, rating tools, recommendations, and scale to assess the level of trust of a health app. New approaches are published regularly, such as the THESIS rating tool [19] but the common point of all these approaches is the difficulty to implement them and to be used

by health apps developers. The common criteria addressed by these rating tools, labels, or guidelines are the transparency, health reliability, technical consistency, security and privacy disclosure, and usability.

Various organizations worked on the issue of security, data privacy, and other criteria related to quality [20]. However, due to the complexity and liability risks to potentially unidentified issues such as the security issue, the assessment of health apps is at its very early stages. A study highlighted that 66% of the health apps certified as clinically safe and trustworthy by the UK NHS apps Library was in fact sending identifying information over the internet without encryption and without disclosure that the app will do so [10]. This has caused the NHS apps service to close for a while. This study has raised three elements of reflection: the current lack of transparency and responsibility of apps related to data usage, storage, and transmission; what can be evaluated reasonably and sustainably; and the risk that no organization assesses health apps as the risk is too important to miss or not be able to check all the necessary elements to guarantee

Table 27.1 Presentation of several labels and guidelines for health apps monitoring—August 2020

Name	Country	Developer	Functioning	Inventory
NHS apps Library	UK	NHS	Registration needed, fee-based evaluation not disclosed. Criteria of evaluation disclosed[a]	95 apps in the NHS Library[b]
Calidad app salud	Spain	Agencia de Calidad Sanitaria de Andalucia	Free 31 recommendations Assesses design, quality, services, and privacy [10]	20 app assessed, 70 under assessment
Just think app	USA	American Health Information Management Information	Brochure to inform and educate users [11]	Education No implementation
MOBILE APPLICATION RATING SCALE	Australia	Queensland University of Technology	23 questions Grading scale from 1 poor to 5 excellent [12]	Self-evaluation
code of conduct on privacy for mhealth app	EU	European Commission	The Code was issued after a research study in 2014 [8]	No implementation
Good practice guidelines on health apps	FRANCE	French Health National Authority	5 categories: Information to users, health content, security, data usage and technical usage [13]	No implementation
mobile app privacy code of conduct	USA	US Government	Privacy notice to disclose their practice related to data storage and usage [14]	Voluntary Not widely used

[a]https://shorturl.at/juFO0
[b]https://www.nhs.uk/apps-library/

security and accuracy. On the other hand, should we rely only on the current model of user rating proposed by the two majors' apps platforms Google Play and iTunes iOS [21] knowing that apps providing measurement of key indicators such as heart rate Blood Pressure readings are commonly downloaded (up to 2.4 million downloads) and rated well?

With the multitude of health apps available today (more than 260,000 health apps), what can be evaluated reasonably and sustainably?

In addition, to assess too many criteria as identified by the HAS will lead to nearly no assessment because the number of apps being assessed will drastically diminish because of high costs and inefficient practices. Transparency and honesty in the production of the apps will engage developers to disclose what is behind the scene and be responsible for what health app it develops. Not all apps need the same attention as they do not imply the same potential risk to consumers. For example, health apps with calculators and algorithms intended to recommend an action or medications may directly impact the user's health [11].

The mHONcode Certification for Mobile Health Apps

Health On the Net Foundation (HON) is a non-governmental organization based in Geneva and in official relations with the WHO (World Health Organization). HON was created to promote the deployment of useful and reliable health information online and to enable its appropriate and efficient use. HON is the oldest online health information standardizing body and was founded in 1995 in Geneva, Switzerland. The Health On the Net Code of Conduct (HONcode), a set of 8 principles used to standardize online health information has been in use for over 20 years for health websites [22]. Two decades on, the HONcode is the oldest and most valued quality marker for online health information. It is a pragmatic solution that has been adopted by more than 8000 websites. This approach has the aim to help consumers to become more efficient at sepa-

rating fact from fiction and at evaluating credibility on the Web in practice.

In 1996, the Health On the Net (HON) Foundation established the HONcode (Boyer et al. 1998) by working with health information editors to come to agreement on typical and common good practice criteria for health information online. This approach involves the external evaluation of health Web pages by experts. The HONcode is a set of ethical, honesty, transparency, and quality standards covering various aspects of health websites, including the disclosure of the qualifications of the authors, the funding sources, references, when the content was created and last updated, the privacy policy, and how data is stored. The HONcode motivates health editors to be transparent in the production process. The commitment of a health information provider to implement or comply with the HON code of conduct is shown by the displaying of a quality label (logo or HONcode seal) on the website. Sites first submit a formal application for HONcode certification. The health website is then manually checked to determine whether or not it meets the principles for compliance. Once HON has determined that the site is committed to and respects the HONcode, it can display the HONcode seal. The site is checked on a regular basis to ensure that it is still compliant and that the health editors are respecting their ethical commitment. However, HON relies on the community to report misuse of the label or non-respect of a principle via an online form. The goal of the HONcode is to guide Internet users and patients towards trustworthy health information by certifying health websites that offer content respecting the HONcode principles. The HONcode is dedicated to the upkeep of the quality of health website, so a new set of principles have been adapted and tailored for the mobile health apps: the mHONcode.

The mHONcode is the new code of conduct of HON, with guidelines adapted to mobile health apps [23]. Apps owners voluntarily request the mHONcode certification, and then their application is evaluated on the one hand on reliability by a medical expert and on the other hand on safety by a member of our IT team. Before any evaluation, a contribution is requested since the processes require between 3 and 5 days of work by experts. This does not in any way guarantee that the certification will be obtained as the application needs to be fully compliant to be certified.

mHONcode Certification and Methodology

The mHONcode is a set of ethical, honesty, transparency, quality, and security standards covering various aspects of health apps, including the disclosure of the qualifications of the authors, the funding sources, references, when the content was created and last updated, what the privacy policy is, and how data is stored and transmitted over the internet (Fig. 27.1). The mHONcode

motivates health apps editors to be transparent in the production process and in the way to use user's data. The commitment of a health information provider to implement or comply with the HON code of conduct for health apps is shown by the displaying of a quality label (logo or HONcode seal) on the website.

Certification process: The health app owner voluntarily applies via the HON website for the mHONcode certification. Upon this application, the app is evaluated manually by an expert medical team and a security officer according to the mHON principles and associated published guidelines[3] (Tables 27.2 and 27.3). In order for this evaluation to take place, the health app editor needs to fill in a self-reporting mHONcode ques-

---

[3]https://www.hon.ch/en/guidelines-mhoncode.html

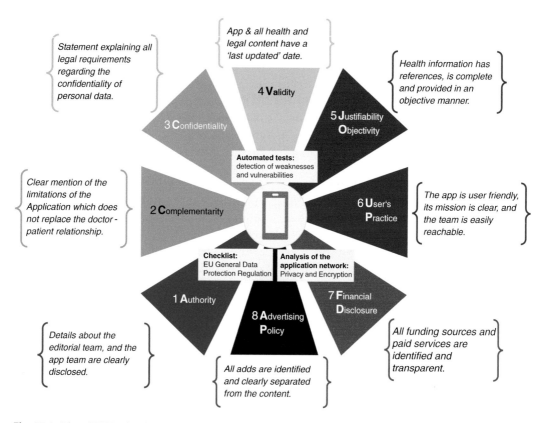

Fig. 27.1 The mHONcode principles dedicated to mobile health apps

Table 27.2   8 principles of the mHONcode regarding the health content of the app

Principles	Description	Examples of questions
1. Authority	Details about the editorial team and the app team are clearly disclosed.	Are the name and qualifications of the editorial manager and the qualifications of writers provided? Who is in charge/responsible for the app?
2. Complementarity	Clear mention of the limitations of the app which does not replace the doctor-patient relationship.	Do you have a statement indicating that the information provided on the application is intended to encourage, not replace, direct relationships between the patient and health professionals?
3. Confidentiality	Statement explaining all legal requirements regarding the confidentiality of personal data.	Does the GPDR apply to your service? Is consent to data collection required for the use of the application? Are data transmitted to third parties?
4. Validity	App & all health and legal content have a "last updated" date.	Does the medical, legal content and app have a last updated date?
5. Justifiability & Objectivity	Health information has references, is complete, and provided in an objective manner.	If app has services with formulae calculating dosage or health scores, are the references/scientific bases of these formulae given? If app has medical content, are the references given and medical information provided in an objective and balanced manner?
6. User's practice	The app is user friendly, its mission is clear, and the team is easily reachable.	What is the mission and audience of the application? Are there any instructions for use? Is a support contact address accessible or is it possible to leave a feedback?
7. Financial disclosure	All funding sources and paid services are identified and transparent.	What are the source(s) of funding? If the application needs an integrated purchase for its use, are there any general conditions available on this subject in the app? Is there a declaration of disclosure of links of interest for health professionals providing content or advice?
8. Advertisement policy	All ads are identified and clearly separated from the content.	If the application displays advertising, is it clearly identified as such and is there a viewable advertising policy on the application? If there are not ads in the app, does a disclaimer indicate that there is none?

tionnaire with 34 questions related to the mHON-code guidelines. The HON's reviewer analyzes the content of the health app and assesses if it conforms or not to the given principle. For any principles that have not been respected, the HONcode reviewer delivers a detailed report at the end of the process with recommendations on how to improve the health app. This resulting evaluation report helps the health app editor to render content that is HONcode compliant and transparent. The evaluation of health apps for the HONcode takes an average of 180 minutes. Once a health app has been validated, it receives a dated, dynamic, and unique logo it can display on the app store to indicate its annual certification and illustrate the trustworthiness of its construction and maintenance. The seal is located on HON servers, so its status can be monitored and adapted. The HONcode seal is linked to its corresponding HONcode certificate. The latter summarizes the result of the certification of the health app—when and why the health app was certified. When a principle does not respect the recommendations (totally or partially), the health app's editor is requested to do the necessary modifications.

Case Study

The mHONcode in Action

HON chose the ten most downloaded free health apps in the two major stores Google Play and Apple with the limitation of the country in the URL of the stores being France, without discrim-

Table 27.3 Technical consistency, security and privacy of the mHONcode for health apps

Technical consistency, Security and privacy	Type	Implementation request
Detection of weakness and vulnerabilities	Improper Platform Usage	Avoid misuse of a platform feature or failure to use platform security controls.
	Insecure Data Storage:	Avoid insecure data storage and unintended data leakage.
	Insecure communication	Avoid poor handshaking, incorrect Secure Sockets Layer (SSL) versions
	Insecure authentication	Ensure authenticating the end-user when needed or avoid bad session management.
	Insufficient Cryptography	Ensure that cryptography is done correctly
	Insecure Authorization	Avoid any failures in the authorization
	Client Code Quality	Feedback for implementation problems in the app
	Code tampering	Avoid dynamic memory modification
	Extraneous Functionality:	Avoid hidden backdoor functionality
Communication, Privacy & Encryption	Communication security	Application requests/queries must be encrypted with SSL protocol. Authentication (login/password) should be encrypted.
	Data minimization	Only required data must be transferred and used. It prevents excessive bandwidth usage and data leaks.
	Permission minimization	Only required access (camera, location, internet access) must be asked and retrieved with explicit consent.
	Data transfer to third party	Transmission of user data (including IP address) to third party should be done after explicit consent of the user.
Data privacy	Self-Assessment General Data Protection Regulation GDPR (EU 2016/679)	Gathered Data (by the app or a tier) must be done with the explicit consent of the User. Data usage should be compliant with the GDPR. Use HON checklist[a] http://shorturl.at/atITV to identify the improvement necessary to the app services in order to be compliant with the GDPR.

[a]GDPR Self-Assessment HONcode Certification http://shorturl.at/atITV

ination of language, mission, functionalities, and rating. None of these apps had voluntarily required the certification or ever been HONcode certified at the time of the study. As we wanted to test if the GDPR[4] was adopted by apps after this new European regulation came into force across the European Union on May 25, 2018, we decided to opt and select the country France. The aim was then to have a representative sample of applications without any further sorting other than choosing the most downloaded applications by users, to obtain results that were limited but representative of the current market of mobile applications as in line with the other publications described below. As the top ten apps is different for either the Apple Store or the Google Play Store, and also because this list changes from day to day, we selected the ten most downloaded apps between the two stores, on May 24, 2019. We also reported the number and the score of ratings as users could base their choice on such criteria. All this information can be found in Tables 27.4 and 27.5.

Ten applications, French and English language-based health-related mobile apps were assessed by two senior expert members of the HON team, following the new guidelines for app certification: the mHONcode (Tables 27.2 and 27.3) [23]. This new code of conduct also includes two security tests: an automated test for detection of weakness and vulnerabilities and a test about privacy and encryption, which analyzes the application's network, they can be found at the end of Table 27.3. Thus, ten apps were manually checked by the IT team regarding the traffic of the data sent by apps on the Internet through differential traffic and network analysis. This

[4]https://ec.europa.eu/commission/priorities/justice-and-fundamental-rights/data-protection/

Table 27.4 Positions, number of downloads for the ten selected apps on May 24, 2019, in France

Application	Versions	Owner	Category	Apple store's positions	GooglePlay store's positions	Downloads in the GooglePlay store
Doctolib	iOS 3.2.1 Android 3.1.9	Doctolib	Appointment booking	#1 Medical	#1 Medical	>one million
Grossesse +	iOS 5.4 Android 5.2	Philips/Health & Parenting	Pregnancy	#2 Medical	#1 Parents	>ten million
Qare	iOS 1.7.65 Android 1.8.85	Qare SAS	Online consultation	#3 Medical	#2 Medical	>100,000
Staying Alive	iOS 6.1.3 Android 6.2.2	AEDMAP	Cartography	#4 Medical	#5 Medical	>500,000
Sauv Life	iOS 2.5.4 Android 2.3.4	Association S.A.U.V.	Cartography	#5 Medical	#7 Medical	>100,000
We Moms	iOS 2.14.17 Android 2.61.07	Globalia SAS	Forum	#6 Medical	#9 Parents	>500,000
Mon Ovulation	iOS 1.4.3 Android 2.7.1	Doctissimo/TF1/ Lagardère	Fertility	#7 Medical	#27 Medical	>500,000
Livi	iOS 3.0.6 Android 3.0.5	Digital Medical Supply France	Online Consultation	#8 Medical	#4 Medical	>100,000
Bébé +	iOS 1.9.4 Android 1.8.4	Philips/Health & Parenting	Baby's health	#9 Medical	#6 Parents	>500,000
Ma Grossesse	iOS 2.6 Android 2.9.0	Doctissimo/TF1/ Lagardère	Pregnancy	#10 Medical	#12 Medical	>one million

Table 27.5 Ratings and number of ratings for the ten selected apps on May 24, 2019

Application	Users's rating for GooglePlay	Numbers of rating for Google Play	User's rating for Apple Store	Numbers of rating for Apple Store
Doctolib	4.8/5	29,000	4.8/5	11,300
Grossesse +	4.6/5	384,000	4.7/5	5800
Qare	4.7/5	567	4.8/5	2000
Staying Alive	4.1/5	2000	4.2/5	2
Sauv Life	3.9/5	786	4.3/5	297
We Moms	4.6/5	9000	4.7/5	129
Mon Ovulation	4.2/5	4000	3.5/5	6
Livi	4.5/5	877	4.9/5	2700
Bébé +	4.5/5	29,000	4.7/5	1300
Ma Grossesse	4.3/5	32,000	4.3/5	34

allowed us to understand (1) the data sharing practice of the apps, how the personal data are transmitted (via a secure link SSL, and how the password and login are transmitted—encrypted or not) and (2) to which third parties personal data are sent with consent or not. These analyses have been done using Mitmproxy, a free open source interactive https proxy[5] allowing to be in between of the app transmission of data over the Internet and the phone. In addition, the Mobile App Security Test,[6] free product by ImmuniWeb, was used to scan the code. For Android, APK or Google play link was used to upload the code, while for iOS an IPA archive was mandatory. This free product provides automated tests regarding six different test types: Static Application Security Testing (SAST); Dynamic Application Security Testing (DAST); Behavior Testing for malicious functionality and privacy; Software Composition Analysis; Mobile Application Outgoing Traffic and Mobile App External Communications. This product was selected as it provides a complete and easy to understand report and is free of charge, with an API or a web version. The results of these tests were analyzed by our team, and major ones are reported in the results section. The ten apps were downloaded to a HUAWEI P20 Android version 9.0.0, Android 8.1.0 and an iPhone 8 iOS version 12.2.Various subjects were covered by the apps assessed: pregnancy, fertility, online consultation, cartography, baby's health, forum. The audience of these apps was the public. Regarding the new code of conduct and especially the eight principles, Table 27.6 shows for each application if it respects each principle. The symbol X means that the principle is not present in the app, while ✓ means that the principle is respected by the app, and NA means that the principle does not apply to the app. For some principles, we separated the results to be more precise, the signification of each initial is indicated below (Table 27.6).

Summary

As demonstrated in the case study described above, there appears to be no correlation between the popularity of an app and the quality parameters laid out by the mHONcode, which demonstrates that the trustworthiness of the app was not

one of the parameters considered by users when choosing it.

It is not surprising, given that mobile apps are still very new. Also, because apps do not provide health information in the traditional sense, like a health website presents pages of health information, it would not be apparent for users to consider trustworthiness as a required characteristic for mobile health apps.

Thus, a way to distinguish trustworthy mobile health apps is required, not only to make them more visible but also to introduce the whole concept of trustworthiness to mobile health app users [24].

As the adaptation of an already proven trustworthy code of conduct of health websites (the HONcode), the mHONcode is well placed to provide guidance for the next generation of health information providers—mobile apps in this case.

Conclusions and Outlook

mHealth is a huge market that provides users the opportunity to have better health and healthcare quality. Health apps support citizen's empowerment through self-management, health promotion, disease prevention, providing personalized health advice and care. However, the risks involved must be considered; the rapid development of the mHealth sector raises concerns about the potential risk of health functions apps providing transmission of health data, the capture of these data via sensors, self-diagnoses, disease management or diagnosis and appropriate processing of the data collected. Since mHealth solutions and devices can collect large quantities of personal information, including personal health information (e.g., data stored by the user on the device and data from different sensors, including location), they can also process them.

The major difficulty for not only general users but also for health professionals who could recommend apps is to discern trustworthy apps from the large pool of apps out there and our list assessment confirms this challenge.

Users, with this new technology in their hands, have direct access to medical and health informa-

---

[5] https://mitmproxy.org/

[6] https://www.immuniweb.com/mobile/#about

Table 27.6 Compliance with each principle for each application—assessment conducted in May 2019

Principles Apps	1. Authority	2. Complementarity	3. Confidentiality Policy	Consent	4. Validity (Dates) M	L	A	5. Justifiability Objectivity R	O	6. User's practice M	A	I	S	7. Financial disclosure	8. Advertisement policy Policy	Identification
Doctolib	X	NA	X	X	NA	X	X	NA	NA	X	X	X	X	X	X	NA
Grossesse+	X	✓	✓	X	X	✓	X	X	✓	X	✓	✓	✓	X	X	X
Qare	✓	✓	✓	X	X	✓	X	NA	NA	✓	X	✓	✓	✓	X	NA
Staying Alive	✓	✓	✓	X	NA	X	X	NA	NA	X	X	✓	✓	✓	✓	NA
Sauv Life	X	NA	✓	X	NA	X	X	NA	NA	✓	✓	X	X	X	X	NA
We Moms	X	✓	✓	✓	X	✓	X	X	✓	✓	✓	✓	✓	X	✓	✓
Mon Ovulation	X	X	X	X	X	✓	X	X	✓	X	✓	X	✓	X	X	X
Livi	X	✓	✓	✓	NA	✓	X	NA	NA	✓	✓	✓	✓	X	X	NA
Bébé +	X	✓	✓	X	X	✓	X	X	✓	✓	✓	✓	✓	X	X	X
Ma Grossesse	X	X	X	X	X	✓	X	X	✓	X	✓	X	X	X	X	X

Principle 4 Validity: M: Medical content/L: Legal content/A: Application
Principle 5 Justifiability & Objectivity: R: References/O: Objectivity
Principle 6 User's practice: MA: Mission & Audience/I: Instructions/S: Support

tion, with no need to take an appointment, straight from their pocket, which of course represents massive advancement in healthcare but also a real danger.

As demonstrated by other studies, our study, based on the ten most downloaded mobile apps in France, has shown clearly that mHealth apps, are sharing data that is far from transparent [14, 15]. The non-conformity with the mHealth HONcode guidelines and issues in terms of privacy or security identified could be easily overcome with guidance to the developing team and the owners of these apps. Given that there is no control, why would app developers decide to conform to strict editorial processes such as security, honesty, and transparency which would cost more without short-term benefit in terms of number of downloads or ranking [25]?

Although, even if only ten apps were used in this study, it should be remembered that the ten chosen were the most popular and thus, a representation of what the public downloads and uses.

mHealth apps are excellent ways to improve your health, in a fast, fun, and accessible way, but only if they are reliable. Otherwise, as was confirmed with this panel of apps, they represent a real public health danger, which can be overcome only with the commitment of the owners/developers of these apps, which the HON Foundation will try to address through its new code of conduct, the mHONcode.

Review Questions
1. What kind of special risks arise from apps on mobile devices compared to websites?
2. Why is it a problem to assess many features of the app as different frameworks suggest?
3. What are the eight principles of the mHONcode?
4. Please describe the mHONcode certification process!

Appendix: Answers to Review Questions

1. What kind of special risks arise from apps on mobile devices compared to websites?

Websites display the data as they are part of the content of this site which is therefore easy to check also in terms of how they are produced. In apps, the algorithms used to analyze the data are kept secret and are not disclosed because they belong to the business model of the app. The privacy and security of transmission and storage is very difficult to test and assess in apps as well. Apps play the role of a "medical device" even if by definition of the relevant laws they are not which is unlike health websites. They do not play a diagnostic role but only an informational role.

2. Why is it a problem to assess many features of the app as different frameworks suggest?

Too many criteria to be assessed may lead to a situation in which developers are reluctant to have their app assessed due to potentially high costs and inefficient practices. This in turn entails a low number of apps being actually assessed. In contrast, transparency and honesty in the production of the apps will engage developers to disclose what is behind the scene and be responsible to what health app it develops. Furthermore, not all apps need the same attention as they do not imply the same potential risk to consumers. For example, health apps with calculators and algorithms intended to recommend an action or medications may directly impact the user's health and must be scrutinized thoroughly, while diary apps just used for documentation are less critical.

3. What are the eight principles of the mHONcode?

   1. Authority.
   2. Complementarity.
   3. Confidentiality.
   4. Validity.
   5. Justifiability & Objectivity.
   6. User's practice.
   7. Financial disclosure.
   8. Advertisement policy

4. Please describe the mHONcode certification process!

Step 1: The health app owner voluntarily applies via the HON website for the mHONcode certification for manual evaluation by an expert medical team and a security officer according to the mHON principles and associated published guidelines.

Step 2: The health app editor needs to fill in a self-reporting mHONcode questionnaire with 34 questions related to the mHONcode guidelines.

Step 3: The HON's reviewer analyzes the content of the health app and assesses if it conforms or not to the given principle.

Step 4: For any principles that have not been respected, the HONcode reviewer delivers a detailed report at the end of the process with recommendations on how to improve the health app. This resulting evaluation report helps the health app editor to render content that is HONcode compliant and transparent.

Appendix: Definitions of Terms in the Text

Digital engagement: Anything that involves a conversation online.

Digital care: An evidence-based software intervention (a program, application, or the like) that is intended to prevent or treat a disease and carries the attributes below.

Data security: Protective digital privacy measures that are applied to prevent unauthorized access to computers, databases, and websites.

e-Health: e-Health is a broad term, and refers to the use of information and communications technologies in healthcare.

Digital health technology: Digital health, which includes digital care programs, is the convergence of digital technologies with health, healthcare, living, and society to enhance the efficiency of healthcare delivery and make medicine more personalized and precise.

Population health: The health outcomes of a group of individuals, including the distribution of such outcomes within the group.

Encryption: The process of converting information or data into a code, especially to prevent unauthorized access.

Algorithms: A process or set of rules to be followed in calculations or other problem-solving operations, especially by a computer.

Cryptography: A method of protecting information and communications through the use of codes, so that only those for whom the information is intended can read and process it.

Data minimization: The principle of data minimization involves limiting data collection to only what is required to fulfill a specific purpose.

References

1. IQVIA Institute for Human Data Science. 2017 The growing value of digital health evidence and impact on human health and the healthcare system. https://www.iqvia.com/insights/the-iqvia-institute/reports/the-growing-value-of-digital-health [Accessed July 2020].
2. Research 2 Guidance. mHealth App Economics 2017/2018 Current Status and Future Trends in Mobile Health Research2Guidance report. USA, 2017, pp 10. https://research2guidance.com/product/mhealth-economics-2017-current-status-and-future-trends-in-mobile-health/ [Accessed May 2019].
3. Business Insider. *10 Ways Mobile Is Transforming Health Care* https://www.businessinsider.fr/us/10-ways-mobile-is-transforming-health-care-2014-6 [Accessed August 2020].
4. Zhang C, Zhang X, Halstead-Nussloch R. Assessment metrics, challenges and strategies for mobile health apps. Issues Inform Syst. 2014;15(2).
5. Day S, Zweig M. Rock health beyond wellness for the healthy: digital health consumer adoption 2018, 2019. https://rockhealth.com/reports/beyond-wellness-for-the-healthy-digital-health-consumer-adoption-2018/
6. Martínez-Pérez B, De La Torre-Díez I, López-Coronado M. Privacy and security in mobile health apps: a review and recommendations. J Med Syst. 2015;39(1):181.
7. Schechner S, Secada M. Feb 2019 You Give Apps Sensitive Personal Information. Then They Tell Facebook. Wall Street J. https://www.wsj.com/articles/you-give-apps-sensitive-personal-information-

then-they-tell-facebook-11550851636 [Accessed August 2020].

8. McKay FH, et al. Evaluating mobile phone applications for health behaviour change: a systematic review. J Telemed Telecare. 2018;24(1):22–30.

9. Carroll JK, et al. Who uses mobile phone health apps and does use matter? A secondary data analytics approach. J Med Internet Res. 2017;19(4):e125.

10. Huckvale K, et al. Unaddressed privacy risks in accredited health and wellness apps: a cross-sectional systematic assessment. BMC Med. 2015a;13:214.

11. Huckvale K, Adomaviciute S, et al. Smartphone apps for calculating insulin dose: a systematic assessment. BMC Med. 2015b;13(1):106.

12. Plante TB, Urrea B, et al. Validation of the instant blood pressure smartphone app. JAMA Intern Med. 2016;176(5):700–2.

13. Wisniewski H, Liu G, Henson P, Vaidyam A, Hajratalli NK, Onnela JP, Torous J. Understanding the quality, effectiveness and attributes of top-rated smartphone health apps. Evid Based Ment Health. 2019;22(1):4–9.

14. Grundy Q, Chiu K, Held F, Continella A, Bero L, Holz R. Data sharing practices of medicines related apps and the mobile ecosystem: traffic, content, and network analysis. BMJ. 2019;364:l920.

15. Huckvale K, Torous J, Larsen ME. Assessment of the data sharing and privacy practices of smartphone apps for depression and smoking cessation. JAMA Netw Open. 2019;2(4):–e192542.

16. DG CONNECT. https://ec.europa.eu/digital-single-market/en/mhealth [Accessed August 2020].

17. Food and Drug Administration (FDA). 2017 Mobile medical applications: guidance for industry and food and drug administration staff. URL: goo.gl/oZGjNE [Accessed August 2020].

18. European Commission. Code of Conduct on privacy for mobile health applications. URL:goo.gl/mFbK47. https://ec.europa.eu/digital-single-market/en/news/code-conduct-privacy-mhealth-apps-has-been-finalised [Accessed August 2020].

19. Levine DM, Co Z, Newmark LP, et al. Design and testing of a mobile health application rating tool. npj Digit Med. 2020;3:74. https://doi.org/10.1038/s41746-020-0268-9.

20. The United States Department of Commerce. Code of Conduct for mobile application ("app") short notices on Application Transparency, 2013. Accessed: 2017-11-14. URL: https://goo.gl/eAKKcf

21. Kumar N, Khunger M, Gupta A, Garg N. A content analysis of smartphone-based applications for hypertension management. J Am Soc Hypertens JASH. 2015;9:130–6.

22. Boyer C, Gaudinat A, Hanbury A, Appel RD, Ball MJ, Geissbühler A, et al. Accessing reliable health information on the web: a review of the HON approach. Stud Health Technol Inform. 2017;245:1004–8. https://doi.org/10.3233/978-1-61499-830-3-1004.

23. Ranasinghe M, Cabrera A, Postel-Vinay N, Boyer C. Transparency and quality of health apps: the HON approach. Stud Health Technol Inform. 2018;247:656–60.

24. Postel-Vinay N, Jouhaud P, Bobrie G, Boyer C. Home blood pressure measurement and mobile health app for pregnant and postpartum. J Hypertens. 2019;37:e280. https://doi.org/10.1097/01.hjh.0000573576.89014.cb.

25. Research 2 Guidance 2018 mHealth Economics – How mHealth App Publishers Are Monetizing Their Apps https://research2guidance.com/product/mhealth-economics-how-mhealth-app-publishers-are-monetizing-their-apps/

Part VI

Privacy, Security, Confidentiality and Ethics in Healthcare

Data Privacy and Security in the US: HIPAA, HITECH and Beyond

28

Joan M. Kiel

Learning Objectives
- Apply the HIPAA Privacy Rule to operational aspects of healthcare.
- Develop a plan to ensure adherence to HIPAA technical, administrative, and physical security standards.
- Evaluate the effect of social media on healthcare data privacy.

Key Terms
- Data privacy
- State confidentiality laws
- Privacy practices
- Administrative security
- Physical security
- Technical security

Introduction

In 2018, the Office for Civil Rights (OCR) saw Health Insurance Portability and Accountability Act (HIPAA) enforcement violations amount to $28.7, the most in one year to date [1]. https://www.hhs.gov/hipaa/for-professionals/compliance-enforcement/agreements/2018enforcement/index.html.Sincethe start of HIPAA in April 2003, there have been 216,195 complaints. This resulted in 39,132 investigations. Seventy percent, 27,225 required corrective action [2].

https://www.hhs.gov/hipaa/for-professionals/compliance-enforcement/data/numbers-glance/index.html#allcomplaints

There is a conundrum for as technology is enhanced, patient health information complaints and settlement dollars abound. With HIPAA though, there is now Federal oversight and complaints are investigated and tracked. In addition, polices, procedures, and formage, guide the organization on keeping patient health information private and secure, while allowing the patients access to their data and having HIPAA-covered entities be very transparent as to how their data are being used. As technology and consumer needs continue to evolve, so too will HIPAA.

HIPAA Privacy

The **HIPAA Privacy Rule** is the piece that most consumers identify with as it directly affects them on each patient encounter that is billed to a third party. Given this, HIPAA regulates three covered entities, healthcare providers who transmit PHI in electronic format, health plans/insurers, and a health care clearinghouse [3] (Privacy: 45CFR160.103). All three of these covered entity types must be compliant with the HIPAA standards to protect **patient health information (PHI)** or individually identifiable health information (IIHI) (Fig. 28.1). It is pertinent to note that

J. M. Kiel (✉)
University HIPAA Compliance, Health Management Systems, Duquesne University, Pittsburgh, PA, USA
e-mail: kiel@duq.edu

© Springer Nature Switzerland AG 2022
U. H. Hübner et al. (eds.), *Nursing Informatics*, Health Informatics,
https://doi.org/10.1007/978-3-030-91237-6_28

427

```
┌─────────────────────────────────────────────┐
│          Operationalizing HIPAA Privacy       │
│                                               │
│ 1. Business Associate Agreements need to be   │
│    signed.                                    │
│ 2. Authorization to Disclose forms must be    │
│    available.                                 │
│ 3. The Notice of Privacy Practices must be    │
│    signed.                                    │
│ 4. The record amendment request process is    │
│    developed.                                 │
│ 5. HIPAA personnel are hired.                 │
│ 6  Complaints and sanctions are handled       │
│    timely.                                    │
└─────────────────────────────────────────────┘
```

Fig. 28.1 Operationalizing HIPAA Privacy

even if one does not say the patient's name, but rather that the person can be individually identified given the information, that would be a HIPAA violation. For example, if one were to say the President of the USA in a particular month and year, everyone would know the person as there is only one President of the USA at one point in time. Whether the information is written, spoken, or electronically sent, it is protected patient health information, and all media must be kept private.

Patient health information, with the exception to a provider for treatment, must be held to the minimum necessary level [4] (Privacy: 45CFR164.502(b)). Those without a need to know cannot have access to the information. Here, the organization must understand the data flow within everyone's role. If the role does not include the use of the particular data, it would be a violation of HIPAA for them to have access to the data. The clear writing of job descriptions becomes paramount as data use and access must be clearly delineated. Permitted uses and disclosures are for treatment, payment, or healthcare operations [5] (Privacy: 45CFR164.502(a)(1)). An organization encounters a **business associate** when a person and or organization in the capacity of their role, external to the organization, involves the use or disclosure of patient health information [3] (Privacy: 45CFR160.103). To ensure that the business associate adheres to the same strict HIPAA standards as the covered entity, the covered entity must have a **business associate agreement.** This document is very specific in how the business associate can use and disclose the data. If the HIPAA Rule were to change, new business associate agreements must be garnered and training on the HIPAA changes must be conducted. This ensures to the public that both those internal and external to the organization who handle data are compliant with HIPAA.

The HIPAA Privacy Rule has its goal to keep private and confidential one's patient health. It is in this venue that an authorization is required for the use and disclosure of patient data. Examples of when an authorization is required are for psychotherapy notes and marketing functions using patient data [6] (Privacy) (45CFR164.508). HIPAA also allows the patient the opportunity to agree to or object to the use and disclosure of their data. Examples here include being listed in the facility directory and for disaster relief [7] (Privacy: 45CFR164.510).

The goal of data privacy must be balanced with the ability of the healthcare system to do its job, that of quality patient healthcare delivery and the corresponding function of payment for that care. Given that, there are several instances where an authorization is not required to use patient health information. Examples here include for public health activities, when the disclosure is required by law, to report to a government authority on a victim of abuse, neglect, or domestic violence, for healthcare oversight activities such as audits, for judicial and administrative matters, and law enforcement [8] (Privacy: 45CFR164.512).

So how does one keep track of how data can be released or not. The answer lies in the **Notice of Privacy Practices.** This critical document outlines how a HIPAA-covered entity, provider, health plan, or clearinghouse, use and disclose patient health information, but also how the patient can get access to their medical record [9] (Privacy: 45CFR164.520). The Notice must be given to the individual on their first visit, but also be available at all times in the event that the patient requests a copy. When HIPAA changes, the changes must be incorporated in the Notice and be given to the patient again. It is paramount that patients understand the Notice as it educates them on their rights to, for example, request to amend their record or the right to request restrictions on certain uses and disclosures [9] (Privacy: 45CFR164.520). I also specify to whom and how a HIPAA complaint can be filed. In this electronic age, a covered entity who has a website must have their Notice on the website [10] (Privacy: 45CFR164.520(c)(3)(i).

In most instances, patients have access to their medical record. In the event of, for example, private psychotherapy notes whereby reading the notes can cause more harm, access would be denied [11] (Privacy: 45CFR164.524(a)(1)(i). When granting access to the medical record, the covered entity has 30 days to fulfill the request, but 60 days if the records are off-site [12] (Privacy: 45CFR164.524(b)(2). Thus it is not an immediate turn around which must be understood by the patient to allay frustration and yet it allows the facility to review the request and proceed in a quality manner. Many times a patient will review their record and then request an amendment. An amendment is not a change in the legal medical record, but rather a notation in the record of new information. An amendment can be denied by the provider if what is requested is not objectively true. The provider must respond to the requested amendment within 60 days [13] (Privacy: 45CFR164.526(b)(2).

Providers, health plans, and clearing houses, all covered entities under HIPAA must ascribe to its many facets. Sometimes a covered entity is already doing what HIPAA requires due to their State confidentiality laws, but many times changes are needed. One of the most important elements is for a covered entity to have a HIPAA Privacy person to manage all of the aspects of compliance to the law [14] (Privacy: 45CFr164.530(a)(1). Employees must know of this person (or people in large organizations) such that when an issue occurs, they know who to contact. This person will facilitate the training on HIPAA for all of its workforce members. This training must be documented in the event of a complaint or an audit [15] (Privacy: 45CFR164.530(2)(b)(1) and (C)(ii). Complaints must be dealt with expeditiously, and the covered entity must have a process that allows people to submit complaints [16] (Privacy: 45CFR164.530(d)(1). The process must be accessible to all and organizations can have multiple methods to submit complaints such as a website, an anonymous telephone line, or even a face-to-face meeting with the designated HIPAA person. All complaints are investigated thoroughly, and then, if necessary, appropriate sanctions are levied [17] (Privacy: 45CFR164.530(e)(1). Documentation must be maintained on complaints and all related HIPAA

business for six years, which again is the responsibility of the HIPAA person [18] (Privacy: 45CFR164.530(j)(2). The organization must have all of the policies and procedures corresponding to each aspect of HIPAA privacy. Thus, HIPAA has brought oversight such that consumers of healthcare can feel confident that their patient health information is private and confidential.

HIPAA Security

Security is the safety of data, whether in transmission or at rest. The HIPAA Security Rule focuses on three areas; **administrative security, physical security, and technical security.** Within these areas are required policies and addressable policies. In this manner, the developers of HIPAA took into account the size, scope, and various situations of covered entities. Required policies must be implemented according to the exact specifications, but addressable policies must be assessed whether the security safeguard is appropriate (Fig. 28.2) [19] (Security: 45CFR164.306)(d). As with HIPAA Privacy, the organization must employ a HIPAA Security personnel who leads the efforts on administrative, physical, and technical security [20] (Security: 45CFR164.308(2)). This position can be combined with another position and or duties of an employee.

Administrative security and safeguards focus on the policies and procedures to keep patient health information secure. Covered entities must conduct a risk analysis and have a robust risk management program in which potential risks are detected and reduced if not eradicated [21] (Security: 45CFR164.308(1). It is here that the entire organization is looked at and personnel are hired with a standard of risk eradication. When employees are hired or their job role changes,

---

Operationalizing HIPAA Security

1. Implement administrative security features
2. Implement physical security features
3. Implement technical security features

Fig. 28.2 Operationalizing HIPAA Security

they are given access to data under specific security controls that allows them to perform within their job role. If an employee were to violate this, sanctions apply [22] (Security: 45CFR164.308(1) (ii)(C)). If a person were to be terminated, their access is to be immediately ended. Data breaches by former employees are a serious matter. An employee who was terminated from a behavioral health organization managed to steal patient health information on 300 clients. Although the analyst received a 30 day jail sentence, the data breach already occurred [23] (Jail Terms). HIPAA requires security training for all employees and it is here that the mission and culture of the organization are imbued with security in mind. The training is to focus on all of the required policies and how the organization responded to the addressable policies [24] (Security: 45CFR164.308(5)(i)). But training is not a one-time event, as the covered entity must have consistent security reminders and awareness. This can be a simple email reminder or an online refresher training or a workshop on a new security technique. Whatever the format, it is pertinent that organizations have security updates [25] (Security: 45CFR164.308(5)(ii)(A)).

Administrative security also involves having the covered entity establish a contingency plan should an emergency occur that could compromise data [26] (Security: 45CFR164.308(7)(i)). Clearly, in healthcare, critical operations must continue in a disaster and thus paired with the contingency plan is a data backup plan, a disaster recovery plan, and an emergency mode operation plan. These will assist the organization in having copies of data, to restore any lost data, and to continue to operate [27] (Security: 45CFR164.308(7)(A–C)).

Lastly, under administrative security is the issue of business associate agreements. Here is where an external entity has access to the covered entity's data to fulfill a business purpose. As data are being shared and transmitted, it is critical that the business associate also ascribes to the HIPAA Security Rule. The covered entity is to have in place a business associate agreement that specifies how the data are to be used and protected [28] (Security: 45CFR164.308.8(b)(1)).

Physical security and safeguards concern barriers that provide security. Those without a need to know are not to have access to the building or storage area of patient health information. A person who is to have legitimate access is to have their identity validated and then gain access to the property [29] Security: 45CFR164.310. The key is to make the access and lack thereof easy for the user such that a hindrance to one's work does not occur. Examples of physical safeguards include locks on door, sturdy file cabinets, and secure workstations. Physical safeguards are not common sense and thus can be overlooked. Workstations are left accessible, locks unlocked, and doors opened, as happened at a California physician's office, which resulted in a laptop with PHI being stolen [30] (Ouellette). Simply by locking the office door that contained the laptop with phi and this situation could have been averted.

Technical security and safeguards involve the information technology systems and one's personal computer and related devices. All of these, per the HIPAA Security Rule, must be accessed by only those with a need to know [31] (Security: 45CFR164.312(a)(1). Here is where the user must have a unique identification to enter into the system [32] (Security: 45CFR164.312(2)(i). This can be the common strong password, a fingerprint, retinal scan, or facial recognition. Whatever the method, it must be unique to the user with role-based access. Other technical security measures can include automatic log-offs after a certain period of inactive time, and encryption and decryption [33] (Security: 45CFR164.312(2)(iii) and (iv)).

HITECH

The **Health Information Technology for Economic and Clinical Health, (HITECH) Act (HITECH),** of 2009 advocated for the adoption of information technology to effectuate the delivery of healthcare and reinforced HIPAA. Business associate agreements became stricter, and reporting of breaches was exacted to here further support the patient and their protected health information. Covered entities are held more accountable for breaches. HITECH requires that individuals be notified when a breach occurs. For example, if an individual's patient health information was breached, the person is to receive a notification within 60 days [34] (HITECH: 45CFR164.404(a) and (b). If the breach is larger than 500 individuals, the covered entity must supply the local media outlet a press release on the circumstances of the breach [35] (HITECH: 45CFR164.406). In addition, to the media, the covered entity must also notify the Secretary of Health and Human Services. In turn, the Department of Health and Human Services will post the breach on their website as public information. So with this more stringent procedure, a covered entity must be transparent in what occurred. No longer can one hide the breach or feign ignorance. Business associates also have to follow the mandates for covered entities when a breach occurs. In this regard, business associates have responsibility for breach notification [36] (HITECH: 45CFR164.410). They cannot blame the covered entity, but they themselves must take responsibility and mitigate the breach. HITECH strengthened the notification process and therefore put covered entities and business associates on alert to be very careful when working with patient data.

Omnibus Final Rule

HITECH was followed up in 2013 by the **Omnibus Final Rule.** This Rule supported the patient in giving them greater access to their medical information and how it can be used. For example, if a patient pays in full for a service, they can restrict that portion of the treatment record from being shared with their insurer [37] (Omnibus: 45CFR164.522). This ascribes to the need to know principle whereby since the health plan is not paying for any of the service, they would not have a need to know the patient health information. With this change, the Notice of Privacy Practices needed to be updated and redistributed to patients. If patient health information is to be sold, an authorization is required hereby giving the patient the right to object [38]

(Omnibus: 45CFR164.508). The same is true for fundraising activities whereby the patient can object to having their information used [39] (Omnibus: 45CFR164.514).

Tangentially to support the patient, penalties for violations increased and thus gave greater incentives to covered entities to protect patient health information. If violations were repetitive or due to willful neglect, penalties reached $1.5 million for the calendar year [40] (Omnibus: 45CFR160.404). A **four-tier penalty system** was enacted, which assessed the following:

a. The number of individuals affected and in what time period.
b. What harm resulted such as physical, financial, reputation, or access to healthcare.
c. The prior record of compliance and violations of the offender.
d. The financial state of the offender, including if its finances affected their ability to comply [41] (Omnibus: 45CFR160.408).

But not only did the Omnibus Final Rule formulate policy on penalties, but it also rendered guidance on administrative safeguards to thus deter noncompliance. For example, a risk analysis is required to be conducted on the covered entity or the business associate. In addition and evaluation must be done when there are environmental or operational changes [42] (Omnibus: 45CFR164.308). So in the twenty-year period since the inception of HIPAA, much has been learned, but what remains uncompromised is the protection of patient health information.

Converting an Entity to a Covered Entity

Healthcare entities follow ethical and legal standards; thus, they want to "do the right thing." From an operational perspective, with the high amount of penalties, healthcare entities must be in compliance and thus be "covered entities." To begin, a key component is selecting a person or persons who will be the HIPAA Privacy Leader and the HIPAA Security Leader as required by law. These positions become the cornerstone for all else that follows in HIPAA, HITECH, and Omnibus. The person must be well-educated to the HIPAA law (although they need not be a lawyer) and its nuances, in addition to understanding the organization and it operations. An immediate duty is to ensure that the Notice of Privacy Practices is updated and if the organization has a website, to post the Notice on the site. Anytime the Notice is substantially updated, it must be distributed to all patients on their first visit after the update. Next, policies and formage must be updated in accordance with the new rules. It is recommended to write directly from the law rather than a secondary source as then there is no misinterpretation. Here, committees on each privacy and security, with even subcommittees on passwords, network security, risk assessments, and even social media use, for example, can be formed. Given that social media is so enculturated, violations are committed as one is not thinking of what they are actually doing with patient health information. The same goes for the business associates. Agreements must be in place with all business associates who are to have a clear understanding of HIPAA and how they must protect patient health information. To remain compliant, all workforce members must be trained on HIPAA and the training documentation be retained in the event that a noncompliance event occurs. As can be seen, HIPAA compliance has many parts, and thus skilled people are crucial to ensuring its success. HIPAA is ongoing and is truly a part of standard operating procedures.

Conclusions and Outlook

HIPAA is continuing to evolve. When HIPAA was instituted in 2003, there was no social media, yet there was email and telephone, No matter the time nor the technology, patient health information must be kept private and secure and the law adhered to. There must be a balance between patients, providers, and insurers having access to the data, yet having it protected from those who do not have a need to know. That is the role of the HIPAA personnel designated to maintain this balance within the confines of the law.

Summary

This chapter will discuss a topic akin to all healthcare professionals, protecting patient health information/data for its intended use and user. The chapter will focus on the highlights of the HIPAA Privacy and HIPAA Security Rules. These highlights include the HIPAA Notice, breaches, disclosures, and the minimum necessary clause under the HIPAA Privacy Rule, and technical, administrative, and physical security under the HIPAA Security Rule. HITECH was instituted to strengthen the above and key factors of the Enforcement Rule will be discussed. Next, the Omnibus/MegaRule will be discussed as to how the changing technologies have given challenges to data privacy and security. Lastly, how an organization transitions to a HIPAA-covered entity will be shown step by step. All of the above will be articulated with a case study on social media, the challenges and opportunities in healthcare. The chapter will end with short answer questions.

Case Study

Memorial Hospital's Unit 5B is a close-knit nursing group. Many of the staff have worked together for over 20 years. The newest member has eleven years in the group; turnover is almost nonexistent. But today, is the retirement luncheon for Sarah James after 37 years working on Unit 5B. She is also very well known throughout the hospital having served on various committees and volunteering for external hospital-related events. It is not surprising that the Unit 5B conference room quickly fills up. The door is opened and additional staff are in the hallway; a few people even say they will stop by later as it is simply too crowded. Food is eaten and gifts are given; now it is time for Sarah to give her farewell address. She thanks everyone as they snap multiple pictures to no end. Everyone is clapping and wishing her well. A few of her family members are in attendance, but others live out of state. Sarah, and a few others, post the pictures on social media. Almost instantaneously, texting ensues and more pictures, and even a video, are taken and posted.

Later that day, the unit manager is checking her social media sites. She immediately freezes on what she sees. In several of the pictures and in the video, patient health information that is written on the conference whiteboard is clearly visible. Given it is on social media sites, she wonders how many people will view it. What is she to do now?

This is a HIPAA breach of the privacy and security of patient health information. Now one must assess that all reverts to being HIPAA compliant.

Useful Resources

1. ahima.org—American Health Information Management Association
2. amia.org—American Medical Informatics Association
3. himss.org—Healthcare Information and Management Systems Society
4. hhs.gov/ocr/index.html—United States Department of Health and Human Services, Office for Civil Rights

Review Questions

1. Per the HIPAA Privacy Rule, discuss what is meant by "minimum necessary."
2. What is a business associate?
3. Who receives the Notice of Privacy Practices and why?
4. Name the three areas of HIPAA Security and how adherence can be achieved in this situation.
5. Name three items that must be done to become a HIPAA-covered entity.
6. What was the effect of social media in this situation?

Appendix: Answers to Review Questions

1. Per the HIPAA Privacy Rule, discuss what is meant by "minimum necessary."

Minimum necessary pertains to only sharing the least amount of patient health information with those people who have a need to know. This is based on the role of the person, and the PHI needed for them to complete their role tasks.

2. What is a business associate?

This is a person or entity external to the covered entity, but in their business dealings with a covered entity, they will encounter patient health information. There must be a signed business associate agreement between the two parties.

3. Who receives the Notice of Privacy Practices and why?

Patients upon their first visit to a provider and when the Notice changes receive one. The Notice specifies the patient's rights in regards to PHI and how their PHI is used.

4. Name the three areas of HIPAA Security and how adherence can be achieved in this situation.

Technical security, administrative security, and physical security.

5. Name three items that must be done to become a HIPAA-covered entity.

  (a) Designate a person to manage HIPAA.
  (b) Develop policies and formage based on the HIPAA law.
  (c) Ensure that business associate agreements are in place.

6. What was the effect of social media in this situation?

Social media created a HIPAA violation as once information is out via a social media site, it cannot be taken back and can be further spread.

References

1. OCR Concludes 2018 with All-Time Record Year for HIPAA Enforcement. https://www.hhs.gov/hipaa/for-professionals/compliance-enforcement/agreements/2018enforcement/index.html. Accessed October 15, 2019.

2. US Department of Health and Human Services. Numbers at a Glance. https://www.hhs.gov/hipaa/for-professionals/compliance-enforcement/data/numbers-glance/index.html#allcomplaints. Accessed October 23, 2019.

3. HIPAA Privacy Law: Standards for Privacy of Individually Identifiable Health Information. U.S. Department of Health and Human Services, Office for Civil Rights. (45CFR Parts 160 and 164) Federal Register, August 14, 2002. 45CFR160.103.

4. HIPAA Privacy Law: Standards for Privacy of Individually Identifiable Health Information. U.S. Department of Health and Human Services, Office for Civil Rights. (45CFR Parts 160 and 164) Federal Register, August 14, 2002. 45CFR164.502(b).

5. HIPAA Privacy Law: Standards for Privacy of Individually Identifiable Health Information. U.S. Department of Health and Human Services, Office for Civil Rights. (45CFR Parts 160 and 164) Federal Register, August 14, 2002. 45CFR164.502(a)(1).

6. HIPAA Privacy Law: Standards for Privacy of Individually Identifiable Health Information. U.S. Department of Health and Human Services, Office for Civil Rights. (45CFR Parts 160 and 164) Federal Register, August 14, 2002. 45CFR164.508.

7. HIPAA Privacy Law: Standards for Privacy of Individually Identifiable Health Information. U.S. Department of Health and Human Services, Office for Civil Rights. (45CFR Parts 160 and 164) Federal Register, August 14, 2002. 45CFR164.510.

8. HIPAA Privacy Law: Standards for Privacy of Individually Identifiable Health Information. U.S. Department of Health and Human Services, Office for Civil Rights. (45CFR Parts 160 and 164) Federal Register, August 14, 2002. 45CFR164.512.

9. HIPAA Privacy Law: Standards for Privacy of Individually Identifiable Health Information. U.S. Department of Health and Human Services, Office for Civil Rights. (45CFR Parts 160 and 164) Federal Register, August 14, 2002. 45CFR164.520.

10. HIPAA Privacy Law: Standards for Privacy of Individually Identifiable Health Information. U.S. Department of Health and Human Services, Office for Civil Rights. (45CFR Parts 160 and 164) Federal Register, August 14, 2002. 45CFR164.520(c)(3)(i).

11. HIPAA Privacy Law: Standards for Privacy of Individually Identifiable Health Information. U.S. Department of Health and Human Services, Office for Civil Rights. (45CFR Parts 160 and 164) Federal Register, August 14, 2002. 45CFR164.524(a)(1)(i).

12. HIPAA Privacy Law: Standards for Privacy of Individually Identifiable Health Information. U.S. Department of Health and Human Services, Office for Civil Rights. (45CFR Parts 160 and 164) Federal Register, August 14, 2002. 45CFR164.524(b)(2).

13. HIPAA Privacy Law: Standards for Privacy of Individually Identifiable Health Information. U.S. Department of Health and Human Services, Office for Civil Rights. (45CFR Parts 160 and 164) Federal Register, August 14, 2002. 45CFR164.526(b)(2).

14. HIPAA Privacy Law: Standards for Privacy of Individually Identifiable Health Information. U.S. Department of Health and Human Services, Office for Civil Rights. (45CFR Parts 160 and 164) Federal Register, August 14, 2002. 45CFr164.530(a)(1).

15. HIPAA Privacy Law: Standards for Privacy of Individually Identifiable Health Information. U.S. Department of Health and Human Services, Office for Civil Rights. (45CFR Parts 160 and 164) Federal Register, August 14, 2002. 45CFR164.530(2)(b)(1) & (C)(ii).

16. HIPAA Privacy Law: Standards for Privacy of Individually Identifiable Health Information. U.S. Department of Health and Human Services, Office for Civil Rights. (45CFR Parts 160 and 164) Federal Register, August 14, 2002. 45CFR164.530(d)(1).

17. HIPAA Privacy Law: Standards for Privacy of Individually Identifiable Health Information. U.S. Department of Health and Human Services, Office for Civil Rights. (45CFR Parts 160 and 164) Federal Register, August 14, 2002. 45CFR164.530(e)(1).

18. HIPAA Privacy Law: Standards for Privacy of Individually Identifiable Health Information. U.S. Department of Health and Human Services, Office for Civil Rights. (45CFR Parts 160 and 164) Federal Register, August 14, 2002. 45CFR164.530(j)(2).

19. HIPAA Security Law: Health Insurance Reform: Security Standards Final Rule. U.S. Department of Health and Human Services, Office of the Secretary (45 CFR parts 160, 162, and 164) Federal Register, February 20, 2003. 45CFR164.306)(d).

20. HIPAA Security Law: Health Insurance Reform: Security Standards Final Rule. U.S. Department of Health and Human Services, Office of the Secretary (45 CFR parts 160, 162, and 164) Federal Register, February 20, 2003. 45CFR164.308(2)).

21. HIPAA Security Law: Health Insurance Reform: Security Standards Final Rule. U.S. Department of Health and Human Services, Office of the Secretary (45 CFR parts 16, 162, and 164) Federal Register, February 20, 2003. 45CFR164.308(1).

22. HIPAA Security Law: Health Insurance Reform: Security Standards Final Rule. U.S. Department of Health and Human Services, Office of the Secretary (45 CFR parts 160, 162, and 164) Federal Register, February 20, 2003. 45CFR164.308(1)(ii)(C)).

23. Jail Terms for HIPAA Violations by Employees HIPAA Journal, March 22, 2018. https://www.hipaajournal.com/jail-terms-for-hipaa-violations-by-employees/. Accessed October 30, 2019).

24. HIPAA Security Law: Health Insurance Reform: Security Standards Final Rule. U.S. Department of Health and Human Services, Office of the Secretary (45 CFR parts 160, 162, and 164) Federal Register, February 20, 2003. 45CFR164.308(5)(i)).

25. HIPAA Security Law: Health Insurance Reform: Security Standards Final Rule. U.S. Department of Health and Human Services, Office of the Secretary (45 CFR parts 160, 162, and 164) Federal Register, February 20, 2003. 45CFR164.308(5)(ii)(A)).

26. HIPAA Security Law: Health Insurance Reform: Security Standards Final Rule. U.S. Department of Health and Human Services, Office of the Secretary (45 CFR parts 160, 162, and 164) Federal Register, February 20, 2003. 45CFR164.308(7)(i)).

27. HIPAA Security Law: Health Insurance Reform: Security Standards Final Rule. U.S. Department of Health and Human Services, Office of the Secretary (45 CFR parts 160, 162, and 164) Federal Register, February 20, 2003. 45CFR164.308(7)(A-C)).

28. HIPAA Security Law: Health Insurance Reform: Security Standards Final Rule. U.S. Department of Health and Human Services, Office of the Secretary (45 CFR parts 160, 162, and 164) Federal Register, February 20, 2003. (45CFR164.308.8(b)(1)).

29. HIPAA Security Law: Health Insurance Reform: Security Standards Final Rule. U.S. Department of Health and Human Services, Office of the Secretary (45 CFR parts 160, 162, and 164) Federal Register, February 20, 2003. 45CFR164.310.

30. Ouellette, Patrick. Health IT Security, Thieves Steal Laptop with phi from California internist, September 9, 2013. Accessed November 5, 2019. https://healthitsecurity.com/news/thieves-steal-laptop-with-phi-from-california-internist).

31. HIPAA Security Law: Health Insurance Reform: Security Standards Final Rule. U.S. Department of Health and Human Services, Office of the Secretary (45 CFR parts 160, 162, and 164) Federal Register, February 20, 2003. 45CFR164.312(a)(1).

32. HIPAA Security Law: Health Insurance Reform: Security Standards Final Rule. U.S. Department of Health and Human Services, Office of the Secretary (45 CFR parts 160, 162, and 164) Federal Register, February 20, 2003. 45CFR164.312(2)(i).

33. HIPAA Security Law: Health Insurance Reform: Security Standards Final Rule. U.S. Department of Health and Human Services, Office of the Secretary (45 CFR parts 160, 162, and 164) Federal Register, February 20, 2003. 45CFR164.312(2)(iii)&(iv)).

34. HITECH: Breach Notification for Unsecured PHI: Interim Final Rule. U.S. Department of Health and Human Services. (45CFR Parts 160 and 164) Federal Register, August 24, 2009. 45CFR164.404(a) & (b).

35. HITECH: Breach Notification for Unsecured PHI: Interim Final Rule. U.S. Department of Health and Human Services. (45CFR Parts 160 and 164) Federal Register, August 24, 2009. 45CFR164.406.

36. HITECH: Breach Notification for Unsecured PHI: Interim Final Rule. U.S. Department of Health and Human Services. (45CFR Parts 160 and 164) Federal Register, August 24, 2009. 45CFR164.410.

37. Omnibus Final Rule: U.S. Department of Health and Human Services, Office of the Secretary (45CFR Parts 160 and 164) Federal Register, January 25, 2013. 45CFR164.522.

38. Omnibus Final Rule: U.S. Department of Health and Human Services, Office of the Secretary (45CFR Parts 160 and 164) Federal Register, January 25, 2013. 45CFR164.508).

39. Omnibus Final Rule: U.S. Department of Health and Human Services, Office of the Secretary (45CFR Parts 160 and 164) Federal Register, January 25, 2013. 45CFR164.514.

40. Omnibus Final Rule: U.S. Department of Health and Human Services, Office of the Secretary (45CFR Parts 160 and 164) Federal Register, January 25, 2013. 45CFR160.404).

41. Omnibus Final Rule: U.S. Department of Health and Human Services, Office of the Secretary (45CFR Parts 160 and 164) Federal Register, January 25, 2013. 45CFR160.408.

42. Omnibus Final Rule: U.S. Department of Health and Human Services, Office of the Secretary (45CFR Parts 160 and 164) Federal Register, January 25, 2013. 45CFR164.308.

Bernd Schütze

Learning Objectives
- To obtain an introduction to the European General Data Protection Regulation (GDPR)
- To understand that any processing of personal data, especially of course patient data, may only be carried out if a legal framework permits it
- To understand the rights that persons can exercise against the companies processing their data
- To understand that personal data must be protected against unauthorized access and that the GDPR also requires a documentation for the processing of personal data

Key Terms
- Data Protection and Data Security from the perspective of the European legislator

Introduction

Since May 25, 2018, the General Data Protection Regulation (GDPR) is the most important legal regulation in Europe with regard to data protection. The GDPR essentially adopts the basic principles of data protection law known from

B. Schütze (✉)
Düsseldorf, Germany
e-mail: schuetze@medizin-informatik.org

Directive 95/46/EC ("Directive 95/46/EC of the European Parliament and of the Council of October 24, 1995, on the protection of individuals with regard to the processing of personal data and on the free movement of such data"): The principles of data minimization, purpose limitation, lawfulness, fairness, and transparency are also reflected in the new regulatory framework. However, since the directive never achieved a harmonization of data protection regulations in Europe, it was replaced by a much more detailed regulation.

But even this regulation does not achieve full harmonization, especially in the area of health care. The European legislator can only regulate cross-border processes; for processes that take place in one member state and do not affect other member states, the European legislator lacks the authority to regulate. For this reason, the legislative competence in health care is primarily the responsibility of the respective national legislators. However, the GDPR imposes conditions on the national legislators, which they must adhere to in their legislation on health data protection.

The most important provisions of the GDPR are therefore presented below. However, this brief presentation cannot, of course, include a complete discussion of all of these regulations, and readers are referred to the relevant commentary literature.

© Springer Nature Switzerland AG 2022
U. H. Hübner et al. (eds.), *Nursing Informatics*, Health Informatics,
https://doi.org/10.1007/978-3-030-91237-6_29

Europe vs. Law of the Member State Law: When Does What Apply?

In European legislation, the most important regulations are the European directives and regulations. According to Article 288(2) Treaty on the Functioning of the European Union (TFEU), regulations are binding legal acts that are directly applicable in all countries of the EU and are binding in all their parts. Directives, in turn, are legal acts in which only one goal to be achieved is specified; directives must first be transposed by the respective legislators of the EU countries into their own legal provisions, whereby the country-specific regulations must, however, implement the goal specified by the EU. Both directives and regulations contain "recitals" [1]. Recitals are non-binding and do not themselves constitute regulations. However, the recitals contain the justification for the actual regulations and are therefore used to interpret what the regulation or directive is intended to achieve.

The GDPR is—as the name suggests—a directly applicable regulation that takes precedence over national law.

Principles Governing the Processing of Personal Data

Article 5(1) GDPR contains principles that must always be guaranteed in any processing of personal data. These principles include:

– Lawfulness, fairness, and transparency (Article 5(1a) GDPR):
  Personal data may only be processed in a lawful manner, in good faith and in a way that is comprehensible to the data subject. This includes:

  1. The processing must serve a legitimate purpose, and there must be a legitimate reason for processing the data. Similarly, if personal data is processed in a third country, the requirements of Chapter V GDPR must be met. If contract processors are used, the specifications for contract processing must

be complied with; if cooperation with partners is involved, a contract for joint processing may have to be concluded.

  2. What exactly the legislator understands by the regulation of "processing in good faith" is not specified anywhere in the GDPR. However, Amendment 38 of Directive 95/46 contains the following [2]:
    "Data processing in good faith requires that data subjects are able to know the existence of processing and to be properly and fully informed about the conditions of collection when data are collected from them."
    This means that the processing must be "fair."

  3. The processing of data must be transparent for the data subjects. This requires in particular that the rights of data subjects as set out in Chapter II GDPR be guaranteed.

– Purpose limitation (Article 5(1b) GDPR):
  Personal data may only be processed within the framework of defined, clear and legitimate purposes. In particular, processing for as yet unknown purposes is therefore ruled out; "data retention" is not compatible with the provisions of the GDPR.

  A change of the purpose again requires a separate permit. Further processing for archiving purposes in the public interest, for scientific or historical research purposes or for statistical purposes is not considered incompatible with the original purpose, which may have to be proven for other changes of purpose.

– Data minimisation (Article 5(1c) GDPR):
  The processing of personal data must be *necessary* for the purpose pursued and be *appropriate*. The processing of personal data is only necessary if the purpose pursued cannot be achieved without such processing. In other words, the data are indispensable for achieving the purposes pursued.

  Adequacy is deemed to exist when there is no "less onerous" means of processing which interferes less with the rights and freedoms of natural persons.

Data minimization therefore does not imply a limitation of the absolute amount of data, it may well be necessary and appropriate to process a very large amount of personal data.

- Accuracy (Article 5(1d) GDPR):
The data must be accurate and, where necessary, kept up to date for the duration of the processing, which runs from the time the data are collected until their deletion ("life cycle" of the data).

All "reasonable" measures must be taken to ensure that personal data which are inaccurate in relation to the purposes of their processing are erased or rectified without delay.

While a correction of incorrect data must always be made, an update of data is only necessary if the update is necessary for the processing of the data. If a patient was under treatment two years ago and this patient moves after two years today, there is no incorrect date, because the address was correct at the time of treatment. Therefore, a correction is not necessary. However, if this patient comes to the hospital for treatment again, the new address must be entered.

- Storage limitation (Article 5(1e) GDPR):
Personal data may only be stored in a form that allows the identification of the data subjects for as long as necessary for the purposes for which they were collected.

Pseudonymized data also allow the identification of a person. Article 5(1e) GDPR therefore requires that personal data be deleted or made anonymous as quickly as possible. This means that anonymization or deletion must take place either directly after the purpose has been achieved or after expiry of the statutory retention obligations, if these exist for processing.

If the processing is carried out solely for archiving purposes in the public interest or for scientific and historical research or statistical purposes, the data may be stored for a longer period if appropriate technical and organizational measures are taken to protect the rights and freedoms of the data subjects. This includes in particular that the processing procedure is developed and implemented in accordance with the requirements of Article 25 GDPR (see Sect. 6.1.1.1).

- Integrity and Confidentiality (Article 5(1f) GDPR):
The integrity of the data and protection against unauthorized access and processing must be guaranteed for each processing operation. This is ensured in particular by implementing the requirements of Article 32 GDPR ("security of personal data").

Article 5(2) GDPR requires that compliance with these principles must be demonstrated. In other words, there is an accountability obligation for every processing operation, which ultimately includes the fulfillment of all requirements of the GDPR.

Authorization

The processing of personal data is generally prohibited under Article 6(1) and Article 9(1) GDPR. Data may only be processed if processing is permitted by law or if the person whose data is to be processed has expressly consented to the processing.

Whenever patient data are processed, the first step to be clarified is why I am allowed to process data.

Legal Grounds for Permission

For data of the special categories according to Article 9(1) GDPR, Article 9(2) GDPR contains permitted offenses, e.g.,

- Occupational medicine: Article 9(2h) in conjunction with Article 9(3) GDPR.
- Legally regulated disease registers (e.g. cancer registers), legal quality assurance: Article 9 (2 h) GDPR.
- Federal health statistics: Article 9(2j) in conjunction with Article 89(1) GDPR.

- Scientific and historical research: Article 9(2j) in conjunction with Article 89(1) GDPR.
- Billing of services: Article 9(2f) GDPR.
- Patient care: Article 9(2h) GDPR.

However, some of these permitting offenses require a national permitting norm under national law, e.g., Article 9(2j) GDPR regarding research. National licensing requirements for research are found, for example, in the German "Arzneimittelgesetz" with regard to research on medicinal products or in the social security codes with regard to research with social data.

Consent

According to Article 9(2a), the processing of special categories of personal data is allowed if the data subject gives his or her consent and Union law or the law of Member States does not prohibit the processing.

For a valid consent, the requirements of the GDPR must be observed. Consent must be given before the collection or processing of the data begins. Consent cannot be used to legitimize processing retroactively. The GDPR describes the "conditions for consent" in Article 7 GDPR. These include, among other things, the verifiability of consent by the responsible body, the clear, unambiguous, and voluntary declaration of intent by the informed consenting party and the possibility of revocation. All the information mentioned in Articles 13 and 14 GDPR must at least be given to the person concerned so that the person can be regarded as informed. Moreover, consent is always earmarked, i.e., it always applies in relation to the processing operations necessary to achieve the specific purpose. The GDPR does not prescribe a specific form for consent. However, the revocation of consent must be as simple as the process of granting consent itself. If the consent is part of a larger document, such as part of another contract, for example, the consent must be clearly distinguishable from the other facts depicted in this contract.

Rights of Data Subjects

The rights of data subjects are defined in Chapter III GDPR (Articles 12–22). The following rights of the data subject and obligations towards the data subject are outlined below:

- Duty to inform when personal data are collected or changed for a different purpose, differentiated according to:
  - Collection from the data subject.
  - Collection not from the data subject ("third-party collection").
- Right of access of the data subject.
- Right of rectification.
- Right of erasure.
- Right to restrict processing.
- Obligation to notify correction, deletion, or restriction.
- Right to data portability.
- Right of objection.
- Limitation of the admissibility of automated decisions in individual cases.

According to Article 12(1), the person responsible must take appropriate measures to comply with these obligations. In other words, a process must be established from the outset to ensure that each person concerned can exercise his or her rights and that the responsible person fulfills his or her obligations without culpable delay.

If a responsible person can *prove that* he or she cannot identify a person, a responsible person may refuse to comply with the data subject's rights (Article 12(2 sentence 2) in conjunction with Article 11(2) GDPR, unless the data subject provides additional information for identification purposes. In cases in which the data controller is unable to carry out the identification and accordingly cannot implement the data subject's rights, he or she must notify the persons exercising their rights.

If, on the other hand, there is only *reasonable* doubt as to the identity of the person, the responsible person may, in accordance with Article 12(6) GDPR, request additional information *necessary* to confirm the identity of the data subject. The

German Data Protection Supervisory Authorities cites a postal address for electronic requests for information as an example of additional information. Ultimately, it is of less interest to the patient whether the processing of personal data is carried out by a processor or by the data controller itself; patients do not have a right of objection. And depending on the number of processors, the idea might arise that other information might be more "hidden" by this information. Finally, it should be borne in mind that there may be changes in the processors used and that without the use of the Internet, the legally required information regarding the list of recipients may prove difficult or even impossible to obtain.

The information must always be communicated in clear and simple language, as required by Article 12 GDPR.

Right to Information

When collecting personal data, the information obligations resulting from Articles 13 and 14 GDPR must be fulfilled.

Ideally, every patient should receive an information letter when treatment is started, in which the necessary details are included in accordance with Article 13 or Article 14 GDPR. This brochure should then also contain a link to the homepage of the person responsible, on which the details of the processors are listed:

– Name of the processor.
– The activity (e.g., support hospital information system).
– When the contractual relationship began.
– If applicable, when the contractual relationship ended (open end date = contractual relationship continues).

In principle, the information can of course also be included in the information letter. But in order to follow the idea of transparency resulting from Article 12 GDPR, it seems appropriate to outsource this information. Ultimately, it is of less interest to the patient whether the data is pro-

vided by a processor or by the person responsible himself or herself; patients do not have a right of objection. And depending on the number of processors, the idea might arise that other information might be "hidden" by this information. Finally, it should be borne in mind that changes may occur in the processors used and that without the use of the Internet, the legally required information regarding the list of recipients may prove difficult or even impossible to obtain.

The information must always be communicated in clear and simple language, as required by Article 12 GDPR.

Right of Access to Personal Data

Every patient has the right to be informed about the data processed or stored about him or her by a responsible person. This must be communicated to him/her as part of the obligation to inform as discussed in chapter "Right to Information". Ideally, this information should include a telephone number as well as a special non-personalized e-mail address, which will therefore be retained even if the responsible person changes.

According to Article 15(3) GDPR, the controller must also provide data subjects with a copy of the personal data, which are the subject of the processing. Accordingly, data controllers should be able to export all data relating to a patient to a pdf file in order to be able to provide this file to requesting patients.

Right of Rectification

According to Article 16, every patient has the right to have incorrect data corrected. Since data is the basis of all medical treatment and research, the correction of incorrect data is of course also in the very own interest of the data processing unit.

However, under Article 16 GDPR, every patient also has the right to have incomplete data completed, if necessary by means of a supplementary declaration. This may lead to different interpretations on the part of the responsible person and the data subject regarding the interpretation of "incomplete." The European legislator therefore requires that this right be exercised "having regard to the purposes of the processing." This means that the assessment of incompleteness must be made from the perspective of the purpose of the processing. In accordance with the requirement to minimize data resulting from Article 5(1c) GDPR, only data necessary for the purpose of processing may be supplemented here. However, it is again in the interest of the controller that this data supporting the processing purpose be supplemented, and that it will therefore be possible at any time.

Every patient must be made aware that these rights exist for him or her. Ideally, this is done in the information letter mentioned in Sect. 1.2.1.

Right to Restrict Processing ("Blocking")

According to Article 18 GDPR, every patient has the right to request the controller to restrict the processing under the conditions of Article 18(1) GDPR. The information letter described in chapter "Right to Information" was intended to inform each patient that he or she has a right to restrict the processing of his or her data. At the same time, he or she should be informed that this right may be restricted by legal provisions.

The person responsible must bear in mind that, according to Article 18(2) GDPR, such a block may only be reversed with the consent of the person concerned. Otherwise, processing, apart from storage, may only take place

- To assert, exercise, or defend legal claims, or
- To protect the rights of another natural or legal person, or
- On grounds of important public interest of the Union or a Member State

take place. Furthermore, in accordance with the requirements of Article 18(3) GDPR, the person responsible must inform the data subject who has obtained a block before the restriction is lifted.

Right of Erasure

According to Article 17 GDPR, every data subject has the right to have data concerning him or her deleted if the circumstances set out in Article 17(1) GDPR apply and the exceptions set out in Article 17(3) GDPR do not apply.

The information letter described in Sect. 1.2.1 should inform each patient that he or she has the right to have his or her data deleted. At the same time, the patients should be informed that this right may be restricted by legal provisions, such as legal retention periods.

Right of Objection

According to Article 21(6) GDPR, every data subject has the right to object, on grounds "arising from his or her particular situation," to the processing of data relating to him or her for the purposes of scientific or historical research. According to Article 21(4) GDPR, every data subject must be expressly informed of this right.

Each respondent or patient should therefore be informed in the information letter mentioned chapter "Right to Information" of his right to object to data processing. It should be taken into account that the respondent or patient is also informed that the right to object may be restricted by legal regulations, e.g., that data must be stored in accordance with legal provisions despite his or her objection.

Right to Data Portability

According to Article 20 GDPR, under the conditions of Article 20(1a,b) GDPR, every patient has the right to

- to be received his personal data from the responsible person a structured, common, and machine-readable format.
  and
- to communicate them or have them communicated to another controller without hindrance by the controller to whom the personal data have been made available.

Each patient should be made aware of these rights in the information letter referred to chapter "Right to Information". However, it should also be pointed out that no recipient of these data is legally obliged to accept these data at all or in the format provided by the data controller.

Data Protection Officer

Obligation to Designate

According to Article 37(1c) GDPR, a data protection officer must be appointed, among other things, if "the core activity consists in the extensive processing of special categories of data pursuant to Article 9." The core activity of persons responsible for health care or medical research consists in the processing of health and/or genetic data, both of which are listed in Article 9(1) GDPR.

Amendments 75 and 91 state that two influencing factors are to be taken into account in the area of the "scope of data processing:" On the one hand, the number of persons, on the other hand, the amount of data processed. According to Amendment 91, the scope of data processing must also take into account whether large amounts of personal data are processed at the regional, national, or supranational level, which ultimately also addresses the volume of data ("large amounts").

The 'Guidelines for Data Protection Officers' [3] issued by the European Data Protection Board (EDPB) recommend that the following factors should be taken into account when determining whether processing operations are substantial:

- The number of persons concerned—either as a specific number or as a proportion of the relevant population.
- The data volume and/or the spectrum of data in process.
- The duration or permanence of the data processing activity.
- The geographical extent of the processing activity.

Information to and Examination by the Data Protection Officer

According to Article 38(1) GDPR, a data protection officer must be "properly and promptly involved in all matters relating to the protection of personal data." This naturally includes the collection of health or genetic data in a clinical register.

In accordance with Article 39(1) a) GDPR, the data protection officer is obliged to monitor compliance with the provisions of all data protection regulations. The Data Protection Officer must therefore not only be informed, but all information must be made available so that the Data Protection Officer can fulfill the inspection duties.

Records of Processing Activities

The records of processing activities is required in Article 30 GDPR by all controllers (Article 30(1) GDPR) and processors (Article 30(2) GDPR) who carry out processing of special categories of data in accordance with Article 9(1) GDPR. Since health data as well as genetic data are covered by this regulation, every clinical register must necessarily keep a register of processing activities. On the subject of "List of processing activities," please refer to bitkom's practical assistance for the interpretation of the legal regulations [4].

The GDPR describes the minimum contents of the directory in Article 30(1) (person responsible) and Article 30(2) (processor); the contents are listed in Table 29.1.

The register shall be kept in writing, including in electronic form.

Data Security

The GDPR contains a risk-oriented approach: the greater the risk of processing, the higher the security requirements.

Table 29.1 Minimum contents of the list of processing activities

Article 30(1) GDPR (controller)	Article 30(2) GDPR (processors)
	The name and contact details of the processor and, where appropriate, the representative of the processor
The name and contact details of the person responsible and, where appropriate, of the person jointly responsible with him/her, the representative of the person responsible	The name and contact details of each controller on whose behalf the processor is acting and, where appropriate, the representative of the controller
The name and contact details of any data protection officer	The name and contact details of any data protection officer of the processor and the controller
Purposes of the processing	Categories of processing operations carried out on behalf of each controller
Description of the categories of data subjects	
Description of the categories of personal data	
Categories of recipients [...], including recipients in third countries or international organizations	Where appropriate, transfers of personal data to a third country or international organization, including an indication of the third country or international organisation concerned, and, in the case of the data transfers referred to in the second subparagraph of Article 49(1), the documentation of appropriate safeguards
The time limits foreseen for the deletion of the different categories of data	
A general description of the technical and organizational measures pursuant to Article 32	A general description of the technical and organizational measures referred to in Article 32

Data Protection Impact Assessment

Article 35 GDPR requires a data protection impact assessment (DPIA) for certain processing operations, whenever a processing operation involves a high risk. As an example, the GDPR also lists the extensive processing of special categories of personal data. In other words, when processing health data, one should always check whether a DPIA is necessary.

A DPIA is a legally required risk management: based on an assessment of the risk to the persons affected by the (data) processing, measures must be taken to minimize the risk. If the risk can be minimized by taking technical and organizational measures to such an extent that it is acceptable from the point of view of the persons concerned, the processing may be carried out. If not, the processing must be waived or coordinated with the competent supervisory authority, which will then decide whether or not processing may take place.

The minimum contents of a DPIA are specified by Article 35 GDPR:

- A systematic description of the planned processing operations.

- A systematic description of the purposes of the processing, including where appropriate the legitimate interests pursued by the controller.
- An assessment of the necessity and proportionality of the processing operations in relation to the purpose.
- An assessment of the risks to the rights and freedoms of data subjects in accordance with Article 35(1) GDPR.
- The corrective actions planned to address the risks.

Both the decision as to whether a DPIA is required or not and the planning and implementation of a DPIA must be documented accordingly in order to meet the legally required obligations to provide evidence.

Privacy by Design and Privacy by Default

Article 25 GDPR requires that appropriate technical and organizational measures be taken to implement the data protection principles (Article 5 GDPR) and to enforce the rights of data subjects (Article 12ff GDPR). This must take place both at the time when the means for processing are determined and at the time of the actual processing. Article 25 GDPR thus requires security of processing from the planning to the deletion of the data; personal data must be protected throughout the entire life cycle.

While Privacy by Design aims already at the conceptual phase, Privacy by Default requires that a data protection-friendly basic attitude always exists at the beginning. The European Data Protection Board (EDPB) published guidelines on the subject in November 2019 [5]; it is advisable to read the text in order to know the view of the EDPB on the subject.

Internationally, the implementation of Ann Cavoukian's "7 Foundational Principles" have gained acceptance with regard to "Privcy by design" [6]:

1. Proactive, not reactive; as prevention and not as remedy.
    The Privacy by Design approach is characterized by proactive, not reactive measures, data protection violations are to be prevented.
2. Data protection as default setting.
    Privacy by Design is intended to ensure the best possible protection of privacy. The objective is that the individual person does not have to do anything for the protection, since the best possible protection is inherent in the system as a standard setting. But of course the individual may reduce the protection.
3. Data protection is embedded in the design.
    Privacy by Design is embedded in the design and architecture of IT systems and business practices. Data protection should be an essential part of the system.
4. Full functionality—one positive sum, no zero sum.
    Privacy by Design meets all legitimate interests and objectives. Privacy by Design must be a satisfactory result for both parties, and there should be no loss of functionality.
5. End-to-end security. Protection during the entire life cycle.
    Privacy by design offers protection from the initial entry to the deletion, i.e., the effect

of Privacy by Design must cover the entire life cycle of the data.
6. Visibility and transparency—ensuring openness.
    Privacy by Design provides security for all parties involved. Individual components and processes remain visible and transparent; equally for users and providers.
7. Respecting the privacy of users: Ensuring user-centered design.
    Privacy by Design demands that the interests of the user come first.

Requirements 1, 2, 4, 5, 6, 7 are always (also) to be considered and implemented in a project/implementation-specific manner. Requirements 3 and 5 also depend on the IT system used: What offers the IT system, what does the manufacturer provide.

Processing Security

Article 32 GDPR requires the taking of appropriate technical and organizational measures to ensure a level of protection appropriate to the risk. With regard to appropriateness, these measures include

- the state of the art.
- the implementation costs.
- the nature, scope, circumstances, and purposes of the processing and
- the likelihood and seriousness of risks to the rights and freedoms of natural persons,

to be considered. The law requires that the measures

- **pseudonymization** and **encryption of** personal data.
- ability to ensure the **confidentiality, integrity, availability and resilience** of systems and services relating to the processing of personal data on a lasting basis.
- the ability to **quickly restore the availability of** and **access** to data in the event of a physical or technical **incident**.

- **a procedure for regular review, assessment, and evaluation of** the effectiveness of the technical and organizational measures to ensure the security of processing,

be taken into account. This means that, where appropriate, reasons must be given if one of these measures cannot be taken. For example, if pseudonymization could pose a risk to patients.

Article 32 GDPR thus requires

- a risk evaluation and assessment of the processing.
- the presentation of a catalog of measures.
- (internal) audits including management evaluation and
- procedures for correction/adjustment of measures taken ("PDCA cycle").

Duty of Proof: Hopefully Everything Documented?

Article 5 GDPR requires proof of compliance with the data processing principles set out therein. The required burden of proof also includes a reversal of the burden of proof: if I cannot provide the legally required proof, the data protection supervisory authority or a court can assume that the person responsible has not complied with the required obligations. In conjunction with the drastic increase in fines, this provides sufficient motivation to comply with the statutory documentation obligations.

The GDPR contains documentation obligations in various places. For example

Proof of the essential requirements (Article 5 GDPR)
Documentation of
- Compliance with legality, transparency (including third country processing),
- Who is the responsible person.
- Purpose(s)/Earmarking.
- Data minimization.
- Correctness.

- Persons concerned (categories).
- Data (categories).
- Recipients (categories).
- Deletion periods/memory limitation.
- Integrity, confidentiality.

Consent (Article 7 GDPR)

"[…] the controller must be able to demonstrate that the data subject has given his or her consent to the processing of his or her personal data;" this includes proof
- Voluntary.
- For the specific case (= earmarking).

Being informed (in particular, being aware of the facts, e.g., also taking into account Articles 12, 13, 14 GDPR)
- An unequivocal expression of will (in the form of a declaration or other unequivocal affirmative act).
- Explicit declaration of intent.

Information obligations (Articles 13, 14 GDPR)
Proof that the person responsible has fulfilled his documentation obligations. I.e., documenting the process, regularly checking the process, and documenting the inspection and inspection results.

Processing security
Proof of the requirements of Artt. 25, 35, and 32 GDPR

Order processing (Article 28 GDPR)

The person responsible must prove
- Criteria for the selection of the processor.
- Compliance with requirements Article 32 GDPR (safety processing).
- Guaranteeing the rights of the data subject.
- Execution and result of an on-the-spot audit (if carried out).
- Conclusion of the contract including compliance with the content requirements of Article 28(3) sentence 2 lit. a-h GDPR.
- Compliance with contractually agreed obligations.

List of processing activities (Article 30 GDPR)

The following must be documented
- Name/contact details of person responsible, if available also data protection officer.
- Purpose(s).
- Persons concerned (categories).
- Data (categories).
- Recipients (categories).
- Deletion periods.
- Third country processing.
- Planned and implemented technical and organizational measures.

Violations of the protection of personal data

The documentation of the data mismatches shall include
- Responsible.
- Name/contact details Data protection officer or other contact person.
- Purpose(s).
- Data subjects (categories), approximate number of data subjects.

- Data (categories).
- Description of the nature of the breach of protection.
- Description of the likely consequences of the breach of personal data protection (risk assessment).
- Obligation to notify.
- Description of the measures taken or proposed to remedy the breach of protection and, where appropriate, measures to mitigate its possible adverse effects.

Documentation for third country processing

- Article 44 GDPR: "[…] shall be permitted only if the person responsible and the processor comply with the conditions laid down in this chapter and the other provisions of this Regulation are also complied with; […]."
  → In particular, the obligation to provide evidence under Article 5 GDPR also applies
- Article 44 GDPR: "All provisions of this chapter shall apply in order to ensure that the level of protection of natural persons guaranteed by this Regulation is not undermined."
  → Proof is required of how the level of protection is maintained.

Procedure for Implementing the Requirements

The implementation of the data protection requirements implies a management process: process description including procedural and work instructions, a regular review of the processes and a corresponding documentation of the review results. This can, for example, be included within the framework of quality management, so it does not necessarily require the introduction of a separate management system.

Using the example of dealing with requests from affected persons, the procedure for establishing structured processes will be demonstrated.

1. Acceptance of a request. This requires:
   – Representation of where requests can be received in the organization.
   – Identification of the "entry points" such as telephone exchange, Internet contact form, e-mail communication addresses of the company, e.g., imprint, etc.
   – Training of the persons receiving the requests.
   – What information must be requested?
   – To whom is the request forwarded?

2. Handling a request.
   2.1 Receiving inspection
   – Verification that the request is indeed a data protection request.
   – Entry of the request in a suitable documentation system.
   – Verification of what is involved
   – (request for information, request for correction, request for cancellation, etc.)
   – Sending an acknowledgment of receipt to the applicant.
   – Verification of the identity of the applicant.
   – Check whether there is respectively there are:
     • An unfounded application within the meaning of Article 12(5) GDPR.
     • Excessive requests from a data subject.
   – Cannot process request immediately: Information to data subject without delay.
   2.2 Content review
   – Checking whether personal data of the data subject are/have been processed.
   – If no data is available: Send negative message to the person concerned.
   – If data are available: Execute.
   2.3 Response
   – Request for information:
     • Compilation of the required information.
     • Immediate reply.
       a. Within one month.

   b. If due to complexity not possible within one month.
      Mandatory implementation within 3 months of application.
      Person must be informed of delay within the first month.
     • Note: Electronic application = information also provided electronically unless the data subject requests otherwise.
   – Correction, deletion, restriction, data transferability.
     • Forwarding to appropriate bodies for implementation.
     • Once implemented → Information to data subject (see request for information).
   – Objection Processing, revocation of consent.
     • Information of the body which
       a. Carries out the processing (e.g., research),
       b. consented.
     • Stop processing.
     • Check whether data must be deleted (Article 17(1b,c) GDPR).
     • Information to the data subject about the measures taken, including, where appropriate, about the deletion (see request for information).

Of course, each processing step involves various elements that need to be documented, e.g., decisions made and, if applicable, their reasons. It is therefore recommended that you use a suitable documentation tool.

Identical information must be documented for different requirements. Here, too, it is advisable to use a documentation tool to ensure uniform documentation, so that, for example, the purpose of processing is documented uniformly and different information is not accidentally found in different places.

Summary

The European General Data Protection Regulation (GDPR) is the fundamental set of rules that constitutes the framework of data protection legislation in Europe. Although national legislators can define the conditions of permission for the processing of health data, the GDPR contains a wide range of requirements that must be fulfilled when processing health data.

The processing of personal data is prohibited. Health data or genetic data may only be processed if processing is permitted by law or if the person whose data are to be processed has expressly consented to the processing. Personal data also includes pseudonymous data. Persons whose data are processed have, in principle, "data protection rights:" they must be informed about the processing and can, for example, request information about the processing or correction, deletion or transmission of the data.

Article 5 GDPR contains principles that must be guaranteed for every processing operation of personal data. In particular, the processing must be transparent for the data subjects, and the data may only be processed within the scope of the previously defined, clear and legitimate purposes. Personal data must be necessary and appropriate to the purposes for which they are processed. It must be specified at the start of processing how long the data will be stored; unlimited storage of data is illegal.

The security of the data must be guaranteed for the entire duration of processing, from the beginning of collection to deletion. The principles "Privacy by Design" and "Privacy by Default" must be applied. Requirements for the implementation of the specifications to be fulfilled with regard to the security of the processing can be found in Article 32 GDPR.

If personal data is processed in a third country, that is, a country outside the EU or EEA, the requirements of Chapter V of the GDPR must be met.

The GDPR contains many other requirements, in particular the need to prove that the requirements of the GDPR are being complied with in processing personal data ("accountability"). Ultimately, this proof can only be provided by describing the process workflows, documenting the processing and checking whether the described processes are complied with.

Conclusions and Outlook

Health data and especially patient data are one of the categories of data with the highest level of need for protection. Accordingly, the processing of this data is generally prohibited and only permitted in exceptional cases. Exceptional cases are legal permissions, such as those that exist for patient care. However, informed and voluntarily given consent can also legitimize the processing of health data.

Since the European legislator may only regulate cross-border processing, the GDPR in healthcare defines only a framework in which national data protection laws for regulating the processing of patient data must operate. Therefore, although the GDPR is applicable, the national regulations of European countries differ in the processing of health data, and a more detailed view of the respective national laws must be taken.

But of course the "framework" of the requirements resulting from the GDPR must also be observed and implemented in the processing of health data. The principles described in Article 5 GDPR obviously also have to be implemented in the processing of health data, the rights of the data subjects must be respected, and the security of the processing must be guaranteed.

Useful Resources
Books
1. Ausloos J. (2020) The Right to Erasure in EU Data Protection Law. Oxford University Press. ISBN 9780198847977.
2. Blokdyk G. (2018) Privacy Impact Assessment A Clear and Con-cise Reference. CreateSpace Independent Publishing Platform. ISBN 978–198,503,949.
3. Foulsham M, Hitchen B, Denley A. (2019) GDPR: How To Achieve and Maintain Compliance. Routledge. ISBN 9781138326170.
4. Gellert R. (2020) The Risk-Based Approach to Data Protection. Oxford University Press. ISBN 9780198837718.
5. Kennedy G. (2020) Data Privacy Law: A Practical Guide to the GDPR. Bowker. ISBN 9780999512722.

6. Kuner/Bygrave/ Docksey/Drechsler (Eds.) The EU General Data Protection Regulation (GDPR). Oxford University Press, 2020. ISBN 9780198826491.
7. Markham K. (2020) A Practical Guide to the General Data Protection Regulation (GDPR) – second Edition. Law Brief Publishing, second ed. ISBN 9781912687763.
8. Slokenberga/Tzortzatou/Reichel (Eds.) GDPR and Biobanking. Springer, 2021. ISBN 9783030493875.
9. Voigt P, von dem Bussche A. (2017) The EU General Data Protection Regulation (GDPR). Springer. ISBN 978–3-319-57,958-0.
10. Wright D. (2012) Privacy Impact Assessment. Springer Verlag. ISBN 978–94–007-2542-3.

European Data Protection Board

1. GDPR: Guidelines, Recommendations, Best Practices. Online, cited on 2019-11-05; Available at https://edpb.europa.eu/our-work-tools/general-guidance/gdpr-guidelines-recommendations-best-practices_en
2. Other documents. Online, cited on 2019-11-05; Available at https://edpb.europa.eu/other-documents_en
3. Opinions. Online, cited on 2019-11-05; Available at https://edpb.europa.eu/our-work-tools/consistency-findings/opinions_en
4. Letters. Online, cited on 2019-11-05; Available at https://edpb.europa.eu/letters_en

Journals

1. Britz T, Indenhuck M. (2019) The Usual Others. Third-Party Data in Contracts. PinG: 44–48.
2. de Jong J. (2020) In Search of Flexibility -Risk, circumstances and context in interpreting the GDPR. PinG: 173–180,
3. Dekhuijzen A. (2019) Policy Rules for Establishing the Amount of Administrative Fines under GDPR. Cri: 70–77.
4. Dove E, Chen J. (2020) Should consent for data processing be privileged in health research? A comparative legal analysis. International Data Privacy Law: 10(2): 117–131.
5. Finck M, Pallas F. (2020) They who must not be identified—distinguishing personal from non-personal data under the GDPR. International Data Privacy Law. 10(1): 11–36.
6. Gellert R. (2018) Understanding the notion of risk in the General Data Protection Regulation. Computer Law & Security Review. https://doi.org/10.1016/j.clsr.2017.12.003
7. Globocnik J. (2020) The Right to Be Forgotten is Taking Shape: CJEU Judgments in GC and Others (C-136/17) and Google v CNIL (C-507/17). GRUR Int.: 380–388.
8. Graef I, Husovec M, van den Boom J. (2020) Spill-Overs in Data Governance: Uncovering the Uneasy Relationship Between the GDPR's Right to Data Portability and EU Sector-Specific Data Access Regimes. EuCML: 3–16.
9. Greze B. (2019) The extra-territorial enforcement of the GDPR: a genuine issue and the quest for alternatives. International Data Privacy Law. 9(2): 109–128.
10. Kindt EJ. (2018) Having yes, using no? About the new legal regime for biometric data. Computer Law & Security Review. https://doi.org/10.1016/j.clsr.2017.11.004
11. Loideain N, Adams r. (2020) From Alexa to Siri and the GDPR: The gendering of Virtual Personal Assistants and the role of Data Protection Impact Assessments. Computer Law & Security Review. https://doi.org/10.1016/j.clsr.2019.105366
12. Mertens T. (2019) On the accountability of the GDPR for EU-based processors. PinG: 186–191.
13. Miño-Vásquez V. (2019) The Protection of Genetic Data under the General Data Protection regulation. DuD: 154–158.
14. Mourby M, Gowans H, Aidinlis S, Smith H, Kaye J. (2019) Governance of academic research data under the GDPR—lessons from the UK. International Data Privacy Law. 9(3): 192–206.
15. Romanou A. (2018) The necessity of the implementation of Privacy by Design in sectors where data protection concerns arise. Computer Law & Security Review. https://doi.org/10.1016/j.clsr.2017.05.021
16. Veale M, Binns R, Ausloos J. (2018) When data protection by design anddata subject rights clash. International Data Privacy Law. 8(2): 105–123.

17. Wagner J. (2018) The transfer of personal data to third countries under the GDPR: when does a recipient country provide an adequate level of protection? International Data Privacy Law. 8(4): 318–337.

18. Wong J, Henderson T. (2019) The right to data portability in practice: exploring the implications of the technologically neutral GDPR. International Data Privacy Law,. 9(3): 173–191.

Review Questions

1. What are the principles mentioned in Article 5 regarding the processing of personal data?
2. What are the rights of data subjects?
3. What information must be included in a list of processing activities under Article 30(1)?

Appendix: Answers to Review Questions

1. What are the principles mentioned in Article 5 regarding the processing of personal data?

   – Article 5(1a): lawfulness, fairness, and transparency.
   – Article 5(1b): purpose limitation.
   – Article 5(1c); data minimisation.
   – Article 5(1d): accuracy.
   – Article 5(1e): storage limitation.
   – Article 5(1f): integrity and confidentiality.
   – Article 5(2): accountability.

2. What are the rights of data subjects?

   – Right of access of the data subject.
   – Right of rectification.
   – Right of erasure.
   – Right to restrict processing.
   – Right to data portability.
   – Right of objection.

3. What information must be included in a list of processing activities under Article 30(1)?

   – Name and contact details of processor and—if exists—of the data protection officer.
   – Purposes of the processing.
   – Description of the categories of data subjects and of the categories of personal data.
   – Categories of recipients.
   – Where applicable, transfers of personal data to a third country or an international organization.
   – Where possible, the envisaged time limits for erasure of the different categories of data.
   – Where possible, a general description of the technical and organizational security measures.

References

1. Joint practical guide of the European Parliament, the Council and the Commission for persons involved in the drafting of European Union legislation. Online, cited on 2019-02-12. Available at https://op.europa.eu/en/publication-detail/-/publication/3879747d-7a3c-411b-a3a0-55c14e2ba732
2. Directive 95/46/EC of the European Parliament and of the Council of 24 October 1995 on the protection of individuals with regard to the processing of personal data and on the free movement of such data. Online, cited on 2019-11-01. Available at https://eur-lex.europa.eu/legal-content/DE/ALL/?uri=CELEX%3A31995L0046.
3. European Data Protection Board: "Guidelines on Data Protection Officers ('DPOs') (wp243rev.01)", taken over from the Article 29 Working Party. Online, cited on 2019-11-05; Available at https://ec.europa.eu/newsroom/article29/item-detail.cfm?item_id=612048
4. bitkom: The Processing Records – Records of Processing Activities according to Article 30 General Data Protection Regulation (GDPR). Online, cited on 2019-11-05. Available at https://www.bitkom.org/Bitkom/Publikationen/The-Processing-Records-Records-of-Processing-Activities-according-to-Art-30-General-Data-Protection-Regulation-GDPR.html
5. EDPB: Guidelines 4/2019 on Article 25 Data Protection by Design and by Default. Online, cited on 2019-11-05. Available at https://edpb.europa.eu/our-work-tools/public-consultations-art-704/2019/guidelines-42019-article-25-data-protection-design_en
6. Privacy Commissioner of Ontario (2009) Privacy by Design: The 7 Foundational Principles. Online, cited on 2019-11-05. Available at Verfügbar unter https://www.ipc.on.ca/wp-content/uploads/Resources/7foundationalprinciples.pdf

Practice and Legal Issues: Clinical Documentation, Data Ownership, Access, and Patient Rights

30

Angelika Haendel and Mervat Abdelhak

Learning Objectives
- Define the Legal Health record.
- List the purposes of the legal health record.
- Identify Medical/Clinical Documentation Requirements that are governed by Laws, Obligations, and Regulations.
- Discuss patient's rights laws and Patient's obligations.
- Discuss laws governing Health Data Ownership and Access.
- Compare and contrast classification systems in use today.

Key Terms
- Health Records
- Content and Documentation Requirements
- Patient's Rights
- Data Access
- Release of Information
- Data Ownership
- Interoperability
- Classification Systems

Introduction

Overview

The Institute of Medicine (IOM) in their published report "Crossing the Quality Chasm-A New Health System for the twenty-first Century" identified six broad aims that should serve as pillars for a quality healthcare system. The report stated that quality healthcare should be safe, patient-centered, efficient, effective, equitable, and timely. This chapter will address selected legal issues, laws, and policies that are within the Health Information Management and Informatics domains and have a direct impact on achieving the six aims as identified by the IOM for quality healthcare.

This chapter will define the legal health record and its purpose. The laws, regulations, obligations, and best practices that govern clinical documentation, health record maintenance, patient rights, data access, and ownership will be presented. The deployment of enabling health information technologies, analytics, virtual care, patient empowerment, and engagement are but some of the factors that are contributing to the deluge of health data and will be addressed in this chapter.

The Origin of Health Records

The origin of patient records can be traced back to the seventeenth century. During that century advances in the natural sciences, including

A. Haendel (✉)
University Hospital Erlangen, Erlangen, Germany
e-mail: angelika.haendel@uk-erlangen.de

M. Abdelhak
University of Pittsburgh, Pittsburgh, PA, USA
e-mail: abdelhak@pitt.edu

© Springer Nature Switzerland AG 2022
U. H. Hübner et al. (eds.), *Nursing Informatics*, Health Informatics,
https://doi.org/10.1007/978-3-030-91237-6_30

human anatomy, which was based on observations from dissection, were evident. These advances impacted the practice of medicine, where physicians systematically began to record case histories primarily for teaching and research.

As the practice of medicine advanced, the maintenance of patient health records also progressed, notably during the 18th and 19th centuries as health-related professional organizations were founded setting higher standards for the education and practice of medicine.

In the USA, the American Medical Association (AMA) was founded in 1847 and the American Hospital Association (AHA) was formed in 1898 with both professional organizations advocating for better care, adopting a code of ethics and promulgating the need for complete and accurate recordkeeping.

During the twentieth century, after World War second, advances in science and medicine were continuing at a faster pace, together with an increasing economic impact for providers and patients alike. This was the time when providers began collecting and recording patient information in a structured format. In addition, individual patient records were created and maintained for each patient.

Such progress in health records maintenance, in the USA, can be attributed to two significant developments that occurred in the twentieth century.

First, the famous Flexner report published in 1910, by Abraham Flexner, identified serious issues in the education of physicians resulting in the closing of many for profit medical schools, a revamping of medical school's curriculum, and the AMA initiating an Accreditation process for medical education. The changes resulting from the Flexner report elevated the requirements for clinical documentation and the maintenance of health records.

The second significant impetus for setting standards for health records came from the American College of Surgeons (ACS), which was founded in 1913. The ACS, to assess the quality of care in hospitals, began collecting data from health records that were found to be in a dire state. In 1917 ACS established the Hospital

Standardization Program, among other standards, which identified minimum standards for health records. The Joint Commission (Previously named "The joint Commission on Accreditation of Healthcare Organizations and The Joint Commission on Accreditation of Hospitals") adopted the ACS Hospital Standardization Program in 1981 and which continues until today to set standards for Health Records and Health Information Management.

Healthcare in the twenty-first century was heralded by many disruptions and breakthroughs in care, informatics, technology, and education. E-Health and the digital transformation continues to impact healthcare, the health information management practice and education as well as the regulations, standards, and requirements for the health record (Fig. 30.1).

The Definition and Purpose of the Legal Health Record

The legal health record is the legal business record of the healthcare facility. The documents to be included in the legal health record, that is created and maintained in the usual course of business, must be defined by the healthcare facility. For example, the healthcare facility must decide whether or not emails or X-rays will be defined as being part of the legal health record. Documents that are created and maintained as part of the usual course of business of the healthcare facility would be included. The legal health record serves as evidence in lawsuits, both civil and criminal cases, and is produced in response to a subpoena. A subpoena dictates to the custodian of the health record to produce certain specific named documents or all the records pertaining to an individual patient and for all admissions. The legal health record can be in paper, electronic, or hybrid format. As the majority of healthcare institutions have implemented electronic health records (EHRs), electronic stored information (ESI) has become admissible and discoverable in litigations, as did paper records, and is referred to as e-discovery.

History of Patient records

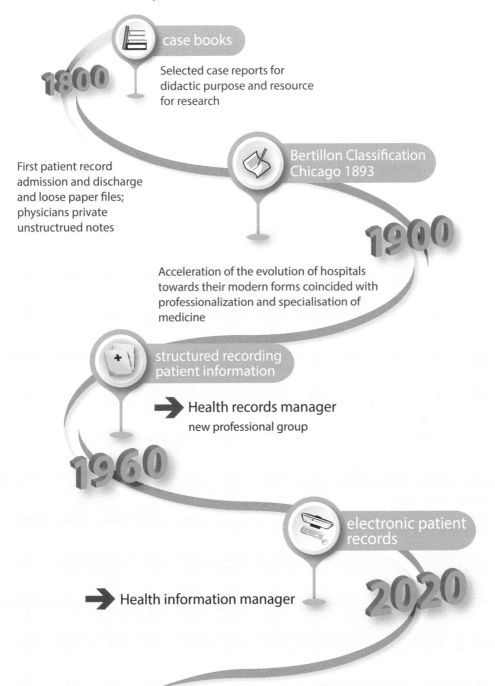

Fig. 30.1 The evolution of patient records

The health information management professional is the custodian and steward of the legal health record (paper and electronic formats), which is the authenticated evidence and declared to be trustworthiness.

While clearly the legal health record is created and maintained as required by law for legal purpose, the primary purpose of health records is to document the treatment and outcomes of care thus facilitating interprofessional communication among the healthcare team and enabling quality and safe patient care.

The legal health record also provides proof of the services rendered and allows the healthcare facility to bill insurance companies and payors for reimbursement. In addition, health records provide individual as well as aggregate data to assess the quality of patient care that was rendered, provide data to achieve accreditation as well as comply with internal and external reporting requirements. Operational information can be extracted from health records, providing data on use of services, market penetration, provider workloads, and patterns of care. Health records are essential for research and education. And last but not least, health records are becoming an integral vehicle to achieve patient engagement and consumer-centered care.

Laws, Obligations, Regulations Governing the Maintenance, Content, and Clinical Documentation Requirements Across the Globe

Overview

The following sections will address the maintenance, content, and documentation requirements of health records in the USA and Europe. It is strikingly evident that the laws, regulations, and obligations that govern the documentation in health records are very much similar across the globe. Laws and voluntary standards have been established to ensure the integrity, completeness, timeliness, authenticity, and accuracy of the data collected in health records.

Health Record Maintenance, Content, and Documentation Requirements in the USA

Health record standards and regulations are established by law by both state and federal agencies. Health record maintenance, content, and documentation requirements are dictated at the federal level by the Department of Health and Human Services (HHS), and the Centers for Medicare and Medicaid Services (CMS). The CMS maintenance, content, and documentation regulations are published in the Conditions of Participation. CMS publishes the Conditions of Participation for a variety of healthcare settings including ones for hospitals, psychiatric facilities, and ambulatory centers.

As an example, the Conditions of Participation for hospitals require that the content of health records contain information to justify admission and continued hospitalization, support the diagnosis, and describe the patient's progress and response to treatment.

In addition to state and federal laws, voluntary accrediting bodies such as the Joint Commission also set standards for the maintenance, content, and documentation requirements for the health record. The Joint Commission publishes standards for health records for a variety of healthcare settings. As an example, The Comprehensive Accreditation Manual for Hospitals covers policies and procedures for record completion, authentication, data access, and the release of information as well as the retention of health records. There are specific requirements regarding the content and data elements to be included in the discharge summary, the history and physical, the operative report and the like.

Another important source of health record maintenance, content, and documentation requirements is the healthcare facilities' own Medical Staff Bylaws. Content requirements that comply with external standards and regulations are included in the medical staff bylaws, including who is permitted to document in the health record, authentication requirements, when records become delinquent, and the facilities record retention policy.

Each team member who is authorized to document in the health record must document factual information, authenticate the note verifying the origin of the information, the person who created the note, and at a minimum sign his or her name and indicate discipline. Healthcare facilities' medical staff bylaws can add additional signature requirements such as requiring the authors' title and credential.

Digital signatures (e-signatures) provide a digital guarantee through encryption, represented by a series of numbers, identifying who performed the encryption that is the provider who is authenticating the entry.

The Medical, Clinical Documentation Obligation in Europe

Overview

The legal obligation for clinical documentation is to be found in the regulations of the Federal Medical Associations. It is part of medical ethics. There is an obligation to keep patient records and to document clinical findings. The medical record serves as a proof and memory aid of all the treatment and measures for each patient. The patient rights have been further strengthened by the new EU General Data Protection Regulation which became effective on May 25, 2018. Healthcare institutions have an obligation to document all significant findings and all measures taken that are relevant to the care of patients. The basic documentation is a uniform, structured database that is used by all service providers in the healthcare system. This documentation is the basis for the transmission of service data to health insurance companies, for the management of a hospital and for official statistics. In Germany, diagnosis codes (ICD-10) need to be transmitted; in the inpatient sector, additionally coded medical procedures (OPS-301), length of stay, and discharge physician must be transmitted. The specialist documentation is specific to certain clinical disciplines. Specialist documentation is often characterized by a high proportion of free text. Special documentation is designed specifically for particular diagnoses and their therapies. They usu-

ally have a high level of structured documentation and are mainly used for quality assurance. A variety of professional groups are involved in clinical documentation: doctors, nurses, MTAs, etc. The authorized persons had to be able to access relevant information promptly at the right place.

The medical documentation obligation is regulated independently of each other by different legal provisions. In Germany, for example, According to 10 para. 1 sentence 1 of the Professional Code of Conduct of the Medical Association of Berlin (BO), physicians must make the necessary records of the determinations made and measures taken in the exercise of their profession.

Sense and Purpose of the Medical and Clinical Documentation

The primary aim of medical documentation is to ensure proper treatment and follow-up of patients. Accordingly, the law governing the medical profession makes it clear that the documentation of treatment is not only a reminder for physicians, but also serves treatment continuity and quality, communication, patient safety, proof of performance, economic efficiency, and scientific purposes. The documentation should make the essential course of treatment comprehensible, avoid unnecessary duplicates, and enable proper communication and interprofessional collaboration for the treatment and betterment of the patient. In addition, patients should always have the possibility of having the medical treatment checked by another doctor on the basis of the documentation. From the physician's perspective, the treatment documentation has an important evidential function. For if medical measures (including information and consent) are not recorded in violation of the duty of documentation, it is assumed, in a medical malpractice suit, at the expense of the physician that he or she did not carry out the measure in question. According to legal aspects, the patient record is a document that serves to make information and knowledge available to authorized persons as completely as possible, at the right time, in the right place, and in the right form. In the case of a legal dispute, e.g., the doctor must prove, on the basis of the clinical documentation, that he has correctly informed the patient about the risks of an intervention. Otherwise, the patient can claim for financial compensation.

Corresponding Professional Duties and Data Protection Regulations

There are a number of laws and regulations that require accurate documentation, e.g., X-ray directive, radiation protection ordinance, transfusion law, infection protection law, and medical devices regulation. For reasons of evidence protection, it is generally recommended to keep patient records for 30 years. It should be noted that data should be deleted or blocked when the period of retention has ended and there is no objective reason for the further storage of the data.

The duty of documentation corresponds to the right of patients to inspect their own medical records. In addition, medical documentation has been close to medical confidentiality with regard to the obligation to preserve treatment documents (and to destroy them after the expiry of the retention period). Thus, both the medical documentation obligation and the applicable data protection regulations must be observed and applied.

The relevant data protection law was completely revised by the so-called General Data Protection Regulation (DSGVO/GDPR) of the EU which became effective on May 25, 2018. The obligations thus applicable to doctors as persons responsible for data must also—but not only—be observed when handling treatment documentation. Violations can result in severe sanctions. The new EU General Data Protection Regulation also further strengthened the patient's rights.

According to the national Patient Rights Act and in accordance with the Regulation 2016/679 of the European Parliament and of the council of 27 April 2016 on the protection of natural persons with regard to the processing of personal data and on the free movement of such data, and repealing Directive 95/46/EC (General Data Protection Regulation) patients have the right to inspect and copy own health-related data, such as diagnoses, examination

results, findings of treating physicians, and details of treatments or interventions.

Scope, Timing, and Form of Documentation

The subject of medical documentation governs all the information and treatment results that are essential from a professional point of view for the current and future treatment of the patient. This includes in particular the medical history, diagnoses, examinations, examination results, findings, therapies, interventions and their effects, consents, and clarifications as well as medical letters from colleagues who have previously treated or co-treated the patient. When a Treatment Content is to be qualified as essential, thus it is covered by the duty of documentation, will depend on the medical aspects and the specific circumstances of the individual case.

The documentation must be made in direct temporal connection with the treatment. The recording should therefore be made during or immediately after the treatment. If this is not possible due to special circumstances, the documentation must be made up promptly. Medical necessities and patient safety are to be taken into account; in particular, the documentation must be made in good time to ensure that any further treatment of the patient that is necessary can be provided without delay. The documentation, while maybe technical in nature, it does not have to be understandable by the patient/layman but must be understood by other physicians and healthcare providers. This documentation standard may need to pivot to accommodate new patient engagement expectations and consumer-centered care. Keyword Information and subject-specific abbreviations are also sufficient if another doctor is able to recognize what is meant and how the procedure was carried out. The prerequisite is always that the documentation is objectively legible and professionally comprehensible. The documentation can be kept both in a paper file and electronically.

Electronic Documentation

In the case of electronic treatment documentation, a number of special features must be taken into account, especially with regard to data security and the evidential value of the records. Key advantages of electronic documentation are availability, readability, flexibility, reusability, and analyzability of patient data.

- Safety and protective measures:

  Electronic treatment documentation requires special security and protection measures to prevent its alteration, destruction, or unlawful use. Doctors must observe the recommendations of the Medical Association. In the interest of patient safety, the special security and protection measures are intended to prevent treatment data from being lost due to hardware or software problems, for example.

  In addition, for reasons of data protection, unauthorized third parties should be prevented from accessing the patient information. For this purpose, access to the data (e.g., by password protection) must be restricted to the physician and the nonmedical staff who are equally bound to secrecy. In addition, the authorship of each entry should be clearly identifiable and all usage should be fully logged. To secure patient data, backup copies should be made daily on suitable media. If patient data are stored externally (outside the healthcare facility), it must be technically ensured that third parties cannot take note of the patient data. If the IT system is maintained by external service providers, the principles applicable to commissioned data processing must be observed (cf. Articles 28 et seq. GDPR); in particular, the service provider must be sworn to secrecy in writing and may only process personal data within the scope of the person responsible for data protection. If the IT system is changed, the electronically documented contents must remain available for the periods applicable for storage.
- "Scanning" of treatment records available in paper form

  Treatment documents in paper form—including, for example, medical letters from colleagues—can be scanned and stored electronically instead of the original. In this so-called "substitute scanning," the electronic document does not have the same evidential value as the original, which can be qualified as a document. Physicians must therefore consider in each individual case whether the documents available in paper form are to be destroyed or retained after scanning.

Classification Systems, Coding, and Revenue Cycle

Classifications systematically arrange terms and bring them together by assigning them to keys (principle of class formation). In this way, for example, unique keys (codes) can be assigned for certain clinical pictures. Classification rules support this unique assignment. Classifications are primarily used for statistical purposes and for the billing of outpatient and inpatient services. Classifications are also used in quality management and clinical research.

International Classification of Diseases

The International Classification of Diseases (ICD) was created by the World Health Organization (WHO) and is used to classify diagnoses. The ICD originally developed from the statistics of causes of death and is now a key standard for national health statistics around the globe.

The tenth revision of the classification, ICD-10, has been in use since 1994 and the ICD in the 11th revision is expected to come into force on January 01, 2022. The ICD-10 is used to code diagnoses in both outpatient and inpatient care worldwide.

International Classification of Functioning, Disability, and Health The International Classification of Functioning, Disability, and Health (ICF) is a classification system for describing a person's functional health status, disability, social impairment, and relevant environmental factors. The ICF enables, that the bio-psycho-social aspects of disease consequences can be systematically recorded. Like the ICD, the

ICF was approved for use by the World Health Organization. The main purposes of the ICF are to provide a scientific basis for understanding and studying health and health-related states, outcomes, determinants, and changes in health status and functioning.

International Classification of Health Interventions

The International Classification of Health Interventions (ICHI), which is currently under development by WHO classifies surgical procedures and health interventions. ICHI is being developed to provide a common tool for reporting and analyzing health interventions for statistical purposes.

Patient Rights: Legal Obligations of Healthcare Providers, Healthcare Facilities, and the Patient

Patients' rights have been predominately established based on laws, rules, and regulations. Some patients' rights have also been established and followed based upon ethical grounding and best practices. Patients' rights are intended to improve patient safety, reduce medical errors, allow for patient-centered care, facilitate transparency of cost and quality data- all of these measures are intended to ultimately improve care coordination and the quality of care. Patients must be given notice of their rights and responsibilities as well as an explanation of the process for bringing grievances against a healthcare provider or a healthcare facility.

Patient's rights are also intertwined with patients' obligations. There are expectations and responsibilities assigned to all parties to patients, to healthcare providers and to healthcare facilities providing protection to each of these entities and to encourage patient engagement in their own healthcare. For example, patients are obligated to provide full and honest information to their healthcare provider and to carry out the agreed upon treatment plans.

The digital transformation, occurring in society as a whole as well as in healthcare, has heightened the importance of patients' rights, patients' expectations as well as their obligations. Patients, as consumers of healthcare, have come to expect speed and quality of service, transparency regarding the cost and quality of care in order for them to make informed decisions. Patients have come to expect the availability of mobile applications, patient portals, and devices for their use, all of these factors have and will continue to change patient and providers' rights, roles, expectations, and responsibilities.

The following are examples of patients' rights that pertain to health data and health information technology. These patients' rights will continue to be front and center in today's digital transformation of healthcare, as we deploy enabling technologies, observe heightened patient expectations, empowerment, and engagement in their healthcare.

1. Collecting and maintaining health information on patients: The duty of healthcare facilities to maintain patient records is imposed by state and federal statutes, as well as by voluntary accreditation standards.
2. Retention, Security, and confidentiality of patients' health information: The healthcare facility and providers have a duty to maintain patients' records according to federal and state record retention laws. Furthermore, these records must be kept secure, safeguarded against loss, destruction, and unauthorized alterations.

    Patients have a right to personal privacy and to the confidentiality of their records.
3. Data ownership: Patients own their health data and have the right to access their health information. They have the right to consent to the release of their health information as well as receive an accounting of where and to whom their health information can or has been released. As patients become more engaged in their healthcare, they become

creators and users of their health data, and they can exercise more control to ensure that their data are neither released nor sold to entities that profit form its use.

4. Data quality and integrity: Healthcare facilities and providers have the duty to ensure that patient data that is collected and maintained is data that is timely, accurate, complete, meaningful to care coordination, and quality patient care. Patient portals, virtual care, telehealth, self-generated patient data, and the collection and use of social data are examples of how the types and sources of data have expanded. Regardless of where and by whom the data is created, collected, maintained, within or external to the physical boundaries of the healthcare facility, the responsibility for data validation, data quality, data integration, and data governance continues to remain with the healthcare provider and the healthcare facility.

Health Data Access, Core Data, and Interoperability

Laws have been introduced to advance interoperability, facilitate the availability, access, exchange, and use of electronic health information (EHI) as well as to deter information blocking.

These laws are intended to improve health data access and interoperability for patients, providers, as well as for EHR and application developers and vendors.

In the USA, The Office of the National Coordinator (ONC) has introduced new rules, under the provision of the twenty-first Century Cures Act, that would allow for the exchange and use of EHI without special effort. These rules would also allow patients to have access to EHI in a single longitudinal format. Furthermore, these rules are intended to prevent healthcare facilities, EHR vendors, and app developers from allowing for intentional or non-intentional information blocking thus impeding nationwide interoperability.

Achieving the goals intended by the 21st Century Cures Act and the ONC Interoperability and information Blocking rules, is a giant leap forward, that would facilitate remote patient monitoring, the integration of patient-generated health data (PGHD) into the EHR's and advancing person-centered healthcare with shared care planning and decisions.

To achieve patient engagement, patients need to have access to a full and complete longitudinal set of EHI, have the ability to contribute and correct that information as well as instruct providers where and to whom to transmit his/her information.

Healthcare providers need to be able to access clinical data about their patients from other providers and healthcare settings. Both patients and providers can access and use structured data and send this data to any health app of their choosing.

To enable nationwide interoperability requires a core data set, a standardized set of data elements to be included in the EHI.

Case Study

Continuity of Care Through Electronic Patient Record

Legal issues in handling a patient record may arise, for example, when patients change their residence and new care providers now taking charge of them require information about previous treatments. This situation is a classic case of continuity of care expected from the patients' perspective. The transfer of any patient information to another doctor or any other third party always requires the patient's consent and must fulfil the demands of data protection, confidentiality, and data security irrespective of how the data are transmitted. In most countries there are legal rights to inspect one's own patient file and there is also a right to have copies made. Copies may be sent directly to other healthcare facilities involved or by the patients themselves. It is relatively easy to retrieve and quickly make printed copies from doctors' letters, reports, discharge summaries, and laboratory findings when the patient record is based on paper form. In such case, the patient receives the printed copy of the data set or the patient can ask the healthcare facility to attach the health data on an offline medium, e.g., on a USB memory stick.

However, also the paper world includes pitfalls concerning access to records or certain parts of the record. The clinician may or may not grant the right to the receiving care provider to see also those parts of the patient record that contain notes reflecting subjective impressions. Another limitation of the access to a patient record could arise when the patient had received psychiatric treatment. In this case, the patient may want to deny access to the psychiatric record which could become a problem for the provider in charge to obtain a complete picture of the patient.

In the course of digitalization and improvements in digital data storage, large amounts of medical data are processed and archived electronically. Consequently, clinical records should be transmitted electronically as well. On top of legal issues, this could lead to problems of interoperability. In most countries, healthcare facilities are free to decide which health IT system they use, which entails a great variety of different systems in use throughout the country. Therefore, seamless exchange of data within and between health information systems is often difficult because of the fragmentation and lack of interoperability of the health information systems involved. In the case of sharing personal health data between different healthcare providers, this can only be achieved if all the involved parties rely on distributed systems with exactly the same health IT standards or on systems with a central database. Health IT standards are not mere technical standards but also composed of standardized vocabularies and terminologies.

Despite existing interoperability issues of health IT systems, the benefits prevail. One major benefit of the use of electronic patient records is that the patient data are available at any time, at any location, and for any authorized person. Implemented properly, an EHR thus can support the transmission of information from one provider to another in case of patients changing their residence.

Summary

eHealth and the digital transformation continue to impact healthcare, the health information management practice, and education as well as the regulations, standards, and requirements for the health record regarding its full spectrum of usage.

The legal health record is the legal business record of the healthcare facility. It serves as evidence in lawsuits, both civil and criminal cases, and is produced in response to a subpoena. While clearly the legal health record is created and maintained as required by law for legal purposes, the primary purpose of health records is to document the treatment and outcomes of care. It is strikingly evident that the laws, regulations, and obligations that govern the documentation in health records are very much similar across the globe. The regulations in the USA and the EU are described to illustrate the details of health records management.

Patients' rights regarding their health data, the ownership, and legal access to the data, are intended to improve patient safety, reduce medical errors, allow for patient-centered care, facilitate transparency of cost and quality data all of these measures are intended to ultimately improve care coordination and the quality of care. In the era of digitalization, laws have been introduced to advance interoperability, facilitate the availability, access, exchange, and use of electronic health information (EHI) as well as to deter information blocking. These laws are intended to improve health data access and interoperability for patients, providers, as well as for EHR and application developers and vendors. They reflect the importance of interoperability including the use of classification systems. As the case study shows legal management of interoperable electronic health records is the foundation of continuity of care.

Conclusions and Outlook

Delivering care in this new healthcare ecosystem, which is influenced by a digital transformation, a myriad of enabling technologies, apps and mobile devices, pandemics, and an accelerated and heightened consumer expectations and engagement, requires more than ever before, quality health data. A shift in care delivery to remote and tele-based care as well as the deluge of health data by expanding the types and sources of clinical and nonclinical data that is collected and shared, exacerbates the need for interoperability.

This new environment is full of both opportunities and challenges. Health Information Management professionals, healthcare providers, and policy makers must leverage health data, one of their most valuable assets, to improve care coordination, patient safety, and individual as well as population health.

Managing the deluge of health data, achieving compliance with applicable laws, rules, regulations, and obligations, minimizing security and privacy risks at the same time allowing for more accessibility and use of data present today's major challenges.

Review Questions

1. List the six pillars for quality healthcare as identified by the Institute of Medicine.
2. Identify the agency of the federal government in the USA that is responsible for setting regulations regarding the content and maintenance of the health record.
3. The health data that is collected and maintained in the health record belong to the healthcare facility or the patient?
4. Define what interoperability means to the patient and the provider.
5. Specify two classification systems and their fields of application.

Useful Resources

1. Berner ES: Ethical and legal issues in the use of health information technology to improve patient safety. HEC Forum 2008 Sep;20(3):243–58.
2. Gillum R: From Papyrus to the Electronic Tablet: A Brief History of the Clinical Medical Record with Lessons for the Digital Age. The American Journal of Medicine (2013) 126, 853–857.

3. Fenton SH, Low S, Abrams KJ, Butler-Henderson K.: Health Information Management: Changing with Time. Year Med Inform 2017 Aug;26(1):72–77.
4. Field RI: Overview: computerized medical records create new legal and business confidentiality problems. Field RI. Health span. 1994 Sep;11(8):3–7.
5. Hoyle P: Health information is central to changes in healthcare: A clinician's view. Health Inf Manag 2019 Jan;48(1):48–51.
6. Institute of Medicine.2001.Crossing the Quality Chasm- a New Health System for the twenty-first Century. Washington, DC: National Academies Press.
7. Mackenzie G, Carter H: Medico legal issues, Stud Health Technol Inform. 2010;151:176–82. Mehta NB, Martin SA, Maypole J, Andrews R: Information management for clinicians. Cleve Clin J Med. 2016 Aug;83(8):589–95.
8. Nymark M: Patients' safety, privacy and effectiveness--a conflict of interests in health care information systems. Med Law 2007 Jun;26(2):245–55.
9. Prideaux A: Issues in nursing documentation and record-keeping practice. Br J Nurs. 2011 Dec 8–2012 Jan 11;20(22):1450–4.
10. Rienhoff O: Digital archives and communication highways in health care require a second look at the legal framework of the seventies. Int J Biomed Comput 1994 Feb;35 Suppl:13–9.

Appendix: Answers to Review Questions

1. List the six pillars for a quality healthcare as identified by the Institute of Medicine.

The six quality aims specified by the Institute of Medicine include safety, patient centeredness, timeliness, efficiency, effectiveness, and equity.

2. Identify the agency of the federal government in the USA that is responsible for setting regu-

lations regarding the content and maintenance of the health record.

The Centers for Medicare and Medicaid Services (CMS) which is a federal agency within the United States Department of Health and Human Services (HHS) is the responsible authority for defining contents and maintenance of health records.

3. The health data that is collected and maintained in the health record belongs to healthcare facility or the patient?

There is no consistent law regarding ownership of medical records; yet it is regulated that the data collected within the health record belongs to the patient whereas the physical form (paper, electronic) belongs to the healthcare facility that is responsible for maintaining and storing the health record in accordance with the current data protection guidelines.

4. Define what interoperability means to the patient and the provider.

Patients who participate, e.g., in a self-monitoring program need to be able to access their own clinical data from each providers and healthcare settings where he or she has been treated. If for example, the patient decides to use a certain data system, but later wants to switch to a different one, he or she must be sure that the data can be migrated without effort, but also other imported data can be transferred from the provider to the patient and back at the click of a button or via a trustworthy service provider.

In order to exchange medical data and information timely and securely between healthcare providers, all systems must be able to communicate with each other unambiguously and in a data-secure manner. Interoperability is the crucial factor for cross-system and cross-sector communication and cooperation, and thus the key to the successful digitization of healthcare. Therefore it is prerequisite to ensure compatibility between the individual systems.

5. Specify two classification systems and their fields of application.

ICD 10

The International Statistical Classification of Diseases and Related Health Problems (ICD) is the international standard of diagnostic classification. The ICD, currently used in the tenth revision is applied to translate diagnoses of diseases and other health problems from words into an alpha-numeric code. The purpose of the ICD are analysis of the general health situation of population groups and the monitoring of the incidence and prevalence of diseases and other health problems. In healthcare settings ICD is also used for financial aspects, such as billing or resource allocation.

ICF

The International Classification of Functioning, Disability, and Health (ICF) is a classification system for describing human functioning and disability. The ICF is applied for understanding and studying health and health-related states, outcomes, determinants, and changes in health status and functioning.

Ethical Issues: Patients, Providers, and Systems

31

Ursula H. Hübner, Nicole Egbert,
and Georg Schulte

Learning Objectives

- To understand the meaning of ethics as a scientific field
- To understand the four ethical principles in biomedicine and their relationship to health IT
- To understand the ethical challenges of big data and artificial intelligence
- To understand ethical questions surrounding smart assistive technologies
- To understand the special ethical questions arising when data are re-used
- To identify and analyze circumstances when patients and clinicians are affected by health IT and to appraise their ethical meaning
- To apply ethical dimensions for the evaluation of health IT

Key Terms

- Ethics
- Moral behavior
- Ethical principles in biomedicine
- Autonomy
- Non-maleficence
- Beneficence
- Justice

- Ethics of data
- Ethics of algorithms
- Ethics of practice
- Informed consent
- Privacy
- Confidentiality
- Model for assessment of telemedicine applications
- Model for the ethical evaluation of socio-technological arrangements

Introduction

What Is Ethics?

Ethics or moral philosophy is the science of studying moral behavior and beliefs as well as how people reason and act. It investigates ethics from a meta-level (metaethics) analyzing the language, concepts, and ways of reasoning that are used to declare and justify moral values, i.e., what is good and what is wrong. While this part of ethics studies inspects the as-is situation and does not set any norms (nonnormative), there is another part called normative ethics that aims at defining what should be. In normative ethics, the questions to be answered are of practical nature. They touch on the principles and guiding rules that should help us to act morally and evaluate our behavior—generally and in specific situations. Normative ethics also provides reasons why these principles should be applied.

U. H. Hübner (✉) · N. Egbert · G. Schulte
University of Applied Sciences (UAS) Osnabrück,
Osnabrück, Niedersachsen, Germany
e-mail: u.huebner@hs-osnabrueck.de;
n.egbert@hs-osnabrueck.de; g.schulte@hs-osnabrueck.de

© Springer Nature Switzerland AG 2022
U. H. Hübner et al. (eds.), *Nursing Informatics*, Health Informatics,
https://doi.org/10.1007/978-3-030-91237-6_31

Legal and ethical issues are often discussed in combination because of various overlaps and inter-relations. In liberal democracies respecting human rights, the ethical discourse usually incorporates the legal norms as a special set of values. While the regulations distinguish legal from illegal behavior, ethics strives to find the best among the legal options based on moral values and preferences. Challenging the existing laws and hereby contributing to the change of laws is a field that Floridi calls hard ethics [1]. An example of hard ethics is when ethics specialists are consulted to help or when they are fighting (as was the case for abolishing apartheid) for shaping new laws and regulations. This may be necessary because the old laws do not provide the instruments to answer new questions that is often the case with new technologies and unprecedented situations. An example would be: How do you prioritize groups of eligible persons in case of scarce resources, e.g., vaccines, devices and drugs needed for treatment? A similar question concerns the liability in case of autonomous driving: who is accountable and who is liable for the consequences of a car crash? Floridi contrasts hard ethics with soft ethics [1] that concerns matters beyond regulations and that should make life or society better. Soft ethics assists in interpreting laws, such as the EU General Data Protection Regulation as well as fosters discourses about the ethically most appropriate solutions, e.g., those that mitigate inequities in society.

Ethics in Healthcare

Ethics has a long tradition in medicine and healthcare, such as the commandments found in the Hippocratic oath and in more recent times in the Declaration of Geneva of the World Medical Association first published in 1948 in the aftermath of the medical atrocities during the time of the Nazi regime. This Declaration is formulated as a pledge that embraces, among others, the dedication to the "service of humanity," the respect of the "autonomy and dignity" of the patient, and of the "secrets that are confided." The full and most current version of this pledge can be retrieved from [2]. In nursing, the Code of Ethics for Nurses was first provided in 1953 by the International Council of Nurses [3]. Today, many professions and specialties in healthcare have a code of ethics to guide their work with patients. Table 31.1 gives an overview of the major documents in medical and healthcare ethics.

With the advent of more advanced methods in biomedicine, first and foremost in genetics, the interest in ethical issues and the need for a framework of principles increased. One of the most influential works in this field is the book "Principles of Biomedical Ethics" by Beauchamp and Childress who propose the following four principles as an overarching framework to serve as a guide: autonomy, nonmaleficence, beneficence, and justice [4]. Although they stand for themselves, they are interrelated in the sense that they can partly overlap or may express conflicting goals, for example, autonomy and justice. Ethical issues do not only apply to patients (including their families) alone. They also apply to any person and with this also to the care providers themselves, e.g., the autonomy of the care providers in making their decisions. In the wake of the increasing influence of technologies, these principles are also tested against the way in which patient care can be practiced by professionals in a digitally supported care delivery system.

Table 31.1 Major documents referring to ethics in medicine and healthcare

Title	Published by	Scope	First published
Declaration of Geneva	World Medical Association	Ethical principles of the medical profession	1948
Code of Ethics for Nurses	International Council of Nurses	Ethical principles of the nursing profession	1953
Declaration of Helsinki	World Medical Association	Medical research involving human subjects	1964
Belmont Report	United States Department of Health, Education, and Welfare	Biomedical and behavioral research involving human subjects	1979

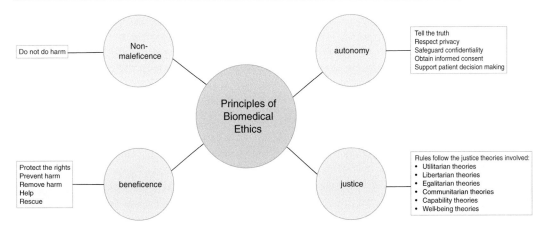

Fig. 31.1 Overview of biomedical ethics following Beauchamp and Childress [4]

Ethical Principles of Biomedicine

Before going into the details of digital ethics, the four principles will be presented and discussed based on Beauchamp and Childress's book [4]. Figure 31.1 provides an overview of these principles and their meaning.

Autonomy is the capacity to decide and act on your own in accordance with your beliefs and values. An autonomous person decides and acts intentionally based on a plan, understands the decision and action, and is free from control by external forces or internal conditions that counteract the self-directedness of the person. The patient's autonomy as a value to be strived for entails that healthcare professionals actively support the patient to be or remain autonomous. The respect for autonomy practically embraces the following:

- Telling the truth to the patients
- Respecting their privacy
- Treating entrusted information as confidential
- Obtaining consent from the patient
- Helping to make decisions when asked to do so

This list exemplifies the active behavior on the part of the health professional. However, it is neither exhaustive nor is it entirely specific to autonomy only, meaning that it could be motivated and justified by other principles as well. Although autonomy of the patient is a state to be aspired it can be challenged by situations where patients do

not want to be autonomous. This can be the case, for example, if they do not want to hear the truth about their illness or cannot act and decide in a self-directed way because they are mentally ill. Cultural differences may lead to different interpretations of the autonomy principle as is extensively discussed in Beauchamp and Childress's book [4]. They also deliberate the issues surrounding patient competencies to make autonomous decisions as well as the prerequisites, the meaning and practice of informed consent in its various manifestations.

Nonmaleficence means that interventions in medicine and patient care shall not harm the patient. It refers to the famous imperative "primum non nocere"—"above all—do not harm" which goes back to Hippocrates. The concept of harming is hereby understood as an activity that in the end leads to an adverse effect on one's interests, mainly physical and psychological interests. It includes thwarting, defeating, or setting back the interests of another person such as inflicting pain, disability, and suffering as well as causing death.

Nonmaleficence is distinguished from beneficence through the concept of avoidance of harmful actions (nonmaleficence) contrasting helping and assisting actions (beneficence). Therefore, nonmaleficence is often expressed as "do not do a certain action," whereas beneficence goes along with preventing or removing evil or harm as well as doing good. Pursuant to Beauchamp and Childress, the rules exemplifying nonmaleficence are ([4] p. 159):

- *Do not kill*
- *Do not cause pain or suffering*
- *Do not incapacitate*
- *Do not cause offense*
- *Do not deprive others of the goods of life*

Good and bad effects (double effects) may result from the same action, e.g., administering medication that reduces pain but may also kill the patient. In order to justify an action as morally permissible, four conditions are discussed ([4] p. 167):

1. *The nature of the act*
2. *The agent's intention*
3. *The distinction between means and effect*
4. *Proportionality between the good and the bad effect*

There is a series of controversial issues in the context of nonmaleficence that cannot be discussed in full length here but should only be briefly listed. They encompass withholding and withdrawing treatments, optional and obligatory treatments, letting or allowing someone to die, and finally assisting in dying. They illustrate the complexity and diversity of this principle.

Beneficence, the complementary principle to nonmaleficence, is defined as all of the activities benefiting people and contributing to their well-being. Beauchamp and Childress distinguish the two principles of beneficence: positive beneficence and utility. Positive beneficence includes the following obligatory rules ([4] p. 219):

- *Protect and defend the rights of others.*
- *Prevent harm from occurring to others.*
- *Remove conditions that will cause harm to others.*
- *Help persons with disabilities.*
- *Rescue persons in danger.*

Hereby, rescuing persons, not only those with whom special relations are entertained, such as family members and patients, is considered as an obligation to be impartially followed. This means that it applies in general (general beneficence), i.e., also to strangers. Rules of specific beneficence, called the duties, are related to specific groups of persons or individuals, such as the patients in healthcare. The obligation to rescue a person in order to prevent the loss or damage of "*basic interests*" ([4], p. 222), such as life and health, is bound to certain conditions. These conditions are that the action is necessary and will be probably successful; furthermore, that the action is not associated with "*significant risks, costs, and burdens*" ([4], p. 222) for the rescuing person nor do these harms, costs, or burdens outweigh the benefits gained for the beneficiary.

Among the justifications for the obligation to benefit others, reciprocity can play a particular role. Based on social interaction, reciprocity means that the benefit gained by the beneficiaries will be returned by them to the one who granted the benefit. As an example, Beauchamp and Childress refer to the concept of the Learning Health System where the health professionals' care for their patients is based on knowledge gained through the most recent patient data. While the patients contribute by consenting to the use of their data to develop new knowledge and thereby allow the care providers to learn, they, in turn, improve their processes and treatments according to these recent findings.

The principle of beneficence may conflict with the principle of autonomy. This is the case when the intent to benefit the patient by some actions, e.g., treatments, clashes with their own ideas and decisions, e.g., not accepting this treatment. Not respecting the autonomy of the patients has been criticized as "paternalism," meaning making decisions over the head of that patient and thereby overriding the patient's preferences.

When there are tensions between equal ethical principles, benefits, risks, and costs of an action have to be balanced. There are various approaches of risk-benefit analyses, cost-effectiveness, or cost-benefit analyses that will not be discussed here.

Justice is understood by many philosophers as "*a fair, equitable, and appropriate treatment in light of what is due or owed to affected individuals or groups*" ([4], pp. 267–268). Such treatment is based on material principles, for example, on needs such as the fundamental needs that are associated with providing basic resources to prevent harm, e.g., developing a disease or becoming malnourished. There is no generally uncontradicted theoretical understanding of what justice means, and the various theories partly reflect diametrically opposed views. Beauchamp and Childress present six theories to show the broad spectrum, particularly with regard to health and healthcare.

- **Utilitarian theories**: Proponents of these theories argue that the rules of justice are rooted in the principle of maximizing utility and social welfare. Healthcare interventions for individuals as well as for the public would thus be justified by improving welfare.
- **Libertarian theories**: These theories revolve around the respecting of individual freedom and property. The principles of justice embrace acquiring, transferring, and rectifying property and are bound by the forces of the free market. By doing so, a just society enables the individual to improve their personal circumstances and make their own arrangements for their health.
- **Egalitarian theories**: Egalitarian theories assert that it is just to treat persons as equals. The amount of liberty permitted to one person is comparable to the amount of another person. Gaining a fair and equal share of opportunities should be achievable for everyone.
- **Communitarian theories**: They emphasize the social relations between individuals and their entrenchment in communities that determine their life. Individual rights that counteract the common good are not worth striving for. In healthcare, such theories would contend that organ donation is generally possible as long as the donor did not object to it explicitly before death.
- **Capability theories**: They belong to a group of theories that strongly consider the value of health. The freedom to achieve a healthy state and a state of well-being depends on the capabilities of a person to lead a life according to one's values. Inequalities can be fought by expanding human capabilities.
- **Well-being theories**: Another group of theories also focusing on health are the well-being theories. In contrast to capability theories, they lay the focus on well-being itself, not on the capability of it. The core six-element

encompass health, personal security, knowledge and understanding, equal respect, personal attachments, and self-determination. A just society ensures that these "states of being" are experienced by all of its members.

Justice theories address discourses about inequalities, disparities, and vulnerabilities as well as how to mitigate or redress them. Countries that have implemented the "right to healthcare" argue on the basis of utilitarian, egalitarian, and communitarian theories. These arguments may apply to the local level as well as the global level.

Beauchamp and Childress's account on ethical principles in biomedicine refers to care and research alike. Ethical concepts and rules in biomedical research in particular were globally described by the World Medical Association in the Declaration of Helsinki [5] that was first issued in 1964 and builds upon the Declaration of Geneva [2]. Meanwhile, many institutional review boards (IRB) work according to its code of ethics. Initiated by severe misconduct in a research study on syphilis, the Belmont Report of 1979 [6] set out the ethical principles and serves as guideline for the protection of human subjects of research. It distinguishes care delivery from scientific research and stipulates that any research taking place in the context of patient care, e.g., assessment of treatment, should undergo special review to ensure the protection of human subjects. The report grounds its explications on the ethical principles of respect of persons, beneficence, and justice. See Table 31.1 for an overview of the relevant documents.

Ethics in Digital Healthcare

While the principles of bioethics as presented hereinabove already give a good overview of what ethics means in medicine, nursing, and healthcare, special challenges arise with:

- The advent of new or elaborated technologies, e.g., machine learning and automation.
- Sharing large amounts of data, e.g., for public health or research.

- Reaching out to patients with digital means and obtaining data outside the healthcare setting, e.g., mobile apps and smart devices.
- Blurring the boundaries between care delivery and research, e.g., multipurpose use of data.
- Changing the provider–patient relationship, e.g., telehealth, social media, and the various digital information sources, just to name a few.

These challenges do not render the existing principles, such as the ones propagated by Beauchamp and Childress (and others), useless—on the contrary. However, they call for special attention to be paid to issues arising from the digitalization of healthcare that not only may be disruptive in many ways but that matters because of scaling effects. Due to the ease of multiplications through digital means, ethical problems can be multiplied as seen when sharing large amounts of data across the healthcare system. A similar situation is observed on the population level where the digital divide may contribute to aggravating the social determinants of health due to poor digital health literacy and reduced access to appropriate equipment. Another example is the case of the ubiquitous monitoring of the elderly suffering from dementia through video or GPS tracking.

These new scenarios embrace technical, organizational, social, behavioral, and mental implications spanning all levels from the individual to society and require a thorough ethical evaluation.

Perspectives on Ethics in Digital Healthcare

Introduction

Different perspectives on outstanding ethical challenges will be taken up in the following subchapters on ethics in digital health (Fig. 31.2). These perspectives will overlap and address recurring moral values and demands for actions. The first part will elaborate on ethical inquiries that are prompted by technologies, including data and algorithms, embracing smart and

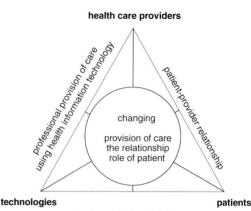

Fig. 31.2 Three perspectives and new ethical challenges due to changes

mobile devices, and social media. The second section focuses on the patients and their right to privacy, confidential treatment of their data, and data ownership. It presents various manifestations of consent and provides an outlook on the opportunities for the participation of patients in research. The third and final perspective represents the healthcare provider which also subsumes the patient–provider relationship.

Technologies

Big Data, Artificial Intelligence, and Machine Learning

With the increasing adoption of electronic patient and health records, patient data that had been confined to paper archives and were only arduously analyzable have become a thing of the past. Interoperable electronic records opened the door to allow the secondary use of the data for quality control, process improvement, decision support, and research. This does not hold only internally within an organization but also externally across organizations. The larger the amount of data is, the better the advanced algorithms of machine learning can be applied. Sharing patient data between organizations on a large scale has, therefore, also becomes attractive for the sake of obtaining results that can be generalized. Big data, data science, and artificial intelligence are

Fig. 32.3 Data ethics

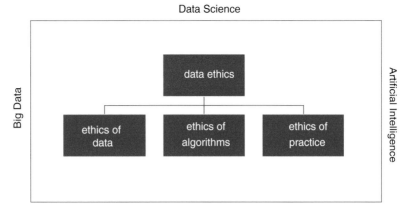

the key concepts that enclose these developments. At their intersection, the use of personal data and the application of so-called black box algorithms have given cause for ethical concerns leading to the development of the concept of data ethics that embraces *ethics of data, ethics of algorithms,* and *ethics of practice* (Fig. 32.3).

Data ethics touches on the moral challenges concerning privacy and anonymity as well as transparency, trust, and responsibility along the pipeline of collecting, curing, analyzing data, and using the results [7]. *Ethics of data* (as a component of data ethics) hereby refers to treating data and the related moral problems:

- Generating and recording data—ensuring the informed consent of the patient, selecting a good data set for training the algorithms.
- Curing the data in case of inconsistencies or missing values, for example.
- Processing them, e.g., adjusting for biases such as the underrepresentation of minorities, anonymizing data, labeling the data so that algorithms can be trained.
- Disseminating, sharing, or any other case of using them, e.g., encrypting data for transportation or storage, using privacy respecting algorithms, or sharing only model parameters, not the raw data.

Ethics of algorithms is concerned with issues arising from the autonomy and complexity of algorithms [7] particularly with the fact that certain algorithms provide results without being able to demonstrate how and why they arrived at this specific result. They are called black box algorithms. Deep learning algorithms as a class of machine learning algorithms belonging to this type. Unlike, for example, regression analysis, they do not come up with coefficients reflecting the contribution of a specific variable to the overall result and as a result of this, explain the meaning of the output. The results can be any kind of output, such as predicting complications under a certain treatment or the classification of patients into groups most susceptible to acquiring a certain condition. Algorithms of such types can be employed in clinical decision support systems. Moral problems related to black box algorithms are a lack of transparency about the way they function and/or the inexplicability of the findings. Given the circumstances wherein health professionals want to rely on these results and ground their clinical decision on them, they cannot explain the rationale to their patients as they should. Therefore, trust can be compromised on the end of the care provider who does not trust the algorithm as well as on the end of the patient who does not trust the provider. Furthermore, issues of responsibility are also concerned: Who is responsible and accountable in case of health complications or death? What roles do the algorithm designers and data scientists play?

Ethics of practice addresses inquiries about professional codes and duties. It includes questions about the responsibilities and liabilities of persons and organizations to ensure the protection of individuals in terms of privacy and to ensure their consent as well as the development of data science and the secondary use of the data [7]. The balance between overprotecting the individual (principle of autonomy) and allowing the social value of data-driven research (principles of beneficence and justice) should guide ethical practice and governance.

Many authors strongly emphasize the paramount importance of data and even "put them before the algorithm" [8] because algorithms can only identify facts in data that are already there. This imposes the obligation to aim for diverse data sets that are representative of the population to avoid biases. Therefore, it is not only the volume but also, first and foremost, the veracity of the data that counts.

Smart Assistive Technologies

Among the many other technologies that raise ethical questions, this chapter will focus on smart assistive technologies, which are also called intelligent assistive technologies (IAT) or ambient assisted living (AAL) technologies. These technologies are primarily developed and implemented to support the elderly to lead a self-determined life. These technologies are often meant to avail persons suffering from self-care deficits or with nursing needs. A particularly challenging group are people with dementia, including those with mild dementia living at home.

IATs embrace video-monitoring and GPS tracking systems, cognitive assistants, and personal robots including companionship robots. Ethical considerations touch on obtaining informed consent, respecting the privacy sphere, protecting from restraint, and the moral problem of deception with the aim of beneficence [9]. Other ethical issues arise when IATs are used for predictive and preventive purposes (e.g., fall prevention) as well as for disease and disability management. These purposes require large amounts of data from almost every aspect of daily life, including the behavior of the patients. Furthermore, for these systems to work efficiently, the extensive use of monitoring, surveillance, and sensor technology in the home environment is necessary. The ubiquitous presence of surveillance technology and the permanent collection of data raises several ethical

issues that can be framed as "4d-risks": the **d**epersonalization of care through algorithm-based standardization, the **d**iscrimination of minority groups through generalization, the **d**ehumanization of the care relationship through automatization, and the **d**isciplination of users through monitoring and surveillance [10].

These new technologies often do not receive a sufficient level of acceptance and adoption because of ethical concerns [11], which demonstrates the increasing importance of ethics in digital health and social care. However, and in contrast to the ethical reservations associated with assistive technologies, particularly IATs for persons with dementia are developed to do good. Ienca and colleagues [9], therefore, investigated what ethical principles guided technical developers. They found that autonomy and independence were the most relevant objectives referred to when designing a system, such as smart home technologies for ensuring independent living. The second and third ranking (almost on tied ranks) were beneficence and nonmaleficence. Enhancing quality of life, establishing well-being, improving self-esteem, and protecting the dignity of the users were mentioned as well as risk reduction in terms of preventing falls while still ensuring mobility. Issues of justice were found less often, although some technologies were deliberately developed with the intent to minimize the cost and other barriers. Interdependence in the sense of social inclusion and exchange and counteracting isolation was the second last ethical value explicitly addressed by the system developers, while ensuring privacy was the one least often mentioned as a positive goal [9].

The study by Ienca and colleagues illustrates the fact that ethical considerations do not only appear in the context of problems of technologies but also as desiderata, i.e., what technologies can contribute to make life better. Meanwhile "Ethics by design" [12] has become an approach considering the ethical values throughout the system life cycle and does not hold for healthcare only. Whether all of these objectives were finally reached and appreciated was beyond the aim of [9] and would be a matter of ex post evaluation scrutinizing the perceived consequences of a technology.

Social Media

Many other technologies have prompted ethical inquiries, such as social media in healthcare, which play an important role because of their widespread use. Due to the limitations of this chapter, we will not be able to cover this field in full depth here and will pick out some issues. When meant to support the patient–provider relationship, social media may lead to severe problems of privacy and confidentiality, as was shown by [13], for the case of mental care for adolescents. Professional ethical rules and the laws define the framework of using social media in patient care, but more education in online professionalism is needed to raise the awareness of problems in a situation where care providers may feel forced to engage in social media [14]. This holds true for the entire spectrum of care provision, research, and academic education [15].

Patients

In reviewing the literature, we showed that informed consent, privacy, and confidentiality sometimes also paired with data ownership were the most often addressed ethical values in the context of clinical and health information systems. This review also included electronic health records, systems for health information exchange, and clinical decision support systems [16]. It also embraced technologies reaching out to patients, in particular mobile devices, health apps, social media, and assistive technologies that are coupled with clinical information systems. This finding illustrates the general conception that topics immediately related to the patient as an individual is of the highest priority. The patients' autonomy as well as their right to exert control over their data and the environment they live in is of utmost importance.

This finding is not new and reflects previous literature reviews. For example, Mittelstadt and Floridi [17] discuss **informed consent** and several alternatives in the context of Big Data research. Informed consent, which rests on the pillars of the information given to the patient, the comprehension of this information by the patient, and the voluntariness of giving consent [18], is the classical way of expressing the approval to use the data for a single-instance and a well-described purpose. In the case of using non-anonymized personal data, it is necessary to obtain consent as it is stipulated in many laws, e.g., the EU General Data Protection Regulation, which defines consent in the following way in Article 4 Definitions [19]:

> Consent of the data subject means any freely given, specific, informed, and unambiguous indication of the data subject's wishes by which he or she, by a statement or by a clear affirmative action, signifies agreement to the processing of personal data relating to him or her.

While the legal foundation is clear, it is discussed how practical it is to obtain the consent for a retrospective analysis of routine data and whether it is feasible at all to obtain consent that would require a special purpose to be described when Big Data analysis as a matter of fact seeks to explore new knowledge in unchartered territories. Excessively high standards for data protection may go along with missed opportunities to develop, for example, new treatment knowledge. These missed opportunities may harm instead of protect the patients [17].

Alternative ways of consent are presented and deliberated with pros and cons. They embrace [18]:

- Broad and blanket consent to preauthorize all of the different types of secondary use.
- Tiered consent that is given to a circumscribed field of uses, e.g., a specific clinical domain.
- Opt-out consent that equals a broad consent unless the patient opts-out.
- Dynamic consent that is given by the patients on a case-by-case basis and is practically implemented via an electronic platform through which the researchers and the patients communicate driven by new analysis options.
- Open consent that is equivalent to the motivation of sharing data as a gift to the public.

Relying on solidarity rather than on autonomy may render consent superfluous because it builds on the willingness of people to support research [17].

New approaches to govern research and ensure the access to the relevant data involve the patients and their representatives (advocate groups). This entails establishing communities consisting of researchers, care providers, and patients to set the agenda. Various roles for patients can be envisioned from just consenting to providing their data or being consulted to setting the research agenda and serving as co-principle investigators [20]. In order to place the patients in the "driver's seat" [p. 788], they must, however, be educated and be able to judge the opportunities and risks of Big Data applications such as precision medicine [21].

Alike informed consent, **privacy and confidentiality** issues relate to the ethical principle of autonomy. From a legal perspective, they are covered by pertinent regulations, such as the GDPR [19]. Ensuring privacy is closely connected to the anonymization of personal data, an ideal and procedure that is increasingly difficult to put into practice due to the possibility of cross-referencing with other data [16]. Similarly, privacy is challenged by linking data from different sectors including settings outside of healthcare, e.g., from fitness and well-being, when data that are otherwise difficult to understand become meaningful through this linkage [22]. Despite a general approval of sharing data from electronic health records, people regarded their privacy at risk, to lose control over their data and be confronted to unintended data leakage, unauthorized access, re-identification, and errors in medical records [23]. Outside big data research and artificial intelligence, privacy is at stake when technologies intrude into the personal and living environment, as is often the case with smart assistive technologies when monitoring persons, particularly those who suffer from dementia. This application portrays the tension between privacy (autonomy) and safety (beneficence) [24]. Privacy and confidentiality issues may also arise in other specific populations, for example, in children and adolescents, as is illustrated by the use of the Australian electronic personal health record MyHR. Children

might not have had the opportunity to decide for themselves as to what information should be visible to others in their MyHR. Furthermore, they might be cautious and reluctant in using the record out of fear that their parents have access to their records. The children's right for privacy (autonomy) thus conflicts with their parents' interest and obligation to take care of their children (beneficence) [25].

Finally, **data ownership**, a topic discussed in the context of informed consent, privacy, and confidentiality, describes both the power to control the data and the right to benefit from the data [16]. Notably, the intellectual property ownership rights in the context of the results derived from patient data, such as in electronic health records, are still an ambiguous issue [26].

Autonomy of patients is a multifaceted area. An important aspect is the twofold role of autonomy when it comes to telehealth and health apps. While these technologies may empower the autonomy of patients through their focus on self-directed actions, these technologies also require a certain degree of autonomy to handle the equipment which can be difficult when (re)building autonomy is a therapeutic goal (e.g., in psychotherapy) [27].

Healthcare Providers and Their Relationship to Patients

Autonomous Decision-Making

While respecting ethical principles when caring for patients traditionally centered around the patients, e.g., their autonomy, new intelligent technologies that are meant to support the care providers turn the spotlight on the providers themselves. One of the groups that have been increasingly confronted with such technologies are radiologists who more and more employ intelligent image analysis tools in diagnosing patients. As they have been actually exposed to Artificial Intelligence technologies and have gained personal experience, they are the ones who, worldwide, raise questions about to what degree can they delegate tasks to such autonomous systems or how can they gird themselves for the automation bias, i.e., the tendency to rather rely on machine results than on human ones [28]. In the same vein, fear is expressed that they would become redundant in light of automatic segmentation (e.g., delineating the tumor), lesion detection, measurements of any kind, and comparison with images of prior encounters [29]. Even if not becoming redundant, it is the radiologist's independent decision-making process that is at stake. Depending on the level of automation, the liability can actually shift from the radiologist to the manufacturer of the AI system [26]. Due to the increasing power of software and its algorithms, software is regarded as a medical device. It is, therefore, subject to the pertinent regulations, e.g., the EU Medical Device Regulation [30] or the FDA Device Regulation [31], which cannot be presented here in-depth. In any case, analyzing the potential risks of intelligent software systems and evaluating their clinical benefit become even more necessary under circumstances wherein software can cause harm.

Harming Clinicians

Digitalization can affect healthcare providers themselves in many ways, not only interfering with their own self-concept as independent health professionals. With the massive adoption of electronic health record systems (and other digital systems) and their use in daily practice in the USA, clinician burnout has become a phenomenon addressed in many recent discussions, e.g., [32–34]. This is a case where digital tools can cause harm to health professionals. The underlying causes could be manifold and include increased workload [32], software poorly integrated into the clinical workflows with bad usability [33], and systems that do not support the intrinsic motivation of clinicians, e.g., autonomy, creativity, and connectedness [34]. Notwithstanding that clinician burnout is a complex condition and relates to an ethical issue, it is not the technology as such that may cause the damage but instances and implementations of a specific real-world system that need to be thoroughly evaluated and improved. For example, over-standardization of patient data without allowing for the narrative of the patient case can be avoided in conceptualizing the EHR with free text sections to account for the documentation of social and behavioral determinants of health, the information of which is often found in the nonstandardized sections of an EHR. In order for healthcare professionals not to be forced to compensate the risk and potential collateral damages resulting from information technologies [35], pertinent skills of physicians as well as nurses have to be enhanced by education and training. "Technomoral wisdom" and leadership have to be developed to overcome the technology-caring gap [36].

Not only are health professionals themselves challenged through the digitalization of care, but it is also their relationship with the patients that faces new scenarios previously impossible. With the advent of health apps and telemedicine, patients are able to collect and share health and fitness data with their care providers. When this happens in a technically well-defined environment based on mutual approval, it can enrich the patient–provider relationship and empower the patient to engage in disease self-management [37]. However, when data are shared in an unsolicited manner and without prior personal contact, respectively, without establishing a patient–provider relationship, many issues including ethical ones can arise. They embrace, among others, obtaining consent, respecting and ensuring privacy and confidentiality, data security, data quality, record keeping, and overall responsibility [38]. While problematic data treatment can be triggered by the patients themselves, as seen in the previous example, the provider's inappropriate data handling can also trigger unethical behavior. Such a phenomenon has become known under the term "patient targeted googling" and refers to cases when psychotherapists search the Internet for the most recent information about their patients without letting them know. Such activities behind the back of patients do not foster an open and trusting relationship [39].

When applied excessively, health apps and devices might produce an exaggerated awareness of one's health condition that may have repercussions on how care providers and patients encounter each other. It may, for example, compromise the trust of the patients in their providers when the information from the device and that of the provider differ. Alike, the trustworthiness of the patients' accounts may be questioned by the providers. Thus, the safe and appropriate use of mobile health devices and the data that looms large calls upon sufficient education on the part of the patients as well as on that of the providers [40]. Education to empower the patients and the providers alike for using the technology in an ethical manner has been recommended in several publications and was summarized in [16]. As a matter of fact, Goodman envisions health information technology as a fulcrum to "invigorate" ethics in medical curricula. General urgent ethical topics, such as "privacy, end-of-life care, access to healthcare and valid consent, and clinician–patient communication," can be exemplified using health informatics [41].

Ethical Evaluation of Health IT

The importance and need to carry out ethical evaluation studies have been stressed at various points in the previous subchapters. Based on the finding that many publications on the ethics of digital healthcare deliberate on the ethical challenges rather than show these issues in practice, empirical studies are urgently required [16]. This means investigating the ethical impact of a particular technical implementation in a selected environment and its practical use in this scenario. Evaluation studies that have been focusing on efficiency and effectiveness in the past need to extend their scope to ethical inquiries. If addressed, ethical matters are often covered by the ELSI complex, i.e., Ethical, Legal, and Social Issues, which then sometimes appears as an addendum to the main research questions.

In the MAST (Model for Assessment of Telemedicine Applications) technology assessment model, ethical, legal, and social aspects are a part of domain 7 "socio-cultural, ethics, and legal aspects." This model was primarily designed for multidisciplinary assessments of an applica-

tion, its safety, clinical effectiveness, the patient perspectives, and the organizational and economic aspects that form the other six domains of the model [42].

In contrast to MAST, the MEESTAR model (Fig. 32.4), which stands for "Model for the Ethical Evaluation of Socio-Technological Arrangements," is specifically meant to support ethical analyses [43]. The fields of application are intelligent assistive technologies. However, the model is also useful outside of this particular area.

The model [43] conceptualizes the following seven dimensions:

- **care**, in the sense of taking care of someone in need.
- **autonomy**, as defined by Beauchamp and Childress [4].
- **safety**, in a wide meaning of the term, including security and the prevention of harm.
- **justice**, here particularly social justice evaluated vis-à-vis various understandings of the concept [4].
- **privacy**, defined as the inviolable zone around a person and derived from autonomy, including solitude, isolation, anonymity, and intimacy with friends and family.
- **participation**, in the meaning of living together with others in society and opposed to exclusion.
- **self-conception**, meaning the way a person perceives and understands himself or herself, for example, as old, ill, or powerful.

These dimensions are relevant on an individual, organizational, and societal level. The technologies to be assessed can be graded according to their perceived potential to do harm into four categories: stage I (no harm), stage II (ethically sensitive), stage III (ethically extremely sensitive), and stage IV (should be rejected from an ethical point of view) [43].

The spectrum of ethical analyses is broad and reaches from early discourses to evaluating a mature technology in a specific environment. As Reijders and colleagues [44] explain, there are various points in time to start the ethical analysis,

Fig. 32.4 The
MEESTAR model based
on [43]

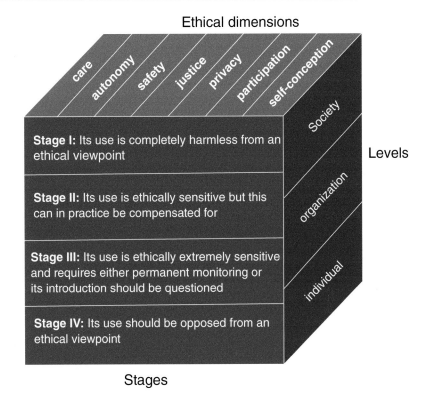

influencing the research methods to be applied. The *ex ante method* investigates technologies in a very early stage, often studies emerging technologies, and aims to anticipate the ethically crucial uses and impacts without looking at a real-world implementation but rather at application scenarios. The *intra method* is applied during the technical design and development process, which then has already become clearer and better defined. Any kind of formative evaluation methods that accompany the realization, such as interactive technology assessment, are suitable in this phase. "Ethics by design" approaches can benefit from *intra method* procedures as they both target the conceptualization and implementation phase. Finally, there is the group of *ex post methods* that seek to identify the ethical impacts of the existing technologies applied in practice [44]. While the MAST and MEESTAR models can be used in any of these phases, they are most valuable when employed in the ex post analysis where the contours of the application are clear and more robust and detailed conclusions can be drawn.

Case Study

The preferred treatment or care at the end-of-life or in case of emergencies that would require resuscitation to save the patient's life are usually expressed in the documentation of the code status or an advance directive. The code status describes the type of resuscitation procedures (if any) that the patient would like the healthcare providers to conduct. Advance directives and code status reflect the intent of the patient and ultimately are statements based on the patient's self-determination and autonomy. However, the hospital staff is not uncommonly confronted with decisions about further treatment or resuscitation despite missing or unclear information about the patient's desire.

This US case study [45], based on the work of the Ethics Committee of the American Medical Informatics Association (AMIA), addresses this ethical issue and illustrates a solution of documenting the patient preferences as code status in a standardized and unambiguous way. In the ideal case, this information would be captured early enough, e.g., at admission, so that no additional emotional stress and burden are put on the patients, their families, or the providers in a life-critical situation. Due to the legal requirements, US hospitals (and those in other countries as well) are obliged to document whether an advance directive exists or has been executed whereby the healthcare providers have to transfer this information into a code status. Despite these requirements, the use of advance directives and code status were reported to be low with only very few healthcare organizations enabling electronic documentation of the code status. Against this background, the AMIA Ethics Committee set up a consensus process for developing a minimum data set to be implemented as a standard in electronic health records.

This data set includes the following mandatory data and corresponding example categories in {} with conditional elements indicated by arrows (→):

- Organization: Where the code status was obtained or documented.
- Patient identifier.
- Patient last name.
- Patient first name.
- Patient date of birth in case of a minor patient → assent of the patient to action in an Advance Directive.
- Date of code status: The date when the code status was obtained, updated, or confirmed.
- Provider recording the code status information: name.
- Provider phone number.
- Provider phone number type.
- Patient ability to consent: {"able to consent," "unable to consent"} in case of "unable" → patient's proxy, surrogate, and/or guardian → relationship of proxy, surrogate, and/or guardian to patient.
- Patient's proxy phone number.
- Code status type: {"full code", "do not resuscitate (DNR)" or "limited resuscitation"} in case of "limited resuscitation" → list of limitations.

There is also a number of optional elements that embrace—amongst others—information about the existence of relevant documents, including a living will and how to obtain these documents. It also allows for information about the name of a witness to the discussion about the code status with the patient or family.

When implemented in electronic health records, this minimum data set would help to provide and communicate detailed information about the code status in emergency or generally in end-of-life situations. It is meant to improve the current practice and help the patients (and their families) to execute their right for self-determination and autonomy.

Summary

This chapter provided an overview of ethics in biomedicine and healthcare focusing on providing care and conducting research in digital environments. A brief historical overview is given relating to milestone declarations after the Second World War. An introduction to the four ethical principles of autonomy, nonmaleficence, beneficence, and justice in biomedicine, according to Beauchamp and Childress [4], is presented. They offer a good foundation for systematizing the ethical inquiries related to the design, implementation, and use of health IT. These ethical questions referring to digitally supported care and research are discussed according to different perspectives.

The first perspective emphasizes the technology investigating the ethical issues raised by big data, artificial intelligence and machine learning, smart assistive technologies, and social media. Data ethics comprising the ethics of data, algorithms, and practice highlights the importance of unbiased and veracious data and their ethically sensitive handling and use as well as the capability of algorithms to provide explanations about how they arrived at their results (explicability). Smart assistive technologies aiming to improve the safety and quality of life of the elderly are checked regarding their initial ethical approach and the concept of "ethics by design." It is argued that the inherent threats to privacy and the confidentiality of information when using social media can only be mitigated by educating the providers and patients alike.

The second perspective is related to the patients covering the nature and foundation of informed consent in the current data protection regulations, alternative ways of obtaining consent, and the threats and risks to privacy and confidentiality. Data ownership is presented as the power to control the data and the right to benefit from the data.

The third and final perspective refers to the healthcare providers and their relationship with the patients. With an increase in autonomy and the pervasion of digital tools, providers are confronted with the risk of losing their independence in decision-making and are themselves becoming victims of poor digital workflows and bad usability of systems. Clinician burnout has become a major issue and is an example of a risk showing that health IT cannot harm patients only but also the providers. Digital media can change the way in which providers and patients used to interact and establish a trustful relationship. Examples of unsolicited data sent by patients to providers and patient-targeted-googling are examples of ethical challenges.

Information technologies are neither good nor bad. It is how they are intended, implemented, and practically used by people that make all the difference. Therefore, assessments and evaluation studies of health IT regarding their ethical impact are required. These studies can be guided by models, such as the MAST and MEESTAR evaluation model.

The case study finally yields an example of what standardized data elements of code status should be implemented in electronic health records to improve the current practice of ensuring the patient's preferences during their end-of-life situation.

Conclusions and Outlook

Several conclusions can be drawn from the current state of affairs and ethical discourses. First, too little is known about the ethical impacts of the real-world applications of health IT. Rigorous methods and evaluation designs have to be employed to gain insights beyond anticipations and case reports. Due to the importance of ethics,

ethical issues must not be hidden in the ELSI complex but must stand out on an equal footing with efficiency and effectiveness.

Second, information technologies become unethical because of their unethical use by people. Various examples in the subchapters herein illustrated this fact and arrived at the conclusion that more education is necessary. Education shall hereby concern providers and patients alike. Practical examples of using technologies in defined situations and relating to theoretical principles and professional ethics code should bridge moral behavior and ethics discourses.

Third, the secondary use of patient data, linking data sets, and analyzing them for purposes outside of the field to which the informed consent was given, all pose ethical tension. This tension between the legal obligation to obtain the patient's consent and the opportunity to develop new crucial medical knowledge from reusing patient data outside of the original purpose for which the consent was given requires new approaches of governance. The voluntary donation of data is a practice that marries the principle of autonomy, particularly self-determination, with that of communitarian justice in the meaning of doing something for the greater good. Involving patients in the research process is another way of ensuring that the voice of the patients, who are granting access to their data, is heard. Other governance structures allow for a process of negotiations with all stakeholders under the guidance of neutral data stewards [22].

New information technologies with new ethical challenges require new approaches. Establishing new governance approaches hereby needs practical advice and concepts from ethics particularly ethics in the sense of a discipline that attends to interpreting and shaping regulations from an ethical perspective. This entails that ethics does not only play the role of asking the right questions but also that of actively developing concepts and schemes for the daily practice of digital healthcare and research.

Review Questions

1. What is ethics?
2. What are the major internationally relevant declarations and their scope?
3. Please sketch the four ethical principles in biomedicine according to Beauchamp and Childress.
4. Please describe and discuss three ethical challenges of big data analysis and artificial intelligence.
5. Please describe and discuss three ethically relevant goals of smart assistive technologies.
6. What is informed consent and what problems arise when data are to be reused?
7. Please describe and discuss three cases of threats to privacy and confidentiality due to health IT.
8. How are care providers themselves concerned regarding the use of artificial intelligence tools and electronic health records?
9. Please illustrate (one example) how the patient–provider relationship can be affected through digital media.
10. Please briefly describe the dimensions captured in the MEESTAR model and the three time points when assessment and evaluation can take place.

Appendix: Answers to Review Questions

1. What is ethics?

Ethics or moral philosophy is a scientific discipline that studies moral behavior and beliefs. Ethical studies can be broken down into nonnormative ethics and normative ethics.

2. What are the major internationally relevant declarations and their scope?

Declaration of Geneva: Ethical principles of the medical profession

Code of Ethics for Nurses: Ethical principles of the nursing profession

Declaration of Helsinki: Medical research involving human subjects

Belmont Report: Biomedical and behavioral research involving human subjects.

3. Please sketch the four ethical principles in biomedicine according to Beauchamp and Childress.

Autonomy is the capacity to decide and act on your own in accordance with your beliefs and values. Decisions and actions are made intentionally based on a plan with an understanding about the decision and action and are made free from control by external forces or internal conditions that counteract the self-directedness of the person.

Nonmaleficence means that interventions in medicine and patient care shall not harm the patient. Related activities are often expressed as "do not do a certain action."

Beneficence, the complementary principle to nonmaleficence, is defined as all activities benefiting people and contributing to their well-being. It includes the protection of others, the prevention and removal of harm as well as helping and rescuing.

Justice is understood by many philosophers as "a fair, equitable, and appropriate treatment in light of what is due or owed to affected individuals or groups." Theories of justice may be classified as utilitarian, egalitarian, libertarian, communitarian in addition to theories specifically related to health.

4. Please describe and discuss three ethical challenges of big data analysis and artificial intelligence.

Ethics of data referring to generating and recording, curing, processing, and disseminating data addresses the challenge to provide unbiased, relevant and meaningful, representative data of high quality that include minorities, are gender-balanced and truthful because they constitute the primary basis for the algorithms.

Ethics of algorithms embraces the explicability of statistical and all other mathematical, and computer science methods for analyzing the data. These methods should demonstrate how they arrived at their result. Otherwise, clinicians cannot justify the use of these findings toward themselves and decisions based on these findings toward their patients.

Ethics of practice is related to defining responsibilities and duties, for example, within the framework of professional ethics code ensuring amongst other the respect for privacy and confidentiality. Ethics of practice is also concerned with the balancing of conflicting ethical values.

5. Please describe and discuss three ethically relevant goals of smart assistive technologies.

Smart assistive technologies are designed and developed with the intention to help and support persons with self-care problems often the elderly. Ethically relevant goals referring to ethical principles are autonomy including independence (e.g., smart home technologies for ensuring independent living), beneficence and nonmaleficence intended to enhance the quality of life, establishing well-being, improving self-esteem and protecting the dignity of the users, reducing risk (e.g., increased mobility through intelligent walkers).

6. What is informed consent and what problems arise when data are to be reused?

Informed consent of the data subject means any freely given, specific, and unambiguous indication of the data subject's wishes that signifies agreement to the processing of personal data relating to him or her. Informed consent rests on information, understanding, and voluntariness. It is related to a single instance and a particular purpose. The problems that arise in the case of secondary use are based on these two requirements because secondary use typically goes beyond that specific purpose and is often connected with multiple analyses.

7. Please describe and discuss three cases of threats to privacy and confidentiality due to health IT.

Ensuring privacy that is closely connected to the anonymization of personal data is jeopardized by the possibility of *cross-referencing* with other data set and thus reversing the de-identification. It is also challenged when data from different sectors including settings from outside of health care, e. g. from fitness and well-being are *linked* and thus attain distinction that was not previously extractable. Privacy is also at stake when technologies intrude into the personal and living environment as is often the case with smart assistive technologies when they are *monitoring persons* via video cameras and or tracking them via GPS. Privacy and confidentiality could be compromised when *parents access* personal electronic health records of their adolescent children who wished that this information is only retrievable by their provider.

8. How are care providers themselves concerned regarding the use of artificial intelligence tools and electronic health records?

Care providers using intelligent autonomous tools and decision support systems, e.g., for automatic image analysis and lesion detection, are facing the threat that their professional decisions are not independent any longer and that their clinical judgment might be replaced by a machine generated diagnosis.

Another issue arises when poor electronic workflows and bad usability of electronic health record systems consume much of the clinicians' time and energy that they experience a feeling of burnout.

9. Please illustrate (one example) how the patient–provider relationship can be affected through digital media.

One example of a misdirected manner of communication between patients and providers is unsolicited data sent to the provider. They are particularly problematic if no prior personal contact had been established. Questions are: What should the provider do with regard to accepting/rejecting this request, checking the identity of the person, ensuring the quality of the data, storing the data, and giving a clinical judgment. What rules should be defined once a personal relationship between the patient and the provider has been established?

10. Please briefly describe the dimensions captured in the MEESTAR model and the three time points when assessment and evaluation can take place.

The ethical dimensions described by the *MEESTAR model* embrace.

- Care, in the sense of taking care of someone in need.
- Autonomy.
- Safety, in a wide meaning of the term including security and prevention of harm.
- Justice, here particularly social justice.
- Privacy, defined as the inviolable zone around a person.
- Participation, in the meaning of living together with others in a society and opposed to exclusion.
- Self-conception, meaning the way a person perceives and understands him- or herself.

    They could be captured ex ante, intra, or ex post regarding product or system development and implementation. The dimensions concern evaluations at the level of the individual person, the organization and the society. Such evaluation would require a statement to be made according to the four stages from "harmless" to "has to be opposed."

References

1. Floridi L. Soft ethics, the governance of the digital and the General Data Protection Regulation. Philos Trans R Soc. 2018;A 376:20180081. https://doi.org/10.1098/rsta.2018.0081.
2. World Medical Association. Declaration of Geneva. Most recent version of 2006. Available from: https://www.wma.net/what-we-do/medical-ethics/declaration-of-geneva/. Accessed June 16, 2021.
3. International Council of Nurses. Code of Ethics for Nurses. 2012. Available from: https://www.icn.ch/sites/default/files/inline-files/2012_ICN_Codeofethicsfornurses_%20eng.pdf Accessed June 16, 2021.
4. Beauchamp TL, Childress JF. Principles of biomedical ethics. 8th ed. Oxford University Press; 2019.
5. World Medical Association. World Medical Association Declaration of Helsinki: ethical principles for medical research involving human subjects. JAMA. 2013;310(20):2191–4. https://doi.org/10.1001/jama.2013.281053.
6. The National Commission for the Protection of Human Subjects of Biomedical and Behavioral Research. The Belmont Report – Ethical Principles and Guidelines for the Protection of Human Subjects of Research. April 18, 1979. Available from https://www.hhs.gov/ohrp/sites/default/files/the-belmont-report-508c_FINAL.pdf. Accessed June 16, 2021.
7. Floridi L, Taddeo M. What is data ethics? Phil Trans R Soc A. 2016;374:20160360. https://doi.org/10.1098/rsta.2016.0360.
8. Cahan EM, Hernandez-Boussard T, Thadaney-Israni S, Rubin DL. Putting the data before the algorithm in big data addressing personalized healthcare. NPJ Digit Med. 2019;2:78. https://doi.org/10.1038/s41746-019-0157-2.
9. Ienca M, Wangmo T, Jotterand F, Kressig RW, Elger B. Ethical design of intelligent technologies for dementia: a descriptive review. Sci Eng Ethics. 2018;24:1035–55.
10. Rubeis G. The disruptive power of artificial intelligence. Ethical aspects of gerontechnology in elderly care. Arch Gerontol Geriatr. 2020; https://doi.org/10.1016/j.archger.2020.104186.
11. Robillard JM, Cleland I, Hoey J, Nugent C. Ethical adoption: a new imperative in the development of technology for dementia. Alzheimers Dement. 2018;14(9):1104–13.
12. World Economic Forum. Ethics by Design: An organizational approach to responsible use of technology. White Paper. December 2020. Available from: http://www3.weforum.org/docs/WEF_Ethics_by_Design_2020.pdf. Accessed June 16, 2021.
13. Sussman N, DeJong SM. Ethical considerations for mental health clinicians working with adolescents in the digital age. Curr Psychiatry Rep. 2018;20(12):113.
14. LaBarge G, Broom M. Social media in primary care. Mo Med. 2019;116(2):106–10.
15. Zimba O, Radchenko O, Strilchuk L. Social media for research, education and practice in rheumatology. Rheumatol Int 2019 Dec 20.
16. Hübner UH, Egbert N, Schulte G. Clinical information systems - seen through the ethics lens. Yearb Med Inform. 2020;29(1):104–14. https://doi.org/10.1055/s-0040-1701996.
17. Mittelstadt BD, Floridi L. The ethics of big data: current and foreseeable issues in biomedical contexts. Sci Eng Ethics. 2016;22(2):303–41. https://doi.org/10.1007/s11948-015-9652-2.
18. Dankar FK, Gergely M, Dankar SK. Informed consent in biomedical research. Comput Struct Biotechnol J. 2019;17:463–74. https://doi.org/10.1016/j.csbj.2019.03.010.

19. European Commission. General data protection regulation. Available from: https://gdpr-info.eu/. Accessed June 16, 2021.

20. Beier K, Schweda M, Schicktanz S. Taking patient involvement seriously: a critical ethical analysis of participatory approaches in data-intensive medical research. BMC Med Inform Decis Mak. 2019;19(1):90. https://doi.org/10.1186/s12911-019-0799-7.

21. Adams SA, Petersen C. Precision medicine: opportunities, possibilities, and challenges for patients and providers. J Am Med Inform Assoc. 2016;23(4):787–90. https://doi.org/10.1093/jamia/ocv215.

22. Laurie GT. Cross-sectoral big data: the application of an ethics framework for big data in health and research. Asian Bioeth Rev. 2019;11(3):327–39.

23. Stockdale J, Cassell J, Ford E. "Giving something back": a systematic review and ethical enquiry into public views on the use of patient data for research in the United Kingdom and the Republic of Ireland. Wellcome Open Res. 2019;3:6.

24. Hall A, Brown Wilson C, Stanmore E, Todd C. Moving beyond "safety" versus "autonomy": a qualitative exploration of the ethics of using monitoring technologies in long-term dementia care. BMC Geriatr. 2017;19:145. https://doi.org/10.1186/s12877-019-1155-6.

25. Meredith J, McCarthy S, Hemsley B. Legal and ethical issues surrounding the use of older children's electronic personal health records. J Law Med. 2018;25(4):1042–55.

26. Jaremko JL, Azar M, Bromwich R, Lum A, Alicia Cheong LH, Giber M, et al. Canadian Association of Radiologists (CAR) Artificial Intelligence Working Group. Canadian association of radiologists white paper on ethical and legal issues related to artificial intelligence in radiology. Can Assoc Radiol J. 2019;70(2):107–18.

27. Rubeis G, Schochow M, Steger F. Patient autonomy and quality of care in telehealthcare. Sci Eng Ethics. 2018;24(1):93–107.

28. Geis JR, Brady AP, Wu CC, Spencer J, Ranschaert E, Jaremko JL, et al. Ethics of artificial intelligence in radiology: summary of the joint European and North American Multisociety Statement. Radiology. 2019;293(2):436–40.

29. Ho CWL, Soon D, Caals K, Kapur J. Governance of automated image analysis and artificial intelligence analytics in healthcare. Clin Radiol. 2019;74(5):329–37. https://doi.org/10.1016/j.crad.2019.02.005.

30. Regulation (EU) 2017/745 of The European Parliament and of the Council of 5 April 2017 on medical devices, amending Directive 2001/83/EC, Regulation (EC) No. 178/2002 and Regulation (EC) No. 1223/2009 and repealing Council Directives 90/385/EEC and 93/42/EEC. Available from: https://eur-lex.europa.eu/eli/reg/2017/745/2017-05-05. Accessed June 16, 2021.

31. US Food and Drug Administration. Software as a Medical Device (SaMD). https://www.fda.gov/medical-devices/digital-health-center-excellence/software-medical-device-samd. Accessed June 16, 2021.

32. Lee MS, Nambudiri VE. Electronic consultations and clinician burnout: an antidote to our emotional pandemic? J Am Med Inform Assoc. 2021;28(5):1038–41. https://doi.org/10.1093/jamia/ocaa300.

33. Dymek C, Kim B, Melton GB, Payne TH, Singh H, Hsiao CJ. Building the evidence-base to reduce electronic health record-related clinician burden. J Am Med Inform Assoc. 2021;28(5):1057–61. https://doi.org/10.1093/jamia/ocaa238.

34. Weir CR, Taber P, Taft T, Reese TJ, Jones B, Del Fiol G. Feeling and thinking: can theories of human motivation explain how EHR design impacts clinician burnout? J Am Med Inform Assoc. 2021;28(5):1042–6. https://doi.org/10.1093/jamia/ocaa270.

35. Rubeis G. Guardians of humanity. The challenging role of nursing professionals in the digital age. Nurs Philos 2021;22(2):e12331. https://doi.org/10.1111/nup.12331.

36. Robichaux C, Tietze M, Stokes F, McBride S. Reconceptualizing the electronic health record for a new decade: a caring technology? ANS Adv Nurs Sci. 2019;42(3):193–205.

37. Veazie S, Winchell K, Gilbert J, Paynter R, Ivlev I, Eden KB, Nussbaum K, Weiskopf N, Guise JM, Helfand M. Rapid evidence review of mobile applications for self-management of diabetes. J Gen Intern Med. 2018;33(7):1167–76. https://doi.org/10.1007/s11606-018-4410-1.

38. Mars M, Morris C, Scott RE. Selfie telemedicine – what are the legal and regulatory issues? Stud Health Technol Inform. 2018;254:53–62.

39. Kuhnel L. TTaPP: together take a pause and ponder: a critical thinking tool for exploring the public/private lives of patients. J Clin Ethics. 2018;29(2):102–13.

40. Ho A, Quick O. Leaving patients to their own devices? Smart technology, safety and therapeutic relationships. BMC Med Ethics. 2018;19(1):18.

41. Goodman KW. Health information technology as a universal donor to bioethics education. Camb Quarterly Healthc Ethics. 2017;26:341–7.

42. Kidholm K, Jensen LK, Kjølhede T, Nielsen E, Horup MB. Validity of the model for assessment of telemedicine: a Delphi study. J Telemed Telecare. 2018;24(2):118–25. https://doi.org/10.1177/1357633X16686553.

43. Manzeschke A, Weber K, Rother E, Fangerau H. Results of the study "Ethical questions in the area of age appropriate assisting systems". Berlin: VDI; 2013.

44. Reijers W, Wright D, Brey P, Weber K, Rodrigues R, O'Sullivan D, Gordijn B. Methods for practising ethics in research and innovation: a literature review, critical analysis and recommendations. Sci Eng Ethics. 2018;24(5):1437–81. https://doi.org/10.1007/s11948-017-9961-8.

45. Lehmann CU, Petersen C, Bhatia H, Berner ES, Goodman KW. Advance directives and code status information exchange: a consensus proposal for a minimum set of attributes. Camb Q Healthc Ethics. 2019 Jan;28(1):178–85. https://doi.org/10.1017/S096318011800052X.

Part VII

Managing Technology and People

Principles of Management: Successfully Implementing Health IT

32

Rachelle Kaye, Reut Ron, Nessa Barry, Andrea Pavlickova, Donna Lesley Henderson, and Haya Barkai

Learning Objectives

This chapter will present key management principles for implementing Health IT derived from the experience of health IT Implementation in Israel and Scotland. After reading this chapter, readers will be able to:

- Identify and list key management principles and critical success factors for implementing health IT.
- Give examples of how these management principles have been successfully implemented in Israel and Scotland.
- Compare the implementation processes in Scotland and Israel—similarities and differences.
- Describe key tools and processes that contributed to the successful implementation of Health IT in both Israel and Scotland.
- Explain the broader context, both historically and in current practice in Europe and the USA, for the Israeli and Scottish experiences.

R. Kaye (✉)
Assuta Medical Centers, Tel Aviv, Israel

R. Ron
Assuta Health Services Research Institute, Tel Aviv, Israel

N. Barry · A. Pavlickova · D. L. Henderson
International Engagement, TEC and Digital Healthcare Innovation, Scottish Government, Edinburgh, UK

H. Barkai
Maccabi Healthcare Services, Tel Aviv, Israel

- Distinguish between the various terms used in the field, specifically, between health IT, eHealth, and digital health and between telehealth, telecare, and telemedicine.

Key Terms
- Health IT
- eHealth
- Tele-care
- Tele-medicine
- Implementation
- Leadership
- Management Principles

Introduction

In 2004, the European Commission issued a Communication to the European Parliament on e-Health that stated that "e-Health can help to deliver better care for less money within citizen-centered health delivery systems. It thus responds to the major challenges that the health sector—which employs 9% of Europe's workforce—is currently facing" [1]. This was echoed by Dr. David Blumenthal in 2010, then director of the US National Coordinator for Health Information Technology who wrote that: "Health information technology (IT) has the potential to improve the health of individuals and the performance of providers, yielding improved quality, cost savings, and greater engagement by patients in their own

© Springer Nature Switzerland AG 2022
U. H. Hübner et al. (eds.), *Nursing Informatics*, Health Informatics,
https://doi.org/10.1007/978-3-030-91237-6_32

health care." [2]. Despite considerable financial investment by both the EU and the USA, implementation of Health IT has proved to be challenging. Clayton Hamilton, Technical Officer, Digitalization of Health Systems, Division of Health Systems and Public Health, World Health Organization (WHO) Regional Office for Europe, noted that: "While a handful of countries in Europe have made significant progress in reorienting their health systems to capitalize upon the advantages which digital health and high-quality data can offer, the reality of the situation across the majority of European countries is a starkly different one. Health systems are still often fraught with piecemeal technology implementations…" [3]. In the USA, there is still uneven implementation of health IT by doctors and hospitals. A major challenge in the United States has been the lack of interoperability among health IT systems that has impeded sharing and exchange of health care data among professionals and among healthcare providers [4].

The objective of this chapter is to share the management principles for implementing Health Information Technology (HIT) that derive from first-hand experience in implementing Health IT in Israel and in Scotland. Both Israel and Scotland have been, and continue to be, leaders in what we now call "digital health," but each approaches it from different vectors due to the differences in context and local challenges. This chapter will also provide some broad historical background on the evolution of Health IT—both in Europe and in the USA—as a context for the Israeli and Scottish journeys in great part because it actually influenced their experiences and decisions.

Case Studies in Brief

Israel

Israel is considered a pioneer in Health IT implementation, having begun its Health IT implementation in the mid-1980s. It is a successful example of a grass-roots bottom-up implementation approach. Israel has a National Health Insurance System, with four competing nationwide HMOs (Health Insurers who are also providers) responsi-

ble for providing the public basket of services to over nine million citizens. In its initial stages, Health IT in Israel was HMO-driven, resulting in the implementation of comprehensive, shared organization-wide Electronic Medical Records in all HMOs by the mid-1990s, followed by one of the first nationwide teleradiology systems in 1997, and patient portals in the early 2000s, enabling citizens online access to their medical information. While initiatives at the HMO and hospital level continue to be drivers for innovation in digital health, during the past decade, the Ministry of Health has assumed increasing leadership, including the development and implementation of a National EHR exchange and the articulation of a national strategy for digital health. Maccabi Healthcare Services, Israel's second largest HMO, was the first to institute an organization-wide EMR and exemplifies the critical management principles necessary to successfully implement Health IT at the organizational level. The critical success factors in the Maccabi Health IT implementation included:

- ongoing innovative and visionary leadership at the helm of the organization,
- commitment of organizational resources,
- establishing and empowering a multidisciplinary inter-departmental working team,
- joint strategic decision-making and co-design with the physicians—who were and remain key stakeholders,
- focusing on practical, tangible, and concrete needs,
- providing incentives,
- providing training and support to clinicians and staff, and
- ongoing collaboration among all of the stakeholders and users, both internal and external, including citizens/members.

At both the organizational and national level, competition has been a major motivator for innovation. The HMOs and hospitals in Israel compete to be the best and the most progressive, with the most advanced digital services for citizens and professionals. Nowhere has this been more evident than in the response of the HMOs and hospitals to the COVID-19 pandemic, resulting in exponential advances in remote care, telemonitoring, and accelerated engagement in digital health for both professionals and patients.

Scotland

From the early 2000s onwards, the implementation of Health IT in Scotland has been grounded in supportive health policy and strategy frameworks. The strategic approach has placed technology at the heart of the quality agenda and provided waves of financial support for IT developments which drive service modernization and (more recently) the integration of health and care.

The National Health Service in Scotland provides healthcare to a population of 5.4 million citizens via 14 geographic (regional) Health Boards, 7 National Health Boards, and 1 Public Health body. The Scottish Parliament and Scottish Government were established in 1999 by an Act of the UK Parliament. Under this Act (Scotland Act 1998), a range of powers, including health and social services, were devolved to Scotland.

Subsequent Scottish eHealth/digital health and care strategies have evidenced a gradual shift away from health IT objectives which focus only on health organizations, towards support for strong citizen engagement and multi-stakeholder leadership to deliver digital solutions and technology enabled care services.

From the mid-2000s, additional investment (and leadership) was provided by the Scottish Government for the use of proven technologies in health and home settings. Technology has been explicitly regarded as a tool to support formal health and social care integration (legislation from 2016). The most recent focus, from 2018, has been the National Education for Scotland Digital Service (NDS) work to create a National Digital Platform for sharing health and social care information.

The critical success factors in the Scottish Health IT implementation journey have included:

- ongoing governmental commitment in policy and resources,

- supportive leadership across health and care, which identifies the role of technology as part drive towards integrated health and care,
- enduring support to work with citizens to develop more user centered services,
- iterative developments, building on success towards implementation at scale.

The current ambition in Scotland is to deliver a national platform that is a truly accessible and integrated system. This exemplifies the "once for Scotland" approach which is most tangibly demonstrated by the work led (since 2018) by National Education for Scotland's Digital Service (NDS) to create a National Digital Platform. Scotland has developed strategies at the national level, relying on shared vision and leadership across stakeholder organizations which engage with citizens.

The Context: Terminology, History, Current Status of Health IT

Terminology and Definitions

As technology has evolved, the associated terminology has also evolved and there is a blurring of the way terms such as Health IT (or ICT), eHealth, and digital health are defined and used.

Health IT (ICT) and health telematics were common terms in the 1980s and the 1990s and referred to the design, development, creation, use, and maintenance of information systems for the healthcare industry. The Electronic Health Record (EHR), a person's official, digital health record, is the central component of the Health IT infrastructure. Other key elements of the Health IT infrastructure are the Personal Health Record (PHR), which is a person's self-maintained health record, and the Health Information Exchange (HIE), a health data clearing house or a group of healthcare organizations that enter into an interoperability pact and agree to share data between their various systems [5].

eHealth made its appearance in the mid to late 1990s as the Internet exploded into public consciousness, and a number of "e-terms" began to appear and proliferate such as: "email" and "e-commerce." Pretlow defined "Ehealth as the process of providing health care via electronic means, in particular over the Internet" [6].

Later definitions became increasingly general such as the World Health Organization (WHO) definition: "Ehealth involves a broad group of activities that use electronic means to deliver health-related information, resources and services: it is the use of information and communication technologies for health" [7].

Digital Health—The European Commission definition of eHealth transitioned into Digital Health and Care as a result of the concept of the Digital Single market—the 2014–2019 strategy of the European Commission [8]. The EC defines digital health and care as the "tools and services that use information and communication technologies to improve prevention, diagnosis, treatment, monitoring and management of health and lifestyle" [9].

The WHO proffered the following definition: The term digital health is rooted in eHealth, which is defined as "the use of information and communications technology in support of health and health-related fields." Mhealth is a subset of eHealth and is defined as "the use of mobile wireless technologies for health." More recently, the term digital health was introduced as "a broad umbrella term encompassing eHealth (which includes mHealth), as well as emerging areas, such as the use of advanced computing sciences in 'big data,' genomics and artificial intelligence" [10].

In summary, the change in terminology has been propelled by the changes in types of technology and what technology enables us to do. Health IT was geared to the computerization of healthcare organizations and systems—the development of health information systems to manage healthcare both administratively and clinically—the foundation of the latter being the Electronic Medical Record, and subsequent technologies for exchanging healthcare data among healthcare providers and for supporting clinical decisions. eHealth came into being with the emergence of the Internet and heralded the inclusion of the patient as a more active participant, generally by enabling him/her to access information from his/her medical record via a portal, make appointments online, and similar activities. The broad

uptake of mobile technology—particularly mobile phones, and medical devices with Bluetooth—propelled us in the direction of patient empowerment and fueled the potential for the "digital revolution in healthcare." This was also driven politically by governments and countries facing challenges of sustainability of healthcare systems due to rapidly aging populations and the increasing burden of chronic disease—demanding greater coordination of care. Digitally enabled integrated care has come to be perceived as the potential solution to these challenges.

An additional set of terms in the context of "digital health" that are often used interchangeably are telehealth, telemedicine, and telecare.

The term **telehealth** is an all-encompassing one. Telecare and telemedicine are generally covered within the broader scope of the term telehealth. Telehealth technology enables the remote diagnoses and evaluation of patients in addition to the ability to remote detection of fluctuations in the medical condition of the patient at home. It also allows for e-prescribing of medications and remotely prescribed treatments [11].

Telecare is the term that relates to technology that enables patients to maintain their independence and safety while remaining in their own homes. Telecare includes electronic devices combined with ICT and professional practices applied to assist and care for people from a distance. Telecare includes services such as monitoring, assistance, information, consultation, and communication [12].

The term **"telemedicine"** has a narrower scope than that of telehealth. Telemedicine refers to the use of information technologies and electronic communications to provide remote clinical services to patients. The digital transmission of medical imaging, remote medical diagnosis and evaluations, and video consultations with specialists are all examples of telemedicine [13]."

Brief History of Health IT and Telemedicine

The roots of the Health Information Management industry can be traced back to the 1920s when healthcare professionals started using medical records to document details, complications, and outcomes of patient care [14].

Dr. Lawrence Weed, a professor of medicine and pharmacology at Yale University, created the first problem-oriented medical record (POMR) to organize the information used in medical records. The POMR was the world's first EMR in 1968.

The introduction of the desktop personal computer really ushered in the modern age of healthcare information technology in the 1980s. HMOs in the USA were among the earliest adopters of Health IT. A study by Kaiser Permanente in 2013 showed that by 2011, 100% of HMOs had implemented Electronic Health records [15]. In Europe, early innovators and adopters were Scandinavian countries such as Sweden, Denmark, and Norway where in the mid-1980s, computer support for medical records really started to emerge [16].

Denmark now has a centralized computer database to which 98% of primary care physicians, all hospital physicians, and all pharmacists now have access. Over 95% of Norwegian GPs have been using an EMR for the past 10 years [17].

Telemedicine—provision of care remotely—has been making its mark on the healthcare community for decades beginning in the United States during the American Civil War with the use of the telegraph to communicate casualty reports, coordinate patient transport, and request medical supplies. In the late 60s and 70s, home monitoring developed more fully in the Mercury space program when the National Aeronautics and Space Administration (NASA) began performing physiologic monitoring over a distance [18].

Rashid L. Bashshur and Gary W. Shannon traced the origin of modern telemedicine applications in Europe beginning with long-distance transfer of ECGs in 1905 by Willem Einthoven, a Dutch physician [19]. The '80s brought telehealth to radiology when images were sent and received for telehealth consultations.

The aging of the population over the past several decades, together with the rapid development of ICT, has led to an increasing focus on telecare. Telecare technology began with social

alarms, graduated to more automatic responses based on sensor information and today, focuses on the generation of integrated systems aimed at enhancing the user's quality of life [20].

The Current Situation in Europe: Gaps and Challenges

"The Communication of the European Commission on eHealth—of 2004 [1] making healthcare better for European citizens: An action plan for a European eHealth Area (eH-AP)," provided the impetus for the widespread development of eHealth in Europe. Member States of the European Union (EU) committed themselves "to develop a national or regional roadmap for eHealth."

A Study of European eHealth Strategies and National eHealth Competence Centres (NeHCs) in Europe in 2018 by EHTEL [21], identified trends in eHealth strategies that signal both the evolution of eHealth technologies and how they are being adopted in National and Regional strategies within the EU.

- The strategies developed between 2004 and 2010 focused on developing the basic infrastructures for implementing electronic health records at the healthcare provider level and exchange of electronic information among providers.
- Strategies published between 2011 and 2013 placed emphasis on moving from organizational and regional systems to National IT systems and setting up central electronic health records at a national level. Strategies placed increasing emphasis on telemedicine and telehealth, patient portals, and Personal Health Records.
- In 2014, strategies began to use the term "digitalization of Healthcare" including digital workflows, patient pathways, and the integration of information from diverse healthcare delivery technology-based systems. There was increasing emphasis on patient-centered care including patients, their carers, and their

systems and the integration of monitoring devices and sensors.

- The most recently updated strategies address the integration between health and social care supported by digital systems. The focus is on patient-centered care, as well as empowering health and social care professionals—using digital tools and apps. Mobile technology is almost taken for granted. The Digital revolution is perceived as a key mechanism for service transformation—bringing care to the citizen—wherever he might be. Many systems have already developed or are developing comprehensive electronic databases and thus we have entered the era of "big data" and strategies for the effective use of data. Cybersecurity has become a key issue and States are setting innovation leadership objectives for themselves in this "brave new world."

On 25th April 2018, the European Commission published the Communication on Digital Transformation of Health and Care in the Digital Single Market [22] that identified three priorities:

- Citizens' secure access to their health data, also across borders.
- Personalized medicine through shared European data infrastructure.
- Citizen empowerment with digital tools for user feedback and person-centered care.

While there is a great deal of strategic discussion across Europe, actual implementation has been variable. Clayton Hamilton, Technical Officer, Digitalization of Health Systems, Division of Health Systems and Public Health, World Health Organization (WHO) Regional Office for Europe, noted that:

"While a handful of countries in Europe have made significant progress in reorienting their health systems to capitalize upon the advantages which digital health and high-quality data can offer, the reality of the situation across the majority of European countries is a starkly different one. Health systems are still often fraught with piecemeal technology implementations, data interoperability across institutional and regional boundaries is poor, governance and financing for digital health is lacking, and health care professionals often feel ill-equipped in their use of the available technologies (in addition to feeling overwhelmed by the burden of data entry). Ensuring that these complex, systemic barriers are appropriately addressed by national digitalization programs requires that the strategic focus remains centered on developing and contextualizing the fundamental building blocks of digital health, that investments are aligned to key health policy objectives, and that the trust of health care professionals and the public in their use of digital solutions is well-established" [3].

Health IT Today in the USA

The Health IT journey in the USA has been significantly different from that in Europe due to the fact that the USA is a highly pluralistic system, dominated by private healthcare providers and multiple payers. In 2004, President Bush signed an Executive Order titled the President's Health Information Technology Plan, which established a ten-year plan to develop and implement electronic medical record systems across the USA to improve the efficiency and safety of care [23].

The executive order signed by President Bush established the Office of the National Coordinator for Health Information Technology. ONC is the principal federal entity charged with coordination of nationwide efforts to implement and use the most advanced health information technology and the electronic exchange of health information.

In addition to setting policy and enacting legislation, a key strategy for promoting the implementation of Health IT in the USA has been financial incentives. The American Recovery and Reinvestment Act, signed into law in 2009 under the Obama Administration, provided approximately $19 billion in incentives for hospitals to shift from paper to electronic medical records. Meaningful Use, as a part of the 2009 Health Information Technology for Economic and Clinical Health Act (HITECH) was the incentive that included over $20 billion for the implementation of HIT alone. The sooner that healthcare providers adopted the system, the more funding they received. As of 2017, nearly nine in ten (86%) of office-based physicians had adopted any EHR, and nearly 4 in 5 (80%) had adopted a certified EHR. In 2017, 96% of all non-federal acute care hospitals possessed certified Health IT.

A major challenge in the United States has been the lack of interoperability among Health IT systems that has impeded sharing and exchange of health care data among professionals and among healthcare providers. Despite the obstacles, the USA has made dramatic advancements in digitizing the care delivery system during the past decade:

- Over one-half of office-based professionals and more than 8 in 10 hospitals are meaningfully using electronic health records (EHRs), which will require them to electronically exchange standardized patient information to support safe care transitions.
- One-half of hospitals are able to electronically search for patient information from sources beyond their organization or health system.
- All 50 states have some form of health information exchange services available to support care.

In 2014 the Office of the National Coordinator for Health Information Technology published a 10-Year Vision to Achieve an Interoperable Health IT Infrastructure in the USA [4].

Health IT Implementation in Israel and Scotland: An In-depth Analysis

Overview

Both Israel and Scotland were among the early adopters and implementers of Health IT. It is valuable to learn from their experience in implementing Health IT as the structures of their healthcare systems are very different and there have been some notable differences in implementation approaches, while at the same time, there have also been commonalities and similar critical success factors.

Implementation of Health IT in Israel

Israel is one of the global pioneers in health information technology, a digital revolution that began in the early 1990s. Israel has a mandatory National Health Insurance system that requires all of Israel's nine million citizens to register in one of four National Health Plans which are obligated to provide their members with all of their healthcare, as defined in the public basket of services (updated annually). Israel's Health Plans (HMOs—both insurers and providers), notably Clalit and Maccabi Healthcare Services, which today serve about 80% of the Israeli population—led Israel's Health IT revolution, which resulted in the implementation of electronic medical records used by virtually 100% of the country's population, the vast use of laboratory and imaging information systems, computerized physician order entries, and e-prescribing [24].

Maccabi Healthcare Services was the first of Israel's four national health plans to develop and implement a comprehensive EHR based IT system and can be considered among the early pioneers in this field, having initiated the development of its system in the mid-1980s [25].

Clalit Health Services was the world's first health plan to implement a health information exchange, enabling the creation of patient files that could include data and information input from various treatment sources, such as clinics and hospitals. Israel was also one of the first countries to use telemedicine, with the initial focus on tele-diagnostics such as teleradiology and tele-ECG, and to introduce electronic clinical decision support systems and online indicators for medical and service quality [24].

Israel prides itself on a quality digital healthcare system and on its technological and enterprising spirit. After a two-decade investment in medical digital documentation, Israel has over 25 years of comprehensive and longitudinal digital medical data and is growing hundreds of start-ups in the health field. Led by the Ministry of Health and the Headquarters for the National Digital Israel Initiative through the Ministry of Social Equality, in collaboration with the Prime Minister's Office, the Treasury, the Innovation Authority, the Planning and Budgeting Committee, and the Ministry of Economy, the Israeli Government set its sights on advancing digital health as a national engine of growth in March 2018. The decision is centered on removing regulatory and infrastructure obstacles hindering collaboration between health data-centric sectors, and on the Mosaic Project, whose objective is the establishment of a genomic clinical database that would enable R&D of products that advance personalized medicine.

A digital health program which was launched as a result of this decision has already begun to operate on several fronts. The national big data infrastructure for R&D in the field of healthcare includes: a telemedicine infrastructure, the Halev infrastructure (the patient at the center) aimed at synchronizing interorganizational processes in the healthcare system (such as making an appointment for a medical procedure which is currently the patient's responsibility), and a new more sophisticated version of medical information exchange between medical professionals within the healthcare system.

With a view to the future, and with suitable processive and regulatory infrastructure, the Ministry is anticipating health services to be based on an integration of capabilities from all these infrastructures. An example is a telemedicine infrastructure that would link devices in possession of patients or their primary medical professionals, to health data in the Eitan EHR exchanges system based on IoT (Internet of Things) capabilities [26].

These capabilities in information, communication, mobile, and cyber technologies, complemented by more than 25 years of experience in implementing Health IT, electronic medical records, and business analytics have created a strong foundation for Israel's ongoing developments in health analytics [27].

One of the defining features of the Israeli healthcare system is the relative autonomy of the Israeli HMOs, within the overall framework of the National Health Insurance Law, and the competition among them. The implementation of Health IT in Israel was HMO-driven. Strategy for Health IT existed at the beginning only at the individual health care organization level. All of the HMOs had fully implemented organization-wide EMRs by the time the Ministry of Health began to take an active role and the Ministry's initial focus was on the implementation of Health IT in hospitals, as the largest owner and operator of hospitals in the country. It is only in the last decade that the Ministry of Health has taken an active leadership role, including the creation of the National EHR exchange to enable medical care data exchange among HMOs and hospitals. Today, the Israeli Ministry of Health has developed a digital healthcare strategy, and is working closely with all of the stakeholders to implement it.

As the foundation of the implementation of Health IT in Israel was HMO-driven, understanding the management strategies and principles at the HMO level is key to understanding the success of the Israeli Health IT system [24, 25, 28, 29].

The Maccabi Story

Maccabi Healthcare Services, the second largest HMO in Israel currently providing services to more than two million people, i.e. 25% of Israel's total population, was the first of Israel's HMOs to implement Health IT. In 1983, Maccabi recognized that the healthcare system of the future would require sophisticated information and communication technology for efficient management, as well as effective and innovative health care services delivery. It aimed to use Information and Communication Technologies (ICT) to create a comprehensive, progressive, and fully computerized system. The idea was to develop a networked infrastructure at all levels (administrative, diagnostic, therapeutic, and preventive) to connect physicians, nurses, therapists, primary carers, and patients.

Maccabi was one of the first healthcare organizations internationally to implement an organization-wide EMR. Maccabi began this process in 1987, and, by 1994, all Maccabi-affiliated physicians were using the Maccabi EMR. Its major objective was to support the clinicians and consequently, as it computerized its medication prescribing, its imaging services and its laboratories, all were integrated with the EMR so that the clinicians had all of the information at their fingertips in real time to support their clinical decisions, supported by a clinical decision support system. The EMR system was expanded to include nurses and healthcare professionals on the same platform. In 2001, this vision was extended to the Maccabi member, who has always been viewed as the center of the system, with the creation of "Maccabi online"—Maccabi's patient portal, giving the patient access to his medical information and other online services. Maccabi's Health IT system has continued to evolve in the ensuing years. The EMR is used by all of the health professionals and relevant administrative personnel and all providers and health services are electronically interconnected online and with continuous clinical data exchange taking place in real time. There is a platform for team coordination and integrated care for complex patients. The system supports a vast array of telemedicine features, for diagnosis, treatment, and patient management. "Maccabi Online"—the patient portal—is highly interactive enabling the patient to request online referrals and prescriptions and receive the referrals and prescriptions online with an electronic signature. In fact, the whole process is now paperless—patients come to the pharmacy or the lab with only their Maccabi card in hand—the prescription or referral is in the system. In addition, patients can ask and receive answers to questions from their doctors. All of this can be done via the "Maccabi online" app as well as by PC. Maccabi doctors also have an app that gives them access to their patients' EMR.

The Maccabi IT story began with a new CEO in 1982—a young and dynamic leader, experienced in the management of public service organizations. He perceived the need for computerized management information systems and set up an IT steering committee (which he chaired) with four subcommittees, reflecting the first priority areas for computerization—members, doctors, hospitals, and finances. Members were the first priority and work on computerization of member information began in 1984. The doctors were next. In 1986, the Maccabi Independent Physicians organization agreed to be a full partner in the implementation of a computerized medical record in all physician clinics. In 1988, Maccabi issued a magnetic membership card to all its members, to be presented at every point of service, thereby enabling the system to capture all of the members' transactions with the healthcare delivery system. The organizing principle of the Maccabi IT system—both administrative and clinical—was the member ID. Maccabi entered into a contract with an Israeli technology company, Rosh Tov and the two organizations set out on the journey to build the Maccabi EMR together—a partnership that continues until today.

What Were the Management Principles That Were Critical Success Factors in the Implementation of Health IT in Maccabi?

Innovative leadership—In Maccabi, innovative leadership included not only vision and commitment, but also hands-on involvement of top management, willingness to step in to solve problems and, of course, willingness to invest and commit organizational resources to the process.

Involving key stakeholders: After an initial planning and evaluation process by professional staff, Maccabi raised the idea of computerizing Maccabi-affiliated independent physicians with the Independent Physicians Organization and it was agreed to set up a multi-disciplinary committee comprised of representatives of the independent doctors and senior staff from the Maccabi Medical Department and IT Department. The committee examined the needs of the organization and the doctors which could be addressed by the system, as well as the barriers and the challenges. The decision to enter into the development of the system was a joint decision of the organization and the doctors.

Assessment—Assessment was done at 3 levels: the steering committees composed of administrative, clinical, and technological staff members, with expert outside consultants, set up in 1983; the above-mentioned assessment of needs together with the doctors, and in 1991, a two-day workshop with the senior multidisciplinary staff of the organization and the physician leadership. In preparation for the workshop, a great deal of effort was invested in research and fact finding and identification of options, so that the assessment and decisions made had a solid foundation.

Clear identification of concrete needs and the goals to be achieved: From the outset Maccabi, as an organization with responsibility for managing its processes and resources, had a clear vision of what it wanted to achieve which was articulated by the steering committee. The essential partner, and potentially the major obstacle, was the doctors. Therefore, it was especially important to make sure that the benefits to the doctors were clear and visible. In Maccabi, the physician was able to perceive four benefits that were realized within a very short time after implementation:

- The magnetic membership card automatically populated the physician's record with the patient's demographic information, saving the physician time in writing or entering the information;
- The membership card generated an online connection to the Maccabi database for verification of the patient's eligibility to receive services, guaranteeing that the doctor would be paid for the visit;
- The opening screen presented the doctor with a summary of the medical information on the patient, including major problems, diagnoses, allergies, and medications;
- Once the doctor entered a diagnosis for the visit, the information was transmitted and the claims adjudication process was initiated, saving additional entry and paperwork for billing.

As the system became more sophisticated, more benefits were realized. For example, e-prescriptions are automatically screened online in real time against the total database by a drug utilization review program, thus helping the doctor avoid adverse drug events; electronic referrals for diagnostic tests ensure that the results are automatically transmitted back to the doctor's computer; online consultation among physicians and between doctors and patients saves time for both doctors and patients.

Integrated responsibility: The designation of an active integrating body responsible for developing and managing the system was a key success factor. In Maccabi, the Director of Organization and Information Systems was designated as the person responsible for developing and implementing the Maccabi Health IT system. He worked with a small dynamic team, including a senior director of the Medical Department, with the complete backing of the CEO and his direct involvement when key decisions needed to be made. There was ongoing liaison and continuous dialogue with leaders in the physician community.

Clear strategy and organizational process—a collaborative process: The strategy for achieving the goals of the project was comprised of the following components and steps:

1. Joint physician/Maccabi medical and IT staff committees were established for every medical specialty to develop the functional specifications needed for each specialty, to oversee the adaptation of the core medical record and to provide ongoing feedback during implementation.
2. A minimum data set was agreed upon, with the gradual addition of new fields and tools over time.
3. It was agreed at a very early stage what the doctor would see first when he opened the EMR—a summary page with the most relevant patient data. The EHR was designed to support his workflow—not change it.
4. In the case of each additional field or tool, the rationale was presented, and the benefits to the doctor, patient, and/or organization were clearly delineated.

5. New networking capabilities were systematically developed and each brought with it relevant changes to the EMR, for example, with the computerization of the lab came electronic referral to the lab and the ability to electronically transmit lab results directly to the doctor's EMR.

6. The uptake of the EMR was also gradual, beginning with doctors who volunteered to pilot the system. After a successful pilot stage, it was agreed that using the EMR would be voluntary for doctors currently under contract but mandatory for new doctors. This continued until the majority of doctors were in the system, at which point it became a condition of "doing business" in Maccabi.

7. Incentives were offered to help persuade existing doctors to start using the EMR. For example, the use of the EMR was linked to more rapid processing of claims and earlier payment to doctors. Through collective procurement, Maccabi reduced the costs of purchasing PCs. Doctors who implemented the EMR received a modest increase in fees. Financial incentives are critical, at least at the beginning of the process. At a very minimum, introducing an EMR-based system into a doctor's clinic should not constitute a financial burden. Maccabi offered a financial incentive and simultaneously reduced the financial burden of computerization.

8. Physician support: At the outset, the physicians did not have to make purchasing decisions on their own and they had a clearly responsible body to turn to in the event of a problem. There was a major investment on the part of Maccabi in training and assisting doctors in developing new skills and making the most of the new technology at their disposal.

The analysis of the Maccabi Healthcare Services experience in developing and implementing an EMR-based health information system identified ten critical success factors.

Five critical success factors fall under the heading of **"innovative leadership"**:

1. vision and making the decisions necessary to implement;
2. clear commitment and involvement of leadership throughout the process;
3. appointment of an authorized health system integrator;
4. addressing tangible, practical needs;
5. establishing an organizational process for implementation and monitoring achievement of objectives.

The second set of critical success factors are grouped together under the heading of **"partnership and collaboration with clinicians and other end users"** and include:

6. establishing a multi-disciplinary working group consisting of managers, clinicians, and IT people at the outset to create a joint vision of the Health IT system upon which the decision to enter into the process is based;
7. financial incentives for clinicians;
8. establishing an ongoing collaborative process;
9. making sure that benefits for clinicians are clear and visible;
10. providing training and ongoing support to clinicians.

Ongoing deployment and expansion of Health IT continued following the initial implementation process described above, which took about four years. Once the basic EMR was in place for all of the medical specialties, the EMR was expanded to include nursing and the other healthcare professions. Additional systems and features were added during the second half of the 1990s, including the Lab and Radiology information systems enabling computerized physician orders and automatic receipt of test results, computerized drug prescriptions, the clinical decision support system, teleradiology, tele-ultrasound, tele-ECG, tele-dermatology, and call centers. In 2001, the patient portal went live and now includes online appointments, online electronic prescriptions, virtual visits. Additional developments have been the secondary use of data for research using an ever growing database, and increasing use of telemedicine. Many of the same management principles continue to be crucial, they just change form. A multi-disciplinary Health IT Steering Committee was formed (that continues to operate today), headed by the CEO, to steer the process, set priorities, evaluate new technologies, and approve the Health IT yearly budget. The IT department expanded as the IT system and functions expanded. A crucial milestone was the creation of the Medical Informatics Department responsible for coding, standards, data quality, the clinical decision support systems, the disease registries, and the ongoing partnership between the clinical departments and the IT department. The expanding role of mobile applications as an integral part of the system has been a game-changer.

From a national perspective, one of the crucial drivers in the ongoing evolution of digital health has been competition, particularly competition among the HMOs in digital innovation. There is also competition for digital excellence at the hospital level. Both HMOs and hospitals partner with Israeli Tech companies and these collaborations are receiving increasing financial support from Israel's innovation Authority.

Implementation of Health IT in Scotland

The National Health Service in Scotland is the publicly funded healthcare system accountable to the Scottish Government. It is comprised of fourteen geographic health boards and seven national health boards and one public health body, which provide services for the population of 5.4 million people.

If you are living in Scotland, you need to register with a local Scottish General Practitioner (GP). The majority of health care provision in Scotland is provided by the public sector (NHS Scotland) and is paid for through taxation. Private healthcare is limited in Scotland, and is paid for through a private healthcare insurance scheme (usually offered to employees by private companies as part of their employee benefit package), or by individuals.

The sociopolitical context in Scotland is relevant to note. In Scotland, the Scottish Parliament and Scottish Government were established in 1999 by an Act of the UK Parliament. Under this Act (Scotland Act 1998) [30] a range of powers including health and social services were devolved to Scotland.

A number of localized IT systems grew across the United Kingdom in the 1990s. In Scotland, this trend towards a proliferation of localized Health IT systems was slowed by a move to unify the number of Health Trusts and Health Boards, resulting in the formation of fourteen geographic health boards and seven national special health boards [31].

Significant early Health IT initiatives in Scotland included the development (from 1984 onwards) of the General Practice Administration System for Scotland (GPASS), a publicly owned electronic health record for primary care [32].

While a single shared electronic health record is not yet in place, the fact that Scottish health organizations can communicate and exchange information by means of the National Information Systems Group (known as the Scottish Care Information (SCI) Gateway) means that significant pieces of the EHR jigsaw are in place [33].

The current ambition in Scotland is to deliver a national platform that is a truly accessible and integrated system. This exemplifies the "once for Scotland" approach which is most tangibly demonstrated by the work led (since 2018) by National Education for Scotland's Digital Service (NDS) to create a National Digital Platform. Scotland has developed strategies at the national level, relying on shared vision and leadership across stakeholder organizations which engage with citizens.

An early step in Scotland's progress towards national connected systems and telehealth was the introduction in 2001 of NHS 24 as a National Special Health Board. NHS 24 began as a telephone-based triage service to cover the out-of-hours period. The triage process out-of-hours has, in turn, been supported by the introduction of the Emergency Care Summary in Scotland. Piloted in 2004, with full national rollout from 2006, the Emergency Care Summary (ECS) is a national information system which hosts a secure central record derived from the GPs' primary care record and automatically updated twice daily [33]. It contains a record of an individual patient's demographic data, medicines prescribed, allergies, etc. In 2012, the Key Information Summary was introduced to allow information to be shared among health workers, doctors, ambulance crews, off-duty doctors, hospitals, pharmacies, and treatment centers.

Critical to the mainstreaming of telehealth in Scotland was the establishment in 2006 (by the Scottish Executive) of the Scottish Centre for Telehealth (SCT) to support NHS Boards to implement telehealth. At that time, Scotland was the only country in Europe that had both a national organization with a specific remit for telehealth and a national strategy for telehealth [34].

In April 2010, SCT was integrated with one of Scotland's 7 special Health Boards, NHS 24 [35], thus providing a national reach for its work. Founded in 2001, NHS 24 is Scotland's national telehealth and telecare organization. This special Health Board operates a national telephone health advice and triage service for Scottish citizens that covers the out-of-hours period. NHS 24 has expanded over the intervening years, with over 1.5 million calls received annually to its 111 service. In addition to its telephone-based services, it provides web-based information resources to connect with and provide health information to citizens.

In 2010, the Scottish Centre for Telehealth took over responsibility for delivery of the national Telecare Program and was rebranded as the Scottish Centre for Telehealth and Telecare (SCTT). The SCTT had the unique remit of supporting stakeholders, across all sectors, with the delivery of the Scottish Government's digital health and care objectives. Working with health, social care, local authority, housing and voluntary sector organizations in Scotland, and facilitating knowledge exchange and research with international partners, created a successful ecosystem to develop and test digital health and care

solutions with a view to implementing successful sustainable services at scale.

Since 2019, the work streams initiated by the SCTT continue to be supported by the Scottish Government's Digital Health and Care Directorate and are now embedded into its work programs [36].

What Were the Principles That Were Critical Success Factors in the Implementation of Health IT in Scotland?

Policy commitment: there has been government support in Scotland since the mid-2000s for what is now referred to as digital health and care. This support, which encourages "tests of change"—iterative developments at local and regional level followed by mainstreaming into routine service, has produced an environment where ICT is viewed as essential to the modernization of health and social care service delivery.

Working in partnership across the health and care landscape: strong relationships and leadership, which recognizes the role of digital solutions by senior organizational stakeholders across the public sector have been reinforced by ongoing support at government level.

Driving integrated services: in Scotland, technology has been explicitly regarded as a tool to support formal health and social care integration (legislation from 2016) and the wider application of digitally enabled solutions in health and care. There exists a clear timeline, in policy terms, for the building of support and integration of digital ambitions into Scottish approaches to health and care.

User centered: looking across the different phases of strategy development in Scotland, similar to the shifting language in other European strategies, there is a recognition of the crucial importance of user-centeredness, citizen empowerment and engagement for sustainable service delivery. The emphasis is on a person-centered approach to service design and improvement using the Healthcare Quality Strategy (2010) [37] as the policy framework that has connected all Scottish Government health and care strategies produced over the past decade.

NHS in Scotland: Stages of Development

In 2004, five years after the first Scottish Parliament was established, the Scottish Government commissioned Professor David Kerr to consider the future shape of the NHS in Scotland. The subsequent report "Building a Health Service Fit for the Future" (2005) [38]—most often referred to as the Kerr Report (2005), was aspirational in terms of the proposals and the timescales included.

The 2005 Report spoke with urgency about the need for a national ICT system, placing ICT at the center of discussions about the future of a high-quality healthcare system and recommended a "complete re-focus of the E-Health strategy" to work towards a single ICT system which included a nationally accessible EHR with functionality to include PACS, e-Prescribing, eBooking, Telehealth and Telecare, and patient access.

The Report also recommended the establishment of what was initially described as a "Telehealth Technology Resource Centre (TTRC)," to develop nationally applicable approaches to telehealth. In 2006, this recommendation became a reality with the establishment of the national Scottish Centre for Telehealth.

In 2005, the Scottish Government produced "Delivering for Health" [39], an Action Plan for the NHS, in part a response to the Kerr Report. Rather than a separate eHealth or Health IT Strategy, the Delivering for Health document accepted many of the recommendations around ICT and was followed in 2007 by the Scottish Government publication "Better Health, Better Care" strategy [40] which referred specifically, and in greater detail, to eHealth initiatives and committed to publishing a dedicated eHealth Strategy.

In 2008, the Scottish Government produced Scotland's first eHealth Strategy [41]. The Strategy covered the period 2008–2011 and marked an essential stage in defining, monitoring, and reporting on eHealth initiatives being delivered nationally (by Government) and

through local health and social care authorities with support from delivery organizations and teams, including the SCTT, across Scotland.

Significant developments included the new GP IT system, finally moving away from GPASS which had been in place since the 1980s, delivered by NHS Scotland to GP practices. A consortium of Health Boards worked on the business case and a framework contract with two commercial products was in place.

In 2010, the Scottish Government produced the Healthcare Quality Strategy which built upon the Better Health, Better Care approach and which is often cited as a formative publication as it describes a unifying approach and a culture that promotes mutuality and participation by all those providing and receiving health and care services.

While the majority of the preceding government documents focused on healthcare, it is important, in the Scottish context, to recognize the work to extend and develop community based telecare systems which was taking place both at the policy level and, more widely, at an operational service level in the 32 local authority settings across Scotland.

In 2008, "Seizing the Opportunity: Telecare Strategy (2008–10)" [42] was published followed in 2011 by "Telecare to 2012: an action plan for Scotland" [43]. The priorities set out for Telecare complimented the eHealth Strategy by identifying areas of service need which, once again, took the iterative approach of building on assets and successes and learning from good practice elsewhere.

Priorities included using technology to:

- support self-management and those living with long-term conditions;
- improve service response, e.g. for people at risk of falling;
- monitor and develop anticipatory approaches which use technology to help keep vulnerable people safe in their own home.

In 2012, reflecting the combined approach of the Scottish Centre for Telehealth and Telecare, "A National Telehealth and Telecare Delivery

Plan for Scotland" (to 2015) [44] was published with support from the NHS, the Scottish Government, and the Convention of Scottish Local Authorities.

The next phase of producing updated and reflective eHealth/Digital health strategies takes us through the period from 2011 to 2020, with the publication of: the eHealth Strategy 2011–2017 [45] and the Digital Health Strategy 2018—present day [46].

The Digital First Service Standards (2016) make it clear that the accepted approach in Scotland for all Scottish Government services and services produced in partnership is to develop services that are consistently: user driven; accessible, and technology enabled. The shift in strategic approaches and definitions outlined earlier in this chapter, from a focus on ICT infrastructures towards a more inclusive understanding of technologies used to support health and wellbeing, is very evident in the Scottish context. The way in which health and social care services are planned and delivered across Scotland was changed by the *Public Bodies (Joint Working) (Scotland) Act 2014*. Local Authorities and Health Boards are required by law to work together to plan and deliver adult community health and social care services, including services for older people. This new way of working is referred to as "Health and Social Care Integration." In total, 31 Health and Social Care Partnerships have been set up across Scotland and they manage almost £9 billion of

health and social care resources [47]. Progress towards shared records systems continues.

The current ambition in Scotland is to deliver a national platform that is a truly accessible and integrated system. This exemplifies the "once for Scotland" approach which is most tangibly demonstrated by the work led (since 2018) by National Education for Scotland's Digital Service (NDS) to create a National Digital Platform. The objective is a Platform approach for building a unified patient-centered record to support digital health and care services.

The main events on the timeline, as described in the chapter, are shown in Fig. 32.1:

Summary

There are two major differences between the implementation of Health IT in Scotland and Israel:

1. Scotland's implementation has been predominantly top-down and Israel's implementation has been bottom-up. Scotland has developed iterative strategies at the national level, whereas Health IT in Israel has been from grass roots, driven by the four HMOs that perceived the need at the organizational level and proceeded to develop and implement.

2. While both countries have implemented both Health Information management systems and

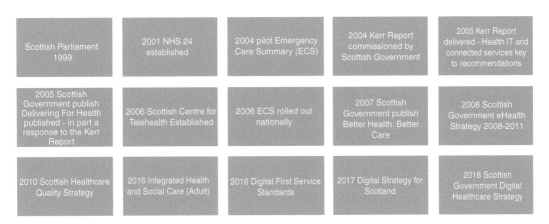

Fig. 32.1 NHS Scotland Stages of development—Main events on the timeline

telemedicine, Scotland placed higher priority on telehealth and telecare and Israel prioritized comprehensive shared electronic medical records supported by clinical decision support systems.

These differences in approach are derived from the structure of the two healthcare systems (Beveridgian vs Bismarkian), geopolitical and cultural differences as well as the maturity of available technology at the various stages of evolution. There is no right or wrong approach. The choice needs to be based on an assessment of the context. This is true regardless of whether the implementation is national, regional, or organizational.

For the most part, the management principles for implementation in both countries are strikingly similar and consistent with well-known change management principles—but also subtly different in the following ways:

1. Leadership—but not just any kind of leadership.
   - In Israel, we see innovative leadership that included thinking "out of the box," vision, appointment of an authorized health system integrator and team, but continued "hands on" commitment and support from the very top, willingness to take risks and willingness to invest and commit organizational resources to the process.
   - In Scotland, there is shared leadership with strong relationships and recognition of the role of digital solutions by senior organizational stakeholders across Scotland, reinforced by ongoing support at government level. There has been clear governmental support in Scotland since the mid-2000s for what is now referred to as the digital health and care agenda. Scotland also appointed digital health and care leadership and through the establishment of the national Scottish Centre for Telehealth and Telecare, and the Technology Enabled Care Program in Scottish Government to support Scottish stakeholders to implement telehealth and telecare.

2. Focusing on compelling needs of the intended users—and addressing these by showing clearly defined benefits. In very practical terms, this means addressing two questions: "where is the pain?" and "what's in it for me?".
   - In Israel, it was clear from the outset that the first primary user would be the doctors. They were frustrated by bureaucracy involved verifying patient eligibility for treatment and billing. They were also frustrated by the lack of clinical information on their patients. The electronic medical record addressed both of these issues and, consequently, the doctors perceived clear benefits from the implementation of the EMR. In addition, Maccabi provided financial incentives for the doctors. Once the bureaucratic issues were addressed, the need for clinical information became the central concern leading to the computerization of the lab system, teleradiology, and computerized prescriptions. Until 2000, the focus was on "IT to support the clinician"—including nursing and healthcare professionals, and it expanded to include the patient leading to the creation of the patient portal with the recognition of the crucial role of the patient in managing his care.
   - In Scotland, the perceived needs and benefits have also changed over time. The initial need was having critical information for the triage process out-of-hours that generated the introduction of Emergency Care Summary. The lack of symmetry between the geographical distribution of the population and healthcare facilities and professionals led to an early emphasis on the development of telehealth that drove the establishment of both a national organization with a specific remit for telehealth and a national strategy for telehealth. It also saw the establishment of a national Telecare Program in 2006 which led to the merging of the telehealth and telecare strategic agenda, led by the Scottish Government's Technology Enabled Care

and Digital Healthcare Innovation Division. The Scottish approach to the **integration of health and social care** was another driver leading to legislation to establish Health and Care Partnerships across Scotland. Technology is seen as an important tool to support the delivery of integration and the wider application of digitally enabled solutions in health and care.

The Covid19 pandemic is an example of compelling need that has driven a quantum leap in telehealth development and implementation in both Israel and Scotland as well as globally.

3. Focused and Concrete Collaboration and Communication.

There are two critical actions that need to take place: building a bridge between management, clinicians, and IT and creating a close working relationship—not just talking to each other but making decisions together; and directly involving users—clinicians and ultimately citizens—in the actual work of design so that the system supports existing processes. By collaboration, we mean not just dialogue but all partners "getting their hands dirty."

- In Maccabi—the decision to implement an EMR was a joint decision of management, clinicians, and IT staff, and the doctors designed the user interface and content of the EMR. There were Working Groups set up for every specialty—they decided on the content and appearance of every screen—as well as rules for the Clinical Decision Support System—a structure which continues to this day. Likewise, the member portal has been designed and redesigned based on active feedback from both clinicians and patients.
- In Scotland, working in partnership across the health and care landscape occurred in successive stages of development of Scottish health and care IT. This is best exemplified by the merging of the Scottish Centre for Telehealth and Telecare within NHS 24. Working in partnership with

health, social care, local authority, housing and voluntary sector organizations in Scotland and facilitating knowledge exchange and research with international partners have created a successful ecosystem to develop and test digital health and care solutions with a view to implementing successful sustainable services at scale.

4. Embedding IT in ongoing organizational processes.

HIT implementation is not an ad hoc activity or a project. It is a way of life. The organizational chart and organizational processes need to support the day-to-day activities of implementation and monitoring achievement of objectives. In Maccabi, the multidisciplinary Steering Committee chaired by the CEO continues to guide the ongoing process of HIT implementation and development. In Scotland, this is reflected in the successive national digital health and care strategies that have been developed, published, legislated, financed, and implemented.

5. Providing training and ongoing support.

Providing training and ongoing support to clinicians and health and care staff is crucial to the ongoing implementation and expansion of Health IT and the accompanying service transformation. In both Israel and Scotland, the doctors in the community are a special challenge as they are independent practitioners—not salaried staff. Maccabi has addressed this challenge using multiple approaches: All clinical staff, including independent physicians, cannot begin to care for Maccabi patients without a training course to use the Maccabi digital systems. When new features are added to the EMR that doctors are expected to use, these features are presented at professional conferences, doctors receive short instructional videos and are also taught how to use them at a time of their choosing by remote access instruction—on their own computers.

In Scotland, the challenge of providing ongoing support to health and care staff is recognized in the 2018 Digital Health and Care Strategy (Domain D: Workforce Capability).

In addition to work-based training on individual systems, the components include: resources, networks, and training opportunities. Online resources provide entry-level content on digital health and care, freely accessible to all health and care staff [48]. More targeted (small group) support is available via the Nursing, Midwifery, and Allied Health Professions Digital Health and Care Leadership Programme hosted by NHS Education for Scotland, now in Cohort 14. Finally, the challenge is also addressed through both clinician specific networks for "eHealth Clinical Leads" and multidisciplinary knowledge exchange networks.

Conclusions and Outlook

There are two major conclusions and recommendations arising from the Israel and Scotland experiences that will impact the successful implementation of Health IT going forward:

1. Changing the semantic—not engagement and not empowerment.

    Human behavior, and particularly organizational behavior, is strongly influenced by the terminology we use and how it is perceived. Part of successful implementation is making sure that everyone involved in the implementation understands clearly what is expected of them and their relationship with others. In the successful implementation of digital health and care, the relationship of management and IT with clinicians and health and care staff is no longer an "engagement"—it is a "marriage" with all that it implies. It is a long-term intimate relationship in which the need for sensitivity to needs and the commitment to develop together is crucial. Likewise, we are not "empowering" patients and citizens—we are partnering them. Patients do not want us to send them home with a "self-care" kit—the therapeutic relationship is an integral part of care. Health IT supports this relationship—it is not a substitute.

2. Never refreezing.

    Implementation of digital health and care is a constantly moving target. In contrast to Lewin's three-stage approach to organizational change management—"Unfreeze, Change, Refreeze" [49] or Kotter's eighth step "establish the new status quo" [50], we cannot allow ourselves to rest on our laurels. The pace of technological change, as well as the advances in medical care and the healthcare needs of the population, is so rapid that we must put into place a process of ongoing transformation and openness. In both Israel and Scotland, successive new strategies driving new health and care innovations exemplify this new reality.

Useful Resources

- **Implementation Management Tools**
  Two key critical factors for successful implementation of Health IT are understanding the context in which we are implementing; identifying the gaps between where we are and where we want to be; and learning as we go—learning from our mistakes and correcting—to make sure we get there. We have found three management tools to be particularly useful: digital maturity assessment, quality improvement, and "Plan Do Study Act"—ongoing implementation analysis with corrective action.

- **Digital Maturity Assessment: The SCIROCCO Tool**
  Integrated health and care, enabled by digital technologies, is a recognized solution to address the challenge of aging population. Yet, regions and countries vary in their success and maturity to drive transformation of their health and social care systems towards more integrated digital health and care services. This was the main rationale for the development of the B3 Maturity Model for Integrated Care [51] as a framework to capture the different ways and rates of how integrated care has been designed and delivered. This work was undertaken as part of the European Commission's initiative European Innovation Partnership on Active and Healthy Ageing (EIPonAHA) [52]. Maturity

Models employ qualitative assessments of progress and may be regarded as a measurement of the ability of a health and care system to progress towards the integration of health and care. The higher the maturity, the higher the chances are that health and care service delivery will lead to improvement in the quality of care and more effective use of the resources. The original B3 Maturity Model was derived from interviews with stakeholders responsible for health and care delivery in 12 European regions [53]. They identified a number of areas that require to be managed in order to effectively deliver digitally enabled, integrated care—these were grouped into 12 "dimensions," each of which addresses a part of the overall transformation process The 12 dimensions are:

- Readiness to Change.
- Structure and Governance.

- Digital infrastructure.
- Funding.
- Process Coordination.
- Removal of Inhibitors.
- Population approach.
- Citizen empowerment.
- Evaluation methods.
- Breadth of ambition.
- Innovation management.
- Capacity-building.

The B3 Maturity Model has been further developed, validated, and tested through the EU Health program funded projects SCIROCCO [54] and SCIROCCO Exchange [55] (Fig. 32.2). The Tool is free to use and can be accessed using the following link: https://scirocco-exchange-tool.inf.ed.ac.uk/en_gb/. Each of the dimensions is further defined in terms of its objectives and assessment scale reflecting different level of maturity one can achieve (Fig. 32.3).

Fig. 32.2 SCIROCCO Self-assessment Tool for Integrated Care

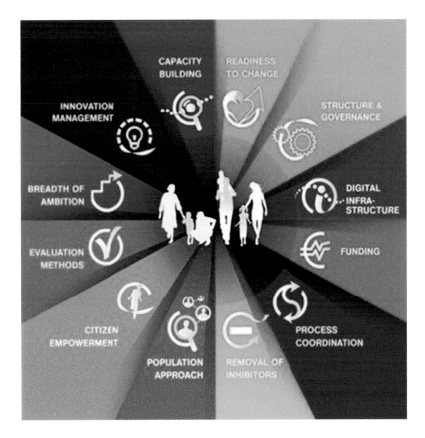

Capturing Maturity Level

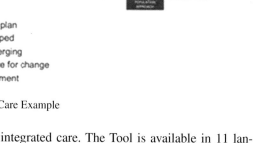

Objectives

If the existing systems of care need to be re-designed to provide a more integrated services, this will require change across many levels, the creation of new roles, processes and working practices, and new systems to support information sharing and collaboration across care teams. This will be disruptive and may be viewed negatively by workers, press and public, so a clear case needs to be made for those changes, including a justification, a strategic plan, and a vision of better care.

Assessment scale

0– No acknowledgment of compelling need to change
1– Compelling need is recognised, but no clear vision or strategic plan
2– Dialogue and consensus-building underway; plan being developed
3– Vision or plan embedded in policy; leaders and champions emerging
4– Leadership, vision and plan clear to the general public; pressure for change
5– Political consensus; public support; visible stakeholder engagement

Fig. 32.3 SCIROCCO Self-assessment Tool for Integrated Care Example

The Tool helps regions and countries to:

- Indicate their readiness and maturity to adopt and scale-up digital integrated care solutions;
- Understand the strengths and weaknesses of their local context for digitally enabled integrated care and inform national, regional and local policy-makers about potential areas of improvement;
- Capture the perceptions of multi-stakeholder teams on maturity of their organizations, regions, and countries to implement digitally enabled integrated care;
- Facilitate multi-stakeholder dialogue on progress towards digitally enabled integrated care.

The SCIROCCO self-assessment tool has been tested and used in more than 82 regions and organizations in Europe and beyond which reflects the needs for, and interest in, frameworks and tools that can support health and social care authorities to better understand how they can improve their progress towards digitally enabled integrated care. The Tool is available in 11 languages (Czech, English, Flemish, German, Hebrew, Italian, Lithuanian, Polish, Slovak, Slovenian, Spanish).

The Quality Improvement Approach

In Scotland, the Quality Improvement approach, which is core to Scotland's Healthcare Quality Strategy (2010), seeks to provide safe, effective, person-centered care [37], a simple objective which is hugely complete to deliver in practice. The methodology employed includes a number of tools and techniques and will include familiar elements:

- clarity about the improvement or change to be achieved;
- understanding the pathway, flow, or process of a treatment or intervention;
- understanding change in a systematic way which includes all those (staff and service users) involved;

- deploying structured tools and techniques to capture, measure, learn from and apply changes.

The techniques used include:

- Plan Do Study Act (PDSA) cycles—PDSA which make it possible to capture and use the results to support continuous improvement [56, 57].
- Process mapping—to map the journey taking into account the experiences of all roles involved [58].

In a progression from the policy and strategic developments outlined in Scotland up to the Healthcare Quality Strategy (2010) the Scottish Government established Healthcare Improvement Scotland in 2011. In addition, to the important work of regulation of independent hospitals and clinics, the remit for this organization includes working with health and care organizations to support continuous improvement as part of service redesign [59].

The Plan Do Study Act Methodology

In Israel, learning as you go and making adjustments along the way is a way of life. The PDSA methodology, articulated by Edward Deming and Walter Shewharts, presents a pragmatic scientific method for testing changes in complex systems [60]. PDSA cycles consist of a systematic series of steps for gaining valuable learning for the continual improvement of a product or process.

Each PDSA cycle consists of four steps [61], as demonstrated in (Fig. 32.4):

1. **Plan**—Plan the intervention, state the objective, and develop a plan to test the change.
2. **Do**—Try out the intervention, and document problems and unexpected observations.
3. **Study**—Analyze the data collected and study the results.
4. **Act**—Refine the change and determine what modifications should be made.

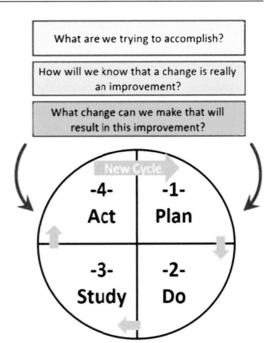

Fig. 32.4 Model for improvement (PDSA)

The PDSA methodology promotes learning through interventional experiments, in recognition of working in complex settings with inherent variability. The PDSA methodology provides overview, ownership, and involvement of stakeholders who at all times have insight on the intervention process. It provides flexibility to develop interventions according to stakeholder's feedback and changing conditions ensuring fit-for-purpose solutions, while providing the opportunity to build evidence for change. In both countries this has been enhanced in recent months due to the COVID crisis by additional processes for managing accelerated technology development such as the Agile methodology [62] in Israel, driving the collaborative effort of self-organizing and cross-functional teams and Rapid Response Tools and Processes in Scotland [63].

These flexible, responsive, and continuous improvement approaches have been used successfully in both Israel and Scotland to advance digitally enabled care for older people and the chronically ill, to support the ongoing digital transformation of health and care and to enable rapid responses to new and unanticipated challenges.

Most Relevant References
Terminology, History, Current Status of Health IT:

1. Rouse M. DEFINITION Health IT (health information technology). Searchhealthit; 2018.
2. European commission website, Shaping the Digital Single Market. Retrieved from: https://ec.europa.eu/digital-single-market/en/policies/shaping-digital-single-market
3. World Health Organization. WHO guideline: recommendations on digital interventions for health system strengthening: web supplement 2: summary of findings and GRADE tables. World Health Organization; 2019.
4. Nesbitt TS. The evolution of telehealth: Where have we been and where are we going. In Institute of Medicine, Board on Health Care Services, & T. A Lustig (Eds.), The role of telehealth in an evolving health care environment: Workshop summary 2012 (pp. 11–16).
5. Kaye R, Kokia E, Shalev V, Idar D, Chinitz D. Barriers and success factors in health information technology: A practitioner's perspective. Journal of Management & Marketing in Healthcare. 2010 Jun 1;3(2):163–75.

Health IT Implementation in Israel and Scotland:

1. Kaye R, Waksman M, Corrigan T. Maccabi Healthcare Services delivers coordinated care to over 1.9 million members. Intel WHITE PAPER Digital health Coordinated Care. 2011.
2. The NHS24 site. https://www.nhs24.scot/
3. Scottish Government. The healthcare quality strategy for NHS Scotland. 2010.
4. Health Foundation (Great Britain). Quality Improvement Made Simple: What Everyone Should Know about Healthcare Quality Improvement: Quick Guide. Health Foundation; 2013.
5. Scottish Government. The Scottish Approach to Service Design (SAtSD). Retrieved from: https://www.gov.scot/publications/the-scottish-approach-to-service-design/

Implementation Management Tools:

1. Deming WE. Out of the Crisis. MIT press; 2018 Sep 21.
2. https://www.scirocco-project.eu
3. https://www.sciroccoexchange.com
4. Moen R, Norman C. Evolution of the PDCA cycle. 2006.

Review Questions

1. What was a key element in the Innovative leadership in Maccabi?
   (a) It focused only on vision and commitment.
   (b) The process completely ignored thinking about organizational resources.
   (c) It did not involve top management at all, but only operational staff members.
   (d) It involved hands-on involvement of top management.
2. According to Maccabi's experience, Involving key stakeholders should:
   (a) Come after an initial planning and evaluation process by professional staff.
   (b) always involve computerizing methods,
   (c) be performed by a multi-disciplinary committee,
   (d) a and c are correct.
3. According to Maccabi's experience, the design of a new EHR should:
   (a) Support the doctor's workflow.
   (b) Begin with a minimum data set.
   (c) should be gradual,
   (d) should not include incentives for the doctors,
   (e) a, b, and c are correct.
4. In Israel, from a national perspective, what is a key driver in the ongoing evolution of digital health?
   (a) Competition.
   (b) Israel's innovation Authority.
   (c) Incentives for the doctors.
   (d) Tech companies involvement.

5. The Scottish government report "Building a Health Service Fit for the Future" in 2005 made explicit the ambition for health IT in Scotland to do what?
   (a) support a competitive approach to identify health IT solutions,
   (b) completely re-focus the E-Health strategy' to work towards a single ICT system,
   (c) promote a variety of different system developments across the NHS,
   (d) seek investment from technology suppliers.

6. Select 2 of the Critical Success Factors identified by the authors in the Scottish deployment of Health IT:
   (a) large-scale investment by technology suppliers,
   (b) policy commitment and clear strategy,
   (c) supportive leadership across health and care,
   (d) financial incentives for health care staff.

7. Why was the publication in 2010 of the Scottish Healthcare Quality Strategy significant for the development of health IT?
   (a) it made clear that Health IT implementation was only the responsibility of hospitals,
   (b) it emphasized that leadership should derive from IT professionals,
   (c) it provides an approach which promotes service quality, mutuality, and participation by all those providing and receiving health and care services.
   (d) it set out the allocation of funding to develop health IT.

8. On reflection (after reading this chapter) do you think that the distinct approaches taken to the development and implementation of health IT in Scotland and Israel stem from:
   (a) sociopolitical differences,
   (b) differences in their readiness to adopt healthcare IT culture differences,
   (c) differences in when suitable technology becomes available,
   (d) differences in leadership approaches,
   (e) All of the above.
   (f) None of the above.

9. What is NOT true?
   (a) Scotland's implementation has been predominantly top-down and Israel's implementation has been bottom-up.
   (b) Both countries placed higher priority on telehealth and telecare.
   (c) Scotland has developed iterative strategies at the national level, whereas Health IT in Israel started at the organizational level.
   (d) Both countries have implemented both Health Information management systems and telemedicine.

10. These differences in approach between the implementation of Health IT in Scotland and Israel are derived from:
    (a) Differences in the healthcare systems (Beveridgian vs Bismarkian).
    (b) Geopolitical and cultural differences.
    (c) The maturity of available technology at the various stages of evolution.
    (d) All of the above.

11. What was learned about Focusing on compelling needs?
    (a) In Israel, the first primary user was the doctors.
    (b) In Scotland, the perceived needs and benefits changed over time.
    (c) In Israel, until 2000, the focus was on "IT to support the clinician".
    (d) All of the above.
    (e) None of the above.

12. What was learned about Embedding IT in ongoing organizational processes?
    (a) HIT implementation is not an ad hoc activity.
    (b) Finance issues should be put aside for proper implementation.
    (c) Multi-disciplinary Stakeholder commitment is a must have component.
    (d) a and c are correct,
    (e) All of the above.

13. What was learned about Changing the semantic?
    (a) Organizational behavior is strongly influenced by the terminology we use.

(b) It is important that everyone involved understands clearly what is expected of them.

(c) The relationship of management and IT with clinicians and health and care staff is crucial.

(d) Health IT supports the therapeutic relationship—it is not a substitute.

(e) All of the above.

14. The SCIROCCO Tool:

(a) Is a Digital Maturity Assessment Tool.

(b) Identified a number of areas that require to be managed in order to effectively deliver digitally enabled, integrated care.

(c) Can help regions and countries.

(d) All of the above.

15. The Quality Improvement Approach:

(a) Is core to Israel's Healthcare Quality Strategy.

(b) Includes a number of tools and techniques.

(c) Focuses only on understanding the pathway, flow, or process of a treatment or intervention.

(d) Is a different name for the PDSA cycle approach.

Appendix: Answers to Review Questions

Correct answers are printed in bold.

1. What was a key element in the Innovative leadership in Maccabi?

(a) It focused only on vision and commitment.

(b) The process completely ignored thinking about organizational resources.

(c) It did not involve top management at all, but only operational staff members.

(d) It involved hands-on involvement of top management.

2. According to Maccabi's experience, involving key stakeholders should:

(a) Come after an initial planning and evaluation process by professional staff.

(b) always involve computerizing methods,

(c) be performed by a multi-disciplinary committee,

(d) a and c are correct,

3. According to Maccabi's experience, the design of a new EHR should:

(a) Support the doctor's workflow.

(b) Begin with a minimum data set.

(c) should be gradual,

(d) should not include incentives for the doctors,

(e) a, b, and c are correct,

4. In Israel, from a national perspective, what a key driver in the ongoing evolution of digital health?

(a) Competition.

(b) Israel's innovation Authority.

(c) Incentives for the doctors.

(d) Tech companies involvement.

5. The Scottish government report "Building a Health Service Fit for the Future" in 2005 made explicit the ambition for health IT in Scotland to do what?

(a) support a competitive approach to identify health IT solutions,

(b) completely re-focus the E-Health strategy' to work towards a single ICT system,

(c) promote a variety of different system developments across the NHS,

(d) seek investment from technology suppliers,

6. Select 2 of the Critical Success Factors identified by the authors in the Scottish deployment of Health IT:

(a) large-scale investment by technology suppliers,

(b) policy commitment and clear strategy,

(c) supportive leadership across health and care,

(d) financial incentives for health care staff,

7. Why was the publication in 2010 of the Scottish Healthcare Quality Strategy significant for the development of health IT?

(a) it made clear that Health IT implementation was only the responsibility of hospitals,

(b) it emphasized that leadership should derive from IT professionals,

(c) it provides an approach which promotes service quality, mutuality, and participation by all those providing and receiving health and care services.

(d) it set out the allocation of funding to develop health IT,

8. On reflection (after reading this chapter) do you think that the distinct approaches taken to the development and implementation of health IT in Scotland and Israel stem from:

(a) sociopolitical differences,

(b) differences in their readiness to adopt healthcare IT culture differences,

(c) differences in when suitable technology becomes available,

(d) differences in leadership approaches,

(e) All of the above.

(f) None of the above.

9. What is NOT true?

(a) Scotland's implementation has been predominantly top-down and Israel's implementation has been bottom-up.

(b) Both countries placed higher priority on telehealth and telecare.

(c) Scotland has developed iterative strategies at the national level, whereas Health IT in Israel started at the organizational level.

(d) Both countries have implemented both Health Information management systems and telemedicine.

10. These differences in approach between the implementation of Health IT in Scotland and Israel are derived from:

(a) Differences in the healthcare systems (Beveridgian vs Bismarkian).

(b) Geopolitical and cultural differences.

(c) The maturity of available technology at the various stages of evolution.

(d) All of the above.

11. What was learned about Focusing on compelling needs?

(a) In Israel, the first primary user was the doctors.

(b) In Scotland, the perceived needs and benefits changed over time.

(c) In Israel, until 2000, the focus was on "IT to support the clinician".

(d) All of the above.

(e) None of the above.

12. What was learned about Embedding IT in ongoing organizational processes?

(a) HIT implementation is not an ad hoc activity.

(b) Finance issues should be put aside for proper implementation.

(c) Multi-disciplinary Stakeholder commitment is a must have component.

(d) a and c are correct,

(e) All of the above.

13. What was learned about Changing the semantic?

(a) Organizational behavior is strongly influenced by the terminology we use.

(b) It is important that everyone involved understands clearly what is expected of them.

(c) The relationship of management and IT with clinicians and health and care staff is crucial.

(d) Health IT supports the therapeutic relationship—it is not a substitute.

(e) All of the above.

14. The SCIROCCO Tool:

(a) Is a Digital Maturity Assessment Tool.

(b) Identified a number of areas that require to be managed in order to effectively deliver digitally enabled, integrated care.

(c) Can help regions and countries.

(d) All of the above.

15. The Quality Improvement Approach:

(a) Is core to Israel's Healthcare Quality Strategy.

(b) **Includes a number of tools and techniques.**

(c) Focuses only on understanding the pathway, flow, or process of a treatment or intervention.

(d) Is a different name for the PDSA cycle approach.

References

1. EU Commission. e-Health-making healthcare better for European citizens: an action plan for a European e-health area. Retrieved August 2004;23:2015.
2. Blumenthal D. Launching hitech. N Engl J Med. 2010;362(5):382–5.
3. Eurohealth—Vol. 25 | No.2 | 2019. Retrieved from: https://apps.who.int/iris/bitstream/handle/10665/326127/Eurohealth-V25-N2-2019-eng.pdf
4. Office of the National Coordinator for Health Information Technology. Connecting health and care for the nation: a 10-year vision to achieve an interoperable health IT infrastructure. 2014.
5. Rouse M. DEFINITION Health IT (health information technology). Searchhealthit; 2018.
6. Pretlow R. eHealth International: A cutting edge company for a new age in health care. Retrieved from: http://www.ehealthnurse.com/ehealthi.html [accessed 2004 June 24]. 2000.
7. European commission website, eHealth. Retrieved from: http://www.euro.who.int/en/health-topics/Health-systems/e-health
8. European commission website, Shaping the Digital Single Market. Retrieved from: https://ec.europa.eu/digital-single-market/en/policies/shaping-digital-single-market
9. European commission website, eHealth: Digital health and care. Retrieved from: https://ec.europa.eu/health/ehealth/overview_en
10. World Health Organization. WHO guideline: recommendations on digital interventions for health system strengthening: web supplement 2: summary of findings and GRADE tables. World Health Organization; 2019.
11. eVisit Resources. Retrieved from: https://evisit.com/resources/what-is-the-difference-between-telemedicine-telecare-and-telehealth/
12. Meidert U, Früh S, Becker H. Telecare: Technology for an ageing society in Europe. Current state and future developments; 2013.
13. McLean S, Protti D, Sheikh A. Telehealthcare for long term conditions. BMJ 342: d120. In Proceedings of the international conference "SCience in TEchnology-SCinTE-2015"; 2011.
14. VertitechIT web site. The History of Healthcare Technology and the Evolution of HER. Mar 11 2020. Retrieved from: https://www.vertitechit.com/history-healthcare-technology/
15. Suarez WG. An Overview of Health IT@. Kaiser Permanente. 2013;
16. Kajbjer K, Nordberg R, Klein GO. Electronic health records in Sweden: from administrative management to clinical decision support. In IFIP conference on history of Nordic computing 2010 Oct 18 (pp. 74–82). Springer, Berlin, Heidelberg.
17. Accenture. Norway – early electronic medical record adoption helped then, But Hurts Now 2015.
18. Nesbitt TS. The evolution of telehealth: where have we been and where are we going. In Institute of Medicine, Board on Health Care Services, & T. A. Lustig (Eds.), The role of telehealth in an evolving health care environment: Workshop summary 2012 (pp. 11–16).
19. Ryu S. History of telemedicine: evolution, context, and transformation. Healthc Inform Res. 2010;16(1):65–6.
20. Turner KJ, McGee-Lennon M. Advances in telecare over the past ten years. Smart Homecare Technol TeleHealth. 2013;1(1):21–34.
21. Kaye R, Kollmann A, Rupp C, Sauermann S, Petersen J, Uffelman J, Laktišová M, Tomášik J, Lange M, Schug S, Whitehead, D. Implementation of the National eHealth Centre in the Czech Republic. Component I.2. Study of European eHealth Strategies and National eHealth Competence Centres (NeHCs) in Europe. 2018.
22. European Commission. Communication on enabling the digital transformation of health and care in the Digital Single Market; empowering citizens and building a healthier society; 2018.
23. RAND Healthcare: Health Information Technology: Can HIT Lower Costs and Improve Quality? Retrieved on July 8, 2006.
24. Peterburg Y. IsraelLs Health IT Industry: What Does the American Recovery and Reinvestment Act Mean for Israeli Collaborative Opportunities. Milken Institute. 2010;
25. Kaye R, Kokia E, Shalev V, Idar D, Chinitz D. Barriers and success factors in health information technology: a practitioner's perspective. J Manage Market Healthc. 2010;3(2):163–75.
26. A digital quantum leap in the healthcare system: The Ministry of Health's vision. Israel Innovation Authority. Retrieved from: https://innovationisrael.org.il/en/article/digital-quantum-leap-healthcare-system
27. Startup Nation Central. Make an in-depth examination of digital health. Retrieved from: https://www.startupnationcentral.org/sector/digital-health/
28. Kaye R, Waksman M, Corrigan T. Maccabi Healthcare Services delivers coordinated care to over 1.9 million members. Intel WHITE PAPER Digital health Coordinated Care 2011.
29. Villalba E, Abadie F, Mansoa F, Rodríguez Mañas L, Peinado I, Sánchez A. Strategic intelligence monitor on personal health systems phase 3 (SIMPHS3). Integrated care programme for older in-and out-

patients University Hospital of Getafe (Spain), case study report. 2015.

30. Parliament UK. Scotland Act 1998 (c. 46). Retrieved from: http://www.legislation.gov.uk/ukpga/1998/46/contents

31. Payne J. eHealth in Scotland-Scottish parliament information centre (SPICe) briefing, 28 p. 2013.

32. Lluch M. Strategic intelligence monitor on personal health systems phase 2 country study. The United Kingdom Joint Research Centre. 2013;

33. Bonomi S. The electronic health record: a comparison of some European countries. Information and Communication Technologies in Organizations and Society 2016 (pp. 33–50). Springer, Champions.

34. Auditor General for Scotland. A review of telehealth in Scotland. Prepared for the Auditor General for Scotland October 2011. Retrieved from: https://www.audit-scotland.gov.uk/docs/health/2011/nr_111013_telehealth.pdf

35. The NHS24 site. https://www.nhs24.scot/

36. The Technology Enabled Care in Scotland site. https://tec.scot

37. Scottish Government. The healthcare quality strategy for NHS Scotland. 2010.

38. Team RA. The National framework for service change in NHS Scotland. Edinburgh: Scottish Executive; 2005.

39. Executive S. Delivering for health. Edinburgh: Scottish Executive. 2005:257–87.

40. Executive S. Better health, better care: action plan. Edinburgh: NHS Scotland. 2007.

41. Executive S. eHealth Strategy 2008–2011. Edinburgh: NHS Scotland. 2008.

42. Team JI. Seizing the opportunity: Telecare strategy 2008–2010. Retrieved November 2008;30: 2010.

43. Team JI. Telecare to 2012: An Action Plan for Scotland. Edinburgh: The Scottish Government St Andrew's House; 2011.

44. Scottish Government. A National Telehealth and Telecare Delivery Plan for Scotland to 2015: Driving Improvement, Integration and Innovation.

45. Scotland NH. eHealth Strategy 2011–2017. Revised 2012.

46. Scottish Government. Scotland's Digital health and care strategy: Enabling, connecting and empowering 2018.

47. Crown Copyright. Public Bodies (Joint Working) (Scotland) Act 2014.

48. Scotland NH. TURAS website. https://turasdashboard.nes.nhs.scot

49. Levasseur RE. People skills: Change management tools—Lewin's change model. Interfaces. 2001;31(4):71–3.

50. Kotter J. The 8-step process for leading change. Kotter International; 2012.

51. Grooten L, Borgermans L, Vrijhoef HJ. An instrument to measure maturity of integrated care: a first validation study. International journal of integrated care. 2018 Jan;18(1).

52. European commission website, EIP on AHA portal. Retrieved from: https://ec.europa.eu/eip/ageing/home_en

53. European commission website, A Maturity Model for Adoption of Integrated Care within Regional Healthcare Systems (B3 Action Group). Retrieved from: https://ec.europa.eu/eip/ageing/repository/maturity-model-adoption-integrated-care-within-regional-healthcare-systems-b3-action_en

54. https://www.scirocco-project.eu

55. https://www.sciroccoexchange.com

56. Deming WE. Out of the crisis. MIT Press; 2018 Sep 21.

57. Health Foundation (Great Britain). Quality improvement made simple: what everyone should know about healthcare quality improvement: quick guide. Health Foundation; 2013.

58. Langley GJ, Moen RD, Nolan KM, Nolan TW, Norman CL, Provost LP. The improvement guide: a practical approach to enhancing organizational performance. Wiley; 2009 Jun 3.

59. Scottish Government. The Scottish Approach to Service Design (SAtSD). Retrieved from: https://www.gov.scot/publications/the-scottish-approach-to-service-design/

60. Moen R, Norman C. Evolution of the PDCA cycle. 2006.

61. Berwick DM. The science of improvement. JAMA 2008;299(10):1182–4.

62. Muslihat D. Agile methodology: an overview. ZenkitBlog. 2018.

63. Digital health and care Scotland. Scotland's digital health and care response to Covid-19. 2020 June. Retrieved from: https://www.digihealthcare.scot/covid-19/scotlands-digital-health-and-care-response-to-covid-19/.

Strategic Information Management: Essential Alignment

33

Susan H. Fenton

Learning Objectives

By the conclusion of this chapter, students will be able to:

- Compare and contrast strategic and tactical management.
- Explain the importance of aligning information management strategy with organizational strategy.
- Describe the strategic management process.
- Create a revised clinical information section strategic plan based on a strategic management case study.

Key Terms

- Critical Success Factor—a methodology, management tool, or design technique that enables the effective development and deployment of a project or process [1].
- Environmental scan—the collection of data and information about the environments, external and internal, to the information organization.
- Mission statement—a formal summary of the aims and values of a company or organization [2].
- Objective—something toward which effort is directed [3].

- Stakeholder—a person or organizational unit that would be involved in or affected by decisions or actions taken.
- Strategy—a plan or a method.
- SWOT—Strengths, Weaknesses, Opportunities, and Threats—a method of analysis designed to assist in objectively assessing an organization or organizational unit.
- Target—a goal or aim that is being worked toward.
- Task Measure—a metric that can be used to determine whether targets and objectives are being met.
- Vision statement—a declaration of the broad, long-term goal of an organization or organizational unit.

Introduction

Clinical and health information technology (HIT) organizational units face many challenges in their day-to-day operations. In fact, sometimes, these units get so caught up in achieving their day-to-day goals, or **tactical management**, that they can lose sight of the "bigger picture" for their unit. This "bigger picture" is more commonly known as **strategic management** for information technology (IT). Strategic management is needed to define how the clinical and HIT units will help the larger organization succeed. This chapter will explore strategic management, including the

S. H. Fenton (✉)
University of TX Health Science Center at Houston, Houston, TX, USA
e-mail: susan.h.fenton@uth.tmc.edu

© Springer Nature Switzerland AG 2022
U. H. Hübner et al. (eds.), *Nursing Informatics*, Health Informatics,
https://doi.org/10.1007/978-3-030-91237-6_33

necessary steps for developing a strategic management plan. It must be noted that strategic management and tactical management must be tied together. For, it is the day-to-day activities and operations and ensuring that those tasks contribute to the strategic plan that supports the entire organizational strategy.

Alignment of Clinical and Health IT Strategy with Organizational Strategy

Clinical and HIT professionals do not perform their work in a vacuum. Generally, IT, even that which is Software-as-a-Service (SaaS), for example, Amazon Web Services, is established to assist an organizational unit or organization achieve their goals. IT services that do not assist the organization to achieve their goals more efficiently and effectively essentially become obstacles to success. Thus, it is imperative that the strategies of the clinical and health IT units align and support the broader organizational strategy.

Strategic Management Process

Environmental Scanning

Environmental scanning is important for the strategic planning process. It involves examining all of the forces, internal and external, that may impact an organization or organizational unit. This will require data and information collection to the greatest extent possible, though often there will be unknown data and information. When considering unknown data and information, it is imperative to keep in mind that there are two types. There are known unknowns, i.e., those where one has the questions or desire the data or information, but it is not available; and unknown unknowns, i.e., those where one has not conceived of the need for the data or information and so cannot seek it out.

External Environmental Scan

The external environmental scan consists of all of the forces outside of the organization or organizational unit. These external forces might include state, federal, and international governmental policies and regulations, societal and cultural values, technological advances, competitors, and stakeholders, among others. For the clinical and health IT units in the United States (U.S.), the external federal governmental policies and regulations would include the current payment regulations, such as the Merit-based Incentive Payment System (MIPS). The goal of this policy is to transition payment for physician services from a volume-based system to a value-based system that incorporates the use of electronic clinical quality measures (eCQMs). For the clinical and health IT units, this transition will require altered data collection and data processing procedures, as well as vastly different data reporting to track performance. Each of these external forces needs to be examined carefully to determine the current and expected future impact.

Internal Environmental Scan

The internal environmental scan consists of all of the forces internal to the organization or organizational unit. The internal forces might include the personnel, financial constraints, technology (either installed or desired), policies and procedures, company culture, etc. For example, in the clinical or health IT unit, the assessment of personnel is extremely important and must be objective. For example, many health care organizations, especially those of any size, would be remiss if they did not employ a certified Chief Information Security Officer (CISO). Other forces such as policies and procedures need to be assessed as they currently exist, not as they are wished to be in the future.

Synthesizing the Environmental Scan

Once the environmental scan is completed and the relevant data and information collected, it is vital to the strategic management process to synthesize the data and information so it can be used

Strengths	Weaknesses
Opportunities	Threats

Fig. 33.1 SWOT Template

for the planning process. A commonly used method for this is to produce a SWOT analysis—Strengths, Weaknesses, Opportunities, and Threats. See Fig. 33.1 for the SWOT template. Those involved in synthesizing the environmental scan will take the data and information collected and insert it in the appropriate block representing the anticipated meaning for the organizational unit. Sometimes, the same item will be included in more than one of the blocks. For example, perhaps the clinical or health IT unit has many employees who have worked in the area for more than a decade. This can be considered a strength for employee loyalty and a strong work culture. At the same time, this might be considered a threat—how can the unit ensure its operations remain current? Thus, every item must be discussed and considered carefully from every perspective.

Vision Statement

Organizations usually initiate their strategic plan by determining their vision for the organization. **Vision statements** are usually very broad and set forth the long-term goal the organization would like to achieve. It can also be thought of as what sets the organization apart or makes it unique. As an example, the vision statement for Southwest Airlines is "To be the world's most loved, most efficient, and most profitable airline." [4] One way to think of a vision is a **stretch goal**—something that is aspired to and something that might even be difficult to measure. How can Southwest ever determine whether or not they are "the world's most loved airline?" The reality is that they probably cannot. There is always likely to be an airline that might contest this claim or stretch goal.

The University of Texas MD Anderson Cancer Center (UT-MDA) vision statement is "We shall be the premier cancer center in the world, based on the excellence of our people, our research-driven patient care and our science. We are Making Cancer History." [5] UT-MDA has taken the last three words of their vision statement and turned into a powerful marketing slogan "Making ~~Cancer~~ History." It can be interpreted two ways. First, their research and treatment advances are making history and, second, they are working to eliminate cancer as an illness, signified by crossing through the word cancer. Similar to Southwest, the second interpretation is a bold stretch goal. While it may be reached at some point, that point is likely far into the future.

While Southwest Airlines and UT-MDA are nationally, even internationally, known and have admirable vision statements, health and clinical IT units should also develop a vision statement. As stated previously, the vision statement of any organizational unit should support the vision statement of the larger organization. Thus, organizational units are bound by the vision statement of the organization, so they may not be free to be as bold as the organization in their proclamations.

Mission Statement

Organizations also need to develop a **mission statement**. A mission statement starts from the vision statement and begins to outline the aims and values that are most important to an organization, as well as describing the organization's purpose. Sometimes, one will see the vision and mission statement combined into a single mission statement. The mission statement of Southwest Airlines is "dedication to the highest quality of customer service delivered with a sense of warmth, friendliness, individual pride, and company spirit." [6] They are specifying customer service and how it will be delivered (warmth, friendliness, etc.).

The mission statement of UT-MDA is "to eliminate cancer in Texas, the nation, and the world through outstanding programs that integrate patient care, research and prevention, and through education for undergraduate and graduate students, trainees, professionals, employees and the public." [5] In this mission statement, UT-MDA has continued their theme of eradicating cancer, only now specifying integrated, outstanding programs. Additionally, they have included their educational mission and listed all of the impacted stakeholders.

For clinical and health IT units, the question becomes how does your mission statement support the mission statement of the organization?

Creating and Implementing an Information Strategy

Once the vision statement and/or mission statement are complete, it is important to develop a **strategy** for achieving the mission and vision. The strategy may include specific actions, such as budgeting, personnel actions, technology acquisition, policy changes, or, in summary, any activities that can help the organization or organizational unit to achieve its goals. The SWOT analysis can be of enormous assistance in creating the information strategy. Those items that are weaknesses or threats will need some type of monitoring or mitigation plan developed. It is not always possible to take steps to directly address weaknesses or threats as they may not be in control of the organizational unit, so sometimes, the best that can be accomplished is monitoring.

Stakeholders

The information strategy will, of necessity, involve multiple **stakeholders**. These stakeholders will be both within the organizational unit, as well as external to the organizational unit. For clinical and health IT units, external stakeholders are expected to include senior management such as the Chief Financial Officer (CFO), Chief Executive Officer (CEO), Chief Nursing Officer (CNO), as well as others such as physicians, pharmacists, patients, patient family members, vendors, and anyone else who interacts with the information systems.

Getting the input from these stakeholders can be accomplished in a variety of ways. Surveys, where questionnaires are distributed across the organization, are useful to a point. However, other methods, such as focus groups or interviews, while not involving all stakeholders, can be used to capture the needs of a representative sample. If workgroups or task forces are established for specific projects, it is a best practice to include a wide range of stakeholders, from housekeeping and front-line clerical staff to the highest levels. Never forget that data entered by the front-line staff feed the reports and decision-making dashboards utilized by senior management.

Objectives

It is impossible to address all needs at one time, so it is important to outline the information strategy **objectives**. Determining the objectives usually requires revisiting the environmental scan and SWOT analysis. Obviously, the objectives should be aligned with any larger organizational objectives, but there should also be objectives specifically designed to focus on the identified weaknesses and threats. Additionally, an organizational unit may want to develop objectives targeting the maintenance of strengths and taking advantage of the opportunities as well. Finally, each objective should have an identified owner, that is, someone who is responsible for monitoring the achievement of the objective. Without accountability, objectives can "fall off the radar," and enjoy little progress.

Once the list of objectives is complete, they must be prioritized, as it is impossible to address all identified objectives at the same time. Available resources, including money and staff time, will always be a constraint. Oftentimes, prioritization may require a risk-benefit analysis of each of the objectives. What is the risk to the organizational unit if the objective is or is not addressed? For example, perhaps the clinical and health IT unit is receiving a growing number of requests to implement decision support software developed using machine learning techniques, yet they have no one on staff with machine learning expertise. Trying to implement new software tools without appropriate expertise could present a significant risk in terms of patient safety and/or provider satisfaction. At the same time, failure to stay current could also present risks if the organization were to become less competitive. Thus, it is important to perform a careful risk-benefit analysis of each objective.

Targets

Once the list of near-term objectives has been decided, **targets** must be established. These are goals and aims that can assist in achieving the objectives, often in a step-wise fashion. For example, if the objective for the clinical and health IT unit is provider satisfaction with services, the unit may set a target of 95% provider satisfaction. However, it is unlikely that 95% will be accomplished immediately. If a target is met from the beginning, it is likely that it can be considered too easy. Reasonable targets should require additional work on behalf of the organizational unit.

Critical Success Factors

Concomitant with the targets are **critical success factors**. Critical success factors are methodologies, management tools, or design techniques that can be used to achieve the targets [1]. For example, when assessing provider satisfaction, it is easy to state that providers tend to be diverse and very subjective, so this is impossible. However, provider satisfaction is important to smooth operations in a health care environment. Therefore, it is important to search for organiza-

tions that have undertaken similar initiatives and evaluate the methodologies, management tools or design techniques. The American Medical Association (AMA) and the RAND Corporation, a national professional association, and an American non-profit global policy think tank and research organization, conducted a literature review and survey that recommended the following for increasing provider satisfaction: (1) Clerical duties should be performed by support staff; (2) Providers should have more authority over their daily schedules; (3) Increase opportunities for interaction with other providers; and (4) Implementing new models for change management, due to a continued need for change [7]. Existing methods, tools, or techniques may not be found depending upon the objective and target; however, one should never try to develop that which is already in existence, especially if it has data proving it to be successful.

Measures

Measures will also be needed for each target. Perhaps it is important to the clinical and health IT unit to have provider satisfaction at 95 percent. This is a great target and would demonstrate significant approval of the operations in question. However, there is also the question of how provider satisfaction is measured. The clinical and health IT unit could develop its own survey, focus group, or interview questions. However, the validity and reliability of the measures are extremely important to (1) be assured that provider satisfaction and not some other construct is being measured; and (2) be certain that the trends over time are consistent. Validity means that one is measuring what one intends to measure, while reliability means that consistent results are obtained under the same conditions. Both must be present for any measures used.

Tasks or Tactics

Tasks, or tactics, must be established to achieve each target. The necessary tasks and tactics may be dependent upon the critical success factors chosen. Now, the person or persons charged with monitoring the objective should determine which tasks are necessary, as well as decide how the tasks associated with meeting the objectives will be carried out and in what order. This is where the strategic planning can sometimes falter. It is all well and good to have an audacious vision and a mission statement, to set objectives and so on, but now the work has to be done. Some tasks may be short term, in that they may only take a week or two to complete, while some may take a year or more.

It is vital to be as complete as possible when specifying the tasks to be accomplished. If essential tasks are left out, not only will it be impossible to meet the stated objectives, it may be discovered that important necessary resources are not available.

Impact/Evaluation

Finally, as the tasks are accomplished, measurements taken, data collected and reported, ongoing evaluation must occur to determine the impact of the strategic plan. Questions to answer in order to craft the evaluation include:

1. What will the timeframe for evaluation be? Weekly, monthly, bi-monthly, quarterly, annually? It could be some combination of all of these depending upon the measures chosen.
2. How often will we revisit the tasks and measures? This is important because failure to meet targets in a given area may be because the wrong measure is being used or the tasks proposed are irrelevant and cannot accomplish what was originally intended.

Evaluating Strategy

At least annually, the organization or organizational unit should undertake an evaluation of the strategy process. This process involves several steps, beginning with assessing the progress made toward achieving the vision. Just because the vision has not been achieved does not mean the vision should be revised. Remember, the vision is a long term, stretch goal that should not be expected to be met in a year. However, if movement has been in the opposite direction, or no progress at all has been made, the vision might need to be re-examined.

The next step should be an assessment of progress made on the objectives that were previously set. Hopefully, some objectives have been met, while partial progress has been made on others. At this time, it might be wise to revisit the environmental scan (Has anything changed?); the SWOT analysis (Again, did something internally or externally change?); and the risk-benefit analyses (Again, has something changed that alters the prioritization?).

Once this is finished, the objectives can be reviewed to determine whether there is a need to revise the list of objectives. For example, the objectives that have been met may be moved from active improvement to maintenance, while others that were prioritized lower can now move onto the list. This review of the objectives should also consider the resources and tasks needed to accomplish any incomplete objectives. It should be determined whether the objectives can still be accomplished or obstacles have been identified making the objective impossible to achieve.

For all objectives, including those that remain incomplete, the process of establishing targets, identifying critical success factors and measures, as well as setting out the necessary tasks begins again. Some may be able to be reused from the previous plan; however, that should not be taken for granted, especially since these items may have been the reason the incomplete objectives were not met in the first place.

Case Study

"Alignment of the Clinical Information Section Strategy with Organizational Strategy."

Background

Susan Martin, MBA, is the enterprise-wide Clinical Informatics Director for an integrated health care delivery system, known here as OneCareSystem (OCS), with 53 hospitals and 212 clinics covering a substantial portion of the southwestern U.S.. Susan reports to the Chief Medical Informatics Officer (CMIO), who directs the Clinical Informatics section and reports to the Chief Information Officer (CIO). In this role, Susan is responsible for all data collection that touches the clinical providers, ensuring that it is integrated into both the Electronic Health Record (her) system and their workflow. She is also tasked with ensuring that all applicable enterprise policies are congruent with federal and state regulations and do not contradict existing enterprise policies.

As the Clinical Informatics Director, Susan has to collaborate with other enterprise directors. For example, clinical data collection is very important for all quality improvement efforts, as well as reporting for national initiatives such as Medicare and state programs, such as Medicaid and public health reporting. In addition, OCS is also exploring using the EHR to recruit subjects for various research studies, including clinical trials.

OneCareSystem

OneCareSystem has grown substantially in the past few years, primarily via the acquisition of hospitals and physician practices. In the most recent reporting year, the 53 hospitals and 212 clinics at OCS reported a total of 175,102 discharges and 5,973,634 ambulatory care visits. This vision statement of OCS is "Helping you to stay healthy." The mission statement is "OCS provides the best diagnostics and care available so our clients remain healthy and regain their health (if needed)."

The core values at OCS are:

C—Care (for Customers and Colleagues)
A—Attention (in All Aspects)
R—Respect (Regardless of the Situation)
E—Enthusiasm (Enjoyment of the Job)

Clinical Informatics Section

The Clinical Informatics Section (CIS) at OCS elected not to develop a vision statement; however, they have adopted a mission statement of "CIS ensures that OCS clinicians and clients have the data and information they require to ensure clients remain healthy and regain their health (if needed)."

CIS adopted the mission statement and core values of OCS. CIS has developed guidance for the CIS workforce to ensure that everyone understands how to apply the values in their day-to-day operations. For C—Care, CIS has specified the usual customers as the persons who are treated by OCS, but they also include everyone who interacts with the clinical information system, i.e., physicians, nurses, pharmacists, etc., as their customers. Colleagues include the many different sections within the Office of Information Technology (IT), as well as others, such as the Business Office and Quality Improvement. For A—Attention, CIS stated that attention to detail, such as when programming is important, but that it is equally important to pay attention to the details of how customers and colleagues interact with the different systems to ensure their experience is as good as it can be. For R—Respect, CIS is clear that this often means respectful interactions in situations when customers or colleagues may be very frustrated with technology that is not working as expected or is not working at all. To assist, all personnel have received customer service training. For E—Enthusiasm, CIS tries to include activities and communications that can bring a sense of engagement and enjoyment to the job. For example, they celebrate "wins," such as when an implementation or upgrade is successful, as well as sharing "testimonials" when positive comments are received about great service.

Currently, the clinical data collection, aggregation, and integration efforts at OCS have been internally focused. They have been very successful as measured by the current critical success factors of system up-time, availability of backup if needed, degree of clinical system integration, average response time, projects completed on-time and within budget, as well as provider satisfaction, among others. Any data collected via the myriad systems, such as the laboratory information system, the pharmacy information system, and so forth, are aggregated into the EHR and made available to clinicians for clinical decision-making. In addition, CIS has created a clinical data warehouse that can be used by clinicians and data scientists to perform analytics for developing dashboards and predictive algorithms to improve patient care. Efforts to integrate data within the organization have been very successful. Those integrating data from other health care organizations have been limited to the data interoperability requirements specified by the Centers for Medicare and Medicaid Services (CMS) and the Office of the National Coordinator for Health Information Technology (ONC).

Change

The OCS Board of Directors and executives recently met in a planning session to determine future directions for OCS. They reaffirmed the vision, mission, and core values; however, they believe that the future of health care is changing drastically. Specifically, they want to see OCS shift from the current focus on delivering in-person care to more delivery via virtual methods and the use of patient-generated data for population health management. This shift in focus is consistent with the stated mission and vision.

Susan has been tasked with leading the CIS work to ensure that their activities and initiatives are supportive of the new direction.

Discussion

This change has profound implications for the personnel and operations in CIS. However, Susan first needs to ensure all efforts are synchronized and moving the organization in the same direction. Consider yourself to be in Susan's position and undertake the following activities.

Activities

1. Perform a SWOT analysis for CIS given the new direction outlined by the OCS Board and executives. Include an approach for performing the SWOT analysis.
2. Make any necessary changes to the mission statement or the core values as implemented by CIS.

3. Determine whether the stakeholders for CIS have changed.
4. Identify three objectives for CIS that are related to the new direction of OCS. Explain why each goal is important to advancing the direction established by the OCS Board and executives.
5. Establish targets and critical success factors for each objective.
6. Compile a list of measures that can be used for each target or critical success factor. Be sure to include the methods by which the data will be collected, as well as whether or not any reliability and validity testing of the measures is needed.
7. Create an evaluation plan that includes the evaluation timeframe, along with the planned review of the tasks and measures.

Summary

Clinical information and related organizational units should have their own strategies guiding their day-to-day operations. This can sometimes be difficult if the larger organization changes its strategic direction without warning or new regulations are promulgated by the government. However, at the same time, having a strategic plan with measures and an evaluation plan can also be used to inform future decisions.

Conclusions and Outlook

Clinical informaticists and related professionals are responsible for the lifeblood of the modern health care organization, the data and information. It is more important than ever that the strategy and hence, the operations, of these units are prepared to support the strategic direction of the larger organization. Following the recommendations in this chapter increases the likelihood that improved care will continue to be delivered, and the leaders of a given organizational unit and the executives or board of directors will have the data and information they need for decision-making.

The future for clinical informaticists has never been better. However, there is a saying "What got you here, won't get you there." [8] Essentially, this means all of the skills that led one to be promoted to a leadership position will not necessarily be sufficient for success as a leader. Understanding the need to be strategic and ensuring operations support the strategy are essential for clinical information professionals.

Useful Resources
Gartner Strategy Template

Review Questions

1. The type of management need for execution of day-to-day operations is:
   (a) Tactical.
   (b) Executive.
   (c) Strategic.
   (d) Business.
2. The clinical informatics section at ABC Hospital decided that they need to create a strategic plan for their organizational unit. As they read about strategic planning, they decided that they need to understand the internal and external forces that might impact their plan. They undertook a(n):
   (a) Literature review.
   (b) Environmental scan.
   (c) Organizational scan.
   (d) Departmental review.
3. There are many types of goals and objectives included in a strategic plan. A goal that is aspired to, but may never be reached is known as a(n):
   (a) Target goal.
   (b) Operational goal.
   (c) Stretch goal.
   (d) Strategic goal.
4. The clinical information system unit has developed a list of objectives based on alignment with larger organizational objectives, as well as the environmental scan and SWOT analysis. The next step in the process is to:
   (a) Determine the measures.
   (b) Establish the critical success factors.
   (c) Get input from stakeholders.
   (d) Assign an owner for each objective.

5. The clinical information system unit is trying to develop measures to determine whether or not objectives are being met. When examining measures for various objectives, it is important to make sure the measures are assessing exactly what is intended. This is known as:
   (a) Validity.
   (b) Reliability.
   (c) Consistency.
   (d) Exactness.

Appendix: Answers to Review Questions

1. The type of management need for execution of day-to-day operations is:
   (a) Tactical.
   (b) Executive.
   (c) Strategic.
   (d) Business.

The correct answer is a—tactical management. Tactical management is used for achieving day-to-day goals. It is not strategic management as that type of management is a plan or methods that are more long-term and support the organizational strategic plan.

2. The clinical informatics section at ABC Hospital decided that they need to create a strategic plan for their organizational unit. As they read about strategic planning, they decided that they need to understand the internal and external forces that might impact their plan. They undertook a(n):
   (a) Literature review.
   (b) Environmental scan.
   (c) Organizational scan.
   (d) Departmental review.

The correct answer is b—environmental scan. The environment in which an organization operates and carries out a strategic plan is comprised of internal and external forces.

3. There are many types of goals and objectives included in a strategic plan. A goal that is aspired to, but may never be reached is known as a(n):
   (a) Target goal.
   (b) Operational goal.
   (c) Stretch goal.
   (d) Strategic goal.

The correct answer is c—stretch goal. A goal that may never be reached is a stretch goal because it usually requires entities (persons, organizational units, and so on) to stretch themselves outside of what they are currently achieving.

4. The clinical information system unit has developed a list of objectives based on alignment with larger organizational objectives, as well as the environmental scan and SWOT analysis. The next step in the process is to:
   (a) Determine the measures.
   (b) Establish the critical success factors.
   (c) Get input from stakeholders.
   (d) Assign an owner for each objective.

The correct answer is d—assign an owner for each objective. Assigning an owner for the objective will help ensure accountability and responsibility. Without an owner, objectives may not be addressed because there is confusion about who is in charge of achieving the objective.

5. The clinical information system unit is trying to develop measures to determine whether or not objectives are being met. When examining measures for various objectives, it is important to make sure the measures are assessing exactly what is intended. This is known as:
   (a) Validity.
   (b) Reliability.
   (c) Consistency.
   (d) Exactness.

The correct answer is a—validity. Validity is when a measure is assessing the concepts or other items intended. This is especially important with satisfaction surveys and similar assessment instruments.

Other questions that could be included are:

• Ranking the steps of the strategic management process in the correct order.
• Matching the different terms to the correct definition.

References

1. Gartner Glossary. Csf (critical Success Factor) [Internet]. Gartner. [cited 2020 May 7]. Available from: https://www.gartner.com/en/information-technology/glossary/csf-critical-success-factor
2. Mission Statement | Meaning of Mission Statement by Lexico [Internet]. Lexico Dictionaries | English. [cited 2020 May 7]. Available from: https://www.lexico.com/definition/mission_statement
3. Definition of OBJECTIVE [Internet]. [cited 2020 May 7]. Available from: https://www.merriam-webster.com/dictionary/objective
4. Purpose, Vision, and The Southwest Way [Internet]. [cited 2020 May 9]. Available from: http://investors.southwest.com/our-company/purpose-vision-and-the-southwest-way
5. About MD Anderson [Internet]. MD Anderson Cancer Center. [cited 2020 May 9]. Available from: https://www.mdanderson.org/about-md-anderson.html
6. About Southwest - Southwest Airlines [Internet]. [cited 2020 May 9]. Available from: https://www.southwest.com/html/about-southwest/index.html
7. Beckers Hospital Review. 4 ways to improve physician satisfaction, practice sustainability [Internet]. [cited 2020 May 10]. Available from: https://www.beckershospitalreview.com/hospital-physician-relationships/4-ways-to-improve-physician-satisfaction-practice-sustainability.html
8. What Got You Here Won't Get You There Quotes by Marshall Goldsmith [Internet]. [cited 2020 Jul 26]. Available from: https://www.goodreads.com/work/quotes/81594-what-got-you-here-won-t-get-you-there-how-successful-people-become-even

Interprofessional Leadership: Innovative Strategies

34

Michelle Troseth and Tracy Christopherson

Learning Objectives
- Define entrepreneurship and intrapreneurship within the context of interprofessional collaborative practice (IPCP) and health information technology (HIT).
- Identify how a polarity mindset supports IPCP entrepreneurship and intrapreneurship.
- Explain the principles of Polarity Thinking™.
- Explain how an interprofessional governance infrastructure supports IPCP, intentional designed HIT, and interprofessional usability.
- Describe the risks of not applying a polarity mindset and leveraging a governance infrastructure.
- Explore the nature of accountability in relationship to interprofessional leadership, HIT implementation, and ongoing evaluation of effectiveness.
- Describe how managing change with a polarity lens can minimize resistance and invite stakeholder engagement.

Key Terms
- Interprofessional Collaborative Practice (IPCP)
- Health Information Technology (HIT)
- Entrepreneurship
- Intrapreneurship

M. Troseth (✉) · T. Christopherson
MissingLogic®, Hudsonville, USA
e-mail: michelle@missinglogic.com;
tracy@missinglogic.com

- Polarity Thinking™
- Polarity Map®
- Interprofessional Governance Infrastructure

Introduction

The past two decades have shown steady progress in implementing health information technology (HIT). Historically, HIT began with design components that were focused on one discipline or profession, more of what is referred to as a unidisciplinary design. For example, physician templates for progress notes or summary notes, as well as a focus on computerized physician order entry (CPOE). Later, as more clinicians embarked on transitioning from paper documentation to electronic documentation, electronic health records (EHRs) began to expand to have each profession documenting their tasks and services in various and separate locations within the EHR, more of what is referred to as a multidisciplinary approach. While EHR adoption has grown exponentially, having a standard design that invites and advances interprofessional collaborative practice (IPCP) has progressed much slower.

To provide context, there have been two major national initiatives that have served as catalysts to speed up the implementation of HIT. The first was in 2004, when former U.S. President George W. Bush established the Office of the National Coordinator of Health Information Technology

(ONC) and declared it the "Decade for Health Information Technology" calling for widespread adoption of interoperable EHRs within 10 years. Within 90 days Dr. David Brailer, the first appointed National Coordinator, completed a Framework for Strategic Action. The Framework was entitled "The Decade of Health Information Technology: Delivering Consumer-centric and Information-rich Healthcare" and included four goals critical to the former President's vision. These goals included: introduction of information tools into clinical practice, electronically connecting clinicians to other clinicians, using information tools to personalize care delivery, and advancing surveillance and reporting for population health improvement. The declaration by former President Bush and the framework drew attention to the need for a national digital health strategy and resulted in moderate progress in the implementation and optimization of EHRs during the next five years.

Another national initiative came in 2009 with the passing of the Health Information Technology for Economic and Clinical Health (HITECH) Act. The HITECH Act was created to stimulate the adoption of EHRs and supporting technology. The Act gave the ONC the authority to manage and set standards for the stimulus program. By 2017, 80% of providers and 96% of hospitals had adopted a federally certified EHR system [1]. Physicians and other health care providers point to the implementation, use, and regulation of HIT and the EHR as a key support tool for care delivery, but also acknowledge it can be a source of frustration. The rapid implementation of EHRs resulted in improvements in quality care and efficiency but has also been associated with negative consequences including increasing EHR-related clinician burden. This increase in clinician burden related to EHRs has been a contributor to burnout as recognized by the National Academy of Medicine's Action Collaborative on Clinician Well-Being and Resilience [2].

The initial effort to address clinician burden was when the twenty-first Century Cures Act (Cures Act) was signed into law in December of 2016. Part of the Cures Act required Health and Human Services (HHS) to articulate a plan of action to reduce regulatory and administrative burden relating to the use of HIT and EHRs. Specifically, the Cures Act directed HHS to: (1) establish a goal for burden reduction relating to the use of EHRs; (2) develop a strategy for meeting the goal; and (3) develop recommendations to meet the goal. After several stakeholder meetings were held jointly with ONC and Center for Medicare & Medicaid Services (CMS) with a wide variety of channels, such as face-to-face meetings, virtual stakeholder feedback sessions, etc., ONC released a draft report open for public comments, and eventually a final report in February of 2020: *Strategy on Reducing Regulatory and Administrative Burden Relating to the Use of Health IT and EHRs* [3].

The National Academies of Practice (NAP) was one of ONC's stakeholder groups providing input on EHRs, clinician burden, and the Cures Act. NAP is comprised of representatives from 14 different health professions and advocates for advancing interprofessional care in the U.S. Health System. In a letter to Dr. Donald Rucker, ONC National Coordinator for Health Information Technology, NAP addressed the need for EHRs to be intentionally designed to support interprofessional care delivery [4]. An interprofessional design enables clinicians to keep the patient at the center of care delivery and engaged in their care (consumer centric) with full contribution of each clinical discipline practicing and documenting care at their full scope of professional practice. The EHR design can move us toward more IPCP by enabling clinicians to coordinate and view the documentation of care delivery through an interprofessional lens. The final ONC report (February 2020) acknowledges that reducing clinician burden is beyond the discipline of medicine and must encompass multiple clinical disciplines' workflows and HIT needs. However, the lack of a true interprofessional EHR design has been impacted by the starts and stops of an interprofessional focus and approach to care delivery.

The value of working collaboratively across health professions has been recognized as an important and necessary strategy for improving the quality of healthcare. However, historically, health professionals have been trained independently within their health profession-specific training programs. The milestone Institute of Medicine (IOM) report, *Health Professions Education: A Bridge to Quality* in 2003 called for a core set of competencies to be shared across all professions and integrated into professional oversight processes. The five core competencies included (1) provide patient-centered care, (2) work in interdisciplinary teams, (3) employ evidence-based practice, (4) apply quality improvement, and (5) utilize informatics [5]. Captured in the report was recognition of the lack of standardized competencies for training health professions and an urgency to prepare the workforce for healthcare delivery in the twenty-first century. In reality, there have been several IOM reports and reports from other organizations such as the Josiah Macy Foundation that have advocated for interprofessional care for many years. For over 50 years, there has been an awareness that interprofessional collaborative care is essential to the consistent delivery of quality care and interprofessional education is a necessity for health profession students to prepare to work in collaborative teams. So, interprofessional education (IPE) and interprofessional collaborative practice (IPCP) are not new concepts. IPE, according to the World Health Organization (WHO), occurs when *students of two or more professions learn with, from, and about each other to enable effective collaboration and improve health outcomes.* IPCP occurs when *multiple healthcare workers from different professional backgrounds work together with patients, families, carers [caregivers], and communities to deliver the highest quality of care* [6].

A newer approach to advance IPE and IPCP is the interprofessional clinical learning environment (IP-CLE). In the fall of 2017, the National Collaborative for Improving the Clinical Learning Environment (NCICLE) held a national symposium to better understand the issues related to enhancing the IP-CLE. IP-CLE is defined as the hospitals, medical centers, and other clinical settings in which new clinicians train [7]. The symposium proceedings acknowledge there is a gap between what is taught through IPE in the academic setting and what is experienced in the clinical setting. In addition, the values taught during IPE are often lost or missing once new clinicians leave the classroom and enter the clinical environment. The proceedings indicate health care leaders need to take a close look at the clinical settings in which clinicians are learning while delivering patient care and consider how existing cultures, structures, and processes can support or hinder interprofessional learning and collaborative practice. Noted in the proceedings were limitations to both the macro-environment (health systems) and meso-environment (hospitals/health clinics) discussions because there were few representatives from executive leadership roles of healthcare organizations (practice stakeholders) at the symposium. Establishing models of distributed leadership was one micro-environment recommendation captured in the proceedings. Distributive leadership invites the voices and work of leadership closer to the frontlines rather than only traditional top-down leadership. We will explore interprofessional governance infrastructures later in this chapter that better demonstrates a shared leadership or partnership infrastructure to understand and advance IPCP. The proceedings concluded with a call for leadership at the macro-, meso-, and micro-environments to take deliberative action steps to optimize IP-CLEs across the country.

The TIGER (Technology Informatics Guiding Education Reform) Initiative has provided great strides in blending the worlds of informatics and interprofessional competencies. Today TIGER's home is the HIMSS organization and it is officially referred to as the TIGER Interprofessional Community. TIGER was originally a grassroots organization of nurses that gathered after Dr. David Brailer convened the first National Health Information Technology Summit in Washington DC and launched the Strategy Framework mentioned earlier in the introduction [8]. A very important observation was made at this first ONC event. There was no mention of nurses who represent the largest section of the healthcare professional workforce. The TIGER Initiative was birthed in 2005 and conducted an invitational summit in 2006 from which a 10-year vision and 3-year action plan emerged. By 2012, the TIGER Initiative had grown and began to widen the participation by forming an Interdisciplinary and Community Engagement committee, recognizing that informatics competencies were applicable across all health professions [9]. By 2016, the TIGER Initiative had expanded its reach both internationally and interprofessionally in committee membership and by launching an international survey and framework of informatics competencies and recommendations across 21 countries [10]. The TIGER International Competency Synthesis Project birthed a framework of global informatics core competencies for all health professions.

To develop and implement HIT that supports IPCP and leads to sustainable outcomes requires innovation. Next, we will share examples of entrepreneurship and intrapreneurship that may stimulate innovative thinking and strategies for interprofessional leadership to lead the way.

Entrepreneurship and Intrapreneurship

Transformation of the healthcare system requires innovation at all levels. Limited financial resources can stimulate creativity and innovation among leaders and clinicians as they search for alternative approaches to meet organizational needs [11]. Patients and families may present with unique challenges and problems that also require clinicians to develop innovative solutions. Organizational challenges and patient and family circumstances provide opportunities for healthcare leaders and professionals to be entrepreneurial or intrapreneurial as they apply their creativity to solving challenges and developing innovative approaches. Health professionals or leaders who are entrepreneurial are self-employed and develop new products, services, or ventures. In contrast, those that are intrapreneurial are employed by an established organization or company and develop an innovative product, service, or venture of some type that has economic value [12].

Historically entrepreneurialism has not been a part of the curriculum for health professionals, but this is beginning to change. Doctoral programs in physical therapy are expanding the curriculum and offering students opportunities to

expand their learning in areas of entrepreneurialism and innovation [13]. Within pharmacy education programs, entrepreneurship has been identified as a key factor driving innovation in pharmacy practice and many schools are incorporating entrepreneurialism into the curriculum [14]. Also, in pharmacy education entrepreneurship has been accepted as an education domain and integrated into accreditation standards for pharmacy programs. In another example, an occupational therapy program expanded its curriculum to include entrepreneurial concepts and interprofessional collaboration by creating an interprofessional learning opportunity for both management students and occupational therapy students [15].

Healthcare organizations are also realizing the unique knowledge and expertise of the clinicians closest to the patient is an asset that can be leveraged to develop innovative solutions. In addition to the unique perspective, knowledge, and expertise entre- and intrapreneurial clinicians have additional characteristics including, self-confidence, courage, integrity, discipline, critical thinking, decision-making, and the ability to take risks and manage failure that support innovation. Some hospitals are developing investment arms and venture capital groups to invest in or be part owners of the intra- and entrepreneurial innovative solutions that are being developed by clinicians at the point of care to solve complex problems.

As mentioned previously, IPCP through IPE is one of the approaches being used to support healthcare transformation. The advancement of IPCP and IPE has required innovative thinking and problem-solving. Many of the IPE and IPCP innovations that are in place today began as grassroots endeavors in both the practice and academic settings. These IPE and IPCP initiatives have had varying degrees of success. It was the need to accelerate the advancement of IPE and IPCP nationally and to measure the outcomes of both that led to an innovative cooperative agreement between the United States Department of Health and Human Services, Health Resources and Services Administration (HRSA), University of Minnesota, and private foundations to establish the National Center for Interprofessional Practice and Education.

Other innovative and collaborative partnerships have been formed to advance IPCP and IPE including the Interprofessional Education Collaborative (IPEC), which is now comprised of 21 institution members representing associations of schools of health professions. IPEC developed and has disseminated IPCP core competencies. The Core Competencies for Interprofessional Collaborative Practice can be accessed at https://www.ipecollaborative.org/. The formation of this collaborative has led to the entrepreneurial development of the IPEC Institute and the Interprofessional Leadership Development Program. An intrapreneurial venture related to IPE is the Educating Health Professions in Interprofessional Care (EHPIC) at the University of Toronto. The EHPIC program rose out of the IPE program at the University of Toronto and now has an international reach serving many countries.

The Clinical Practice Model (CPM) established by Bonnie Wesorick, a nurse, is an example of intrapreneurialism in the practice setting. The CPM Framework was established within a larger tertiary hospital in the early 1980s and implementation of the framework expanded to over 450 hospitals across North America. The framework provided point of care clinicians with the tools, resources, and infrastructures to support IPCP and evidence-based practice through intentionally designed health information technology. What was initially an intrapreneurial effort became entrepreneurial when Wesorick established the Clinical Practice Model Resource Center (CPMRC).

When thinking about examples of HIT entrepreneurialism the most widely known example is the development of Epic Systems by founder Judy Faulkner. She developed the HIT system in her basement with one other individual and today more than 250 million patients have a health record in Epic.

Innovation is at the heart of intra- and entrepreneurialism. This innovation represents the desire of healthcare leaders and health professionals to solve a problem or fill a gap to move beyond current circumstances. When it comes to IPE and IPCP the innovations are related to how we work together, tools that support our collaboration and learning with, from, and about each other in new ways. When it comes to HIT, innovations are aimed at improving quality, efficiency, and the cost of healthcare.

The first step in innovation is to fully understand the challenge you face. What healthcare leaders and clinicians do not often recognize is that not every challenge, gap, or circumstance is a problem that can be solved. Some of these challenges are polarities. Polarities are interdependent pairs of values or points of view, that appear to be unrelated, opposite, or conflicting, (i.e., individual and team) but need each other over time to achieve a greater purpose or outcomes neither could achieve alone [16, 17]. Polarities are also known as dilemmas, paradoxes, dualities, tensions wicked problems, and interdependent pairs [18, 19]. The ability to differentiate between a problem and a polarity is a key skill for healthcare intrapreneurship and entrepreneurship because a polarity misdiagnosed as a problem leads to failure over time.

The Polarity Thinking™ Model

In his book, *Polarity Management: Identifying and Managing Unsolvable Problems*, Dr. Barry Johnson, an organizational design consultant, describes the Polarity Thinking™ Model which includes a set of principles and a diagrammatic or visual representation called a Polarity Map®. Bonnie Wesorick, a nurse and health care visionary, applied Polarity Thinking™ to the health care ecosystem. Her book *Polarity Thinking in Healthcare: The Missing Logic to Achieve Transformation* identifies and maps common health care polarities.

One way to differentiate between a problem and a polarity is to ask yourself the following questions: (1) Is the problem ongoing? (2) Is there an endpoint? (3) Is there a single solution? Below is a simple table to differentiate between a problem and a polarity. If the answer to these questions is yes, then you are dealing with a problem. If the difficulty has persisted over time, has no endpoint and the alternatives to choose from are interdependent then this is a polarity that needs to be managed or leveraged.

If a polarity is approached as if it is a problem, it is like only seeing half of a picture. The portion of the picture you see is accurate but incomplete, which leads to an incomplete solution or action strategy. Figure 34.1 illustrates this point.

What do you see when you look at this illustration? When individuals look at this illustration, they typically see two faces *or* a vase. Both the face and the vase exist within the illusion, but when looked at separately, they provide an incomplete picture. The perspective that the vase exists is correct, but not more correct than the perspective that the faces exist. Each view is accurate but incomplete. If you do not alternate

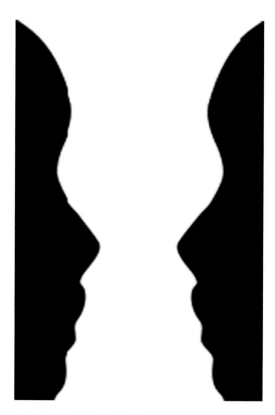

Fig. 34.1 Face and Vase Illusion developed by Danish Psychologist. Edgar Rubin (1886–1951)

your attention between both, you will fail to see the whole picture. The face and the vase represent an interdependent relationship; both are needed to complete the picture. If you take away the faces you will not see the vase and if you remove the vase you will not see the faces. If the illustration represented technology and practice, it is easy to see that attention to both is necessary to see the complete picture. If the current state of HIT is only examined from the perspective of technology, it is possible national leaders and those in healthcare organizations may only see and address half of the issue.

The Polarity Map® (Fig. 34.2 above) developed by Johnson makes all the elements of a polarity visible. The Polarity Map® is comprised of twelve basic components:

An interdependent pair: Placement of the names of each pole of the interdependent pair.

The infinity loop: The loop visualizes the natural tension/energy around each pole.

Greater purpose statement (GPS): A goal or outcome that neither pole can "reach" alone. It answers the question *Why leverage this polarity?*

Greater fear: The failure to achieve the greater purpose if action is not taken or is ineffective to support one or both poles.

Virtuous cycle: This arrow shows that tension/energy is moving toward the greatest purpose.

Vicious cycle: This arrow shows the tension/energy is moving toward the greater fear.

Upside quadrants (2): These spaces are reserved for the lists of positive/upside outcomes (one space for each pole).

Downside quadrants (2): These spaces are reserved for the lists of negative/downside outcomes (one space for each pole).

After identifying and mapping the components of the polarity, action steps can be established to achieve the positive outcomes of both poles. Early warning signs can also be identified to indicate when efforts have over-focused on one pole to the neglect of the other or to indicate ineffective action strategies. Being vigilant about monitoring and measuring

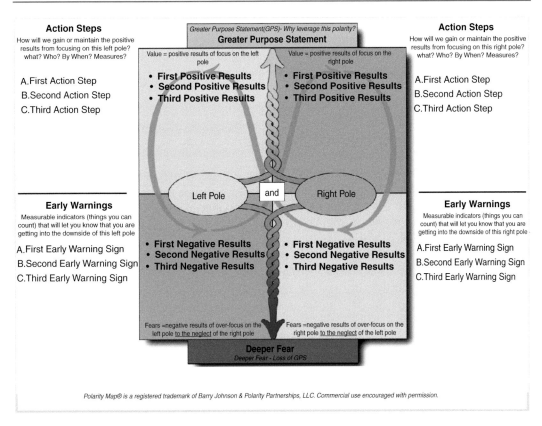

Fig. 34.2 The Polarity Map®

progress over time is an essential step to effectively leveraging a polarity to sustain the desired outcome. We will discuss this in more detail later in the chapter.

There are some basic principles that describe how polarities work. One of the most powerful facts about polarities is that they all work in the same way, which makes polarities predictable. The polarity principles include:

- Both poles of a polarity are equally important.
- Polarities never go away.
- Both poles must be strong to reach a greater purpose neither can achieve alone.
- Each pole has associated positive outcomes or an upside.
- Because the poles are interdependent, they have a potential downside.
- Polarities are unavoidable, unsolvable, indestructible, and unstoppable.

- There is 100% predictability that, over time, negative outcomes will be experienced if one pole is neglected.

Polarities can show up as unsustainable outcomes experienced as the same difficulty persisting over time. The reason IPE and IPCP have not been sustained, despite 50 years of attempts to have both be the status quo in healthcare for more efficient, effective, and integrated care, is because the approach has been to treat both IPE and IPCP as a problem to solve rather than a polarity to be managed. The Polarity Thinking™ Model and the Polarity Map ® provide an organized way to consider the interdependent relationship between IPE and IPCP (Wesorick, 2016, pg. 111–115). One organization that leveraged the Polarity Thinking™ Model to examine the interdependent relationship between IPE and IPCP with their constituency was the Association of Schools Advancing Health Professions (ASAHP).

ASAHP hosted a summit on Healthcare Workforce Readiness for Interprofessional Collaboration in July of 2018. The summit was planned by ASAHP's Leadership Development Program members in collaboration with the chapter authors and included an Institutional Review Board (IRB) approved study aimed to measure the interdependency between IPE and IPCP using the Polarity Thinking Assessment™ tool. The tool was designed to provide real-time metrics as reported by the participants that reflect the reality of each of the positive and negative outcome statements identified on the Polarity Map® [20]. The IPE-IPCP Polarity Map® content was developed based on a current literature review and validated by the AHAHP Leadership Development program members. As a result, the summit participants were able to visually see how they were experiencing both poles via mean scores and a visual infinity loop from the assessment data results. From the results, they were able to identify actions steps and early warning signs to support both IPE *and* IPCP to reach the greater purpose of efficient, effective, and integrated care. The summit outcomes were published as an 18-page summit report and in the Journal for Interprofessional Care [21, 22] and can be accessed at: http://www.asahp.org/summit.

The IPE and IPCP polarity map in the report shows each pole has an action step to implement structural support. One way to provide structural support for both poles is a partnership infrastructure, a type of interprofessional governance infrastructure, described in the next section. Developing a partnership infrastructure between academic and practice partners can bridge the gap between academia and practice to advance IPE and collaborative practice in pursuit of sustainable, efficient, effective, integrated care for patients, families, and communities. Practice settings that have interprofessional unit-based/department partnership infrastructure can more easily cultivate a safe environment where health professionals can come together to own their practice, deepen their understanding of IPCP and embrace students participating in the IP-CLE activities.

Interprofessional Governance Infrastructure

To advance and sustain IPCP in practice environments we recommend organizations create and sustain an interprofessional governance infrastructure. This infrastructure is one that invites shared interprofessional leadership and decision-making through a consistent structure, processes, and outcomes across an organization. A detailed charter supports the infrastructure with operational guidelines including roles and accountabilities, guiding principles, decision-making guidelines, and a visual representation of the unit/departments included within the interprofessional governance infrastructure. A consistent infrastructure helps to assure that multiple healthcare workers from different professional backgrounds "work together," but they also have the infrastructure to foster interprofessional collaboration, shared decision-making, role clarification, alignment with organizational priorities, and equal accountability to quality outcomes. The following represents interprofessional governance infrastructure best practices based on over 25 years of experience in assisting healthcare organizations committed to culture and clinical transformation implement interprofessional shared governance infrastructures referred to as partnership councils from this point on [23].

Unit/Department Based Interprofessional Partnership Councils

We recommend that councils be implemented at the unit or department level. Each unit/department council (i.e., intensive care, respiratory therapy, radiology, pediatrics, emergency care, etc.) should meet frequently and routinely (i.e., monthly). Each council is best supported by a chair and co-chair in a staff role and supported with strong partnerships with the management and professional development leaders. The make-up of the councils should "mirror" the unit/department with representation from all the different roles and enough representation to assure the voice of every member of the unit/department is heard and represented by the council members. The representation should also include all the health professions that practice in that area (i.e., physicians, nurses, dietitians, physical therapy, etc.). Council agenda items will vary and are a combination of items that represent or connect the organization goals/needs as a whole (global) to the goals/needs of the unit/department (local). Having a strong partnership council infrastructure at the unit/department level can help advance HIT and IPCP because the clinicians at the local level need to know how to accurately utilize the technology and own their professional practice as an individual discipline and an interprofessional team. Suggested areas of focus to advance HIT and IPCP are developing and using one patient story, one plan of care, interprofessional rounds, and leadership dyads and/or triads [24]. Together, strategic goals can be set and processes put in place for implementation and continued optimization of both HIT and IPCP with the greater goal of safe, efficient quality care.

Central Partnership Council

One of the greatest strengths of partnership councils as an organizational infrastructure is the powerful connection of all their work to the central partnership council. The centralized council meets once a month and membership consists of all the partnership council chairs/co-chairs throughout the organization/system. The purpose of the centralized partnership council is to continue and connect the work of unit/department level partnership councils to the global/organizational work and initiatives. The centralized partnership council also provides a way to communicate global learnings or changes back to each partnership council throughout the organization/system. The central council is typically led by two unit/department council chairs each representing different professions (i.e., a nurse and a physical therapist, a pharmacist, and an occupational therapist, etc.). The central partnership council is also the place where members from key organizational tracks are represented such as

operation/management, research, education/professional development, quality, and clinical informatics. An example of a leadership triad is at the organizational level executive sponsorship and partnership between practice, informatics, and quality with each track having representation at the central partnership council. Decisions to change or optimize the EHR can be coordinated through the interprofessional governance infrastructure to minimize fragmentation, redundancies, and added clinician burden to the documentation of professional services. The central partnership council provides a strong reminder and anchor to the *why* of HIT and IPCP.

Core Partnership Council Skills and Competencies

It has been our experience that providing common training and setting the intention to create a safe place to meet and deepen interprofessional practice and coordination of care can create a thriving healthy work environment. Teaching the essential skills of partnership and dialogue fosters new ways of thinking, being, and relating necessary to develop transformational interprofessional relationships that lead to sustainable outcomes. Having a common place to introduce, discuss and learn together the HIT and IPCP core competencies provides great momentum for an organization/system to advance technology and practice. A core leadership competency of the interprofessional governance leaders and members is Polarity Thinking™. Having a common understanding and "common language" to discern and make decisions based on knowing the difference between problems to be solved and polarities to be managed is a game changer. Understanding the underlying polarities at play in our work environments and culture is the root of understanding continuity and transformation that is supported by the principles and structure of the Polarity Thinking™ Model. Without a polarity mindset and lens, we continue to see initiatives come and go and yet still have the same issues arise over time. It also explains why leaders and health professionals experience unintentional consequences of over focusing efforts on one pole to the neglect of the other pole in an interdependent pair. Some of the key polarities members of the interprofessional governance infrastructure manage include hierarchical relationships and partnering relationships; individual and team; candor and diplomacy; individual competency and team competency; task and scope of practice; directive decision-making and shared decision-making; evidence-based care and autonomous care; and the technology platform and practice platform.

We think you will agree that these chronic tensions (polarities) are ones that healthcare leaders and interprofessional teams deal with on an ongoing basis. These are common crux polarities that are never going to go away and require monitoring over time for any course correction that might be necessary. We are going to close the chapter with a significant polarity that has touched everyone in the field of informatics and interprofessional practice, the *Technology Platform-Practice Platform Polarity* that was first identified by Wesorick (2013 [25], 2015 and 2016).

Wesorick framed the tension between technology and practice around the platforms that are necessary to scale and standardize both poles. Technology is not just widgets and practice is not just clinical documentation. A *technology platform* establishes and maintains technology for the digital delivery of care (think of the telephone standards where we can exponentially scale and connect over multiple devices). A *practice platform* establishes and maintains an infrastructure for the delivery of interprofessional professional practice. This calls for common evidence-based practice standards that can be scalable as well as a positive work culture to support the care experience between the practitioners and patients.

It is logical to understand why the rapid rollout of EHRs with the HITECH Act caused negative, unintended consequences such as clinician burden and in one statewide study by McBride, Tietz, Hanley, and Thomas in 2017, signs of dissonance or distress [26]. The frustrations and experiences are represented in the downside of the left pole (technology platform) due to the over-focus on technology during the rapid rollout of EHRs. The clinician burden and distress are also represented in the map as the loss of the valuable outcomes of having a strong practice platform. The benefits and value of implementing a technology platform to advance interprofessional and profession-specific practice was often not part of the mandatory preparation for technology implementations. The current call for shifting our focus to "optimizing the EHR" still lacks the understanding of the interdependency between the technology platform and practice platform amongst leaders accountable for HIT and professional practice. One nursing informatics article pointed out the constant "tug of war" between practice and technology [27]. The constant tug is representative of the underlying polarity of the technology platform and practice platform. The chapter authors had the opportunity to dig deeper into this polarity with the article author, Dr. Catherine Ivory, on Healthcare's MissingLogic Podcast. During our conversation, we identified some key action steps to support both technology *and* practice [28]. Having Polarity Thinking™ as a leadership competency would help healthcare leaders in informatics, practice, quality, and operations understand the need to *course correct* to strengthen the practice platform to minimize the negative consequences of technology and improve the positive outcomes of experiencing a strong practice platform on a large-scale.

Risks and Accountability

Now that you know what a polarity is and how polarities work, it is time to discuss how to leverage a polarity to achieve sustainable outcomes. When we say leverage the polarity, we are referring to leveraging the natural tension/energy that flows between the two poles. The first step in leveraging a polarity is to identify the polarity. The next step toward leveraging a polarity is to create a polarity map (Fig. 34.2), so you can visualize the polarity and the energy flow represented by the infinity loop. During this step, you are identifying the names of the neutral poles, the greater purpose or reason for leveraging the polarity and the deeper fear, and you also identify the positive outcomes for each pole as well as the negative consequences associated with each pole, as in Fig. 34.3 with the Technology Platform-Practice Platform Polarity.

Because polarities are not automatically leveraged; the next step is to identify and implement action steps to achieve the positive outcomes associated with each pole and keep both poles strong. Specific action steps are added to the right and left of the upper quadrants as shown in Fig. 34.3. The action steps are interventions that are necessary to consistently achieve the positive outcomes described in the upper quadrants of each pole. Remember the poles are interdependent, so the action steps must be implemented *simultaneously* to keep the energy/tension moving between the upsides of each pole in a virtuous cycle and avoiding the downsides. If one pole is

neglected, in other words, actions are not taken or are ineffective; it will result in the energy/tension moving downward into the lower quadrant and the experience of the negative consequences of the pole that is focused on. The action steps support the achievement of the greater purpose and minimize the experience of the negative outcomes of each pole.

Another essential step in leveraging polarities is to identify early warning signs for each pole. These warning signs specific to the polarity are located next to the downsides or lower quadrant of each pole, as in Figs. 34.3. The early warning signs are measurable indicators that there is an over-emphasis on one pole to the neglect of the other and the energy/tension is starting to shift into the downside. These early warning signs enable individuals or teams to course correct and take actions to strengthen the neglected pole before the energy/tension slips too far into the

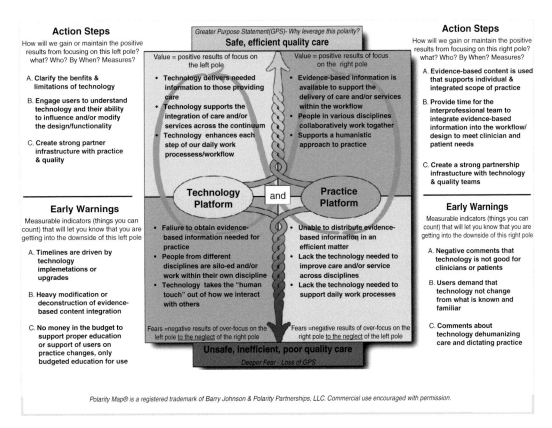

Fig. 34.3 The Technology Platform & Practice Platform Polarity Map®. Map adapted with permission from Wesorick (2016, p. 79)

downside of the pole they are focused on and a vicious cycle of negative consequences are experienced. Here it is important to emphasize the warning signs should be the very *earliest of indicators,* so that course correction can occur immediately, and the energy/tension can be pulled back up into a positive flow.

Interprofessional shared governance members are essential to the polarity mapping process and to identifying action steps and early warning signs. As an example, the members have a unique knowledge and perspective of the realities associated with interprofessional practice and the utilization of HIT. It is essential to have the voices and perspectives of all stakeholders represented in the process to have an accurate and complete picture and understanding of the current realities.

Leveraging a polarity is supported by the completed Polarity Map® in three ways. First, the completed Polarity Map® makes the polarity visible. Second, it organizes your wisdom about polarity and how to leverage it and helps you see the whole picture including the positive and negative consequences of leveraging polarity. Last, it provides you with a documented strategic plan for leveraging the polarity. The final step in leveraging a polarity is to *vigilantly* monitor the polarity *over time*. Polarities never go away, and things can change quickly in the environment, so what was an effective intervention previously may not be effective today. Therefore, you must assess for the presence of early warning signs and evaluate to what degree you are experiencing the positive outcomes of each pole on an ongoing basis. Evaluating the effectiveness of the action steps and making modifications (i.e., adding new interventions, modifying current interventions, eliminating ineffective interventions) is one way to keep the energy/tension between the poles flowing in a positive and virtuous cycle.

A final critical point to remember: Polarities are unstoppable. Polarities do not have an endpoint and therefore are always at work, meaning the energy/tension is always flowing, always moving, automatically. All polarities behave the same way. The outcomes are 100% predictable. When you can intentionally monitor the flow of the energy/tension and take the necessary actions to keep the energy flowing in a virtuous cycle you will achieve sustainable positive outcomes and a greater purpose. When you neglect to monitor the energy/tension and take the necessary simultaneous actions you will experience a vicious cycle of negative outcomes and not achieve your greater purpose but eventually experience your deepest fear.

Leveraging Polarities to Manage Resistance to Change

We would be remiss in this chapter if we did not address the role that polarities have in understanding resistance to change and the need to rethink traditional change management theories. As mentioned above, polarities are unstoppable and never go away. All change comes with resistance for a very good reason! Change is not a "problem" that gets fixed and goes away. Change is continuous and it is only evident because it is a part of an interdependent pair and the opposite value is stability. This polarity is often referred to as Stability *and* Change or Continuity *and* Transformation.

Individuals are resistant to change because they fear the loss of the positive outcomes of stability. Most change management strategies do not incorporate maintaining some stability at the same time. Think back to the face/vast picture in Fig. 34.1 earlier in the chapter and the key points made about only seeing half of the picture if we do not see the entire polarity. It is the same in this instance; if we only focus on change we are missing half of the picture.

Change management strategies are part of evidence-based practice changes, organizational infrastructure changes and HIT implementation/upgrade processes. Many change management strategies and implementation plans typically include some form of assessment and gap analysis, in which you determine "current state" and create a vision for the "future state" and lay out the strategy to bridge the gap. We refer to this as the "Going From and Going To" approach to change. This approach to implementing change represents a problem-solving approach to filling the gap. When the situation is a problem this approach is effective but when you are dealing with a polarity it results in failure or lack of sustainable outcomes because you are neglecting the opposite pole. When resistance is present it is a good indicator that the situation you are dealing with is a polarity. It is a call to listen to and evaluate the positive benefits or outcomes associated with what you are "moving away" from. Appreciating the "wisdom in resistance" can help guide action steps to preserve the positive outcomes associated with "current state" while getting the best out of a new and better "future state". The Stability *and* Change or Continuity *and* Transformation polarity is at play in many change efforts. It is important not to adopt a change management approach that over-focuses on change to the neglect of stability when the challenge or issue you face is a polarity. When operating from a Polarity Thinking™ perspective the "change management strategy" includes simultaneous or dual action steps that support the positive outcomes of both the current and future state.

A key strategy to leading change leveraging a polarity lens is to engage all key stakeholders, especially those that are resistant to the change. It is safe to assume that there will be wisdom in the resistance to change. Polarity Thinking™ principles also inform us that the fewer the resistant voices (the "stability or continuity" voices), the more important it is to listen to those stakeholders because they hold a perspective/knowledge that is critical to achieving the greater purpose or reason for managing the polarity. Only by listening closely to the voices and perspectives of all stakeholders represented do you develop an accurate and complete picture and understanding of the current realities. Another essential strategy is to have stakeholder input on the priority dual-action steps and early warning signs to keep what is good strong and what must be transformed accomplished. Lastly, it is important to remember polarities are unstoppable and have no endpoint, therefore the never-ending energy between Stability *and* Change/Continuity *and* Transformation must be leveraged. Having a core competency in Polarity Thinking™ and a com-

mon language amongst the stakeholders will expedite the change or transformation and with less effort.

Intrapreneur and Entrepreneur Case Study

This case study provides an exemplar of a visionary nurse intrapreneur and entrepreneur who has made significant contributions to advance interprofessional collaborative practice by leveraging health information technology.

Long before the Institute of Medicine's *Crossing the Quality Chasm* Report was published to improve the safety and quality of care in the USA and the Health Information and Technology for Economic and Clinical Health (HITECH) Act was established to accelerate electronic health record (EHR) adoption, one nurse leader was already acting on her vision to engage health professionals and healthcare organizations to co-create the best places to give and receive care.

Bonnie Wesorick, MSN, RN, DPNAP, FAAN began her intrapreneurial journey in 1983 after being challenged by one of her nursing students who had recently graduated. This previous student challenged Wesorick to recognize the wide gap between what nursing students were taught in nursing school and what was the reality in "real world" clinical practice settings. The new graduate threatened to quit the profession from exhaustion and disillusionment, exclaiming to Wesorick, *"you are living a lie!"* At that moment, Wesorick's purpose became clear. She left her role in academia and set out to change the realities in the healthcare setting and live a legacy.

Wesorick began her intrapreneurship at a large hospital in the Midwest of the U.S. in the role of Clinical Nurse Specialist (CNS) for Professional Practice. Wesorick demonstrated an intrapreneurial vision and spirit when she asked for volunteers to begin the work of establishing a nursing professional practice environment and forty volunteers showed up to the first meeting. When asked what her new work was to be called, she intuitively said, "the Clinical Practice Model" and the "CPM" was born. Sometime later, Wesorick invited other hospitals from across North America to join in a collective effort to co-create the best places to give and receive care using a common model to grow and learn together as a consortium. This collective of healthcare organizations became known as the CPM Consortium. As the CPM Consortium grew, Wesorick eventually formed the first nurse-hospital joint venture called the Clinical Practice Model Resource Center (CPMRC) at which time she became an entrepreneur.

The CPMRC and its consortium of rural, community, and academic healthcare settings worked diligently on strengthening the fundamental elements of an evolving professional practice framework. In the 1990s, the CPMRC led two fundamental advancements of the CPM: (1) expansion from a nursing practice model to a true interprofessional practice model and (2) transition from a standardized evidence-based paper documentation system to developing the first "pre-configured" evidence-based clinical documentation system via a unique clinical practice-technology partnership with technology vendors. Both efforts had a significant impact on healthcare delivery. Fundamental components of the advancements included extensive work in clarifying the scope of practice of multiple different health professions, translating evidence into meaningful clinical workflow, and establishing interprofessional partnership infrastructures.

Wesorick recognized there were no quick fixes to healthcare's many issues. In studying the patterns across the CPMRC consortium, Wesorick realized transformational work at the organization level was not only difficult but challenging to sustain over time. In 2001, the CPMRC established a partnership with Dr. Barry Johnson and Polarity Management Associates to begin the work of learning at a deep level how polarities could be applied to healthcare to achieve sustainable outcomes. Wesorick became the first Polarity Thinking™ Master, in healthcare. Johnson eventually created a web-based survey tool to provide real-time diagnostics of how polarities are managed over time. Wesorick was the primary developer and investigator on the research conducted

to test the reliability and validity of the CPM Polarity Assessment™ for Healthcare (CPAH). In 2016, she authored the book, *Polarity Thinking in Healthcare: The Missing Logic to Achieve Transformation.*

Wesorick's legacy and intrapreneurial and entrepreneurial spirit lives on at *The Bonnie Wesorick Center for Healthcare Transformation.* The center was created at Grand Valley State University, Allendale Michigan to honor and expand Wesorick's legacy work. The Center was created and is also the home of *The Interprofessional Institute for Polarity Thinking in Healthcare.*

Summary

The past two decades have seen an unprecedented focus on automating the healthcare system and an increased focus on improving the nature of interprofessional healthcare delivery. We have experienced enormous financial incentives from the federal government in the establishment of the ONC (2004) and later the HITECH Act (2009) that have resulted in rapid adoption of EHRs for providers and hospitals. While there have been improvements in quality care and efficiencies, there have also been negative unintended consequences. A primary complaint from providers is the increasing burden of documentation, billing, and coding for clinical care. This burden was called out in the Cures Act (2016) when congress required ONC to investigate the cause of clinical burden and to make recommendations for a strategy to reduce clinician burden when using HIT. The ONC Report (2020) *Strategy on Reducing Regulatory and Administrative Burden Relating to the Use of Health IT and EHRs* acknowledged the strategy is inclusive of all professions. An interprofessional approach to care is critical when leveraging HIT to decrease siloes of care, improve care coordination, and support the WHO's definitions of IPE and IPCP in a digital world.

To implement HIT to advance IPCP will require innovation. Innovation can come from entrepreneurship and intrapreneurship efforts and a polarity mindset. Several examples of entrepreneurship and intrapreneurship are given and why problems to solve must be differentiated from polarities to be leveraged for sustainability.

An introduction to the Polarity Thinking™ Model sets the context as to how the principles of polarities work and how the Polarity Map® helps to visualize the invisible energy that binds two poles together. The example of the IPE-IPCP Polarity Map demonstrates the "and/both" approach to manage IPE and IPCP at the local level. The Technology Platform-Practice Platform Polarity Map demonstrates why we have been experiencing the negative unintended consequences of the technology platform and provides insights into course correcting to strengthen the practice platform while not letting go of the focus on technology.

To leverage the HIT and IPCP advantage requires an interprofessional governance infrastructure that is consistent and focused on constantly improving the technology and practice platforms over time. Best practices for establishing an interprofessional partnership council infrastructure that includes both the local (unit/department) and global (central/organizational) levels were offered. Critical skillsets including competency in Polarity Thinking™ were shared along with the most common crux polarities that members of an interprofessional governance infrastructure measure and monitor. Finally, we explored how leaders can leverage polarities to manage risks and accountabilities. A Polarity Map® is a wisdom organizer offering an innovative strategy and approach interprofessional leaders can use to identify and manage crux tensions or polarities associated with advancing IPCP and the development and utilization of HIT across the interprofessional team.

Conclusions and Outlook

The implementation of electronic health records has been a heavy lift for the healthcare industry. National incentives have helped move the US health system to high technology adoption rates.

Much of the design of the technology and the incentives for adoption focused on problem solving, which has led to positive outcomes regarding adoption rates but poor clinician satisfaction and increased clinician burden associated with using the technology. Since care is not provided for by any one discipline, having technology designed to support interprofessional collaboration practice is of utmost importance for care coordination, burden reduction and patient safety. This requires interprofessional leaders, to be competent in Polarity Thinking™ in order to have the ability to accurately differentiate between problems to solve and polarities that must be leveraged within the context of IPCP and HIT. Adoption of a polarity mindset will then lead to identifying and vigilant monitoring of polarities over time by leveraging Polarity Maps® and Polarity Thinking Assessment™ tools to determine actions that lead to sustainable positive IPCP and HIT outcomes.

Useful Resources

1. *Polarity Thinking in Healthcare: The Missing Logic to Achieve Transformation* by Bonnie Wesorick.
2. Healthcare's MissingLogic Podcast is available on Apple Podcast, Spotify, and Stitcher.
3. MissingLogic, LLC YouTube Channel
4. Bonnie Wesorick Center for Health Care Transformation: https://www.gvsu.edu/wesorick/visionary-stories-26.htm

Review Questions

1. True or False: Intrapreneurial individuals develop or create innovative solutions, services, or products while being employed by an established organization.
2. True or False: It is important to have a polarity mindset as an entrepreneur or intrapreneur because without the ability to differentiate between a problem and a polarity you may develop a solution or service that will ultimately fail to solve the challenge it is intended to.
3. Which of the following are principles of Polarity Thinking™?

(a) Both poles of a polarity are equally important.
(b) Because the poles are interdependent they have a potential downside.
(c) Polarities are unavoidable, unsolvable, indestructable, and unstoppable.
(d) The tension associated with a polarity will eventually go away.
(e) a, b, c,
(f) All of the above.

4. True or False: An interprofessional governance infrastructure supports IPCP, intentional design of HIT, and interprofessional usability by providing consistent structures and processes to support shared interprofessional leadership and decision-making.

5. True or False: If you misdiagnose a polarity as a problem, you are 100% guaranteed to fail over time.

Appendix: Answers to Review Questions

1. True or False: Intrapreneurial individuals develop or create innovative solutions, services, or products while being employed by an established organization.

The answer is True. This is the definition of intrapreneur.

2. True or False: It is important to have a polarity mindset as an entrepreneur or intrapreneur because without the ability to differentiate between a problem and a polarity you may develop a solution or service that will ultimately fail to solve the challenge it is intended to.

The answer is True. When we approach a challenge as a problem we are looking for an independent alternative or solution to address the challenge and eliminate the consequences associated with the challenge. We choose alternative a or b and the problem is solved. If the challenge is not a problem, and instead is a polarity it cannot be solved because the alternatives used to address the challenge are interdependent and you need to apply both. You must choose both a and b to man-

age the challenge. Based on the principles of how all polarities work, applying only one alternative will lead to failure or negative consequences over time.

3. Which of the following are principles of Polarity Thinking™?
(a) Both poles of a polarity are equally important.
(b) Because the poles are interdependent they have a potential downside.
(c) Polarities are unavoidable, unsolvable, indestructable, and unstoppable.
(d) The tension associated with a polarity will eventually go away.
(e) a, b, c,
(f) All of the above.

These are the fundamental principles described previously in the chapter that apply to all polarities.

4. True or False: An interprofessional governance infrastructure supports IPCP, intentional design of HIT, and interprofessional usability by providing consistent structures and processes to support shared interprofessional leadership and decision-making.

The answer is True. In our 25 years of experience establishing and coaching others as they established interprofessional shared governance infrastructures we found those with the best results had a consistent structure, members, and processes that enabled meaningful conversation, relationship building across health professions and roles, and shared decision-making.

5. True or False: If you misdiagnose a polarity as a problem, you are 100% guaranteed to fail over time.

The answer is True This is a fundamental principle of how polarities work and how the energy flows between the two poles. To successfully manage or leverage a polarity you need to take simultaneous actions to support the positive outcomes of both poles. If one pole is neglected or the actions are ineffective it is guaranteed, 100%

of the time, you will experience the negative consequences of the pole that was over-emphasized.

References

1. ONC website: Dashboard Analytics. https://dashboard.healthit.gov/apps/health-information-technology-data-summaries.php?state=National&cat9=all+data&cat1=ehr+adoption#summary-data. (2017). Accessed 21 April 2020.
2. Ommaya AK, Cipriano PF, Hoyt DB, Horvath KA, Tang P, Paz HL, et al. Care-centered clinical documentation in the digital environment: Solutions to alleviate burnout. NAM Perspectives. Discussion Paper, National Academy of Medicine, Washington, DC. 2018. https://nam.edu/care-centered-clinical-documentation-digital-environment-solutions-alleviate-burnout
3. ONC website: Strategy on reducing regulatory and administrative burden relating to the use of health IT and EHRs. 2020. https://www.healthit.gov/topic/usability-and-provider-burden/strategy-reducing-burden-relating-use-health-it-and-ehrs Accessed 28 April 2020.
4. National Academies of Practice (NAP): https://www.napractice.org/comments Accessed 28 April 2020.
5. Institute of Medicine. Health Professions Education: A Bridge to Quality. Washington, DC: The National Academies Press; 2003. https://doi.org/10.17226/10681.
6. World Health Organization. Framework for action on interprofessional education & collaborative practice. 2010. https://www.who.int/hrh/resources/framework_action/en/ Accessed 28 April 2020.
7. National Collaborative for Improving the Clinical Learning Environment (NCICLE) Report: Achieving the Optimal Learning Interprofessional Clinical Learning Environment: Proceedings from an NCICLE Symposium. 2017. https://www.ncicle.org/documents Accessed 28 April 2020.
8. Troseth M. The TIGER initiative. In: Saba VK, McCormick KA, editors. Essentials of nursing informatics. New York: McGraw Hill; 2011. p. 633–40.
9. Schlak SE, Troseth MR. TIGER initiative: advancing health IT, Nursing Management. 2013;44:19–20.
10. Hübner U, Shaw T, Thye J, Egbert N, Marin H, Ball M. Towards an international framework for recommendations of core competencies in nursing and interprofessional informatics: the TIGER Competency Synthesis Project. Stud Health Technol Inform. 2016;228:655–9.
11. Darbyshire P, Downes M, Collins C, Dyer S. Moving from institutional dependence to entrepreneurialism. Creating and funding a collaborative research and practice development position. J Clin Nurs. 2005;14:926–34.
12. Parker, Simon C. (2009): Intrapreneurship or entrepreneurship?, IZA Discussion Papers, No. 4195, Institute for the Study of Labor (IZA), Bonn, http://nbn-resolving.de/urn:nbn:de:101:1-20090615104   doi:https://doi.org/10.1097/01.NUMA.0000424025.21411.be
13. Tepper DE (Ed.). March, 2020. Institutionalizing Inventiveness, *PTinMOTIONmag.org.*
14. Mattingly II TJ, Mullins CD, Melendez DR, Boyden K, & Eddington ND. A systematic review of entrepreneurship in pharmacy practice and education. Am J Pharm Educ 2019; 83. Article 7233.
15. Lachter LG, Szymanska I. Teaching entrepreneurship through interprofessional collaboration. Am J Occup Ther. August, 2016. https://doi.org/10.5014/ajot.2016.70S1-PO3066.
16. Johnson B. Polarity management: identifying and managing unsolvable problems. HRD Press. 1992;
17. Wesorick B. Polarity thinking in healthcare: the missing logic to achieve transformation. HRD Press. 2016;
18. Smith WK, Lewis MW. Toward a theory of paradox: a dynamic equilibrium model of organizing. Acad Manag Rev. 2011;36:381–403.
19. Johnson B. Reflections-a perspective on paradox and its application to modern management. J Appl Behav Sci. 2014;50:206–12.
20. Wesorick B, Shaha S. Guiding healthcare transformation: a next-generation diagnostic remediation tool for leveraging polarities. Nurs Outlook. 2015;63:671–702. https://doi.org/10.1016/j.outlook.2015.05.007.
21. ASAHP Summit Report on Healthcare Workforce Readiness for Interprofessional Collaborative Practice. 2018. http:/www.asahp.org/summit. Accessed 8 May 2020.
22. Adams EM, Breitbach AP, Dutton LL, Talbert PY, Christopherson T, Troseth MR, Butler AJ. Looking though a new lends, exploring the interdependent relationship between interprofessional education and collaborative practice with Polarity Thinking™. J Interprof Care. https://doi.org/10.1080/13561820.2019.1697218.
23. Wesorick B, Shiparski L, Troseth M, Wyngarden K. Partnership council field book: strategies and tools for co-creating a healthy workplace. Grand Rapids, MI: Practice Field Publishing; 1997.
24. Troseth M. Interprofessional collaboration through technology. Nurs Manag. August 2017;15–17.
25. Wesorick B. Essential steps for successful implementation of the EHR to achieve sustainable, safe, quality care. In EHealth Technologies and Improving Patient Safety: Exploring Organizational Factors. Ed by Mountzoglou A, Kastania A. PA: IGI Global; 2013.
26. McBride S, Tietz M, Hanley M, Thomas L. Statewide study to assess nurses' experiences with meaningful use-based electronic records. CIN – Computers, Informatics, Nursing 2017;35(1):18–28. https://doi.org/10.1097/CIN.0000000000000290.
27. Ivory C. The tug of war between practice and technology. Nurs Manag January 2019, 7–9.
28. Healthcare's Missing Logic Podcast Episode 29: The tension between technology and practice: Where we started, where we are now, and what's at risk without both/and choices. January 28, 2020. Missinglogic.com/new-podcast.

Disrupting Healthcare: Innovations in Information and Communications Technology

35

Beth L. Elias, Cory Stephens, and Jonathan Pitts

Learning Objectives: Please Share up to Five Here

Upon completion of this chapter the learner will be able to:

- Define the concept of disruptive innovation.
- Describe disruptive innovation in the context of healthcare.
- Examine examples of disruptive healthcare innovations being seen today.
- Compare current healthcare delivery models and innovative models.
- Summarize the drivers of disruptive healthcare information technology innovations.

Key Terms
- Disruptive innovation
- Value-based healthcare
- Wearable technology
- Smartphones and devices
- Healthcare business model

- Telehealth
- Healthcare consumers
- Information and communication technologies

Introduction

Healthcare in 2022 and beyond will continue to see a shift toward value-based care for consumers whose expectations are, in part, shaping and being shaped by disruptive innovations (DIs) in information and communication technologies (ICT) [1]. DIs, such as smartphones and the Medical Internet of Things (MIoT), are playing a large role in propelling us on this journey. Estimates show that 3.5 billion people, nearly half of the world's population, owned a smartphone in 2020 [2]. With their explosion of application (app) offerings and real-time communication features, smartphones are changing when and how consumers access a multitude of services. People can do their banking and their grocery shopping with a few simple taps on their phones, wherever and whenever they choose.

Additionally, wearable devices such as Fitbit and Apple Watch enable consumers to monitor their own health and wellness and share data with their healthcare professionals. As vendors respond to this increasing demand by developing a wider offering of wearables and medical apps, healthcare consumers will begin to see a new market that is increasingly oriented to their own

B. L. Elias (✉)
Panuska College of Professional Studies, University of Scranton, Scranton, PA, USA

C. Stephens
Clinical Center – Department of Clinical Research Informatics, National Institutes of Health, Bethesda, MD, USA

J. Pitts
Population Health Solutions, UNC Health Care, Chapel Hill, NC, USA

© Springer Nature Switzerland AG 2022
U. H. Hübner et al. (eds.), *Nursing Informatics*, Health Informatics,
https://doi.org/10.1007/978-3-030-91237-6_35

preferences and expectations. The services provided by healthcare organizations must also adapt to this shifting market and to the evolving demands of the consumers they serve.

In this chapter, we will examine who or what is driving disruptive ICT innovations in healthcare, and why healthcare across the world seems to be ripe for this type of disruption. We will also examine how disruptive ICT innovation is affecting healthcare and consumers. Finally, we will imagine how disruptive ICT innovation can carry us into the future.

Disruptive Innovation

DIs have occurred throughout human history, from the wheel to the development of personal computers in the 1980s. Released in 1984, the Apple Macintosh 128K was one of the very first portable personal computers, weighing in at over 16 pounds, and came equipped with its own carrying bag [3]. The seeds of the modern Internet were also sown in the 1960s, when U.S. Defense Advanced Research Projects Agency (DARPA) scientists developed packet switching communication networks, rather than the circuit switching communication networks used by telephones at that time [4].

These new network models would give us the modern Internet, replacing previous limited telephone-based computer-to-computer communication tools, such as File Transfer Protocol (FTP) and Unix-to-Unix Copy (UUCP). Ultimately, the Internet would foster disruptive replacements in our preferences for communicating, such as email over physical mail and texting over phone calls. With the evolution of cellular phones to smart mobile devices in the 2000s, the DI of convenient, portable, and perpetually accessible computing power was now in place. This rate of change in ICT would become rapid, and then explosive, leaving many existing products and business models behind.

With any DI, change can necessitate a thoughtful consideration for the pros, cons, and other surrounding issues, such as standardization. This can also highlight the need to be aware of ethical considerations, winners and losers, as well as the requirement for devices to be safe and reliable. This is evidenced today in the digital divide, which leaves those without resources, such as broadband Internet access, without access to this new world of Internet and smart device-based resources [5].

Defining Disruptive Innovation and Business Models

The term *disruption* can be defined as "a break or interruption in the normal course or continuation of an activity or process" [6]. The term *innovation* can be defined as "a new idea, method, or device" [7]. Taken together we can see the outline of the concept of DI, proposed by Clayton M. Christensen in 1997, which he described as a "process by which a product or service takes root initially in simple applications at the bottom of a market and then relentlessly moves up market, eventually displacing established competitors" [8].

The concept of DI was proposed by Christensen to explain market behaviors that were not previously well understood. As Christensen explained, DIs target dominant existing business models. Over time, the new business model behind the DI grows in popularity and pushes existing models aside, becoming the new dominant model. The disruption to the existing market and value network, therefore, becomes complete and a new market and value network are created. The device, tool, or process that were seen as the innovation, are in fact simply the means by which this business model change occurs. It is the new business model behind the innovation that is the actual disruption.

Christensen also explains that a DI can be identified by 4 key characteristics:

- They are low cost and highly accessible.
- They have lower gross margins than their contemporaries or the incumbent.
- They serve a smaller low-end target market at first, before expanding to a vast market due to their accessibility.

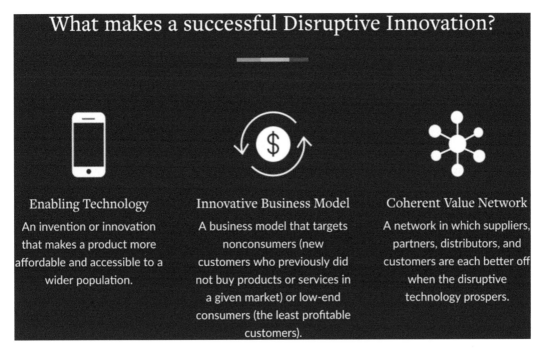

What makes a successful Disruptive Innovation?

Enabling Technology

An invention or innovation that makes a product more affordable and accessible to a wider population.

Innovative Business Model

A business model that targets nonconsumers (new customers who previously did not buy products or services in a given market) or low-end consumers (the least profitable customers).

Coherent Value Network

A network in which suppliers, partners, distributors, and customers are each better off when the disruptive technology prospers.

Fig. 35.1 Disruptive Innovation Business Model. Reproduced with the permission of Jason Hwang, MD

- They are difficult to see coming and is not taken seriously at first.

Current well-known examples of innovations that have been largely categorized as being disruptive include video downloads and streaming which replaced physical video rentals, online education which is overtaking attending a "brick-and-mortar" university, and smartphones and tablets, which have become a substitute for desktop personal computers. All of these DIs also play a part in healthcare consumer expectations. The DI process is illustrated in Fig. 35.1.

Positive vs Negative Impact

The effects of DIs can seem positive to some and negative to others. One can imagine that displaced market leaders may not feel that the responsible innovation is positive. Thus, every DI should be evaluated with an eye toward who or what it will impact positively and/or negatively. One example may be vendor apps for healthcare services like TelaDoc®(https://www.teladoc. com) and 98point6® (https://www.98point6. com), where healthcare consumers can have an affordable, nearly immediate consultation with a physician using their smartphone or other device, from wherever they are. Of course, these innovations can be seen as contributing to the digital divide for those who do not have access to high speed Internet or the necessary smartphone connectivity.

While these healthcare services are convenient and oriented to the healthcare consumer, local providers will lose the healthcare dollars they would have received from charging for an office visit and any associated testing or diagnostic services. One could also see how this sort of healthcare service could contribute to denying affordable access to healthcare services to those who may not be able to effectively use ICT devices or afford the associated data charges.

These seemingly positive and negative effects of DI are reflected in Joseph Strumpeter's concept of creative destruction in which he describes the free market in terms of how progress is both chaotic and unpredictable [9]. There are both winners and losers within this concept; some jobs are lost, others are created as the market lurches forward, toward what the consumer hopes is an increased availability of better products and services.

Stakeholders in the Disruptive Innovation of Healthcare

To apply Christenson's theory of DI in this age when data, information, and technology are becoming the currency of healthcare, it is important to understand the many faces of the healthcare community since they are at the heart of any business model. There are healthcare consumers who have been predominant in modern healthcare, and there are some types who have come to the forefront recently as a result of DI. As with many innovations, consumers are in fact stakeholders. The concept of a healthcare consumer is expanding to mean more than a user of a healthcare service or product.

In thinking about healthcare consumers, a patient often comes to mind first. Historically, patients seek information or a service and a fee is paid to consume that information or service. However, the way in which patients consume healthcare is changing thanks to DI. With smartphone apps and wearables, patients are increasingly turning to vendor provided care for health and wellness monitoring. They are also using it for preventive care, and treatment for minor ailments, often skipping a trip to the clinic altogether. Patients are now being linked directly to vendors as the consumers of new technologies created to support wellness and provide healthcare. When a patient chooses to seek care via an app or wearable, the vendor becomes the holder of the data collected. This is significant because the patient's primary care provider (PCP) can easily miss out on this useful patient data, leaving them with an incomplete picture of their patient. Data is further fragmented, isolated, and often monetized in this situation.

As we have seen, new health IT (HIT) vendors are becoming more powerful actors in this evolving healthcare ecosystem. Small innovative DI services are collecting more patient data than ever before, while also providing more information, technology, and services directly to patients. In this emerging direct vendor-to-patient business model, the vendor consumes patient data collected from apps and wearables and delivers new or improved technology for patients, targeting their preferences and needs. The data itself can then be analyzed to help the vendor improve their services or be marketed in other ways. Traditional HIT vendors that cater to healthcare organizations will soon face the problem of integrating different, external, sources of data from these vendors or from patient's health and wellness devices. With current electronic medical records (EMRs) and electronic health records (EHRs) still struggling to share data across healthcare organizations, additional pressure will look to un-silo these products allowing for greater health information exchange (HIE) and data sharing.

Traditionally, a nurse completes an admission assessment for a patient, the nurse collects the patient history and records it in an EHR. As the nurse completes this task, they are consumers of the technology being used. The nurse's preferences and needs become important to vendors who develop the technology and to the healthcare executives who do the decision-making. Additionally, paid home care providers, as consumers, are increasingly making use of apps that support them in caring for their client, providing them with relevant information and trending analytics. Family caregivers are also able to make use of apps and patient portals to help manage their loved-one's healthcare needs. HIT vendors, therefore, need to consider the preferences and needs of the nursing profession and home care providers in developing their DI.

Healthcare executives are also consumers of HIT products and services, though typically through purchase decisions and the use of these products and services by their healthcare organizations employees. Currently they are fairly isolated from the DI explosion of new vendors and direct-to-consumer services, but the impact will soon be felt. Understanding how to become competitive in this new landscape requires that executive leadership sees itself as a consumer who can evaluate and integrate these new services, adapting their business model to do so. Innovative vendors also need to understand that marketing to this group must include education and support for change. An executive's failure to educate themselves about new trends could mean that their business model will likely be replaced by a model developed by those who have been more successful in adopting the evolutionary steps that the DI is forcing. Organizations such as the Healthcare Information and Management Systems Society (HIMSS) can provide resources and opportunities for executives to be exposed to DI in a setting that provides the educational information needed to inform decision-making.

Finally, healthcare IT professionals constitute a consumer type as one that traditionally has had responsibility for the design, development, installation, maintenance, security, and privacy of HIT products used in healthcare organizations. As such, the HIT professional has knowledge and experience that can support successful DI and also support the evolution of the existing healthcare business model. Vendors can market to this consumer group as part of their DI business model and also make use of the knowledge base to help develop successful DI. With the explosive growth of new vendors marketing directly to consumers, HIT roles and opportunities are expanded and are rapidly changing. For example, dashboards developed for IT monitoring of cybersecurity risks seem to be made with the HIT professional in mind, allowing for the rapid visualization of threats in real-time [10].

Today's Healthcare Business Model Ecosystem

Current U.S. Healthcare Business Model

Within the United States (U.S.) healthcare system, the primary business model is a private payer fee-for-service model where healthcare consumers are charged a fee for each service provided to, resource used for, and interaction with a patient [11]. The main payer for healthcare services are private insurance companies, where the insurance is provided to employees as a benefit by employers. Some discounted and public options exist for those in lower income groups, those with disabilities and for those over 65 years of age.

While some efforts to change to capitated payment models are being made in the U.S., through pay for performance initiatives at the federal level, fee-for-service stands today as the primary model [12]. Many of these efforts to develop different payment models are intended to bring the spiraling cost of healthcare in the U.S. under control and to improve the consistency and quality of care [13, 14]. However, with a fee-for-service model, providers and healthcare organizations have little incentive to change and potentially reduce their income.

The provision of healthcare in the U.S. and elsewhere, is traditionally a physician-led hierarchy with patients often at the periphery of decision-making. Physicians, and more recently nurse practitioners, can directly bill for their services, putting them on the credit side of the healthcare ledger. Other healthcare professionals such as registered nurses provide services that cannot be billed directly to the patient or the patient's insurer, putting them on the debit side of healthcare's ledger.

Though some efforts are being made to explore other models of care such as patient-centered interprofessional team-based care, partly to improve outcomes, healthcare consumers today have little control over the services they receive, how much they cost, or when and where they receive them [15]. The U.S. healthcare system primarily requires that consumers visit a clinic or a healthcare organization to receive care. Patients must make appointments, wait, and then travel to receive care when, where, and how they are instructed. With some exceptions for limited use of telemedicine, services are still predominantly provided face-to-face. The regulatory and legal environment that impacts healthcare organizations and vendors hinders change and, in the past, has stifled innovation, contributing to the persistence of the existing model.

Publicly Funded and Public/Privately Funded Healthcare Systems Globally

Even with publicly funded healthcare systems, such as those in England, Canada, Norway, and India, fee-for-service is also the dominant payment model [16]. These systems provide scheduled or walk-in face-to-face services to consumers who visit a clinic or a larger healthcare organization. The lack of adequate funding is a constant challenge for these publicly funded systems given the challenges of containing healthcare costs [17].

Healthcare consumer choice and control are most often attained through the purchase of private health insurance policies. Due to this, private payers are also a component of many of these publicly funded healthcare systems, typically purchased by consumers to reduce the length of time to receive services as well as to provide access to services that may not be covered by the publicly funded system. However, the model is still physician-led, though many primary care services are provided by nurse practitioners, who have prescribing authority and who can work autonomously, to reduce the workload on primary care physicians [18].

In Germany, the business model is a combination of statutory healthcare insurance for low-income people and private insurance for those who make over a certain income in a fee-for-service model [16]. However, while there are similar wait times for access to services between the required and private insurance, older people, those with the required healthcare insurance and those in eastern Germany experience higher chances of increased wait times [19]. Consumers must also seek services at clinics and hospitals.

The current healthcare system in Germany is physician-led, though other more team-based interdisciplinary models are being experimented with, particularly for complex patients [20]. These efforts are, in part, an attempt to address a shortage of physicians and nurses in a system that has become fragmented. The role of nursing in the German healthcare system does not include advanced practice nursing. Registered nurses are also less autonomous than in other countries, with nurses providing services that are prescribed by a physician, either at a clinic, hospital, or the patient's home, if necessary (personal interview with Professor Ursula Hübner, 2020 Apr 1; unreferenced). The shortage of nurses is exacerbated by the relatively low pay, which further reduces the applicant pool.

Countries such as Kenya and other sub-Saharan areas in Africa are studying different methods of providing care as well as different insurance-payer models to improve the health of vulnerable and often disenfranchised people, such as HIV+ women [21]. These efforts are, in part, intended to help relieve strain on the National Healthcare Insurance Fund (NHIF), which is committed to providing free healthcare services to Kenyans through payroll deductions and private premiums. Initiated in 1966, the NHIF has struggled to maintain adequate funding to provide services due to the HIV/AIDs crisis, which has significantly impacted the sub-Saharan region. To try and provide cost-effective healthcare services the NHIF is increasingly making use of nurses to manage some aspects of healthcare delivery, also trained health care workers are being used to bring health and wellness services to more remote villages and populations.

Vendor Focus

Previously, health informatics vendors have marketed their products to healthcare organizations and healthcare professionals, primarily physicians. EMR vendors, point-of-care testing device manufacturers, and health informatics consultants have traditionally focused on the needs of the healthcare organization or professional in developing, marketing, and implementing their products, typically at significant financial costs. The patient has not been a major part of the equation, other than as a source of data or as the focus of a service.

Innovative vendors are now marketing new healthcare products and services, built around information technology such as smartphones and tablets, directly to consumers, transforming them from patients into customers. Fitting into Christensen's concept of a DI, the products and services are low cost, highly accessible, have lower gross margins, and are serving a low-end target market. The business model behind these products and services bypasses the current healthcare business model, depending on increased direct sales of units or services to customers at a lower cost to be profitable.

Additionally, in the current healthcare business model, pricing of services is not transparent, often varying widely in the same geographic region. This lack of clarity around cost prevents patients from comparing prices when shopping for healthcare services, putting them in a near powerless position. This lack of transparency is complicated by insurance companies that often require a patient to stay within their given network of healthcare organizations and professionals, as well as restricted formularies and services. As a result, patients who try to be informed consumers are often faced with an impossible task. In contrast, innovative web-based healthcare services vendors are ensuring pricing information is readily available on websites or when you sign up for the service [22, 23]. This gives the patient a level of control, as an informed healthcare consumer, allowing them to compare prices, convenience, accessibility, and insurance coverage before purchasing the product or services from the vendor of their choice. Given the relative impossibility of evaluating cost within the traditional healthcare system, particularly in the U.S., this level of customer control would be hard to implement in the traditional healthcare business model.

Ripe for Disruptive Innovation?

With few exceptions, the current models of healthcare globally are now being seen as inefficient, overly costly, and often having low levels of quality, consistency, and consumer satisfaction. Efforts to improve these levels through the use of ICT have not resulted in significant change and healthcare is still seen as lagging behind in innovation around the provision of care particularly. In addition, changing consumer expectations of what services these models deliver and how innovations such as smartphones, which have the potential to enable anytime-anywhere services with cost comparison, is still a challenge.

These devices also have the potential for developing countries to improve healthcare by leapfrogging over the traditional clinic or hospital-based delivery of services to services delivered where the consumer lives. With smart mobile devices able to function as glucometers, otoscopes, microscopes, portable ultrasound, and ECG monitors, health workers can function as virtual traveling clinics. In a recent study in Kenya, community health workers were able to use mobile technology to administer audiology and otoscopic screenings in semi-rural areas, identifying children with hearing loss or otoscopic abnormalities [24]. Being able to bring healthcare services to people in more remote or rural areas can significantly improve their health and wellness through identification and intervention, as well as reducing healthcare costs.

In the U.S., innovations such as CVS's MinuteClinic®, Walmart's Health Centers, Walgreens' Healthcare Clinics, and Urgent Care Centers provide walk-in services that reduce wait times and can be less expensive than a traditional physician's office or Emergency Department visit. In addition, new preventive health screening services provide a variety of options from wellness screenings to carotid artery ultrasound exams [25]. In part these services, which are being marketed directly to consumers, offer a game-changing level of convenience, control, and cost savings. Since many make more effective use of advanced practice nurses, they can also redistribute the demand for healthcare professionals, increasing access in underserved areas. The new business model of these DIs is disrupting the current business model and creating new value, as shown in Fig. 35.2.

Disruptive Innovations of Today

Information and Communication Technologies in Healthcare Today

The U.S. healthcare system, as with many others, has not kept pace with other industries in the integration of information technology to reduce costs, increase efficiency, customer satisfaction, and improve service delivery. In spite of these potential benefits, resistance on the part of healthcare organizations and professionals reluctant to change the status quo and current business models have slowed the adoption and development of health informatics tools [26]. As noted by the authors, the groundwork is being laid for significant changes to be made in the near future as healthcare organizations and HIT vendors move toward more integrated information systems and devices. This integration is often taking place within a healthcare system or between systems that adopt the same vendor's products.

Adoption of tools such as telehealth to reach underserved rural populations struggled to move forward pre-pandemic, in part due to high cost and a lack of health insurance in the population that the services are expected to reach [27]. This lack of health insurance has been complicated by a lack of willingness on the part of payers, for those who do have health insurance, to reimburse healthcare organizations for telehealth services. However, recently in the U.S., the Centers for Medicare and Medicaid Services has greatly expanded the number of billing codes available for reimbursements, making this an area that will likely change more rapidly now [28]. With the COVID pandemic we have seen this rapid change accelerate an an almost unbelievable rate. The question now is how much of this progress will remain post-pandemic.

In Australia, a lack of Internet infrastructure in remote rural areas has contributed to telehealth services not reaching those who would benefit from the access to care that they can provide [29]. Adding to that is the lack of insurance billing codes for telehealth services, reducing incentive for healthcare organizations and governments to improve access. Some positive signs of development have started in Germany where, as a means to reduce the burden on physicians, a health telematics infrastructure is seeing an increase of use, in part to help support communications between physicians (personal interview with Professor Ursula Hübner, 2020 Apr 1;

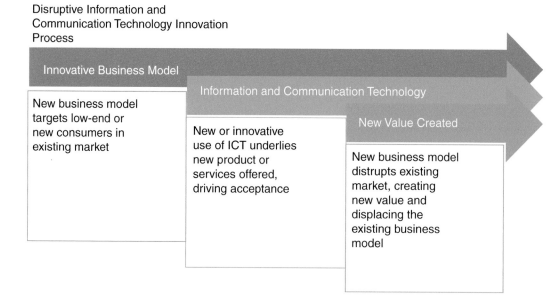

Fig. 35.2 Disruption Creates New Value

unreferenced). More recently, the Federal Ministry of Health in Germany has started promoting apps to help patients self-manage chronic diseases and mental health conditions, and to improve communication between physicians and patients. However, these apps must be prescribed by a physician for patient use.

The slow adoption and integration of HIT across countries has been complicated by a lack of defined HIT competencies required for different healthcare professional roles. There is also a persistent lack of informatics training in the curricula of healthcare professionals, due in part to a lack of trained faculty who can teach the content adequately [30–32], though work has been done recently to gain a more global understanding of this phenomenon and to engage in conversations around this issue [33].

What Is Being Disrupted and Why

Today, in many global healthcare systems, a prospective customer must call for an appointment, wait until the appointment time, drive or travel to a clinic, be seen by a healthcare provider, then travel home. This system seems antiquated when a few taps on our smartphone or other device can give us access to a world of services, such as Teladoc® or 98point6®, which provide access to healthcare services at any time, from anywhere, in moments. However, the regulatory environment around these innovations is unclear, though in the U.S., the Food and Drug Administration (FDA) is working to find a way to protect healthcare consumers while not stifling the innovations that can empower them [34]. While temporary allowance have been made for telehealth during the COVID pandemic, the longer term regulatory future remains unclear.

While in the past, and still commonly today, insurance reimbursement for teleservices has been a barrier to the innovation, recent analyses are suggesting that this trend is changing and that teleservices are now being seen as a viable business model [35]. We can also see in other studies that patient expectations are changing. In a recent study from Iran, patients are begin-

ning to expect the same sort of customized experience in healthcare that they experience in other service sectors [36]. As previously discussed, there is also evidence suggesting that the physician-led model in the U.S. is changing with the advent of convenient walk-in clinics that are staffed by nurse practitioners and physician assistants, such as CVS's MinuteClinic® and UrgentCare Clinics [37]. Certainly COVID has opened consumer's eyes to the convenience and safety offered by virtual services, a change that may be difficult for the traditional model of care delivery to roll back.

Additionally, recent studies are also seeing an ICT driven paradigm shift away from "reactive medicine" to a more preventive model, with more information and self-tracking options for healthcare consumers [38]. However, these shifts and changes are not happening in a vacuum. The current healthcare ecosystem needs to be successfully integrated with this new model, with technical challenges and legal issues also needing to be identified and addressed for healthcare systems to successfully evolve [39].

Case Study: Disruptive Innovation Case Study: Singapore and TraceTogether

Abstract

Individual countries are engineering innovative solutions to combat the ongoing coronavirus disease (COVID-19) pandemic. Singapore, which learned many valuable lessons with its own experience of SARS in 2003, has been leading the way in innovating to support effective contact tracing. The difficulties of relying on interviews and the memories of infected individuals as the existing method for comprehensive contact tracing helped inspire the development of the TraceTogether digital application by the Singapore Ministry of Health (SMOH). Singapore was among the first countries to deploy a national coronavirus contact tracing app. With only a third of the population downloading the app, Singapore fell short of the majority the SMOH was aiming for. This prompted the development of a wearable dongle, called a TraceTogether Token. Dongles are small hardware devices that can be plugged into a computer to download the data they collect, in this case contact with someone identified as COVID-positive. Both the app and Tokens raise concerns over individual privacy and the potential for governments to abuse the technology in the future.

Technical Approach

Contact tracing prevents the spread of a disease by identifying infected people and those who they have been in contact with. Currently, in order to curtail spreading diseases, public health officials rely on contact tracing interviews (CTI) to identify and isolate those who have come in contact with infected persons [1]. Providing a list of contacts during a CTI is fundamentally a task of memory. Patient's recalling their contacts are vulnerable to well-established weaknesses in human memory, exacerbated when ill.

This was a concern for epidemiologists at the SMOH, as there were numerous instances of interviewees not remembering all their contacts, or not knowing whom they had been in contact with [2]. On March 20, 2020, the Government Technology Agency of Singapore, in collaboration with the SMOH, announced the launch of the TraceTogether mobile app. The smartphone app was developed as a means to help support and supplement current contact tracing efforts to reduce the spread of COVID-19.

The App Process, illustrated in Fig. 35.3

- The free TraceTogether app works by exchanging short-distance Bluetooth signals between phones to detect other participating TraceTogether users in close proximity.
- Records of such encounters are stored locally on each user's phone for 25 days.
- If a user is interviewed by SMOH as part of the contact tracing efforts, they can consent to send their TraceTogether data to SMOH.
- This facilitates the contact tracing process, enabling contact tracers to rapidly notify TraceTogether users who are close contacts of COVID-19 cases.
- The TraceTogether app can be downloaded from the Android Google Play or Apple App Store.

App Analysis

Although over two million had downloaded the app, it fell far short of the national target of 75% of the population. Several issues can account for the low adoption rate. The app was known to have usability and reliability issues on iOS devices, deterring those using iPhone devices from downloading the app [3]. For the app to work properly, it has to be turned on and be on a user's front screen, which can pose a significant drain on battery life. Various measures were put

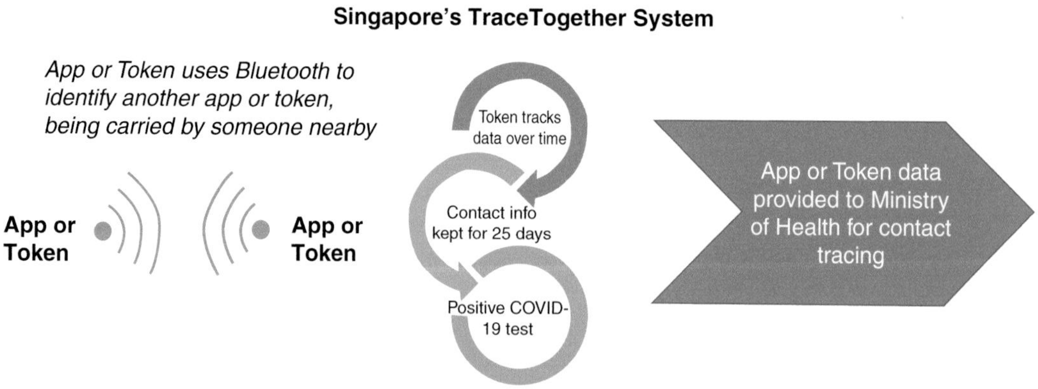

Singapore's TraceTogether System

App or Token uses Bluetooth to identify another app or token, being carried by someone nearby

App or Token   App or Token

Token tracks data over time

Contact info kept for 25 days

Positive COVID-19 test

App or Token data provided to Ministry of Health for contact tracing

Fig. 35.3 TraceTogether Contact Tracing System

in place to protect user privacy, such as decentralized privacy-preserving proximity tracing (DP-3T) in which an individual phone's contact logs are only stored locally. Although reassurances made by developers and the SMOH to protect privacy, users continued to express concerns over privacy [4]. Also, the app does not currently cover the digitally excluded populations such as the elderly and young children who may not have smartphones [5]. Lastly, downloading the app is not mandatory for every citizen, only for Singapore's migrant workers, who have accounted for the majority of Singapore's COVID-19 infections due to the density of their living and working conditions [6].

The Dongle Process

- Citizens must provide their national ID and phone numbers to acquire a free dongle, which is encoded with their national ID for contact identification purposes.
- The device uses Bluetooth technology to identify other users who are either connected to the TraceTogether app, or wearing a dongle, then exchanging IDs. Contact ID logs are stored locally on the dongle for 25 days [5].
- The token has a long battery life, which can last up to nine months without needing a recharge.
- If dongle users test positive for the disease, they physically hand their device to the SMOH so their contact log can be accessed. Unlike the app, the dongle cannot transmit data over the Internet [7].

Dongle Analysis

The government contracted with electronics manufacturer PCI to manufacture an initial run of 300,000 of these contact tracing wearables. The first dongles were prioritized (with seniors given priority) and given out by volunteers to individuals who do not have phones capable of running the TraceTogether app. The government plans to continue generating more awareness about the TraceTogether Tokens among their prioritized populations, through telephone and other opportunistic engagements. They have also publicly stated that there will not be a global positioning system (GPS) tracking chip or any mobile connectivity in the tokens at any point.

Business Models and Value

The current business model, of public health officials using CTI for contact tracing, is ripe for disruptive innovation (DI) due to the weaknesses around relying on human memory. Therefore, the value to public health is limited. The DI of using smartphone apps or wearables that can automatically log each contact can replace this model and allow for accurate and comprehensive contact tracing. The value to public health cannot be underestimated. However, concerns around privacy and abuse of data, now and in the future, are endangering this innovation and the value it could bring.

Lessons Learned

- Not relying on the memory of interviewees is a significant improvement for contact tracing. Because the data on the app is digital it can also be available more quickly, decreasing the time to contact potentially infected individuals.
- Voluntary adoption by the public is key to success. TraceTogether has struggled, due in part to poor usability as well as privacy concerns. The wearable TraceTogether Tokens are meant to be a response and solution to these concerns. Poor usability and battery life are not issues. The dongle remains offline and only makes its stored data available when a medical professional physically requests access to the device. Yet even though the device is not connected to the Internet, it is "always on" in terms of logging Bluetooth contacts. This continues to raise concerns over privacy, even inspiring an online petition against its use, which garnered over 50,000 signatures by the end of June 2020 [8].
- With this technology being so new, there has been very little time to study its social effects or the ramifications it may have for the future. As of now, no definitive policies or regula-

tions are in place and the potential for their abuse by both individuals and governments is of concern.

Case Study Summary

Singapore's Bluetooth-based contact tracing app and dongles, TraceTogether, were the first of their kind, with the potential to disrupt the current contact tracing model. Due to issues of privacy and usability, TraceTogether has struggled to garner the rate of adoption needed to have the impact on contagion control that it was designed for. The impact on the current business model of CTI is yet to be determined and due to the identified issues may not become clear in the foreseeable future. The value that could be created is similarly in flux.

Case Study Discussion/Debate/ Essay Questions

1. Is the loss of privacy that some fear acceptable to achieve control of the virus?
2. What control should the individual have over data on who they have been in contact with?
3. What adding GPS tracking unacceptably increase the potential risk of hacker abuse and government control of its citizens?

Summary

Healthcare business models all over the world are ripe for disruption through innovations in ICT. While generally late to adopt ground-breaking ICT solutions when compared to other industries, the healthcare industry now has an opportunity to integrate DIs and adapt to the rapidly changing landscape of consumer expectations. As individuals make the transition from patient to consumer, they are now being given a variety of options by more nimble vendors that traditional healthcare organizations have not been able to offer. When viewing all stakeholders as consumers of healthcare, it is clear that chang-

ing consumer expectations will continue to drive DI in healthcare.

Conclusions and Outlook

While it remains to be seen which innovations will be disruptive and which will yield positive and/or negative effects, the rate of change does not appear to be slowing. The current COVID-19 pandemic has forced the unprecedented use, for the time being, of telehealth services by traditional healthcare organizations and providers, however, it remains unclear what the longer-term impact of this will be. Will this solidify the use of information technology as a means to provide services or will we return to the traditional in-clinic model once the virus is under more control? What role will the consumer/patient's preferences have, once they have experienced telehealth services from their providers?

At the time of this writing, the American Medical Association and other physician groups are beginning to advocate for pandemic-forced changes to rules, in part around telehealth, to be rolled back once the pandemic is over, to return to the traditional model of healthcare delivery. Will they be successful in turning back the clock? Though the answer will not be known for some time, healthcare will experience many changes as it endeavors to survive and thrive in the Information and ongoing or post-pandemic age; where data, information, and technology are motivating forces shaping consumer and healthcare systems' behaviors.

Useful Resources

The following links are to resources and vendor services discussed in the chapter:

1. Bank My Cell: https://www.bankmycell.com
2. Defense Advanced Research Projects Agency (DARPA): https://www.darpa.mil
3. Internet Society: https://www.internetsociety.org/internet/history-internet/brief-history-internet/
4. Clayton Christensen website: http://clayton-christensen.com/key-concepts/

5. Teladoc: https://www.teladoc.com
6. 98point6: https://www.98point6.com
7. The Library of Economics and Liberty's Creative Destruction page: https://www.econlib.org/library/Enc/CreativeDestruction.html
8. Health IT News Cybersecurity Dashboard: https://www.healthcareitnews.com/news/cio-guide-building-dashboard-cybersecurity
9. U.S. Centers for Medicare & Medicaid Services: https://www.cms.gov
10. The Commonwealth Fund's International Health Care Systems Profiles: https://international.commonwealthfund.org/countries/
11. CVS Pharmacy's Minute Clinic: https://www.cvs.com/minuteclinic/services/price-lists,
12. https://98point6.zendesk.com/hc/en-us/categories/360000063423-Personal-Plans
13. Life Line Screening: The Power of Prevention: https://www.lifelinescreening.com
14. Training Leader Healthcare: https://healthcare.trainingleader.com/2019/07/medicare-telemedicine-policy/
15. U.S. Food & Drug Administration's (FDA) Digital Health landing page: https://www.fda.gov/medical-devices/digital-health

Review Questions

1. The digital divide can be said to reduce access to innovative services for those who do not have access to resources such as
   (a) Broadband Internet
   (b) Fitbit
   (c) Information and communication technologies (ICT)
   (d) File Transfer Protocol (FTP)
2. The concept of disruptive innovation (DI) was proposed by Clayton Christensen and can be defined as
   (a) The process by which a product or service takes root initially in simple applications at the bottom of a market and then relentlessly moves up market, eventually displacing established competitors.
   (b) To explain market behaviors that were not previously well understood about the diffusion of an innovation.
   (c) The device, tool, or process that were seen as the innovation and how it works in better ways than the older device, tool, or process.
   (d) The new business model behind the innovation that is disruptive taking a large market share immediately.
3. True or False: DIs serve a smaller low-end target market at first, before expanding to a vast market due to their accessibility.
   (a) True
   (b) False
4. The U.S. healthcare system is primarily a public or private payer model that is physician or healthcare team led? Please select more than one:
   (a) Private
   (b) Public
   (c) Physician
   (d) Healthcare team led
5. Currently innovative vendors are beginning to market new healthcare products and services, built around information technology such as smartphones and tablets, directly to consumers. Describe one new healthcare product that you have encountered and discuss what the service provides. (Open Answer).

Acknowledgement We are grateful to Franky, BPharm(Hons), BCGP, CAHIMS, Senior Pharmacist, Woodlands Health Campus, Singapore, for his insights into contact tracing as an information and communication technology means to control the spread of COVID-19.

Appendix: Answers to Review Questions

1. The digital divide can be said to reduce access to innovative services for those who do not have access to resources such as.
   (a) Broadband Internet
   (b) Fitbit

(c) Information and communication technologies (ICT)
(d) File Transfer Protocol (FTP)

The correct answer is a: Broadband Internet. Those left without resources, such as broadband Internet access, will be left without access to this new world of the Internet and smart device-based resources.

2. The concept of disruptive innovation (DI) was proposed by Clayton Christensen and can be defined as.
   (a) The process by which a product or service takes root initially in simple applications at the bottom of a market and then relentlessly moves up market, eventually displacing established competitors.
   (b) To explain market behaviors that were not previously well understood about the diffusion of an innovation.
   (c) The device, tool, or process that were seen as the innovation and how it works in better ways than the older device, tool, or process.
   (d) The new business model behind the innovation that is disruptive taking a large market share immediately.

The correct answer is a: The process by which a product or service takes root initially in simple applications at the bottom of a market and then relentlessly moves up market, eventually displacing established competitors. The term disruption is defined as "a break or interruption in the normal course or continuation of an activity or process." The term innovation is defined as "an idea, method, or device." Coupled together outlines the disruptive innovation (DI) proposed by Clayton M. Christensen in 1997.

3. True or False: DIs serve a smaller low-end target market at first, before expanding to a vast market due to their accessibility.
   (a) True
   (b) False

The answer is true. Christensen explains that DI can be identified as one of four characteristics: (1) They are low cost and highly accessible; (2) They have lower gross margins than their contemporaries or the incumbent; (3) They serve a smaller low-end target market at first, then expanding to a vast market due to their accessibility (the answer); and (4) They are difficult to see coming and is not taken seriously at first.

4. The U.S. healthcare system is primarily a public or private payer model that is physician or healthcare team led? Please select more than one:
   (a) Private
   (b) Public
   (c) Physician
   (d) Healthcare team led

The correct answers are a and c. The U.S. healthcare system is primarily a private payer fee-for-service model where healthcare companies are charged a fee for each service provided to, resources used for, and interaction with patient. The provision of healthcare in the U.S. and elsewhere, is traditionally a physician-led hierarchy with patients at the periphery of decision-making.

5. Currently innovative vendors are beginning to market new healthcare products and services, built around information technology such as smartphones and tablets, directly to consumers. Describe one new healthcare product that you have encountered and discuss what the service provides. (Open Answer).

The answer to this question is open. Suggestions include: The Internet of Things (IoT), The Medical IoT, EHRs, Remove Care, 3D Printing, LASIK, Retail Clinics, Augmented Reality, Precision Medicine, and more.

References

1. Faiola A, Papautsky EL, Isola M. Empowering the aging with mobile health: a mhealth framework for supporting sustainable healthy lifestyle behavior. Curr Probl Cardiol. 2019;44(8):232–66.

2. O'Dea S. Number of smartphone users worldwide from 2016 to 2021 [Website]. 2020 [cited 2020 19 June, 2020]. Available from: https://www.statista.com/statistics/330695/number-of-smartphone-users-worldwide/.

3. Macintosh 128K: Technical Specifications: Apple Inc.; [cited 2020 19 June, 2020]. Jul 26, 2017: Available from: https://support.apple.com/kb/SP186?locale=en_US.

4. Leiner BM, Cerf VG, Clark DD, Kahn RE, Kleinrock L, Lynch DC, et al. Brief History of the Internet: Internet Society; 1997 [cited 2020 19 June, 2020]. Available from: https://www.internetsociety.org/internet/history-internet/brief-history-internet/.

5. Zhao JY, Song B, Anand E, Schwartz D, Panesar M, Jackson GP, et al. Barriers, facilitators, and solutions to optimal patient portal and personal health record use: a systematic review of the literature. AMIA Annual Symposium proceedings/AMIA Symposium AMIA Symposium. 2017;2017:1913–22.

6. Disruption: Merriam-Webster, Inc.; 2020 [cited 2020 19 June, 2020]. Available from: https://www.merriam-webster.com/dictionary/disruption.

7. Innovation: Merriam-Webster, Inc.; 2020 [cited 2020 19 June, 2020]. Available from: https://www.merriam-webster.com/dictionary/innovation.

8. Christensen C. Disruptive Innovation: Clayton Christensen 2020 [cited 2020 19 June, 2020]. Available from: https://claytonchristensen.com/key-concepts/.

9. Alm R, Cox WM. Creative Destruction: The Library of Economics and Liberty; 2020 [cited 2020 19 June, 2020]. Available from: https://www.econlib.org/library/Enc/CreativeDestruction.html.

10. Siwicki W. A CIO guide to building a dashboard for cybersecurity: HIMSS Media; 2018 [cited 2020 19 June, 2020]. Available from: https://www.healthcareitnews.com/news/cio-guide-building-dashboard-cybersecurity.

11. Slotkin JR, Ross OA, Newman ED, Comrey JL, Watson V, Lee RV, et al. Episode-based payment and direct employer purchasing of healthcare services: recent bundled payment innovations and the Geisinger health system experience. Neurosurgery. 2017;80(4S):S50–S8.

12. Anumudu SJ, Erickson KF. Physician reimbursement for outpatient dialysis care: past, present, and future. Semin Dial. 2020;33(1):68–74.

13. Smith SP, Elias BL. Shared medical appointments: balancing efficiency with patient satisfaction and outcomes. Am J Manag Care. 2016;22(7):491–4.

14. Elias B, Barginere M, Berry PA, Selleck CS. Implementation of an electronic health records system within an interprofessional model of care. J Interprof Care. 2015;29(6):551–4.

15. Kuziemsky C, Vimarlund V. Multi-sided markets for transforming healthcare service delivery. Stud Health Technol Inform. 2018;247:626–30.

16. Tikkanen R, Osborn R, Mossialos E, Djordjevic A, Wharton GA. International Health Care System Profiles: The Commonwealth Fund; 2020. [cited 2020 19 June, 2020]. Available from: https://www.commonwealthfund.org/international-health-policy-center/countries.

17. van Leersum N, Bennemeer P, Otten M, Visser S, Klink A, Kremer JAM. Cure for increasing health care costs: The Bernhoven case as driver of new standards of appropriate care. Health Policy. 2019;123(3):306–11.

18. Kruth T. Advanced practice nursing in the United Kingdom: International Advanced Practice Nursing; 2013 [Available from: https://internationalapn.org/2013/10/07/united-kingdom/.

19. Luque-Ramos A, Hoffmann F, Spreckelsen O. Waiting times in primary care depending on insurance scheme in Germany. BMC Health Serv Res. 2018;18(1):191.

20. Ulrich LR, Pham TT, Gerlach FM, Erler A. Family health teams in Ontario: Ideas for Germany from a Canadian Primary Care Model. Gesundheitswesen. 2019;81(6):492–7.

21. Were LPO, Were E, Wamai R, Hogan J, Galarraga O. Effects of social health insurance on access and utilization of obstetric health services: results from HIV+ pregnant women in Kenya. BMC Public Health. 2020;20(1):87.

22. How Much Does 98point6 Cost? : 98point6 Inc.; 2020 [cited 2020 19 June, 2020]. Available from: https://98point6.zendesk.com/hc/en-us/articles/360043139171-How-much-does-98point6-cost-.

23. Price List: CVS Pharmacy Inc.; 2020 [cited 2020 19 June, 2020]. Available from: https://www.cvs.com/minuteclinic/services/price-lists.

24. Jayawardena ADL, Kahue CN, Cummins SM, Netterville JL. Expanding the capacity of otolaryngologists in Kenya through mobile technology. OTO Open 2018;2(1):2473974X18766824.

25. Preventive Health Test & Screening: Life Line Screening; 2020 [cited 2020 19 June, 2020]. Available from: https://www.lifelinescreening.com/.

26. Mitchell M, Kan L. Digital technology and the future of health systems. Health Syst Reform. 2019;5(2):113–20.

27. Lee S, Black D, Held ML. Factors associated with telehealth service utilization among rural populations. J Health Care Poor Underserved. 2019;30(4):1259–72.

28. Updated 2019 Medicare Telemedicine Policy: Healthcare Training Leader; 2019 [cited 2020 19 June, 2020]. Available from: https://healthcare.trainingleader.com/2019/07/medicare-telemedicine-policy/.

29. St. Clair M, Murtagh D. Barriers to telehealth uptake in rural, regional, remote Australia: what can be done to expand telehealth access in remote areas? Stud Health Technol Inform 2019;266:174–182.

30. Bove LA. Integration of informatics content in baccalaureate and graduate nursing education: an updated status report. Nurse Educ. 2019.

31. Champagne-Langabeer T, Revere L, Tankimovich M, Yu E, Spears R, Swails JL. Integrating diverse dis-

ciplines to enhance interprofessional competency in healthcare delivery. Healthcare (Basel). 2019;7(2)

32. Pontefract SK, Wilson K. Using electronic patient records: defining learning outcomes for undergraduate education. BMC Med Educ. 2019;19(1):30.

33. Hübner U, Thye J, Shaw T, Elias B, Egbert N, Saranto K, et al. Towards the TIGER international framework for recommendations of core competencies in health informatics 2.0: extending the scope and the roles. Stud Health Technol Inform. 2019;264:1218–22.

34. Digital Health: Federal Department of Agrictulture, United States Food & Drug Administration; 2020 [cited 2020 19 June, 2020]. Available from: https://www.fda.gov/medical-devices/digital-health.

35. Lin JC, Kavousi Y, Sullivan B, Stevens C. Analysis of outpatient telemedicine reimbursement in an integrated healthcare system. Ann Vasc Surg. 2019;

36. Minvielle E. Toward customized care comment on "(re) making the procrustean bed? standardization and customization as competing logics in healthcare". Int J Health Policy Manag. 2018;7(3):272–4.

37. Bartsch SM, Taitel MS, DePasse JV, Cox SN, Smith-Ray RL, Wedlock P, et al. Epidemiologic and economic impact of pharmacies as vaccination locations during an influenza epidemic. Vaccine. 2018;36(46):7054–63.

38. Moerenhout T, Devisch I, Cornelis GC. E-health beyond technology: analyzing the paradigm shift that lies beneath. Med Health Care Philos. 2017;

39. Fourneyron E, Wittwer J, Rachid Salmi L, Groupe de recherche Eva TSN. Health information technology: current use and challenges for primary healthcare services. Med Sci. 2018;34(6–7):581–6.

Project Management: Enabling Communication and Healthcare IT Implementations

36

Rebecca Nally and Ginny Waters

Learning Objectives
- Identify the five process groups that every project should have.
- Define why communication is important in project management.
- Identify reasons why the Closing phase is generally skipped and why project managers should make a point to complete the phase.
- Describe how project management is important in Healthcare IT projects.

Key Terms
- Scope Creep
- Communication
- Project
- Process Groups
- Stakeholder
- Scope
- Risk
- Lessons Learned

Introduction

Healthcare is one of the most important business industries in the world today. It has the fastest-growing average of new jobs compared to any other industry [1]. There are life and death situations, and whether you are a provider on the front lines or a relative of a patient, every person will experience the healthcare system at some point in their life. Given the continuous changes in the healthcare industry, healthcare professionals must stay informed and adapt to the new changes. When a patient is in a crisis, they expect the healthcare professionals to know what to do and be able to give them information. To do this, healthcare professionals need to stay informed. By staying informed, making changes, and being flexible, healthcare facilities can stay at the top of their game and ahead of their competitors. Information Technology (IT) is at the forefront of healthcare changes. Healthcare IT improves the quality of healthcare, reduces medical errors, and reinforces the relations of patient and provider [2]. Technology is ever expanding and physicians can do so much more with the technology than ever before. Although new technology can be a major investment, healthcare facilities can grow their profits exponentially with its use [3]. All of these changes certainly involve IT and require a project manager to understand the impact of the change and lead the project team to a successful implementation by keeping all the tasks and milestones on time and under budget [4].

R. Nally (✉) · G. Waters
Deaconess Health System, Evansville, IN, USA

© Springer Nature Switzerland AG 2022
U. H. Hübner et al. (eds.), *Nursing Informatics*, Health Informatics,
https://doi.org/10.1007/978-3-030-91237-6_36

Importance of Project Management in Healthcare IT

Through the history of time, projects have always existed; think of the Great Pyramids, the Olympics, building massive skyscrapers, or implementing a railway system across the United States. In fact, it is believed that NASA first used the concept of project management and project managers, as we know them today [5]. A project is anything that has a beginning and an end; it is temporary in nature. The official definition of a project is "a temporary endeavor undertaken to create a unique product, service or result" [6]. Some projects last a few days, and some last a few years, but to be considered a project, it must close at some point.

Project management is used across the world in every discipline, so why is it so important in Healthcare IT? As the healthcare industry continues to expand, the demand for improved and more advanced technology also grows. Most Healthcare projects have some type of technology component within them, making the need to manage and coordinate those resources vital to the overall success of the project. As an example, when new electronic medical record systems are being implemented, regulations must be followed, quality must stay high, and costs must decrease [7]. Healthcare IT projects can be very involved and have a lot of pieces and parts to them. Having someone to keep track of the logistics and timelines of the project is very important. Many things can go wrong, and project managers evaluate risks and mitigate the effects while keeping everything on track. Project managers are responsible for planning, managing, and engaging team members to execute the project [7].

Project managers also need to work with the project sponsor and project stakeholders, all while keeping the patients and their safety at the forefront. In Healthcare IT, the list of stakeholders involved with the project could include people from various backgrounds, including doctors, nurses, CEOs, CFOs, managers, analysts, and billers, for example.

The Project Management Book of Knowledge (PMBOK) is a book that the Project Management Institute began to show project managers the best practices and standards for leading projects. It highlights skills and techniques that are vital in project success. The PMBOK is not specific to any particular industry, but instead can be used by project managers of any industry. The PMBOK lists five project process groups that every project needs to have. These include Initiating, Planning, Executing, Monitoring and Controlling, and Closing [6] (Exhibit A, Fig. 36.1).

Initiating

- Create the Project Charter
- Define Scope
- Communicate
- Discovery

The Initiation phase of a project includes many essential steps to getting your project off on the right foot in the beginning. To begin, you will want to create a Project Charter. The Project Charter formally authorizes the existence of a project [6]. It also provides the project manager with the authority to use resources on activities related to the project [8]. Generally, the project sponsor creates the Charter, but the Project

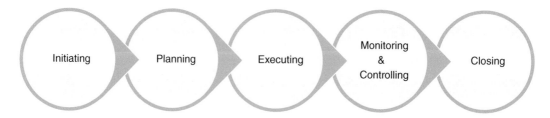

Fig. 36.1 The five project process groups as defined by the Project Management Institute in the PMBOK

Manager should provide input as well. There may be times that the sponsor needs assistance in drafting the Charter, and the project manager can help as needed. The sponsor would review the content, make any additional edits, then approve and authorize the final version. During the drafting of the Project Charter, you may not know all of the information regarding the project, such as budget or scope. The Charter should be written with the information known at the time [8]. Project Charters are high level and should show how the project will contribute to the overall strategic plans of the organization.

As a project manager, you must define the scope of your project. The project manager should have a clear understanding of everything included in the project from the beginning and throughout the extent of the project. This prevents scope creep, which is when tasks and milestones that were not originally in the plan end up as part of the project. These tasks were not budgeted nor planned for, therefore, they have the potential to cause significant issues, including a failed project. According to a recent study, 52% of projects experience scope creep [9]. Avoiding scope creep is a vital part of the project manager's job.

Communication with stakeholders from the start and creating a scope document that is shared with everyone involved in the project is key. Identifying what is out of scope early in the project is also important, so it is known from the beginning and there is no confusion by any of the parties involved.

During Discovery, project managers and their team determine what their portion of the project will look like. They may sit through meetings and ask specific questions about what the company currently does and what they want it to look like at project completion. The team may also physically visit the location where the project will take place. In terms of IT projects, this could mean visiting the unit in the hospital, or the physician's office, or the server room. Speaking to stakeholders is critical and communication is vital. Discovery may bring out additional tasks that were unknown before it occurs. If any other tasks were revealed during Discovery, they would then

need to be vetted to determine if they need to be in scope for the project or out of scope, which can lead to another project later.

Planning

Successful projects always involve a great deal of planning [10] as planning activities and research into the project can reduce risk and save stakeholders money. The project managers need to do a few things in the Planning phase, such as create a schedule, a project plan, and a detailed budget. They also need a list of milestones and dates associated with them, an outline of the critical path deliverables, a list of stakeholders, and team members that will be working on the project. Ideally, the list of team members will also have their assignments and tasks for which they are responsible. Of course, these items correlate to the scope that was defined in the Initiating phase.

Project plans are important in any project. It keeps everything on track and lets everyone, including the project team and stakeholders, know what task is coming next and if the project is on track or at risk. Project plans are not set in stone and will need to be fluid to adapt as the project progresses. It is up to the project manager to make sure that changes are documented and communicated to the team. The Project Plan should include all tasks associated with the project, start dates and end dates for each task, and who is responsible for each task. Critical Path items should be highlighted and called out in some fashion. An Executive Summary is also helpful for showing the highlights of the Project Plan. Not every stakeholder will want to see each individual task of a project; they just want the highlights and to know the significant milestones. All stakeholders should approve the project plans, and each member should approve the areas that affect them and their work [11]. Each time a project plan is revised or changed, review, and approval by the stakeholders should occur.

Project Plans for projects within Information and Technology (IT) are especially important given that there are a lot of unique factors involved. Devices have to be budgeted for, procured, delivered, and deployed. If using these with an Electronic Medical Record (EMR), they will need to be mapped within the EMR to work correctly. If there is any delay in procurement or delivery, this could delay the project significantly. At times there are shortages of certain technologies within the market that can cause delays, potentially significant.

Planning also includes creating a list of stakeholders and team members. This should include contact information and tasks that each person is directly responsible for completing. This would be part of the Communication Plan. Since communication is such an essential piece of any project, having a plan surrounding this is extremely important. Anytime there is a change to the project plan or timeline, this needs to be communicated to all stakeholders and team members.

Often, there are questions regarding what is in scope or if something can be added. Communication in these instances is vital to keeping a project on track and ensuring its success. Effective communication keeps all parties up to date, keeps the project within scope, and keeps the team motivated and engaged [12]. If everyone involved in the project understands how important communication is to the success of a project, they would make time to do it effectively to ensure the project is a success (See Fig. 36.2).

Ineffective communication is to blame for more than half of projects that fail to meet business goals [12]. One out of five projects is unsuccessful due to ineffective communications [12].

Risk management is also a key element in the Planning phase. Risk should be monitored throughout the project, but planning for risks

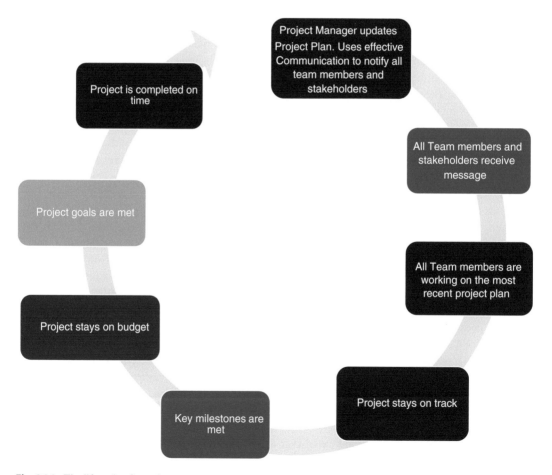

Fig. 36.2 The lifecycle of a project

should start in the Planning phase. Every project will contain some amount of risk. A poorly planned project adds to that risk [13]. Risks to a project cannot always be eliminated, but they can be reduced.

Executing

The execution phase is where most of the work on deliverables is completed. It is also usually the longest phase of a project. After teams know the scope of the project and their milestones and deadlines, work can begin on each task. The project team is usually busy completing their milestones in this phase. This is the stage where the project plan is executed, so it is important that all team members know what their tasks are when they are due, and how they may impact other team members' tasks. Project managers must manage the team members in this phase and communicate with them constantly. Team members need to be held accountable for any delays [14]. They should be communicating all issues to the project manager as soon as they arise, so a plan can be put in place to resolve the issue. Updates to project plans and the schedule sometimes need to be made, which means adjusting and managing risks. Project managers must also monitor milestones and make sure the project team is staying on track. If there is an unforeseeable change or missed deadline, the project manager must adjust future steps to accommodate this.

The budget is also watched closely during this phase and adjusted as needed. Constant communication between the project manager, project team, and stakeholders is extremely important in this part of the project to ensure the budget stays on track. As an example, if the project involves opening a new wing in a hospital; beds, devices, chairs, décor, etc. will all need to be procured before opening. All of these items and details will need to be outlined in the budget and managed carefully.

At times, tasks can get off track and diverge from the project plan. The goal of the project manager is to make sure any adverse effects are minimized, and future steps are adjusted to account for the change [7]. The success or failure of a project will show in the execution stage. If the team has a lack of understanding, this will cause significant problems for everyone. If the executive sponsors are not engaged, this could also lead to a lack of communication on needed items, and therefore, the project will fail. If the project does not truly meet the strategic goals of the company, the project could be pulled at any time. The project manager should work to create action plans for all of these possible gaps to help fix any issues as they arise [14]. One of the most important things for a project manager is to be open and flexible [14]. Every project is different, and every team is different. Project managers must be able to be flexible and make changes as needed.

Another important success strategy that project managers should utilize is to celebrate achievements. Whether it is a small milestone or a large one, keeping the team's morale up is very important, especially during this phase, since it will be the most time-consuming for everyone. Acknowledging the team members and their hard work is important to keep the team working at optimal levels.

Monitoring and Controlling

As a project manager, you need to always know the status of your project. Communication between your project team and stakeholders is extremely important here. Knowing how the project is going and where it is in terms of the timeline are crucial in knowing if there is a problem or not. There will be a lot of status updates to executives during this time, so you want to make sure your statuses are as up to date as possible and be ready to explain each piece, in case there are questions. Project managers use Key Performance Indicators (KPIs) to help turn the information gathered, such as the scope statement, into objectives to measure the project's success [15]. The KPIs should be selected by determining what the stakeholders want.

Everyone should agree on what the KPIs will be for the project, and they should be reflective of the goals and objectives of the project.

During the monitoring and controlling phase, project managers may also need to make decisions on if a change is necessary. If there is a change to the project plan, the project manager will need to identify any risks that could be associated with that change or update. It must also be known that one change could significantly impact another task. The illustration in Fig. 36.3 shows how actions to one task can affect others.

W. Edwards Deming's Plan-Do-Check-Action (PDCA) Cycle (Fig. 36.4) is a good tool to help

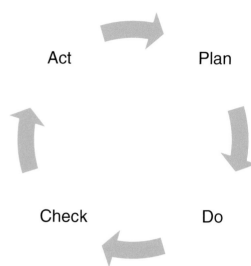

Fig. 36.4 W.Edward Deming's Plan-Do-Check-Act Cycle

understand the impacts of changes to the project. If part of the project is going to change, you must first plan. You should check to see if the change will positively or negatively affect the rest of the project. The next step is to test the change before implementing it. After testing occurs, it must be decided if this change will work. If it will, the change can go into effect after communication to the team members and stakeholders has been completed. However, if the change testing does not work, other options must be explored, and the process will have to start over.

As stated earlier, a common theme in projects is frequent communication. It is vital to a project's overall success. In monitoring and controlling, team members must be aware of any change that is potentially going to happen. Team members then have the responsibility to communicate with the project manager of any potential adverse effects that they see that could occur. Leadership and stakeholders need to be aware of any changes as well to help determine what the best plan of action would be. Projects cannot be run in a silo as the tasks being completed stretch out to many areas and impact the work of many groups of people.

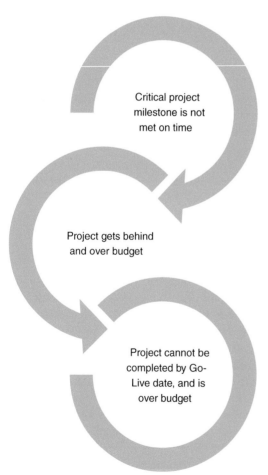

Critical project milestone is not met on time

Project gets behind and over budget

Project cannot be completed by Go-Live date, and is over budget

Fig. 36.3 Tasks and actions affect the next task and action

Closing

In the closing phase, all agreed-upon deliverables are delivered to the customer. The new process is implemented, the software updates to the system are completed, and/or the new facility opens its doors. During the Closing phase, it is also the ideal time to compile Lessons Learned (Fig. 36.5). These include both positive and negative experiences of a project [16]. These help project managers and project team members know what worked well, what did not, and can then be used to improve upon future projects. Lessons Learned help the project manager grow and improve as well as incorporate new ideas and processes into future projects. Lessons learned prevents teams from making the same mistakes on project after project. Many times identifying lessons learned is done in a session with all team members, but surveys or templates can also be made for the team to share their information.

The closing phase is also a time to compare the hours projected and budgeted for the project to the actual number of hours spent working. Completing this analysis will help with future capacity planning and timeline planning for similar projects that arise in the future. Budget and timeline summaries need to be created to show where the project ended up when deliverables were delivered [7].

The closing phase is an important phase in a project; however, many times, it is forgotten or skipped. There are many reasons for this, such as another project is starting and there just is not time to do all of the Closing tasks and/or team members are not as accessible, so it is difficult to gather their feedback. Many project teams can be stretched thin and may be worried about the deadlines of the next project. After all the deliverables are delivered to the customer, the project team generally moves on. However, the closing phase really needs to be completed fully before putting that project aside. There are so many valuable lessons and items that come out to this phase [17].

Case Study

Overview

Jones Primary Care office is currently using an outdated EMR system that is no longer able to meet Meaningful Use requirements. They have a desire to update their technology, make their office workflows more standard and efficient, and

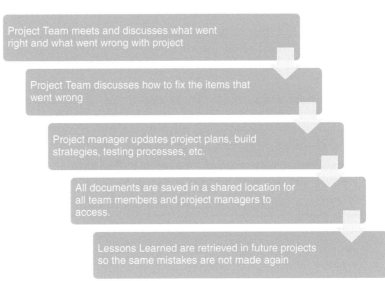

Fig. 36.5 Lessons Learned

LESSONS LEARNED

Project Team meets and discusses what went right and what went wrong with project

Project Team discusses how to fix the items that went wrong

Project manager updates project plans, build strategies, testing processes, etc.

All documents are saved in a shared location for all team members and project managers to access.

Lessons Learned are retrieved in future projects so the same mistakes are not made again ideally streamline their communication with the local hospital. Their preferred solution would provide integration between scheduling, clinical documentation, billing, and medical records management functionality.

Implementation Process

- EMR search and selection.
  - Three different EMR vendors were reviewed and evaluated. Feature comparisons were completed. Interoperability options were investigated. Implementation and annual maintenance costs were compared. Selection made!
- Kick-off meeting.
  - To ensure staff was engaged and communication about the new EMR implementation was shared, a kick-off meeting was held to review the timeline and major milestones. Representatives from the EMR vendor were present to answer any questions providers, administrators, and staff may have.
- Discovery Sessions.
  - Once the Kick-off meeting was complete, the EMR system representatives spent time learning about the needs of the office and completing observations of each areas workflow. Scheduling details, document samples, list of in-office procedures, charge codes, and KPI metrics were collected to make sure the data was included in the new EMR system.
- Build Phase.
  - The EMR representatives use the data that was collected during discovery to customize the new EMR system for the Jones Primary Care office. When needed, follow-up discussions occurred with the office staff to clarity configuration options and decisions.
- System Testing.
  - All build was tested in an integrated manner. The EMR system team worked together to ensure the testing demonstrated efficient workflows that could be standardized across the office. User Acceptance Testing was also completed by a few members of the office staff to ensure the new EMR system would meet their needs for scheduling, clinical documentation, and revenue cycle completion.
- End-User Training.
  - Approximately 3–4 weeks before the new EMR was to be implemented, all office staff members were required to complete training. It included both online lessons as well as face-to-face classroom time with a qualified trainer. After passing an assessment, each end-user was provided their own unique ID and Password to access the new EMR system.
- Pre-Go Live Milestones.
  - To prepare for the Go Live event, the following milestones were completed approximately 1–2 weeks before implementation: Device Testing, Appointment Conversion, Clinical Data Conversion, and Dress Rehearsal.
- Go Live Event.
  - On this day, the Independent Primary Care office began using the new EMR system. Support staff from the EMR vendor were on-site with the end-users for 2 weeks to assist them with workflow questions, system updates, and general support with the transition.
- Post Live Support.
  - Representatives from the EMR system revisit the office approximately 30 days post Go Live to see how the office staff are doing with the new system. They re-evaluate workflows and present KPI metric data pre and post-implementation.

Benefits

- Improved coordination of care across the clinic and overall community.
- Standard workflows for end-users to follow.
- Avoid financial penalties by meeting Meaningful Use metrics and quality requirements.

Case Study Conclusion

By implementing a new EMR system, the Jones Primary Care office was able to meet all of their goals in a reasonable timeline and within their desired budget. The local hospital uses the same EMR system so clinical data for their patients can be shared across both organizations, thus improving the continuity of care in their community.

Summary

Project management in healthcare IT is vital to the success of projects. IT projects are complex and extremely important to the success of healthcare facilities. Healthcare IT projects are constantly changing, which means healthcare is changing as well. Project managers need to keep projects on task, on schedule, organized, and communicated. Without communication between all members of the project team and stakeholders, projects fail. Communication is probably the most important piece of any project, and the project manager needs to have a plan to make sure it is continually occurring. There are five critical processes of every project and communication is important in every single one. The five processes are Initiating, Planning, Executing, Monitoring and Controlling, and Closing. Usually, these processes overlap each other, meaning the project manager is doing more than one process at a time. Each process is vital to every project, and it is crucial not to skip any of them.

Conclusions and Outlook

Project management is an ever-changing field. IT projects are becoming more sophisticated and healthcare is undoubtedly changing. Project managers need to be able to adapt to changes and be flexible throughout the life of a project. Project managers need to continue to learn and grow in their field, learn how to communicate effectively, educate team members and users, and be flexible to changes.

The outlook of project management is bright and continues to grow and prosper as industries, including healthcare, will continue to come up with new and innovative projects. With so many complex tasks involved in big projects, leaders are relying on project managers to keep everything organized and on schedule. Several different types of project management styles have evolved over time, such as Waterfall, Agile, Scrum, and Kanban; with Agile Project Management currently becoming more popular than traditional methodology. Agile project management breaks the project into smaller increments and is much more iterative than the conventional one. The project plans are reassessed often, and changes are made much more frequently. This is not to say that conventional project management will go away. Many businesses or industries prefer one over the other; therefore, both traditional and Agile project management styles will continue to be in demand as long as companies keep to rely on project managers.

Useful Resources

1. www.pmi.org
2. www.projectmanagement.com
3. www.healthcareITnews.com
4. www.heatlhIT.gov
5. www.kff.org
6. www.himss.org

Review Questions

1. What are the five process groups of every project?
2. What is scope creep?
3. What is the definition of a project?
4. Why is collecting lessons learned so important?
5. Why is communication so important in a project?

Appendix: Answers to Review Questions

1. What are the five process groups of every project?

Initiating, Planning, Executing, Monitoring and Controlling, and Closing.

2. What is scope creep?

Scope creep is changes or uncontrolled growth to the scope of a project after the project begins. Scope creep is a huge risk to the success of a project and the project budget.

3. What is the definition of a project?

The definition of a project is a temporary endeavor undertaken to create a unique product, service, or result.

4. Why is collecting lessons learned so important?

Lessons learned are important because they show the negative and positive aspects of the project. They teach project managers and the team what works and what does not, so they know what to repeat and make sure what to not repeat in future projects.

5. Why is communication so important in a project?

Communication is important because it keeps everyone up to date on all aspects of the project. The project manager needs to have a communication plan in place and needs to make sure that all team members and all stakeholders are aware of the plan and any changes that are made.

References

1. Healthcare Occupations: https://www.bls.gov/ooh/healthcare/home.htm
2. The Importance of Health Information Technology in Developing Areas. Openmrs.org
3. Why the Evolving Healthcare Services and Technology Market Matter: https://healthcare.mckinsey.com/why-evolving-healthcare-services-and-technology-market-matters/
4. Aziz L. Managing change in healthcare information technology projects: the role of the project manager. In: Paper presented at PMI® Global Congress 2007—North America. Atlanta, GA. Newtown Square, PA: Project Management Institute; 2007.
5. Shirley D. Project Management for Healthcare. Boca Raton: CRC Press; 2011. https://doi.org/10.1201/b10853.
6. PMBOK® Guide – Sixth Edition (2017).
7. https://www.hsph.harvard.edu/ecpe/a-primer-on-project-management-for-health-care/
8. Brown AS. The charter: selling your project. Paper presented at PMI® Global Congress 2005—North America. Toronto, Ontario, Canada. Newtown Square, PA: Project Management Institute; 2005.
9. Elton C. Scope patrol: scope creep is on the rise as stakeholder expectations increase; Here's how to keep projects within bounds. PM Netw. 2018;32(7):38–45.
10. Serrador P. The importance of the planning phase to project success. Paper presented at PMI® Global Congress 2012—North America. Vancouver, British Columbia, Canada. Newtown Square, PA: Project Management Institute; 2012.
11. Whitten N. Project planning: frequently asked questions — part 2. PM Netw. 2000;14(10):21.
12. Communication: The Message is Clear (2013). *PMI White Papers.*
13. Signore AA. Conceptual project planning from an owner's perspective. Proj Manag J. 1985;16(4):52–8.
14. Projectmanager.com/blog/preoject-execution
15. Hayes Munson KA. How do you know the status of your project?: Project monitoring and controlling. In: Paper presented at PMI® Global Congress 2012—North America, Vancouver, British Columbia, Canada. Newtown Square, PA: Project Management Institute; 2012.
16. Rowe SF, Sikes S. Lessons learned: sharing the knowledge. Paper presented at PMI® Global Congress 2006—EMEA. Madrid, Spain. Newtown Square, PA: Project Management Institute; 2006.
17. Martin PK, Tate K. The forgotten phase. PM Netw. 2000;14(2):29.

Process Management: Designing Digital Workflows

37

Bernhard Breil and Thomas Lux

Learning Objectives
- The aim of this chapter is to understand supply processes in the health care system and to optimize them through the sensible use of IT. Process management helps to analyze processes, model workflows and therefore make them more efficient and effective.
- For this purpose, the most important terms of process management will be introduced, and a typical hospital process will be presented using important points of time during the process. Furthermore, two modeling tools, the Electronic Process Chain (EPC) and the Business Process Model Notation (BPMN), will be presented and the former will be applied to this hospital process.
- In addition, the perspectives of the involved stakeholders are to be taken into account when supporting the care process from admission to discharge or rehabilitation measures. A case study then brings all the elements together and uses the example of pain management to show how the various stakeholders use the process management tools to optimize this typical process from nursing care.

Key Terms
- Process view
- Core processes in health care
- Interprofessional processes
- Process view and decision making
- Process re-engineering
- Introduction of IT systems
- IT support of processes
- Case study: pain management
- Patient perspective
- Integration of outpatient care

Introduction

Definition and General Aspects Processes

A process is an ordered sequence of activities or tasks that are directly related to each other. In the context of corporate management, processes are called business processes if they are directly involved in the value creation of the company. They are either production or service processes. The term process is used colloquially in various areas. In most cases, its meaning in these areas is self-explanatory, e.g., a legal process, a chemical reaction process or a production process. The term process always denotes a sequence of activities that are linked together. A business process is a specific type of process. It describes a process for adding value from an economic perspective.

B. Breil (✉)
University AS Niederrhein, Krefeld, Krefeld, Germany
e-mail: bernhard.breil@hs-niederrhein.de

T. Lux
Hochschule Niederrhein, Krefeld, Germany
e-mail: thomas.lux@hs-niederrhein.de

© Springer Nature Switzerland AG 2022
U. H. Hübner et al. (eds.), *Nursing Informatics*, Health Informatics,
https://doi.org/10.1007/978-3-030-91237-6_37

Processes delivering directly value are called main core businesses or core business processes. Processes that are not directly involved in value creation or are not part of a value-adding area, although they are crucial to the activities of the company, are called supporting processes. For example, personnel management as well as facility management play a key role in value creation, but neither business area is directly involved in the value chain. Management processes, such as controlling or business planning, are presented as another separate process area. Both support and management processes have cross-divisional or supporting functions for the company (see [14]).

The process view forms an important link between the strategic level and the application or software/data level. It is necessary to translate the strategic decisions of the management into concrete processes. This requires a high degree of flexibility of the processes in order to be able to constantly adapt them to new customer or environmental requirements. A transformation of the corporate strategy to the process level therefore takes place. Applications are used to support the processes, e.g., workflow management systems. Due to the demands of agility on the processes, it is obligatory for the application systems to be flexible in order not to prevent or block changes in the process flows. The storage and processing of data used by the process-oriented applications is taking place on the software or data level. A component-oriented structure enables suitable IT structures and is usually applicable in the long term. The quality of IT is largely determined by the degree of IT process support, which can be used for benchmarking purposes (see [13]).

Core Processes in the Healthcare Sector

The essential core processes in the health care system and especially in hospitals is divided into the areas of admission, diagnostics, treatment, and discharge (see [3]). The starting point for inpatient care processes is the *admission* of patients to hospitals. However, outpatient service providers, rescue services or the patient may already be involved in the care process prior to admission (Hübner et al.). In the prototypical process that follows admission, the patient's *medical history* is typically the anamnesis, in which the doctor asks about the history of the underlying hospital visit. This is followed by *diagnostics*, which are used to make a diagnosis in imaging procedures or laboratory analyses. After a diagnosis is being made the *therapy* follows. This is followed by *treatment*, for example, surgery or the administration of medication. At the end of the inpatient process chain, the patient will be *discharged*. The hospital stay may be followed by outpatient *follow-up treatment* or a *rehabilitation measure*.

Admission (Elective/Emergency)

The path of a patient in hospital starts with the admission. A fundamental distinction is obligatory between the following types of admission:

The patient is scheduled for elective surgery, which is not urgent and often cannot be performed immediately, sometimes even after waiting for a long time for an appointment (e.g., with an end prosthesis). The person arrives unplanned as an emergency. It has to be checked whether inpatient treatment is necessary or only outpatient care. Emergency patients must be treated by the hospital as quickly as possible all the time. The urgency of treatments is often determined by triage. Hospitals to be scheduled to treat emergencies can only unsubscribe from emergency care in exceptional situations

Diagnostics and Treatment

Treatment management includes all activities that take place during the in-patient stay and serve to treat and care for the patient. It also includes:

- Diagnostic and therapeutic measures (including special diagnostics, operations, interventions)
- Patient care and monitoring
- Measures to control and optimize the length of stay

Good treatment quality requires an efficient and structured organization within the framework of ward management.

Discharge Management

Discharge management includes all processes that prepare or facilitate the discharge of an inpatient. In order for patients to be discharged quickly, various aspects must be considered. For example, it is necessary the doctor's letter to be completed timely on the day of discharge. Treatment/diagnostics, such as taking blood samples, should be avoided on the day of discharge if possible, unless there are medical arguments against it. Relatives must also be informed within a reasonable time about when the patient will be picked up or transported. Accommodation must be arranged through the social services.

Interfaces to post-operative care are also important for the success of treatment (outcome). For example, these are further medical care (outpatient or inpatient), rehabilitation care, nursing care, but also advice and information provided by social services (see [11]).

Modeling

Business Process Management refers to the entire systematic procedure for recording, designing, executing, documenting, measuring, monitoring, and controlling processes (see [11]). However, before a process can be improved, it must be analyzed. Process models have established themselves as the basis for these analyses, which enable a standardized mapping of processes. Process modeling is a method that can be used sensibly in various application scenarios. On the one hand, it can be used as a tool for reorganization when existing processes need to be optimized (process re-engineering). In addition, process modeling supports the introduction of new IT, as this is often accompanied by corresponding process changes. Finally, process modeling can be used to analyze and visualize direct IT support (workflow management). Essentially, process modeling is about mapping a chronological and logical sequence of activities (cf. [11]). The two best-known representatives are Event-driven Process Chains (EPC) and the Business Process Modeling Notation (BPMN).

Event-Driven Process Chains (EPC)

Basically, event-driven process chains comprise the three basic elements such as function, event, and connector. Functions are used to describe the activities or operations performed. Examples of functions are activities "Admit Patient" or "Make Booking." Functions are characterized by measurable time periods and can be divided into subfunctions (subsystems) during modeling. Depending on the level of detail or granularity, one can differentiate between functions, subfunctions, and elementary functions (activity).

Events are triggers and the result of functions. They describe the occurrence of a business-relevant event. For example, the function "Admit Patient" could lead to an event called "Patient is admitted." Functions describe periods of time, whereas events refer to a state.

Operators control the logical linking of functions and events if an event or function has more than one input or output. A distinction is made between the three connectors AND, OR, and XOR. For example, a patient could arrive as an elective case (event: elective patient arrives) or as an emergency case (event: emergency case arrives). In both cases (AND connector), you must first enter the patient data (Function: Enter Patient Data) (see [2]).

Business Process Management Notation (BPMN)

The BPMN distinguishes between three different flow elements. *Activities* indicating what happens or must be done in a process step. *Activities* therefore have a duration. In addition, there are *events* that can be used to make decisions and *gateways* that indicate certain conditions. These three basic elements are connected by *connecting objects* such as maintenance (for *sequence* or *message flows*) or dashes (*associations*). Associated objects are usually data that is generated, processed, or stored in the respective process steps.

The BPMN is useful and well applicable both for the business modeling of non-IT-savvy people and for precise specification within IT. Clear definitions and rules enable a clear modeling in which validation rules can also be implemented. Further advantages arise in BPMN by modeling exceptions and interactions of several processes.

Support of the Supply Process

The care process should be defined in a patient-centered manner and reflect the views of the user groups involved. Only the participation of the three different user groups (patients, nursing staff, doctors) directs the focus to the interprofessional treatment process and ensures a high process quality. In the following, IT support possibilities are shown from the respective perspectives. Looking at the process from prevention to rehabilitation, the focus is on different actors in the different phases. In prevention, the patient is the main focus, in diagnostics the doctor and in therapy the nursing staff (see [6]).

IT Support from the Perspective of the Doctors

An essential process support of medical activities is the electronic service point management by CPOE systems. They support all request and documentation processes in which several service points or several persons are involved. Studies indicate that electronic drug prescription can reduce medication errors and thus significantly improve patient safety. The positive effects include reduction of the time required to distribute and complete orders, while increasing efficiency by reducing transcription errors and eliminating duplicate order entry, while simplifying inventory management and billing.

Overall, CPOE systems can thus effectively support the medication process and improve medication safety. Other studies point to potential problems in the planning, introduction, and use of CPOE systems. The problems and risks include lack of usability and training

IT Support from the Perspective of the Nursing Staff

Advantages such as time savings are not only due to the nursing documentation, but also to IT systems that support organization and processes in nursing homes and outpatient care services. These include the support of time-consuming activities such as the management of sickness-related absences and the short-term search for adequate replacements, taking into account competencies (skills, language, training level). The complete process mapping and control from admission to discharge ensure transparency through uniform, prompt and complete medical and nursing documentation using individualize terminology such as SNOMED CT. In case of personnel change or change of wards, information exchange is realized efficiently and securely without loss.

IT Support from the Patients' Perspective

Thanks to current IT support, the patient can be involved in the process at many points. The first symptoms can be entered into a diagnostic app, where an AI already names possible diagnoses and specialists for validation. The subsequent contact and appointment search is carried out by online comparison with the appointment calendar of the respective doctor or hospital. In the hospital, the waiting time from the doctor's appointments can be used for the digital completion of patient questionnaires (e.g., on quality of life or on anxiety/depression), which are then available in the information system in electronic form and can be evaluated [5]. In rehabilitation, the exercises to be completed are displayed on the smartphone in an individualized way for the respective patient and the patient is given an individualized description.

Requirements for Workflow Management

In order to take advantage of process orientation, the processes must be digitally supported. This has long since ceased to apply to a single system, but rather to a large number of different systems in the health care system. For example, in hospitals, information from referring doctors is merged with patient data.

In order to implement these elements in a meaningful way, requirements for workflow management must be defined. One of these requirements is the (semantic) interoperability of the systems involved. Interoperability is the ability of different systems to work together as closely as possible (see [4]). This means that users usually do not notice when system boundaries are crossed during information exchange.

Case Study: Pain Management in Nursing Care

Pain and its consequences are increasingly becoming a social problem. Adequate care can hardly be guaranteed, especially in nursing. The many actors and professions involved in the therapy require a very high level of coordination, which is usually hardly possible. The development of integrated treatment processes and IT support of the processes with suitable methods and concepts of e-health enable a better quality of care. In the context of this contribution, the various facets of pain (management) are briefly introduced and also suitable solutions through the design of integrated cross-actor processes and their support through e-health applications. The process of pain management in nursing and its potential for networking is shown as an example.

Case Study: Expert Standard Pain Management

Painlessness is the central goal of pain therapy and the basic prerequisite for the patient's well-being. ([10], p. 4) The pain therapy of the German Society for Pain Research (DGSS) even declares freedom from pain to be a fundamental human right. According to this, all people have "the same right to adequate pain relief" ([16], p. 11).

This goal can only be achieved on the basis of comprehensive pain management. The nursing staff plays a key role in this process, as they not only coordinate the activities between the doctor, nursing staff and the interdisciplinary team, but also promote communication between the patient and all those involved in the process. Pain therapy includes the targeted and structured recording of pain and pain-related care problems, the planning and coordination of suitable pain therapy measures, and the monitoring of therapy measures and their effects and side effects. A continuous review of the measures in a therapeutic team as well as the early information of the physician in case of changes in the pain condition are as much a part of the pain treatment as the consultation and training of the patients and their relatives ([1], p. 692). Figure 37.1 shows the four phases of pain therapy.

In phase 1, pain is systematically assessed and evaluated using appropriate assessment tools. The documentation of pain (phase 2) serves to explicate the patient's subjective sensation and thus make it communicable. In phase 3, pain is measured using reliable and simple methods. The pain therapy (phase 4) of chronic pain serves primarily to improve the patient's function.

Mapping of the Expert Standard as a Process (EPC)

Pain patients in inpatient care are usually undersupplied. Only every fifth patient receives adequate care [6]. In particular, the role of care (and care by relatives in home care) must be redefined

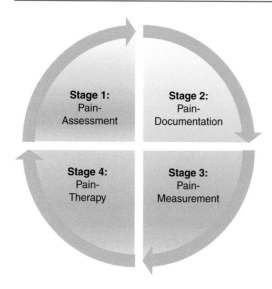

Fig. 37.1 Four phases of pain therapy

here. Although there is regular close interaction with the patient here, the potential room for varying the pain therapy is rather small, and the uncertainty that abilities will be exceeded is high. By networking the actors, considerable improvements could be achieved by improving the exchange of information and by describing the roles and tasks in the individual treatment scenario of the patient in a concrete and reliable way.

The process chain in Fig. 37.2 shows the exemplary conception of a networked pain management by using an IT solution as a result of various projects in this environment with an exemplary pain management process [8].

IT Support of the Process

Actors involved in the treatment of pain, e.g., in-patient care facilities are the responsible nursing staff, general practitioners and specialists as well as the affected residents and their relatives. The team is supplemented by other therapists and actors such as physiotherapists, occupational therapists and psychotherapists, who are involved

in the pain therapy depending on the pain situation and the condition of the resident. The role of the main actors is briefly explained below.

Nursing professionals play a decisive key role, especially in the care of residents with chronic pain, since they usually have regular and intensive contact with the affected persons and are also contact persons. They are responsible for pain assessment and thus for determining the state of pain. In addition, they are responsible for "initiating interventions in consultation with the affected persons in the event of a pain assessment of more than 3/10 at rest or more than 5/10 on the NRS [Numerical Rating Scale] during stress/movement, and for communicating with all those involved in pain care, such as medical and therapeutic staff, employees of supplying pharmacies [...] or other members of the treatment team" ([15], p. 530).

Especially in the inpatient care sector, it is important to create defined communication channels with the actors involved in care, due to the fact that the care areas are remote from doctors. Nursing staff form an important interface between the treating physician and the residents. The most important nursing tasks in drug therapy include, among other things, determining the need for painkillers, informing the attending physician about pain, changes in pain conditions and about the implementation and, above all, monitoring the progress of therapeutic measures in order to ensure their effectiveness and also to detect side effects of measures at an early stage. In addition, a comprehensive knowledge of pain and therapy is an important prerequisite for adequate pain management, especially for nursing staff. This is because they are responsible for ensuring that as many of the intervention options as possible are used to the full and that the nursing staff are informed about pain management and involved in the course of the therapy. In all the areas mentioned above, IT-supported networking holds great potential for ensuring an almost optimal care process ([9], p. 51 and [15], p. 530).

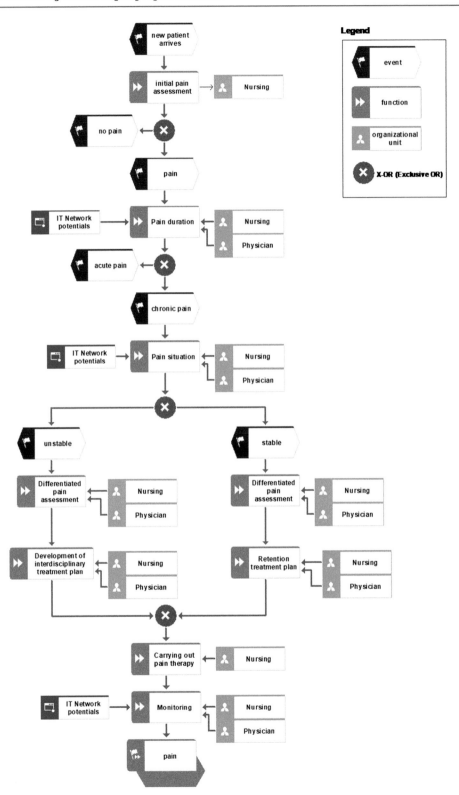

Fig. 37.2 EPC of the pain management process

Summary

A process is a systematic sequence of activities. This general principle can also be applied to the hospital care process from admission to discharge. To understand it, such a process can be modeled and analyzed using modeling tools like the presented EPC and BPMN. Thus, the perspective of the different stakeholders involved as well as technical interfaces (process interaction) become clear. Using the example of pain management in nursing, it will be shown how modeling (in this case with the EPC) allows a holistic view of the process and can also be used to map expert standards.

Once a process has been optimized, IT support can be checked. This sequence is important, because otherwise you run the risk of adapting the process to the IT tools at an early stage, which can lead to problems, especially when interfaces to other tools are created or when systems are replaced.

Conclusions and Outlook

Within the hospital, doctors often already have adequate IT solutions in place, which are particularly good at mapping processes of internal service point communication. CPOE is already standard in the vast majority of hospital information systems and helps to design request processes effectively. However, advantages are not only created for doctors but also for nursing staff and increasingly for patients. Two developments will inevitably change the IT support of supply processes in the future.

1. Increasing outpatient care will make it necessary to consider and model care processes not only within one institution but across institutions. This makes analysis more complex and it requires the use of modeling tools. In addition to the organizational complexity, the technical side must also be considered. Cross-sector documentation and communication across system boundaries require seamless networking of the respective information systems. In order to guarantee this technically, the requirements mentioned above regarding technical and semantic interoperability must be considered.

2. Furthermore, the patient will play an increasingly important role in the care process. Especially with regard to the abovementioned example of pain management, diary entries with the current pain sensation would be a helpful support for the attending physician, if he can access them directly in his file. For this purpose, the technical and organizational prerequisites must be created to transfer such data from the patient-related electronic patient or health record.

Useful Resources
BPMB
1. Current BPMN specification (http://www. bpmn.org/)
2. BPMN Tools (https://bpmnmatrix.github.io/)
3. https://www.omg.org/spec/BPMN/

EPK
1. ARIS-Tool: https://www.ariscommunity.com/ aris-express
2. http://www.bflow.org/

Review Questions
1. What are the core processes in a hospital?
2. What are the four main phases of a pain therapy?
3. How can process views contribute to good decisions?
4. Which perspectives are important in the support of the supply process
5. What is a function in an event-driven process chain (EPC)? Explain and give an example!

Appendix: Answers to Review Questions

1. What are the core processes in a hospital?

The essential core processes in hospitals are divided into the areas of admission, diagnostics, treatment, and discharge.

2. What are the four main phases of a pain therapy?

The four phases are assessment, documentation, measurement, and therapy.

3. How can process views contribute to good decisions?

Process view forms an important link between the strategic level and the application or software/data level and help to translate the strategic decisions of the management into concrete processes. Therefore, Process view is a benchmarking tool.

4. Which perspectives are important in the support of the supply process

The perspective of the doctors, the perspective of the nursing staff and the patients' perspective.

5. What is a function in an event-driven process chain (EPC)? Explain and give an example!

Functions are used to describe the activities or operations performed. Functions are characterized by measurable time periods and can be divided into subfunctions (subsystems) during modeling. Examples of functions are the activities "Admit patient" or "Make booking."

References

1. Baumgärtel F, Al-Abtah J. I care – Pflege. Stuttgart: Thieme Verlag; 2015.
2. Becker J, Kugeler M, Rosemann M. Prozessmanagement, Ein Leitfaden zur prozessorientierten Organisationsgestaltung. 6. Auflage ed. Berlin/Heidelberg: Springer; 2008.
3. Breil B, Fritz F, Thieman V, Dugas M. Mapping Turnaround Times (TAT) to a generic timeline: a systematic review of TAT definitions in clinical domains. 2011. BMC Med Inform Decis Mak. May 24, 2011;11:34. https://doi.org/10.1186/1472-6947-11-34.
4. Breil B. Technische Standards bei eHealth-Anwendungen. In: F. Fischer und A. Krämer (Hrsg.), eHealth in Deutschland; 2016. https://doi.org/10.1007/978-3-662-49504-9_8
5. Fritz F, Balhorn S. Riek M, Breil B, Dugas M. Qualitative and quantitative evaluation of EHR-integrated mobile patient questionnaires regarding usability and cost-efficiency; 2011. https://doi.org/10.1016/j.ijmedinf.2011.12.008
6. Grobe T, Steinmann S, Szecsenyi J. Barmer GEK Arztreport 2016, Schriftenreihe zur Gesundheitsanalyse, Bd 37. Berlin: Barmer GEK; 2016.
7. Lux T. Prozessorientierte Krankenhausinformationssysteme. In: F. Fischer und A. Krämer (Hrsg.), eHealth in Deutschland. 2016; https://doi.org/10.1007/978-3-662-49504-9_8.
8. Lux T. Vernetztes Schmerzmanagement durch E-Health in der Pflege. In: Pfannstiel MA, Krammer S, Swoboda W, editors. Digitale Transformation von Dienstleistungen im Gesundheitswesen IV. Berlin: Springer; 2018. p. 165–18.
9. Menche N, Brandt I. Pflege konkret. Innere Medizin, Pflege konkret, Bd. 4, 6. Aufl. Elsevier und Urban & Fischer Verlag, München; 2013
10. Osterbrink J. Vorwort zum aktualisierten Expertenstandard. In: Deutsches Netzwerk für Qualitätsentwicklung in der Pflege (Hrsg.), Expertenstandard Schmerzmanagement in der Pflege bei akuten Schmerzen, 1. Aktualisierung, Schriftenreihe des Deutschen Netzwerk für Qualitätsentwicklung in der Pflege, Osnabrück,S. 3–6; 2011.
11. Rücker B. Praxishandbuch BPMN
12. Schlüchtermann J. Betriebswirtschaft und Management im Krankenhaus, Berlin, Medizinisch Wissenschaftliche Verlagsgesellschaft; 2. Auflage, 2016.
13. Thye J, Straede MC, Liebe JD, Hübner U. IT-Benchmarking of Clinical Workflows: Concept, Implementation, and Evaluation. Stud Health Technol Inform. 2014;198:116–24.
14. Weber P, Gabriel R, Lux T, Schroer N, Menke K. Basics in Business Informatics. Springer Nature Campus-Verlag. 2019;1:Auflage.
15. Wulff I, Könner F, Kölzsch M, Budnick A, Dräger D, Kreutz R. Interdisziplinäre Handlungsempfehlung zum Management von Schmerzen bei älteren Menschen in Pflegeheimen. In: Gerontologie und Geriatrie. 2012;45(6):505–44.
16. Zenz M. Ethik-Charta der DGSS: Schmerz in Deutschland. Köln: Deutscher Schmerzverlag; 2007.

The TIGER Initiative: Global, Interprofessional Health Informatics Workforce Development

38

Toria Shaw Morawski and Man Qing Liang

Learning Objectives
- Share about TIGER's evolution from a grass-roots initiative focused on nursing to a global community embracing an interprofessional approach.
- Describe the role TIGER is playing—from identifying core health informatics competencies and developing resources—to enhancing global workforce development.
- Understand how TIGER works as a conduit, both as an initiative and interprofessional community, to support the clinical workforce toward the common goal of improving patient care.

Key Terms
- Case studies
- Competency attainment
- Competency development
- Digital health
- Digital skills
- eHealth
- Information and technology

- Interdisciplinary
- Multiinterdisciplinary
- Recommendations
- Virtual learning environment

Overview of the TIGER Initiative

In 2004, President Bush established a goal that every American would have an electronic health record (EHR) by 2014 [1]. In January 2005, a core group of prominent nursing leaders dubbed the 'TIGER Team' for *Technology Informatics Guiding Educational Reform*, agreed that "utilizing informatics" is a core competency for healthcare professionals in the twenty-first century, as acknowledged by the Institute of Medicine (IOM) [2]. There was also agreement amongst the emerging nursing informatics community that a majority of nurses lacked information technology (IT) skills and the use of informatics competencies in their roles. Health informatics education for the nursing workforce was identified as instrumental for driving innovation in healthcare, facilitating proper adoption, and achieving the meaningful use of health IT by improving the quality of care [3]. Indeed, innovation, which includes the development of new products, processes, and organizational approaches, cannot take place within the health IT space without the profound involvement of health professionals and educators that comprises the global workforce [3].

T. Shaw Morawski (✉)
Healthcare Information and Management System, Chicago, IL, USA
e-mail: tori@torism44.com

M. Q. Liang
TIGER Intern, HIMSS, Montréal, Québec, Canada
e-mail: man.qing.liang@umontreal.ca

© Springer Nature Switzerland AG 2022
U. H. Hübner et al. (eds.), *Nursing Informatics*, Health Informatics,
https://doi.org/10.1007/978-3-030-91237-6_38

TIGER was formalized as a grassroots initiative within the nursing community in 2006, supported by over 70 contributing organizations, including the Robert Wood Johnson Foundation, the National Library of Medicine, and several private donors. TIGER's original goal was to engage and prepare the nursing workforce in using technology and informatics to improve the delivery of patient care. Since its creation 15 years ago, the TIGER cause has been carried by hundreds of volunteers, organizations, and activities around the world. TIGER's rich history is summarized in Figs. 38.1 and 38.2 and presented in detail in a previous publication by Shaw Morawski, Sensmeier, and Anderson [4].

Today, TIGER is a stable, grassroots global initiative focused on education and reform, fostering community development and workforce development using an interprofessional approach. TIGER "offers the global community tools and resources designed for learners to advance their skills and for educators to develop technology and health informatics curricula" [5].

As a grassroots initiative, TIGER not only encourages its community members to identify practical health informatics issues in the field (e.g., developing projects based on its members' needs), it also serves as a bridge to provide evidence-based recommendations to allow for an easy translation from theory to practice. By providing the necessary resources to integrate technology and health informatics into education, clinical practice and research, the TIGER Initiative helps prepare the next generation of global healthcare professionals to improve patient care [5]. This chapter will detail TIGER's evolution from nursing to an interprofessional perspective, from formulating global competency recommendations to leveraging recently developed recommendation frameworks for competency attainment applicable to all disciplines. As reflected in Table 38.1, TIGER's interprofessional audiences comprise academic professionals, students, early careerists/adult learners, clinical educators, and a hybrid of one or more.

TIGER Initiative and Interprofessional Community: Strategies, Resources, and Tools

TIGER's Transition into HIMSS

The TIGER Foundation (2009–2014) was incorporated in 2011 to help prepare nurses and interprofessional colleagues to use informatics and emerging technologies to make healthcare safer, more effective, efficient, patient-centered, timely, and equitable.

The TIGER Foundation was, however, not able to maintain sufficient funding. In 2014, TIGER transitioned into the Healthcare Information and Management Systems Society (HIMSS) and is currently supported by the Professional Development department. As TIGER prepared to transition into HIMSS, pioneers of the initiative recognized the work that began to benefit the nursing community was applicable to informatics—regardless of discipline. With this transition, TIGER began embracing an interdisciplinary approach with a global perspective woven into every project, resource, and tool created. TIGER pioneers, such as Dr. Marion J. Ball, Joyce Sensmeier, Michelle Troseth, Diane Skiba, and countless nursing informaticists, recognized the critical need to enter into an interprofessional space while upholding and learning from its rich nursing history.

HIMSS, a global, cause-based, not-for-profit organization focused on better health through information and technology [6], provided the perfect foundation for the TIGER Initiative to expand upon. HIMSS leads efforts to optimize health engagements and care outcomes using information *and* technology. With a unique depth of expertise and capabilities, HIMSS works to improve the quality, safety, and efficiency of health, healthcare, and care outcomes. The HIMSS vision is to realize the full health potential of every human, everywhere; the HIMSS mission is focused on reforming the global

TIGER's History: Past to Current

2004

The National Mandate for Healthcare Informatics

- Creation of the **Forerunner of the Office of the National Coordinator (ONC)** of Health Information Technology by U.S. President George W. Bush
  - Strategy: **Electronic health record within a 10-year** timeframe
- **Lack of nurse representation** at the first ONC National Health IT conference

2005

The Birth of the TIGER Initiative

- A group of leaders in nursing called the 'TIGER Team' for *Technology Informatics Guiding Educational Reform* began a **grassroots effort** to ensure **nursing** would be integrated into the nation's healthcare delivery systems and academic programs with other key stakeholders/ advocates of health IT.

TIGER Pioneers include:
- Marion J. Ball
- Joyce Sensmeier
- Patricia Hinton Walker
- Diane Skiba
- Michelle Troseth
- Brian Gugerty

2006 - 2014

The TIGER Summit
&
Publication of Landmark Reports from Collaborative Workgroups (see **Section 4.1**)

- **TIGER Summit 2006**: Consensus on a 10-year vision and a 3-year action plan[1]
- TIGER's Recommendations for Integrating Technology to Transform Practice and Education[2]
- **Summary Report**[3]
- Identification of nine key "collaboratives" and publication of workgroups **landmark reports**, including:
  - Informatics Competencies[4]
  - Usability & Clinical Application Design[5]
  - Leadership Development
  - Consumer Empowerment & Personal Health Records
  - Education and Faculty Development
  - Usability & Clinical Application Design
- The TIGER Initiative became established as the **TIGER Foundation**, with more than 1500 volunteers

2009

Launch of the TIGER Virtual Learning Environment (see **Section 3.1**)

- **Web-based education portal** designed to expand health IT/informatics knowledge and skillset in a self-paced format Courses tied to certificates of completion
  - Resource library
  - Webinar events archive
- First major relaunch in 2015
- Second major relaunch in 2019

2011

Publication of Nursing Informatics: Where Technology and Caring Meet (4th edition) (see **Section 5**)

- The 4th edition of this world-renowned book was dedicated to the over 1,000 volunteers who have contributed to the TIGER cause since formalizing in 2005.
- This edition has gone on to sell over 80,000 copies and was translated into six languages.

2012

International Expansion

- TIGER launches the **TIGER International Committee** to support the global health informatics workforce

Fig. 38.1 TIGER's beginnings as a grassroots nursing initiative . [1]TIGER Summit Consensus available at http://www.tigersummit.com/uploads/TIGERInitiative_Report2007_Color.pdf. [2]TIGER's Recommendations for Integrating Technology to Transform Practice and Education available at http://s3.amazonaws.com/rdcms-himss/files/production/public/FileDownloads/the-leadership-imperative.pdf. [3]Summary Report available at http://www.tigersummit.com/uploads/TIGER_Collaborative_Exec_Summary_040509.pdf. [4]Informatics Competencies report available at http://www.tigersummit.com/uploads/3.Tiger.Report_Competencies_final.pdf. [5]Usability & Clinical Application Design report available at http://www.tigersummit.com/uploads/Tiger_Usability_Report.pdf

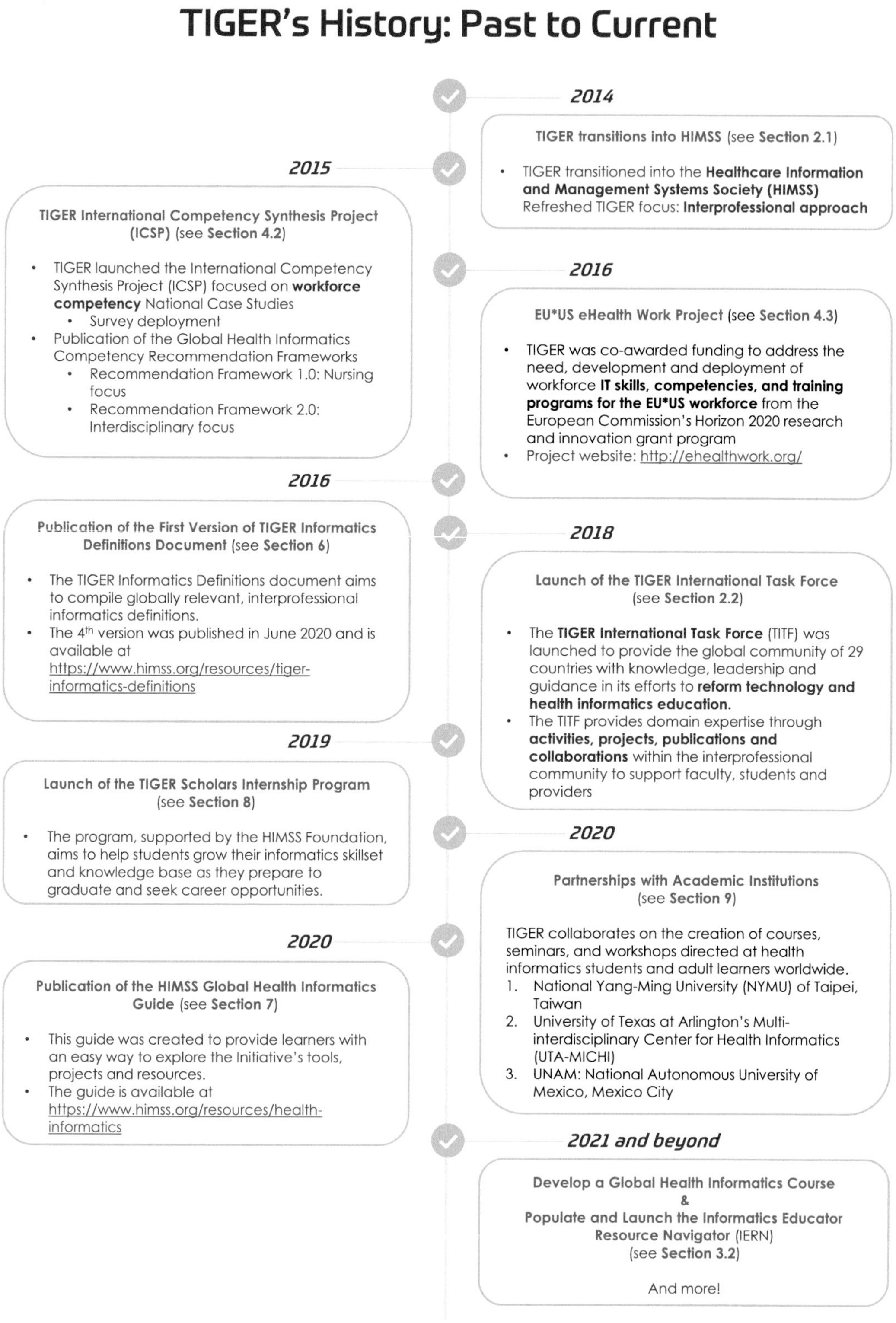

TIGER's History: Past to Current

2014

TIGER transitions into HIMSS (see Section 2.1)

- TIGER transitioned into the **Healthcare Information and Management Systems Society (HIMSS)** Refreshed TIGER focus: **Interprofessional approach**

2015

TIGER International Competency Synthesis Project (ICSP) (see Section 4.2)

- TIGER launched the International Competency Synthesis Project (ICSP) focused on **workforce competency** National Case Studies
  - Survey deployment
- Publication of the Global Health Informatics Competency Recommendation Frameworks
  - Recommendation Framework 1.0: Nursing focus
  - Recommendation Framework 2.0: Interdisciplinary focus

2016

EU*US eHealth Work Project (see Section 4.3)

- TIGER was co-awarded funding to address the need, development and deployment of workforce **IT skills, competencies, and training programs for the EU*US workforce** from the European Commission's Horizon 2020 research and innovation grant program
- Project website: http://ehealthwork.org/

2016

Publication of the First Version of TIGER Informatics Definitions Document (see Section 6)

- The TIGER Informatics Definitions document aims to compile globally relevant, interprofessional informatics definitions.
- The 4th version was published in June 2020 and is available at https://www.himss.org/resources/tiger-informatics-definitions

2018

Launch of the TIGER International Task Force (see Section 2.2)

- The **TIGER International Task Force** (TITF) was launched to provide the global community of 29 countries with knowledge, leadership and guidance in its efforts to **reform technology and health informatics education.**
- The TITF provides domain expertise through **activities, projects, publications and collaborations** within the interprofessional community to support faculty, students and providers

2019

Launch of the TIGER Scholars Internship Program (see Section 8)

- The program, supported by the HIMSS Foundation, aims to help students grow their informatics skillset and knowledge base as they prepare to graduate and seek career opportunities.

2020

Partnerships with Academic Institutions (see Section 9)

TIGER collaborates on the creation of courses, seminars, and workshops directed at health informatics students and adult learners worldwide.
1. National Yang-Ming University (NYMU) of Taipei, Taiwan
2. University of Texas at Arlington's Multi-interdisciplinary Center for Health Informatics (UTA-MICHI)
3. UNAM: National Autonomous University of Mexico, Mexico City

2020

Publication of the HIMSS Global Health Informatics Guide (see Section 7)

- This guide was created to provide learners with an easy way to explore the Initiative's tools, projects and resources.
- The guide is available at https://www.himss.org/resources/health-informatics

2021 and beyond

Develop a Global Health Informatics Course & Populate and Launch the Informatics Educator Resource Navigator (IERN) (see Section 3.2)

And more!

Fig. 38.2 TIGER's transition toward a global and interprofessional community

Table 38.1   TIGER's core target audiences

Type of audience	Objective
Academic Professionals	Seek to find and easily integrate resources and modules into classroom curricula and supplemental materials
Students	Seek to expand their informatics knowledge base and skill set as they prepare to graduate, secure an internship, etc.
Early Careerists/ Adult Learners	Seek to expand their informatics knowledge base to advance their career trajectories or gain inroads into the field
Clinical Educators	Seek resources and courses to support their staff as they evolve informatics knowledge base and skillset
Hybrid of two or more	Many fall into one or more of these buckets. They are short on time allocated to finding tools and resources to expand their informatics foundation.

healthcare ecosystem through the power of information and technology [6]. With more than 350 employees located around the world, HIMSS is headquartered in Chicago, IL, with operations in North America, the Asia Pacific, Europe, Latin America, the Middle East, and the UK.

TIGER International Task Force

While TIGER's grassroots efforts formalized in the USA, international expansion began in 2012, with the launch of the TIGER International Committee, with the goal of supporting the health informatics workforce and scientific community. Since 2018, all volunteer groups have been merged into one under the TIGER International Task Force (TITF).

The TITF "is charged with providing domain expertise, leadership and guidance to activities, projects and collaborations within the global health informatics community" [7]. Work streams

aligned to defined scopes of work and goals further support the TITF with actualizing the vision refined on an annual basis.

As of 2021, the TITF was comprised of 96 members representing 34 different countries (Australia, Austria, Brazil, Canada, Chile, China, Denmark, Finland, Germany, Ghana, India, Iran, Ireland, Japan, Mexico, New Zealand, Nigeria, Pakistan, Panama, Peru, the Philippines, Portugal, Qatar, Saudi Arabia, Singapore, South Korea, Spain, Switzerland, Taiwan, Turkey, United Kingdom (UK-England, Scotland), United Arab Emirates (UAE), and the USA).

The TITF is divided into two core volunteer streams:

- Active volunteers serving on the Task Force with a two-year term.
- Global TIGER Network (GTN): The GTN was created to keep emeritus volunteers and pioneers of the initiative still engaged when formal volunteer terms conclude.

The interprofessional TIGER landscape at HIMSS is two-fold: The Initiative's staff at HIMSS collaborates with volunteers via the TITF to co-create educational resources (events, projects, publications, tools, etc.) that the interprofessional community consumes. The community members benefit from the development of resources outlined above to assist with educational gaps, clinical practice, and research, focusing on preparing the next generation of global healthcare professionals.

In addition to the volunteer streams, the TIGER interprofessional community opt-in for HIMSS members was created to "engage and prepare the global workforce in using technology and health informatics to improve the delivery of patient care" [8]. The TIGER Initiative contributes to the community by developing tools and resources to aid clinical practice, educational needs, and research focused on expanding knowledge base and skillset to help advance the career trajectories of the global healthcare workforce.

Those interested in getting involved with TIGER are encouraged to reach out via email at tiger@himss.org.

Emergence of the TIGER VLE: Web-Based Education Portal

TIGER Virtual Learning Environment

The TIGER Virtual Learning Environment (VLE) emerged as a web-based education portal in 2009.

The mission and vision of the education portal encompass the true essence of the TIGER spirit [9]:

- **Mission:** To maintain an accessible educational portal that meets the ever-changing knowledge development needs of the global health IT workforce.
- **Vision:** To support students, adult learners, and educators in their efforts to grow and learn in the ever-changing health information technology (IT) industry by decreasing barriers and increasing access to current, high quality, resources focused on health informatics topics and expert content through relevant webinar events.

Powered by HIMSS, the TIGER VLE is an interactive, online learning platform containing:

1. Courses tied to certificates of completion
2. A globally relevant *Resource Library* and
3. Archived webinar events designed to expand health IT/informatics knowledge and skillset in a self-paced format

Courses Tied to Certificates of Completion

The education portal's first major relaunch took place in 2015, shortly after moving from a stand-alone foundation to HIMSS. With this relaunch, the first course was aligned and tied to a certifi-

cate of completion: *Health Information Technology (IT) Foundations (HITF)*. HITF is a foundational course housed by Carnegie Mellon University's (CMU) Open Learning Initiative (OLI) focused on interprofessionals who are new to the health IT field. This course offers an overview of healthcare, health I.T., and health information management systems. The focus is on the role and responsibilities of entry-level health IT specialists in each phase of the health information management systems lifecycle. The course curriculum is aligned to the Certified Associate in Healthcare Information and Management Systems (CAHIMS) certification administered by HIMSS. For more information about HIMSS certification, please visit https://www.himss.org/resources-certification/overview.

TIGER VLE Resource Library

In preparation for a complete overhaul of the VLE, TIGER relaunched a VLE Workgroup in fall 2018. Workgroup members, led by Dr. Jennifer (Jenna) Thate of Siena College, helped keep the online learning platform up to date, streamlined and intuitive for those seeking to evolve their knowledge base. A priority of the group was to increase access to current, high-quality technology and informatics resources for the interprofessional community. The education portal was fully reimagined and relaunched to streamline the look and feel of the HIMSS Learning Center. The most recent VLE refinement took place in July 2020 to align the TIGER VLE to the new HIMSS branding. The *Resource Library* is useful for keeping up with current and emerging trends with multidisciplinary offerings that are globally applicable. There, learners will easily find content that reflects the ever-changing and expansive state of the health IT industry within 18 diverse categories such as AI/machine learning, innovation, interoperability, privacy and security, and more.

By highlighting the work of open source collaborators, TIGER sifts through information from around the world to curate content for our subscribers. Educators can then easily integrate these resources and modules into classroom curricula and beyond.

Webinar Events and Archive

In 2016, the TIGER webinar series debuted within the VLE with events focusing on emerging trends and hot topics in the health informatics field. Today, TIGER hosts a free interprofessional webinar series available to all who desire to attend. Event recordings are then archived for on-demand listening within the VLE. CA/CPHIMS enduring credits are available for one hour per event. The *Webinar Archive* is also useful for keeping up with current events and topics of interest, such as the COVID-19 pandemic. Event recordings are tied to 11 distinct content categories such as health informatics, health information management (HIM), nursing, telehealth, amongst others, along with a collection of recorded EU*US eHealth Work Project-related events.

TIGER VLE Educational Resources Under Development

TIGER VLE's robust offerings will be further strengthened with the development of new tools and resources currently underway.

Informatics Educators Resource Navigator

The TITF is working to curate and launch the Informatics Educators Resource Navigator (IERN). The development workstream is led by Drs. David Marc and David Gibbs. IERN is intended to be a valuable resource within the VLE to support health informatics education while also striving to be "educate the educators" about the ever-changing and expanding field of informatics. Informatics-focused educators from academic and clinical settings will have access to up-to-date documents, best practices, case studies, tutorial videos, and templates to leverage in educational efforts and curricular development. These resources will be tied to recommended competencies with the goal of designing resources aligned to competency attainment (*see Sect. 4.1—TIGER International Competency Synthesis Project for more information about Recommendation Frameworks 1.0 (nursing centric) and 2.0 (interprofessional)*).

In Chap. 12 titled *The Educator's View: Global Needs for Health Informatics Education and Training*, the authors shared a few of the pain points educators face when it comes to teaching informatics. IERN's goal is to have readily available resources for informatics educators that showcase "state of the art" resources valued in education and training based on "what works" in the real world.

These curated resources also seek to address the 10 gaps identified during the EU*US eHealth Work Project [10]:

1. Health informatics knowledge and skills of healthcare professionals
2. Health informatics knowledge and skills of informal caregivers
3. Knowledge and skills of teachers and trainers
4. Availability of courses and programs at various levels and for various professions
5. Quality and quantity of eHealth training material
6. Adaptation of job descriptions, training on the job, staff development
7. eHealth infrastructure
8. eHealth usage
9. Acceptance and usability of systems
10. Shortage of health professionals and gender disparities

Global Health Informatics Course

In partnership with the University of Texas at Arlington's Multi-Interprofessional Center for Health Informatics (UTA-MICHI), TIGER will co-develop a global health informatics course (GHIC) focused on the fundamentals of health informatics and digital health. This marks the first time that TIGER is venturing into curriculum development.

Global Activities: From Recommendations to Actionable Partnerships

TIGER Informatics Competencies Collaborative

As a nursing informatics grassroots initiative, TIGER pioneered the development of core nursing informatics competency frameworks. This work began in 2010 when the TIGER Informatics Competencies Collaborative (TICC) was formed to develop informatics recommendations for all practicing nurses and nursing students. The group published a landmark report titled *Informatics Competencies for Every Practicing Nurse: Recommendations from the TIGER Collaborative* [11].

To this day, the TIGER Initiative continues to innovate globally by defining and standardizing core competencies across multiple health informatics disciplines. TIGER's competency frameworks have notably been featured and leveraged in many publications and have informed curricula found in the literature [12].

Competency Recommendation Frameworks: Priorities for Health Informatics Professionals

Since 2011, TIGER's emphasis has shifted from solely working in the benefit of the nursing workforce to interprofessional with a global focus and the conversation around competency development was catapulted forward through the launch of the **TIGER International Competency Synthesis Project (ICSP)**. "In a changing and dynamic (health informatics) environment, TIGER continues to encourage the adoption of informatics competencies through existing education, research, and work from practice groups" [13]. The ICSP is dedicated to highlighting core recommended informatics competencies and recognition of the role of education as a powerful enabler and change agent. The project's initial objective was "to empirically define and validate a framework of globally accepted core competency areas in health informatics and to enrich this framework with exemplar information derived from local educational settings" initially focused on the nursing domain [14].

In 2015, TIGER began comprehensive activities to compile recommended core competencies reflective of many countries, scientific societies, and research projects. This project initially comprised three phases:

1. Deployment of a survey to evaluate and prioritize a broad list of core competencies. Based on the survey results, core informatics competencies of health care professionals within the five domains were identified: (1) nursing management, (2) IT management in nursing (e.g., nurse informatics officer), (3) quality management, (4) interprofessional coordination of care, and (5) clinical nursing. The survey yielded participants from 21 countries to capture a global perspective.

2. Next, a compilation of national case studies from Australia, Brazil, China/Taiwan, Finland, Germany (inclusive of Austria and Switzerland), Ireland, New Zealand, the Philippines, Portugal, Scotland, and the USA focused on integrating local perspectives and needs.

3. Development of a *Recommendation Framework* outlining both shared and country-specific competencies derived from the survey results, case studies, and stakeholder input. Framework 1.0 was developed in collaboration with the University of Applied Sciences Osnabruck, Germany, and the Competency Development for Health Professionals in the Context of Lifelong Learning (KeGL) project (German: *Kompetenzentwicklung für Gesundheitsfachberufe im Kontext des lebenslangen Lernens*). The KeGL project was funded by the German Federal Ministry of Education and Research (BMBF). As an "open education project", KeGL encourages interdisciplinary learners to support continuing education course for professionals in the healthcare field.

Insights gathered from national case studies, survey findings, and stakeholder input served as building blocks of information to populate *Recommendation Framework 1.0*. National case study discoveries were matched to survey competency areas with expert stakeholder input cementing the conclusions before being reassembled into a "Framework." Framework 1.0 showcases the top 10 competency areas within the five nursing roles outlined above, with relevance ratings derived from global stakeholders and workshop attendees gathered throughout the project's evolution.

Framework 1.0 is directed at nurses, providing a grid of knowledge for teachers and learners alike that is instantiated with knowledge about informatics competencies, professional roles, priorities, and practical local experience. It also provides a methodology for developing frameworks for other professions/disciplines. Finally, this framework lays the foundation of cross-country learning in health informatics education for nurses and other health professionals.

Based on the project findings, the priorities found in this framework strived to help health care professionals better meet the requirements of an interprofessional process and outcome-oriented way of providing modern care. Overall, the project aimed to develop a framework for core informatics competencies, to derive recommendations for education, and finally, to show best practice examples on how to make use of these recommendations.

The project findings and case studies were leveraged as the foundation to begin the EU*eHealth Work Project, which is discussed in detail within Sect. 4.2.1.

EU*US eHealth Work Project

In September 2016, the TIGER Initiative via the HIMSS Foundation was co-awarded funding to address the need, development, and deployment of workforce IT skills, competencies, and training programs from the European Commission's Horizon 2020 research and innovation grant program. The EU*US eHealth Work Project worked on measuring, informing, educating, and advancing the development of a skilled eHealth workforce throughout the European Union (EU), USA and globally with its Consortium members and a larger stakeholder community. The overall project goal was to create a legacy of digitally empowered health care professionals. More specifically, the Consortium aimed to describe and validate *Recommendation Framework 2.0*, meant to augment nursing focus to a series of other professional roles, i.e., direct patient care, health information management, executives, chief information officers, health IT specialists, researchers, and educators. Insights were extracted from survey input across 51 countries and from 22 global case studies [15]. Table 38.2 summarizes the top 10 health informatics core competency areas for healthcare and health informatics professionals that were identified in the survey [16, 17].

TIGER was an ideal partner for several reasons: many volunteers and collaborators reside in Europe and the initiative was able to capitalize on the ICSP work that began in 2015. Moreover, TIGER's global network is far-reaching, with strong global alliances with healthcare professionals rooted in the heart of care delivery, education, and training.

The project presented a unique opportunity for both HIMSS and TIGER to collaborate with European partners on an international level. As a Consortium member, the HIMSS Foundation, via the TIGER Initiative, worked to transform health through information and technology to benefit global workforce development. By mapping, quantifying, and projecting the need, supply, and demand for competencies and development of IT skills, the Consortium worked to realize a trained and skilled transatlantic eHealth workforce. The project focus also benefited health care workers on a global scale.

This Consortium and its stakeholders formed a network of partners from academia, healthcare providers, and industry, providing access to a rich wealth of experience and knowledge in health informatics education and training to heighten skills and knowledge. More specifically, the Consortium's mission was to (1) map skills and competencies, (2) provide access to knowledge

Table 38.2 Top 10 health informatics core competency areas for health professionals and other roles as identified by TIGER International Competency Synthesis Project (ICSP)

	Nurses, physicians and other patient care providers	Health information management	Executives (clinical and administrative)	Chief information officers (CIO) (clinical and technical)	Engineering or health IT specialist	Science and education
1	Communication	Communication	Leadership	Leadership	Communication	Communication
2	Documentation	Documentation	Communication	Communication	Care processes & IT integration	Teaching, training & education in health care
3	Information & Knowledge management in patient care	Data analytics	Quality & safety management	Care processes & IT integration	Information & communication technology (applications)	Leadership
4	Quality & safety management	Leadership	Information & knowledge management in patient care	Principles of management	Leadership	Learning techniques
5	Leadership	Data protection & security	Strategic management	Quality & safety management	Project management	Ethics in health IT
6	Learning techniques	Information & knowledge management in patient care	Principles of management	Strategic management	Data protection & security	Documentation
7	Teaching, training & education in healthcare	Ethics in health IT	Legal issues in health IT	Process management	Ethics in health IT	Information & knowledge management in patient care
8	Ethics in health IT	Principles of health informatics	Process management	Change & stakeholder management	Interoperability & integration	Principles of health informatics
9	Information & communication technology (applications)	Care processes & IT integration	Resource planning & management	Ethics in health IT	Documentation	Quality & safety management
10	Care processes & IT integration	Learning techniques	Ethics in health IT	Resource planning & management	Process management	Data analytics

tools and platforms, and (3) strengthen, disseminate and exploit success outcomes for a skilled transatlantic eHealth workforce. Not looking to recreate the wheel, the Consortium executed this project by undertaking research, available resources and tools such as the Health IT Competencies Tool and Repository known as HITComp, and leveraged previous dissemination efforts related to the eHealth/health IT workforce. Figure 38.3 details milestones in TIGER's competency development work in collaboration with HOS and the EU*US eHealth Work Project findings.

The EU*US eHealth Work Project encompassed five major work plans (WP) as detailed in Fig. 38.4. TIGER, with the University of Applied Sciences in Osnabrück Germany (Hochschule Osnabrück (HOS)) were responsible for large segments of the WPs that included:

- **White paper** publication detailing the project titled *EU*US eHealth Works to Improve Global Workforce Development* [18];
- **Survey** that served as the flagship of the project as findings informed the development of all project deliverables that followed. The survey helped to identify global health IT/eHealth workforce development needs, trends, and gaps to help the Consortium to create the big picture of how to achieve a highly skilled workforce regionally, across borders, and on a global scale. The survey also captured information about health IT skillset, available curricula and/or workplace training programs, and skill assessment tools along with educational needs and trends to inform future state mapping for the transatlantic workforce. Overall, 1080 participants from 51 countries shared their insights;
- **Gap analysis findings**, formulated based on the survey results, identified 10 major gaps in skills, training, funding, and other areas of eHealth workforce preparation, development, and advancement;
- **Compilation of 22 global case studies** that speak to survey and gap analysis findings: disparities in health IT skillset; available curriculum and/or workplace training programs and

skills assessment tools; educational needs, trends, and future state mapping for the transatlantic workforce.

In addition to the work plans listed above, additional resources developed by the project include:

- Interactive Website Platform (IWP) to locate eHealth tools, resources, information, and education (TRIE)
- Educator Demonstrator Modules (EDM) are instruction videos focused on cybersecurity and how to leverage HITComp and the foundational course.
- Stakeholder Engagement Event Recordings
- Skills Knowledge and Assessment Development Framework (SKAD)

The ICSP is ongoing. In the near future, HOS and TIGER will explore the development of *Recommendation Framework 3.0* dedicated to the patient perspective and their empowerment through the newly awarded project, eHealth4All@ EU—an interprofessional European eHealth program rooted in higher education.

Funded by ERASMUS+, the European Commissions (EC)'s program, which supports education, training, youth, and sports, brings TIGER partners from academic institutions located in Finland, Germany, and Portugal together to solve problem-based learning, develop interdisciplinary, open-access online courses and host an in-person summer school session in the future. As eHealth remains a priority throughout EU member states, developing interdisciplinary digital education will address pressing barrier issues such as lack of awareness, comprehension, and technology confidence to benefit the interprofessional workforce [19].

Moreover, the eHealth4All@EU project will integrate the 2.0 Framework's top competency categories aligned to curricula and summer school offerings. This project, coupled with TIGER's resources under development, will act as incubators to further apply and validate the framework.

TIGER's Work in Competency Development
From TIGER's International Competency Synthesis Project (ICSP) to the EU*US eHealth Work Project and beyond

TIGER's International Competency Synthesis Project (ICSP)

In 2015, TIGER began compiling core recommended international informatics competencies reflective of many countries, scientific societies and research projects.

 National Case Studies

Compiled national studies from the global TIGER community

 Survey deployment

Deployed a survey composed of 24 core competencies within five domains

 Recommendation Framework 1.0 – nursing centric

Creation derived from case studies, survey results and global stakeholder input.

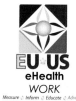

The EU*US eHealth Work Project
2016 – 2019

TIGER was co-awarded funding from the European Commission's Horizon 2020 to **measure, inform, educate and advance** development of a skilled eHealth workforce throughout the EU, US and globally.

 Survey & gap analysis

1,080 professionals participated from 51 countries; 10 gap areas identified

 Global case studies

22 studies compiled to highlight and enrich the survey and gap analysis findings
Available: https://www.himss.org/resources/developing-skilled-transatlantic-ehealth-workforce-case-studies-report

 Foundational course

Global introductory online course in eHealth
Available: http://hitcomp.org/education/

 Recommendation Frameworks 2.0 - interdisciplinary

TIGER joined forces with the EU*US eHealth Work Project to describe and validate the framework
Available: https://www.himss.org/resources/global-health-informatics-competency-recommendation-frameworks

eHealth Competency Repository: http://hitcomp.org/competencies/

Fig. 38.3 Project components from the ICSP and the EU*US eHealth Work Project that populated Recommendation Frameworks 1.0 and 2.0

EU*US eHealth Work Project —Five Major Work Plans

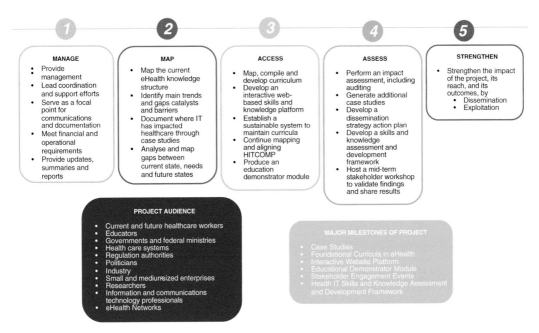

Fig. 38.4 Five major work plans tied to the EU*US eHealth Work Project. Adapted by Man Qing Liang. Original figure from the EU*US eHealth Work Project Consortium

Publication of the Fourth Edition of the Nursing Informatics: Where Technology and Caring Meet Book

The fourth edition of *Nursing Informatics: Where Technology and Caring Meet* was edited by pioneers of the TIGER Initiative (Marion J. Ball, Judith V. Douglas, Patricia Hinton Walker, Donna DuLong, Brian Gugerty, Kathryn J. Hannah, Joan Kiel, Susan Newbold, Joyce Sensmeier, Diane Skiba, and Michelle Troseth). This book served as a definitive guide to the informatics transformation led by hundreds of nurse advocates through the TIGER Initiative [20]. The book also showcased the work accomplished by the nine key collaboratives that have been identified following the first TIGER summit in 2007: (1) Education and faculty development, (2) Staff development, (3) Informatics competencies, (4) Standards and interoperability, (5) Usability and clinical application design, (6) Leadership development, (7) National health information technology agenda, (8) Virtual demonstration center, and (9) Consumer and personal health record.

The current edition, the fifth edition, has been updated to align each chapter to the TIGER International Competency Synthesis Project (ICSP) categories (see Sect. 4.3).

Illuminating Health Informatics Terminology

In 2015, the HIMSS TIGER Initiative began compiling interprofessional informatics definitions, which became publicly available in 2016. The catalyst for creating the document was to collaboratively define and document core informatics terminology to provide context to the TIGER interprofessional community. The document initially strived to serve as a reference for consideration when the terms were included in newly created resources, official documents, and throughout the TIGER VLE. Over time, this document took on more meaning in the benefit of the global informatics-focused workforce. Rather than creating new definitions, TIGER aimed to curate global definitions that have been defined by world experts in the field and leading institutions. When strung together, these definitions form the story of how health informatics has evolved over the last decade.

The fourth edition of the document, published in 2020, was refined to embrace a global focus inclusive of an informatics timeline, with a revised statement of purpose and updated infographics. The re-focused iteration includes cross-discipline informatics terms that are applicable locally, nationally, and globally [21]. In an increasingly virtual environment, the unprecedented need to facilitate data and knowledge sharing at the international level requires definitions relating to informatics that extend beyond geographic borders and regions [21].

Not only does this document provide context to the interdisciplinary informatics community, it also defines these terms, which are critical for helping new specialties and professions within the informatics field take shape and "illuminate different health professions and their specialties, especially when it comes to those related to health informatics" [21].

You can access and download the fourth version of TIGER's *Global Informatics Definitions* document at https://www.himss.org/resources/tiger-informatics-definitions.

Health Informatics Guide Focused on TIGER's Competency Development Work

The HIMSS Health Informatics guide "aims to acquaint those learning about the field with a direct conduit on where to locate and how to leverage the tools and resources available" within the global competency development and attainment domain [18]. Inspired by TIGER and other leading institutions around the world tied to competency development work published in recent years, the guide focuses on the growth of global informatics competencies related to:

- **Aligning core health informatics competencies:** Numerous health professional associations have identified proficiency with informatics solutions as an essential competency to develop as a health professional. Due to the rapidly changing and evolving informatics landscape, informatics educators are having a hard time keeping up with the required skills necessary to not only understand informatics but teach it to their target audiences. The guide expands upon the core competencies required in nursing, medicine, pharmacy while addressing gaps in education and training and sharing possible solutions and resources to remedy gaps and pain points.

- **Understanding basic health informatics competency terminology:** This section outlines core competence categories identified in the TIGER ICSP and describes how "core competencies can be understood as a broadly specialized system of skills, abilities or knowledge necessary to achieve a specific goal [22]. Healthcare organizations, health informatics educators, and students are encouraged to use the recommendation framework as a compass to identify competence areas relevant to their local setting [17].

- **Workforce development needs to be tied to health informatics branches:** Health informatics is a multidisciplinary field that weaves together technology, healthcare, computer science, research, and information. By exploring the informatics competencies showcased throughout the guide, professionals may be inspired to pursue a career in one of the many branches of health informatics, which include:

1. Clinical Informatics
2. Consumer Health Informatics
3. Nursing Informatics
4. Pharmacy Informatics
5. Public Health Informatics

The guide also emphasizes the importance of supporting interprofessional cooperation with a focus on the importance of leadership and communication amongst occupational groups. This concept is essential as clinicians working in direct patient care (nurses, physicians, allied health professionals) share overlapping competencies, and there is much to be learned from one another [14].

With an ever-increasing amount of data generated in healthcare, the last decade has created many new promising career opportunities at the intersection of healthcare and informatics. Aspiring health informatics professionals are encouraged to develop a mix of competencies in diverse domains, such as technology, computer science, management, ethics, communication, and patient care, to meet the increasing demand for a competent informatics healthcare workforce in the years to come [23].

Launch of the TIGER Scholars Informatics Internship Program

The TIGER Scholars Informatics Internship Program was formally launched across the enterprise in 2020. The program's vision is to advance the spirit of TIGER as an interprofessional initiative by contributing to the future interdisciplinary, informatics-focused workforce. The mission is for TIGER to mentor and help advance future healthcare leaders by establishing a global scholars program directed at undergraduate students and those seeking advanced level degrees (master and doctoral levels). This program contributes to TIGER's enduring legacy and honors the countless individuals and organizations instrumental in the initiative coming into existence and transforming over the last 16 years.

Every year, two interns (one domestic, one international) seeking a healthcare master's degree or doctorate are selected to participate in the program which the HIMSS Foundation financially supports. The program's goal is to help students grow their informatics skillset and knowledge base as they prepare to graduate and seek career opportunities. Program components include (1) Mentorship and professional coaching via the global TIGER volunteer network; (2) the opportunity to serve as a Program Assistant at the HIMSS global health conference; (3) complimentary HIMSS student membership; and (4) complimentary access to the TIGER VLE and courses aligned to certificates of completion. All interns participate in the program remotely.

This unique internship program offers the opportunity for students to enhance their understanding of health informatics education and practice; grow their global professional networks; cultivate relationships with leading informatics subject matter experts; engage in activities that promote the informatics profession via advocacy and educational opportunities; learn firsthand about the opportunities and services offered by HIMSS and TIGER for career advancement, certification, professional development; and finally, to contribute to the TIGER interprofessional community at HIMSS by serving as a member of the TIGER International Task Force (TITF) through conferences, meetings, webinar events, workstreams, etc.

The open call to apply for the program goes out every spring. Candidates are selected to interview in the summer before two students are onboarded for the yearlong academic internship to begin at the end of August into early September through May of the following year.

TIGER's Partnerships with Academic Institutions

National Yang Ming University (Taiwan)

In March 2020, TIGER executed its first academic partnership with National Yang-Ming University (NYMU) located in Taipei, Taiwan. The partnership focuses on developing courses, seminars and workshops hosted at the university and throughout mainland China inspired by TIGER ICSP recommendation frameworks and publications. The goal of this partnership is to support the expansion of informatics education and knowledge for interdisciplinary healthcare professionals at all career stages. Each offering is tied to a certificate of completion from HIMSS, NYMU, and TIGER.

Recent training sessions and workshops focus on basic informatics competencies, workflow analysis, mobile health, documentation, analytics, hospital systems, and information systems inclusive of hands-on experience and demonstration of how to integrate these concepts into the nursing process, applications for documentation, analytics, etc. Site visits are also woven into the training process when applicable.

The University of Texas at Arlington's Multi-Interprofessional Center for Health Informatics

Focused on preparing the next generation of global healthcare professionals with expanded health informatics knowledge and skillset, the HIMSS Professional Development (PD) Center of Excellence and the University of Texas at Arlington's (UTA) Multi-Interprofessional Center for Health Informatics (MICHI) seek to establish a dynamic partnership focused on providing academic professionals, students, clinical educators, and adult learners with courses and educational events that will yield continuing education credits and certificates of completion that align to certification exams offered by HIMSS.

The TIGER Initiative and UTA-MICHI will work together to promote existing courses and develop new curricula and workshops inspired by the EU*US eHealth Work Project and this textbook. The first offering, a Global Health Informatics Course (GHIC), is anticipated to be market-ready/available for purchase in August 2021. Course access will be available via the TIGER VLE. In 2022, the partnership will focus on developing additional courses and hosting in-person and digital workshops aligned to the chapters reflected in this textbook in collaboration with the University of Applied Sciences Osnabrück Germany (HOS).

National Autonomous University of Mexico

The National Autonomous University of Mexico's (UNAM) Biomedical Informatics department is working on translating and providing the foundation course from the EU*US eHealth Work Project in Spanish. During the translation process, the course is being custom-ized to address content gaps and interweave country and local eHealth priorities and needs to benefit the University's target audiences (faculty, staff, and students). This course will also be aligned to a certificate of completion. Finally, UNAM and TIGER will work together to translate additional courses as they become market-ready to translate into Spanish. Moving into 2022 and beyond, the partnership's goal is to make Spanish-translated health informatics-focused courses and additional resources available to the public.

Case Study

Nursing Informatics Competency Development in China and Taiwan

Polun Chang, Chiao-Ling Chelsey Hsu, Yuan Chen, Qian Xiao, Meihua Ji, Jiwen Sun, Yu Qian, Wenyi Luo, Peipei Xue, Hong Lu and Cuihong Liu

National Yang-Ming University, Taipei, Taiwan
Xiamen Cardiovascular Hospital Xiamen University, Xiamen, China
School of Nursing, Capital Medical University, Beijing, China
Shanghai Children's Medical Center, Shanghai, China
Affiliated Eye Hospital of Shandong University of Traditional Chinese Medicine (TCM), Jinan, Shandong, China

TIGER's work in identifying key competency development for the healthcare informatics workforce has been leveraged around the world, notably in China and Taiwan. This case study provides insights into the informatics-focused training efforts in China and Taiwan led by staff from National Yang-Ming University (NYMU), in concert with the HIMSS TIGER Initiative. The efforts began in 2013, when the TIGER competency framework was introduced to Taiwan (Fig. 38.5). Subsequently, the framework was also adapted to reflect the professional and organizational culture in China.

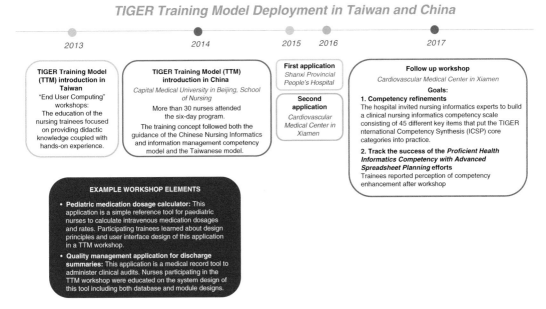

Fig. 38.5 Timeline of TIGER Training Model Deployment in Taiwan & China

The Taiwan model followed a "End User Computing" strategy: Nursing trainees focused on providing didactic knowledge coupled with hands-on experience. End-User Computing is a method leveraged to make non-informatics specialists acquainted with general principles of information systems and their development. Trainees learn to use applications that are commonly used in multiple settings, such as learning to use spreadsheets. This method encourages trainees to feel confident working with information systems, lowers the threshold to get started, raises clinician motivation, and often leads to enhanced self-efficacy.

This competency development program aimed to empower nursing staff to design, lead, and create innovation and, ultimately, improve care safety and effectiveness [24]. The application of the Taiwanese model and the nursing informatics educational component were successful and offered a cost-effective tool. Health care institutions and their corresponding clinical staff were well equipped to deal with challenges associated with innovation and information and communication technologies (ICT).

Following the Taiwanese example, China later embraced the TIGER Training Model (TTM) as well. In 2014, the first training cohort was held at the *School of Nursing, Capital Medical University*

in Beijing. The six-day training concept followed both the guidance of the Chinese Nursing Informatics and information management competency model and the Taiwanese model. Similar to the Taiwanese objective of improving nurses' informatics competencies, the Chinese model also included a nursing information system needs assessment, programming language foundation, process reengineering, form design, application design, data information system application, and interface design [25].

Examples of workshop elements, described in Fig. 38.6, showcase how the TTM workshops are set up to educate nurses about informatics with the goal of building skillsets and capabilities tailored to everyday care practice. The workshops also contribute to the empowerment of learners to assist with the development of future nursing informatics-focused applications.

Hospital Applications and Effects

In practice, the China TIGER Model (CTM) was first applied in a hospital program located at the *Shanxi Provincial People's Hospital* in 2015. In 2016, the model was leveraged at the Cardiovascular Medical Center in Xiamen to develop a strategy focused on hospital informatics competencies development.

In 2020, a workshop was conducted in follow-up to competency refinements and to track the success of the efforts named *Proficient Health Informatics Competency with Advanced Spreadsheet Planning*. In all, 43 nurses attended and 38 successfully completed the training. The hospital invited nursing informatics experts to build a clinical nursing informatics competency scale consisting of 45 different key items that put the TIGER International Competency Synthesis (ICSP) core categories into practice. Table 38.3

provides an excerpt of the results. After the workshop, trainees reported competency confidence in the areas ranked from no. 1 (*Team Work*) to no. 5 (*Interface Design*). Two-thirds of the trainees agreed that these top five computer competency categories were beneficial [26].

Case Study Conclusion

This case study highlighted the application of the TTM to educate nurses in the field of informatics throughout Taiwan and mainland China.

Table 38.3 Top 10: Trainee's self-perception of competency enhancement after the workshop (excerpt) (based on study by Yuan et al. [26])

Rank	Item	Agree/strongly agree to be competent after workshop ($n = 43$)	Related TIGER competencies from Framework 2.0
1	Team Work Having an effective internal cooperation model to complete information management	86%	Communication
2	Nursing Informatics Education Taking the education in Nursing Informatics	79%	Teaching, training & education in healthcare
3	Facilitation Quality Improvement Monitoring the quality indicators, using computers to facilitate statistical analysis and clinical quality improvement	77%	Quality & safety management
4	System Functions and Structures Understanding the nursing-related systems functions and structures	74%	Information & communication technology (applications)
5	Interface Design Knowing good interface design principles and user experiences	72%	Information & communication technology (applications)
6	Feasibility Study Be capable of doing feasibility assessment (e.g., safety, effectiveness, cost impacts)	72%	General competency to become confident designing and implementing a small system via feasibility assessment[a]
7	Clinical Systems and Hardware Understanding clinical information systems (e.g., nursing information system), hardware devices (e.g., monitors, PDA, barcode scanners)	70%	Information & communication technology (applications)
8	Design and Study of Information System Having information system design and research capabilities	70%	Information & communication technology (applications)
9	System Requirement and Communication Being able to propose a feasible clinical system needs by effective communication with IT professionals and users	67%	Communication and Leadership
10	System Feedback and Improvement Being able to doing a routine evaluation, feedback and continuous improvement on information systems	67%	Quality & safety management

[a]Competency not explicitly mentioned in the TIGER Framework 2.0

As presented above, Taiwan led the adoption of the TTM, followed by China. The TTM is applicable in various settings, as illustrated in this case study. The exemplary follow-up assessment from the *Cardiovascular Medical Center* in Xiamen points to crucial and meaningful improvements for nurses expanding their skill set and application of informatics in the field. In particular, trainees reported in multiple areas that their competencies were enhanced and that the acquired skills were valuable. This case study demonstrates how the TTM can be applied in different settings and research opportunities. Finally, it is important to point out the need to modify the TTM for the benefit of other global healthcare systems and the targeted clinical workforce.

Summary

Over the last seven years, TIGER's projects, resources, and tools have been created to serve as building blocks to one another. Since the beginning of 2005, when nursing pioneers first began organizing to birth TIGER, the initiative has continuously blossomed as a grassroots movement. At its core, TIGER represents a network of networks that mirrors the intergenerational, multidisciplinary workforce. As a global network, TIGER works with volunteers (current and Emeritus), community members, and collaborating partners to develop practice resources and tools that can be quickly adopted. The initiative also informs individual practice as a vehicle for digital health/health informatics knowledge expansion. Together, the global TIGER network and its partners create a web of resources; the tighter the weave, the stronger and more resilient the network becomes.

One of the initiative's priorities is connected to the need for updating interprofessional competency recommendations that serve as a conduit to develop curricula and training materials to assist the global health informatics workforce with competency attainment. Competency attainment is a building block to upskilling and career advancement.

Another pressing priority is to educate health informatics educators by curating content that fosters curricula and supplemental resource creation with ease. By supporting informatics educators regardless of where one is located, TIGER strives to address pain points and offer remedies.

As TIGER continues to expand its collaborative catalog of health informatics resources, tools, and soon, curricula, the global network will undoubtedly positively impact how future healthcare leaders are taught and trained to ultimately better patient outcomes.

Conclusions and Outlook

Health information and technology cannot be appropriately adopted or used meaningfully without involving healthcare professionals in the decision-making process. This understanding will require organizational and academic leadership to consider how they can better acquaint staff, clinicians, and educators with digital tools and methods while raising awareness regarding the impact and consequences of health IT integration—the positive as well as negative. Digital literacy must be woven into the onboarding process, upskilling practices, and educational offerings. While scientific societies and associations have issued recommendations within their communities for many years, a lack of approach motivated by the practice and interprofessional coordination in providing patient care remains. TIGER seeks to fill this gap by providing competency recommendations coupled with tools and resources tied to attainment and serving as a connector to volunteer opportunities, community development, and resource creation as the global TIGER network works to expand the interprofessional, intergenerational community at HIMSS. Through this lens, TIGER continues to foster international community development and strives to work as a bridge-builder and conduit for translating what is occurring within the health informatics field into practice. TIGER's expansion beyond international borders and interprofessional silos to integrate health informatics into daily practice to benefit patient care has never been more relevant or important.

As shared in this chapter, one crucial area of focus for TIGER has been global competency development and recommendations to support nurses and the interdisciplinary communities alike post-transition to HIMSS in 2014. The authors recognize that digital literacy for patients and citizens is paramount. TIGER will continue to refine the core competencies as reflected on *Recommendation Frameworks* 1.0 and 2.0 for clinicians while also exploring the compilation of necessary competencies geared toward the patient to empower and recognize patients as an official member of the care coordination team.

Useful Resources

1. eHealth4All@EU Program: https://www.uas7.org/en/ehealth4alleu-interprofessional-european-ehealth-programme-higher-education
2. EU*US eHealth Work Project: http://ehealthwork.org/
   - *EU*US eHealth Works to Improve Global Workforce Development* white paper: https://www.himss.org/sites/hde/files/d7/eu-us-ehealth-workforce-development.pdf
   - The Health IT Competencies Tool and Repository (HITComp): http://hitcomp.org/
   - Skills knowledge assessment and development framework (SKAD): http://ehealthwork.org/Skills%20and%20Knowledge%20Assessment%20and%20Development%20Framework/index.html
   - Compilation of global case studies: https://www.himss.org/resources/developing-skilled-transatlantic-ehealth-workforce-case-studies-report
   - Interactive website platform (IWP): http://ehealthwork.org/IWP/index.html
   - Interactive education demonstrator modules (IEDM):
     Cybersecurity: http://ehealthwork.org/Cybersecurity_FINAL_020617.mp4
     Foundational curriculum: http://ehealthwork.org/Foundational_curricula_video.mp4
     Health IT Competencies Tool and Repository (HITComp): http://ehealthwork.org/hitcomp.mp4

3. HIMSS Certification: https://www.himss.org/resources-certification/overview
   - HIMSS Foundation: https://foundation.himss.org/
   - HIMSS Learning Center: https://www.himsslearn.org/
   - HIMSS TIGER's Global Informatics Definitions v4: https://www.himss.org/resources/tiger-informatics-definitions

4. HIMSS Health Informatics Guide: Inspired by TIGER's global projects and scopes of work over the last six years: https://www.himss.org/resources/health-informatics

5. *The Evolution of the TIGER Initiative* publication in Computers, Informatics, Nursing (CIN): https://journals.lww.com/cinjournal/Citation/2017/06000/The_Evolution_of_the_TIGER_Initiative.2.aspx

6. TIGER Virtual Learning Environment: https://www.himss.org/tiger-virtual-learning-environment

7. TIGER International Competency Synthesis Project: https://www.himss.org/tiger-initiative-international-competency-synthesis-project
   - Recorded project education sessions delivered at HIMSS19: https://www.youtube.com/watch?v=WnmPkcVD97U

8. University of Applied Sciences Osnabrück Germany: https://www.hs-osnabrueck.de

Review Questions

1. In 2014, the TIGER Initiative transitioned from a standalone foundation into which organization?
   (a) AMIA
   (b) HIMSS
   (c) IMIA
   (d) MIE
2. To date, how many recommendation frameworks has the TIGER ICSP created?
   (a) One
   (b) Two
   (c) Three
   (d) Four
3. In 2020, which version of the *HIMSS TIGER Global Informatics Definitions* document was released?

(a) First
(b) Second
(c) Third
(d) Fourth

4. Which of the following was not one of the major working plans defined in the EU*US eHealth Work Project?
   (a) Map
   (b) Assess
   (c) Apply
   (d) Strengthen

5. Which TIGER resource would you recommend for a learner who wishes to become familiar with global health informatics terminology?
   (a) TIGER Health Informatics guide
   (b) TIGER Global Informatics Definitions document
   (c) TIGER International Competency Synthesis Project
   (d) TIGER Virtual Learning Environment

Appendix: Answers to Review Questions

1. In 2014, the TIGER Initiative transitioned from a standalone foundation into which organization?
   (a) AMIA
   (b) HIMSS
   (c) IMIA
   (d) MIE

In 2014, the TIGER Initiative transitioned from a standalone foundation into the HIMSS enterprise. With this move, TIGER shifted its focus from solely nursing informatics to embracing an interdisciplinary, interprofessional approach. TIGER pioneers realized that the work they were doing was applicable regardless of discipline.

2. To date, how many recommendation frameworks has the TIGER ICSP created?
   (a) One
   (b) Two
   (c) Three
   (d) Four

To date, the TIGER International Competency Synthesis Project (ICSP) has released two rec-

ommendation frameworks: 1.0 focused on nursing and 2.0 focused on a broad range of global healthcare professionals and interprofessional collaboration.

3. In 2020, which version of the *HIMSS TIGER Global Informatics Definitions* document was released?
   (a) First
   (b) Second
   (c) Third
   (d) Fourth

In July 2020, TIGER released the fourth version of the Global Informatics Definitions document. The first version was released in 2016. The fourth version embraces a global focus which also includes an informatics timeline, revised statement of purpose, and updated infographics.

4. Which of the following was not one of the major working plans defined in the EU*US eHealth Work Project?
   (a) Map
   (b) Assess
   (c) Apply
   (d) Strengthen

There were five major work plans that were part of the EU*US eHealth Work Project: (1) Manage; (2) Map; (3) Access; (4) Assess; (5) Strengthen. Since the completion of the EU*US eHealth Work Project, TIGER and HOS have continuously worked to apply and publish the project results.

5. Which TIGER resource would you recommend for a learner who wishes to become familiar with global health informatics terminology?
   (a) TIGER Health Informatics guide
   (b) TIGER Global Informatics Definitions document
   (c) TIGER International Competency Synthesis Project
   (d) TIGER Virtual Learning Environment

The *HIMSS TIGER Global Informatics Definitions* document is the recommended resource for learners that wish to learn more about global core informatics terminology.

References

1. The TIGER Initiative. Collaborating to integrate evidence and informatics into nursing practice and education: an executive summary [internet]. Chicago; 2012 [cited 2020 Nov 13]. Available from: https://www.himss.org/sites/hde/files/media/file/2020/03/10/the-evolution-of-tiger-competencies-and-informatics-resources-final-10.2017.pdf

2. Institute of Medicine (US) Committee on the Health Professions Education Summit. health professions education: a bridge to quality [internet]. Greiner AC, Knebel E, editors. Washington (DC): National Academies Press (US); 2003 [cited 2020 Dec 19]. Available from: http://www.ncbi.nlm.nih.gov/books/NBK221528/

3. The TIGER Initiative Foundation. The leadership imperative: TIGER's recommendations for integrating technology to transform practice and education [Internet]. 2014. Available from: http://s3.amazonaws.com/rdcms-himss/files/production/public/FileDownloads/the-leadership-imperative.pdf

4. Shaw T, Sensmeier J, Anderson C. The evolution of the TIGER initiative. CIN Comput Inform Nurs. 2017 Jun;35(6):278–80.

5. HIMSS. Technology Informatics Guiding Education Reform (TIGER) [Internet]. 2020 [cited 2020 Dec 19]. Available from: https://www.himss.org/tiger

6. HIMSS. Who we are [Internet]. 2019 [cited 2021 Jan 9]. Available from: https://www.himss.org/who-we-are

7. HIMSS. TIGER International Task Force [Internet]. 2018 [cited 2021 Jan 9]. Available from: https://www.himss.org/tiger-international-task-force

8. HIMSS. Technology Informatics Guiding Education Reform (TIGER) Interprofessional Community [Internet] 2019 [cited 2021 Jan 9]. Available from: https://www.himss.org/membership-participation/technology-informatics-guiding-education-reform-tiger-interprofessional-community

9. HIMSS. Virtual Learning Environment | TIGER Education Reform | HIMSS [Internet]. [cited 2021 Jan 9]. Available from: https://www.himss.org/tiger-virtual-learning-environment

10. Hübner U, Shaw Morawski T, Elias B, Bell S, Blake R. Developing a skilled transatlantic ehealth workforce case studies report [internet]. 2019 [cited 2021 Feb 25]. Available from: https://www.himss.org/resources/developing-skilled-transatlantic-ehealth-workforce-case-studies-report

11. The TIGER Initiative. Informatics competencies for every practicing nurse: recommendations from the TIGER collaborative [internet]. 2009 [cited 2021 Mar 1] p. 34. Available from: http://www.tigersummit.com/uploads/3.Tiger.Report_Competencies_final.pdf

12. Davies A, Mueller J, Moulton G. Core competencies for clinical informaticians: a systematic review. Int J Med Inf. 2020 Sep;141:104237.

13. Shaw T, Blake R, Hübner U, Anderson C, Wangia-Anderson V, Elias B. The evolution of TIGER competencies and informatics resources: executive supplemental report [internet]. HIMSS; 2017 [cited 2021 Jan 9]. Available from: https://www.himss.org/sites/hde/files/media/file/2020/03/10/the-evolution-of-tiger-competencies-and-informatics-resources-final-10.2017.pdf

14. Hübner U, Shaw T, Thye J, Egbert N, Marin H de F, Chang P, et al. Technology informatics guiding education reform – TIGER. Methods Inf Med 2018 May;57(S 01):e30–42.

15. HIMSS. TIGER international competency synthesis project [internet]. 2020 [cited 2020 Dec 19]. Available from: https://www.himss.org/tiger-initiative-international-competency-synthesis-project

16. HIMSS. Global health informatics competency recommendation frameworks [internet]. 2020 [cited 2020 Nov 5]. Available from: https://www.himss.org/resources/global-health-informatics-competency-recommendation-frameworks

17. Hübner U, Thye J, Shaw T, Elias B, Egbert N, Saranto K, et al. Towards the TIGER international framework for recommendations of core competencies in health informatics 2.0: extending the scope and the roles. Stud Health Technol Inform. 2019 Aug;21(264):1218–22.

18. Blake R, Shaw T, Blake A, Hübner U, Kaye R, Schug S, et al. EU*US eHealth works to improve global workforce development [internet]. 2017 p. 12. Available from: https://www.himss.org/sites/hde/files/d7/eu-us-ehealth-workforce-development.pdf

19. UAS7. eHealth4all@EU – Interprofessional European eHealth Programme in Higher Education [Internet]. [cited 2021 Feb 11]. Available from: https://www.uas7.org/en/ehealth4alleu-interprofessional-european-ehealth-programme-higher-education

20. Ball MJ, Douglas JV, Walker PH, DuLong D, Gugerty B, Hannah KJ, et al., editors. Nursing informatics: where technology and caring meet [internet], 4th ed. London: Springer; 2011 [cited 2021 Mar 5]. (Health Informatics). Available from: https://www.springer.com/gp/book/9781849962773

21. Shaw Morawski T, Fanberg H, Pitts J. Responding to the need to curate global informatics definitions. Nurs Manag (Harrow). 2021 Jan;52(1):52–4.

22. Thye J. Understanding health informatics core competencies [internet]. 2020 [cited 2020 Dec 19]. Available from: https://www.himss.org/resources/health-informatics

23. HIMSS. Health Informatics [Internet]. 2020 [cited 2020 Dec 19]. Available from: https://www.himss.org/resources/health-informatics

24. Chang P, Kuo M-C. Taiwan model: nursing informatics training. In: Nursing informatics: where technology and caring meet. 4th ed. London: Springer; 2011. p. 411–28. (Health Informatics).

25. Gugerty B, Delaney C. TIGER Informatics Competencies Collaborative (TICC) final report 2009 p. 17.

26. Chen Y, Yan L, Zheng W, Lin B, Wu L, Wu Z, et al. Establishment of nursing informatics competency evaluation index system of clinical nurses. Chin Nurs Manag. 2020;20(6):921–4.

Preparing the Health Informatics Workforce for the Future

39

JoAnn Klinedinst

J. Klinedinst (✉)
HIMSS, Chicago, IL, USA
e-mail: joann.klinedinst@himss.org

Learning Objectives
- Examine and appreciate the various definitions of professional development
- Define characteristics of the employees engaged in the workforce of the future
- Identify the intent of the professional development plan framework
- Discover resources identified that will support the development and sustainment of the workforce of the future.

Key Terms
- Advancement
- Career development
- Career roadmap
- Continuing professional development
- Certification
- Certificate
- Credential
- Designation
- Digital education
- Informatics
- Lifelong learning
- Professional association
- Professional development plan
- Self-directed learning
- Talent development
- Workforce development

Preparing the Health Informatics Workforce for the Future: An Introduction

Because there is an abundance of opportunities across the health informatics ecosystem, a career in this field can be both exciting and rewarding. The environment is fast-paced, stressful, and rewarding, all at the same time. Opportunities abound locally, regionally, nationally, and internationally. Many healthcare professional certifications and credentials are recognized globally as are many professional associations. This chapter will serve as a roadmap for establishing, preparing, and maintaining a framework for one's career not only today but also in the future.

To prepare the health informatics workforce for the future, we will draw on concepts experienced from the perspective of the United States (US) but are universally applicable to regions around the world. And to aid our discussions internally to healthcare, we look externally to research focused across America, where "building the workforce of the future" involves community interventions like training, investment in workforce training, creating partnerships between educators, a focus on lifelong learning, and strengthening K-12 education [1].

What are the characteristics of a prepared workforce of the future? For employees to excel, there are multiple characteristics that one should be aware and consider: some are obvious, others are not. Many are common sense. While the following list may change over time, its components represent sound advice for those interested in a health informatics career:

- Be resourceful;
- Be respectful of others;
- Be responsive to organizational needs;
- Be adaptable, flexible, and nimble;
- Engage in lifelong learning;
- Appreciate and respect the cultural diversity of the workplace;
- Embrace change enthusiastically and wholeheartedly;
- Create a professional development plan (see information that follows) that is as complete as possible while being updated on a periodic basis;
- Be present and engaged;
- Be passionate;
- Be the best that you can be;
- Say "please" and "thank you", always;
- And be sure to invest in yourself.

The language of health informatics can be found in the health informatics body of knowledge (HIBOK^sm) of sorts, a vast compilation of resources that spans topics like applied artificial intelligence (AI) and machine learning (ML), to cybersecurity, data and analytics, innovation, user experience, and others. The concepts can be as straightforward as change management processes or as complex as accelerating interoperability among disparate systems. One source of global thought leadership, the Healthcare Information and Management Systems Society (HIMSS), serves a global audience by delivering tools and resources that address challenges and opportunities across the health ecosystem. A great place to immerse oneself into the language of health informatics, through education, exhibition, and networking, is at a HIMSS Global Health Conference where topics will display the breadth, depth, and importance of this critical area. The main topic categories of the 2021 HIMSS Global Health Conference and Exhibition are:

- Academic Preparation, Professional Development, Workforce

- Applied Artificial Intelligence and Machine Learning
- Bioinformatics or Healthcare Informatics Research
- Change Management
- Consumers, Caregiver, or Patient Experience
- Cybersecurity, Information Security, Privacy
- Data and Analytics
- Digital Health Transformation Leadership
- Health Information Exchange or Interoperability
- Healthcare Applications and Technologies
- Innovation, Entrepreneurship, Venture Investment
- Pandemic Response
- Population Health, Public Health, SDOH
- Precision Health and Medicine
- Telehealth, Connected Health, Virtual Health
- User Experience, Usability, User-Centered Design
- Volume to Value, Quality, Patient Safety

They are explained and described in more detail in the following paragraphs (permission to use these descriptions is provided by HIMSS).

Academic Preparation, Professional Development, or Workforce

Description: When delivering patient care in today's complex healthcare environment, executive leadership faces a multitude of health informatics professional development or workforce challenges and opportunities across administrative, financial, operational, and technical areas. To meet the pressures of maintaining clinical excellence and technical competence, healthcare leaders must define, attract, and develop the right mix of talent for today and the future. Academicians and others must ensure the right education, tools, resources, and experiences exist to support and grow a diverse and inclusive health informatics workforce, and continuing professional development opportunities must exist so that professionals may maintain and advance their practice.

Applied Artificial Intelligence and Machine Learning

Description: Topics in this category address how solutions like artificial intelligence and machine learning provide the promise and, more recently, the reality of revolutionizing the way healthcare data is analyzed and delivered. By leveraging the power of reasoning, knowledge representation, planning, learning, natural language processing, and other methods, AI and ML can positively enhance efficiencies, reduce risk, increase value, improve outcomes, and reduce clinical variation. The proposal would ensure that these solutions are working or have been tested in clinical environments and have delivered clear, evidence-based healthcare outcomes.

Bioinformatics or Healthcare Informatics Research

Description: This category focuses on case studies, lessons learned from implementation, strategies, research, best practices, or other formats that discuss information, technologies, innovations, and methodologies that impact patient care. Clinicians engaged in biomedical informatics strive to improve knowledge access and contributing guidance on effective strategies to engage clinicians in embracing technology and optimizing health information and technology. Health informatics topics also address the interdisciplinary study of the design, development, adoption, and application of IT-based innovations in healthcare services delivery, management, and planning.

Change Management

Description: To truly transform care processes, critical organizational capabilities such as process improvement, change management, and workflow analysis and design are essential for today's healthcare information and technology professional. By focusing on the design, installa-tion, and improvement of integrated systems of people, culture, material, facilities, information, equipment, and energy, internal to both the IT organization and the organization as a whole, organizations anywhere can realize transformative change in the delivery of care. Evaluating the art and impact of organizational change management processes, methods, and models is important for the development of the profession.

Consumers, Caregiver, or Patient Experience

Description: Topics in this category focus on tools, technologies, programs, and strategies designed to embrace consumers (patients and their families) in becoming active partners with providers and other professionals in managing their health and wellness. Payers and clinical organizations must provide tools that encourage healthy behaviors and help patients manage their conditions. These tools are necessary to enable patients and their families to be partners with clinicians in their own health and in making appropriate healthcare decisions.

Cybersecurity, Information Security, and Privacy

Description: Healthcare organizations must diligently protect the privacy and security of information. This information may exist in many places, such as in the cloud, on a device, within an application, on stored media, or within a database. Ensuring that confidentiality, integrity, and availability of this information is essential for the safe and efficient operation of the healthcare organization, assets, and devices within. Information is the lifeblood of all healthcare organizations. As a result, this information must be rigorously protected to help facilitate normal and efficient operations of organizations and to provide a solid foundation for clinical care of patients.

Data and Analytics

Description: As an essential tool for healthcare stakeholders across the continuum of care, data and analytics can provide insight and intelligence for health systems pursuing clinical transformation while dramatically improving clinical performance aligned with the quadruple aim.

Digital Health Transformation Leadership

Description: The environment of healthcare information and technology is fast-paced, dynamic, global, and ever changing. Leading organizations through disruptive changes brought about by digitization of data and information present both challenges and opportunities across many administrative, clinical, and financial aspects. Leaders in today's digital health environment must constantly adapt in order to understand and leverage the interdependencies of people, culture, and technology to drive optimal value from data and what it reveals about delivering better, cost-effective care to all.

Health Information Exchange or Interoperability

Description: Topics in this category will examine all aspects of information exchange, interoperability, and standards across technical and administrative strategies that contribute to sustaining the healthcare enterprise regardless of the size and enabling a positive individual and clinician experience. Critical to this topic are experiences with connecting individuals and their data with clinicians at the local, regional, state, national levels, and global levels while also supporting advanced care models, demonstrating value by increasing quality and reducing costs, and implementing services that add value to a clinician's workflow.

Healthcare Applications and Technologies

Description: This category focuses on the results of technologies implemented that lead to recorded improved outcomes with the use of administrative, clinical, and financial and patient-focused applications. Proposals in this category should show methodologically sound and statistically measured impact of applications and technologies that will lead to these results. Proposals should have quantitative results.

Innovation, Entrepreneurs, or Venture Investment

Description: Proposals in this category should examine the entire lifecycle of all aspects of healthcare information and technology innovation and investment that positively affect healthcare by improving the care experience, individual and population health, and reducing costs. Strategies and tactics to do so, including, but not limited to, the emerging business landscape, funding trends, barriers to investment and provider technology adoption, and new market and sector opportunities. By exploring the challenges and opportunities of taking viable ideas and new products to market more efficiently, as well as novel collaborations and partnerships between entrepreneurs, investors, and providers for designing, evaluating, validating, funding, and adopting emerging tech-enabled solutions that meet clinical needs, quality of care delivered can be greatly enhanced. Proposals would include projects/investments that have been implemented with predetermined outcomes, rather than ideation of possible technologies in clinical settings.

Pandemic Response

Description: According to The World Health Organization, a pandemic is defined as the "worldwide spread of a new disease". With COVID-19, the virus that causes the disease, we all are experiencing an unprecedented time for our healthcare community, our nation, and our world. And as history may repeat itself, this may not be the last pandemic that we experience. With global disruption across every aspect of patient care, proposals in this category will emphasis how technology has enabled the healthcare ecosystem to navigate this new, global normal.

Population Health, Public Health, SDOH

Description: According to the CDC, public health works to protect and improve the health of communities through policy recommendations, health education and outreach, and research for disease detection and injury prevention, and population health provides an opportunity for health care system, agencies, and organizations to work together in order to improve the health outcomes of the communities they serve. This category addresses how information and technology support collective, collaborative societal efforts to both assure the conditions in which people can be healthy and the provision of care that promotes health and wellness of the population. Both public health and population health provide critical insights that can inform ways in which community-based organizations, healthcare providers, and public health institutions address specific health risks and needs, optimize health status, protect groups from harm, perform essential health tasks, allocate resources to overcome systemic challenges that drive chronic health conditions, and support physical, mental health, and wellness in that population. This topic also addresses disparities and equity in treatment and research based on gender, race, ethnicity, sexual orientation, and other demographic characteristics. The challenge of addressing disparities may be exacerbated by inequities in social determinants of health (e.g., stable housing, balanced meals, reliable transportation, access to healthcare services,

and social isolation) and silos between physical health services and social determinants from rural areas to densely populated urban centers. Facilitated on a foundation of people and culture, business and financial functions, and data, information, technology, and actionable analytics, stakeholders can identify ways to equitably allocate resources to overcome the challenges and opportunities of managing the population and/or public health of a community and larger areas and eliminate or reduce disparities in care.

Precision Medicine and Health

Description: This category addresses a developing area in healthcare with the goal of providing the most effective and individualized care for each patient through omic-informed personalized care. Facilitated by evidence-based medicine, precision health is an emerging approach for disease treatment and prevention. It also encompasses research and development to accelerate biomedical research using very large sets of health and disease-related data including genotypic, phenotypic, and lifestyle data. Tools and solutions employed can include molecular diagnostics, imaging, and analytics/software. Combining new informatics approaches that enable access and integrate many kinds of data with omic data in disease research allows researchers to better understand the genetic bases of drug response and disease. Novel technology and process solutions to support and accelerate advances in gene therapy, vector development, and/or omic predictive analytics should be included in proposals.

Telehealth, Connected Health, Virtual Health

Description: Telehealth, or the provision of care via information and communications technology (ICT) across time and space, is transforming healthcare operations of all types. From bringing specialty provider expertise to rural and remote areas to offering clinicians flexibility to better balance their lives, telemedicine use is growing rapidly through integration into the ongoing operations of hospitals, specialty departments, home health agencies, private physician offices, as well as consumer's homes and workplaces. Telemedicine is the natural evolution of healthcare in the digital world since it greatly improves the quality, equity, and affordability of healthcare throughout the world.

User Experience, Usability, User-Centered Design

Description: There is a vast and increasing array of spaces, systems, and devices used by providers and patients to diagnose, treat, and manage disease states and wellness activities. The experience patients and providers have while interacting with those spaces, systems, and devices has direct impact on clinical, operational, and financial outcomes. This category explores the effect that product and process design choices have on the user experience and its implications for quality, safety, satisfaction, and operational efficiency. Abstract submitters for this category are encouraged to propose interactive presentations to engage the audience in innovative approaches to improving UX, usability, and user-centered design.

Volume to Value, Quality, Patient Safety

Description: Topics in this category focus on the thoughtful application of information and technology required to shift from volume to value while also leveraging data to identify opportunities for improved safety and care delivery. The intent is to help healthcare professionals measurably improve clinical outcomes, enhance patient safety, and address the business aspects of care delivery. This topic also incorporates initiatives to develop robust quality measurement and out-

comes improvement programs along with guidance for designing, installing, and improving integration of systems, including but not limited to people, material, facilities, information, equipment, and energy all designed to improve the care delivered to patients.

In order to prepare the health informatics workforce for the future, we turn to generally accepted definitions to guide our path. According to HIMSS, health informatics is defined as the "interdisciplinary study of the design, development, adoption and application of IT-based innovations in healthcare services delivery, management and planning" [2]. The American Medical Informatics Association (AMIA), another health care services globally focused professional association, describes informatics as "the science of how to use data, information and knowledge to improve human health and the delivery of health care services" [3].

As the global non-profit association for the health information management (HIM) professional, the American Health Information Management Association (AHIMA) defines health informatics as "a science that defines how health information is technically captured, transmitted, and utilized" [4]. And the HIMSS Technology Informatics Guiding Education Reform (TIGER) Interprofessional Community, a global network of over 60 participants representing over 29 countries (as of August 2020), defines health informatics as "the discipline that researches, formulates, designs, develops, implements, and evaluates information-related concepts, methods, and tools (e.g., information and communication technology (ICT)) to support clinical care, research, health services administration, and education" [5].

The Meaning of Work: An Overview

In today's work environment, the term workplace has taken on new meanings: not only may the workplace be located in either an in-place setting such as an office or at home but also it can occur virtually anywhere one has access to a WiFi connection. While this flexibility can be a welcomed addition to one's busy lifestyle, others may feel overburdened by the temptation and the very real possibility of being "always on".

In addition to the location of the workplace, the term "work" has also embodied new and different meanings: terms like re-skilling (enhancing one's existing skillset to accommodate for next-generation thinking), up-skilling (adding tools to one's professional toolbox that will supplement and enhance one's existing skillsets), and future-skilling (preparing for a workplace of the future which continues to evolve) are now part of the workforce's vernacular. Gratten explains that "every conceivable job will have new technologies to learn and new personal relationships to navigate as those roles fit and refit into a changing economic landscape" [6]. Therefore, by understanding these terms, employees entering the workforce of the future can plan to adapt to ensure a successful career in health informatics. And to emphasize the differences, the terms re-skilling, up-skilling, and future-skilling are best viewed in tandem. An example follows.

A director of clinical education at a healthcare organization is currently engaged in "re-skilling" her department's approach to designing and delivering clinical education assets. While in-person training resonates with many adult learners in the health information and technology sector, the director must identify new formats and delivery methods for her staff that will continue to appeal to a wide variety of adult learners, particularly since the workforce encompasses multiple generations, defined by Brandman University as "Traditionalists (born in 1945 and before); Baby Boomers (born between 1946 and 1964); Generation X (born between 1965 and 1976); Millennials (born between 1977 and 1995); and Generation Z (born in 1996 and after)" [7], as well as those may work remotely or at satellite facilities. By engaging in re-skilling, the director can be assured that her organization will continue its competitive advantage by appealing to the changing needs of the workforce, as identified above. From an up-skilling perspective, the director encourages her team to develop coursework that incorporates learning design techniques (also referred to as instruc-

tional design), like storyboarding, expanded design templates, and enhanced ways of embedding interactivity, into learning objectives. By developing these new tools with a focus on re-skilling and up-skilling, the director will ensure that the organization's investment in digital learning will continue to evolve and be more inviting and engaging to adult learners.

From a future-skilling perspective, the director of clinical education recognizes access to digital learning, across multiple platforms, will continue to appeal to learners. Added to this, the increased focus on innovation in healthcare resulting from pitch competitions, hack-a-thons, tech challenges, and other activities will accelerate the development and release of emerging technologies, requiring and even greater need in delivering education at the right time and the right place. With these formats, facilitators succeed "in making education more engaging and interesting to students" [8]. And it is only through the director's active and persistent involvement with re-skilling and up-skilling, and a focus on future-skilling, that the organization will be positioned to adapt education rapidly and effectively to the future of digital learning.

To prepare the health informatics workforce of the future, there is no doubt that continuous engagement in lifelong learning is both a critical and a strategic comparative, enabled by organizations, and for the benefit of both. [Continuing] professional education is "any learning, formal or informal, structured or self-directed, live or electronic, voluntary or required (for certification or any other reason) to help you grow professionally OR in your job or career", offers Albert and Dignam [9].

Talent development refers to the "efforts that foster learning and employee development to drive organizational performance, productivity, and results" [10]. Viewed as a collaborative effort between the employee and the employer, developing future leaders in the workforce of the future is both a responsibility and a requirement as we strive to prepare our future generations for the workforce. Paine notes 10 characteristics of the future learning leader, which include "focusing, above all, on business impact", "being aware of the horizon (the day-to-day business processes and procedures)", and "showing general optimism about the future, and the future of learning, delivering, and influencing at the highest level in the organization" [11]. Because the world is constantly changing, Kippen states that "it is through this wired and global lens that we [must] evaluate future challenges and opportunities" [12] to benefit our workforce of the future.

When taking responsibility to develop one's talent, engaging in activities that contribute to a professional development plan, either encouraged by a supervisor or self-identified by the employee, one can feel a sense of satisfaction and empowerment, while feeling energized and excited about learning new things that can be applicable to one's responsibilities. And the supervisor who encourages an employee to engage in professional development activities, and allows them time to do so, is actually preparing the workforce of the future, today. With health informatics, technology changes so rapidly that keeping up-to-date with industry trends requires a focus on lifelong learning. For the employer who already has competent staff applying process improvement tools, like a SWOT (strengths, weaknesses, opportunities, threats) analysis or six sigma techniques have been available for quite some time, he or she could continue to develop employee talent by encouraging them to keep up-to-date with the latest developments. By doing so, the employee could supplement one's toolkit with design thinking tools that have gained great popularity recently for change management activities. By a supervisor encouraging an employee to learn more about these types of tools not only benefits the employee but the employer too.

Professional Development: A Definition

Professional development, as described by Wittnebel, is "the vehicle that keeps practitioners informed of the latest developments in their respective fields" [13]. Professional development is critical in any professional, technical, or tactical position. Also referred to as "lifelong learn-

ing", employees, regardless of their position, must be given opportunities to grow in knowledge and skill. Maintaining one's professional competency is no longer a luxury but rather a competitive advantage in today's rapidly changing, fast-paced, and dynamic global workplace.

HIMSS defines professional development as not only embodying the technical aspects of one's work (workforce development) but also focusing on building competency throughout one's career (career development). Therefore, one engages in professional development, through activities involving career development and workforce development, all of which lead to lifelong learning. Added to this, Daiker discusses that "continuing professional development is a learner-driven, lifelong journey. It doesn't start with formalized education and it doesn't end when the coursework is over, it is a continuous process" [14].

Professional Development: Taking Advantage of Endless Possibilities

While there has been increased focus on health and healthcare as essential functions as we experience the COVID-19 pandemic, there is an entire ecosystem in the background that is supporting the front-line clinician. But as one contemplates the potential for a career in healthcare for the glamor, excitement, or job security, be aware that not everyone can tolerate the very real characteristics of a healthcare environment. While it may appear glamourous, a healthcare environment's pace can be frantic, one that is laced with stress, and one where burnout is associated with administrative, clinical, financial, or technical burdens. In addition, one may be exposed to hazardous materials, chemicals, or body fluids as well as being physically attacked when caring for patients. However, for those with a passion for embracing truly meaningful work, either delivering direct patient care or supporting those who do will find a rewarding opportunity in health informatics as a great way to contribute.

What exactly encompasses a health and healthcare ecosystem? There is no doubt that the health and healthcare ecosystem is vast. Stakeholders include, but are not limited to, providers from both organizational and independent perspectives; payers; hardware and software market-suppliers; telecommunications providers; consulting services; legal perspectives; strategic partner perspectives; community-based organizations; local, regional, and national governmental organizations; pharmaceutical and life sciences organizations; patient advocate groups; and others. Because "the patient now constitutes the focus of the healthcare system, so any individual, profession or organization whose work supports that focus is part of the healthcare network" [15].

Professional Development: Creating a Professional Development Plan (Career Roadmap)

To determine where your interest may be the strongest in a health informatics career, creating a professional development plan, or career roadmap, is paramount. Planning is a critical task necessary in virtually every aspect of one's life, and one's career is no exception. Benjamin Franklin said, "by failing to prepare yourself, you are preparing to fail" [16]. And when planning, Covey reminds us to "Be patient with yourself. Self-growth is tender; it's holy ground. There's no greater investment [then in you]" [17].

When creating a professional development plan, it is best to approach it as a living plan that should be updated on a periodic basis, perhaps annually. Depending upon one's career level, whether an emerging leader with 5 or less years of experience, or, perhaps a mid-level professional with 10 to 15 years of experience, the components of one's plan may differ slightly from another. For example, to determine whether the health informatics industry is a fit, one will want to devote considerable time to explore positions in the field.

Table 39.1 provides a recommended framework for creating a personalized professional development plan. The plan may follow this format specifically or sections may be added,

updated, or even deleted. The important point is that one must be comfortable with the plan that he or she has created since it will serve as to identify a personal journey for one's professional life. The framework identifies five sections: I. All about Me; II. All about Finding a Position; III. All about My Career; IV. All about My Education; and V. All about Engaging with My Industry. To complete the plan, use a narrative to describe responses to the various sections that explain the actions to take to address the item. When developing a plan, authors should not only be as complete as possible but also consider soliciting feedback from others, like a colleague, friend, mentor, or other trusted advisor to review a draft of the plan. Comments from objective contributors can be well worth the effort by helping to identify both gaps and responses to gaps that may not be obvious to the plan's author. By adopting this approach, mentors and influencers, for example, one's supervisor who encourages the employee to grow and to stretch through professional development opportunities, can offer objective feedback worthy of inclusion.

1. Jones-Smith, V. Creating a personal brand. In: The handbook of continuing professional development for the health IT professional. Boca Raton: CRC Press; 2017. p. 17–24
2. Skills Knowledge Assessment and Development Framework. Accessed on 22 July 2020 at https://ehealthwork.org/SKAD/index.html
3. Health Information Technology and Competencies. Accessed on 22 July 2020 at http://hitcomp.org/
4. HIMSS Nursing Informatics Survey. Access on 22 July 2020 at https://www.himss.org/sites/hde/files/media/file/2020/06/19/nursinginformaticsworkforcesurveyexectivesummary-final.pdf
5. AHIMA Career Map. https://my.ahima.org/careermap. Accessed 14 July 2020
6. Beich E. ATD's Foundation of Talent Development. "Develop your talent development staff". Alexandria: ATD Press; 2018. p. 395

Table 39.1 Professional development plan

A. All About Me

1. Conduct a SWOT (strengths, weaknesses, opportunities, and threats) analysis to identify your likes, dislikes, and other characteristics of you
2. Create a response to items identified in the SWOT analysis
3. Articulate your personal brand, as defined by William Arruda as "your unique promise of you" [1]
4. Identify your desired work–life balance
5. Express your interest in using a mentor or a professional coach
6. Create your moral compass by articulating your morals, values, and ethics, statement
7. Determine the comfort of your health informatics work setting: Clinical or non-clinical; provider or market-supplier setting; for-profit or non-profit setting; administrative or financial
8. Conduct a skills assessment to determine your familiarity with certain tools and resources. Tools available include the Skills Knowledge Assessment and Development Framework [2], the HITCOMP [3], or the HIMSS Nursing Informatics Survey [4].

B. All About Finding a Position

1. Search for positions of interest across multiple job posting databases like the HIMSS JobMine, Indeed, LinkedIn, and others; review resumes posted that highlight open positions of interest
2. Develop a plan on how to achieve attributes of resumes you reviewed
3. Prepare application materials, that is, identify where to gather transcripts, request letters of recommendation, a resume, points of interest for a cover letter
4. Before applying, review the guidance provided by the employer of interest
5. Review tactics to land a job interview
6. Research and prepare interviewing skills and techniques
7. Thoroughly prepare for the interview, that is, review the job description, research the industry, study the organization, research who you will be interviewing with
8. Reflect on the interview once it has been completed: what worked, what did not, what you would do differently, and other items to prepare for the next interview
9. Anticipating an offer: Determine your negotiable and non-negotiable requirements
10. Receiving an offer: what to expect with salary, benefits, working conditions; identifying "must haves"
11. Negotiating the offer: create your guidelines to follow
12. Accepting the offer: determining your requirements
13. Envision and prepare for your first day of work: what you need

C. All About My Career

1. Identify your professional aspirations such as an individual contributor or people manager
2. Determine the type of position you would like to pursue (access the AHIMA Career Map to learn more about health information management (HIM) careers in general [5])
3. Examine ways that you can diversify your skillset by combining passion with profession
4. Create an individual development plan that identifies "short-term goals, developmental opportunities, and a timeline with milestones and required resources" [6]

D. All About My Education

1. Create a learning plan that will supplement structured learning with on-the-job training
2. Identify a certificate program to learn more about a particular area without investing in an advanced degree
3. Determine what type of professional certification that you would like to pursue
4. Identify a plan to continue your academic career
5. Determine post-graduate work that can contribute to your profession

E. All About Engaging with Your Industry

1. Identify and join a professional association(s) that aligns with your professional goals
2. Develop a plan to become engaged in the professional association(s) you identified
3. Determine whether to pursue advancement opportunities with the professional association(s) you identified
4. Identify a plan to give back to your professional association through volunteering

Establishing and Nurturing Your Career

Establishing and Nurturing Your Career: The Role of the Professional Society

To build a workforce of the future, membership within a professional association, is an excellent way to become immersed in an industry-specific topic. One is never too new or too advanced in a career to engage with an association (or even multiple ones).

Associations help members connect, advance, and learn. Members who engage with one another in volunteer activities have the opportunity to connect with other professionals who can share the same challenges, opportunities, and interests, across one's personal or professional life. Activities that help members engage include, but are not limited to, virtual activities like webinars and digital learning, as well as in-person events like leadership summits, conferences, or workshops. By actively connecting and learning, members can accumulate advancement points that can lead to senior, fellow, or life fellow member status. These activities all contribute to one's lifelong professional development. Not only are professional societies a great source of information but also they are a great way to engage with other like-minded professionals at the local, regional, national, or international level.

Professional societies are excellent sources for up-to-date industry resources spanning publications, news, white papers, (e)books, blogs, and other media. They also provide information on certification, advancement, events, job boards, career centers, membership directories, policy and advocacy perspectives, product and services buyer's guides, and more. Essentially, associations are a convening point for all things: education, networking, market-place, and research across an industry. While there are dozens of health informatics-related membership associations (see Appendix Table 39.2), finding one that is aligned with your professional goals and objectives, as well as your interests, may take some work; however, it is well worth the time invested in doing so. Think of a professional society as your professional home.

Membership types vary within a professional society and may encompass emerging leaders, or those new to the industry, through individual, organizational, or corporate levels; tiered packages like professional or professional plus membership plans where fee-based content may be made available as a member benefit; and membership types based on years of service such as life member. Dues vary based on the membership type selected; however, significant savings can be offered to affiliate-type organizational or academic group membership offerings. Many times, professional associations offer student members significant savings on many of the same benefits offered to those who are actively involved in the industry.

While joining a professional society is an excellent step toward preparing oneself for the workforce for the future, volunteering with the professional society is an excellent way to maximize one's membership investment. The importance of volunteering cannot be overstated. By engaging with other professionals, either virtually or in-person, one can expand one's professional (and personal, too!) competencies while giving back to the industry. Many associations have volunteer opportunities for serving on committees, holding leadership positions at chapter or international levels, involvement in advocacy initiatives, and other ways to enhance developing one's career. Table 39.2 (Appendix) identifies health informatics-related professional associations across the globe.

This table is original material adapted from *The Handbook of Continuing Professional Development for the Health IT Professional*, JoAnn Klinedinst, published by HIMSS and CRC Press, Taylor and Francis Group, copyright 2017, ISBN: 9781138033238. Permission granted from HIMSS and CRC Press, Taylor and Francis Group.

Attributes of a Professional Society

Professional societies provide excellent resources, both complimentary and fee-based, for its members. As a trusted partner to the member, professional societies or thought leadership organizations, as is the case with HIMSS, provide many of the benefits that contribute to lifelong learning. Imagine a partner who has your best interest in mind; couple that with like-minded peers and a collective desire to advance one's industry's goals and body of knowledge, and one has many elements that can contribute to professional (and personal, too!) success.

Attributes of a professional society can vary among organizations; however, the following exemplifies a robust member benefit's offering. Investing your time and resources, while also engaging with the organization, will enhance your professional development.

Content An excellent indicator of a worthy professional association is its attention to the development of thought leadership by employing subject matter experts, also known as SMEs. These SMEs, many who have years of industry experience aligned with the mission and vision of the professional association, facilitate activities for members to engage in by conducting research both individually and collectively, as well as providing access to industry-recognized luminaries to develop thought leadership, benefiting both the member and the association. Additionally, many organizations publish a member-driven peer-review journal, or access to independent journals, while also offering publications by and for members through bookstores. And some organizations provide member access to internationally respected online libraries such as EBSCO to aid in member- and association-generated thought leadership.

Advocacy Another important area of service to membership and the industry in general is advocacy work conducted by professional societies. Government Relations teams are indispensable members of the organization since they work tirelessly to solicit and organize public comment periods involving members on pending legislation, facilitating education and training for recently enacted regulations, and keeping the membership appraised of developing topics. Many times, the professional association is guided by Legislative Principles, developed jointly by the professional association and volunteers, which are updated annually.

Educational Programming Many professional societies offer a full complement of educational programming featuring thought leaders, SMEs, industry luminaries, and others that contribute to the subject matter. Delivery mechanisms may include in-person education occurring at the local, regional, national, or international level; virtual events like conferences, webinars, or previously recorded conference sessions aggregated into one portal for easy access; and courses that may occur synchronously (together with an instructor and students) or asynchronously (self-directed learning). Additionally, professional societies may also have arrangements with "approved education partners", also referred to as AEPs, who can also contribute yet another source of educational programming through non-credit courses, certificate programs, or all levels of degreed programs.

Career Development and Workforce Development Professional societies are an excellent source of activities that contribute to continuous professional development and life-long learning for career advancement. To demonstrate one's grasp of a body of knowledge, many professional associations offer tools and resources to help candidates achieve an introductory- or advanced-level certification, which are usually based on experience and/or education. And once a candidate earns a certification, professional societies provide education and training to help certificants maintain one's credential. With abundant opportunities in the health information and technology sector, members can find a rich source of job listings, career advice, mentorship opportunities, or virtual job fairs to help identify what may be next in one's career. And by engaging in volunteer activities, many organizations allow members to earn points toward advancement to senior, advanced, fellow, or life status. With recognition being a major component of professional societies, there are ample opportunities for advancement, scholarships, awards, and other mechanisms to recognize exceptional service, leadership, and engagement.

Establishing and Nurturing Your Career: The Importance of Volunteering

Giving back to others, whether it be from a personal or professional perspective, is immensely rewarding. If chosen thoughtfully, engaging as a volunteer can help to provide an outlet beyond one's chosen area of expertise. Or, you may decide to supplement your work life experiences and volunteer with organizations that closely mirror your employment responsibilities. Whatever one's approach, be sure to include volunteering in your professional development plan.

Professional associations are excellent sources for many types of volunteer activities. By working next to peers, not only can you contribute to a cause but also you can get to know others: one may even identify a way to engage in an area that closely aligns with your employment and your passion.

Establishing and Nurturing Your Career: Earning a Professional Certification

Earning a professional certification is a great way to communicate to others about your comprehensive understanding of a body of knowledge. In health informatics, there are multiple certifications from which to choose: it just depends upon your interest, whether one is qualified to take the exam since many certifications are based on both experience and education; one's ability to prepare for the exam; one's willingness to sit for the exam since they can be many hours in duration; and one's ability to maintain the credential since most, if not all, certifications require a continuing education (CE) component. In a health informatics setting, one can choose from technical certifications, like those associated with hardware, infrastructure, or cloud-based services; software applications, either enterprise-related or specialty applications that serve a product line or business unit; project-related certifications, including risk, portfolio, agile, or business processes; clinical certifications; financial certifications; or others. The opportunities are many but your selection should be few.

After earning a certification, the credential holder must create a plan for earning continuing education (CE) to maintain the credential. One could choose not to participate in CE but rather re-take the exam. By all means, continuing education is the preferred means of maintaining a credential because one continues to learn over time. By doing so, the certificant is engaging in learning that can benefit one's skillset, as well as the industry.

The Importance of Lifelong Learning.

The Importance of Lifelong Learning: Earning an Advanced Degree

After one identifies an area of interest in health informatics and determines that it is worthy of investing the time and energy into furthering one's focus, earning an advanced degree will greatly enhance one's knowledge of the chosen field. While many equate earning an advanced degree with an increased salary or promotion in an existing organization, many times, that is not the case. An advanced degree will, however, provide one with many opportunities to use the workplace setting as a source of papers, projects, and even a thesis topic. Of course, one may identify in his or her professional development plan that an advanced degree is a pathway to engagement and employment with other organizations.

The Importance of Lifelong Learning: Engaging Socially

Engaging socially is an excellent way to remain active and knowledge about current trends in a specific industry. There are many social media outlets like Twitter, LinkedIn, Instagram, and others that provide highly credible socialized content. In addition, choosing to follow various social media influencers who lead with thought leadership and research, as identified through Symplur and other social media curators, is a wise decision.

The Importance of Lifelong Learning: Self-Directed Learning

Because health informatics is a rapidly evolving discipline, the need for independent, self-directed learning is critical to ensure that one's knowledge keeps pace with the changes in the industry. Of all the recommendations in this chapter, most critical is one's ability to establish a self-directed learning plan that not only extends over time but also is flexible and adaptable as one's professional interests evolve. While learning in an academic setting may be a preferred method, that's only one component of a self-directed learning plan. Components may focus on traditional academic institutions (brick-and-mortar, convened at a distance, or a hybrid of both) where fee-based coursework could lead to earning a certificate at the same time as earning an advanced degree; academic-focused consortiums like edX that offer thousands of free courses across hundreds of academic institutions available through massive open online courses (MOOCs); continuing professional development with professional associations that include certificates of completion that may also contribute to maintaining a professional certification; publications available, again, through professional associations like the HIMSS Bookstore with savings passed onto members; eBooks, focused on thought leadership and education, many times published by the professional association; research organizations (non-commercial influencers) like the Robert Wood Johnson Foundation, where research-focused topics like healthcare quality and value, disease prevention and promotion, health disparities, and others abound; the World Health Organization (WHO), with hundreds of topics that include fact sheets, facts in pictures, publications, and other resources; the Bill and Melinda Gates Foundation, which is focused on enhanced education through innovation; and finally, research organizations (commercial influencers) which are focused on health-related topics like Deloitte© Insights Center for Integrated Research that offers "fresh perspectives on critical business issues" where multiple industries are of focus [18]; the McKinsey Global Institute, whose mission is to "help leaders in the commercial, public, and social sectors develop a deeper understanding of the evolution of the global economy and to provide a fact base that contributes to decision making on critical management and policy issues [19]"; and the Rand Corporation, where their research focus is on "critical issues of particular relevance to the public policy debate" across research that spans decades [20]. All contribute to development of health informatics professionals through thought leadership designed to complement self-directed learning.

Case Studies

Based on the longevity of the author's career, JoAnn Klinedinst offers two case studies for review. The first is entitled "Establishing a Career in Health Information and Technology", which details her journey in a community hospital setting where employed in the health information and technology discipline. The second case study, entitled "Health Information and Technology: Focusing on the Continuing Professional Development of Health Information and Technology Professionals" details her journey that ensures the health informatics workforce of the future has the tools, resources, education, and training to succeed now and into the future.

Case Study #1: Establishing a First Career in Health Information and Technology: A Member Case Study

(The following case study appeared in 2017 in *The Handbook of Continuing Professional Development for Health IT Professionals* and is used with permission.) This case study is original material from *The Handbook of Continuing Professional Development for the Health IT Professional*, JoAnn Klinedinst, published by HIMSS and CRC Press, Taylor and Francis Group, copyright 2017, ISBN: 9781138033238.

[21] Permission granted from HIMSS and CRC Press, Taylor and Francis Group.

My involvement with professional associations has been pivotal in my development as a health information technology (IT) professional. While working in the Management Information Systems (MIS) Department of a local hospital, I realized that healthcare was the place for me. At the time (early 1990s), a career in health IT was not viewed as positive since the industry lacked advanced technology and offered lower pay than the IT industry in general. However, I welcomed the family-like atmosphere among many of the departments in this small, community hospital setting.

After being hired in the MIS Department for my knowledge of PC-based applications for word processing, database, and spreadsheet applications, I started getting more involved in the technical aspects of implementing MEDITECH through report writing, dictionary building, and other activities. While my degree was in business management, I had little knowledge of the hospital setting. As a result, I began exploring various professional associations that could provide additional education and training to supplement my healthcare knowledge.

After a search of many different types of organizations, I joined HIMSS in 1991. I did so because of the thought leadership that was available through peer-reviewed themed journals which allowed me to expand my knowledge in the areas of telehealth, clinical systems applications, the computer-based patient record, and many others. Further, HIMSS held an annual conference that combined education, exhibition, and networking. For me, this was a great start on my journey to begin my understanding of health IT. (And that journey still exists today.)

Much to my surprise, my involvement in HIMSS was not only accessing thought leadership journals but much more. I attended my first conference in 1995 (San Antonio, TX) and was immediately captivated. After a few years, I decided that I too had experiences to contribute and responded to my first call for proposal on a poster session entitled "Critical Success Factors of Application Upgrades". I was accepted and actually earned recognition for the best poster session overall.

In addition to speaking at HIMSS over the course of three times over 10 years, I also served as a paper reviewer for many years. In fact, opportunities still exist today to become involved as a peer-reviewer volunteer with HIMSS and without a long-term commitment. Through this experience, I decided that I wanted to serve on the Annual Conference Education Committee (ACEC) so I also applied for a Board appointment. There were no guarantees that I would get appointed but I wanted to try. Much to my surprise, I was selected for a two-year term (1999–2000) and served as chair in 2000. This was an absolutely amazing experience. To think that someone from a small community hospital could be recognized for her skillsets and abilities was just amazing to me.

And this is true today as well: HIMSS welcomes the involvement of individuals from all different types of stakeholders. The only differentiating factors are a willingness to serve the health IT sector.

As my appointment came to an end on the ACEC, I applied for an appointment to the Advocacy Committee. I too was accepted for a two-year term. By this point, I was very much engaged in my local DVHIMSS (Delaware Valley) chapter and served on the State Advocacy Committee. It was I who set up the appointments for attendees to meet with their legislative representatives: all 110 attendees. While advocacy was a different area for me, I learned quite a lot which helped me to become even better-rounded as a health IT professional.

As I progressed in my volunteer efforts with HIMSS, I realized that I may not always want to work in healthcare so I diversified my professional association involvement and joined the Project Management Institute (PMI). Because so much of what I did in healthcare was project-focused, I decided that PMI was a good fit for me. I served in a variety of capacities for the PMI Healthcare Special Interest Group (SIG). While I wanted to diversify the places I worked, I kept coming back to healthcare. At the same time, I became involved in various SIGs with HIMSS: the Supply Chain Management SIG, Long-Term Care SIG, and the Project Management SIG. All provided an opportunity to engage but without the commitment of a Board appointment.

One advantage to becoming involved with a professional society as an active volunteer is that one can earn points for advancement. HIMSS has advancement opportunities for Senior Members and Fellows. Many of these activities contributed to my overall advancement score and I became a Fellow in 2000.

After I earned the Fellow member (FHIMSS) designation of HIMSS, a new certification was being launched by HIMSS called the Certified Professional in Healthcare Information and Management Systems (CPHIMS). I decided to study and then sit for that exam. Again, my involvement in HIMSS definitely prepared me to understand the vast body of health IT knowledge. So, with 200 of my closest friends on a Sunday morning at the HIMSS Annual Conference and Exhibition 2002 (HIMSS02) in Atlanta, we were the first to be seated to take the exam. I passed, adding the CPHIMS designation to accompany my FHIMSS designation.

As an engaged volunteer, one has the opportunity to work with peers both nationally and internationally. And this recognition sometimes results in an industry or service award nomination, as it did for me. I was nominated and selected for the HIMSS Leadership Award based on my many years of involvement with HIMSS. While I never expected anything like this, professional associations do recognize their well-deserving members. And I happened to be one who was recognized. And a moment I still remember to this day.

While still involved with PMI and HIMSS jointly, I decided to earn the Project Management Professional (PMP) certification. I had the experience needed to apply and had also enrolled in Villanova University's Masters Certificate in IS/IT Project Management (which is still available today). Based on three modules, the third was devoted to preparing for the PMP exam. I completed the certificate and then sat for the exam. Although I failed the first time, I decided to try again. This exam was (and still is) highly rigorous but I felt I had the competencies to succeed. And I passed on my second try.

With my time approaching an end on the Advocacy Committee, I decided that I would apply for membership on the Ambulatory Information Systems Committee. Since I had moved from the acute setting to the ambulatory setting, this made sense to me. At the same time, HIMSS was hiring subject matter experts (SMEs) like myself and others. I interviewed for and was selected as the Director of Enterprise Information Systems. Fortunately for me I was hired; however, my volunteer involvement with HIMSS came to an end as a paid employee.

While my experience may be atypical, one never knows where an engagement with a professional association may lead. To this day, I see vendors that I worked with at my community hospital who also exhibit at the HIMSS Annual Conference and Exhibition. While some may have retired, I still seem to find a person or two who I worked with some 20 years previously.

Case Study #2: "Health Information and Technology: Focusing on the Continuing Professional Development of Health Information and Technology Professionals"

After leaving the community hospital IT setting, I accepted a position as an SME with HIMSS. This was a bold step for me since I was leaving a familiar setting of 16 years for one that was somewhat unfamiliar and would require a major adjustment: not because I didn't know the organization, content, or the staff, but rather because I would be held responsible for revenue generation across multiple product lines.

Realizing that I was a team of multiples with a revenue achievement plan, I accepted the position. Starting as an SME in the Enterprise setting by serving as a staff liaison to the Enterprise Information Systems IS Steering Committee and the Management Engineering Community. With HIMSS volunteers, I facilitated meetings, curated content development, coordinated legislative Notice of Proposed Rule Making (NPRM) for comment, and other tasks driven by mission and vision. Similar to a healthcare setting, HIMSS provided opportunities for advancement. After being promoted to a Senior Director level, I had the opportunity several years later to interview for the position of Vice President of Education. I was offered the role and accepted. Some 18 months later, my role expanded to my current position of Vice President, Professional Development.

In my current role at HIMSS, I am responsible for all aspects of continuing professional development that leads to the lifelong learning and engagement of health information and technology professionals. Although I had strong SME for this role and continue to nurture it, I lacked an advanced degree, particularly in the educational discipline. To address this gap, I entered a masters of adult education program at The Pennsylvania State University's World Campus. Graduating several years later, I earned a M.Ed. and a Certificate of Completion in distance education.

Upon graduation, I began searching for a professional association that could provide me with the critical tools and resources that would help me grow in my new profession, within the health information and technology environment. However, it was difficult for me to find an organization that addressed my role of developing and executing educational programming: I did not work in an academic setting nor was my role centralized in a corporate HR department. While I found several organizations focused on workforce development, of which was also an area of interest and responsibility, the fit was not quite right: I was not focused on workforce investment boards nor was I interested in engaging with a professional association whose website was sorely out of date. After continuing my search, I decided that association executive management was too restrictive for me since I enjoyed being a specialist and not a generalist. Engaging as an association executive would prepare me to lead any association, but I wanted to maintain my specialization of health information and technology. After six years of searching, I identified and joined the Association of Talent Development (ATD).

The benefits I receive as a member of ATD are very worthwhile in my role as creating and implementing professional development resources for HIMSS' 85,000+ members. From a content perspective, I benefit from multiple publications which define the talent management body of knowledge. These resources are particularly helpful since I have qualified to sit for the Certified Professional in Talent Development (CPTD) professional certification. From a course perspective, I am currently up-skilling my skillset and recently participated in a 12-hour, online certificate course entitled "Designing Virtual Events". Since so many events, including HIMSS20, pivoted to a virtual presence due to the COVID-19 pandemic, I took advantage of attending this workshop and I am currently evaluating others. Further, I have participated in the ATD 2020 virtual conference, including on-demand access, and I have attended various webcasts on topics of interest to my role. From a publication perspective, I am able to access electronically the most current association journal issue while also accessing archived content, all in my Member Portal. With three membership levels to choose from, I was able to join as a "Professional" member while I explored my membership. When I renew, I will advance to the "Professional Plus" membership level since I will

gain access to even more resources. The resources that I can access are exceptional: I am able to gain seamless access to peer-reviewed journals and other resources from EBSCO which helped inform this chapter.

Based on my two different career opportunities, I share applicable attributes of my journey. I have earned multiple certifications along my health information and technology journey that compliment my various interests. As a long-time, engaged member of HIMSS, I have participated in various initiatives that have allowed me to advance to a HIMSS Fellow and soon-to-be-life Fellow (30 years of continuous membership). In addition, I hold the HIMSS certification, the CPHIMS™. For these, and many other reasons, HIMSS is my most important membership that I hold because health information and technology is my passion and my purpose: I would never be without its membership.

Following HIMSS, I also maintain membership in the Project Management Institute (PMI). As a member for the past 16 years, I became a certified project manager (PMP®) in 2005. I maintain this membership because of my respect and dedication to the project management competency. In addition, I am also a member (through HIMSS' organizational membership) of the Professional Convention Managers Association (PCMA) which is the organization where I earned the digital event strategist (DES). Events management is critical to my role, whether it be in-person or from a distance. The connections that I make with PCMA is priceless, especially during our industry's pivot to virtual events. I am also a member of the American College of Healthcare Executives (ACHE) where I also earned the board certification as a Fellow of ACHE (FACHE). This credential is important to me since it demonstrates my grasp and understanding of healthcare management while also giving me the competencies to serve as a member of the Commission on the Accreditation of Healthcare Management Education (CAHME) Site Visit Team (and previously as a Board member and member of the Accreditation Council).

My second most critical membership is through the Association for Talent Development (ATD) as discussed in detail above. While my professional association memberships may seem excessive, each one has a strategic importance that supports my professional development plan. I encourage you to identify what is important to you and seek out a professional association(s) that will enable you to grow in your career, wherever the health informatics workforce of the future may take you.

Summary

Preparing the health informatics workforce for the future is exciting, challenging, and rewarding, not only for the candidate but also for the employer. But the key to being prepared is to have a plan: one that is living and not stagnant; one that is periodically reviewed and updated; one that is shared with a mentor or other trusted adviser; and one that is realistic. While a plan is critical to guide one's journey, the contents of the plan must be realistic, reasonable, reachable, and relevant. And there is no better resource than a professional society to help guide you along this journey. In fact, you may find that multiple professional societies are not only needed but also required. I have found this to be true based on my vast amount of interests and work experience.

Conclusions and Outlook

There has never been a better time to embrace a career in health informatics. With a focus on technology, innovation, and data science, as well as many other topics, the advances made each and every day are benefiting patients and their families. According to the McKinsey Global Institute "all employers will need to make adept decisions about strategy, investment, technology, workflow redesign, talent needs and training, and the potential impact on the communities in which they operate" [1].

Useful Resources

1. American College of Healthcare Executives: www.ache.org/
2. American Health Informatics Management Association: www.ahima.org/
3. American Medical Informatics Association: www.amia.org/
4. Association of Talent Development: www.td.org/
5. Bill and Melinda Gates Foundation: https://www.who.int/
6. Board Certification: FACHE https://www.ache.org/fache
7. Certification: CAHIMS and CPHIMS: https://www.himss.org/resources/certification
8. Certification: Certified Professional in Talent Development: https://www.td.org/certification/cptd/eligibility
9. Certification: PMP https://www.pmi.org/certifications/types
10. Deloitte: www.deloitte.com/
11. EBSCO: https://www.ebsco.com/
12. eBooks: https://www.himss.org/resources/himss-insights-ebook-series-educational-and-thought-leadership-driven-content
13. Free online courses offered by Harvard, MIT, and many others: https://www.edx.org/
14. HIMSS COVID-19 Resources: https://www.himss.org/news/covid-19
15. HIMSS Global Health Conference and Exhibition: https://www.himssconference.org/
16. HIIMSS Healthcare Information and Management Systems Society: www.himss.org/
17. HIMSS JobMine: https://www.himss.org/resources/himss-jobmine
18. Indeed (Job Search): https://www.indeed.com/
19. LinkedIn Jobs: https://www.linkedin.com/jobs/
20. McKinsey and Company: www.mckinsey.com/
21. Professional Conference Managers Association: https://www.pcma.org/
23. Project Management Institute: www.pmi.org/
24. Rand Corporation: www.rand.org/
25. Robert Wood Johnson Foundation: https://www.rwjf.org/
26. Skills Knowledge Assessment and Development Framework: https://ehealthwork.org/SKAD/index.html
27. Social Media Channel: https://www.instagram.com/

27 Social Media Channel: https://www.linke-din.com/feed/
28. Social Media Channel: https://twitter.com/home
29. Social Media Influencers and related resources: https://www.symplur.com/topic/health-informatics/
30. The World Health Organization: https://www.who.int/
31. TIGER Initiative for Technology and Healthcare Informatics: https://www.himss.org/tiger-initiative-technology-and-health-informatics-education

Review Questions

1. In the workplace, the term "work" has embodied new and different meanings like re-skilling, up-skilling, and future-skilling. Which one of the following is an example of an employee engaging in an "up-skilling" activity?
   (a) Learning a new skill that is unrelated in one's current position
   (b) Earning a second professional certification that enhances one's current position
   (c) Developing a business plan to implement a yet-to-be developed product
   (d) Earning a professional certificate to determine whether a new career is feasible or not

2. Because health informatics is a rapidly evolving discipline, the need for independent, self-directed learning is critical to ensure that one's knowledge keeps pace with the changes in the industry. Which one of the following is not an example of self-directed learning?
   (a) Taking a hybrid course from a university located several thousand miles away
   (b) Earning a certificate of completion from an association
   (c) Having a causal conversation with a friend about the challenges and opportunities in your industry
   (d) Reading and implementing concepts from an eBook on a topic related to your industry

3. Characteristics of the workforce of the future involve many concepts that are deemed as common sense. Which one of the following is not a characteristic of an employee of the workforce of the future?
   (a) Be adaptable, flexible, and nimble

   (b) Engage in lifelong learning
   (c) Appreciate and respect the cultural diversity of the workplace
   (d) Avoid change at all costs

4. One engages in professional development, through activities involving career development and workforce development, all of which lead to lifelong learning. Which one of the following is an example of activities related to workforce development?
   (a) Receiving orientation on the use of a newly acquired infusion pump
   (b) Earning a professional certification
   (c) Receiving continuing medical education units for attending a seminar
   (d) Writing a chapter for a new publication on health informatics

5. Professional societies provide excellent resources, both complimentary and fee-based, for its members, including many benefits that contribute to lifelong learning. Which one of the following is not a typical example of a professional society's benefits?
   (a) Providing public comment on a proposed legislative rule
   (b) Attending an educational event at a discount
   (c) Receiving reimbursement for a parking violation
   (d) Earning a life-time designation, for example, for continuous years of service

Appendix: Answers to Review Questions

1. In the workplace, the term "work" has embodied new and different meanings like re-skilling, up-skilling, and future-skilling. Which one of the following is an example of an employee engaging in an "up-skilling" activity?
   (a) Learning a new skill that is unrelated in one's current position
   (b) **Earning a second professional certification that enhances one's current position**
   (c) Developing a business plan to implement a yet-to-be developed product
   (d) Earning a professional certificate to determine whether a new career is feasible or not

Earning an additional, but related, professional certification is an excellent example of engaging in up-skilling or enhancing one's existing skills and abilities. By doing so, one not only gains additional skills that serve to add to existing knowledge but also contributes to enhancing the quality of work delivered due to acquiring additional skills.

2. Because health informatics is a rapidly evolving discipline, the need for independent, self-directed learning is critical to ensure that one's knowledge keeps pace with the changes in the industry. Which one of the following is not an example of self-directed learning?
   (a) Taking a hybrid course from a university located several thousand miles away
   (b) Earning a certificate of completion from an association
   (c) Having a causal conversation with a friend about the challenges and opportunities in your industry
   (d) Reading and implementing concepts from an eBook on a topic related to your industry

Self-directed learning is an excellent way to proactively identify resources that will contribute to lifelong learning as indicated in one's professional development plan. While engaging in a conversation with a friend may be helpful, it lacks the structure that courses, journal articles, and other tasks provide when engaging in self-directed learning.

3. Characteristics of the workforce of the future involve many concepts that are deemed as common sense. Which one of the following is not a characteristic of an employee of the workforce of the future?
   (a) Be adaptable, flexible, and nimble
   (b) Engage in lifelong learning
   (c) Appreciate and respect the cultural diversity of the workplace
   (d) Avoid change at all costs

Avoiding change at all costs is just not in the vernacular of a health informatics professional of either today's environment or the workplace of the future.

4. One engages in professional development, through activities involving career development and workforce development, all of which lead to lifelong learning. Which one of the following is an example of activities related to workforce development?
   (a) Receiving orientation on the use of a newly acquired infusion pump
   (b) Earning a professional certification
   (c) Receiving continuing medical education units for attending a seminar
   (d) Writing a chapter for a new publication on health informatics

One example of the technical training, as a component of workforce development, involves receiving orientation on the use of a newly acquired infusion pump.

5. Professional societies provide excellent resources, both complimentary and fee-based, for its members, including many benefits that contribute to lifelong learning. Which one of the following is not a typical example of a professional society's benefits?
   (a) Providing public comment on a proposed legislative rule
   (b) Attending an educational event at a discount
   (c) Receiving reimbursement for a parking violation
   (d) Earning a life-time designation, for example, for continuous years of service

Professional societies offer typical benefits like preferred member pricing on education, advanced notice on product offerings, life insurance, car insurance, and other items; however, paying for a personal parking violation is not typical and should not be expected, even if attending a professional association event.

Appendix: Table 39.2

Table 39.2 Appendix: professional associations in the US and around the globe

Professional association name	Focus	Website
Academy of Nutrition and Dietetics	Food and nutrition informaticists, US	https://www.eatrightpro.org/
AcademyHealth Health Information Technology Interest Group	Health Care Delivery and Management, US	http://www.academyhealth.org/index.cfm
Alliance for Nursing Informatics	Nursing, US	http://www.allianceni.org/
American Dental Association Center for Informatics and Standards	Dental, US	https://www.ada.org/en
American Academy of Pediatrics	Physicians	http://www.aap.org/
American Association for Physician Leadership	Physicians	www.physicianleaders.org
American Association for Technology in Psychiatry	Psychiatry, US	http://www.techpsych.org
American Association of Nurse Practitioners	Clinicians	www.aanp.org
American Bar Association	Legal	http://www.americanbar.org/aba.html
American College of Cardiology	Cardiologists	www.acc.org
American College of Clinical Engineering	Biomedical Engineers	http://accenet.org/
American College of Healthcare Executives	Healthcare Executives, US	http://www.ache.org/
American Health Information Management Association	Health Information Management, US	http://www.ahima.org/
American Heart Association	Clinicians	www.heart.org
American Immunization Registry Association	Registries	http://www.immregistries.org/
American Medical Association	Powerful Patient Care Ally Composed of Physicians	https://www.ama-assn.org/
American Medical Informatics Association	Medical Informatics, US and International	https://www.amia.org/
American Nurses Association	Nursing, US	www.nursingworld.org
American Nursing Informatics Association	Nursing Informatics, US	https://www.ania.org/
American Society of Health-System Pharmacists	Pharmacy Informatics, US	http://www.ashp.org/
Association for Clinical Data Management	Clinical Data Management, US	http://www.acdm.org.uk/
Association for Healthcare Documentation Integrity	Health Records Professionals	https://www.ahdionline.org/
Association for Pathology Informatics	Pathology Informatics, US	http://pathologyinformatics.org/
Association for the Advancement of Medical Instrumentation	Clinical Engineers	http://www.aami.org
Association for Veterinary Informatics	Veterinary Informatics, US	https://avinformatics.wildapricot.org/
Association of Medical Directors of Information Systems	Medical Directors, US	http://www.amdis.org
Association of State and Territorial Health Officials	Public Health Agencies in the US, US Territories, and Washington, DC	www.astho.org
Association of University Programs in Health Administration	Undergraduate Health Management Education	www.aupha.org
Australian Institute of Digital Health	Digital Health Transformation, International	https://digitalhealth.org.au/

(continued)

Table 39.2 (continued)

Professional association name	Focus	Website
Belgian Society for Medical Informatics	Medical Informatics for Physicians, Belgium	http://www.bmia.be/en/home/
CAQH	Health Plans and the Business of Healthcare, US	www.caqh.org
College of Healthcare Information Management Executives	Healthcare Information Management Executives	https://chimecentral.org/
Digital Health Canada	Digital Healthcare, Canada	https://digitalhealthcanada.com
ECRI Institute	Safety and Quality, International	www.ecri.org
Electronic Health Record Association	Adoption of EHRs, US	https://www.ehra.org/
Health Informatics New Zealand	Digital Healthcare association for events, networking, and education, New Zealand	http://www.hinz.org.nz/
Health Informatics Society of Ireland	Digital Healthcare association for events, networking, and education, Ireland	https://www.hisi.ie/
Health Information Management Association of Australia Limited	Health Information Management, Australia	http://www.himaa2.org.au/
HealthCare Executive Group	Healthcare Executives and Thought Leaders	www.hceg.org
Healthcare Financial Management Association	Healthcare Financial Management Executives, US	https://www.hfma.org/
Healthcare Information and Management Systems Society	Health Information and Technology, Global	http://www.himss.org/
Indian Association for Medical Informatics	Medical Informatics, India	http://www.iami.org.in/index.aspx
Information Technology Association of Canada	Technology, Canada	http://www.itac.ca/
Integrating the Healthcare Enterprise, US	Standards Adoption, US	https://www.iheusa.org
International Association of Healthcare Security and Safety	Healthcare Security, International	http://www.iahss.org
International Health Terminology Standards Development Organisation	Data Standardization, International	http://www.ihtsdo.org/
International Medical Informatics Association	Physicians, International	http://www.imia-medinfo.org/new2/
Medical Group Management Association	Physician Practices	www.mgma.com
Medical Library Association, Medical Informatics Section	Medical librarians, Health Professionals, Information Sciences Professionals, US	http://www.mlanet.org/p/cm/ld/fid=532
National Association of Community Health Centers	Community-Based Health Centers, US	http://www.nachc.org/
National Association of County and City Health Officials	Local health departments, US	www.naccho.org
National Association of Health Services Executives	Minority and underserved communities, focusing on the black health care leaders	www.nahse.org
National Association of School Nurses	Student health, safety, and learning	https://www.nasn.org/
National Association of State Chief Information Officers	State Chief Information Officers, US	http://www.nascio.org/
National Council for Prescription Drug Programs	Data interchange standards for medications, supplies, and pharmacy services sector	http://www.ncpdp.org/
National Cyber Security Alliance	Cybersecurity awareness	https://www.staysafeonline.org/
National Health IT Collaborative for the Underserved	Underserved populations in the development and use of health information technology (HIT)	http://www.nhitunderserved.org

Table 39.2 (continued)

Professional association name	Focus	Website
North Carolina Healthcare Information and Communications Alliance	Healthcare Data Exchange, US	http://nchica.org/
Physicians EHR Coalition	Physician education on EHRs	http://www.pehrc.org
Scottish Health Information Network	Healthcare, Scotland	http://www.shinelib.org.uk/
Society for Imaging Informatics in Medicine	Biomedical imaging, US	http://siim.org/
Strategic Health Information Exchange Collaborative	Health information exchange	https://strategichie.com
The Cyprus Society of Medical Informatics	Physicians, Cyprus	http://www.csmi.org.cy/
Workgroup for Electronic Data Interchange	Healthcare Information Exchange, US	http://www.wedi.org/

References

1. Lund S, Manyika J, Hilton Segel L, Dua A, Hancock B, Rutherford S, Macon B. The future of work in America. https://www.mckinsey.com/~/media/McKinsey/Featured%20Insights/Future%20of%20Organizations/The%20future%20of%20work%20in%20America%20People%20and%20places%20today%20and%20tomorrow/The-Future-of-Work-in-America-Full-Report.pdf. Accessed 13 July 2020.
2. Hudak C, Ozanich GW. In: HIMSS Dictionary of health information and technology terms, acronyms and organizations. 5th ed. 2019. https://www.routledge.com/HIMSS-Dictionary-of-Health-Information-and-Technology-Terms-Acronyms-and/HIMSS/p/book/9780367148645. Accessed 13 July 2020.
3. AMIA. What is informatics? https://www.amia.org/fact-sheets/what-informatics. Accessed 13 July 2020.
4. AHIMA. Health informatics. https://www.ahima.org/careers/healthinfo. Accessed 13 July 2020.
5. HIMSS TIGER Interprofessional community. Global informatics definitions. https://www.himss.org/sites/hde/files/media/file/2020/07/20/tiger_informaticsdefinitions-v4-final.pdf. Accessed 23 July 2020.
6. Gratton L. New frontiers in up-skilling and re-skilling. In MIT Sloan Management Review. https://sloanreview.mit.edu/article/new-frontiers-in-re-skilling-and-upskilling/. Accessed 23 July 2020.
7. Brandman University. Overcoming the challenges of a multi-generational workforce. https://www.brandman.edu/news-and-events/blog/multigenerational-workforce. Accessed 23 July 2020.
8. Nandi A, Mandermach, M. Hackathons as an informal learning platform. In: Proceedings of the 47th ACM Technical Symposium on Computing Science Education (SIGCSE'16). New York, NY: Association for Computing Machinery; 2016. pp. 346–351. https://doi.org/10.1145/2839509.2844590
9. Albert LR, Dignma M. Who are the learners? In: The decision to learn: why people seek continuing education and how membership organizations can meet learners' needs. Washington, DC: Association Management Press; 2010. p. 14.
10. Association for Talent Development. Talent development body of knowledge. Alexandria: ATD Press; 2020. p. 627.
11. Paine N. Guiding your organization's future. In: The learning challenge. Alexandria: ATD Press; 2018. p. 525.
12. Kippon K. The future of learning: one size fits one. In: Biech E, editor. ATD's foundations of talent development. Alexandria: ATD Press; 2018. p. 464–9.
13. Wittnebel L. Business as usual? A review of continuing professional education and adult learning. In: Journal of adult and continuing education. Manchester: Manchester University Press; 2012. p. 80–8.
14. Daiker, M. Continuing professional development and its greater rewards. 2019. https://www.himss.org/resources/continuing-professional-development-and-its-greater-rewards. Accessed 13 July 2020.
15. A leadership resource for patient and family engagement strategies. Health Research & Educational Trust, Chicago: July 2013. http://www.hpoe.org/resources/ahahret-guides/1407. (Appears in Preparing for Success in Healthcare and Information Systems: The CAHIMS Review Guide, Chicago: 2015). Accessed 14 July 2020.
16. Franklin B. https://www.forbes.com/quotes/1107/. Accessed 17 July 2020.
17. Covey S. https://www.awakenthegreatnesswithin.com/40-inspirational-stephen-covey-quotes-on-success/. Accessed 17 July 2020.

18. Deloitte Center for Integrated Research. https://www2.deloitte.com/us/en/pages/about-deloitte/solutions/center-integrated-research.html. Accessed 17 July 2020.
19. McKinsey Global Institute. Mission. https://www.mckinsey.com/mgi/overview. Accessed 17 July 2020.
20. Rand Corporation. https://www.rand.org/research.html. Accessed 17 July 2020.
21. Blash A, Klinedinst J. The role of the professional association. In: The Handbook of Continuing Professional Development for the Health IT Professional, JoAnn Klinedinst, published by HIMSS and CRC Press, Taylor and Francis Group, copyright 2017, ISBN: 9781138033238

Health Informatics Education: Standards, Challenges, and Tools

40

Jennifer Thate and Robert G. Brookshire

Learning Objectives

Readers will be able to:

- Compare and contrast the various programs and standards for health informatics education.
- Describe curricular threads in health informatics education.
- Support an interprofessional and interdisciplinary approach to health informatics education.
- Discuss challenges in health informatics education.
- Evaluate different technologies, digital tools, and approaches used in healthcare education.
- Explain how the TIGER VLE resources can be used to deliver health informatics education and training.

Key Terms

- Accreditation
- Competencies
- Interprofessional
- Interdisciplinary
- Massive Online Open Course (MOOC)
- Virtual learning environment
- Virtual reality
- Augmented reality

- Simulation
- Gaming

Introduction

While the discipline of health informatics (HI) has grown and matured over the years, there is not one degree or educational path that prepares one for a career in HI. Furthermore, HI is just one term used to describe the interrelated specialty or discipline encompassing the use of information science, computer science, the knowledge of various healthcare disciplines, and technology.[1] Future refinement of the HI discipline would benefit from consensus and clarity regarding terms, educational preparation, and standards or competencies. Much work has been done to achieve this by initiatives such as Technology Informatics Guiding Educational Reform (TIGER) (see Chap. 38). Additionally, the International Medical Informatics Association (IMIA) has provided recommenda-

[1] In this chapter, we have used health informatics (HI) to refer to the discipline. HI is defined in the HIMSS TIGER Interprofessional Community Global Informatics Definitions document as "the interdisciplinary study of the design, development, adoption, and application of information technology (IT)-based innovations in healthcare services delivery, management, and planning." We recognize that there is overlap and variation globally in terms and that eHealth may also be used to refer to this field. Please see the HIMSS TIGER Interprofessional Community Global Informatics Definitions document for further information on related terms.

J. Thate (✉)
Siena College, Albany, NY, USA
e-mail: jthate@siena.edu

R. G. Brookshire (✉)
University of South Carolina, Columbia, SC, USA
e-mail: rbrook@mailbox.sc.edu

© Springer Nature Switzerland AG 2022
U. H. Hübner et al. (eds.), *Nursing Informatics*, Health Informatics,
https://doi.org/10.1007/978-3-030-91237-6_40

tions for educational programs in Biomedical and Health Informatics (BMHI). Such efforts provide guideposts for educators in preparing clinicians and the global HI workforce to leverage technology and informatics to improve the health of people and communities around the world.

In addition to the lack of consensus regarding terms, educational preparation, and standards or competencies, there are several challenges facing the development and delivery of HI education. One challenge is ensuring programs reflect appropriate standards or competencies and competencies that keep pace with current and future trends in healthcare *and* informatics. Furthermore, there is an ongoing need for faculty with expertise in the rapidly changing field of HI. Educators also face the challenge of preparing students to navigate the complexity of this highly interdisciplinary and interprofessional field. Finally, HI education must have a global reach to promote universal fluency in the field.

One way to augment and expand HI education is through the use of technologies and digital tools. Technology and informatics tools have a long history of use in higher education. They have also been widely used in health professions programs, such as nursing and medicine, to prepare clinicians for clinical care with a significant focus on simulation. When digital tools and distance modalities are used to augment educational programs designed for those pursuing degrees in HI, technology and informatics are both the subject of study and the means by which the content is delivered and learned.

Educational Programs Related to Health Informatics

There is a wide variety of educational programs related to HI due to the scope of professions within and ancillary to healthcare and the diverse disciplines needed to support the development and application of information and communication technologies (ICT). All healthcare professionals need to have proficiency in the use and application of ICT in order to provide effective quality care, so content related to HI must be incorporated into all educational programs pre-

paring students for healthcare professions. Other disciplines relevant to the field of HI include computer science; information technology (IT), information science, and information systems; business and information management; engineering, biomedical informatics, data science, and many others. The names of these disciplines may vary globally, but they all address two general areas: the technical components and development of ICT and the use of these technologies in the healthcare system by clinicians and administrators. Educational programs are thus aligned with these different disciplines. Additionally, some programs provide opportunities for healthcare professionals to seek specialization in an aspect of HI after obtaining a degree in their selected profession. In summary, there are two broad categories of focus within HI education, the ICT or IT user and the HI or BMHI specialist [1].

Box 40.1 Key Acronyms in Alphabetical Order

AACN: American Association of Colleges of Nursing

AMIA: American Medical Informatics Association

ANIA: American Nursing Informatics Association

BMHI: Biomedical and Health Informatics

CAHIIM: Commission on Accreditation for Health Informatics and Information Management Education

CCNE: Commission on Collegiate Nursing Education

EFMI: European Federation of Medical Informatics

HI: Health Informatics

HIMSS: Healthcare Information and Management Systems Society

HIT: Health Information Technology

ICT: Information and Communication Technologies

IMIA: International Medical Informatics Association

TIGER: Technology Informatics Guiding Educational Reform

Several organizations and associations support informatics practice related to specific specialties within the field of HI. They provide starting points for exploring educational programs that prepare graduates for careers in HI. The American Medical Informatics Association (AMIA) provides a repository for academic and training programs in biomedical, health, and nursing informatics (NI). The programs contained on the AMIA website range from baccalaureate programs to doctoral programs and include certificate programs and fellowships. Programs may be identified as HI, health information management (HIM), biomedical informatics, bioinformatics, data science, or simply informatics. This is a sampling of programs and degree options, as posting program information on the site is voluntary, but it signifies the varied academic and training programs related to HI. The American Nursing Informatics Association (ANIA) includes a list of educational partners on their website; however, they do not provide a repository for NI programs. Similarly, the Healthcare Information and Management Systems Society (HIMSS) provides a list of approved education partners which encompasses continuing education or training as well as degree-granting programs through institutions of higher education. Beyond the U.S., the European Federation of Medical Informatics (EFMI) provides an online catalog of biomedical and HI programs across Europe including 30 countries and 1900 higher education institutions. Unfortunately, there is currently no repository or catalog of educational programs globally. These examples not only illustrate the breadth of pathways and opportunities but also highlight the potential for varied standards. See the *Useful Resources* section for weblinks to organizations with information on education programs.

Accreditation and Standards Guiding eHealth and Health Informatics Education

Accreditation is a process whereby educators and administrators of degree-granting programs demonstrate to the public their adherence to a set of standards reflecting their programs' academic quality. This process includes regular self and peer assessment of a program in collaboration with the accrediting body. This ongoing and continuous process ensures adherence to current and evolving standards. For example, programs in HIM seek accreditation through the Commission on Accreditation for Health Informatics and Information Management Education (CAHIIM). At this writing, there are 350 CAHIIM-accredited programs in HIM or HI. Of these, 252 offer associate degrees, 73 offer baccalaureate degrees, and 26 offer master's degrees. Of these programs, 273 can be taken online and 205 can be taken on-campus, with many offering programs in both modalities.

International accreditation has also begun to be offered through IMIA in collaboration with representatives from EFMI [2]. International accreditation offers unique benefits and challenges. The benefits include the evaluation of a program's global relevancy by demonstrating alignment to international standards and competencies. This promotes global fluency in HI as well as international mobility for graduates [3]. The challenges include addressing language barriers when providing guidance for program administrators on submitting self-assessment reports and for reviewers when reviewing program materials; navigating the diversity of cultural practices when establishing policies and processes for site visits; and identifying suitable reviewers to facilitate the peer-review site visit and analysis [3]. IMIA's development and refinement of the international accreditation process have the potential to further coalesce the global field of HI.

In the U.S., while programs in HI may seek accreditation through CAHIIM, specific disciplines or professions within healthcare may also have informatics-specific standards as a part of their accreditation process. This addresses the imperative for informatics competency for all health professionals. In nursing, there are informatics standards for preparation of the nurse generalist at the baccalaureate level that are distinct from standards for the NI specialist requiring a graduate degree. The U.S. Commission on

Collegiate Nursing Education (CCNE) is an example of a national nursing accreditation agency that has identified HI competencies as a necessary part of the professional standards guiding curriculum development for an accredited baccalaureate nursing program. In the American Association of Colleges of Nursing (AACN) *Essentials of Baccalaureate Education for Professional Nursing Practice*, which are required standards for programs seeking CCNE accreditation, there are nine areas describing expected outcomes for programs. One area, "Information Management and Application of Patient Care Technology," focuses on knowledge and skills related to information management and the use of technology to deliver quality patient care. This demonstrates that all nurses prepared at the baccalaureate level to obtain licensure as a registered nurse (RN) need to achieve a level of competency in HI. At this writing, the *Essentials* are being reviewed and updated, including revisions to the informatics-focused area, to further specify key aspects of preparation for nurses in HI. The challenge explored in the next section is the preparation or availability of faculty to guide students in obtaining the outcomes to support this crucial area.

IMIA has also recognized the need for informatics competencies for all practicing clinicians, who, by nature of their roles, will be at least users of information systems and ICT. The term **competency** is used to describe possessing knowledge or skill in a particular area and having the ability to apply one's knowledge and skill. Many standards for informatics education are written as learner outcomes including skills and knowledge by domain. IMIA emphasizes required skills and knowledge in biomedical HI for all healthcare professionals as part of their preparation for practice. This is aligned with the *Essentials of Baccalaureate Education for Professional Nursing Practice*, described above. To further delineate the knowledge and skills required for nurses, IMIA put forth educational recommendations for NI for both nurse generalist and NI specialist programs [4].

Other sources providing a framework for the education and practice of nursing informaticists include the American Nursing Association's (ANA) Nursing Informatics Scope and Standards of Practice. The first version of ANA's standards of practice was published in 1995, with the most recent edition appearing in 2015. This document outlines the elements of the specialty of NI including the role of the informatics nurse and the informatics nurse specialist (INS). The informatics nurse is distinguished by board certification offered through ANCC. While this certification does not require a graduate degree, it does include practice requirements, continuing education, and experience in informatics nursing. In contrast, an INS is a nurse who holds a graduate degree with a specialty in NI. IMIA similarly distinguishes among groups within the field of HI: the specialized healthcare practitioner (nurse, physician, etc.) with additional training in informatics; the computer scientist or ICT specialist; and the health informatician [4]. Some would consider the health informatician as equivalent to the specialized healthcare practitioner who has additional training in informatics. Thus, another example of the continued need for clarification of terms. These distinctions highlight the varied pathways to a career in HI and the range of ways to contribute to the field.

In an analysis of existing HI education programs across Europe and the U.S., Herzog and colleagues [5] categorized programs on how they aligned to three professional groups within HI: healthcare, engineering, and management. These groups were identified as necessary areas of expertise to meet the challenges of increasing interoperability in HI, specifically recognizing the essential role of management. For academic programs in Europe, they found the majority of offerings were in engineering or management, while in the U.S., the majority of offerings were programs for healthcare professionals, followed by programs for engineers. They also found that varied terminology was used to describe courses and content in these programs; however, core concepts were identified and consolidated for comparison. Understanding the interdisciplinary and interprofessional nature of this field is paramount to developing educational programs that successfully prepare graduates for their unique roles.

Educators must consider both where program outcomes and standards should have commonalities and where they should be distinctive.

Curricular Threads and Interdisciplinary Competencies

Due to the multidisciplinary nature of HI, we need to consider common threads running through the various curricula that prepare students to work in this field. Identifying interprofessional or interdisciplinary competencies in HI highlights the intersection of the various professions and disciplines and prepares graduates to communicate effectively among the HI team. **Interprofessional** refers to the interface of two or more professions (i.e. nurse, physician, or pharmacist), whereas **interdisciplinary** refers two or more disciplines (i.e. computer science, medicine, or engineering). These terms are often used interchangeably; however, interprofessional collaboration is something specific to practice, while interdisciplinary courses, programs, or projects occur within academic institutions that prepare students for interprofessional practice. Several projects have been carried out to describe common informatics competencies across disciplines, some of which are described later in this chapter as well as in Chap. 11: The Educator's View [6]. IMIA's revised recommendations on BMHI education includes a table with various organizations publications related to HI competencies [1].

IMIA identified three knowledge and skill domains necessary for educational programs related to BMHI regardless of profession or discipline (Table 40.1). They include (1) BMHI core knowledge and skills; (2) medicine, health and biosciences, health system organization; and (3) informatics/computer science, mathematics, and biometry [1]. In the IMIA recommendations, the extent of focus in each area depends on the program type. For example, an informatics/computer science program should place more emphasis on health and biosciences and the health system organization, as these topics are not innate to the field of computer science. A key takeaway from the IMIA recommendations is the need to tailor the breadth, depth, and focus of the learning outcomes to meet the needs of different program types, educational institutions, and healthcare systems. One cannot over-emphasize the team-based approach needed to meet the challenges of improving health and care using ICT. Establishing a common framework for the field of BMHI contributes to the development of competent individuals within the field and enhances communication among the healthcare/HI team. Common frameworks also support global cooperation in HI. The IMIA document provides a solid foundation and comprehensive framework to guide the development of educational programs in the complex interdisciplinary and interprofessional field of HI [1].

Challenges in Health Informatics Education

The first challenge in HI education is having a clear understanding of the scope and standards of the profession. As Hersch [7] notes, this is essential for the profession to exist. Educators will be challenged to prepare students for their roles in and related to HI if the end goal is fuzzy. Defining key competencies for the global HI workforce is one of the primary means to accomplish this end. As noted above, much work has been done to identify and define these competencies. However, as evidenced in the call by CAHIIM for a clearer, more coordinated career path model, this work must continue as the field evolves and matures.

The second challenge is the development of academic leaders and educators in health professions and HI programs equipped to prepare students to fulfill these competencies. This depends upon clarity in workforce roles and competencies in the field, as well as ensuring that the leaders and educators utilize these standards when developing educational programs. Accreditation is one way to encourage adherence to these standards.

In spite of the consensus on the need for BMHI education for those who will work in healthcare, there remain hurdles to providing educational programs that align with the recommendations for all the IMIA knowledge and skill

Table 40.1 Recommended and optional learning outcomes in terms of levels of knowledge and skills for professionals in healthcare either in their role as IT users or as BMHI specialists. Additional recommendations, specific for a certain educational program, will be added in Sects. 4 and 5. Recommended level of knowledge and skills: + = introductory. ++ = intermediate. +++ = advanced

Knowledge/skill—Domain		Level	
		IT user	BMHI specialist
(1) Biomedical and Health Informatics Core Knowledge and Skills			
1.1	Evolution of informatics as a discipline and as a profession	+	+
1.2	Need for systematic information processing in healthcare, benefits and constraints of information technology in healthcare	++	++
1.3	Efficient and responsible use of information processing tools to support healthcare professionals' practice and their decision making	++	++
1.4	Use of personal application software for documentation, personal communication including Internet access, for publication and basic statistics	++	++
1.5	Information literacy: library classification and systematic health-related terminologies and their coding, literature retrieval methods, research methods, and research paradigms	++	++
1.6	Characteristics, functionalities, and examples of information systems in healthcare (e.g. clinical information systems, primary care information systems, etc.)	+	+++
1.7	Architectures of information systems in healthcare; approaches and standards for communication and cooperation and for interfacing and integration of component, architectural paradigms (e.g. service-oriented architectures)		++
1.8	Management of information systems in healthcare (health information management, strategic and tactic information management, IT governance, IT service management, legal and regulatory issues)	+	+++
1.9	Characteristics, functionalities, and examples of information systems to support patients and the public (e.g. patient-oriented information system architectures and applications, personal health records, sensor-enhanced information systems)	+	++
1.10	Methods and approaches to regional networking and shared care (eHealth, health telematics applications, and interorganizational information exchange)	+	++
1.11	Appropriate documentation and health data management principles including ability to use health and medical coding systems, construction of health and medical coding systems	+	+++
1.12	Structure, design, and analysis principles of the health record including notions of data quality, minimum data sets, architecture, and general applications of the electronic patient record/electronic health record	+	+++
1.13	Socio-organizational and socio-technical issues, including workflow/process modeling and reorganization	+	+++
1.14	Principles of data representation and data analysis using primary and secondary data sources principles of data mining, data warehouses knowledge management	+	++
1.15	Biomedical modeling and simulation		+
1.16	Ethical and security issues including accountability of healthcare providers and managers and BMHI specialists and the confidentiality, privacy, and security of patient data	+	++
1.17	Nomenclatures, vocabularies, terminologies, ontologies, and taxonomies in BMHI	+	++

Table 40.1 (continued)

Knowledge/skill—Domain		Level	
		IT user	BMHI specialist
1.18	Informatics methods and tools to support education (incl. flexible and distance learning), use of relevant educational technologies, incl. Internet and World Wide Web		+
1.19	Evaluation and assessment of information systems, including study design, selection and triangulation of (quantitative and qualitative) methods, outcome and impact evaluation, economic evaluation, unintended consequences, systematic reviews and meta-analysis, evidence-based health informatics		++
(2) Medicine, Health and Biosciences, Health System Organization			
2.1	Fundamentals of human functioning and biosciences (anatomy, physiology, microbiology, genomics, and clinical disciplines such as internal medicine, surgery, etc.)	+	+
2.2	Fundamentals of what constitutes health, from physiological, sociological, psychological, nutritional, emotional, environmental, cultural, spiritual perspectives, and its assessment	+	+
2.3	Principles of clinical/medical decision making and diagnostic and therapeutic strategies	+	++
2.4	Organization of health institutions and of the overall health system, interorganizational aspects, shared care	+	+++
2.5	Policy and regulatory frameworks for information handling in healthcare		+
2.6	Principles of evidence-based practice (evidence-based medicine, evidence-based nursing)	+	+
2.7	Health administration, health economics, health quality management and resource management, patient safety initiatives, public health services, and outcome measurement	+	++
(3) Informatics/Computer Science, Mathematics, Biometry (continued)			
3.1	Basic informatics terminology like data, information, knowledge, hardware, software, computer, networks, information systems, information systems management	+	+++
3.2	Ability to use personal computers, text processing and spread sheet software, easy-to-use database management systems	++	+++
3.3	Ability to communicate electronically, including electronic data exchange, with other healthcare professionals, Internet/intranet use	++	+++
3.4	Methods of practical informatics/computer science, especially on programming languages, software engineering, data structures, database management systems information and system modeling tools, information systems theory and practice, knowledge engineering, (concept) representation and acquisition, software architectures		+++
3.5	Methods of theoretical informatics/computer science, for example, complexity theory, encryption/security		++
3.6	Methods of technical informatics/computer science, for example, network architectures and topologies, telecommunications, wireless technology, virtual reality, multimedia		++
3.7	Methods of interfacing and integration of information system components in healthcare, interfacing standards, dealing with multiple patient identifiers		++
3.8	Handling of the information system life cycle: analysis, requirement specification, implementation and/or selection of information systems, risk management, user training	+	+++

(continued)

Table 40.1 (continued)

Knowledge/skill—Domain		Level	
		IT user	BMHI specialist
3.9	Methods of project management and change management (i.e. project planning, resource management, team management, conflict management, collaboration and motivation, change theories, change strategies)	+	+++
3.10	Mathematics: algebra, analysis, logic, numerical mathematics, probability theory and statistics, cryptography		++
3.11	Biometry, epidemiology, and health research methods, including study design		++
3.12	Methods for decision support and their application to patient management, acquisition, representation, and engineering of medical knowledge; construction and use of clinical pathways and guidelines	+	+++
3.13	Basic concepts and applications of ubiquitous computing (e.g. pervasive, sensor-based, and ambient technologies in healthcare, health-enabling technologies, ubiquitous health systems, and ambient-assisted living)		+
3.14	Usability engineering, human–computer interaction, usability evaluation, cognitive aspects of information processing		++
(4) Optional Modules in BHMI and from Related Fields			
4.1	Biomedical imaging and signal processing		+ − +++
4.2	Clinical/medical bioinformatics and computational biology		+ − +++
4.3	Health-enabling technologies, ubiquitous health systems, and ambient-assisted living		+ − +++
4.4	Health information sciences		+ − +++
4.5	Medical chemoinformatics		+ − +++
4.6	Medical nanoinformatics		+ − +++
4.7	Medical robotics		+ − +++
4.8	Public health informatics		+ − +++

From Mantas J, Ammenwerth E, Demiris G, Hasman A, Haux R, Hersh W, et al. Recommendations of the International Medical Informatics Association (IMIA) on Education in Biomedical and Health Informatics. Methods Inf Med. 2010;49(2):105–20. Table 2: p. 112. Copyright © by IMIA. Reprinted with permission from IMIA

domains. Even with guiding documents from IMIA, TIGER, AMIA, AHIMA, ANA, and others, the integration of informatics content into, for example, baccalaureate nursing programs remains varied [8]. Some programs do not sufficiently distinguish between computer skills and informatics competencies. While computer skills and digital literacy are important, they do not represent the inclusion of informatics in a curriculum. Increasing academic nurse educators' and nursing program administrators' exposure to these guiding documents coupled with evidence of the necessity of HI for all clinicians in order to provide high-quality care is needed. This most commonly is accomplished by HI champions in nursing programs and their involvement in key standard setting organizations for nursing education, such as AACN.

There is also a need to evolve medical education to prepare physicians to practice in healthcare systems inextricable from ICT and the broader application of HI. In a review of the inclusion of health information technologies (HIT) content in medical education within the European Union, it was noted that only approximately one-third of schools included HIT courses in their curricula [9]. In response to the need to enhance informatics competency for physicians in the U.S., the American Medical Association (AMA) established the *Accelerating Change in Medical Education Initiative* in 2013. Incorporation of HI content and experiences was a significant aspect of this initiative.

This somewhat recent focus on the integration of informatics in medical education suggests, just as in nursing, the identified need for informatics knowledge and expertise in academic medical educators to prepare future clinicians. An effort in the U.S. that will help in this regard is the formation of the new medical subspecialty in clinical informatics which began in 2013. These programs are accredited by the Accreditation Council for Graduate Medical Education (ACGME), which recognizes clinical informatics as a subspecialty within 9 of its 28 medical specialties: anesthesiology, emergency medicine, family medicine, internal medicine, medical genetics and genomics, pathology, pediatrics, preventive medicine, and radiology. These physicians will plausibly lead future growth in the incorporation of HI into medical education.

Some nursing programs have also noted a lack of access by students to information systems in clinical practice or during clinical experiences at healthcare organizations [8]. This prevents students from engaging in and learning to maximize the benefit of ICT to support practice. Overcoming this lack of access in the clinical setting requires buy-in from healthcare system leaders who recognize that using clinical information systems during training is vital to preparing students for practice in the highly technical and information-dependent system.

Educators are further challenged by the required intersection of the many professions and disciplines encompassing the complex systems of healthcare *and* IT (see Fig. 40.1). Reviewing the IMIA recommendations for knowledge and skills required for the IT user and the BMHI specialist,

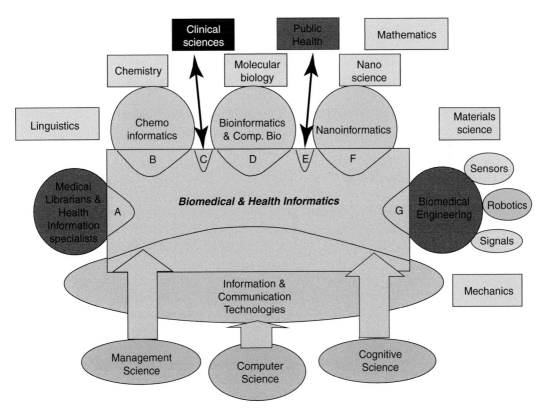

Fig. 40.1 Biomedical and health informatics and related fields. Overlapping areas: (**a**) Medical information science, (**b**) Medical chemoinformatics, (**c**) Clinical informatics, (**d**) Medical (translational) bioinformatics, (**e**) Public health informatics, (**f**) Medical nanoinformatics, (**g**) Medical imaging and devices (From Mantas J, Ammenwerth E, Demiris G, Hasman A, Haux R, Hersh W, et al. Recommendations of the International Medical Informatics Association (IMIA) on Education in Biomedical and Health Informatics. Methods Inf Med. 2010;49 (2):105–20. Figure 2: p. 110. Copyright © by IMIA. Reprinted with permission from IMIA.)

it is evident that a team of educators with extensive and varied backgrounds is needed. Identifying individuals equipped to assist students in meeting the learning outcomes to achieve these competencies depends on a concerted effort to mentor and prepare individuals for the role of HI educators and academics. Those administering HI programs need to curate teams of educators with backgrounds in a variety of disciplines and identify liaisons who can serve as bridges or translators on the team, just as is done in industry.

An additional obstacle facing HI education is the disparity in available technologies and the supporting infrastructures between well-resourced and resource-limited communities. These disparities result in a "digital divide," whether within a country such as the U.S. or between global regions such as Europe and sub-Saharan Africa. Although resource-limited communities may have sufficient access to certain technologies such as cellular telephones, they may lack access to the more complex technology infrastructure needed to implement electronic health records (EHR) or patient monitoring systems. This lack of technological infrastructure impacts not only the delivery of healthcare but also the delivery of healthcare and HI education.

Ways to Address the Challenges

Leaders across the globe have recognized that coalescing efforts to establish clear competencies and standards to define the profession is key to meeting the challenges in HI education. This is difficult due to the variety of professions, disciplines, and specialties necessary to develop, design, and apply ICT to support high-quality care, but as described in Sect. 1, progress is being made. Establishing and implementing these standards will benefit both students and faculty, and ultimately the global HI workforce, better equipping them to leverage ICT to improve care. HI champions who collaborate through organizations such as TIGER will be integral to these efforts.

As the field of HI matures, we see increasing evidence that ICT facilitates safe, quality care, but more research is needed. Evidence derived from research about the impact of HI must reach key decision makers and leaders in healthcare systems to drive demand for quality education in HI and provide funding where needed. Continued development of academic and industry leaders depends on partnerships and information sharing between these two sectors.

One of the simplest solutions is *increasing access* to high-quality courses and programs, regardless of location, for both students and future HI faculty, that adhere to the standards and recommendations discussed thus far. This will contribute to a well-prepared workforce and increase the number of future educators. One way this can be accomplished is by leveraging technologies and tools to deliver and enhance HI education.

Tools Used in Health Informatics Education

Technologies used in HI education derive from two rich sources: those used in higher education in general and those specifically used in healthcare education and training. In this section, we describe the principal computer-based or digital tools used in HI education. As will become apparent, many of these technologies are combined to deliver training effectively, efficiently, and engagingly.

Computer-Based Training

Computer-based training (CBT), also known as computer-assisted instruction, computer-assisted learning, computer-based instruction, or computer-based testing, is the oldest form of digital training, having first appeared with PLATO (Programmed Logic for Automated Teaching Operations) at the University of Illinois in 1959 [10, 11].

CBT provides a linear sequence of instructions guiding learners through content with frequent checks on their understanding and feedback. It may include multimedia and interactive exercises. If the goal of instruction is to certify or credential the learner, a testing component may be incorporated. The goal is that learners teach themselves with little or no help from an instructor. CBT is widely used by human resource departments to train employees on policies and procedures.

In healthcare education, CBT is available to teach HIPAA or Institutional Review Board (IRB) regulations for clinicians, administrators, and others. Under the U.S. Health Information Technology for Economic and Clinical Health (HITECH) Act of 2009 [12], the Office of the National Coordinator (ONC) for HIT contracted with several universities to develop training on EHRs and meaningful use. These CBT resources are available with open access through the ONC website [13].

A specialized type of CBT is the performance support system, providing just-in-time training or assistance in the context of a particular piece of software. This may include online help, tutorials, databases of frequently asked questions, expert systems, and multimedia. One example is the help system built into the Microsoft Office software suite.

Performance support systems organize information around processes or tasks rather than subject matter, making training available when it is needed. Performance support systems are presented to learners when they are most highly motivated to learn in order to accomplish a certain goal. They can provide training at different levels of detail depending on the learners' needs, from simple suggestions to complex instructions.

Online Instructor-Led Training

Online instructor-led training, whether synchronous or asynchronous, is the most widely used digital learning method for universities, companies, and healthcare institutions. With asynchronous delivery, lessons can be accessed anywhere, anytime from desktop or mobile devices. Online instruction provides flexibility to design any kind of instruction, from short tutorials to complete degree programs. Online instruction can be as effective as classroom-based instruction. Online teaching, enhanced with multimedia and interaction, can keep learners' interest and increase their motivation. Learners can pause lessons and continue later or repeat lessons until they have achieved mastery. Online learning can be faster than traditional face-to-face instruction, as learners can move at their own pace and take alternative pathways through the material.

Online learning is often supported by learning management systems (LMSs), such as Blackboard, Moodle, or Canvas, that help to deliver, track, and assess learning [14]. An LMS can expand the capability and reduce the complexity of creating and handling learning material. An LMS is particularly important in delivering massive open online courses (MOOCs).

An MOOC is massive because it serves hundreds or thousands of learners; open, as learners can enroll without prerequisites or fees; online, as it is accessible worldwide through the Internet; and a course because it teaches a specific subject. Siemens and Downes coined the term "MOOC" in 2008 for their online course, "Connectivism & Connective Knowledge," at the University of Manitoba, with 25 on-campus and 2300 online participants [15]. By 2019, more than 900 universities and several independent organizations around the world offered MOOCs, delivering more than 11,000 courses for more than 100 million students.

Medical MOOCs are a fairly recent development. Healthcare providers must keep up with advances in medicine, and medical certification authorities require them to complete a number of continuing medical education credits annually. Until recently, healthcare professionals earned those credits primarily by attending conferences, but MOOCs have expanded into this area. Several programs are approved by the Accreditation Council for Continuing Medical Education (ACCME). The "Class Central" database contains 1219 health and medicine MOOCs, among which 888 were certificate courses. Coursera and edX, a joint venture between Harvard and the Massachusetts Institute of Technology (MIT), are the major MOOC platforms. At this writing, Coursera is delivering a free MOOC developed by Johns Hopkins University to teach COVID-19 contact tracing.

MOOCs can provide excellent instructional materials, the ability to engage with instructors and other learners globally, and greatly reduced cost. However, many learners enrolled in MOOCs fail to complete their courses. Language challenges, course difficulty, low engagement with the material, and poor motivation contribute to the high drop-out rate.

Tools to Enhance Learning

Recently, educators and trainers have been introducing technologies such as virtual reality (VR), augmented reality (AR), and gamification to enhance the learner's experience. VR uses computer technology, sound, and animation to immerse the learner in an artificial setting that may or may not closely mimic reality. AR is the introduction of computer-generated content into a real-life setting. Gamification is the introduction of game elements or concepts into the design of the learning experience.

VR has been used in healthcare education since the 1990s. It is widely employed to teach surgical and diagnostic techniques. For nursing students, VR has been used to teach anatomy, childbirth education, decontamination, intravenous catheterization, phlebotomy, spinal anesthesia, ultrasound skills, and many other topics. AR is being used to train surgeons using real surgical tools on simulated patients. These technologies allow learners to gain hands-on practice in realistic settings without endangering patients. They also can provide clinical experiences in situations where there is limited availability of placement sites or with specialized techniques or procedures not frequently encountered in practice.

It is estimated that, worldwide, people spend 3 billion hours a week playing computer and video games. Because games are so engaging, teachers and course developers are introducing gamification into the learning experience. Challenges, competition, and rewards are used to enhance the learner's engagement. Gamification takes advantage of the four freedoms of play: freedom to fail—the power to make mistakes without serious consequences; freedom to experiment—the ability to invent new approaches; the freedom to fashion different identities; and freedom of effort—being able to alternate intense and relaxed activity [16].

The use of games has grown dramatically in healthcare education and training, including games with multiplayer options promoting team learning, problem-solving, and management. A few examples of successful serious medical games include "Emergency Birth!" for obstetrics, "Elderquest" for geriatrics, and "Skinquizition" for dermatology.

Online Digital Learning Resources

Used on their own or in combination with the technologies we have described, digital education resources have made learning easier and less expensive. Libraries have converted texts and articles to digital formats accessible on tablets, computers, and smartphones. Computer-based resources are the primary source of clinical information for medical professionals in the U.S. and Canada, replacing paper texts. Digital reference works not only reduce costs but also are more frequently updated.

Academic databases provide access to peer-reviewed articles and conference proceedings for research. Google Scholar, for example, is a freely accessible database of scholarly literature. Other databases such as CINAHL, Scopus, Web of Science, and PubMed are available by subscription. A growing assortment of Web-based resources such as WebMD, MayoClinic.org, and others are increasingly popular with patients as well as clinicians and may even be linked to a hospital or other healthcare provider's patient portal.

Digital audio and video resources such as YouTube, TED talks, podcasts, and webinars have become important tools in medical education and training. YouTube contains hundreds of thousands of videos aimed at medical training used by medical professionals across the globe. TED (Technology, Entertainment, Design) Conferences is a media company that posts short talks online for free distribution. TEDx, a local version, is a network of self-organized events bringing individuals together to share TED-like presentations. TEDMED is an independent health and medicine edition of the TED conference. TED talks help to spread and popularize innovative medical ideas.

Webinar software such as GoToWebinar by GoToMeeting, Easy Webinar, Adobe Connect, Webex, and Zoom enable seminars to be delivered to large audiences regardless of location. Many of these webinars are recorded for future use. These platforms can be tools to acquire technical expertise in a variety of disciplines. Social networks can also provide digital learning content. In online communities, participants can exchange ideas and share files, videos, web links, or multimedia.

Blogs (originally weblogs) began as online diaries, but have evolved to serve a number of purposes, including education. Blogs provide web pages where teachers can discuss topics, post articles and other content, provide links to online content, and solicit responses from learners. They can also be used to distribute training or communicate within an organization.

A wiki (Hawaiian for "fast" or "quick") is a website for the submission and editing of content by a user community. The largest, Wikipedia, contains over 6 million articles. Wikipedia hosts a tremendous amount of information on healthcare topics, but there are medical wikis specifically focusing on healthcare. Some, like WikiDoc and Radiopaedia, do not require contributors to have medical credentials, while others, like Clinfowiki, HemOnc.org, and WikEm (The Global Emergency Wiki), are limited to contributions from healthcare professionals. Wikis are also used within organizations, or even with classes, to develop knowledge bases for particular situations or topics. The Blackboard LMS, for example, allows students and teachers to create wikis for individual classes.

Computers and IT have redefined education, making it more widely available, less expensive, more effective, and more efficient. Technology helps learners find the content they want when they want it and at a reasonable price. Increased access is critical to efforts to further educate the global HI workforce. At the same time, technology has contributed to the digital divide, in which wealthier learners have greater access to educational resources than resource-limited ones. Digital content is not always friendly to learners with visual or other impairments, though the wider adoption of universal design principles is helping to reduce these barriers. Some learners will achieve better results in more highly structured environments or with more personal attention from a tutor or teacher. However, as supplements to, rather than replacements for, more traditional learning environments, digital technologies have a great capacity to enrich the learning experience.

The HIMSS TIGER Virtual Learning Environment

The HIMSS TIGER VLE is an online resource containing HI training and educational material, including MOOCs, games, augmented and virtual reality, webinars, podcasts, and more. This learning environment is designed to help academic professionals, students, adult learners, and clinical educators increase their knowledge and expand their skills in a personalized, self-paced format. The VLE enables learners to take courses tied to certificates of completion, get to know leaders in HI through live and archived webinars on demand, and earn continuing education credits. Educators can easily integrate VLE resources into their classroom or online curricula.

Background

The TIGER Initiative is a component of HIMSS, an international health technology nonprofit organization whose membership includes more than 80,000 individuals, 480 healthcare provider organizations, 470 nonprofits, and 650 health services organizations from around the world. The TIGER International Task Force directs the activities of the TIGER community and comprises 60 members from 29 countries. TIGER began as a grassroots initiative within the nursing community in 2006, gradually extending its scope to include other clinical disciplines moving into the interprofessional arena in 2014. Today, TIGER focuses on HI education reform and fostering community and global workforce development using an interdisciplinary approach to improve the delivery of patient care. One way TIGER accomplishes this is through the development of resources like the VLE.

Summary of VLE Offerings

The VLE includes a Resource Library with content organized into 18 subject categories reflecting the ever-changing and expanding state of the global health IT industry. Users can search the Resource Library by topic such as AI/Machine Learning (ML) interoperability and mHealth. These topics and resources are updated and refined on an ongoing basis. Learners can also search the Resource Library by type of resource, including blog post, course/MOOC, podcast/webinar, publication, white paper, or other tool/resource. See Box 40.2 for the complete list of topics and resource types.

Box 40.2 TIGER VLE Topics and Resource Types

1. Augmented Reality
2. Artificial Intelligence (AI)/Machine Learning (ML)
3. Blog Post
4. TIGER International Competency Synthesis Project (ICSP)
5. Courses/MOOC
6. Social Determinants of Health (SDoH)
7. eHealth/Health Informatics
8. Health Information Management (HIM)
9. Innovation
10. Interoperability
11. mHealth
12. Nursing
13. Pharmacy
14. Podcast/Webinar
15. Publication
16. Population Health
17. Physician
18. Privacy and Security
19. Report/White Paper
20. Telehealth
21. TIGER Historical
22. Tool/Resource
23. Global Workforce Development

Among the courses and MOOCs in the VLE is the Health Informatics Forum's "Introduction to Health Informatics," containing 17 modules on such topics as EHRs, computerized provider order entry (CPOE), clinical decision support systems (CDSS), and patient monitoring systems. Another MOOC is an introduction to AR, including how to develop AR experiences. A third MOOC provides quality and safety education for nurses, developed by the France Payne Bolton School of Nursing at Case Western Reserve University. In addition to these MOOCs, there are curriculum resources for health IT developed by the ONC and another set developed for pharmacy educators. There are also two self-paced courses: the Health IT Foundations Course and the IT in HealthCare Course. Both courses include a comprehensive assessment and lead to certificates of completion and enduring education credits.

The podcast and webinar offerings include a number of healthcare topics such as e-prescribing, smart pumps, telehealth, and other more general subjects such as AR, ML, and AI. The publications section includes refereed articles on HIT topics and links to journals in HI. The white papers not only focus mostly on the TIGER community and its work products, but also include a survey of AR and VR technologies.

An additional resource is the Webinar Theater. This section contains dozens of webinar recordings on topics such as AI, AR, global health workforce development, nursing, privacy and security, and telehealth. The webinars include events showcasing international case studies from Israel, Ireland, Canada, Portugal, Norway, Australia, New Zealand, and the U.K. as well as the U.S.

Finally, there are additional resources accessed through the VLE born out of the EU*US eHealth Work Project Consortium, of which TIGER was a member. This consortium was formed in 2016 to quantify and project the supply of and demand for HI workforce skills and competencies in the U.S., the European Union, and globally. An outcome of this effort was the development of a training program and tools to address the need for workforce skill development. One such tool is the Skills and Knowledge Assessment and

Development (SKAD) Framework, a survey that assesses the learner's basic IT competencies and identifying gaps that might be addressed through further training. Another is the HIT Competencies Tool and Repository (HITComp), an interactive online tool for identifying the IT skills needed by healthcare professionals in Europe and the U.S., with links to online courses where instruction on these skills can be obtained. There are also toolkits on health information privacy and security by HIMSS and the American Health Information Management Association (AHIMA) and the ONC's training games on contingency planning and information privacy and security. Video courses on cybersecurity and an introduction to eHealth are in this section, as well as, links to job postings through the HIMSS JobMine, a website listing positions in healthcare informatics (https://jobmine.himss.org).

The TIGER VLE is repository of HI resources demonstrating how a range of digital tools can be collected to provide an inclusive collection for those looking for training and professional development. The VLE exhibits the international scope and applicability of these tools. As such, it provides a valuable resource for educators and those seeking to expand their knowledge of HI.

Case Study

Curriculum Adoption of the TIGER VLE in an RN to BS Health Informatics Course: Leveraging Digital Tools to Meet Standards in Nursing Informatics Education

Background

Nursing faculty teaching in an undergraduate nursing program were tasked with creating and teaching an HI course for RNs seeking to complete a bachelor's degree in nursing. The nursing program was part of the State University of New York system and was uniquely situated within a branch campus on the grounds of a community college, extending the university's offerings to another region of the state. Providing a Bachelor of Science in nursing program on the community college's campus contributed to efforts to increase the number of baccalaureate prepared nurses, which has been called for in the U.S. to improve safe, quality care. Baccalaureate programs accredited by CCNE have required curriculum standards, one of which includes "Information Management and Application of Patient Care Technology."[1] Such additional content in HI has the potential to further prepare RNs to meet the challenges of providing safe, quality care.

Program Specifics

The nursing program at the branch campus offered all classes on one day a week, in a hybrid format, to accommodate the schedules of working RNs. Classes met every other week in person, with an online component on the alternating weeks. During online weeks, the focus was on asynchronous content delivery and student preparation for the in-person activities. The in-person activities involved the application of learned concepts. Because the program is geared toward the working RN, students had at least some exposure to clinical practice, which enhanced the application of course material.

Major Course Elements

1. **Addressing attitudes and values**

   The first activity in the HI course was designed to explore student attitudes regarding the need for RNs to demonstrate competency in HI. Students were asked to review the outline of the course concepts and reflect on the relevancy of HI to their nursing practice. Students shared their thoughts in an online discussion board in the LMS. This activity set the stage for learning and promoted the formation of values and attitudes that influence the integration of HI knowledge and skill into nursing practice. This activity also addresses the Quality and Safety Education for Nurses (QSEN)[2] competencies that include student learning outcomes in three domains: knowledge, skills, and attitudes. One outcome in the attitude domain states that learners will "[v]alue nurses' involvement in design, selection, implementation, and evaluation of information technologies to support patient care."

2. **Adoption of the TIGER VLE in lieu of a standard textbook**

   The adoption of the VLE was to meet several identified needs in preparing the HI course. One factor in selection of this resource was the desire to get students to engage with current publications and conversations in the field of informatics and encourage them to read from a variety of sources. The VLE provided this through curated resources and the ongoing posting of webinars featuring thought leaders in HI.

   A second need was a comprehensive presentation of foundational concepts covering the multi- and interdisciplinary field of informatics. Capably presenting on such a variety of topics posed a challenge for faculty, and the Health IT Foundations Course offered within the VLE provided a means to meet this challenge. In each in-person class period, students and faculty would discuss concepts learned in the Health IT Foundations course and further apply concepts specifically to nursing practice.

3. **Using technology as a tool**

   A final element of the course design was ensuring that all of the learning activities not only introduced informatics concepts but also aided students in developing computer skills and digital literacy. Therefore, each assignment required the students to leverage technology to achieve the course outcomes.

Key Assignments

1. Self-assessment of computer skills using the Pretest for Attitudes Towards Computers in Healthcare (PATCH) assessment scale[3] followed by online discussion where students shared strengths and areas for improvement with their classmates. This set the stage for peer assistance where strengths and needs matched across students.

2. Use of a wiki for students to create a shared document with information regarding Standardized Nursing Languages and their use in HI.

3. Patient Case exercise where students had to respond to a patient inquiry via email. The students also had to recommend an app and a website to their "patient" after using standards to assess an app and a website. This provided an opportunity for students to apply concepts related to privacy and security when communicating via email.[4]

4. Student-led interactive presentations leveraging digital tools on selected HI topics. Students used resources from the VLE to develop these presentations.

Evaluation of Course and Key Takeaways

- Assessment of student attitudes at the beginning of the course demonstrated that many students recognized the value in HI in a nursing curriculum. Their responses also reflected insight about how nurses should be involved in HI. This was encouraging! However, some students felt content should be integrated and HI should not constitute an entire course in the program.

- Empowering students to assist their classmates with computer-related technical skills increased confidence and promoted further engagement in HI content. Increasing nurses' confidence and providing a foundation in HI concepts through a dedicated course have the potential to encourage nurses to contribute to HI projects in their practice settings. One student indicated they were now eager to volunteer to serve on their institution's Informatics Committee.

- In course evaluations, students overwhelmingly supported the use of the TIGER VLE in lieu of a traditional textbook. Furthermore, using the VLE provided a significant savings to students in comparison to purchasing a textbook.
- With regard to the Health IT Foundations course, the students preferred this content delivery modality compared to a traditional textbook. They felt it was a better way to engage with the material as the course had interactive quizzes integrated within different learning activities. All students took and passed the exam at the end of the course to obtain a certificate of completion.
- The VLE and the interactive assignments appealed to and accommodated a variety of learning styles.

Discussion Questions

1. What role do attitudes and values play in HI education?
2. How do you distinguish between digital literacy or technology skills and HI? How do the concepts relate to each other?
3. What do you think are the benefits of leveraging an online education portal versus a traditional textbook?
4. What are some issues you might encounter if using an online education portal versus a traditional textbook?
5. Do you think the benefits or issues differ globally? Explain.

1. American Association of Colleges of Nursing (AACN) *Essentials of Baccalaureate Education for Professional Nursing Practice*
2. https://qsen.org/competencies/pre-licensure-ksas/#informatics
3. http://nursing-informatics.com/niassess/plan.html

4. Adapted from a presentation given by D. Skiba at a New York League for Nursing (NYLN) Conference

Summary

The chapter content is organized into four sections. The first section includes examples of HI-related programs, the standards for these programs, and key curricular threads. The second section of this chapter explores the challenges facing HI educators and begins a discussion on ways to address them. The third section describes technologies and digital tools supporting healthcare and HI education. The final and fourth section highlights one resource, the TIGER Virtual Learning Environment (VLE), and how it can be used to support HI education and skills attainment. This section also includes a case study describing the adoption of the TIGER VLE in an undergraduate HI course for nurses returning to school to complete a baccalaureate degree in nursing.

Conclusions and Outlook

HI is one of the fastest changing disciplines in healthcare. Its interdisciplinary and interprofessional nature encompasses subjects from every technology field and every health profession. Although there is a lack of clarity about many aspects of the field, significant progress is being made through the efforts of many organizations, both in the U.S. and internationally. Through the work of the global TIGER network of volunteers, new initiatives such as the Informatics Educators Resource Navigator (IREN) intend to make resources available to informatics educators showcasing "state-of-the-art" approaches in education and training based on what works in the real world. Such initiatives will support the work of current and future HI educators as they seek to align their teaching and training with globally relevant learning outcomes and competencies. TIGER also makes yearly updates to a document with key informatics definitions providing clarity and consistency regarding global HI terminology. This document demonstrates the evolution of the field and provides consistency of terms across disciplines, professions, and regions of the world. Additionally, TIGER is developing a global HI mini-course tied to the courses and tools created by the EU*US eHealth Work Project, to increase the availability of globally applicable content. There are still many challenges to overcome in the delivery of HI education, including defining and refining the competencies needed, the development of expertise among faculty and practitioners, and surmounting the digital divide, both at home and globally. The field is fortunate, however, to have a variety of digital tools to meet the challenge of delivering education and training that is informative, engaging, and stimulating, preparing learners to deliver efficient healthcare that enhances the well-being of patients and communities.

Useful Resources

1. Web Link to the HIMSS TIGER Interprofessional Community: Global Informatics Definitions
   https://www.himss.org/resources/tiger-informatics-definitions
2. Web Links to organizations with information on education programs and accreditation

IMIA Academic Institution Members
https://imia-medinfo.org/wp/academic-institutional-members/
EFMI listing of Educational Programmes
https://efmi.org/accreditation-and-certification/educational-programmes/
http://efmi-ac2.bmhi-edu.org/
AMIA Informatics Academic & Training Programs
https://www.amia.org/education/programs-and-courses
CAHIIM Program Directory
https://www.cahiim.org/programs/program-directory
CAHIIM Health Informatics Accreditation
https://www.cahiim.org/accreditation/health-informatics
HIMSS Approved Education Partners
https://www.himss.org/find-approved-education-partner
The Essentials of Baccalaureate Education for Professional Nursing Practice
http://www.aacnnursing.org/portals/42/publications/baccessentials08.pdf

3. **Web Links to online learning sites, courses, and competencies**

Database of MOOCs
https://www.classcentral.com/
Health IT Resources for Educators
https://www.healthit.gov/topic/onc-programs/workforce-development-programs
HITComp
http://hitcomp.org/
TEDMED Talks
https://www.tedmed.com/
TIGER Virtual Learning Environment
https://www.himss.org/tiger-virtual-learning-environment

Review Questions

1. True or False: IMIA sets the standards for health informatics education around the world.
2. True or False: Clinical informatics is recognized as a medical specialty for physicians by the AMA.
3. Which of the following is a method of online instructor-led training?
   (a) A wiki
   (b) A blog
   (c) Asynchronous instruction
   (d) Virtual reality
4. Which of the following kinds of resources can be found in the TIGER VLE?
   (a) Courses
   (b) Blogs
   (c) Webinars
   (d) All of the above
5. According to the Case Study, what is a benefit of using a VLE that includes a variety of content delivery modalities?
   (a) It encourages the teacher to expand their digital literacy.
   (b) It appeals to and accommodates a variety of learning styles.
   (c) It is less likely to have errors in content.
   (d) It adheres to standards for Health Informatics education.

Appendix: Answers to Review Questions

1. True or False: IMIA sets the standards for health informatics education around the world.

False: Many different bodies in the U.S. and internationally have recommended standards for health informatics education.

2. True or False: Clinical informatics is recognized as a medical specialty for physicians by the AMA.

False: Clinical informatics is recognized as a sub-specialty in nine medical specialties by the ACGME.

3. Which of the following is a method of online instructor-led training?
   (a) A wiki
   (b) A blog
   (c) Asynchronous instruction
   (d) Virtual reality

Asynchronous instruction. The other terms describe tools that may or may not be used in online instruction.

4. Which of the following kinds of resources can be found in the TIGER VLE?
   (a) Courses
   (b) Blogs
   (c) Webinars
   (d) All of the above

All of the above and more.

5. According to the Case Study, what is a benefit of using a VLE that includes a variety of content delivery modalities?
   (a) It encourages the teacher to expand their digital literacy.
   (b) It appeals to and accommodates a variety of learning styles.
   (c) It is less likely to have errors in content.
   (d) It adheres to standards for Health Informatics education.

The variety of content delivery modalities available in a virtual learning environment appeal to and accommodate a variety of learning styles. The other answer choices were not discussed in the case study and may or may not be a benefit of using a virtual learning environment.

References

1. Mantas J, Ammenwerth E, Demiris G, Hasman A, Haux R, Hersh W, et al. Recommendations of the International Medical Informatics Association (IMIA) on education in biomedical and health informatics. Methods Inf Med. 2010;49(2):105–20.
2. Hörbst A, Winter A, Stoicu-Tivadar L. EFMI working and project groups – overview and current activities. Yearb Med Inform. 2017 Aug;26(1):311–22.
3. Jaspers MW, Mantas J, Borycki E, Hasman A. IMIA accreditation of biomedical and health informatics education: current state and future directions. Yearb Med Inform. 2017;26(1):252–6.
4. Mantas J, Hasman A. IMIA educational recommendations and nursing informatics. Stud Health Technol Inform. 2017;232:20–30.
5. Herzog J, Pohn B, Forjan M, Sauermann S, Urbauer P. Education for eHealth – a status analysis. eHealth2014-Health Informatics Meets eHealth; 2014. p. 10.
6. Ahonen O, Kinnunen U-M, Lejonqvist G-B, Apkalna B, Viitkar K, Saranto K. Identifying biomedical and health informatics competencies in higher education curricula. Stud Health Technol Inform. 2018;251:261–4.
7. Hersh W. Health and biomedical informatics: opportunities and challenges for a twenty-first century profession and its education. Yearb Med Inform. 2008;2008:157–64.
8. De Gagne JC, Bisanar WA, Makowski JT, Neumann JL. Integrating informatics into the BSN curriculum: a review of the literature. Nurse Educ Today. 2012;32(6):675–82.
9. Giunti G, Guisado-Fernandez E, Belani H, Lacalle-Remigio JR. Mapping the access of future doctors to health information technologies training in the European Union: cross-sectional descriptive study. J Med Internet Res. 2019;21(8):e14086.
10. Lowe J. Computer-based education: is it a panacea? J Res Technol Educ. 2001;34(2):163–71.
11. Alpert D, Bitzer DL. Advances in computer-based education. Science. 1970;167(3925):1582–90.
12. Blumenthal D. Launching HITECH. N Engl J Med. 2010;362(5):382–5.
13. Workforce Development Programs | HealthIT. gov [Internet]. [cited 2020 Jun 26]. Available from

https://www.healthit.gov/topic/onc-programs/
workforce-development-programs

14. Stone DE, Zheng G. Learning management systems in a changing environment [Internet]. Handbook of research on education and technology in a changing society. 2014 [cited 2020 Jun 26]. Available from www.igi-global.com/chapter/learning-management-systems-in-a-changing-environment/111885

15. Cormier D, Siemens G. Through the open door: open courses as research, learning and engagement. Educause Rev. 2010;45(4):30–9.

16. Osterweil S, Klopfer E. Are games all Child's play? In: De Freitas S, Maharg P, editors. Digital games and learning. London: Bloomsbury Publishing; 2011 Mar 31.

Interprofessional Practice and Education: Core Data Set and Information Exchange Infrastructure

41

Connie White Delaney, Laura Pejsa, and Barbara F. Brandt

Learning Objectives
- Identify key contextual factors contributing to the health care transformation of interprofessional practice
- Describe state-of-the-art information exchange and communication to support interprofessional health care
- Explain the National Center for Interprofessional Practice and Education (NCIPE) as a resource to advance interprofessional cooperation and cooperation
- Outline the National Center interprofessional core data set and information exchange infrastructure to advance interprofessional care

Key Terms
- Interprofessional
- Education
- Practice
- Nexus
- Data
- Informatics
- Essential
- Quadruple
- Interdisciplinary
- Digital

C. W. Delaney (✉)
School of Nursing, University of Minnesota, Minneapolis, MN, USA
e-mail: delaney@umn.edu

L. Pejsa
National Center for Interprofessional Practice & Education, MN Northstar GWEP, University of Minnesota, Minneapolis, MN, USA
e-mail: pejsa@umn.edu

B. F. Brandt
National Center for Interprofessional Practice & Education, University of Minnesota, Minneapolis, MN, USA
e-mail: brandt@umn.edu

Introduction

Health care concerns have proliferated over several decades, including alarms about effectiveness, quality, patient safety, access and inequities, patient and health system outcomes, and costs. Enthusiasm for interprofessional practice and education (IPE) to address these concerns has been renewed [1, 2]. While the complexity of IPE creates challenges in measuring its ultimate impact on outcomes, it is clear that systems thinking, team approaches, and the synergy between practice and education are required to improve health and health care. It is also apparent that generating knowledge and informing best practices in clinical care and education needs to address the lag time between educational interventions and patient outcomes, robust educational design and evaluation, and comparability of findings enhanced by the inclusion of descriptions of research methods [3, 4]. While collaboration is inherent in IPE and has the capacity to advance team-based research [4], there is a "dearth" of robust studies specifically designed to link IPE and health outcomes [4, 5]. Moreover, despite health care and education being key drivers of the growth of big data science, there is an absence of capacity and, thus, the engagement of IPE.

The science of IPE and collaborative practice was the beneficiary of a public-private partnership in 2012 when the University of Minnesota was selected to create the National Center for Interprofessional Practice and Education (National Center). Funded by the United States (U.S.) Health Resources and Services Administration, the National Center was designed to advance the field of IPE and collaborative practice to achieve Triple/Quadruple Aim outcomes (improving the patient care experience, improving the health of populations, and reducing the per capita cost of health care; plus provider experience) [6–8]. The National Center (N.C.) established the Knowledge Generation approach, intentionally designed to address the long-standing gaps in IPE and recognized challenges through collecting comparable, sharable data developed by teams of interdisciplinary and interprofessional researchers, scholars, and clinicians. IPE Knowledge Generation advances the use of a variety of data sources and leverages contemporary "big data" approaches that employ large datasets [4].

The National Center adopted the Institute of Medicine's (IOM) Interprofessional Learning Continuum Model (IPLC Model) [4] (Fig. 41.1) as the framework for identifying essential data and information to advance understanding of IPE. This IPLC Model incorporates the foundation, graduate, and professional education learning continuum; interprofessional education and collaborative practice learning outcomes [5, 9, 10]; individual and population health outcomes, organizational changes, systems efficiencies, cost-effectiveness and system outcomes; and the enabling and interfering factors that influence processes and outcomes.

After further examination, the National Center Knowledge Generation team developed the National Center Expanded Interprofessional Learning Continuum Model (NC-EIPLCM) (Fig. 41.2) that also includes the focus on the Quadruple Aim, more appropriately positions the enabling and interfering factors as important moderating negative, positive, or neutral forces between interprofessional education and collaborative practice, and recognizes the ability to simultaneously achieve both learning and Quadruple Aim (health and system) outcomes.

The capacity for interprofessional cooperation and communication (including digital information exchange & sharing) was further enriched when the N.C. created the Nexus Innovation Network in 2013. The original Nexus Innovation Network was composed of nine higher education institutions that had leadership and investments that were committed to IPE and had a large-scale vision for healthcare, communities, and education [7, 8]. This Network has grown to represent more than 70 sites implementing over 100 IPE programs [7, 8], and it was an essential source for Knowledge Generation through sharing knowledge and experience informing the identification, testing, and validation of essential comparable and shareable data to advance IPE scholarship. Additional expertise informed the Knowledge Generation initiative includes (a) the diversity of the Knowledge Generation Team itself, which represents professional expertise in education and practice, including health professions educators, clinicians, and researchers in informatics, health services, research methods, statistics, and measurement expertise; (b) the national Knowledge Generation Advisory Council, and (c) shared knowledge and experience with the U.S. national CTSA and CORI networks including the big data and associated infrastructure at the University of Minnesota.

Knowledge Generation Vision, IPE Core Data, Information Infrastructure

Knowledge Generation envisions advancing best practices for the care of individuals and communities through the synergy among clinical practice and education, collection of comparable and scalable data using a common

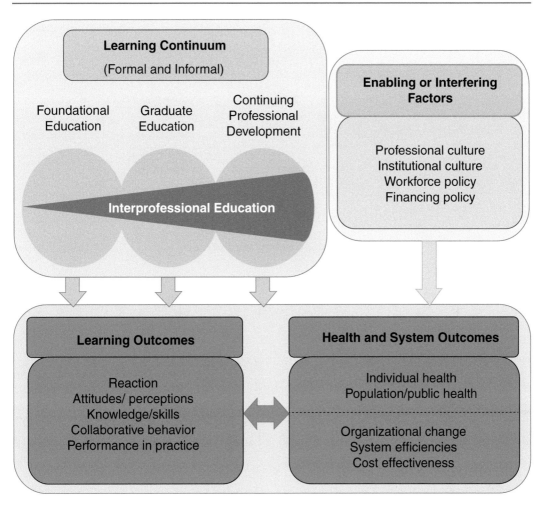

Fig. 41.1 Institute of Medicine Interprofessional Learning Continuum Model (IPLC Model). Institute of Medicine. 2015. *Measuring the Impact of Interprofessional Education on Collaborative Practice and Patient* *Outcomes.* https://doi.org/10.17226/21726. Reprinted with permission the National Academy of Sciences, Courtesy of the National Academies Press, Washington, DC

information infrastructure, and incorporating the science of big data and big data analytics. By collecting and sharing data, IPE Knowledge Generation supports collaboration through linking locally generated data on individual programs to additional data across programs. This approach represents a significant shift in how data is used, including the use of data sampling or the use of the entire population [11]. Thinking shifts from a focus only about correlation and causality and a static collection of information on one program at a point in time to thinking about data as a reusable resource within and across IPE programs over time.

There are six categories of the IPE Core Data Set that outline essential shareable, comparable data: (1) interprofessional competencies, (2) interprofessional educational learning environment, (3) interprofessional clinical learning environment, (4) critical events of IPE, (5) teamness, and (6) health and system outcomes (Fig. 41.3). Each category and specific data elements are described.

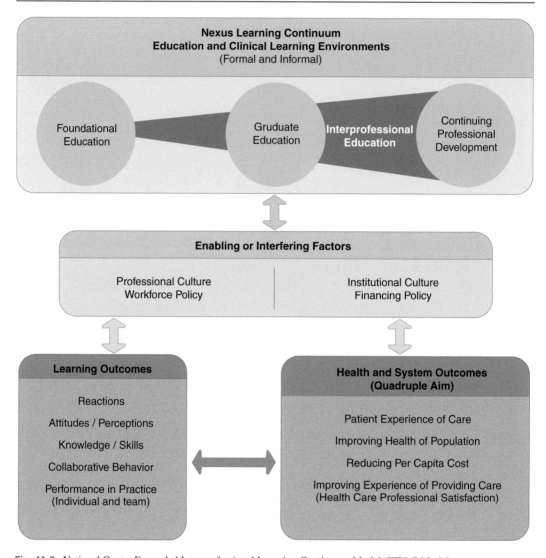

Fig. 41.2 National Center Expanded Interprofessional Learning Continuum Model (EIPLC Model)

Interprofessional Competencies

The Interprofessional Collaborative Competency Attainment Survey (ICCAS) measures interprofessional competencies across the NC-EIPLCM from foundational education, graduate education, and continuing professional development. These are self-reported competencies of interprofessional care in interprofessional education programs in a retrospective pretest/posttest design [12]. The ICCAS allows comparisons across sites and programs, demonstrates strong validity, and has been used across the learning continuum in Canada, New Zealand and the U.S. [13]. Moreover, the ICCAS is closely aligned to the IPEC competencies, and the IPLCM Modified Kirkpatrick Model supports the use of this standardized measure to assess IPE learning outcomes.

Interprofessional Educational and Clinical Learning Environments

Two instruments about learning environments provide information about key variables influ-

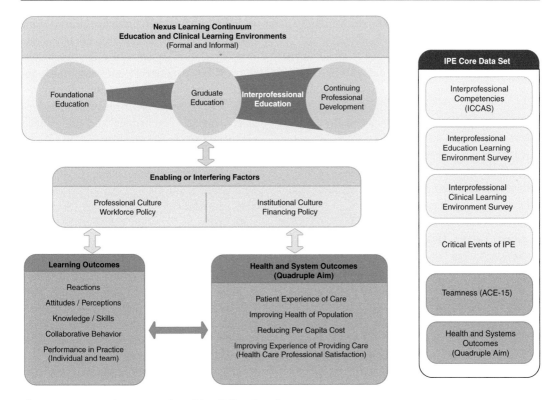

Fig. 41.3 National Center EIPLCM with IPE Core Data Set

encing impact and outcomes of interprofessional practice and education: Interprofessional Educational Learning Environment Survey (IELES) and the Interprofessional Clinical Learning Environment Survey (ICLES). The two instruments, which are mirror measures of the education and practice learning environments, include six domains of data: (1) Organizational Structure for IPE, (2) Organizational Culture for IPE, (3) Organizational Investment in IPE, (4) Nexus Program Team and Processes, (5) Professional Development Opportunities, and (6) Managing the Nexus Program.

Critical Events of IPE Instrument

The Nexus Innovation Network was a key informant in creating the Critical Events of IPE Instrument. The critical events of IPE serve as a record of the challenges and positive forces having an impact on the IPE program. Following extensive data gathering and analyses processes, seven categories of critical events were identified: (1) The need to change program strategy/plan significantly, (2) Key staff member left or was added, (3) Change in key educational organization partner, (3) Change of key practice organization partner, (4) Unforeseen external forces, (5) Money and resources, and (6) Difficulty collecting data for evaluation purposes.

Teamness

The Knowledge Generation team selected a rapid assessment instrument suitable for a broad range of clinical environments to measure Teamness, the Assessment for Collaborative Environments (ACE-15). This 15-item instrument measures perceptions of team environments and measures a single factor for interprofessional clinical teamwork, or "teamness." The ACE-15 is applicable as IPE moves from classrooms to practice to ensure interprofessional clinical learning environments [14].

Quadruple Aim Outcomes

The Knowledge Generation team maintained sensitivity to data collection burden and consequently elected several widely-used and validated instruments already used in the health systems for measuring perceived health and health-related quality of life, and the patient experience of care, much of which is already collected in health systems. Outcome data for the N.C. is de-identified before submission. Sources of outcome data include the following.

- **Short-Form Health Survey** (SF-36 or SF-12). Core data for population health includes measures for general health, recent changes in health, and deaths in the past year. The 36-item short-form and 12-item short health surveys (SF-36 and SF-12 respectively), developed by the RAND Health Insurance Experiment have been extensively tested and been found reliable for measuring functional health (physical and mental) and well-being [15]. Both instruments are designed to monitor population health and can be used to compare and analyze disease burden, as well as estimate potential medical expenses. Patient-reported data collected periodically at the time of the clinical experience is used to evaluate patient-perceived health and changes in health status in the past year. In combination with mortality, these measures could be used to compute quality-adjusted life-year measures [16].
- **Consumer Assessment of Health Care Providers Surveys** (CAHPS). The U.S. Agency for Health Research and Quality (AHRQ) has developed a series of instruments designed to capture patient experiences and satisfaction with their health care providers and services. Several different surveys exist for different provider settings (e.g., clinics, home health care, dental, adult, and child hospital) [17]. If CAHPS are not appropriate for an IPE setting, or it is difficult to obtain this in a setting, a subset of four questions from CAHPS can be substituted. These four questions comprise the core measures for patient experience: a global measure asking about patient experience, an endorsement of the care experience, how much the patient was helped through the experience, and how much the patient improved in handling their daily problems. These items are readily standardized across diverse populations and are patient-completed and easily understood [18].
- **Use of Health Services**. This information comprises office visits, home health care, emergency room visits, hospitalizations, etc. Service usage constitutes a proxy for cost, as well as disease burden. Usage is best measured through the extraction of patient data using nationally accepted administrative codes in the U.S., such as the International Statistical Classification of Diseases and Related Health Problems (ICD) and Diagnostic Related Groups (DRGs). Programs should identify and select only those codes that reflect the Program's IPE intervention.
- **Health Care Professional Satisfaction.** The final component of the Quadruple Aim concerns improving the experience of providing care (health care professionals including provider, clinician, and staff satisfaction). The National Center has adopted health care professional satisfaction, measured by site-specific determined standardized instruments, to be the current proxy.

In summary, the Knowledge Generation team has adopted multiple commonly used instruments to measure outcomes. In addition, customized data collection to serve individual program needs related to a specific patient population or locally driven interest such as using a specific IPE measurement instrument or patient data are accommodated.

National Center IPE Information Exchange

The National Center IPE Information Exchange (NCIIE), supporting the collection and analyses of core data and program management, is designed to (1) facilitate capture, access, and flow of study and operational data within an IPE implementation site or program, their own institution and beyond; (2) serve as a local program management tool for individual IPE sites and programs to track their own progress and reporting; (3) support use of informatics to catalyze discoveries across the spectrum of IPE at the National Center and its network partners; and (4) share contributions with the national consortium, the Nexus Innovation Network. The NCIIE supports four functions: National Center Data Repository (NCDR), IPE Core Data Set, Informatics-Driven Dashboard, and Program Management.

The NCIIE (Fig. 41.4) utilizes protected health information (PHI) compliant infrastructure (NCDR) that ensures the implementation of best data practices and national standards. This infrastructure supports: (1) secure and encrypted data exchange and storage; (2) role-based user authentication management that allows for local control of data access based on role; (3) data de-identification methods that ensure no PHI data are uploaded; (4) regular secure data backups; (5) use of PHI compliant tools for data extraction and delivery, and (6) various additional security measures (e.g., firewalls, password requirements, data retention and destruction).

Data use agreements governed the relationship between the National Center and the individual sites or programs along with security model and data management policies governed by the University of Minnesota Health Sciences Technology Data Protection Services. Agreements and policies are regularly (at least annually) reviewed by all relevant privacy, compliance, Institutional Review Board (IRB), and Health Insurance Portability and Accountability Act of 1996 (HIPAA) entities. The NCIIE is also a secure HIPAA-and Family Educational Rights and Privacy Act (FERPA) compliant state-of-the-art environment. This platform ensures both data privacy and security provisions for safeguarding health information (HIPAA) and protection of the privacy of student education records (FERPA). This collaborative work across local practice and education settings, a single system, and national and international environments, meets the state-of-the-art information exchange infrastructure to advance the collective understanding of what works and what does not work in interprofessional practice and education.

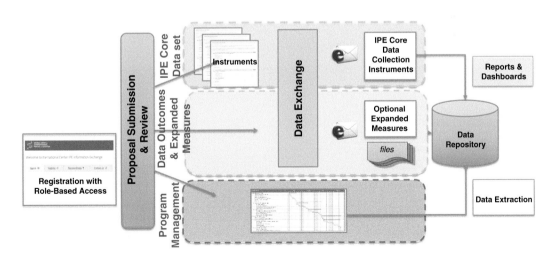

Fig. 41.4 National Center IPE Information Exchange

Instrument and Report Examples

The following examples illustrate an excerpt for the Critical Incident core data component within the NCIIE. Figure 41.5 demonstrates one element of the instrument.

The NCIIE contains programmed data dictionaries and can generate standardized reports for each of the IPE Core Data Set instruments (e.g., ICCAS, ACE-15) to enable program leaders to access data on their own programs at any time and request reports. The individual program

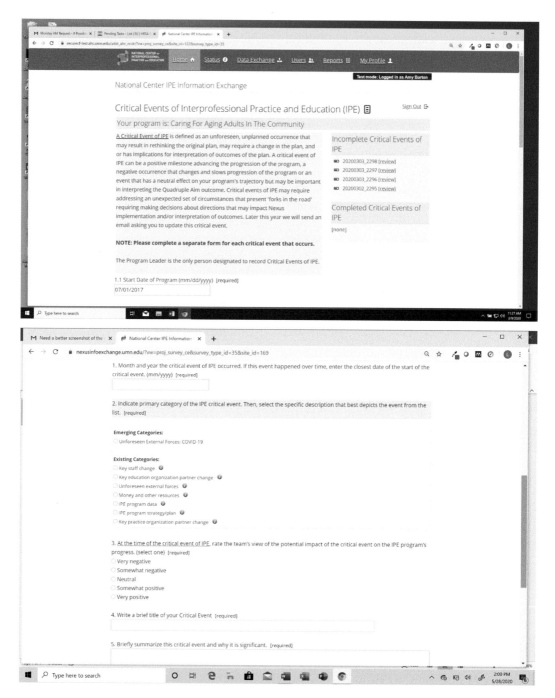

Fig. 41.5 Critical Events of Interprofessional Practice and Education in the NCII

standard reports provide information about how their results change over time. As data is submitted from multiple programs and sites, the National Center will be able to provide aggregate reports that compare findings across programs and sites and eventually for all components of the NC-EIPLC Model. Figure 41.6 is one sample report for Critical Incidents and shows the capacity to demonstrate current time status, as well as the capacity to compare data to other programs in the Network. The ultimate goal is advancing the evidence base for IPE learning and organizational and health care outcomes.

Case Study

The case study selected for this chapter illustrates the key objectives of this chapter. It demonstrates the application of the National Center IPE Core Data Set in practice. The MN Northstar Geriatrics Workforce Enhancement Program at the University of Minnesota Department of Family Medicine and Community Health Case Study is described prepared by Laura Pejsa, Director of Evaluation &

Organizational Learning, and National Center for Interprofessional Practice & Education. The Minnesota Northstar GWEP is a five-year, $3.74 million program funded by the Health Resources & Services Administration (HRSA). The MN GWEP is implementing 13 distinct projects under the grant program's umbrella, incorporating eight community partners and faculty and learners from dentistry, family medicine, internal medicine, nursing, pharmacy, physical therapy, public health, and social work. The 13 projects and associated activities:

- Bring together Minnesota's best minds in geriatrics care and education
- Educate current and future health professionals in Age-Friendly care
- Transform primary care clinics for Age-Friendly care and learning
- Offer public education and support for families and direct care workers, and
- Focus on dementia care, support, and safety

Through this extensive programming, MN GWEP hopes to make significant strides toward

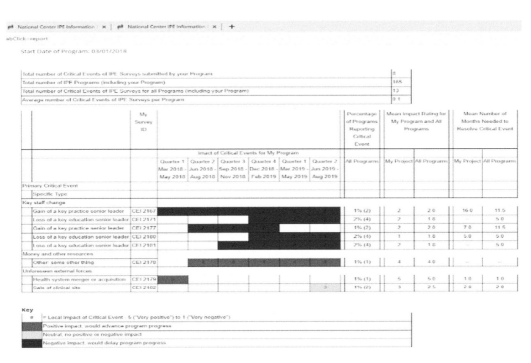

Fig. 41.6   Sample Report of Critical Events of IPE for One Program

closing the gap when it comes to Age-Friendly care. The ultimate goal is for all Minnesotan geriatric patients to receive treatment that faithfully adheres to the 4M framework: what matters in their lives, their medications, their mobility, and their mentation.

The National Center for Interprofessional Education and Practice (National Center) is a key partner for MN GWEP, leading both the grant evaluation and contribution to IPE knowledge generation. In its grant application to HRSA, the MN GWEP stated its intent to utilize the National Center IPE Information Exchange to plan, track, and report data on educational and health systems outcomes. This includes HRSA-required data on geriatrics-related interventions and MIPS measures. The program committed to joining the national network to contribute data using the IPE Core Data set as well, expanding the potential impact of collected data beyond accountability reporting. As MN GWEP implements its 13 projects, the grant team continuously revisits how each programmatic element will be evaluated and share data in line with this framework.

For example, the MN GWEP offers a compelling case study in Critical Events of IPE during the COVID-19 pandemic. This case demonstrates how the National Center Critical Events of IPE tool is being used by the MN GWEP program evaluator to document and track in real-time the rapid, disruptive events that impacted the program on a daily, or even hourly, basis during spring 2020.

The program was in its first year of funding from the Health Resources and Services Administration (HRSA) and was just beginning to implement the proposed and approved programming when the pandemic hit. Immediately, all planned activities needed reassessment as learners left campus, clinic partners shifted to pandemic care teams, and faculty were redirected to patient care and University crisis management.

This situation was prime to use the National Center the Critical Events (component of the IPE Core Data Set) of the IPE tool. The MN Northstar GWEP began tracking key programmatic shifts in the midst of COVID-19 in real-time to provide information and data for real-time decision-making. The grant program coordina-

tor interviewed all faculty and staff about their planned adaptations to the approved work plan, and updates are shared during weekly virtual meetings and team emails. The following are examples of critical events and the program's initial assessments of their impact:

1. The first annual Interprofessional Geriatrics Case Competition, a 3-week competitive experience for the University of Minnesota learners, was scheduled to begin in mid-March 2020. As learners were instructed to leave campus and all in-person instruction was suspended, the event was canceled. The initial assessment of this event was that it was somewhat negative. Many months of planning, volunteer judge and coach recruitment, and marketing were lost. This event has been rescheduled for the fall semester in a virtual format, and the evaluator will continue to document the resolution of this issue in the system.

2. Because of COVID-19, an annual Caring for Persons with Memory Loss conference, scheduled for June 2020, was canceled. The audience for this conference (250–300 people) consists mainly of caregivers and family members caring for people with dementia. Many have difficulty even registering online, so offering a virtual event was not feasible. The initial assessment of this event was that it was somewhat negative.

3. Because the annual conference could not be offered, the Principal Investigator reallocated some of the funds earmarked for in-person conferences to offer a free webcast entitled "COVID-19 and Living with Dementia: Maintaining Well-Being and Purpose" (April 17, 2020), the M.N. Northstar GWEP partnered with the Minnesota Gerontological Society to develop and deliver a free webcast. Over 1600 people—professionals, caregivers, family members, and people with dementia— attended the webcast. The attendance was record-breaking for both organizations and surpassed grant goals. This was very positive for the program.

4. Cancelations and timeline changes for in-person activities left the program with unal-

located money and faculty time for year one. After reviewing the entire work plan and budget, the program shifted focus and funds to initiatives that could proceed amid closures and stay-at-home orders. The timeline for curriculum development—including geriatrics care modules and preceptor training materials—has accelerated significantly. The program will surpass its goals for developing and disseminating these educational materials. The initial assessment is that this event is somewhat positive.

5. Plans to implement age-friendly interventions in partner clinics (with interprofessional healthcare teams, including learners) were postponed. The clinical leaders and care teams needed to focus on responding to the crisis— treating patients, keeping healthcare workers safe, and reimagining clinical processes for COVID-19. The program assessed this event as somewhat positive. Although the timeline for age-friendly care was altered, a plan was put in place to observe and record significant interactions and care adaptations with older adults during this time. As the clinical partners return to planning the age-friendly interventions for the Fall, they are doing so with new perspectives and knowledge about: how to prevent and treat the virus in older adults; how to incorporate an age-friendly care initiative that is immediately impactful with the lowest burden for providers; how telehealth can be effectively utilized for instruction and care; and innovative ways to incorporate learners to add value in the clinical environment.

6. In summer 2020, HRSA announced an allocation of CARES act funds to each of the 44 GWEP programs in the United States. The funds were earmarked for activities that increased preparation for and access to COVID-19 prevention and care for adults over 65. The MN GWEP is leveraging these additional funds to develop a 14th project under the grant umbrella, focused on access for Somali elders at high risk for contracting and spreading the virus. This opportunity to reach an underserved population in response to an urgent community need represents a significant, unplanned critical event for the MN GWEP team.

Because of successfully navigating the significant, disruptive "forks-in-road," Minnesota Northstar GWEP has boldly stated that, by the conclusion of the 5-year grant, it will have trained thousands of learners in I.P. geriatrics team care, transformed 9 primary care training clinics and 56 community primary care clinics into age-friendly sites, and promoted dementia-friendly systems and communities to thousands of older adults, families, caregivers, health professions learners, and clinicians. Using the Critical Events of IPE tool, the program is: monitoring progress toward these goals in an unprecedented time; driving team reflection; supporting informed, real-time decision-making; and creating a historical record for both reports to funders and IPE knowledge generation. By using the National Center IPE Information Exchange and an IPE Core Data Set tool to record these events, the MN GWEP is contributing to IPE Knowledge Generation.

Summary

While health care concerns have proliferated over several decades, including alarms about effectiveness, quality, patient safety, access and inequities, patient and health system outcomes, and costs, this chapter has lifted up the empowerment of the Knowledge Generation initiative through a first of its kind national public-private partnership creating the National Center for Interprofessional Practice and Education. This chapter provides information and invitation to leverage local innovations into national transformation through the power of collaborating, team scholarship, and transparency of sharable, comparable data. The inaugural national IPE Core Data was described and included (1) interprofessional competencies, (2) interprofessional educational learning environment, (3) interprofessional clinical learning environment, (4) critical events of IPE, (5) teamness, and (6) health and system outcomes. Moreover, the NCIIE is a robust, safe, secure infrastructure to support local to national collaboration and enable IPE to enter the contemporary state of the scientific methods of big data science. The call for IPE and its potential to engage all providers and foster functioning at the top of license determined through data and most significantly to empower outcomes that address the individuals, families, and communities we serve now.

Conclusions and Outlook

We live in times of perhaps unprecedented visibility of the heath and heath care divide and the visibility of the underserved. We live in times of perhaps unprecedented visibility of the strengths and challenges of our health care and public health systems. And despite this reality, we live at a time of unprecedented innovation and opportunity to step up as a community and accept nothing less than the rapid adoption of strategies supporting collaboration, dissolve of barriers and maintain the practice and education synergy where boundaries have vanished during the pandemic to address these divides. You are invited to explore and engage in the IPE informatics empowerment.

Useful Resources
1. National Center for Interprofessional Practice & Education
   https://nexusipe.org/
2. N.C. Partners & Centers
   https://nexusipe.org/informing/about-national-center/news/two-new-collections-announced-nexusipeorg-resource-center
   https://nexusipe.org/connecting/ipe-centers
3. IPE Core Data Set
   https://nexusipe.org/advancing/nexus-innovations-network/webinars
4. **Delaney, C.**, Weaver, C., Warren, J., Clancy, T., & Simpson, R. Editors. (2017). Big Data-Enabled Nursing: Education, Research and Practice. Springer. ISBN: 978-3-319-53299-8
5. **Delaney, C.**, Kuziemsky, Craig, & Brandt, B. (Guest Editors) (2015). Interprofessional Informatics (Special Themed Section).

Journal of Interprofessional Care, Vol 29, No 6, 525-651 ISSN: 1356-1820

Review Questions
1. Describe the importance and impact of a national IPE essential core data set on health and health care delivery.
2. Outline barriers to implementing comparable, sharable core data at (a) your local site, (b) nationally, and (c) globally.
3. Select one of the six components of the IPE Core Data Set, and discuss how that component would be implemented on one clinical/education partnership.

Appendix: Answers to Review Questions

1. Describe the importance and impact of a national IPE essential core data set on health and health care delivery.

The IPE essential core data set is important as it enhances a collective understanding of interprofessional practice and education by fostering essential shareable, comparable data in the following domains: (1) interprofessional competencies, (2) interprofessional educational learning environment, (3) interprofessional clinical learning environment, (4) critical events of IPE, (5) teamness, and (6) health and system outcome. This national resource contributes to better health and health care delivery outcomes that address the individuals, families, and communities we serve now.

2. Outline barriers to implementing comparable, sharable core data at (a) your local site, (b) nationally, and (c) globally.

Each learner will use own examples.

3. Select one of the six components of the IPE Core Data Set, and discuss how that component would be implemented on one clinical/education partnership.

Each learner will select one component and discuss.

References

1. Cerra F, Brandt BF. Renewed focus in the United States links interprofessional education with redesigning health care. J Interprof Care. 2011;25(6):394–6. https://doi.org/10.3109/13561820.2011.615576.
2. Maloney S, Reeves S, Rivers G, Ilic D, Foo J, Walsh K. The Prato statement on cost and value in professional and interprofessional education. J Interprof Care. 2017;31(1):1–4. https://doi.org/10.1080/13561820.2016.1257255.
3. Cox M, Cuff P, Brandt B, Reeves S, Zierler B. Measuring the impact of interprofessional education on collaborative practice and patient outcomes. J Interprof Care. 2016;30(1):1–3. https://doi.org/10.3109/13561820.2015.1111052.
4. Institute of Medicine. Measuring the impact of Interprofessional education on collaborative practice and patient outcomes. New York: The National Academies Press; 2015. https://doi.org/10.17226/21726.
5. Reeves S, Goldman J, Gilbert J, Tepper J, Silver I, Suter E, Zwarenstein M. A scoping review to improve conceptual clarity of interprofessional interventions. J Interprof Care. 2011;25(3):167–74. https://doi.org/10.3109/13561820.2010.529960.
6. Berwick DM, Nolan TW, Whittington J. The triple aim: care, health, and cost. Health Affairs (Millwood). 2008;27(3):759–69. https://doi.org/10.1377/hlthaff.27.3.759.
7. Pechacek J, Cerra F, Brandt B, Lutfiyya M, Delaney C. Creating the evidence through comparative effectiveness research for Interprofessional education and collaborative practice by deploying a National Intervention Network and a National Data Repository. Healthcare. 2015;3(1):146–61. https://doi.org/10.3390/healthcare3010146.
8. Pechacek J, Shandling J, Lutfiyya MN, Brandt BF, Cerra FB, Delaney CW. The National United States Center Data Repository: core essential interprofessional practice & education data enabling triple aim analytics. J Interprof Care. 2015;29(6):587–91. https://doi.org/10.3109/13561820.2015.1075474.
9. Barr H, Koppel I, Reeves S, Hammick M, Freeth D. Effective interprofessional education: argument, assumption and evidence. Oxford: Blackwell; 2005.
10. Kirkpatrick DL. Techniques for evaluation training programs. Journal of the American Society of Training Directors. 1959;13:21–6.
11. Delaney CW, Simpson RL. Why big data? Why nursing? In: Delaney CW, Weaver C, Warren JJ, Clancy TR, Simpson RL, editors. Big data-enabled nursing: education, research, and practice. New York: Springer; 2017. p. 3–10. https://doi.org/10.1007/978-3-319-53300-1_23.
12. Archibald D, Trumpower D, MacDonald CJ. Validation of the interprofessional collaborative competency attainment survey (ICCAS). J Interprof Care. 2014;28(6):553–8. https://doi.org/10.3109/13561820.2014.917407.
13. Schmitz CC, Radosevich DM, Jardine P, MacDonald CJ, Trumpower D, Archibald D. The Interprofessional collaborative competency attainment survey (ICCAS): a replication validation study. J Interprof Care. 2016;31(1):28–34. https://doi.org/10.1080/13561820.2016.1233096.
14. Tilden VP, Eckstrom E, Dieckmann NF. Development of the Assessment for Collaborative Environments (ACE-15): a tool to measure perceptions of interprofessional 'teamness.'. J Interprof Care. 2016;30(3):288–94. https://doi.org/10.3109/13561820.2015.1137891.
15. Ware JE, Sherbourne CD. The MOS 36-item short-form health survey (SF-36) I. Conceptual framework and item selection. Med Care. 1992;30(6):473–83.
16. Nichol MB, Sengupta N, Globe DR. Evaluating quality-adjusted life years: estimation of the health utility index (HUI2) from the SF-36. Med Decis Mak. 2001;21(2):105–12. https://doi.org/10.1177/0272989X0102100203.
17. Agency for Healthcare Research and Quality (AHRQ). CAHPS surveys and guidance. 2018. http://www.ahrq.gov/cahps/surveys-guidance/index.html
18. Crofton C, Lubalin J, Darby C. Consumer assessment of health plans study foreword. Med Care. 1999;37(3):MS1–MS9.

Digital Professionalism: Digital Learning and Teaching Techniques

42

Oliver J. Bott, Marianne Behrends,
Nils-Hendrik Benning, Ina Hoffmann,
and Marie-Louise Witte

Learning Objectives
- The chapter conveys the basics of online teaching with the relevant theoretical foundations of learning, methods and tools.
- Readers get familiar with a concrete five-phase didactical framework that conveys the basics of designing activating online courses especially for smaller learning groups.
- After reading the chapter, readers will know the basic functions of learning management systems (LMSs) and are able to select suitable digital learning tools for teaching corresponding to the phase model.
- Readers know relevant frameworks that describe digital competences for online teaching and learning and can name sources to determine their own digital competencies.
- After reading this chapter, readers will be familiar with the essential characteristics of continuing education (CE) and factors for the successful design of digital CE offers.

Key Terms
- Five-phase didactic framework
- Socio-constructivist learning theory
- Access and Motivation
- Online Socialization
- Information Exchange
- Knowledge Construction
- Development
- E-tivities
- Activating input
- Previous knowledge
- Different types of learning
- Promoting an in-depth examination
- Knowledge reflection
- Self-assessment tests
- Netiquette
- Formative assessments
- Formative evaluation
- Summative assessmen
- Written exams
- Information security and legal security
- Community of Inquiry questionnaire
- Learning analytics
- Fears of losing control
- Continuing education (CE)
- European Framework for Digital Competence of Educators (DigCompEdu)

O. J. Bott (✉) · M.-L. Witte
Faculty III - Media, Information and Design,
University of Applied Sciences and Arts,
Hannover, Germany
e-mail: oliver.bott@hs-hannover.de

M. Behrends · I. Hoffmann
Peter L. Reichertz Institute for Medical Informatics
of TU Braunschweig and Hannover Medical School,
Hannover Medical School, Hannover, Germany

N.-H. Benning
Institute of Medical Informatics, Heidelberg
University, Heidelberg, Germany

© Springer Nature Switzerland AG 2022
U. H. Hübner et al. (eds.), *Nursing Informatics*, Health Informatics,
https://doi.org/10.1007/978-3-030-91237-6_42

Definitions

- The *five-phase didactical framework* is intended to serve as a pragmatic introduction in digital learning and teaching on the basis of selected pedagogical theories.
- To cover the theoretical background very briefly and to set expectations correctly, it is worth noting that the introduced concept is based on a *socio-constructivist learning theory and the 5-stage model for online learning by Salmon.*
- Phase 1 is called *Reception and Introduction* and ensures, that all learners have an easy and unhindered entry into the course.
- Phase 2, *Presentation of Learning Objectives and Course Organization,* includes the presentation of the learning objectives and the planned process of the online course, which plays an essential role in the field of e-learning as well as in traditional face-to-face teaching.
- In Phase 3, *Processing of Learning Units*, the course is broken down into thematically defined learning units according to the learning objectives.
- Phase 4, *Summative Assessment*, not only allows formal certification of learning success, but also promotes learner motivation.
- Phase 5, *Completion and Evaluation*, allows learners to give feedback as an essential part of quality assurance in (digital) teaching.
- The didactical framework makes intensive use of the proccessing of tasks and the moderation of the collaborative processing of these tasks based on the *e-tivities* concept by Salmon.
- The aim of offering material in phase 3 should not only be pure knowledge transfer. Rather, the learning material should also represent an *activating input* that builds on the *prior knowledge* of the learners, takes into account *different types of learners* and *promotes an in-depth examination* of the topic.
- E-tivities aiming at *knowledge reflection* can have a positive influence on the learning process, just like the task to write a brief summary, since the passively receiving learning attitude is interrupted in favor of an active examination of the subject.
- The didactical framework can easily be implemented with modern *learning management systems (LMSs).*
- In order to ensure good communication, it is helpful to agree on rules of conduct for communication with the learners (a so-called *netiquette).*
- For *formative assessments*, i.e. the diagnostic use of assessments to provide feedback to educators and learners concerning the learning success, for example results presentations of *group work*, *e-portfolios* or *tests* can be used. Especially the *self-assessment tests* can easily be implemented with modern LMSs that also offer features for an *automated evaluation* of the test results.
- A *formative evaluation* involves a systematic reflection of the course by educators and learners.
- After completing a *summative assessment*, the course usually concludes with a *certificate of successful participation* or *a certificate of attendance.*
- Summative assessments can be carried out in different forms. *Written exams*, final *tests* in form of *answer-choice procedures*, *oral exams* or *homeworks* and *degrees theses* are possible.
- Establishing *information security and legal security* in summative assessments is a particular challenge that needs specific IT expertise or support by commercial providers of online assessment systems.
- To specifically measure the achievement of the didactic concept's objectives in phase 5, the *Community of Inquiry questionnaire* is particularly recommended.
- Another option for evaluating courses is *learning analytics* as a data-driven approach.
- Educators' negative attitudes towards online teaching can be the result of *fears of losing control* of the teaching process in a digital environment and should be addressed in training programmes for online educators.
- *Continuing education* refers to educational activities that usually build on existing voca-

tional training and deepen, expand or update it.

- The *European Framework for Digital Competence of Educators* (DigCompEdu) describes educator-specific digital competences. In order to determine the *personal level of digital competence*, DigCompEdu offers a *self-assessment tool.*

Introduction

Digital learning enables the transfer of knowledge across institutional boundaries and even across physical distances. Therefore, new formats are utilized, being based on digital tools and considering the changed setting of a virtual classroom. However, neither educators nor learners are used to these settings, as these are used rather rarely in academia. Many educators still see themselves as a lecturer and follow a traditional understanding of teaching through giving lectures, which mainly consist of a monolog in front of passive learners, consuming the monolog. Modern concepts of teaching understand the role of educators rather as someone who accompanies and supports learners during their learning process. The challenge of this role understanding of an educator and the lack of experience with digitally supported virtual learning settings often prevent an intensification of digital learning in academia.

To overcome these obstacles, this chapter provides educators with a knowledge base and pragmatic recommendations for designing didactic sound digital courses. These recommendations focus on small courses, allowing personal interaction with learners to facilitate skill acquisition, and not on organizational structures in a curriculum. For this, we introduce a basic *five-phase didactical framework*, intended to serve as a pragmatic entry into such formats based on selected pedagogical theories. This chapter is not intended to provide a well-founded introduction to learning theories, but rather to enable a practical, didactically sound start to e-learning.

To cover the theoretical background very briefly and to set expectations correctly, it is worth noting that the introduced concept is based on a *socio-constructivist learning theory*. This means that interactions between learners and their collaboration are considered as a fundamental step toward understanding and acquiring competences in a course. Thus, the didactic concept mostly focuses on the definition of tasks, so-called *e-tivities*, and the moderation of the collaborative processing of these tasks.

All course activities shall be aligned with the competences, supposed to be acquired in the course. The competence-oriented description of learning goals should be interpreted as a functional understanding, describing what learners should be capable of, after they participated in a course. In other words, a *competence* describes if a learner is prepared to handle a given challenge [2]. This competence orientation is not just a reliable mechanism to align the course with, for example, a university's module description but also an important mechanism to align with requirements of national and international professional societies. For example, in the field of Medical Informatics (MI), the International Medical Informatics Association (IMIA) defines competences, which should be covered in such curricula. In the field of Nursing Informatics (NI) examples are the TIGER Initiative (Technology Informatics Guiding Education Reform) and the recommendations by GMDS, ÖGPI and IGPI [3]. The use of such competence catalogs goes beyond designing university modules: After completing university education, virtually all professions in healthcare require lifelong learning by *continuing education*. For this, competence catalogs help to select skills, which should be acquired or updated.

To enable efficient utilization of the presented didactical framework, it assumes a very slim set of equipment: Basic content production tools like presentation graphics software, a web cam and a *learning management system* (LMS), offering basic collaboration features like forums or wikis. For the LMSs, a variety of ready-to-use solutions exist, ranging from open-source tools (e.g. Moodle, ILIAS) and custom solutions for teaching consortiums (e.g. in Germany oncampus.de, vfh.de) to commercial and non-commercial *Massive Open Online Courses (MOOC) platforms* (e. g. coursera.org, edx.org or open.hpi. org) that focus on courses with a potentially very large number of participants without any particular access or admission restrictions. Virtually all of these tools offer a mobile version, meaning courses can be accessed on mobile devices like smartphones and tablets and thus enable *mobile learning*.

Based upon selected didactic fundamentals, the following sections describe the five-phase-based didactical framework in detail and introduce each phase in a separate section. Afterward, digital learning tools will be introduced, including typical use cases. Then, necessary skills for educators and learners in online settings and the specifics of digital teaching in continuous education are discussed. Last, two case studies from the German Medical Informatics Initiative (MII) [4], more specifically, the HiGHmeducation teaching consortium [5], will show how the didactic framework can be realized in practice. The chapter ends with a summary, conclusions and an outlook.

Didactical Framework

The following Section Fundamentals of the Five-Phase Didactical Framework for Online Courses introduces the didactic fundamentals of a learning phase-oriented *five-phase didactical framework* for online courses that is presented in Section Five-Phase Didactical Framework for Online Courses. The didactical framework aims at organizing online courses with a focus on collaborative learning using an LMS. It is based upon a corresponding framework of the HiGHmeducation subproject of the HiGHmed consortium that is part of the Medical Informatics Initiative (MII), an initiative funded by the German Federal Ministry of Education and Research (BMBF) that, among others, focuses on solutions to address the growing demand of online education in the field of medical informatics [6]. The framework forms the basis for 12 online learning modules respectively courses developed by

HiGHmeducation until June 2020, some of which were implemented and evaluated for the first time in the 2019/20 winter semester.

Fundamentals of the Five-Phase Didactical Framework for Online Courses

The five-phase didactical framework is based upon different phases, allowing participants to go through course contents autonomous and in their own pace, while being accompanied by the educator as a kind of e-moderator. These phases are derived from, but due to their mapping to a course design within an LMS not equal to the *five-stage model* by Salmon [7]. Salmon's model distinguishes five stages that a group goes through in pure online learning and which represents different levels of cooperation and knowledge acquisition. Each of Salmon's stage is named by a characteristic task and defines technical tasks for the educators as well as e-moderating tasks. Stage 1 is called *Access and Motivation*, defining the setup of a digital learning environment, typically an LMS, as a technical task, including ensuring that all learners have access to the environment. In terms of e-moderating, the stage proposes welcoming and encouraging the participants. Stage 2, *Online Socialization*, aims at building a community of learners through developing appropriate ways of communication and interaction as well as the familiarization of different social environments within the course that may differ in cultural and social aspects. Stage 3 is meant to establish effective *Information Exchange* through offering methodical and technical support for searching for and working with information relevant for the course. From an e-moderating point of view, educators have to offer tutoring and also support learners in using available learning materials. *Knowledge Construction*, achieved in Stage 4, should be technically supported by an opportunity for conferencing and e-moderated with the aim to facilitate the process of knowledge construction within the cohort. Finally, Stage 5, *Development*, expands the course to resources outside of the LMS: Technical support consists of providing links to references outside the learning environment. Educators should e-moderate very passively in this stage by supporting and responding to learner inquires.

The didactical framework, which is introduced below, shows how Salmon's five-stage model can be mapped to a time-oriented course structure in an LMS. The proposed time-based course structure should not be interpreted as a fixed template but as an example that can be flexibly adapted to specific course requirements. The framework suggests different digital learning tools to be used in the phases, including learning materials such as literature or lecture videos, but especially including tasks to be conducted by the learners. The latter are a crucial part of the socio-constructivist learning environment aimed for and thus have their own structure and name: *e-tivities*. The concept of e-tivities was defined by Salmon [8]. The following didactical framework adapts the concept of e-tivities and suggests to describe and organize e-tivities the following way:

- *Name*: A short name that arouses curiosity and invites to take part, ideally referring to the content or topic of the e-tivity.
- *Spark*: An introduction that creates the setting for the e-tivity. This includes to explain the embedding in the course's topic(s). The spark should be authored creatively and aim for motivating the learners' collaboration.
- *Purpose*: A description what the learner will take home by conducting this e-tivity. This description should be based on verbs and make very clear what impact the e-tivity has on the learner's individual competencies: "If you complete the e-tivity, you will be able to…".
- *Task*: Precise and clear description of the contributions expected from each participant. This includes requirements on how the results should be organized: media (forum, wiki, etc.), deadline (date and time) and expected length.
- *Dialogue begins*: Ask learners to response to the results of other learners. This is the crucial

part to create a social learning environment. Make sure to create a motivational message that clearly defines when learners should reflect on whose results and in what way.
- *Support*: Describe clearly what the e-moderator's interventions will be and when learners can expect them.
- *Schedule and Time*: Provide the participants with an estimate for the total time needed to conduct the e-tivity. If the e-tivity time should be organized over a given time corridor in a specific way, provide corresponding details at this point (e.g. complete individual contributions until day X and consolidate all contributions until day Y).
- *Next*: Put a link to the next e-tivity here, to make it easy for participants to navigate within the course. This is also a good place for further materials. If these are included, make clear which ones are mandatory and which are not.

Five-Phase Didactical Framework for Online Courses

Based on the five-stage model of Salmon, online courses should aim at fostering active engagement and collaboration of the learners when working with the learning material to prevent frustration induced by isolated learning. Sufficient opportunities for learners for reflection, questions, practice and testing are important and should be included explicitly when planning an online course.

To support this kind of communication and collaborative learning in an online course setting, the didactic process can be divided into five phases forming the *five-phase didactical framework for online courses*. The phases of this framework aim at activation of the learners, knowledge transfer, self-directed processing of learning tasks, learning success control and feedback. In each phase, digital learning tools can be used to promote a sustainable learning success by motivating learners to interact with the subject matter and by enabling communication and collaboration between learners. A significant aspect

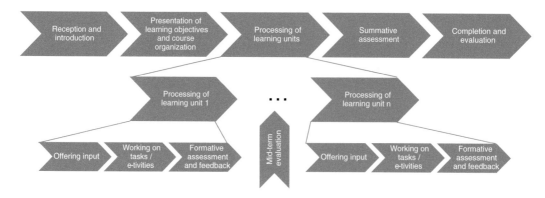

Fig. 42.1 The five-phase didactical framework for collaborative online courses

of the approach, especially incorporated in phase three but also in other phases of the didactical framework, is the use of e-tivities (s.a.). The five phases are (see Fig. 42.1) as follows:

1. Reception and introduction
2. Presentation of learning objectives and course organization
3. Processing of learning units

This phase encompasses processing of one to many learning units composing of

   (a) offering input
   (b) working on one or more tasks, respectively, e-tivities
   (c) formative assessment and feedback

4. Summative assessment
5. Completion and evaluation

   E-tivities are mainly used in phase 3 but also in phases 1 and 2 to get the learners gradually familiar with the concept of e-tivities. After processing the first learning units, a formative mid-term evaluation of the course is recommended to adjust the course concept based on feedback of the learners.

   The didactical framework for collaborative online courses can be used to address two typical online teaching scenarios:

1. Educating a smaller group of up to about 25 learners which enables intensive collaboration between the learners supervised individually by one or more educators. A small group size or a high support rate makes it easier for the course participants and the educators to form

a *"Community of Inquiry"* according to Garrison [9] that actively and collaboratively develops knowledge and skills. E-tivities in this type of online course typically can be moderated and accompanied with sufficient intensity by the educator(s).

2. In online courses with larger study groups, in which the educators cannot supervise the course participants as intensively as in scenario 1, the learners have to learn with a higher degree of autonomy. Collaboration is possible also in this scenario, but in contrast to scenario 1, peer review and electronic assessment typically replace the supervision by the educator in the e-tivites. The course organization and the use of e-tivites have to reflect the group size, for example, through a more structured and distributed organization of the feedback and/or by subdividing the group into subgroups.

   The following sections describe the five phases in more detail.

Phase 1: Reception and Introduction

For a successful implementation of online learning, it is important to ensure at the beginning of the course that all learners have an *easy and unhindered access* to the learning objects. Additionally, it should be clear to the learners which LMS functions are available for processing a task and how they can use them. Therefore, the educator should make *precise instructions* for working within the LMS available. These instructions can be presented, for example, in the form of a video that explains the functions of the system using screen recordings or by an illustrated text file that can be printed out. Since there are different types of learners with variable depth of experience in the use of an LMS, it makes sense to provide various guidance materials in different levels of detail in order to offer users a choice. While experienced users are rather annoyed by long and detailed introductions, others feel insecure if they do not have access to detailed descriptions concerning the LMS functions they do not know yet. The offers can be supplemented with a collection of frequently asked questions and a forum where open questions and problems concerning the use of the system can be raised. The educator answers the questions in the forum, but support from other learners is also very welcome and should be explicitly encouraged.

Initial working tasks during the introduction phase can be used to *check that all participants have access* to the course and are able to use its main functions. For this purpose, it can be valuable to conduct a survey or set up an e-tivity on learners' expectations and previous knowledge. For small learning groups, for example, a first task for the learners could also be to use a forum or even a wiki to introduce themselves personally or to answer an introductory question. With early feedback, educators can also obtain important information about the learners like their level of previous knowledge as well as their motivation. A personal *presentation of the participants* in a forum or wiki may be especially appropriate if the learners come from different universities or areas of expertise or if it is important that small groups are formed for further learning phases. By getting to know each other, the communication between the participants, which is important for the learning success, can be improved.

Besides clarifying the *technical questions* and introducing the learners and their expectations, a *welcome message* of the educator(s) is also an important aspect in this phase. Each educator should introduce him/herself as well as his/her role within the course and should give a concise overview on the topics of the course. The main aims of this introduction are to create a good atmosphere, to arouse pleasure in the course and to motivate the learners to participate actively. This introduction can take the form of a video or text. A face-to-face online meeting via a web-based video conference tool at the beginning of the course is also a good way to achieve these goals. There are numerous tools for conducting online meetings, often directly integrated into the LMSs.

Phase 2: Presentation of Learning Objectives and Course Organization

Learning objectives play an essential role in the area of e-learning, just like in traditional classroom teaching. They are an important means of designing a course and help to promote the learning performance and motivation of the learners. Clear *competence-oriented learning objectives* based, for example, on the revised taxonomy of Bloom [10] make it easier for learners to build on previous experiences and to understand the objectives of the course as their own. They support the personal selection of learning material, the design of one's own learning activities and the monitoring of the individual learning progress.

If previous knowledge and skills are required to successfully complete the course, these *prerequisites* must be plainly communicated by the educator in this phase of the course at the latest. In order to communicate these requirements clearly, the same taxonomy can be used that is used to describe the competency-based learning objectives, for example, "A prerequisite for a good start to the course is that you are able to use the basic commands of SQL effectively". An effective mean to prevent learners from frustration because of missing required competencies is to offer a short test that allows learners to self-assess their competencies. *Self-assessment tests* can easily be implemented with modern LMSs that also offer features for an automated evaluation of the test results. If the test detects missing competencies, tips should be given for, for example, other courses that convey the missing competencies.

In addition to the presentation of the content based on learning objectives, the *organizational structure and expected workload* of the course should also be described in this phase. The participants should get a clear idea of what to expect in the course. In addition to the duration of the course, this includes, for example, information about (virtual) attendance times and online phases. The expectations placed on the course participants in the course must also be clearly stated: for example, processing of at least 90% of the learning tasks, participation in the (virtual) events, weekly feedback, or documentation of the learning status for more complex exercises. It should also be shown which learning materials (software, own folders, group work areas, etc.) have to be used and which assessments must be taken in order to successfully pass the course.

A separate forum in the LMSs should be set up for *organizational issues*, with a defined time frame in which feedback is given by the educator. The use of forums prevents the same questions from having to be answered again and again. A list of frequently asked questions (FAQ) could also be helpful, whereby a wiki or a glossary can be used as an object of an LMS for a collection of FAQs. A defined, reliable process for feedback on questions in the forum gives learners security and relieves the educators. To ensure good communication, it will be helpful, possibly together with the learners, to determine an agreement on rules of conduct for communication issues that can counteract this uncertainty (a so called *netiquette*). Uncertainty about the mode of direct personal addressing can negatively affect the communication between learners among themselves and with the educator.

During this phase, an online meeting via a video conference tool might be a good way to personally clarify all relevant issues.

Phase 3: Processing of Learning Units

According to the learning objectives (see phase 2), the course should be divided into thematically defined learning units. The aim of each learning unit is the acquisition of the competences defined by the respective learning objectives. Corresponding learning activities enable an intensive and in-depth examination of the learning material. Each learning unit should have a similar and obvious structure and should consist of the following three phases:

a. offering input,
b. working on one or more tasks,
c. formative assessment and feedback.

Furthermore, a formative evaluation can be carried out in the middle of the course period:

d. Mid-term evaluation of the course

Offering Input

This phase of the course includes the provision of online material such as self-written texts supplemented, for example, by images, videos, podcasts, journal articles or book chapters. Talk or lecture recordings have become a widely used method of making learning material available in a digital form. Simple recording tools, and sometimes even the presentation tools themselves, enable educators to record presentations themselves with little effort. Many universities already offer lecture recording as standard. However, the aim of the input should not only be a pure transfer of knowledge, rather the learning material should also represent an *activating input*, building on the *previous knowledge* of the learners, considering *different types of learning* and *promoting an in-depth examination* of the topic. Conceivable here are, for example, expert interviews, case presentations or problem descriptions with corresponding accompanying materials. Other forms to make the knowledge transfer stimulating and exciting can be explanatory videos, gamification approaches or simulations. Although the structure of the learning units should be similar and easy to understand, the input should be varying and demanding.

Working on One or More Tasks

In addition to the learning material offered in the previous phase, the tasks based on it are of essential importance for the learning success. They should *motivate and activate learners* to deal with the topic according to the learning objectives. If the offering input phase takes place without an online meeting of the educator with the course participants, it is even more important to promote the activating learning processes through suitable and ideally cooperative work tasks.

E-tivities are a suitable mean to define such tasks. An example is that learners shall comment on and evaluate interviews with experts, afterward learners discuss their comments and evaluation results with each other moderated by the educator. E-tivities aiming at *knowledge reflection* can have a positive influence on the learning process, just like the task to write a brief summary, since the passively receiving learning attitude is interrupted in favor of an active examination of the subject. Work tasks and work instructions in e-learning should be formulated as clearly as possible in order to avoid queries about the task as far as possible. In a research-oriented teaching setting, this phase can be designed by means of *inquiry-based learning* which means that learners develop their own questions based on source material, which they then work on their own or in small groups.

Besides learning materials and tools for working on the tasks, *virtual workspaces* should also be made available, especially if cooperation between learners is desired and educators wish to accompany, support or evaluate the learning processes. There are various objects in LMSs to support *collaborative learning* (see Section Digital Learning Tools of Learning Management Systems (LMSs)), especially in groups: learners can upload objects and work on it together, create shared content with wikis or discuss topics in forums.

The combination of the "Offering input" phase and the "Working on one or more tasks" phase is comparable to the *inverted classroom method* [11] (also called flipped classroom method). The inverted classroom method is a blended learning approach in which the classroom sessions are preceded by an online self-learning phase comparable with the "Offering input" phase. During the online learning phase, learners acquire the necessary factual knowledge, which serves as the basis for application and consolidation in the following classroom session. Passive learning thus takes place in an online self-learning phase. The presence phase in the classroom (comparable with the "Working on one or more tasks" phase) is used specifically for activating learning with communicative and collaborative learning processes.

Formative Assessment and Feedback

Each learning unit should end with *feedback from the educator* and, if applicable, the learners (*peer group feedback*) concerning learning performance and status. This feedback is important for both educators and learners: Educators recognize whether and which deficits still exist among the learners and if everyone can follow the course. Learners receive information about their own learning status. Feedback on the results of the work tasks also increases motivation and willingness to participate actively.

For so-called *formative assessments,* that is, the diagnostic use of assessment to provide feedback to educators and learners concerning the *learning success*, for example, results presentations of group work, e-portfolios or tests can serve as proof of individual learning performance. In digital learning settings, feedback is also possible by comparing the learner's solutions with sample solutions that were previously created by the educators. It has not yet been scientifically proven whether static feedback through a sample solution or individual feedback from an educator promotes better learning success. In many cases, the number of participants and the personnel resources of supervising educators will drive the decision which form of feedback is offered.

Mid-Term Evaluation of the Course

To identify improvement potential already while the implementation phase of a course, an evaluation in the middle of the course period is recommended. This involves a systematic reflection of the course by conducting a *formative evaluation.* Based on the results of the evaluation of the course participants about the experienced teaching quality and learning situation as well as the course concept, educators can identify opportunities for improvement at an early stage and optimize the course already during its implementation. In addition, the formative evaluation serves to keep the learners motivated. In order to obtain a general picture of the course atmosphere, a formative evaluation in the form of a questionnaire with the possibility of making constructive suggestions is recommended. This can be done very well with an appropriately designed e-tivity.

Phase 4: Summative Assessment

To assess if learning objectives are met by the course participants is important not only for motivation, but also for formally certificating the learning success. After completing a *summative assessment*, the course usually concludes with a *certificate of successful participation* or *a certificate of attendance*. While the didactic goal of the formative assessment is to support the learner in his learning process with feedback concerning his or her learning success, the summative assessment always represents a *final performance assessment*.

Summative assessments can be carried out in different forms. *Written exams*, final *tests* in form of *answer-choice procedures*, *oral exams* or *homeworks* and *degrees theses* are possible. Dedicated digital assessment systems also as modern LMSs support the implementation of different types of summative assessment tasks and especially of tests in the answer-choice procedure, whereby different types of questions can be used, such as multiple- or single-choice questions, matching questions, long menu questions or numerical questions.

If tests are not evaluated automatically, they are usually not suitable for assessments in learning settings with a large number of participants. Here tests in the answer-choice procedure, mapping tasks or simple computation tasks can be used, which can be evaluated automatically. In addition to these types of tasks, much research has been done to automate assessment for more complex types of tasks such as programming or math tasks or modeling tasks. The extent to which such functions can be used depends on the LMSs and the number of available corresponding plug-ins.

Oral exams can be conducted online, as part of a video conference. To organize the submission of individual work as proof of performance, LMSs usually offer suitable objects in form of exercises in ILIAS or as tasks in Moodle. A fixed schedule can be defined for the submission of the work and feedback on the assessment can also be given via the system. This way the submission and processing status is transparent for educators and learners. Exercises or tasks can of course also be used for formative assessments.

If these systems are used for summative assessment, it must be checked whether there is sufficient legal certainty for conducting summative assessments using these assessment functionalities. Regarding the organizational context of the assessment, the respective examination rules and regulations have to be considered. Fraud opportunities by learners should be prevented as far as possible. Legal security is preceded by a corresponding level of information security to be ensured in the LMSs or assessment systems. Depending on the legal significance of the assessment, ensuring the necessary legal and information technology requirements for the examination system can be a challenge. This is particularly the case if an exam is not carried out on-site on the computer and monitored by supervisors, but online at the learner's home. Establishing *information security and legal security* in this assessment scenario is a particular challenge that is addressed by commercial providers of online assessment systems.

An important analysis function that usually is included in sophisticated LMSs or assessment systems addresses the quality of tests and test questions through *offering test statistics*. Besides information, for example, about the average score achieved, the standard deviation of scores achieved or a histogram of scores, these test statistics allow the assessment of the difficulty of a task or its discriminatory power. As a result, a test question might be excluded from the assessment or might be improved before used the next time.

Phase 5: Completion and Evaluation

Feedback from learners is a crucial part of quality assurance in (digital) teaching. This feedback can be collected by interpreting results from formative and summative assessments and by explicit evaluation formats. The latter ones can be organized in different ways: Qualitative methods are considered to deliver more accurate insights into teaching quality but considering effort and feasibility, quantitative methods are typically preferred. These methods are mostly based on standardized instruments (i.e. questionnaires), which can be easily used within an LMS.

There are several dimensions the educator can examine in a course cohort [1]:

- *Social presence*
  (Measures the ability of participants to identify with the course cohort)
- *Cognitive presence*
  (Measures the ability of participants to construct knowledge through reflection and discourse)
- *Teaching presence*
  (Measures the ability to facilitate the social and cognitive processes in the course to realize meaningful and worthwhile learning outcomes)

To specifically measure the achievement of the didactic concept's objectives, the *Community of Inquiry questionnaire* is particularly recommended [1]. It measures the socialization of the cohort and their attitude toward online learning with regard to the specific course. Supplemented by optional free text questions for comments and suggestions for improvement, this questionnaire is an efficient tool to gain meaningful insights into the learners' perception of the course, enabling educators to optimize the course for further iterations.

Another option for evaluating courses is a data-driven approach: *Learning analytics*. This discipline refers to the interpretation of automatically collected data from LMSs and other systems used for teaching. These data especially include log data of learners like access times to course objects, participation in interactive components like tests and finally public communication data (e.g. in forums). These data are interpreted with the help of statistic methods in order to generate knowledge on specific course objects, on collaboration between learners or on the learning process as a whole. Evaluations range from simple indicators such as access counts for single course objects to complex analyses of learners' communication networks [12]. Many LMSs are configured to record basic log data of all users by default, so it is possible to perform simple analyses in many environments without preparing data collection. Such analyses can often be performed by using the user interface of the LMSs, by graphically presenting recorded data. In case an LMS does not offer this function, it might offer an export functionality, exporting a file, which can be analyzed within a spreadsheet program. In more sophisticated environments, organizations might use a *learning record store (LRS)*, which is a dedicated system to store data from learners that will be used by other applications. These applications might conduct more complex calculations such as the aforementioned network analyses and present the results to educators. However, for educators who are new to e-learning, we recommend expanding the questionnaire-based evaluation by using access numbers for course objects as a first step. It is obvious that this type of analysis has to be carried out in accordance with the respective data privacy regulations.

Digital Learning Tools of Learning Management Systems (LMSs)

Even if the development of a digital learning content is primarily influenced by didactic decisions, nevertheless a lot of technological challenges need to be solved:

- How can password-protected access to the learning materials be ensured?
- Is the learning material displayed in different browsers correctly?
- Which aspects of usability have to be considered for navigation and design?
- Are backups be carried out regularly?
- What should be considered in relation to data protection? Who will manage the user accounts?

These are only some of the questions needed to be clarified when creating web-based learning offers. Since educators will be overwhelmed by this, *learning management systems* (LMSs) have been established in all areas of teaching. In schools and universities as well as in continuing education, digital teaching is carried out with the help of LMSs. Thereby LMSs support digital teaching and learning processes by managing user data and learning materials and by enabling the provision of learning content via Internet, the organization of learning processes in courses and groups and the communication and interaction between educators and learners. LMSs also offer *authoring tools* to create learning materials without programming knowledge. Further typical *LMS functionalities* relate to the administration of users, courses and learning content as well as the communication and interaction of users within the system. By enabling the organization of digital teaching, LMSs differ from *content management systems* (CMSs), which only allow to provide learning materials.

For educators, however, the question arises how well LMSs also support didactic aspects. Therefore, different digital learning tools are presented here, which are available in common LMSs. Representatively for many other systems, the two learning management systems *ILIAS* (https://www.ilias.de) and *Moodle* (https://moodle.org) will be examined more closely. Both systems are *open-source systems* published under the GNU General Public License. The technical infrastructure of both systems is implemented as a client-server architecture with PHP and MySQL. Thereby the content is stored on a central server that can be accessed by computers or mobile devices via the Internet. The user interaction with the system is logged, so that, for example, learning process can be monitored.

ILIAS stands for "Integriertes Lern-, Informations- und Arbeitskooperations-System" (German for "Integrated Learning, Information and Work Cooperation System"). The version 1 of ILIAS was published in 1998 and has been continuously developed since then (at the time of publication version 7 will be available). ILIAS is one of the first LMSs and one of the most widespread in Germany.

Moodle is the world's most popular learning platform and was originally an acronym for Modular Object-Oriented Dynamic Learning Environment. The founder and chief developer of Moodle, Martin Dougiamas, grew up in the Australian outback, started in 1999 experimenting with an early prototype of a new LMS. Moodle was first released as an open-source platform in 2001 and has also been continuously developed since then (the release of Moodle 3.11 should be available at the time of this publication). All courses and learning objects can also be accessed directly on a mobile device via a Moodle app, both online and offline.

The following tables contain an overview of typical digital learning tools that LMSs offer and their representations in Moodle and ILIAS separated by semicolons. The tools are presented

according to their main field of application in an online course:

1. *Content provision or compilation*
2. *Communication*
3. *Collaboration*
4. *(Formative or summative) Assessment*
5. *Feedback/evaluation*
6. *Organization*

1. *Content provision or compilation*

Description	Definition
File storage; file [ILIAS 5.3.7; Moodle 3.5]	Learning or working material can be uploaded as digital file, including, for example, word-processed documents or slideshow presentations. Certain file types are combined with special viewing software. Especially for presenting videos (e.g. recorded lectures), often tools/plug-ins are integrated that allow a convenient navigation through a presentation.
e-Portfolio; portfolio template [ILIAS 5.3.7]; portfolios [Moodle 3.5]	Practice or learning results are submitted by learners by uploading files or linking to work results. This includes, for example, word-processed documents, spreadsheets, and images, audio and video clips.
Glossary [all]	List of definitions or a collection of links, like a dictionary. Can be used for FAQs, which can be continued and administered by the learners and/or the educator(s).
Learning module; learning module [ILIAS 5.3.7]; lesson [Moodle 3.5]	A learning module is a digital textbook that typically can be created with an integrated authoring environment of the LMSs. A learning module is structured by chapters and pages and can contain text, graphics, tables and pictures as well as questions or videos. Lessons in Moodle present a series of pages to the learner who is usually asked to make some sort of choice or test underneath the content area. The choice or test result will redirect them to a specific page in the lesson.
SCORM learning module; learning module SCORM [ILIAS 5.3.7]; SCORM package [Moodle 3.5]	SCORM (Shareable Content Object Reference Model) is a collection of specifications that enable interoperability, accessibility and reusability of web-based learning content. With SCORM learning modules, content can be shared with other LMSs. SCORM modules are textbook-like presentations of multimedia learning content (see learning module).

Description	Definition
Link; web link [ILIAS 5.3.7]; link/URL [Moodle 3.5]	Links to existing information sources or learning materials on the Internet. Links can be set up in various ways, for example, to enable opening a webpage in a new window so the learner can access and use the link independent from the LMSs.
List of literature; ditto [ILIAS 5.3.7] [unavailable in Moodle]	The literature list object in ILIAS is used to represent a given literature list. The common formats of literature management are supported: .ris, .bib or .bibtex.
Data collection; ditto [ILIAS 5.3.7]; database [Moodle 3.5]	Allows the educator and/or learners to build, display and search a set of record entries about any conceivable topic. Can include objects in various formats, such as text, images, numbers, URLs, dates and files.

2. Communication

Description	Definition
Notification function; system news [ILIAS 5.3.7]; messaging [Moodle 3.5]	Notification of participants via automatic e-mail transmission, including storage of accumulated notifications. This can be triggered, for example, by new learning units, forum posts, etc.
Blog [all]	Online diary to present content or to communicate with other learners. The contributions are presented in chronological order. Blogs usually are written by one person, although some blogs can be authored by groups.
Video-conferencing system (or web-conferencing system); typically a plug-in [all];	Online meetings can be held using a video conferencing system (VCS) that allows the sharing of the screen of the educator or a learner to present applications, documents or other learning materials. Modern VCS allows the management of VCS-groups to emulate group-based practice sessions.

3. Collaboration

Description	Definition
Chat; chat room [ILIAS 5.3.7]; chat [Moodle 3.5];	In a chat, learners can also discuss with each other and the educator in real time, for example, to clarify open questions, exchange opinions and perspectives on a course topic.

Description	Definition
Forum [all]	Forums are a text-based time- and location-independent opportunity to exchange thoughts, opinions and experiences and to discuss asynchronously. Educators and/or learners can ask questions parallel to event topics, which can be discussed in the form of text contributions.
Grouping; group [ILIAS 5.3.7]; group choice [Moodle 3.5]	The educator creates groups of learners and determines the maximum group size. Afterward the course participants can register themselves in these groups or are registered by the educator. Group members typically have authoring rights only in their group.
Student folder; my work space [ILIAS 5.3.7]; student folder [Moodle 3.5];	With a student folder, learners can upload documents and files. This enables learners to collect own learning material and to share documents with other users. Deployment scenarios are group work based on the division of labor, documentation and presentation of work results, knowledge sharing, delivery of materials and creation of an (own) knowledge pool.
Wiki [all]	A wiki is a collection of collaboratively authored web documents. Basically, a wiki page is a web page that everyone in the course can edit in the browser, without needing to know HTML. A wiki starts with one front page. Each learner can add other pages to the wiki by simply creating a link to a page that does not exist yet. Wikis can be a powerful tool for collaborative work on content. The process of editing is logged so that educators can see who has been involved in editing the wiki.

4. Assessment

Description	Definition
Assignment with submission; exercise [ILIAS 5.3.7]; task [Moodle 3.5]	Learners submit their results to an assignment, which is then evaluated by the educator. The submission can consist of one or more files that are uploaded by the learners (e.g. the result of a homework). The solution of an assignment can also be entered directly online using a text editor.
Test [all]	Educators use tests as an objective measure to assess the learning success. Tests can be created with a variety of different question types (e.g. multiple choice, true/false questions, various drag-and-drop and short answer questions).

5. Feedback/evaluation

Description	Definition
Vote [all]	Votes are questions with predefined answer options. A vote is suitable, among other things, to pose an introductory question for a certain topic, to get an opinion on a certain question or to check the general understanding or to find an appointment.
Survey; ditto [ILIAS 5.3.7]; feedback [Moodle 3.5]	Surveys can be used to query learners' experiences and opinions or for the creation of own surveys and/or evaluation forms. There are typically various types of questions to choose from.

6. Organization

Description	Definition
Structuring element; categories, folders, object block [Ilias 5.3.7]; directory [Moodle 3.5]	Allows to combine several objects, such as folders.
Calendar [all]	The calendar can display site, course, group, user and category events in addition to assignment and quiz deadlines, chat times and other course events. A calendar may be included in a course or the site front page.
Desk; personal desk [ILIAS 5.3.7]; dashboard [Moodle 3.5]	A desk is an individually adaptable overview page that provides users with links to their profile information, messages, the calendar, their own learning progress, etc.

Digital Skills of Educators and Learners

The availability and use of digital applications in all areas of life and work raise the question of what knowledge and skills are needed to act actively and self-determinedly in the process of digital transformation. Therefore in 2013, the European Commission developed a *Digital Competence Framework for Citizens* (DigComp), the current revised version is available since 2016 [13]. DigComp describes knowledge, skills and abilities that are neces-

sary to ensure that people can use digital technology

- to search and find digital information as well as manage and evaluate digital data,
- for communication and collaboration,
- to create digital content,
- to protect personal devices, data, environment and health,
- to solve problems regarding digital technologies [13].

Neither technical skills about concepts of *information and communication technology* nor knowledge about structure or function of digital systems and applications are described in DigComp, it focuses rather on core competencies for using digital technologies. In the professional context, there are also different profession-specific competence models which supplement and extend these digital core competences. The International Medical Informatics Association (IMIA) recommends necessary competences for health care professionals and for Biomedical and Health Informatics [14]. Competencies for nursing were described by organizations in Austria, Germany and Switzerland [15] or by the TIGER Initiative [16]. The database created within the framework of the project HITComp (Health Information Technology Competencies) (http://hitcomp.org/) enables a structured search in over 1000 competencies needed for a variety of healthcare roles, levels and areas of knowledge.

The different frameworks show how important it is, that healthcare professionals can acquire *digital competencies in education and training* — particularly through digital teaching. Thereby on every level of education, the competences of educators play an important role — not only to impart technological knowledge, but also to enable learners to gain experience in using digital tools in different contexts. For this reason, the European Framework for *Digital Competence of Educators* (DigCompEdu) captures 22 educator-specific digital competences in six areas [17]. Like DigComp, DigCompEdu does not focus on technical skills but addresses digital competencies on different didactic areas and teaching contexts [17]:

1. Area: *Professional Engagement*
   Area 1 describes four competencies regarding the use of digital technologies to communicate with learners, to collaborate with other educators, to reflect digital pedagogical practice and for continuous professional development.
2. Area: *Digital Resources*
   Area 2 includes three competencies to select, create, modify and manage digital resources for teaching and learning regarding pedagogical as well as legal requirements.
3. Area: *Teaching and Learning*
   Area 3 focuses on planning and implementing digital devices and resources in the teaching process, especially to enhance the interaction with learners, to foster and enhance learner collaboration and to support self-regulated learning processes.
4. Area: *Assessment*
   In area 4, competencies regarding the use of digital technologies for formative and summative assessments, for analyzing evidence on learner activity, performance and progress and for feedback are described.
5. Area: *Empowering Learners*
   Area 5 focuses on skills of educators to ensure accessibility to learning resources and activities for all learners, including those with special needs, to address personal needs of learners and to use digital technologies within pedagogic strategies that foster learners' transversal skills, deep thinking and creative expression.
6. Area: *Facilitating Learners' Digital Competence*
   Area 6 includes competencies of educators to incorporate learning activities, assignments and assessments which require learners to train their own digital skills regarding information literacy, digital communication and collaboration, creation of digital content, protecting own wellbeing, and to identify and solve technical problems, or to transfer technological knowledge creatively to new situations.

DigCompEdu is only one reference model for digital competencies. There is a number of national initiatives and approaches to describe digital competences for educators. Even if DigCompEdu and DigComp do not describe technical skills, the authors consider, for example, that a basic understanding of underlying concepts is important for creative and critical use of digital technologies.

For a successful acquisition of competences, however, the personal attitude of the learners toward the content is a critical factor. For educators, openness toward digital teaching methods and curiosity to get new teaching experiences are necessary to recognize and to implement the opportunities of digital learning for their own teaching. A fundamental critical attitude of digital teaching complicates the development of appropriate digital teaching skills. Negative attitudes can be the result of *fears of losing control* over the teaching process in a digital environment but need to be overcome.

In order to determine the personal level of competence, DigCompEdu offers a *self-assessment tool* (https://ec.europa.eu/jrc/en/digcompedu/self-assessment). The tool enables educators to reflect personal attitudes toward digital teaching and individual needs for further training. Based on that, it is possible to choose training courses that meet one's owns expectations and needs. Many educational institutions offer a wide range of further training regarding digital competencies.

Didactical Principles in Digital Continuing Education and Workforce Development in Health Care

Continuing education (CE) refers to educational activities that usually build on existing vocational training and deepen, expand or update it. This deepening, expansion or updating is usually carried out through solitary courses or a series of courses that require a comparably small amount of time up to continuing education programs of universities that may last several semesters. In addition to the question of whether a CE program is carried out purely digitally, digitally supported or classically in presence, there are further distinguishing features, that is, whether the training is carried out full-time or part-time and whether it is an internal CE program, i.e. a program organized and carried out by the employer, or a training offer offered by an external training provider. The target group addressed with regard to their intra- or interprofessional heterogeneity also influences the design of a CE training offer. In order to distinguish from university CE study programs or long-term CE programs and the concepts of digital teaching that are suitable for this kind of programs, this section focuses on the special features of CE programs that are carried out part-time in a rather shorter time.

The general question of whether digital teaching formats have advantages over conventional teaching formats for such programs is not clearly answered in the scientific literature. Some reviews document mostly positive effects [18] or the tendency that digital offers are at least as effective as traditional learning approaches [19]. Other reviews document no or only slight differences [20].

When making comparative assessments, it must be taken into account that the effects of digital CE training courses can lie at different levels. One prominent model that can be used for the assessment and evaluation of CE training offers is the *Kirkpatrick model* [21]: It differentiates between four levels: first *reaction* (reactions of the learner to the CE training offer), second *learning* (to what extent does the CE training offer improve the level of knowledge and the attitude of the participant to a topic), third *behavior* (to what extent does the CE training offer influence the thinking and acting of the participant) and fourth *results* (to what extent does the CE training offer have effects, for example, on treatment costs or quality).

A CE training offer should ideally have positive effects on all four levels. Levels 1 and 2 are of particular interest with regard to cues on the design of digital CE education offers. The review by [18] brings together the following study results:

- Level 1: *Reaction*. Positive factors are the quality of the content, the quality and amount of social interaction and active learning, the flexibility or possibility of self-directed, time-saving learning, the effectiveness and ease of use of the technology and the quality of the support. Negative factors include technical difficulties, a lack of computer and online/Internet experience and a slow exchange of information.
- Level 2: *Knowledge*. Various subject areas in which knowledge could be improved with e-learning are identifiable, but also areas are shown in which purely digital teaching has achieved worse results than traditional classroom teaching. The examples mentioned focus on the handling of medical devices and the learning of haptic-motor skills, which underlines that the purely digitally supported teaching of such skills is a particular challenge.

In this respect, the success factors of digitally supported CE training do not appear to be much more specific than the success factors of digitally supported training in general. However, the higher inter- and intraprofessional heterogeneity of the target group can be challenging for the didactical concept of an online-based course offer, whereby particular attention should be paid to overcoming technical and communicative barriers to the use of digital learning tools. Another crucial success factor for an effective digital CE course is the provision of enough time for the learners to align the course with everyday work and family life. In digital CE courses, the participants typically do not yet know each other, thus special attention must be paid to phase 1 (reception and introduction) of the five-phase didactical framework.

Case Studies

This chapter presents two examples on how a course can be implemented digitally in different LMSs based on the presented five-phase didactical framework.

Course 1: Digitalization of Medicine—Data Literacy for Clinical Research and Health Care

Background	The digitalization of medicine has a strong influence on the work of health professionals. An essential aspect of these changes is the digital collection, management and analysis of medical data. The acquisition of basic skills in handling digital data is therefore necessary for all current and future health professionals.
Target group	Medical students, physicians, nursing staff and other persons working in health care as well as students of medical information management or medical informatics.
Learning objectives and content	The learning objectives are based on the five core concepts of data literacy from Ridsdale et al. [22]: • *Conceptual framework*: Learners can define and reflect different terms and concepts regarding data literacy. • *Data collection*: Learners can collect activity and health data using mobile sensors and know various sources of medical data. • *Data management*: Learners know functionalities and tasks of data integration centers and know approaches to data modeling. • *Data evaluation*: Learners are able to analyze and visualize data. • *Data application*: Learners can discuss their role as well as ethical and legal aspects regarding a cross-sectoral collection and use of medical data. An essential aspect of the module is to promote an active engagement of the learners. The module is implemented at the Hannover Medical School as elective subject and comprises 28 h.
Implementation of the five-phase didactical framework	Within the course, learners work in 5 weeks on 14 e-tivities regarding the five core concepts of data literacy: conceptual framework, data collection, data management, data evaluation and data application. All learning material is offered in the LMS ILIAS of the university. In addition to the asynchronous learning phases, four online meetings are conducted using a separate video conferencing tool. Alternatively, these live online meetings can take place also as classroom event. The didactic sequence of the course follows the didactical framework presented above. As an introduction to the course, the learners work on an e-tivity in which they formulate their own expectations. As "spark" of the e-tivity, the metaphor of a joint research trip is used, inviting the learners to formulate what they would take with them on a research trip. In another e-tivity, learners introduce themselves and describe their role in the research team. The educators also introduce themselves in this form (Phase 1). In the first online meeting, the learning objectives, the course structure and workflow as well as the expected workload are presented (Phase 2). Phase 3 consists of five learning units according to the core concepts of data literacy. For each topic, a separate folder with the related two or three e-tivities was created. Each e-tivity contains different "sparks" such as images, videos or screen recordings. For collaborative work, the learners use forums. In addition to the classical structure of an e-tivity, learners have to summarize their results in a wiki (Phase 4 with summative assessment). The evaluation takes place at the end of the course.

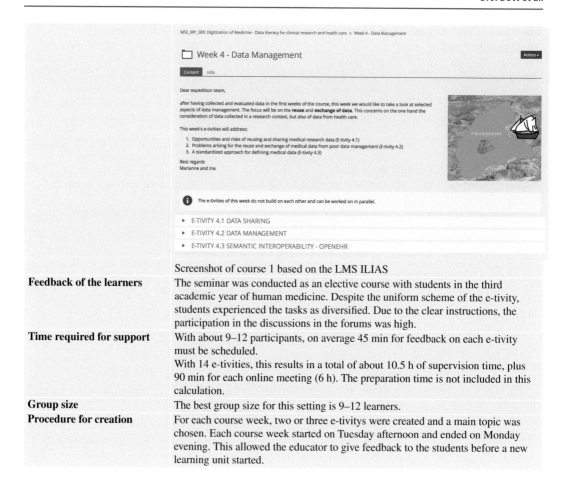

	Screenshot of course 1 based on the LMS ILIAS
Feedback of the learners	The seminar was conducted as an elective course with students in the third academic year of human medicine. Despite the uniform scheme of the e-tivity, students experienced the tasks as diversified. Due to the clear instructions, the participation in the discussions in the forums was high.
Time required for support	With about 9–12 participants, on average 45 min for feedback on each e-tivity must be scheduled. With 14 e-tivities, this results in a total of about 10.5 h of supervision time, plus 90 min for each online meeting (6 h). The preparation time is not included in this calculation.
Group size	The best group size for this setting is 9–12 learners.
Procedure for creation	For each course week, two or three e-tivitys were created and a main topic was chosen. Each course week started on Tuesday afternoon and ended on Monday evening. This allowed the educator to give feedback to the students before a new learning unit started.

Course 2: Advanced Concepts of Data Analytics and Curation—Business Intelligence, Data Warehousing and Data Mining in Health Care and Research

Background	Competencies in data analytics and curation have become a key success factor for all research and care processes in medicine.
Target group	Master students of medical information management or medical informatics, scientists with CE training needs in data integration and analysis in the context of medical research.
Learning objectives and content	The course offers an introduction to the concepts and methods of (clinical) data warehouses (DTW) and data mining analysis methods (machine learning, ML). The learning objectives of the course are:

- Learners know and understand basic concepts and typical application scenarios of data warehouses in medicine and clinical research and data mining analysis procedures in the context of business intelligence (BI) and knowledge discovery. Also they are aware of data quality and curation issues in these fields.
- Learners understand the use and creation of multidimensional data models and the concept of data cubes. They are able to implement Online Analytical Processing (OLAP) methodologies.
- Learners know typical use cases and the limitations of machine and statistical learning. They can apply these methods and algorithms in typical application scenarios in medicine and clinical research.

The module is implemented at the University of Applied Sciences and Arts, Department of Information and Communication in Hannover and comprises 180 h.

Implementation of the five-phase didactical framework	All learning materials were offered in the LMS Moodle. In addition to the asynchronous work in the learning phases, five online meetings are held with a video conference system integrated in Moodle, where break rooms were set up for group work.

The didactic sequence of the course follows the didactical framework presented in Section Didactical Framework. The course begins with a first introductory section to welcome the learners and to explain the technical and organizational framework of the LMS Moodle as well as the recommended rules of conduct for online communication. A first e-tivity for the presentation and expectations of each course participant takes place in this section to introduce this new format of an exercise. The second section focuses on organizational matters and explains the content of the course. Learning objectives and general information as well as work tools and corresponding tools for successful course participation are also explained in this section. In the learning units phase, the key topics of the course are taught to learners in a *uniform structure*. Each learning unit follows the same structure:

1. Introductory text to describe the topic
2. Learning objectives (text page)
3. Lecture slides (PDF file) and lecture recording (video) or learning video
4. E-tivity (forum) with materials/tools for the respective e-tivity (Access, Excel, SQL Server, etc.)
5. Questions on the topic (forum)
6. Reflection (forum)

The summative assessment consists of the processing of the individual e-tivities and a final submission in the respective forum. Active participation in the form of participation in discussions and constructive feedback is also expected.

Finally, the evaluation is carried out using a standardized electronic form generated with an external evaluation system.

Week 2 - Data-Warehouse-Architecture

At the beginning of a data warehouse development, it is necessary to know which architecture concept is to be used for its subsequent development. There is no simple standard design for a data warehouse, but the size and appearance vary according to the intended use and different company-specific requirements. Therefore, in the second week, we deal with the following topics, among other things: Requirements for the data warehouse architecture, a given reference architecture, the individual development phases of a data warehouse and the various components and layers that have to be created so that a complete data warehouse system can be created.

📘 SLIDES - WEEK 2: DATA-WAREHOUSE-ARCHITECTURE

📄 LEARNING GOALS - WEEK 2

📄 LECTURE RECORDING: DATA-WAREHOUSE-ARCHITECTURE UP TO AND INCLUDING E-TIVITY 2.1

🎥 VIDEO TUTORIAL ON PIVOT ANALYSIS (E-TIVITY 2.1)
Check out this video before editing Etivity 2.1.

💬 E-TIVITY 2.1: PIVOT TABLES

📊 SOLUTION TO E-TIVITY 2.1: PIVOT TABLES

💬 QUESTIONS ON TOPIC - WEEK 2

💬 REFLECTION - WEEK 2

Screenshot of course 2 based on the LMS Moodle

Feedback of the student	The learners found the new blended learning concept as a new challenge, but they enjoyed being able to work from home and to organize their time more flexibly. They found the learning videos helpful as a preparation for the e-tivities.
Time required for support	On average, 30 min for each feedback on an e-tivity must be scheduled. With 47 learning e-tivities, five of which are optional, there is a total supervision time of 23.5 h, plus 2 h for each online seminar ($2 \times 7 = 14$ h). Thereby, the preparation time is not calculated.
Group size	The maximum number of participants is 35.

Summary

Digitalization changes learning and teaching. The development and use of new information technologies create opportunities and chances to make teaching and learning more attractive, more customizable and more flexible. But the transition from traditional classroom-based structures to online teaching also poses challenges. Suitable digitalization strategies are rare. This chapter dealt with concepts and techniques of digital teaching and learning in academic and continuing education, which should serve as a recommendation for the successful implementation of online courses. It presented a didactical framework consisting of a five-phase model starting from welcoming of the learners and the processing of learning units to the summative assessment and course completion. Furthermore, the chapter linked the didactically motivated framework for designing online teaching with suitable LMS tools to support the teaching and learning activities of the phases. Two real life course examples illustrated how online courses can be set up based on the presented framework using the LMS Moodle and ILIAS. The chapter also addressed necessary skills for educators and learners for successful digital learning and discussed the specifics of digital teaching in continuous education.

Conclusions and Outlook

In addition to the numerous potentials of e-learning, challenges for educators and learners should not be ignored. Digital teaching and learning is not only about the use of technologies but needs the inclusion of suitable didactical concepts to successfully implement online courses. Learning in online courses is particularly effective when it includes successful communication and cooperation between learners and with the educator. Thus, educators have to intensify and adapt their ways of communicating to ensure effective online socialization of the course participants and to keep the motivation for communication and collaboration among learners on a high level [23]. But also the technical aspects of online teaching and learning need to be mastered by both educators and learners. In addition to sending e-mails and exchanging files, todays LMSs such as Moodle or ILIAS offer much more options to support activating teaching methods such as problem-based learning, project learning, research-based learning or group work. For this, both the learners and the educators must have a sufficient degree of digital competence. In addition to mature and ergonomically designed learning technologies, this is a prerequisite for that the used technologies do not hinder the learning processes but support it effectively.

As a result of advancing digitalization, further digital learning and teaching techniques are emerging. A major technological trend is the use of mobile devices like tablets or smartphones and apps for mobile learning [24]. For example, the LMS Moodle is already available as a free app for mobile devices. Other trends of digital teaching and learning focus on concepts like gamification, 3D interfaces and interactive tutorials. Incorporating such trends depends on the interests and abilities of the educators and their available resources, as these approaches are sometimes complex to implement. In addition to these trends, the evolving research field of "learning analytics" also offers valuable methods and tools to improve the quality of digital teaching [12].

All authors are members of the HiGHmed consortium, a program funded by the Federal Ministry of Education and Research (BMBF) as part of the Medical Informatics Initiative (MII).

Useful Resources

1. Self-assessment tool that enables educators to reflect personal attitudes toward digital teaching and individual needs for further training. Link: https://ec.europa.eu/jrc/en/digcompedu/self-assessment
2. References to the open-source learning management systems (LMSs) named in the chapter:
   - https://www.ilias.de/en/
   - https://moodle.org/?lang=en
3. Some open-source web conferencing systems for online learning: BigBlueButton (BBB:

https://bigbluebutton.org/), Apache OpenMeetings (http://openmeetings.apache.org/), jitsy (https://jitsi.org/)

4. Open-source solution for automated video capture, management and distribution: Opencast (https://opencast.org/)

5. Open-source software for video recordings (e.g. lecture recordings) and live streaming: https://obsproject.com/

6. Open educational resources (OER) are free to use learning materials often managed by national and international OER initiatives and platforms (e.g. https://www.oercommons.org/)

7. Introduction to test statistics and item analytics: https://www.washington.edu/assessment/scanning-scoring/scoring/reports/item-analysis/

8. Gilly Salmon is working for more than 30 years on the topic of digital learning in higher education. Her website focuses on different aspects on e-learning.
Link: https://www.gillysalmon.com/

9. Further information concerning the Kirkpatrick model for evaluating the effectiveness of training.
Link: https://www.kirkpatrickpartners.com/Our-Philosophy/The-Kirkpatrick-Model

Review Questions

1. What are the central functions of a learning management system?
   (a) Administration of users
   (b) Supporting organization of learning processes
   (c) Enabling the provision of learning content via Internet
   (d) Supporting communication and interaction between educators and learners
   (e) Provision of authoring tools to create learning materials

2. Which two learning management systems (LMSs) are examined more closely in this chapter?
   (a) Moodle
   (b) Open edX
   (c) ILIAS

(d) Canvas
(e) OpenOLAT

3. Which of the following tools of a learning management system (LMS) does not fit into the subject area collaboration?
   (a) chat
   (b) test
   (c) forum
   (d) wiki
   (e) grouping

4. The beginning of an e-learning course has a decisive influence on its successful implementation. Therefore, in the phase "reception and introduction" the educator should …
   (a) … offer a forum where open questions and problems concerning the use of the LMSs can be raised
   (b) … provide various kinds of instructions for working within the LMSs addressing different types of learners with variable depth of experiences
   (c) …ensure that all learners have easy and unhindered access to the learning objects
   (d) …present learning objective-related working material
   (e) …motivate learners to actively participate in the course

5. Which sub-phases should each learning unit consist of?
   (a) Welcome and introduction
   (b) Formative assessment and feedback
   (c) Farewell and outlook
   (d) Offering input
   (e) Working on one or more tasks

6. Which phase of the five-phase didactical framework is characterized by an intensive use of e-tivities?
   (a) Reception and introduction
   (b) Presentation of learning objectives and course organization
   (c) Processing of learning units
   (d) Summative assessment
   (e) Completion and evaluation

7. Which kind of evaluation of an online course is recommended by the presented five-phase didactical framework to adjust the course concept based on feedback of the learners?
    (a) Evaluation after the first and the second third of the course
    (b) Evaluation in the middle of the course
    (c) Evaluation after the second third of the course
    (d) Evaluation at the end of the course
    (e) Evaluation in the middle and the end of the course

8. Which answer concerning the European Framework for Digital Competence of Educators (DigCompEdu) is correct?
    (a) DigCompEdu is the only reference model for digital competencies.
    (b) DigCompEdu focus on technical skills and data protection.
    (c) DigCompEdu captures educator-specific digital competencies.
    (d) DigCompEdu is a competence framework for all citizens in Europe.

9. Which of the following is no phase of the Kirkpatrick model of training evaluation?
    (a) reaction
    (b) learning
    (c) behavior
    (d) experiences
    (e) results

10. Which dimensions of presence can be examined while evaluating online courses and what are they about?

Appendix: Answers to Review Questions

1. What are the central functions of a learning management system?
    (a) Administration of users
    (b) Supporting organization of learning processes
    (c) Enabling the provision of learning content via Internet

    (d) Supporting communication and interaction between educators and learners
    (e) Provision of authoring tools to create learning materials
    Correct answer: The five functions described are all central to a learning management system. Learning management systems should support the learning process on an organizational, communicative and social level and enable the provision of learning materials in an easy way.

2. Which two learning management systems (LMSs) are examined more closely in this chapter?
    (a) Moodle
    (b) Open edX
    (c) ILIAS
    (d) Canvas
    (e) OpenOLAT
    Correct answer: The open-source LMSs Moodle and ILIAS have been presented.

3. Which of the following tools of a learning management system (LMS) does not fit into the subject area collaboration?
    (a) chat
    (b) test
    (c) forum
    (d) wiki
    (e) grouping
    Correct answer: Tests are one mean to implement formative or summative assessments. The other tools are used to support collaboration especially in groups.

4. The beginning of an e-learning course has a decisive influence on its successful implementation. Therefore, in the phase "reception and introduction" the educator should …
    (a) …offer a forum where open questions and problems concerning the use of the LMSs can be raised
    (b) …provide various kinds of instructions for working within the LMSs addressing different types of learners with variable depth of experiences

(c) …ensure that all learners have easy and unhindered access to the learning objects

(d) …present learning objective-related working material

(e) …motivate learners to actively participate in the course

Correct answer: Learning objective-related working material should be offered in phase 3 "Processing of learning units". The other four answers are correct and are supplemented by a collection of FAQs, the educator's self-presentation and initial working tasks.

5. Which sub-phases should each learning unit consist of?
   (a) Welcome and introduction
   (b) Formative assessment and feedback
   (c) Farewell and outlook
   (d) Offering input
   (e) Working on one or more tasks

   Correct answer: Every learning unit should consist of the following three sub-phases:

   • Offering input
   • Working on one or more tasks
   • Formative assessment and feedback

6. Which phase of the five-phase didactical framework is characterized by an intensive use of e-tivities?
   (a) Reception and introduction
   (b) Presentation of learning objectives and course organization
   (c) Processing of learning units
   (d) Summative assessment
   (e) Completion and evaluation

   Correct answer: Processing of learning units

7. Which kind of evaluation of an online course is recommended by the presented five-phase didactical framework to adjust the course concept based on feedback of the learners?
   (a) Evaluation after the first and the second third of the course
   (b) Evaluation in the middle of the course

(c) Evaluation after the second third of the course

(d) Evaluation at the end of the course

(e) Evaluation in the middle and the end of the course

Correct answer: Evaluation in the middle and the end of the course

8. Which answer concerning the European Framework for Digital Competence of Educators (DigCompEdu) is correct?
   (a) DigCompEdu is the only reference model for digital competencies.
   (b) DigCompEdu focus on technical skills and data protection.
   (c) DigCompEdu captures educator-specific digital competencies.
   (d) DigCompEdu is a competence framework for all citizens in Europe.

   Correct answer: DigCompEdu captures educator-specific digital competences.

   The European Framework for Digital Competence of Educators (DigCompEdu) describes educator-specific digital competences. Starting with competencies to engage the own professional development regarding digital technologies three competence areas focus on using these technologies in learning processes. These are providing digital learning resources, integration of digital technologies to enhance interaction and collaboration as well as realizing formative and summative assessments. Based on this, competencies to empower learners and to facility learners own digital competence are addressed in the framework.

9. Which of the following is no phase of the Kirkpatrick model of training evaluation?
   (a) reaction
   (b) learning
   (c) behavior
   (d) experiences
   (e) results

   Correct answer: Experiences are no phase of the Kirkpatrick model.

10. Which dimensions of presence can be examined while evaluating online courses and what are they about?

Social presence (ability of participants to identify with other participants), cognitive presence (participants' ability to construct knowledge through reflection/discourse), teaching presence (ability to facilitate social and cognitive process to realize learning outcomes)

References

1. Arbaugh JB, Cleveland-Innes M, Diaz SR, Garrison DR, Ice P, Richardson C, et al. Developing a community of inquiry instrument: testing a measure of the Community of Inquiry framework using a multi-institutional sample. Internet High Educ. 2008;11(3–4):133–6. https://doi.org/10.1016/j.iheduc.2008.06.003.

2. Klieme E, Hartig J, Rauch D. The concept of competence in educational contexts. In: Hartig J, Klieme E, Leutner D, editors. Assessment of competencies in educational contexts. Ashland, OH: Hogrefe & Huber Publishers; 2008. p. 3–22.

3. Hübner U, Egbert N, Hackl W, Lysser M, Schulte G, Thye J, et al. What nursing informatics core competencies are needed by nursing professionals in Austria, Germany and Switzerland? Recommendations by GMDS, ÖGPI and IGPI. GMS Med Inf Biom Epidemiol. 2017;13(1):Doc02. https://doi.org/10.3205/mibe000169.

4. Knaup P, Deserno TM, Prokosch HU, Sax U. Implementation of a National Framework to promote health data sharing. Yearb Med Inform. 2018;27(01):302–4. https://doi.org/10.1055/s-0038-1641210.

5. Haarbrandt B, Schreiweis B, Rey S, Sax U, Scheithauer S, Rienhoff O, et al. HiGHmed – an open platform approach to enhance care and research across institutional boundaries. Methods Inf Med. 2018 Jul 17;57:e66–81. https://doi.org/10.3414/ME18-02-0002.

6. Witte ML, Behrends M, Benning NH, Hoffmann I, HiGHmeducation Consortium, Bott OJ. The HiGHmed didactical framework for online learning modules on medical informatics: first experiences. Stud Health Technol Inform. 2020 Jun;26(272):163–6. https://doi.org/10.3233/SHTI200519.

7. Salmon G. E-moderating: the key to teaching and learning online. 3rd ed. New York: Routledge; 2011.

8. Salmon G. E-tivities: a key to active online learning. 2nd ed. New York: Routledge; 2013.

9. Garrison DR. E-learning in the 21st century: a community of inquiry framework for research and practice. 3rd ed. New York: Routledge; 2016.

10. Anderson LW, Arasian PW, Cruikshank K, et al. A taxonomy for learning, teaching, and assessing: a revision of Bloom's taxonomy of educational objectives. New York: Longman; 2001.

11. Tolks D, Schäfer C, Raupach T, Kruse L, Sarikas A, Gerhardt-Szép S, et al. An introduction to the inverted/flipped classroom model in education and advanced training in medicine and in the healthcare professions. GMS J Med Educ. 2016;33(3):Doc46. https://doi.org/10.3205/zma001045.

12. Ammenwerth E, Hackl WO. Monitoring of students' interaction in online learning settings by structural network analysis and indicators. Stud Health Technol Inform. 2017;235:293–7. https://doi.org/10.3233/978-1-61499-753-5-293.

13. Kluzer S, Pujol PL. DigComp into action - get inspired, make it happen. A user guide to the European digital competence framework. In: Carretero S, Punie Y, Vuorikari R, Cabrera M, O'Keefe W, editors. JRC Science for Policy Report, EUR 29115 EN. Luxembourg: Publications Office of the European Union; 2018.

14. Mantas J, Ammenwerth E, Demiris G, Hasman A, Haux R, Hersh W, et al. Recommendations of the international medical informatics association (IMIA) on education in biomedical and health informatics. First revision. Methods Inf Med. 2010;49(2):105–20. https://doi.org/10.3414/ME5119.

15. Egbert N, Thye J, Hackl WO, Müller-Staub M, Ammenwerth E, Hübner U. Competencies for nursing in a digital world. Methodology, results, and use of the DACH-recommendations for nursing informatics core competency areas in Austria, Germany, and Switzerland. Inform Health Soc Care. 2019;44(4):351–75. https://doi.org/10.1080/17538157.2018.1497635.

16. The TIGER Initiative. Informatics Competencies for Every Practicing Nurse: Recommendations from the TIGER Collaborative. [cited 2020 September 29]. Available from: http://s3.amazonaws.com/rdcms-himss/files/production/public/FileDownloads/tiger-report-informatics-competencies.pdf

17. Redecker C. European framework for the digital competence of educators: DigCompEdu. In: Punie Y, editor. JRC science for policy report, EUR 28775 EN. Luxembourg: Publications Office of the European Union; 2017.

18. Rouleau G, Gagnon MP, Côté J, Payne-Gangnon J, Hudson E, Dubois CA, et al. Effects of E-learning in a continuing education context on nursing care: systematic review of systematic qualitative, quantitative, and mixed-studies reviews. J Med

Internet Res. 2019;21(10):e15118. https://doi.org/10.2196/15118.

19. Sinclair PM, Kable A, Levett-Jones T, Booth D. The effectiveness of internet-based E-learning on clinician behaviour and patient outcomes: a systematic review. Int J Nurs Stud. 2016;57:70–81. https://doi.org/10.1016/j.ijnurstu.2016.01.011.

20. Vaona A, Banzi R, Kwag KH, Rigon G, Cereda D, Pevoraro V, et al. E-learning for health professionals. Cochrane Database Syst Rev. 2018 Jan 21;1(1):CD011736. https://doi.org/10.1002/14651858.CD011736.pub2.

21. Kirkpatrick DL, Kirkpatrick JD. Evaluating training programs: the four levels. 3rd ed. San Francisco, CA: Berrett-Koehler Publishers; 2006.

22. Ridsdale C, Rothwell J, Smit M, Ali-Hassan H, Bliemel M, Irvine D et al Strategies and best practices for data literacy education: knowledge synthesis report; 2015. https://doi.org/10.13140/RG.2.1.1922.5044

23. Serdyukov P, Serdyukova N. Effects of communication, socialization and collaboration on online learning. ESJ [Internet]. 2015 Jun 23 [cited 2020 Sep 29]; 11(10). Available from: http://eujournal.org/index.php/esj/article/view/5756

24. Uther M. Mobile learning—trends and practices. Educ Sci. 2019;9(1):33. https://doi.org/10.3390/educsci9010033.

Part IX

Global Perspectives in Health Informatics

Bangladesh: eHealth and Telemedicine

43

Rafiqul Islam Maruf, Ashir Ahmed, Fumihiko Yokota, Kimiyo Kikuchi, Rieko Izukura, Yoko Sato, Mariko Nishikitani, Yasunobu Nohara, and Naoki Nakashima

Learning Objectives
- To understand primary healthcare services as a form of population health management to the unreached rural communities of Bangladesh
- To obtain an understanding what a Portable Health Clinic (PHC) based on a telemedicine system means

- To be able to appraise the PHC for supporting aging communities in urban areas

Key Terms
- Telemedicine
- Mobile healthcare
- Population health management
- Triage system
- Preventive healthcare
- Unreached communities

R. I. Maruf · R. Izukura · M. Nishikitani
N. Nakashima (✉)
Medical Information Center, Kyushu University Hospital, Kyushu University, Fukuoka, Japan
e-mail: islam.rafiqul.072@m.kyushu-u.ac.jp;
ochamame@info.med.kyushu-u.ac.jp;
makorin@info.med.kyushu-u.ac.jp;
nnaoki@info.med.kyushu-u.ac.jp

A. Ahmed
Graduate School of Information Science and Electrical Engineering, Kyushu University, Fukuoka, Japan,
e-mail: ashir@ait.kyushu-u.ac.jp

F. Yokota
Institute of Decision Science for Sustainable Society, Kyushu University, Fukuoka, Japan

K. Kikuchi · Y. Sato
Department of Health Sciences, Faculty of Medical Sciences, Kyushu University, Fukuoka, Japan
e-mail: kikuchia@hs.med.kyushu-u.ac.jp;
satyoko@hs.med.kyushu-u.ac.jp

Y. Nohara
Faculty of Advanced Science and Technology, Kumamoto University, Kumamoto, Japan
e-mail: nohara@cs.kumamoto-u.ac.jp

Introduction

Portable Health Clinic: A Tool for the SDGs in Bangladesh

Background

A PHC is a *remote healthcare service delivery platform*. It was jointly developed by Kyushu University in Japan and Grameen Communications in Bangladesh for primary healthcare of the *unreached communities* with a special focus on non-communicable diseases (NCDs) and so far served 43,000 people since 2010. Through this platform, we can achieve multiple goals listed in the SDGs.

This chapter focuses on Goal #3 of the SDGs, which is to *"Ensure healthy lives and promote well-being for all at all ages."* It also describes the current status of Bangladesh and how PHCs can contribute to achieving these goals in a cost-

© Springer Nature Switzerland AG 2022
U. H. Hübner et al. (eds.), *Nursing Informatics*, Health Informatics,
https://doi.org/10.1007/978-3-030-91237-6_43

Table 43.1 Major SDG 3 indicators and status in Bangladesh [1]

No.	SDG indicators	2015	2016	2017	2018	2030
SDG 3.1.1	3.1.1 Reduce the maternal mortality ratio to 70 per 100,000 live births	181	178	172	169	70
SDG 3.2.1	3.2.1 Reduce the under-5 mortality rate to 25 per 1000 live births	36	35	31	29	25
SDG 3.2.2	3.2.2 Reduce the neonatal mortality rate to 12 per 1000 live births	20	19	17	16	12
SDG 3.4.1	3.4.1 Mortality between 30 and 70 years of age from cardiovascular diseases, cancer, diabetes, or chronic respiratory diseases (%)		21.6			
SDG 3.4.2	3.4.2 Suicide mortality rate (per 100,000 population)		5.9			
SDG 3.5.2	3.5.2 Total alcohol per capita (age 15+ years) consumption		<0.05			
SDG 3.6.1	3.6.1 Mortality rate from road traffic injuries (per 100,000 population)	13.6		15.56		

effective manner without compromising the quality of healthcare delivery. The UN has defined 13 targets and 28 indicators for SDG 3. The targets specify the goals and the indicators represent the metrics by which the world aims to track whether these targets are achieved (Table 43.1).

The indicators have been developed, but not all the data are ready for monitoring the status of SDG 3 in Bangladesh. Of the 28 indicators of SDG 3, data for 12 indicators are readily available, data for 10 are partially available, and data for 4 are unavailable. Bangladesh continues to grapple with the existing issues of increasing access to, improving the quality of, and achieving equity in healthcare services for all. The increasing burden of NCDs, such as diabetes, cardiovascular diseases, and cancer, has contributed to increased morbidity and mortality. Table 43.2 identifies the major indicators and status.

The project seeks collaboration and funding to effectively implement and achieve SDG 3.

Basic Structure of the Portable Health Clinic System

The PHC system (Fig. 43.1) has been developed as a *Remote Healthcare System* (RHS) for unreached communities with a special focus on NCDs [2–5]. A health worker visits a patient with the PHC box to measure their vital information and uploads the data with the patient's medical history to an online server using the *GramHealth Client Application* installed in a smartphone or tablet PC inside the PHC box. The remote doctor accesses this data and makes a video call to the patient for further verification. Finally, the doctor creates an online prescription and enters it into the online server under each patient's profile. The health worker accesses the system to print the prescription and instantly passes it to the patient with a detailed explanation. The entire process takes approximately 15 to 30 min per patient. The PHC system introduces a *triage protocol* to classify the subjects into four categories: (i) green (healthy), (ii) yellow (suspicious), (iii) orange (affected), and (iv) red (emergent), based on a gradually increasing risk of health status. The subjects classified as orange and red are those primarily diagnosed as high risk and require a doctor's consultation.

The PHC service is delivered by a trained healthcare worker and a remote doctor connected by a video conferencing system. Services include basic health checkups and regular monitoring. Basic health checkups include (a) a set of demographic questions, (b) 14 clinical measurements, and (c) consultation with a doctor for prescriptions. The 14 clinical measurements include (1) blood pressure, (2) pulse rate, (3) body temperature, (4) blood oxygenation (SpO$_2$), (5) arrhythmia, (6) BMI, (7) waist, hip, and waist-to-hip ratio, (8) blood glucose, (9) blood cholesterol, (10) blood hemoglobin, (11) blood uric acid, (12) blood grouping, (13) urinary sugar, and (14) urinary protein.

Table 43.2 Major areas of SDG 3 in which the PHC system can contribute

No.	Objective	How PHCs can contribute
SDG 3.4	By 2030, reduce premature mortality from non-communicable diseases by one-third through prevention and treatment and by promoting mental health and well-being.	PHCs have a set of sensors to diagnose non-communicable diseases. The software tool can triage populations in four colors ranging from green to red to demonstrate their status of illness and the remote doctor provides necessary consultancy accordingly.
SDG 3.8	Achieve universal health coverage, including financial risk protection, access to quality essential healthcare services, and access to safe, effective, quality, and affordable essential medicines and vaccines for all.	PHCs are designed to serve unreached populations where usual healthcare facilities (doctors, health workers, clinics, primary screening tools) are not available. PHCs include additional features to work where electricity and Internet connectivity are not stable.
SDG 3.c	Substantially increase health financing and the recruitment, development, training, and retention of the health workforce in developing countries, particularly in the least developed countries and small island developing states.	One of the important features of PHCs is that every PHC box is owned and operated by one trained healthcare worker. We developed schemes to train both the healthcare workers and the trainers.
SDG 3.d	Strengthen the capacity of all countries, particularly developing countries, for early warning, risk reduction, and management of national and global health risks.	We recently developed a C-logic (corona logic) that can ultimately reduce the transmission risk from patients to medical staffs.

Every patient has a health account to access their past health history and health trends. The patients and their authorized family members or doctors can access the health account.

Expansion of Portable Health Clinics Services

PHCs have been used in Bangladesh for purposes other than NCDs, for example, to produce pathological reports (Tele-Pathology), provide eye-care services (Tele-Eye), and provide maternal and child health (MCH) care [4, 6, 7]. The following types of communities have been served thus far: (a) rural unreached communities, (b) urban aging communities, (c) urban small- and medium-sized corporate communities, and (d) urban morning walker communities.

Geographical Expansion of Portable Health Clinics

We have developed and added features to the PHCs to adapt to community needs. The system can be easily installed and deployed in low-resource settings where medical facilities (doctors, healthcare workers, clinics, primary screening tools) are not adequate. However, RHSs are not free from *medical errors*. We identified the sources of errors and introduced tools to detect and remove anomalies to improve system efficiency. We also developed an extended *Technology Acceptance Model* to measure and increase its use and the consumers' trust.

The PHC concept has been introduced in several other countries including Cambodia, China, India, Indonesia, Liberia, Malaysia, Pakistan, and Thailand. The PHC operation team has trained staffs in India, Liberia, Malaysia, Pakistan, and Thailand. Besides, PHCs have been piloted in Cambodia, India, Malaysia, and Pakistan, and the results among these countries should be compared.

Personal Health Record Service in Portable Health Clinics

Why Personal Health Records?
Currently, PHCs are conducted by a local health worker and serve as a tool for population/individual health management, provide a database of time series health/medical data, and coordinate telemedicine between patients and doctors in call centers. However, daily self-management is one of the most important factors for preventing and/or improving NCDs. If we can involve patients/

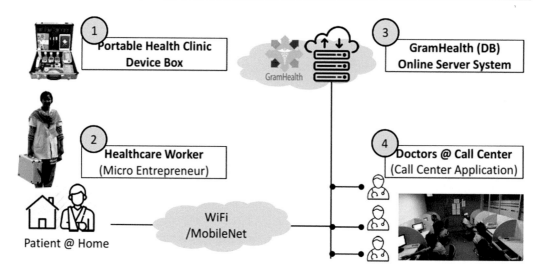

Fig. 43.1 System diagram of a portable health clinics

citizens as users of PHCs, and they use it for their daily self-management, the role of PHCs can be expanded tremendously.

Currently, there are smartphone applications that help patients manage their personal daily health data or clinical data on NCDs. We generally call these applications "*Personal Health Records* (PHRs)." PHRs data are generated from health checkup sites, clinics, and drug-dispensing pharmacies. We also expect that a PHR can manage information regarding an individual's location, vital signs, exercise patterns, and behaviors at home or at the office using built-in sensors in the smartphone or using sensor networks based on Internet of things technology.

Therefore, PHCs are a suitable data source for PHRs because PHCs contain data from health checkup sites and clinics and connect many vital sensors with mobile networks.

The benefits of patient engagement enabled by the technology include enhanced communication, better care and improved outcomes, increased satisfaction, and lower costs [8].

The World Health Organization (WHO) has promoted the installation of patient engagement, particularly for developing countries, because it is a cost-effective way to make people healthier. PHRs are considered an indispensable tool for patient engagement [9].

Patient engagement enables NCD patients to access their personal health/medical data using the PHR, monitor the disease, and determine the treatment policy. This not only increases the rate of concordance regarding the treatment policy between the physician and patient but also provides the physician a trigger to change the policy and intervene [10].

Patient-reported outcome (PRO) is another area for which there are smartphone applications. PHRs function in coordination with PROs for a greater generation of data and accuracy [11]. Because of the rapid increase in communication with patients and families, the application and service system should be considered before they are developed and implemented to ensure that they do not place too much of a burden on the healthcare/medical staff.

Data items in PHRs for specified diseases such as NCDs should be standardized before use of the smartphone application for maintaining data sustainability. For example, six *Japanese academic clinical societies* determined the "recommended configuration for PHR" by creating minimum data item sets for diabetes mellitus, hypertension, dyslipidemia, and chronic kidney diseases [12]. PHC items should also be considered from the perspective of creating standardized items to link to PHRs.

Personal Health Record System in Portable Health Clinics

Like many other developing countries, public healthcare facilities in Bangladesh do not currently maintain any *Electronic Health Records* (EHRs). Some private hospitals that are only accessible to high-income individuals have their own EHR system. However, PHRs are not yet widely utilized in Bangladesh. In this context, when the PHC system was designed in 2010, EHRs were present from the onset; patients' vital information was preserved in electronic format to the online server, and the patient's feedback was obtained via survey format [2–4]. Later, the PHR service was added as a personal service for the patients. The patients can access their own data on a smartphone and monitor and share their feedback with physicians [4]. The concerning physician can access the patients' data to provide consultations with better assessment. The patients can also access their password-protected PHRs at anytime and anywhere using an online application and share this information with doctors when necessary.

The PHR configuration recommended by the Japanese academic clinical societies can be considered a pioneer work in this research area [12]. Because no global standard currently exists, this should be considered a reference for the standardization of PHR. They proposed a total of 41 general items for the PHRs with specified units and expressions. However, the *Self-Management Item Sets* (SMIS) for different diseases including diabetes mellitus, hypertension, dyslipidemia,

and chronic kidney disease are different and specified. The item set of the PHR system of PHCs covers almost all mandatory items of the Japanese proposal, and it includes some additional items based on local disease patterns (body temperature, blood oxygenation, arrhythmia, pulse rate, and uric acid). After introducing the Eye-Care and MCH modules in the PHC system, additional new clinical data have been added. This combined clinical data set will enable the PHC system to maintain new SMIS for additional diseases.

The data units used in this PHR system are those commonly used in Bangladesh. For example, (1) body temperature is reported in degree Fahrenheit, (2) blood glucose is reported in mmol/dl, and (3) hemoglobin is reported in g/dl. These units vary in other countries, and there is a need to standardize these items and units to ensure interoperability with other systems.

The graphical analysis of the PHR data in the PHC system is very easy for patients and doctors to understand, and the patients become anxious if there is any irregularity in the data (Fig. 43.2). This is very helpful as the patients become more conscious of their data and communicate with the health workers. Thus, patient engagement contributes to ensuring better and timelier service.

Variation of Portable Health Clinics Service Modules and ICT System

Requirement of Modular Expansion of Portable Health Clinics

The PHC services were initially designed to provide primary healthcare to rural communities that are suffering from a shortage of healthcare facilities. However, when the primary service was initiated by the PHC system, it became evident that these communities were not happy with only receiving primary healthcare. The prevalence of NCDs such as diabetes mellitus and hypertension has increased to a concerning level in Bangladesh. *Approximately 70% of all deaths are caused by*

Patient Profile

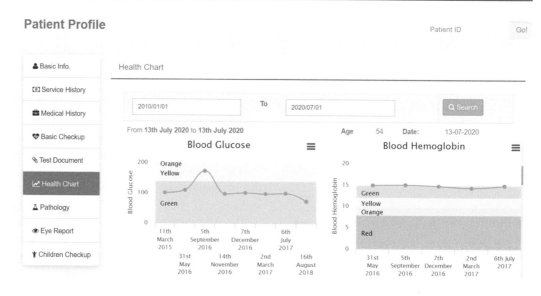

Fig. 43.2 Graphical interface of PHRs in PHCs

NCDs. Therefore, many NCD patients require expert consultancy with further investigation. Given the need to provide further investigation and better assessment by remote doctors through telemedicine, the demand of pathological support has been noted by both patients and doctors. Consequently, the PHC system added a new module called *"Tele-Pathology"* [4, 6].

Additionally, village women have fewer opportunities to see doctors in the city when necessary because they mostly stay at home and manage the household. Sometimes local culture and religious faith act as barriers for women to see a doctor in clinics or hospitals located in distance. Therefore, most village women depend on unskilled traditional quacks or rural midwifes for any issues and particularly for Ob-Gyn care. This results in many unwanted health issues and death. Therefore, PHC services found a huge need for MCH care support in the village and subsequently added another new module for MCH care. Similarly, the "Tele-Eye" care module was added in response to the need for ophthalmic care. Thus, the PHC system must gradually expand and create new modules based on the community requirements. One such development work is now underway called "Tele-Dental" care module to respond the needs of dental problem.

Tele-Pathology System in Portable Health Clinics

Introduction

The PHC system with telemedicine services is very much suitable for providing primary health care in remote communities. However, this service cannot be limited to primary health care because rural people do not have alternative options for secondary or tertiary levels of treatment. Therefore, the PHC system must be expanded to provide some sort of secondary level of treatment. Because doctors must provide teleconsultancy on critical cases in this secondary treatment level, the doctors require further details on the patients' health information, that is, pathological reports, to reduce the risk of diagnosis without physical investigation. A Tele-Pathology module has been added to the PHC system in response to this issue [6].

To respond to the growing needs of medical diagnosis, many small pathological laboratories called diagnosis centers have been developed in rural Bangladesh. In most cases, they are run by young *laboratory technologists* with 2–3 years of diploma certification in pathology. Officially, they are permitted to perform sample collections and conduct some specific primary tests. They require support from a pathologist to prepare advanced pathological reports. However, because there is a huge shortage of pathologists in Bangladesh (0.26 pathologists for every 10,000 individuals, while the USA, Canada, and Japan have rates of 3.94, 4.81, and 1.89, respectively) and they mostly remain in the cities, the rural laboratory technologists need to prepare the final reports by themselves. This causes many problems. The PHC system established the idea of Tele-Pathology to support these laboratory technologists and empower them by virtually connecting with remote pathologists. Thus, they can jointly produce authentic reports for rural patients (Fig. 43.3).

Tele-Pathology System and Service Delivery Process

When a rural patient receives PHC services, if the remote doctor feels that a pathological report is necessary for better diagnosis, the patient is referred to the nearest Tele-Pathology-supported diagnosis center. Then, the laboratory technologist (1) collects the sample, prepares the physi-

cal report, produces the test slides, takes several microscopic images of the slides in various positions, and then uploads the images together with the physical report to the online server (Fig. 43.3). The remote pathologist then (2) diagnoses the sample based on the cell counts of the microscopic slide images with the physical report for reference, finalizes the pathology report, and uploads the data to the online server. Finally, the remote doctor can access the pathological report of the patient from the online server and use it as a reference for a better diagnosis.

This system uses the Optima G-302 microscope (Eyepiece: WF10x; Objective: 4x, 10x, 100x; Light source: 6v20w halogen; Power Supply: 220v), which is commonly used in local pathology laboratories. Microscopic images are taken with a SONY Cyber-shot DSC-W320 camera (14.1 mega-pixel camera with 4x optical zoom lens; starting at a wide 26 mm equiv. and a 2.7-inch screen). However, other commonly available devices were also tried and were found to be significantly workable.

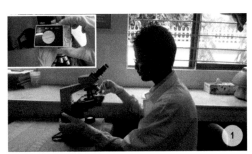

Laboratory Technologist ↑

Remote Pathologist ↓

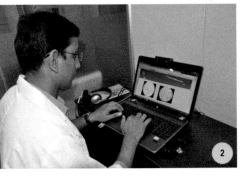

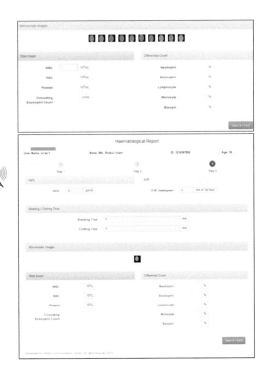

Fig. 43.3 Tele-Pathology system in PHC

Service Statistic

This Tele-Pathology system has been used in four pilot sites in Bangladesh in 2016. During this time, among others, hematological reports, routine urine examination reports, and routine stool examination reports were primarily produced by this system with the support of the remote pathologist. The hematological reports included 1012 complete blood counts (CBCs) performed by the remote pathologist using the Tele-Pathology system (29% of patients were male and 71% were female). In this study, the overall prevalence of anemia was 77%. Of these patients, 83%, 17%, and 0% had mild, moderate, and severe anemia, respectively. The *highest prevalence of anemia was found in female patients (78%)*, and the prevalence was 66% among reproductive-aged (15–49 years) patients. The following characteristics were reported among the anemic patients: high white blood cell count (16%), low red blood cell count (86%), high platelet count (12%), high erythrocyte sedimentation rate (ESR, 48%), high total eosinophil count (27%), low neutrophil level (2%), and high neutrophil level (22%).

Maternal and Child Health System in Portable Health Clinics

Introduction

Low levels of access to MCH services have been reported in medical resource-limited settings such as low- and middle-income countries. However, health checkups of mothers and children are important to detect health problems in the early stages. To improve access to care, in such areas, remote health checkups are required so that the patients can receive care at their homes. Therefore, we launched a trial to apply PHCs to MCH care.

To implement this trial, we selected a rural area in the district of Shariatpur in Bangladesh. According to our baseline analysis, only *9.5% of women had received continuous antenatal care four times or more, facility delivery, and postnatal care*. Consequently, this area has room to

improve health checkup rate and mortality rate of mothers and children.

In the following sections, we introduce the PHC system for providing MCH care in Bangladesh and show the findings observed during the follow-up of health checkups. This section is written based on the previously presented conference proceedings [7].

MCH Care System Structure in Portable Health Clinics

The target population for remote health checkups using PHCs to provide MCH care was pregnant/parturient women and their newborns. A local pharmacy operator and a traditional birth attendant collect health data of the women and newborns using the PHC's medical devices. If the health data indicate a triage color of orange or red, the women are connected to a doctor at a call center in Dhaka using an Internet video communication system. The doctor remotely diagnoses the health problems of the women and newborns based on the collected data and consultation. Then, the doctor issues prescriptions to the women via the Internet. *Health checkups are conducted at 4, 6, 8, and 9 months of pregnancy and at 2–3 days, 6 days, and 6 weeks after delivery/birth.*

Expected Outcome of the MCH Care System

These remote health checkups are expected to improve the uptake rate of antenatal and postnatal care. This may also allow the early detection and treatment of *pregnancy-induced hypertension and diabetes* and contribute to the reduction of maternal and newborn mortality/morbidity.

Findings from MCH and Child Health Follow-Up Services

We started using the PHC for MCH care in June 2019, and the follow-up is currently underway. The findings presented in this article represent the cross-sectional aggregation based on the 94 women who had been regularly monitored by March 2020. The frequency of maternal checkups of each woman varies because their week of pregnancy varied at the entry point of this survey. Of the 94 subjects, 32 (34%) had a postnatal checkup (from after delivery until 21 days or more after delivery).

The mean age of the monitored women was 24 years old (range, 15–45 years) at the time of receiving the maternal health checkup. The mean number of maternal checkups was 2.2 (range, 1–4). Two miscarriages and one neonatal death were observed. Although most of the women did not display any symptoms, we found some abnormal values, as described below.

Anemia in Pregnancy

The WHO defines blood hemoglobin (Hb) levels <11 g/dL as anemic during pregnancy. The prevalence of anemia during pregnancy is reported to be high worldwide, particularly in South Asia (52%) and Central and West Africa (56%) [12]. In Bangladesh, 42% of women of childbearing age are anemic, and anemia during pregnancy is also predicted to occur with a high prevalence [13]. In this study, the percentage of subjects with anemia during pregnancy ranged from 45% to 54% (varied depending on the gestational weeks). Sixty-three pregnant subjects (67%) experienced Hb levels <11 g/dl more than once during pregnancy. Among 32 postnatal subjects who received health checkups more than 21 days after delivery, 9 subjects (28%) who had experienced pregnancy anemia at least once during pregnancy could not recover to normal levels of Hb (≥12 g/dL) at this point.

Above results could not be grasped unless PHC is introduced in this area, and PHC is considered to be an important intervention especially in Bangladesh where the prevalence of anemia is high. Anemia during pregnancy is known to be associated with a low birth weight and preterm birth. Furthermore, the *perinatal mortality rate* and *neonatal mortality rate* have been reported to significantly increase in anemic pregnant women [14]. In the future, we will analyze anemia in pregnancy and perinatal prognosis in these subjects.

Pulse Rate (Heart Rate)

In general, the pulse rate (heart rate) (normal range: 60–80 bpm) begins to increase around the eighth week of pregnancy and reaches its maximum around 28–32 weeks of pregnancy. The maximum is about 15% (about 10 bpm) increase of normal level. However, approximately 20%–40% of subjects had abnormal pulse rate (tachycardia, heart rate ≥ 100 bpm). The tachycardia rate was relatively high in our study. However, among those who had tachycardia, only two had a body temperature of ≥99.5 °F, and no one experienced rupture. The higher *prevalence of tachycardia* in the subjects may have been associated with physical activity or mental tension before the measurement or at the measurement. And, we also need to consider the effect of the race and the climate.

Blood Pressure

In our study, two (2.1%) women had systolic blood pressure ≥ 130 mmHg and diastolic blood pressure ≥ 80 mmHg, but both had negative urinary protein results. No women were suspected to have severe hypertensive disorders of pregnancy. During pregnancy and postpartum, no subjects had abnormal systolic hypertension (≥140 mmHg) or mean blood pressure values. During pregnancy, 4% of women had diastolic hypertension (≥90 mmHg), whereas 12% displayed this condition after delivery, and the percentage tended to increase. This may be due to the amount of blood loss during delivery and physical fatigue from delivery and childrearing. Since the women had a mean age of 24 years old and only seven (7%) were over 35 years old, the incidence of hypertension during pregnancy and postpartum was not high.

Blood Glucose

Blood glucose levels were measured as random plasma glucose levels, and values ≥100 mg/dL were judged to be concerning. Every gestational period, 50% of the subjects had a random plasma glucose level ≥ 100 mg/dL, and 11 subjects (12%) reported at least one measurement of 126 mg/dL or more. No subjects had random plasma glucose levels ≥200 mg/dL during pregnancy, and no subjects were suspected of having overt diabetes during pregnancy. However, some subjects who had random plasma glucose levels ≥100 mg/dL during pregnancy experienced postnatal levels of ≥200 mg/dL.

In 2019, the prevalence of gestational diabetes in Bangladesh was 18.1%, which was higher than that reported in Japan (4.2%) and China (8.3%). Thus, managing gestational diabetes during pregnancy is as important as managing anemia [15]. Since definitive diagnoses of gestational diabetes mellitus (75 g OGTT) were not performed, it is not possible to ascertain the exact prevalence of gestational diabetes mellitus. Further research should be performed to predict the prevalence of gestational diabetes based on blood glucose level and on risk factors such as age, BMI, and family history of diabetes.

Perspective and Future Considerations for Applying the Maternal and Child Health System of Portable Health Clinics to Nursing Informatics

PHCs for providing MCH care with data collection using ICT and teleconsultation with doctors are useful tools for nursing personnel who engage in maternity health services in developing countries. However, a variety of challenges, as described below, are unavoidable to effectively apply the MCH system. As those factors are intricately involved, MCH should involve multidisciplinary approaches across various fields and perspectives. We examine the nursing efforts necessary to promote the MCH system through MCH experiences in rural Bangladesh.

1. Financial issues

   • Although some pregnant women were triaged as an abnormal, they did not buy the medications prescribed by the doctor via teleconsultation.

2. Educational/sociocultural issues

   • The elderly are the decision-makers regarding childbirth in the family, not the mother of the child.
   • Pregnant women are prone to believe community-based superstitions and experience-based advice via community members including *traditional birth attendances* (TBAs) rather than evidence-based advice.

3. Infrastructural issues/sociocultural issues

   • Some pregnant women did not answer the phone at the appointment time because they did not have their own mobile phone and shared one within the family.

In this context, two types of nursing efforts will be required. First, educational programs should be redesigned to involve family members to recognize the importance of MCH activities and the risks of pregnancy-induced complications. Second, childbirth-related advice in MCH care should be collaborative with TBAs. Over 50% of deliveries are still assisted by TBAs who engage strongly in the rural community [16]. Rural residents with a strong sociocultural relationship may consider TBAs' advice as more reliable information than that of outsiders. Although the effectiveness of government-led-training programs for TBAs that ended in 1997 remains controversial, TBA training programs that focus on maternal health education must be designed for rural residents [16].

In the future, PHCs for MCH care are expected to be utilized as a primary resource for providing maternal health care not only in rural areas but also in various environmental settings such as disasters and accidents.

Portable Health Clinic: COVID-19 System

Introduction

PHCs, even in their present form, can be effectively deployed to eliminate the risk of transmission among frontline healthcare staffs and contribute significantly toward reducing pressure on healthcare services and resources. With considered re-alignment of its technical configuration, PHCs can be deployed as ancillary resources supporting large-scale public health emergencies, exemplified by the COVID-19 pandemic. NCDs are positively correlated with the severity of symptoms and fatality from COVID-19. In both cases, RHS may help minimize the risk of transmission.

We have already established an algorithm describing the *post-disaster operation* of PHCs [17]. Based on this algorithm, we have added an emergency mode in our PHC system for addressing communicable diseases such as COVID-19 (Table 43.3).

Portable Health Clinic: COVID-19 System Structure

Figure 43.4 explains how PHCs will operate during COVID-19-like contexts. Unlike the conventional PHCs for NCDs, the local health worker collects the primary symptoms of a patient through a standard questionnaire. If the patient is identified as a potential patient, the PHC COVID-19 box will be sent to the patient's home temporarily together with an operation manual so that they can check themselves under the guidance of the health worker.

If a patient is identified as a potential COVID-19 carrier (red category) through this primary screening using the triage system, the patient will be immediately advised to see a nearby hospital for further investigation and follow-up as needed. Otherwise, the health worker will provide guidelines for remaining at home

under quarantine. Since the patients already know the community health workers, the patients feel more comfortable and safer under their guidance. The privacy of sensitive information of patients will be protected and secured because it is required by an increasing body of legislative provisions and standards.

Although the original PHC box contains various medical sensors, only COVID-19-related sensors will be used in this box, which include the following: (i) thermometer (OMRON) for measuring body temperature; (ii) pulse oximeter (OXI METER) for measuring blood oxygenation; (iii) digital BP machine (A & D) for measuring blood pressure, pulse rate, and arrhythmia; and (iv) glucometer (TERUMO) for measuring blood glucose in diabetic patients. After taking the measurements, the triage algorithm at the PHC client device classifies the patients into four categories.

Online Survey Using COVID-19 Triage in Portable Health Clinics

We conducted a telephone-based survey to PHC-registered general patients ($N = 1116$) in both rural and urban areas. The patients were asked whether they had any concerns about COVID. The results indicated that 27% ($N = 312$) had potential symptoms. We applied our c-logic (corona logic, based on *Japanese standard triage*) to classify the patients ($N = 300$, 12 people were unavailable) into 5 groups in early June 2020 as follows: green (220), light yellow (45), yellow (2), orange (30), and red (3). According to the protocol, the *red patients* were advised by the health worker to visit a hospital immediately to see a doctor and take a *PCR test*. The *orange patients* were advised to contact the call center doctors, and the doctors advised those who were considered highly suspect to have COVID-19 based on the investigation data to receive a PCR test. The other patients were advised to remain at home under quarantine. These home-quarantined *orange patients* and the *yellow patients*, who were also advised by the health workers to remain at home under quarantine, were followed-up by the health workers regularly. If a

Table 43.3 PHC functionalities during general and emergency modes

Activity	General mode	Emergency mode
Symptom collection	Health worker	Mobile phone or app
Clinical measurements	Health worker	Patients self-test or health worker
Medical consultancy	Remote doctor	Remote doctor
e-prescription	GramHealth application, printed by e-health worker	GramHealth application or medical facilities

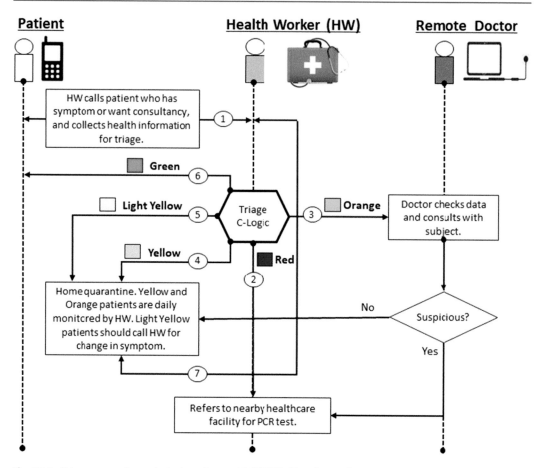

Fig. 43.4 Primary screening and triaging of potential COVID-19 patients using the "PHC COVID-19" system

patient's situation worsened, the patient was advised to contact the call center doctors for consultation. *Light yellow patients* were also advised by health workers to remain at home under quarantine, but they were asked to report to the health worker if their situation worsened. Only the *green patients* were set free with basic advice, that is, wear a mask, wash hands with sanitizers, maintain social distancing, etc., to keep them safe.

Usability of the Portable Health Clinic COVID-19 System

The PHC system can be effective in providing:

1. A primary-level screening mechanism that can demonstrably reduce the burden of NCD-related complications among COVID-19 patients and directly contribute to the reduc-

tion of the incidence of NCDs by providing timely advice and treatment.

2. A primary healthcare service platform for under-served populations in remote regions of developing countries. PHCs are now mature enough to be adapted to respond to large-scale public health emergencies such as COVID-19 to reduce associated mortality and morbidities.

3. A reliable platform for the early detection of NCDs and associated comorbidities among target populations and the ability to effectively contribute to a tangible reduction in the burden of disease.

4. A key ancillary mechanism for controlling *patient-to-caregiver transmission* of COVID-19 by creating physical distance between all except diagnosed cases and attending clinical staff.

5. Evidence for health authorities to choose e-Health technologies, such as PHC services, to provide primary healthcare services simultaneously for COVID-19 and NCDs, including video consultation with physicians, preventive health education and awareness at the grassroots, and encouraging well-being behaviors.

6. An effective outreach tool for controlling NCDs and decreasing the burden of disease in the target community.

7. A new approach to respond to large-scale public health emergencies like COVID-19 and contribute directly to building adaptive resilience among populations at risk.

Case Studies

The PHC system has been adapted to three different modules: Tele-Pathology, MCH, and PCH COVID-19.

Similar to the basic PHC protocol, the Tele-Pathology system, as explained in section "Pulse Rate (Heart Rate)", uses simple, low-cost, and available devices for its operation. Due to this simplicity, PHCs are very useful systems for wide use in low-income rural communities in a sustainable way. This module of PHC significantly improves health care by ensuring quality diagnosis and virtual consultations with doctors for remote patients.

PHC for MCH care, as explained in section "Blood Pressure", is a system designed to administer regular checkups of pregnant/postnatal women and newborns in rural areas where there are shortages of Ob-Gyns and pediatric experts. These regular checkups significantly increase the confidence of the village women regarding both their own health and their ability to give birth to healthy babies. The newborn babies receive regular checkups during their mothers' postnatal service period, which extends until the end of the second week of life and is very important. By offering these opportunities, we can expect a significant reduction in maternal and newborn mortality and morbidity.

PHCs introduce an affordable and usable set of sensors with the transmission ability to convey the clinical data of a COVID-19 patient to a remote doctor so that the doctor can make an accurate decision. PHC with its new triage algorithm (*corona logic*) classifies the patients based on whether the patient should visit a clinic for a PCR test. As mentioned in the previous section "Blood Glucose", the new model can reduce the risk of transmission and psychological stress on frontline healthcare staff, and it also optimizes healthcare resources for more patients who need them the most. The consultancy service mostly refers to nearby hospitals, provides doctor appointments, and interprets prescriptions. This is considered a very valued service in rural communities where there are no facilities for COVID-19 suspects or patients.

Summary

The extreme shortage of medical resources and the deficit of people's knowledge about health and diseases still exist, particularly in the countryside in many developing countries. However, poverty and immature legislation including medical insurance systems prohibit the growth of healthcare and medical businesses in such areas.

We are conscious about SDGs when we promote PHC activity. The purpose of this project is to improve health care, eliminate poverty by establishing a business model, improvement of status of females, etc. Thus, PHCs are related to SDG 1, 2, 3, 5, 6, 9, 13, and 17 (Table 43.4).

PHCs consist of (1) the accumulation of time series questionnaire data and biometric sensor data in cloud storage, (2) risk stratification (triage) by our original algorithm, created from standard diagnosis guidelines, and (3) online medical consultation to high-risk subjects including online prescription. This technology is useful for both *population management* and *individual management*.

In the beginning, we initiated PHC activity with a focus on NCDs and then spread to the

Table 43.4 How PHCs can contribute to achieving the SDGs

No.	Objective	How does it relate
SDG 1	No poverty	Establishes businesses and employment
SDG 2	Zero hunger	Creating employment opportunity for the poor
SDG 3	Good health and well-being	Population and individual health management
SDG 5	Gender equality	Creating business opportunities for females
SDG 8	Decent work and economic growth	Establishes a business model
SDG 9	Industry, innovation, and infrastructure	Establishes a collaborative platform where the device vendors, software solution providers, and researchers can find their incentives
SDG 13	Climate action	Establishes a post-disaster service
SDG 17	Partnerships for the goals	Creates partnerships between Japan and Bangladesh and other countries

MCH field. We also added Tele-Pathology and Tele-Eye care as service options to increase the functions of PHCs. We developed PHRs in PHCs to improve communication between health workers and users (citizens) and to promote patient engagement, which the WHO has promoted since 2015.

Currently, PHCs are spreading from countryside models to urban models and to other countries outside of Bangladesh.

Additionally, we have established a new COVID-19 module to manage PCR testing in 2020 and have now started to use it in Bangladesh.

Conclusions and Outlook

The global expansion of new broad area mobile networks including in countryside areas in Bangladesh and other developing countries is a new social infrastructure that can be used for new social service and business models. Services can be provided by this infrastructure to all 7 billion citizens on earth, including the poorest citizens, and it has the potential to change their lives.

PHCs are a type of intervention that uses this broad area mobile network to promote the SDGs and creates platforms for various services and/or devices for practical use.

Furthermore, with an effective platform, active projects such as PHCs have a huge potential to yield a variety of innovations that not only improve health care, poverty, and gender equality in developing countries but also change lives worldwide including in advanced countries, particularly during the "with-Corona" and "beyond-Corona" era.

Useful Resources

1. Since the PHC research project began in 2010, many peer-reviewed related journal articles have been published as of June 2020. In addition to peer-reviewed journal articles, three book chapters and more than 10 conference proceedings and non-peer-reviewed articles related to PHC research activities in Bangladesh, India, Cambodia, Pakistan, China, and Japan have been published. Table 43.5 below summarizes the key findings of 15 selected PHC-related journal articles.

Table 43.5 List of PHC-related peer-reviewed articles with key findings

No.	Year of publication	Title of article	Name of journal	Key findings
1	2020	A predictive model for height tracking in an adult male population in Bangladesh to reduce input errors	*International Journal of Environmental Research and Public Health*	Analyzed data on 40,391 patients collected from PHCs in Bangladesh from 2010 to 2019 to predict the acceptable height range for male patients. Key findings indicated that height for the 20–49 age group showed no significant change, those aged 50–64 showed a pattern of slight height decreases, and those aged 65–100 showed a drastic decrease in height
2	2020	Influence of factors on the adoption and use of ICT-based e-Health technology by urban corporate people	*Journal of Service Science and Management*	Analyzed 264 urban corporate individuals who received PHC services in Dhaka, Bangladesh, in 2018. They identified the three most important factors associated with PHC utilization: (1) perceived usefulness, (2) intention to use, and (3) health awareness
3	2019	Growth characteristics of age and gender-based anthropometric data from human-assisted remote healthcare system	*International Journal of Advanced Computer Science and Applications*	Analyzed 13,069 male participants who received PHC services in Bangladesh from 2010 to 2019. They found that male height does not significantly change in men 20–49 years old, declines slightly in men 50–79 years old, and declines sharply after the age of 80. Male weight increases until the age of 49 and decreases after that. Male waist and hip measurements show similar growth characteristics as weight
4	2019	Portable Health Clinic: An advanced tele-healthcare system for unreached communities	IOS Press (Med-Info Publication)	Describes (1) the PHC system, (2) the progress of serving 41,000 people by 2019, (3) a simple analysis of regional health status, and (4) a simple expansion of PHCs in the areas of Tele-Pathology and Tele-Eye care
5	2018	Lessons learned from co-design and co-production in a Portable Health Clinic research project in Jaipur District, India (2016–2018)	*Sustainability*	The study identified eight key factors that were effective for co-designing and co-implementing PHC research projects with multiple stakeholders in India: (1) mutual stakeholder agreement, (2) harmonizing research objectives, (3) stakeholder's commitment and sense of ownership, (4) stakeholder trust, (5) effective coordinators, (6) personality type and characteristics of leaders, (7) capacity building and the empowerment, and (8) continuous efforts to involve stakeholders

(continued)

Table 43.5 (continued)

No.	Year of publication	Title of article	Name of journal	Key findings
6	2018	The relationship and risk factors associated with hypertension, diabetes, and proteinuria among adults from Bheramara Upazila, Bangladesh: findings from Portable Health Clinic Data, 2013–2016	*International Journal of Medical Research and Health Sciences*	Analyzed 2890 participants who received PHC services in the Bheramara sub-district in Bangladesh from 2013 to 2016. A logistic regression model found significant associations between diabetes and proteinuria and between hypertension and diabetes. Participants older than 40 years had higher odds of having diabetes or having hypertension than participants aged 15–39 years old
7	2018	Factors influencing rural end-users' acceptance of e-Health in developing countries: a study on Portable Health Clinic in Bangladesh	*Telemedicine and e-Health*	Analyzed 292 randomly selected rural respondents in the Bheramara sub-district in Bangladesh between June and July 2016. The most significant influencing factors for accepting PHC e-health services were (1) social references, (2) advertisements, (3) attitude toward the system, (4) access to a cellphone, and (5) perceived system effectiveness
8	2018	Factors affecting rural patients' primary compliance with e-prescription: a developing country perspective	*Telemedicine and e-Health*	Analyzed 95 randomly selected rural patients who received e-prescriptions from PHC services in the Bheramara sub-district in Bangladesh. Out of the 95 who received e-prescriptions, 74.7% ($n = 71$) reported that they purchased the medicines recommended by the e-prescriptions. Females, those who visited health facilities frequently, had a mid-high level of education and traveled a shorter distance to healthcare facilities were significantly more likely to comply with e-prescriptions
9	2018	Postnatal care could be the key to improving the continuum of care in maternal and child health in Ratanakiri, Cambodia.	PLoS One.	Analyzed data from 377 women in Ratanakiri, Cambodia. The study indicates the needs for efforts to reduce the number of women who discontinue the continuum of care and who do not receive any care to avoid neonatal complications. Findings also suggested the need for MCH care PHC services for women who live a long distance from health facilities in remote rural areas.

Table 43.5 (continued)

No.	Year of publication	Title of article	Name of journal	Key findings
10	2018	School-based educational intervention to improve children's oral health-related behaviors in rural Bangladesh	*South East Asia Journal of Public Health*	Analyzed data collected from 52 students at the intervention primary school and 37 students at a control school in the Tangail district in Bangladesh. The intervention group who received face-to-face dental exercises and a group seminar showed significant improvements in brushing their teeth two or more times per day and brushing their teeth before bed after 6 months compared with the control group. The study identified needs for PHCs to provide dental checkups for school children
11	2017	Mobile healthcare system for health checkups and telemedicine in post-disaster situations	*Stud Health Technol Inform*	Described an adopted PHC system to fit post-disaster conditions and the new algorithm. They tested the operability and turn-around time of the adapted system at the debris flow disaster shelters in Hiroshima
12	2015	Health checkup and telemedical intervention program for preventive medicine in developing countries: verification study	*Journal of Medical Internet Research*	Described a PHC system and the logic in Bangladesh. Analyzed 16,741 participants who received PHC services in Bangladesh and 2361 participants who returned to receive their second PHC services after 1 year. Systolic blood pressure was significantly decreased from an average of 121 mmHg to an average of 116 mmHg. Proposed a cost-effective method using a machine-learning technique including medical interviews, subject profiles, and checkup results
13	2015	Improvement of hemoglobin with repeated health checks among women in Bangladesh	*Stud Health Technol Inform*	Hemoglobin level of Bangladesh women who received PHC services increased from the first checkup to the second visit after receiving iron supplements prescribed at the first checkup
14	2015	Targeting morbidity in unreached communities using portable health clinic system	*IEICE Transactions on Communications*	Tested the effectiveness of the PHC system to target morbidity by analyzing 8690 patients in rural and urban areas of Bangladesh during September 2012 to January 2013. They also identified the intensity of morbidities and reexamined the morbid patients 2 months later
15	2014	An affordable, usable, and sustainable preventive healthcare system for unreached people in Bangladesh	*Studies in Health Technology and Informatics*	Described the results of pilot PHC health checkup projects. Analyzed 791 patients who attended baseline PHC health checkups. Of the 791 patients, 154 were classified as orange or red at baseline. Ninety-six of the 154 patients returned to receive their second PHC health checkup

Review Questions

1. What are the primary components for designing a remote healthcare (e.g., Portable Health Clinic) system?
2. In PHC project, we show the contents to users (healthy subjects and patients) by smartphone. We call this system "personal health record, PHR." What is the benefit of this PHR function in PHC?
3. How does a village laboratory technologist prepare a standard hematology report for a patient in village using Tele-Eye care system?
4. What should be considered in advance before exploring the activities or conducting the intervention relative to the nursing informatics in the community?
5. What is the difference between the PHC treatment process of light yellow and yellow patients identified by COVID-19 triage system?

Appendix: Answers to Review Questions

1. What are the primary components for designing a remote healthcare (e.g., Portable Health Clinic) system?

There are four major components to design a human-assisted remote healthcare system. (1) A box containing healthcare sensors, (2) A certified health worker, (3) An online server, and (4) A doctor call center.

2. In PHC project, we show the contents to users (healthy subjects and patients) by smartphone. We call this system "personal health record, PHR." What is the benefit of this PHR function in PHC?

Accessibility to their personal health/medical information is one of the key elements of "patient engagement" which WHO has recommended. PHR allows users to access their personal health/

medical information and increase users' interests about it. Patient engagement enhances patient/family participation to medical policy/decision and increases patient satisfaction and medical cost-effectiveness also.

3. How does a village laboratory technologist prepare a standard hematology report for a patient in village using Tele-Eye care system?

The village laboratory actually prepares the report with the support of a city pathologist using the PHC online system. First, the village laboratory technologist collects blood sample from the patient in village. Then s/he prepares a glass slide with the sample, takes several microscopic images from different significant positions, and upload to the online server together with a physical report. Finally, the city pathologist checks these, prepares the hematology report, and preserves to the online server for the laboratory technologist to be delivered to the patient.

4. What should be considered in advance before exploring the activities or conducting the intervention relative to the nursing informatics in the community?

The local potential and capacity might be investigated in advance and need to consider collaborating with them. For example, a traditional birth attendant is usually trusted by the community people and knows very well what a local pregnant woman wants or doesn't want. She could be a competent collaborator and could be a key person who is able to disseminate your activities or intervention in the field.

5. What is the difference between the PHC treatment process of light yellow and yellow patients identified by COVID-19 triage system?

Both light yellow and yellow patients should go under home quarantine and keep records of the health status using self-checking devices in the

PHC box. In case of yellow patients, the PHC health worker will follow up the progress of the status and take necessary actions accordingly. However, in case of light yellow patients, the patients will notify the health worker if needed due to any significant progress.

References

1. "SDG Tracker, Bangladesh", http://www.sdg.gov.bd/page/indicator-wise/5/427/2/5#1. Accessed 14 June 2020.
2. Ahmed A, Rebeiro-Hargrave A, Nohara Y, Islam RM, Ghosh PP, Nakashima N, Yasuura H. Portable health clinic: a Telehealthcare system for unreached communities. In: Smart sensors and systems. New York: Springer; 2015. p. 447–67.
3. Nohara Y, Kai E, Ghosh P, Islam R, Ahmed A, et al. Health checkup and telemedical intervention program for preventive medicine in developing countries: verification study. J Med Internet Res. 2015;17(1):e2.
4. Islam R, Nohara Y, Rahman JU, Sultana N, Ahmed A, Nakashima N. Portable health clinic: an advanced tele-healthcare system for unreached communities. Stud Health Technol Inform. 2019;264:416–9.
5. Yokota F, Ahmed A, Kikuchi K, Nishikitani M, Islam R, Nakashima N. Diabetes, obesity, and hypertension in Bheramara Kushtia District, Bangladesh - results from Portable Health Clinic Data, 2013-2016. In: Proceeding of Social Business Academia Conference, 2016.
6. Islam R, Rahman MJ, Ahmed A, Nakashima N. GramHealth: tele-pathology system for PHC telemedicine service. In: Proceeding of the 4th Digital Pathology Congress: ASIA, 2018.
7. Kikuchi K, Sato Y, Izukura R, Nishikitani M, Islam R, Kato K, Morokuma S et al. Portable health clinic for sustainable care of mothers and newborns in rural Bangladesh. In: Conference Proceeding of Asia-Pacific Association for Medical Informatics, 2020.
8. Roberts S, Chaboyer W, Gonzalez R, Marshall A. Using technology to engage hospitalised patients in their care: a realist review. BMC Health Serv Res. 2017;17(1):650. https://doi.org/10.1186/s12913-017-2314-0.
9. World Health Organization (2015). Technical series on safer primary care; patient engagement. https://apps.who.int/iris/bitstream/handle/10665/252269/9789241511629-eng.pdf?sequence=1
10. Bombard Y, Baker GR, Orlando E, et al. Engaging patients to improve quality of care: a systematic review. Implement Sci. 2018;13(1):98.
11. Bae WK, Kwon J, Lee HW, et al. Feasibility and accessibility of electronic patient-reported outcome measures using a smartphone during routine chemotherapy: a pilot study. Support Care Cancer. 2018;26(11):3721–8. https://doi.org/10.1007/s00520-018-4232-z.
12. Nakashima N, Noda M, Ueki K, et al. Recommended configuration for personal health records by standardized data item sets for diabetes mellitus and associated chronic diseases: a report from a collaborative initiative by six Japanese associations. Diabetol Int. 2019;10(2):85–92.
13. Rahman MM, Abe SK, Rahman MS, et al. Maternal anemia and risk of adverse birth and health outcomes in low- and middle-income countries: systematic review and meta-analysis. Am J Clin Nutr. 2016;103(2):495–504.
14. Matias SL, Mridha MK, Young RT, Hussain S, Dewey KG. Daily maternal lipid-based nutrient supplementation with 20 mg iron, compared with iron and folic acid with 60 mg iron, resulted in lower iron status in late pregnancy but not at 6 months postpartum in either the mothers or their infants in Bangladesh. J Nutr. 2018;148:1615–24.
15. International Diabetes Federation: Diabetes Atlas, 9th edition 2019. https://diabetesatlas.org/data/en/indicators/14/. Accessed 29 May 2020.
16. Sarker BK, Rahman M, Rahman T, Hossain J, Reichenbach L, Mitra DK. Reasons for preference of home delivery with traditional birth attendants (TBAs) in rural Bangladesh: a qualitative exploration. PLoS One. 2016;11(1):e0146161.
17. Hu M, Sugimoto M, Hargrave AR, Nohara Y, Moriyama M, Ahmed A, Shimizu S, Nakashima N. Mobile healthcare system for health checkups and telemedicine in post-disaster situations. Stud Health Technol Inform. 2015;216:79–83.

Brazil: Information Communication and Technology for Nurses and Patient Care Delivery

44

Heimar Marin and Heloisa Helena Ciqueto Peres

Learning Objectives
- Demonstrate basic understanding and use of the information and communication technology is being applied for nursing care in Brazil to support nursing knowledge work, health care delivery, and the advancement of nursing knowledge.
- Describe the adoption of ICT to support nursing care delivery across the country.
- Demonstrate the use of a standardized terminology in a care environment that reflects nursing's unique contribution to patient outcomes.

Key Terms
- ICT adoption in Brazilian healthcare system
- ICT adoption in Brazilian healthcare system
- ICT adoption of Brazilian nurses
- IData collection
- data quality
- Outcome measures
- Nursing terminologies
- NANDA
- NIC
- NOC
- ICNP
- Effectiveness
- Efficiency

- User satisfaction
- Software usability
- Evaluation

Definition

Nursing Informatics: "Nursing Informatics science and practice integrates nursing, its information and knowledge and their management with information and communication technologies to promote the health of people, families and communities worldwide" (available in: https://imianews.wordpress.com/2009/08/24/imia-ni-definition-of-nursing-informatics-updated/).

Effectiveness: precision and integrity with which users achieve specified objectives [1].

Efficiency: resources used (time, human effort, costs, and materials) in relation to the results achieved [1].

H. Marin (✉) · H. H. Ciqueto Peres
Universidade Federal de São Paulo, São Paulo, Brazil

© Springer Nature Switzerland AG 2022
U. H. Hübner et al. (eds.), *Nursing Informatics*, Health Informatics,
https://doi.org/10.1007/978-3-030-91237-6_44

Statements

To achieve the best outcome technology can provide to support health population, it is mandatory to consider digital and health literacy as high complex theme that demands clearly articulation among all subjects involved.

• *Education is a continuous life event. Only through research using real data from nursing practice, recorded at the point of care, we can evaluate our profession and enrich our capabilities.*

Introduction

Brazil, officially Federative Republic of Brazil occupies half the continent's landmass. It is the fifth largest country in the world facing the Atlantic Ocean along 4600 miles (7400 km) of coastline and shares more than 9750 miles (15,700 km) of inland borders with every South American country except Chile and Ecuador. Brazil encompasses a wide range of tropical and subtropical landscapes, including wetlands, savannas, plateaus, and low mountains. The country contains no desert, high-mountain, or arctic environments. The population is over 211 million people (available in https://www.ibge.gov.br/estatisticas/sociais/populacao.html. Accessed on March 4, 2020).

The healthcare workforce relies on physician and nurses. The nursing profession comprises technicians (1293.873), auxiliary (451,148), and nurses (551,751) according to the Brazilian Federal Council of Nurses (http://www.cofen.gov.br/enfermagem-em-numeros). Nurses are the leader of the team, but it is evident that the number of nurses across country is not sufficient to cover all population needs. Thus, technology plays an important role on the education and nursing assistance.

As a pillar of the nursing care, information is a key factor to improved health conditions and prevention of diseases and can be used to provide the population with information and knowledge, considering the dimension and geographical and development economy of the country. The range of Information Communication Technology (ICT) healthcare strategies comprises the creation of website, portals, social network, and synchronous and asynchronous communication. Many of these strategies are low-cost and not complex processes. These tools brought about a significant change in the daily lives of individuals and families and represent a significant change in healthcare delivery and patient engagement and empowerment. These tools are important supports for health promotion and supporting the coordinated work of social sectors and the population, consistent with personal, family, and communities' environments [2].

ICT represents a strong power to support healthcare, education, management as much as it is present at all human activities. Although, in Brazil, healthcare delivery is traditionally being focused on acute conditions, it is necessary today to design models and systems according to the contemporaneous conditions of living, and being health, recovering health, dealing with chronic diseases, facing endemics, and having a dignified end of life. Seeing patient care as a collaboration between providers and patients around patient's health and life conditions enables nurses to understand how to transform health care by focusing on non-visit-based care, patient engagement, and new models of care delivery.

Among all healthcare strategies being implemented by countries, ICT is a priority. As a priority to reach high quality of information for evaluation and healthcare planning, most countries must invest on affordable technology and deploy resources that enable the provision of provide care and expertise at a distance.

For several countries and populations, ICT adoption has been slow due to cost, infrastructure, conception models, architecture, integration, usability, and public policies implementation. Adoption and deployment are also dependent on training and education. It is mandatory to influence government leaders about the importance of education and preparation as fundamental to ensuring that patients and families can engage effectively in the ways that they want and need to achieve optimum health status as possible.

The components of basic nursing are uncomplicated and self-explanatory. We can initiate to explore how technology can help us to support the patient to achieve health or getting independent. As nurses we all know how important is to be fed, to sleep, to rest, to breathe, to select suitable clothes, to move. Most important, nurses are the largest population on any healthcare system and the primary user of any ICT on health. We can make a difference on the continuous care of persons. Even the best surgeon in the world would not succeed if a high-quality nursing care does not follow the procedure. A good technique is not enough to bring those patients at the same or better conditions as before. Patients need nurses. The healthcare systems need nurses.

To achieve the best outcome technology to support health population, it is mandatory to consider digital and health literacy as high complex theme that demands clearly articulation among all subjects involved. Individuals must know what should be known, where the best information is available, what is reliable, and where to find information as needed. Providers should welcome the opportunity to partner with their patients and encourage them to access health information. Organizations must be sensitive to combine common values, vision, policies, attitudes, behaviors, and beliefs, as well as different cultures with different defining characteristics.

Effective operation requires strong leadership at the national, regional, and organizational level. The government regulatory and supervisory role is imperative for successful implementation. The deployment of ICT in health services is a major infrastructural investment and the adaptation by health service providers to this infrastructure should be supported [3].

All nursing care must be implemented based on physiological principles, age, cultural background, emotional balance, and physical and intellectual capacities. Quality of care is affected by the competencies, abilities, and preparation of the nursing personnel rather than the number of hours we spend doing things.

Leadership skills that will be required of nurses to appropriately respond to emerging technology include being able to use technology to facilitate mobility, communication, and relationships, having expertise in knowledge information, acquisition, and distribution. We are in a profession where knowledge acquirement demands full commitment since the advance of science and technology is fast and complex. At nursing profession, we must become the master of knowledge management. We need to master the process to use technology to improve population health strategies and ICT to improve population health outcomes.

Education is a continuous life event and we must be engaged. We must provide educational environment; we must stimulate our colleagues to study, to learn. We must educate and be educated.

Considering all tendencies in the modern world, the globalization process, and the awareness that everything must be documented to exist, nurses have dedicated more attention to make visible their contribution to the health of population. Important aspects to be considered include not only strategies to store and retrieve information but also the way the information can better characterize and build nursing knowledge.

ICT in Healthcare: Nurses' Adoption Across the Country

The Organization for Economic Cooperation and Development (OECD) states that the inefficiency of healthcare systems is related to deficits in the transmission of information, which can be improved using technologies. The potential benefits of the application of ICT can increase the quality of treatments and efficiency, reduce operating and administrative costs, and offer possibilities for new treatment approaches and models [4].

The establishment of indicators that can be used by countries is necessary to evaluate the results and benefits of ICT. However, the consolidation of internationally recognized indicators requires efforts and researcher's involvement. The first comprehensive study to collect and analyze information on e-Health to ascertain a group of internationally comparable indicators was coordinated by the European Commission. The survey identified 4400 theme-related indicators in the countries of the European Union, Iceland, Norway, Canada, and the United States [5].

Considering the international scenario and the Brazilian development in health informatics and technological resources, a national study has been conducted to pursuit consistent indicators to measure the impact of the use of information and communication technology for the health of the population. Thus, the overall objective of this study was to identify the existing infrastructure of information and communication technologies available in healthcare facilities, including the stage of implementation by these facilities and its adoption by health professionals [6].

The study is a descriptive research being conducted annually since 2012. The sample comprised Executive and ICT Directors (CEO and CIO), physicians, and nurses included at the National Record of Healthcare Establishments (CNES), maintained by the Department of Informatics of the Ministry of Health (DATASUS, Ministry of Health). It was excluded isolated clinics, mobile units, and establishments with non-physician and non-nurses. The sample was selected by probability sampling technique considering the country region and the type of establishment (outpatient, diagnosis and therapy services, inpatient up to 50 beds, and inpatient with more than 50 beds), including both private and public facilities [6].

Data collection was done by a questionnaire with 37 questions to understand the adoption of ICT in their daily nursing duties. As an annual investigation, the questions bring up data and information related to the last 12 months of implementation and adoption of ICT-based systems and services. The last edition published in 2019 interviewed 2716 nurses. The results showed that the use of computers by nurses while caring for patients has increased in recent years, from 79% in 2016 to 87% in 2018 [7].

Considering professionals who reported referring to patient data electronically, password-protected access was the most commonly used security tool by 90% of nurses in 2018. On the other hand, approximately 27% said they had used digital certificates, and only 4% of nurses mentioned using biometrics-protected access to electronic systems [7].

In 2018, nurses used electronic system functionalities less often compared to the physicians who used for prescription and surgery report. Nurses used more functionalities related to administrative activities, such as generating requests for materials and supplies and booking appointments, tests, or surgeries. Functionalities used during patient care were also among those most used by nurses, such as listing medications being taken by a specific patient and listing lab test results for a specific patient [7].

The results of the 2018 survey also showed the persistence of low availability of decision support functionalities in healthcare facilities. Clinical guidelines and protocols were the most mentioned, available to half of nurses (52%).The second-most used, also by approximately one-third of professionals, were drug allergy alerts and reminders, drug dosage alerts and reminders, and alerts and reminders for drug interference with lab results [7].

According to the assessment of professionals, in general, the available electronic systems were not considered adapted to their needs and daily tasks: only 37% of nurses agreed that the electronic systems were well adapted to their needs. This finding may reflect the low involvement of these professionals in the development and implementation of electronic systems in facilities, considering that 46% of nurses agreed that they had participated in this development. Furthermore, approximately half of the professionals from both categories agreed that they were trained and motivated to use the facilities' electronic systems [7].

The perception of nurses about the impact of the use of electronic systems in their activities is an important indicator to understand ICT appropriation by these professionals. In 2018, the greatest benefits of using electronic systems were related to security and confidentiality of information, as mentioned by 63% of nurses. The possibility of exchanging information among the electronic systems of different healthcare facilities was identified by 34% of nurses. However, among both types of professionals, a low percentage agreed that the financial resources for investment in electronic systems were adequate to meet facility needs (29% of nurses), which can point to difficulties faced by them when using the available systems. Furthermore, 47% of nurses agreed that governmental policies encouraged the implementation and use of electronic systems in the facilities [7].

Regarding the impact of the adoption of computerized systems in health, the survey results showed that, in general, professionals perceived neither an increase nor a decrease in the workload with the use of computers and the Internet (58% of nurses). Moreover, considering the objective impacts of the use of electronic systems, the most commonly mentioned were improvement in the efficiency of teamwork processes (92%) and the perception that the electronic systems led to greater efficiency of service (89% for nurses) [7].

The data indicate that, despite an increase in ICT in Brazilian healthcare facilities, electronic systems still need to be better adapted to the needs of nurses. The assessment of professionals corroborates the fact that few of them are involved in the development and implementation of electronic health systems in the facilities in which they work. The participation of these professionals in the stages of planning and implementing electronic systems could

result in those systems being better adapted to their needs, improving system usability and appropriation of the resources during patient care and service management activities.

According to the survey results, the overall information security scenario in healthcare facilities is still very critical: only one-quarter (23%) had information security policies. Furthermore, the low diversity of information security tools used indicates that there is very little use of more complex tools, such as biometrics-protected access to electronic systems and data encryption. This reality causes even more concern when considering the Brazilian General Data Protection Law [8], which provides for the protection and processing of personal information, including data available electronically, based on the fundamental rights of freedom and privacy. The impact of the LGPD in the health area has given rise to intense debates among experts in the field because the document values patient data confidentiality and privacy and regulates the level of data security that healthcare facilities must provide. Thus, all public and private institutions must invest in protection and security solutions, in addition to developing and implementing information technology governance. Thus, strategies in the area must aim both to provide better patient care, preserving the privacy of their information and protecting their personal data, and to expand healthcare services, so that they reach all citizens, ensuring quality and safety of care.

From Data Collection to Outcome Measurements

Nursing practice is based on health information. Thus, quality of information demands quality of data collection. The best computerized system will not support patient care delivery with lack of quality on data collected, recorded, and analyzed. Consequently, aware of the importance of data quality to assure nursing care, professionals in the country develop initiatives to use standardized terminologies on nursing process (NP). The most used over decades were the International Classification of Nursing Interventions (ICNP®) [9], NANDA-International structures [10], Classification of Outcomes (NOC) [11], and Classification of Interventions (NIC) [12].

ICNP has been implemented in several computerized systems. A bibliometric study to identify the use of ICNP in Brazil found 136 scientific productions of theses from 1999 to 2016, of which 108 used ICNP® and 23 cited ICNP®. The authors also demonstrated that the use of ICNP is implemented in different geographic regions. The Northeast and Southeast presented, respectively, 41 (37.9%) productions of theses followed by the South region with 25 (23.1%) and 1 (0.9%) in the Center-West region [13].

The use of the ICNP in the country also analyses the potential of the terminology to support nursing documentation on specific disease protocols such as myocardial infarction, leprosy, AIDS, impaired skin integrity, among others [14–16]. As example, considering the utility of terminological subsets to facilitate the implementation of protocols, a study elaborated a terminological subset for patients with acute myocardial infarction using the Activities of Living Model. The authors identified 22 [17] diagnoses and 22 nursing outcomes. Of these, 17 nursing diagnosis statements and 17 nursing outcome statements presented content validity index (CVI) ≥ 0.80. Of the 113 elaborated nursing interventions, 42 reached a CVI ≥ 0.80 and 51 interventions made up the terminological subset [18].

Analyzing the use of NANDA, NIC, and NOC terminologies, one example is a study conducted after 10 years of deployment of a computerized system at the Teaching Hospital of University of São Paulo, denominated PROCEnf-USP® System. The main objective was to evaluate the contribution of this system so that users of different levels of nursing education including undergraduate students, residents, and nurses could identify moderate- and high-accuracy nursing diagnoses, the accuracy for selecting appropriate interventions that

lead to achieving better results for patients. Among the benefits in the use of technology, it can be highlighted the support to ascertain the accuracy of diagnoses, in the indication of the best evidence-based interventions, supported by clinical reasoning and decision-making process [19].

Recently, the system was also evaluated in terms of effectiveness, efficiency, and satisfaction [20]. Effectiveness refers to the "precision and integrity with which users achieve specified objectives" [1]. Efficiency refers to the "resources used (time, human effort, costs and materials) in relation to the results achieved" [1]. It is usually measured by the average time taken to complete the task. Thus, time spent to perform a task is a general measure of efficiency. In the evaluation, it was assumed that the less time the user spends to complete the task, the less resource the task consumes, and the better result will present by the product [21].

Satisfaction is defined as "the extent to which the physical, cognitive and emotional responses resulting from the use of a system, product or service meet the needs and expectations of the user". In other words, satisfaction measures the user experience when using the system. Satisfaction should be measured using a standardized questionnaire, using measures that provide easy-to-interpret data [1, 21].

In evaluating the effectiveness of the system, the instrument Quality of Diagnoses, Interventions and Outcomes (Q-DIO) Brazilian Version was used [22]. According to the data from this research, users documented the nursing process with greater efficiency in the system, evidenced by the increase in the accuracy and integrity of the records, according to the Q-DIO score. Factors that contributed to this result were attributed to the training of the team and the implementation of more advanced functionalities [20].

Efficiency was assessed by surveying the time spent by nurses to document the nursing assessment in the system. The average time spent was 12.5 min, with a standard deviation of 11.2 min and a median of 8.9 min. Time was correlated with the number of diagnostics, outcomes, indicators, interventions, and evaluation activities. A positive correlation was observed between the time and the number of items in the evaluation. It can be inferred that the greater the complexity of the patient health situation, the greater the time spent on the evaluation [20].

To assess the satisfaction of nurses and nursing technicians, the Software Usability Measurement Inventory—SUMI® questionnaire was used. The SUMI *questionnaire* comprises five scales: efficiency, affect, helpfulness, control, and learnability. It is a proprietary tool, developed by Jurek Kirakowski, protected by copyright. SUMI® is currently marketed by the HFRG (Human Factors Research Group) of University College Cork (Ireland) in printed format (packages containing 50 questionnaires) and in electronic format [17, 23].

The SUMI® Learning scale obtained the highest average among nursing technicians. The task of checking the prescription and nursing annotation of the care provided seems to them quite simple and the interface is very intuitive. In addition, there is no need to use manuals to use the system [20].

The satisfaction of nurses and nursing technicians with the usability of the PROCEnf-USP® system was assessed and the average on most SUMI® scales was above the international reference database. This finding demonstrated that users are satisfied with the PROCEnf-USP® system. However, users have also indicated critical areas that need to be worked on to enhance user satisfaction [20].

The main reasons for nurses' dissatisfaction related to the PROCEnf-USP® system, according to the answer to the SUMI® questionnaire, were associated with the speed of the software, high number of clicks to perform the scheduling, and screen freezing that considerably increases the downtime of the system. These practices force the user to wait for the system to be loaded [20].

These results are like the evaluation of the quality of the software product carried out in 2012 in the PROCEnf-USP® system, in which

the characteristic performance efficiency obtained only 46% of positive responses [24]. The comparison between the results of the two surveys pointed out needs for improvements related to usability, demonstrating that health software developers need to be more proactive and critical in improving the performance of these systems and the experience of clinical users. The meaning of the PROCEnf-USP® system for nursing technicians can be configured as digital inclusion, updating, knowledge, learning, and the possibility of documenting the care provided in a clear, legible, and organized manner [20].

Usability problems related to efficiency can have a notable impact on the workflow and on nurses' satisfaction, requiring areas to be redesigned to optimize NP documentation. It is believed that the factors that contributed to the user's satisfaction with the implementation of PROCEnf-USP® are linked to the importance that professionals attribute of the nursing process in the institution, strongly consolidated since its foundation, and to the continuous investments in training and development of the company. Nursing team was continuous training in clinical reasoning, critical thinking, and the use of Standardized Nursing Language (SNL) to document nursing care delivered.

The SUMI® Control scale also obtained the lowest average among the scales, in the assessment of nursing technicians. They also reported problems with the software related to usability such as slowness in response time, many clicks to perform simple tasks, difficulty finding data, and lack of ordering of the nursing prescriptions dates [20].

It was also observed that the greater the software skills and knowledge on the part of users are nurses or nursing technicians, the higher the averages of the SUMI® scales. The scores of the SUMI® Global Usability scale was lower for users who thought they had little competence and skill with the software in general. The importance of health system developers, designers, educators, nursing managers, and policy makers is important to expend efforts to minimize usability problems in Electronic Health Record (EHR) [20].

It is pointed out that investments in health software are necessary to increase the effectiveness of the clinical user, reducing time spent on documentation, and improve the satisfaction of the end user. To achieve success, it is fundamental to involve the user since the first step of development or selection of a system to assure that functionalities will be useful and consistent with the care delivery workflow.

Case Study

The PROCEnf-USP System

Over more than three decades, nurses in the Nursing Department at the University Hospital of the University of São Paulo (HU-USP) have based the care delivery and educational practice on the nursing process [25]. The Nursing Department, aware of the advancement of information technologies in health systems and the importance of ensuring that nursing was prepared, not only to document in electronic systems, but also to have an effective participation in technological development, included in its strategic goals the computerization of clinical nursing documentation [26]. In 2003, faculties of the School of Nursing—University of São Paulo (EEUSP) at the Departments of Professional Guidance (ENO) and Medical-Surgical Nursing (ENC) initiated the project to develop a customized nursing system to support nursing documentation using standardized terminology. The project received financial support from the National Council for Technological and Scientific Development (CNPq), which made it possible to increase the project including a Clinical Decision Support System (SADC) for nursing documentation to facilitate bedside records and student learning for undergraduate and graduate courses [26].

The system was named as the Electronic Documentation System of the Nursing Process at the University of São Paulo (PROCEnf-USP®). Its adoption had as its main premise the continuous improvement of the nursing process (NP), the clinical reasoning of nurses and undergraduate students, building evidence bases for the profession and promoting the development of research [26]. Thus, the PROCEnf-USP® system was organized according to a knowledge base anchored in the definitions of diagnoses and their components, following the hierarchy of domains, classes, and diagnoses, proposed by the unification of NANDA-International structures [10], Classification of Outcomes (NOC) [11], and Classification of Interventions (NIC) [12]. This unification of structures is known as NANDA-NOC-NIC Linkages or NNN Linkages [27].

PROCEnf-USP® was built to integrate the core information systems of the hospital. Thus, the nursing process for documentation includes data collection, nursing diagnosis, care plan and evolution of patient outcomes. The terminologies are applied as Nursing Outcomes Classification (NOC) and Nursing Interventions Classification (NIC). Outcomes Indicators, patient evolution, nursing notes and scheduling of the nursing orders are considered to analyse and measure nursing care outcomes [15]. It was an agreement among the professionals involved in the system development that the system should provide better resources to the nursing care delivery emphasizing a humanized care with a system centered on the patient and family [26]. Consequently, it was considered as important functionality the support for documenting the nursing process contributing to the formulation of accurate diagnoses and effective interventions, which can lead to highly significant and clinically relevant results for the patient, contributing to the nursing base knowledge underpinning the evolution of Evidence Base Practice (EBP) in nursing care [28] (Fig. 44.1).

PROCEnf-USP® allows access to intervention protocols associated with EBP, included in the selection stage of nursing interventions. Thus, it can conveniently offer nurses a list of activities during the documentation of the nursing process in the system. These protocols were built from the refined search for the best studies, the result of a partnership between the Center for Evidence-Based Nursing (NUEBE) at the University Hospital of the University of São Paulo and the Brazilian Center for Health Care Informed by Evidence: Center of

Excellence Joanna Briggs Institute of EEUSP [29] (Fig. 44.2).

From the data documentation in the Data Collection phase (History and Physical Examination), the PROCEnf-USP® system

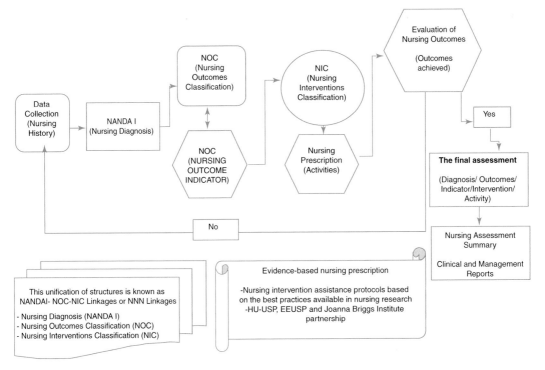

Fig. 44.1 Framework of the support system for clinical decision for the nursing process at the University Hospital of the University of São Paulo—PROCEnf-USP®.

Source: Screen taken by the authors on October 10, 2020. São Paulo. The University Hospital of the University São Paulo. Brazil

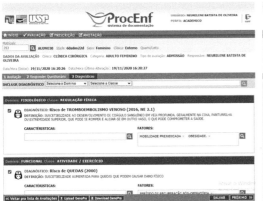
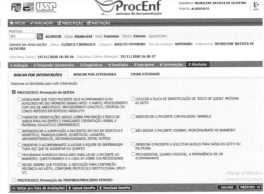

Fig. 44.2 Support system for clinical decision, PROCEnf-USP®. The selection stage of Nursing Diagnosis and access to intervention protocols associated with EBP, included in the stage of nursing intervention.

Source: Screen taken by the authors on October 10, 2020. São Paulo. The University Hospital of the University São Paulo. Brazil

presents the diagnostic hypotheses generated automatically (calculated diagnoses), which can be confirmed or refuted by the nurse. After selecting the diagnoses, it presents possible connections to support the choice of outcomes and nursing interventions. The outcomes allow the evaluation of the quality and effectiveness of the care plan, being possible to demonstrate that the intervention was more effective to achieve the desired results. Those results or outcomes are based on the use of indicators that are standardized measures, with a Likert scale from 1 to 5, where 1 is always the worst situation and 5 the best situation. Upon admission, after choosing the outcomes, the nurse selects the indicators, establishing the status and the goal to be achieved, reassessing each assessment [12, 20] (Fig. 44.3).

Nursing interventions can be selected for each outcome. An intervention is considered as any treatment, based on judgment and clinical knowledge, performed by a nurse, to improve the patient's results. The nurse after selecting the nursing interventions can select the activities for each intervention. Nursing activities are specific actions to implement an intervention that help patients to progress toward the desired outcome. The system provides a list of activities related to the interventions, helping nurses to make clinical decisions [13, 20].

Once the interventions are select, the next phase is the implementation by the nursing team (nurse and nursing technician) of the activities prescribed in the assistance planning stage, that is, the record of compliance with the nursing prescription.

The nursing assessment recognized as a deliberate, systematic, and continuous process of verifying the results achieved because of nursing actions or interventions, representing the timeframe to verify the need to change or redesign the nursing care plan [30]. At HU-USP, this step is performed every 24 h. In the PROCEnf-USP® system, nursing assessment begins with the reassessment of the goals established in the NOC outcomes indicators. If pertinent, the nurse returns to the diagnosis stage to add new diagnostics and outcome or remove resolved diagnoses. To approve the final assessment, the nurse goes through the intervention, activities, scheduling of the nursing prescription phases, and the system automatically generates the nursing assessment summary.

Summary

Technology resources represent important instruments to facilitate access to information and, gradually, it can be identified more and

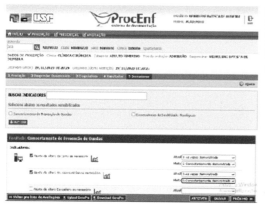 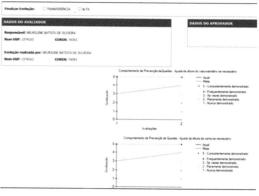

Fig. 44.3 Support system for clinical decision, PROCEnf-USP® The selection stage of Nursing Outcomes. The nurse selects the indicators, establishing the status and the goal to be achieved. Source: Screen taken by the authors on October 10, 2020. São Paulo. The University Hospital of the University São Paulo, Brazil

more possibilities to apply the resources to dynamize care activities. It is worth remembering that the more specific information we have, the better decision can be made. This statement is essential for nursing and all health professions, which are dependent on information to be able to carry out any action with quality to deliver patient care and citizen maintenance health status.

Nursing information systems are increasingly acting as catalyst agents to restructure the profession, forcing nurses to explore the nature of the profession, the essence of the practice, the body of scientific knowledge, leading them to acquire increasingly specialized skills to provide a better level of healthcare patients and citizen. The data collection and information analysis are based on quality of data collection. It is also important to emphasize that quantity does not mean quality. In fact, all data collected should provide information. Otherwise, why to spend time and resources on data collection.

Standardized terminologies are supposed to provide rationality on the nursing process. The description of this chapter summarizes few experiences on the use on terminology integrated in the nursing system.

However, the evolution in nursing informatics scenario represents a great opportunity for nursing. Adoption of technological resources in practice will make nurses see trends in the health system more clearly as a challenge and unique opportunity for growth. Thus, new roles and new careers demand specialized knowledge. The opportunities are ample for those who decide to incorporate technological resources in daily practice and to make them an instrument for improving the quality of patient care and the infrastructure to exercise the profession with dignity and the perspective of growth and development.

Since there is no single and comprehensive system as a solution to meet all the needs of the health and nursing area and innovative solutions need to be developed to respond to the increasingly complex demands of providing nursing care, it is essential that nurses are involved in the development and/or selection of computerized systems, providing knowledge and experience for planning, management, teaching, and health care. The systems must have a behavioral component, that is, one must choose a system that presents the information in an easy way for understanding and handling. Consequently, all the information and communication technology resources deployed have as main goal to assist in the provision of health care, which is assumed to be humanized, comprehensive, and effective and that meets the needs, providing relief, improvement, and dignified conditions to face the situation that imposes itself.

Conclusions and Outlook

We do need engagement to consolidate science on our field. We do need to name and to describe and to measure all phenomena we are involved to. We do need to realize that technology brings a lot of resources to support our activity. However, there is the other side of applications—the overwhelming, the adverse effect, the iatrogenic technology. Do not forget that patient is the most important—patient must be the center of our attention and subject of care. He/she is our biggest and highest interest.

Using technology we can be with our patients at distance, we can communicate, we can interact, we can prevent sudden episodes without control, we can keep on track of their health conditions, and we can also promote comfort, joy moments, and social integration. Robots are being used by researchers to analyses the possibility to control risks at home.

We need more and better analytics tools to promote continuous quality improvement; we need better clinical decision support systems and more intelligence on the electronic health records. We need to identify better use of ICT tools to support learning and education. We need better ready to respond to emerging technology. We need leaders well prepared and aware about possibilities and proactively addressing any skill set deficits of the nurse team.

With the ICT resources, we can create systems that could give strong support for nursing practice, systems that can be used to show our commitment to the health care of the population, systems that could be used to analyze our efficiency and effectiveness and verify what modifications need to be made for changing or improving our tasks as providers, researchers, and educators. Only through research using real data from nursing practice, recorded at the point of care, we can evaluate our profession and enrich our capabilities. Moreover, we can also drive the tendencies of political decisions in the professional area.

Useful Resources

1. American Medical Informatics Association – NIWG: AMIA NI-WG
2. American Nursing Informatics Association: ANIA
3. International Medical Informatics Association: IMIA
4. IMIA—Nursing Informatics Special Interest Group: IMIS NI SIG
5. *International Journal of Medical Informatics*: IJMI—https://www.journals.elsevier.com/international-journal-of-medical-informatics

Review Questions

1. Describe how the use of the information and communication technology are being applied for nursing care in Brazil to support nursing knowledge.
2. How can ICT adoption be measured?
3. Cite some indicators to support nursing system evaluations and deployment.

Appendix: Answers to Review Questions

1. Describe how the use of the information and communication technology is being applied for nursing care in Brazil to support nursing knowledge.

- Considering the international scenario and the Brazilian development in health informatics and technological resources, a national study has been conducted to pursuit consistent indicators to measure the impact of the use of information and communication technology for the health of the population. Thus, the overall objective of this study was to identify the existing infrastructure of information and communication technologies available in healthcare facilities, including the stage of implementation by these facilities and its adoption by health professionals [6].
- The study is a descriptive research being conducted annually since 2012. The sample comprised Executive and ICT Directors (CEO and CIO), physicians, and nurses included at the National Record of Healthcare Establishments (CNES), maintained by the Department of Informatics of the Ministry of Health (DATASUS, Ministry of Health). It was excluded isolated clinics, mobile units, and establishments with non-physician and non-nurses. The sample was selected by probability sampling technique considering the country region and the type of establishment (outpatient, diagnosis and therapy services, inpatient up to 50 beds, and inpatient with more than 50 beds), including both private and public facilities [6].
- Data collection was done by a questionnaire with 37 questions to understand the adoption of ICT in their daily nursing duties. As an annual investigation, the questions bring up data and information related to the last 12 months of implementation and adoption of ICT-based systems and services. The last edition published in 2019 interviewed 2716 nurses. The results showed that the use of computers by nurses while caring for patients has increased in recent years, from 79% in 2016 to 87% in 2018 [7].

- Considering professionals who reported referring to patient data electronically, password-protected access was the most commonly used security tool by 90% of nurses in 2018. On the other hand, approximately 27% said they had used digital certificates, and only 4% of nurses mentioned using biometrics-protected access to electronic systems [7].
- In 2018, nurses used electronic system functionalities less often compared to the physicians that use for prescription and surgery report. Nurses used more functionalities related to administrative activities, such as generating requests for materials and supplies and booking appointments, tests, or surgeries. Functionalities used during patient care were also among those most used by nurses, such as listing medications being taken by a specific patient and listing lab test results for a specific patient [7].
- The results of the 2018 survey also showed the persistence of low availability of decision support functionalities in healthcare facilities. Clinical guidelines and protocols were the most mentioned, available to half of nurses (52%). The second-most used, also by approximately one-third of professionals, were drug allergy alerts and reminders, drug dosage alerts and reminders, and alerts and reminders for drug interference with lab results [7].
- According to the assessment of professionals, in general, the available electronic systems were not considered adapted to their needs and daily tasks: only 37% of nurses agreed that the electronic systems were well adapted to their needs. This finding may reflect the low involvement of these professionals in the development and implementation of electronic systems in facilities, considering that 46% of nurses agreed that they had participated in this development. Furthermore, approximately half of the

professionals from both categories agreed that they were trained and motivated to use the facilities' electronic systems [7].
- The perception of nurses about the impact of the use of electronic systems in their activities is an important indicator to understand ICT appropriation by these professionals. In 2018, the greatest benefits of using electronic systems were related to security and confidentiality of information, as mentioned by 63% of nurses. The possibility of exchanging information among the electronic systems of different healthcare facilities was identified by 34% of nurses. However, among both types of professionals, a low percentage agreed that the financial resources for investment in electronic systems were adequate to meet facility needs (29% of nurses), which can point to difficulties faced by them when using the available systems. Furthermore, 47% of nurses agreed that governmental policies encouraged the implementation and use of electronic systems in the facilities [7].

2. How can ICT adoption be measured?

ICT adoption can be measured by:
- Identify the existing infrastructure of information and communication technologies available in healthcare facilities, including the stage of implementation by these facilities and its adoption by health professional.
- Research on the perception of professionals in relation to the impact of adopting computerized systems in increasing or decreasing the workload with the use of computers and the Internet; improving the efficiency of teamwork processes; in the perception that electronic systems have led to greater service efficiency.
- Evaluate the quality of health information and nursing process records. To this end, computerized systems can support patient

care through the quality of data collected, recorded, and analyzed. Professionals from various countries develop initiatives to use standardized terminologies in the nursing process. The most used over the decades were the International Classification of Nursing Interventions (CIPE®), the NANDA-International structures, the Classification of Results (NOC), and the Classification of Interventions (NIC).

3. Cite some indicators to support nursing system evaluations and deployment.

- The system can be evaluated in terms of effectiveness, efficiency, and satisfaction;
- Effectiveness refers to the "precision and integrity with which users achieve specified objectives";
- Efficiency refers to the "resources used (time, human effort, costs and materials) in relation to the results achieved";
- Efficiency was assessed by surveying the time spent by nurses to document the nursing assessment in the system. Time was correlated with the number of diagnostics, outcomes, indicators, interventions, and evaluation activities. A positive correlation was observed between the time and the number of items in the evaluation. It can be inferred that the greater the complexity of the patient health situation, the greater the time spent on the evaluation;
- Satisfaction is defined as "the extent to which the physical, cognitive and emotional responses resulting from the use of a system, product or service meet the needs and expectations of the user". In other words, satisfaction measures the user experience when using the system;
- The perception of nurses about the impact of the use of electronic systems in their activities is an important indicator to understand ICT appropriation by these professionals.

References

1. ISO 9241:11. Ergonomics of human-system interaction – Part:11 Usability: definitions and concepts. Switzerland; 2018. Available www.iso.org/standard/63500.html
2. Marin HF, Delaney C. Patient engagement and digital health communities. In: Marin HF, Massad E, Gutierrez MA, Rodrigues RJ, Sigulem D, editors. Global health informatics. New York: Elsevier; 2017. p. 218–31.
3. Kem ZG. Searching for an integrated strategy in chronic disease management: a potential role for information and communication technologies. Manag Health. 2011;15(4)
4. World Health Organization. Global Observatory for eHealth Featured Project, 2010. Available from: http://www.who.int/goe/en/. Accessed 03 Apr 2020.
5. European Commission. eHealth benchmarking (phase II). Final Report. European Commission, Empirica. 2010.
6. Brazilian Internet Steering Committee – CGI. BR. Survey on the use of information and communication technology in Brazilian Healthcare Facilities – ICT health 2013. São Paulo: CGI; 2014.
7. Brazilian Internet Steering Committee – CGI. BR. Survey on the use of information and communication technology in Brazilian Healthcare Facilities – ICT health 2018. São Paulo: CGI; 2019.
8. Brazilian General Data Protection Law – LGPD. Law no. 13.709, of August 14, 2018 (2018). Addresses the processing of personal data, including in digital media, by natural or legal persons, of public or private law, with the goal of protecting the fundamental rights of freedom and privacy and the free development of the personality of natural persons. Brasília, DF. Retrieved on August 15, 2019. Available from http://www.planalto.gov.br/ccivil_03/_Ato2015-2018/2018/Lei/L13709.htm
9. International Council of Nurses. International classification for nursing practice version 1. Geneva: The Association; 2005.
10. Nursing Diagnoses: Definitions and Classification 2018-2020. 11th New York: Thieme; 2017, 512p.
11. Moorhead S, Swanson E, Johnson M, Maas M. Nursing outcomes classification (NOC): measurement of health outcomes. 6th ed. Philadelphia: Elsevier; 2018. p. 671.
12. Butcher HK, Bulechek GM, Dochterman J, Wagner CM. Nursing interventions classification (NIC). 7th ed. Philadelphia: Elsevier; 2018. p. 512.
13. Beserra PJF, Gomes GLL, Santos MCF, Bittencourt GKGD, Nóbrega MML. Scientific production of the international classification for nursing practice: a bibliometric study. Rev Bras Enferm [Internet]. 2018;71(6):2860–8. https://doi.org/10.1590/0034-7167-2017-0411.

14. Oliveira MDS, Roque e Lima JO, Garcia TR, Bachion MM. Termos úteis à prática de enfermagem na atenção a pessoas com hanseníase. Rev Bras Enferm [Internet]. 2019;72(3):744–52. https://doi.org/10.1590/0034-7167-2017-0684.

15. Souza Neto VL, Costa RTS, Belmiro SSDR, Lima MA, Silva RAR. ICNP® Diagnoses of people living with AIDS, and empirical indicators. Rev Bras Enferm. 2018;72(5):1226–34. https://doi.org/10.1590/0034-7167-2017-0850.

16. Meneses LBA, Medeiros FAL, Oliveira JS, Nóbrega MML, Silva MAD, Soares MJGO. Revista Brasileira de Enfermagem jun. 2020;73(4):e20190258. https://doi.org/10.1590/0034-7167-2019-0258

17. Kirakowski J, Corbett M. SUMI: the software usability measurement inventory. Br J Educ Technol. 1993;24(3):210–2. https://doi.org/10.1111/j.1467-8535.1993.tb00076.x.

18. Passinho RS, Primo CC, Fioresi M, Nóbrega MML, Brandão MAG, Romero WG. Elaboration and validation of an ICNP® terminology subset for patients with acute myocardial infarction. Rev Esc Enferm USP. 2019;53:e03442. https://doi.org/10.1590/S1980-220X2018000603442.

19. Diogo RCS. Evaluation of the accuracy of nursing diagnoses determined by users of a clinical decision support system. [Thesis]. São Paulo: School of Nurse. University of São Paulo; 2019.

20. Oliveira NB. Usability evaluation nursing process-clinical decision support system [Thesis]. São Paulo: School of Nurse. University of São Paulo; 2020.

21. ISO/IEC 14598-6:2004: engenharia de software: avaliação de produto -Parte 6: documentação de módulos de avaliação. Associação Brasileira de Normas Técnicas Rio de Janeiro; 2004.

22. Linch GFC, Rabelo-Silva ER, Keenan GM, Moraes MA, Stifter J, Müller-Staub M. Validation of the quality of diagnoses, interventions, and outcomes (Q-DIO) instrument for USE in Brazil and the United States. Int J Nurs Knowl. 2015;26(1):19–25.

23. Kirakowski J. Background notes on the SUMI questionnaire. Available from http://sumi.uxp.ie/about/sumipapp.html

24. Oliveira NB, Peres HHC. Evaluation of the functional performance and technical quality of an Electronic Documentation System of the Nursing Process. Rev Latino-Am Enfermagem. 2015;23(2):242–9. Available from https://doi.org/10.1590/0104-1169.3562.2548

25. Melleiro MM, Fugulin FMT, Rogenski NMB, Gonçalves VLM, Tronchin DMR. A evolução do sistema de assistência de enfermagem no Hospital Universitário da Universidade de São Paulo: uma história de 30 anos. In: Cianciarullo TI, DMR G, Melleiro MM, Anabuki MM, editors. Sistema de assistência de enfermagem: evolução e tendências. 5th ed. São Paulo: Ícone; 2012. p. 85–102.

26. Peres HHC, Cruz DALM, Lima AFC, Gaidzinski RR, Ortiz DCF, Trindade MM et al. Development electronic systems of nursing clinical documentation structured by diagnosis, outcomes and interventions. Rev Esc Enferm USP. 2009; 43(spe2):1149–1155. Available from https://doi.org/10.1590/S0080-62342009000600002

27. Johnson M, Moorhead S, Bulechek G, Butcher H, Maas M, Swanson E. NOC and NIC linkages to NANDA-I and clinical conditions: supporting critical thinking and quality care. 3th ed. Philadelphia: Elsevier; 2011. p. 432.

28. Müller-Staub M, de Graaf-Waar H, Paans W. An internationally consented standard for nursing process-clinical decision support systems in electronic health records. Comput Inform Nursing. 2016;3411:493–502.

29. Maia F, Cruz D, Shimoda G, Sichieri K, Inaba SL (2018). Falls prevention strategies for adult inpatients in a university hospital of São Paulo, Brazil: a best practice implementation project. JBI database of systematic reviews and implementation reports. 1720–1736. https://doi.org/10.11124/JBISRIR-2017-003556

30. Brasil. Conselho Federal de Enfermagem. Resolução n° 358 de 15/10/2009. Diário Oficial da União. Brasília, 23 out. 2009, Seção 1, p.179.

Health IT Across Health Care Systems: Finland, Germany and the U.S.

45

Laura Naumann and Hendrike Berger

Learning Objectives

Introducing Health IT is a challenge for politicians, health care professionals, and decision makers across the globe. Thus, learning from the experiences in other health care systems is a common strategy. This chapter offers an overview of how a country comparison on Health IT might look. In this context, readers of this chapter will learn about the following aspects:

- Differences in health care systems across the world
- Typical procedures and measurements of how to compare Health IT across countries
- Differences in Health IT in selected countries with different health care systems
- Limitations and strengths of country comparisons on Health IT

Key Terms

- Health IT
- Global health IT
- Typology of health care systems
- Health care system comparisons
- Health policy
- Finland
- Germany
- United States

L. Naumann · H. Berger (✉)
University AS Osnabrück, Osnabrück, Germany
e-mail: l.naumann@hs-osnabrueck.de;
h.berger@hs-osnabrueck.de

Introduction

Overview

Policy makers across the world are facing the challenge of keeping up the pace in Health IT developments. Approaches to tackling Health IT differ, as do the circumstances in which Health IT is introduced, set up, and used. Even though each country has to meet its specific needs in terms of Health IT, looking at other countries' experiences can be an interesting focal point for reflections on one's own path as well as for new ideas and alternate approaches. In order to conduct a country comparison on Health IT, readers of this chapter will learn about relevant country-specific features (such as size, population density, extent of health care funding). With currently 193 different sovereign states listed within the United Nations, this chapter can only present a brief excerpt of the full picture, mostly relying on aggregated data from global institutions like the WHO (World Health Organization) or the OECD (Organisation for Economic Co-operation and Development). Nevertheless, we hope to give the reader an understanding of how Health IT can be studied globally and how to put the international findings into context:

1. Measuring Health IT across countries: How is it done and what does the research reveal?

2. Exemplary cases: The lessons learned so far will be demonstrated referring to selected countries, illustrating the history, specific challenges, progress, and setbacks, as well as a short overview of recent developments.
3. Limitations and strengths: Cross-country comparisons alone have their confines, which need to be considered in interpretation and deriving implications.

To address these topics and questions some prior additional information and explanations may help. Therefore, this introductory paragraph will elaborate on health care systems and how to compare them. It will also provide introductory explanations on Health IT in this specific context.

Health Care Systems in Comparison

Health care system comparisons are a relatively common approach in health economic research. Country-specific regulations affected by history, culture, geography, demographics, economy, and so on play a major role in a country's understanding of welfare and, related to this, a country's understanding of how health care is provided for its society. Comparing health care systems across the world reveals a great amount of heterogeneity in the designs of health care systems. Nevertheless, commonalities can also be identified, and health care systems can be clustered.

Typologies of Health Care Systems
There are many health care system typologies and proposals for health care classifications [1]. For the sake of simplicity, we will rely on the following three health care system types [2] (Fig. 45.1).

Private Health Insurance Systems
Private Health Insurance (PHI) systems rely primarily on a competitive market. Providers of health insurance are organized as private companies, insurances can be purchased by individuals or employers. Insurance fees are calculated based on the individual risk of getting sick and likely costs of health care provision. The public regulations are of minor importance as compared to the other types of health systems. The government may set the framework, but there may be no legal requirements for citizens to purchase health insurance, nor an obligation to contract for insurance (meaning individuals can be rejected when they apply for insurance). Consequently, the consumer sovereignty is high in these systems. For example, the US health care system in large part is considered a PHI system.

Social Health Insurance Systems
In Social Health Insurance (SHI) systems it is mandatory for citizens to sign up and hence be covered by public (statutory) health insurance. The health system is funded by insurance fees, typically collected from employers and employees based on salaries. Within these systems the aspect of solidarity in the society plays an important part. Therefore, an insurance fee is not determined by the individual risk of getting sick but rather by the person's income level. The provision of care can be supplied by public or private providers. The system is organized via a self-government of relevant stakeholders and supervised by the central government. For instance, Germany, Austria, France, and Japan are typically characterized as SHI systems.

Health System Types

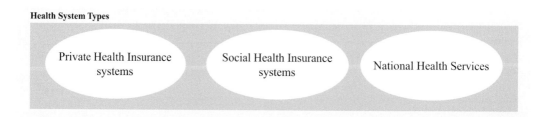

Private Health Insurance systems

Social Health Insurance systems

National Health Services

Fig. 45.1 Simplified systematic of health system types [2]. Own illustration

Health System Institutional Characteristics

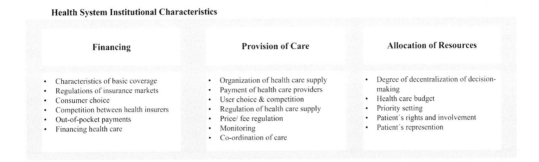

Financing	Provision of Care	Allocation of Resources
• Characteristics of basic coverage	• Organization of health care supply	• Degree of decentralization of decision-
• Regulations of insurance markets	• Payment of health care providers	making
• Consumer choice	• User choice & competition	• Health care budget
• Competition between health insurers	• Regulation of health care supply	• Priority setting
• Out-of-pocket payments	• Price/ fee regulation	• Patient´s rights and involvement
• Financing health care	• Monitoring	• Patient´s represention
	• Co-ordination of care	

Fig. 45.2 Institutional characteristics of health care systems (cf. [4]). No claim for completeness. Own illustration

National Health Services

In health care systems which are described as National Health Services (NHS) the responsibility for providing and organizing health care lies directly in the hands of the government. Tasks involving implications for the whole population (such as Health IT or planning of tertiary care) lie with the central government, while other tasks with a more regional impact are looked after by regional or communal governments (such as the organization of community care). The following characteristics are typical of National Health Services. The health care system is funded through tax revenues and is controlled by the government. There is no need for health insurance because health care is provided by the government for all citizens. Consequently, there is relatively equal access to publicly provided health care and equal scope of available services. In NHS systems, health care providers such as doctors and nurses are commonly employees of public institutions. For instance, the health systems in Great Britain, Finland, and New Zealand are considered NHS systems.

It is worth noting that the depicted health care system types are rather simplistic classifications which might not adequately describe every health care system in the world. For our purposes, however, this classification will suffice. For more sophisticated approaches and discussions on how to classify health care across the globe, please see the following articles: [1, 3], European Observatory on Health Systems and Policies 2020.

Organizing the Delivery of Care

In addition to typology, health care systems can differ in their institutional structure. This applies to (a) financing, (b) provision of care, and (c) allocation of resources [4] (Fig. 45.2).

Financing

Health care services can be financed through different schemes: taxes, social insurance contributions, private insurance contributions, medical saving accounts, and out-of-pocket payments are all sources of financing health care. Different countries use different methods of financing or combine different methods. Based on the financing model there may be different incentives which may lead to different patterns of behavior on the side of stakeholders of a health care system (payers, providers, patients, politicians). This can influence the adoption of new technologies or Health IT, for instance.

Provision of Care

Health care services can be provided by public or private organizations, or by a combination of the two. Also, there are differences in the freedom to choose between health care providers; for instance, access to specialized care may be gated in one health care system which is not common in other health care systems (patient autonomy). Finally, there is the question as to whether purchasers and providers are organizationally separate ("purchaser-provider split") or whether purchaser and provider act as one entity.

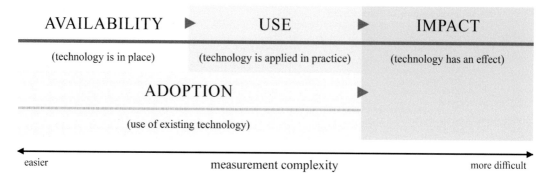

Fig. 45.3 Key terms of Health IT. Own illustration

Allocation of Resources

Finally, the organization of health care may differ in terms of the allocation of resources. Four different organizational forms are possible: (a) direct payment principle (health care providers are directly paid by patients for services rendered), (b) reimbursement of expenses (health care providers are directly paid by patients for services rendered, and the patient is later reimbursed by his/her health insurance), (c) benefit-in-kind-principle (health care providers are directly paid by health insurances or the NHS, no payment from the patient is required), or (d) cost sharing principle (the patient pays a share of the cost for services rendered (deductibles) while the rest is paid for by insurance or the NHS; this can be combined with (b) and/or (c). Hence, there are various options for the design of a health care system. Depending on the chosen model and practices, Health IT must fit in versatile settings, which may be unique to each country.

Health IT: Availability, Adoption, Use, and Diffusion

Literature sometimes reveals a lack of clear distinctions between terms such as *availability* and *use* [5]. Additionally, the term *adoption* commonly occurs. According to Villumsen and colleagues, *adoption* is utilized as a proxy for actual use when the availability of Health IT is measured. For instance, successful adoption was defined as the status when an adopter recognizes an innovation and is able to implement and use it

meaningfully [6]. As a short overview, Fig. 45.3 systematizes the central terms of Health IT.

In research practice, the most frequently applied approach is to focus on the availability or adoption of Health IT [7]. A study by Greenhalgh and colleagues identified "key attributes" which may explain why individuals may adopt one innovation and ignore another:

- Relative advantage: clear advantage, e.g., regarding cost-effectiveness or effectiveness
- Compatibility: in relation to values, norms, and perceived needs
- Trialability: innovations, offered to the user for testing
- Observability: visible benefits
- Reinvention: options to adapt, refine, or modify according to individual needs
- Fuzzy boundaries: "soft periphery" of innovations, adaptiveness

Research suggests that innovations are adopted more easily if they fulfill these attributes [8].

A similar question arising in this context is: How do information technologies enter everyday care practice? In related research, Rogers' theory of "Diffusion of innovations" [9] is usually consulted to describe how innovations spread. Greenhalgh et al. studied the diffusion of innovation in health care organizations (by conducting a systematic literature review). In their study they used the following distinction for the different terms to describe the field more accurately, which are useful for a better understanding:

Diffusion:	Diffusion is defined as a passive spread of innovations.
Dissemination:	Dissemination is described as an active, planned effort aiming to make target groups adopt innovations.
Implementation:	Implementation is defined as an active, planned effort to maintain an innovation within an organization.
Sustainability:	Sustainability is considered as the integration of an innovation as a routine until it is outdated.

Greenhalgh et al. [8]

These definitions highlight the fact that Health IT encompasses various facets and different levels of involvement. Related research in this context may focus on particular IT innovations [10] or on the macro level, comparing different countries [11, 12].

However, diffusion theories are not flawless and limitations need to be considered: diffusion of innovation may be influenced by multiple factors, and it is not likely that one diffusion theory can incorporate all of those factors adequately. Also, most theories are displayed as linear, which does not necessarily reflect reality [8, 9, 13]. Beyond the mere availability, adoption, or use of an IT solution it is also interesting to take on the actual usage in practice. However, these kinds of studies are less common [7].

Challenges in the Process of Introducing Health IT

Introducing Health IT into existing health care structures and processes poses a challenge. There are many small and big stories on failure [14]. Systemizing this complexity, Greenhalgh et al. [15] offer a comprehensive framework for Nonadoption, Abandonment, and Challenges to the Scale-Up, Spread, and Sustainability of Health and Care Technologies, (NASSS) [15]. This theory acknowledges different settings, for different solutions, and summarizes the challenges within health care systems at micro, meso, and macro level:

1. **Condition**: Field of application (for which illness, conditions, considering sociocultural factors)

2. **Technology**: Features of the technology (material, required data, needed support/knowledge)
3. **Value Proposition**: Beneficiaries of the technology (developer perspective: financial aspect vs patient perspective: e.g., safety)
4. **Adopters**: Adoption and continued use of staff or patients or caregivers
5. **Organization**: Capacity and readiness for a technology, disruption of routines, implementation work
6. **Wider System**: Political, legal, professional, sociocultural context
7. **Embedding and Adaption over time**: Scope and organizational resilience [15].

Also, health care systems should not be regarded as a monolithic block: even within one national context, Health IT can show different levels of progress. For instance, differences between privately and publicly funded health care providers or urban vs rural areas may occur [16].

International Efforts

As indicated, studying Health IT is a comprehensive endeavor [5]. Benchmarking across country borders is a common phenomenon in research: the Nordic countries in Europe, the OECD, and the World Health Organization (WHO) are prominent players in this context offering comprehensive methodological recommendations for monitoring Health IT in a comparable way. The most common method to collect data is via surveys [5].

Nordic eHealth Benchmarking

The *Nordic eHealth Benchmarking* is carried out through a cooperation between the Nordic countries (i.e., Denmark, Finland, Iceland, Norway, Sweden, the Faroe Islands, Greenland, and Åland). It is a regional partnership. These countries set up the Nordic eHealth Research Network in 2012 to measure the Health IT developments with a set of common indicators. The Nordic countries exhibit similarities in their health care systems, which makes a comparison easier, and experiences from one country may be more applicable or interesting to another one. This cooperation aims for cross-country learning [17]. The network has a mandate from the Nordic Council of Ministers for conducting their research. Three mandates with the following topics have been carried out so far and were published by the research network [18]:

1. **2012–2013:** Developing/testing of common eHealth indicators [17]
2. **2013–2015:** Extension of the common indicators, lessons learned, benchmarking between the Nordic countries [19]
3. **2015–2017:** Long-term study of the development ("from piloting towards established practice") [18]

The most recent Nordic eHealth Benchmarking [18] showed in all Nordic countries a trend toward governance (establishment of policies and monitoring of their implementation) and patient empowerment (e.g., by enabling patients to access and manage their own health data). Formerly there was a greater emphasis on establishing the technical infrastructure. The Nordic eHealth Benchmarking is also working together with the European Union, the OECD, and the WHO.

OECD: ICT Benchmarking

Within the OECD efforts to measure Health IT date back to 2008 (OECD). The OECD decided to approach the benchmarking to measure Health ICTs (Information and Communication Technologies) across countries as a "continuum": the concept starts with measuring availability of Health IT, followed by its effective use, and finally by measuring the impact of Health IT [20]. Also, the OECD chose to design a model survey framework to offer a tool for countries to measure Health IT in a comparable way [21]. The framework consists of core and add-on-modules, which allows countries to adjust the survey according to their national needs, yet remain within an internationally comparable scope.

The survey includes four broad categories, which can be surveyed [21]:

1. **Provider-centered electronic records**
2. **Patient-centered electronic records**
3. **Health Information Exchange**
4. **Telehealth**

A study by Zelmer and colleagues assessed in a pilot the use of the OECD guide to measure ICTs in the health care sector in 38 OECD and non-OECD countries. The research showed that the OECD guide can be applied to different countries, offering an opportunity to collect comparable data across borders. Among other things, this study identified as a similarity across countries that progress in a distinct care setting (either primary or secondary) was more easily achieved than in cross-sectional settings; in other words, providing Health IT that connects different care settings (i.e., Health Information Exchange, e.g., from out-patient to in-patient care or vice versa) seems to be a greater challenge [22].

The goals of the OECD align with the objectives named by the Nordic eHealth Benchmarking [21]: The OECD is striving to identify best practice examples, drawing attention to barriers and facilitators experienced by countries while trying to promote Health IT. Also the OECD provides assistance during the introduction of Health IT and corresponding programs [22].

WHO: Atlas of eHealth Country Profiles

The WHO provides an atlas of eHealth country profiles which are considered a "snapshot" of the current Health IT situation based on selected, comparable indicators. The data for the country profiles were collected through expert surveys by WHO Global Observatory for eHealth; 125 member countries participated [23]. Besides country context information (such as population size or economic status) the survey covers the following topics:

1. **eHealth foundation**: Policies/strategies, funding, multilingualism, capacity building
2. **Legal framework**: Policies and legislation
3. **Telehealth**: Operating level of telehealth services (from international to local) and types of programs (informal, pilot, or established telehealth services)

4. **Electronic Health Records (EHR)**: State of adoption, existing national EHRs, level of use (in which care setting, in what proportion)
5. **Use of eLearning in health science**: Pre-service education for students, or self-training for professionals
6. **mHealth**: Level of mHealth Services from international to local and types of programs (informal, pilot, or established mHealth services)
7. **Social media**: Policies/strategies to use social media by health care providers, individuals, or communities
8. **Big Data**: Policies/strategies of the government to include Big Data

This survey is the third report by the WHO Global Observatory for eHealth. In comparison to the 2010 survey, the WHO noted an uptake on eHealth across its members. The atlas of eHealth country profiles is complemented by another WHO report which does not focus on the distinct country developments, but rather on specific Health IT topics (Nr. 1–8) [24].

Considering the three depicted approaches to monitoring Health IT across country borders (the Nordic eHealth Benchmarking, the OECD ICT benchmarking, and the WHO atlas of eHealth country profiles), they reveal some similarities and differences. On the one hand, the scope of included countries is the most obvious difference. Besides this factor there are also slightly different thematic emphases. However, the methods and goals used are quite similar.

The OECD and the Nordic eHealth Benchmarking encompass high-income countries. The majority of publications in this specific field originate from Europe (especially Northern Europe) and North America (especially the United States) [5]. Health IT is also of relevance in low- and middle-income countries and may offer a potential to improve health care delivery [25] but this is not addressed in this chapter.

In summary, international research offers a range of methods for gathering data in a comparable manner. Furthermore, research offers explanations and insights on how Health IT is studied across countries. Usually the situation in a coun-

try cannot be explained through linear, single factors and coherencies. To describe the challenges at hand in a more tangible way, the following case study will illustrate and compare the circumstances in selected countries.

Comparing the Health IT Developments in Finland, Germany, and the United States

General Features of the Three Selected Countries

This chapter highlights the above-mentioned research efforts by focusing on three selected countries: Finland, Germany, and the United States. As an overview, Table 45.1 gives a first brief idea about the key features of the countries and their respective health care systems.

The information provided in Table 45.1 indicates similarities and differences across Finland, Germany, and the United States. To point out one aspect: the health care systems in the three countries are responsible for different numbers of people and the people are distributed differently across the country (see Population: total number and density). The common denominator is that all of these countries are considered high-income countries and that they spend relatively large sums on health care (see Health expenditure; the average value in the OECD is 8.8% of the GDP). Since these figures do not reveal how the different health care systems are constructed and organized, Table 45.2 offers an overview of the three systems:

The information in Table 45.2 provides a brief overview of the three different health care systems in Finland, Germany, and the United States. Health care systems have grown over time and are shaped by the distinct societal, political, and economic conditions. These circumstances can lead to complex structures and mechanisms. In addition, this is not a complete process: health care systems are often subject to change due to health care reforms. For our topic—Health IT—this means that the introduction of technological innovations to the health care systems is

Table 45.1 General characteristics of the selected countries

	Population, total (2018)[a]	Land area, sq. km[b]	Population density, per sq. km (2016)[a]	Population + 65 years (2018)[c]	GDP per capita (2018)[a]	Health expenditure (% of GDP) (2018)[c]	Hospitals per m. population (2017)[c]
FIN	5,5 m	338,000	18.1	21.4%	50,152 USD	9.0%	44.8
GER	82,9 m	357,000	236	21.4%	47,603 USD	11.5%	37.3
USA	326, 7 m	9,700,000	35.4	16.0%	62,794 USD	16.9%	19.1

[a]https://databank.worldbank.org
[b]https://www.hspm.org/
[c]https://stats.oecd.org/

Table 45.2 Description of the health care systems of the selected countries

	Type	Financing	Provision of care	Allocation of resources
FIN	NHS	There are two sources of financing: (1) municipality financing based on taxes and (2) compulsory insurance fees (National Health insurance, NHI), e.g., for outpatient drugs and transportation cost. There is no clear purchaser-provider split in the health care provided by the municipalities.	Municipalities are obliged to maintain primary care health centers for their residents (on their own or with other municipalities). Specialized care is provided through 21 hospital districts. Municipalities can purchase services from other municipalities. Municipalities can also purchase services from private health care providers.	Since a reform in 1993 the Finish health care system is highly decentralized. Health care is weakly regulated by the central government, and the municipalities are mainly responsible for health care. There is a strong focus on health promotion. However, new reform projects are aiming for greater privatization in the Finnish health care system as well.
GER	SHI	Financing mostly comes from insurance fees. Health insurance is mandatory: (1) either via social health insurance (covering approximately 85% of the population) or (2) via private health insurances (covering approximately 11% of the population). Taxes as a source of funding play only a minor role.	Traditionally, there is a clear institutional separation between the different care sectors. A mix of public, private, and church-based institutions provide health care services. Public health services (such as health education and promotion) are provided by approximately 350 public health offices (regional differences).	It is described as a "self-regulated" system: the decision-making power is distributed between the state, federal level and legitimized "self-governing bodies" (corporatist associations representing different players, such as health care providers). These institutions are required by law to ensure the provision of care for the population. The scope of services is legally defined.
USA	PHI	Coverage of health care services through private health insurance (health insurance is not mandatory; often insurance is obtained through the employer) Out-of-pocket costs for patients are common. Payments differ depending on the service provided. There is also public financing (at federal, state, and local level), e.g., for Medicare or Medicaid. The care system for the military/veterans is detached from the PHI system and is funded through federal public funding.	The private sector plays a stronger role. Public and private payers can purchase services from health care providers. The largest public purchaser is Medicare (for Americans +65 years). Insured patients usually enter the system through their primary care physician; uninsured patients usually enter the system through community health clinics or emergency rooms.	Decentralization: the power is divided between federal and state governments. There is relatively limited regulation, planning, and coordination for the entire US health care system. Public health is organized through local health departments and they can operate independently to some extent; however, these departments depend on public funding (state or federal).

See: https://www.hspm.org/

confronted with a variety of different framework conditions (which can evolve over time); this poses individual challenges for each country.

Health IT in the Three Selected Countries

How Finland, Germany, and the United States perform in the described international comparisons is displayed in Tables 45.3 and 45.4. This overview includes only the data from the OECD and the WHO. The Nordic eHealth Benchmarking does not offer information on Germany and the United States—therefore, it would not add value to this comparison.

In summary, the data presented in Tables 45.3 and 45.4 from the OECD [22] and the WHO [23] indicate a better performance of Finland in comparison to Germany and the United States. The data also show a wide range of Health IT solutions that have appeared in health care systems. The data from these two selected studies indicate different levels of progress, depending

on the respective health sectors and Health IT applications in question. The data from Tables 45.3 and 45.4 also highlight the confines of consulting international comparisons like these: the given data may be incomplete, either because not every question was answered or because not every country participated in a study. Therefore, international efforts like the ones presented are a useful starting point but for details and specific information about the situation, latest progress, and coherencies, additional sources must be consulted. The following brief examples will give you an idea about the country-specific Health IT contexts and developments.

Finland: Status Quo and Perspective
As suggested by the previous data, Finland has made progress in implementing Health IT services. A report from 2019 summarizes the situation in Finland (Vehko et al. [26]): first steps toward introducing Health IT on a national scale in the health care system date back to 1995. Since then strategies have been updated to fit new requirements. As indicated in the segment on the

Table 45.3 Synthesis of the OECD data by [22] (selected indicators)

	% of primary care practices that use electronic systems to store and manage patient health information	% of acute care facilities that exchange radiology results/ images electronically with outside organizations	% of acute care facilities that have synchronous telehealth capabilities	% access to test results online	% e-appointment booking	e-request for prescription renewal/ refill	Secure messaging (asynchronous)
FIN	75–100%	75–100%	<50%	<50%	<50%	<50%	<50%
GER	75–100%	50–74%	<50%	<50%	<50%	<50%	<50%
USA	75–100%	50–74%	n.a.	n.a.	n.a.	n.a.	<50%

n.a. no data available

Table 45.4 Synthesis of the WHO atlas of eHealth country profiles for Finland and the United States (selected indicators)

	National eHealth policy or strategy	Tele-radiology (program type)	National EHR system	Primary care facilities with EHRs	Secondary care facilities with EHRs	Laboratory information systems	Mobile telehealth (program type)
FIN	Yes	Established	Yes	>75%	>75%	Yes	Established
USA	Yes	Not applicable	No	Un-answered	Un-answered	Not applicable	Established

Germany did not participate in this WHO survey [23]

Nordic eHealth Benchmarking, Finland collaborates in international efforts to measure and monitor Health IT. Beyond availability and use of IT applications, Finland also shows efforts to study user experiences. The latest report from 2019 shows that digitalization has spread extensively in the Finnish health care system: there is an adequate infrastructure to connect care sectors and regions, and the use of Health Information Exchange (e.g., the data exchange between inpatient and out-patient health care providers) revealed better results. Electronic patient records (for professional health care providers) are applied in practice. Also, services for citizens (e.g., electronic appointment booking, advisory services, and access to and viewing of test results) have increased. However, the study also identified the need to improve Health IT services for citizens.

Germany: Status Quo and Perspective
Germany's first eHealth initiatives date back to 2003 and have been followed by a series of laws ever since. A lot of the efforts were concentrated on the electronic health card (eGK); however, the experiences were accompanied by controversies, delays, and setbacks [27]. In 2015 a new E-Health Act passed to foster the Health IT infrastructure and Health IT applications. The Act was accompanied by concrete deadlines, incentives, and sanctions [28]. The digitalization of the German hospital sector has been monitored and measured repeatedly with the *IT-Report Healthcare* [29]. While progress in Health IT in the hospital sector is notable, the development of diffusion of hospitals' EHRs slowed down in Germany [11], and Health Information Exchange across providers and also the electronic communication with patients were identified as fields which leave room for improvement [30]. The lack of a successful central digitalization strategy and the necessary funding of a well-connected IT infrastructure may in part be explained by the many stakeholders that are responsible for decisions in the German health care system. However, the current Covid-19 pandemic seems to be accelerating digitalization efforts, e. g.,. in public health offices or by setting up—on short notice—a central electronic register to track the availability of intensive care beds including ventilators across Germany.

United States: Status Quo and Perspective
The development of Health IT in the United States is marked by the HITECH Act (*Health Information Technology for Economic and Clinical Health* Act) and its *Meaningful Use* incentive program from 2009. In the course of this program, physicians and hospitals could receive financial incentives when they adopted electronic health records. As a result, EHR adoption increased [28]. Yet, the developments across the hospital sector are heterogeneous, and while there is an increase in EHR adoption in hospitals, the use of advanced EHR functionalities is lagging behind [16]. The HITECH Act has been acknowledged as beneficial for the Health IT development; however, for the future there are calls for a greater focus on user needs and collaboration [31] or stronger policies and more incentives for Health IT [32]. Currently, the debate on Health IT in the United States is concentrated on Health Information Exchange between care sectors as a next priority [28].

Synopsis: Health IT in Finland, Germany, and the United States
The examples highlight the different emphases in the three selected countries: while Finland is directing its Health IT efforts toward citizens' needs, the tasks at hand in Germany and the United States have a different focus: the digitalization of the hospital sector is receiving a lot of attention, and the ongoing fostering of Health Information Exchange has been identified as an upcoming task. Even though the near future priorities may differ between Finland on the one side and Germany and the United States on the other, these insights may be of relevance: the experiences from Finland may sketch out prospective challenges.

Limitations and Strengths

Comparing health care systems has certain limitations and strengths that should be considered. The following case study highlights and illustrates the advantages and limitations of such an approach.

Self-reporting

Conducting surveys is a common way to gather data in this research context. There may be a risk of biases: recall bias may occur or participants may answer in a socially desirable way [5]. It is also important to consider which experts were surveyed and if they were able to provide country-representative answers. The WHO, for instance, explicitly acknowledges these problems [23]. However, surveys are cost-efficient tools to gather a lot of data in a standardized way from many countries.

Different Understandings

Research shows there are inconsistencies in the literature referring to the terms Health IT availability, adoption, and use [5]. Due to its nature, the field of Health IT is changing and evolving over time; however, for the synonym eHealth, which is often used to refer to the field, there is no universally accepted definition of what is covered by the term and what is not [33]. Nevertheless, international efforts by the Nordic countries, the OECD, the WHO, etc. are under way to help to establish a more uniform language.

Available Data

The given data from the major international efforts like the OECD or the WHO can be ambiguous. The data has the advantage that it usually covers a breadth of information from many countries. Usually this data is available for free and often the homepages of the institutions offer search engines to modify and specify the query. Accordingly, these services are easily accessible, user friendly, and provide a lot of information. Yet, the given data is usually supplied in aggregated form: therefore, one has no insights into the raw data, and it is not always clear how an aggregated value is composed. Still, the aggregation of data offers an opportunity to compare values across countries in a feasible manner.

Beyond aggregation, an incomplete dataset can pose a problem. As shown in the case study of Finland, Germany, and the United States (Sect. 2.1), no matter how comprehensive the international studies are, there is always the possibility that individual countries are not included or did not participate and that questions are not answered. Depending on the selected countries, selected parameters, and the availability of data, the comparability can be extremely limited in some cases. Therefore, for a more realistic view, we recommend seeking information from local health and IT professionals. Interviews, surveys with representatives, or even site visits may be associated with additional work, but will provide solid and tangible insights.

Comparability

In addition, the issue of comparability needs to be kept in mind. As the comparative case study of Finland, Germany, and the United States indicated, health care systems can operate in vastly different circumstances. Solutions that fit one health care system—with its distinct population, organization of care, structures, and processes—do not necessarily apply in another country. However, lessons learned from other countries can be very insightful: Especially issues like avoiding common mistakes or identifying areas for improvement can be useful points to look at.

Longitudinal Efforts

The Nordic eHealth Benchmarking, the OECD, and the WHO have chosen procedures to study the development of Health IT by repeating the studies and by extending the Health IT indicators. Besides cross-country comparisons this allows for analysis and tracking over time and to adjust the research measures to new developments accordingly. Due to the dynamics of the field this approach seems appropriate, offering many insights into the evolution of Health IT.

Case Study

Guideline "How to Compare Health IT Across Countries"

We provide this guideline because we think this approach can lead readers through a complex topic in a simple way: even though it's a multi-layered topic, conducting country comparisons on Health IT can be a feasible task. This guideline may help to systemize and structure the process and tailor it according to your research questions; also, it points out limitations for reflection. The outlined steps correspond with the procedures in Sects. 2.1–2.3 (comparison between Finland, Germany, and the United States). The following is our recommendation:

HEALTH IT COUNTRY COMPARISON SCHEME

(1) Country selection: Q: Which countries would you like to compare and why?	In Sect. 2 we included Finland, Germany, and the United States because for this chapter's purpose we thought a variety of health care systems (PHI, SHI, NHS) would be more interesting for readers. Also, a lot of research exists on these countries, which makes a comparison easier.
(2) Country comparison: Q: What are relevant differences or similarities across the countries?	We included the following aspects: • Health care type and health care features (e.g., role of the government or hospital density) • Population (e.g., number, density, percentage of elderly) • Country size (e.g., land area) • Economic situation (e.g., GDP) Additional aspects may also be relevant.
(2) Health IT comparison: Q: On what level would you like to compare the countries and on which aspects of Health IT would you like to concentrate?	We suggest first taking a look at the established international research efforts, i.e., from the WHO or the OECD, for an initial orientation. However, for more detailed information a closer look to the literature/selected studies may be necessary. We recommend interviews/surveys with stakeholders and/or site visits to gain insights about the status quo in practice.
(3) Concluding assessment: Q: What kinds of limitations do you have to consider, putting your findings into perspective?	We pointed out a few limitations (Sect. 2.3) you should keep in mind for your conclusion from a cross-country comparison on Health IT: aspects such as self-reporting as a common method for data collection, different understandings of key terms, or insufficient data should be taken into consideration.

Summary

This chapter covers Health IT from a global perspective. Therefore, it provides background information on relevant Health IT terms, on classifications of health care systems, and on international efforts to study Health IT from a cross-country perspective. For clarification purposes, an exemplary comparison between Finland, Germany, and the United States is provided in this chapter. The comparison of the three selected countries, their national health care systems, and their adoption of Health IT gives an idea of how cross-country comparisons on Health IT might look and what advantages and limitations may be associated with such an undertaking. Summarizing the chapter, the case study provides a model for how to proceed when comparing Health IT adoption and use between different countries.

Conclusions and Outlook

From a global perspective, policy makers are faced with similar challenges when it comes to introducing Health IT into an established health care system. Therefore, a glance across national borders can be interesting to study lessons learned from other countries. This chapter provided background information and examples on "Comparing Health IT Across Different Health Care Systems." Also, this chapter shows that there is ongoing, large-scale research on this subject. Despite its limitations, cross-country comparison highlights how valuable it can be for politicians, health professionals, researchers, and other stakeholders to change the perspective once in a while.

Useful Resources

1. The Health Systems and Policy Monitor: see https://www.hspm.org/. The platform offers information on health care systems in different countries, including a search engine to compare different countries based on selectable indicators.
2. The publications from the Nordic Cooperation (Nordic eHealth Benchmarking) are available here: https://www.norden.org/en/publication/nordic-ehealth-benchmarking-0.
3. Information on the efforts by the OECD and their model survey to measure ICTs in health care is available here: https://www.oecd.org/els/health-systems/measuring-icts-in-the-health-sector.htm
4. You can find the WHO atlas of eHealth country profiles here: https://www.afro.who.int/publications/atlas-ehealth-country-profiles-use-ehealth-support-universal-health-coverage

Review Questions

1. How can you classify different health care systems?
2. Health IT: Please differentiate between Health IT availability, adoption, use, and impact.

3. International efforts: What are similarities and differences between the Nordic eHealth Benchmarking and the efforts from the OECD and the WHO?
4. Compare and assess the Health IT status between Finland, Germany, and the United States based on the information provided in this chapter.

Appendix: Answers to Review Questions

1. How can you classify different health care systems and what difference does this make for patients/citizens?

A simple classification categorizes different health care systems into Private Health Insurance (PHI) systems, National Health Services (NHS)systems, and Social Health Insurance (SHI) systems. The health care system types reveal different roles and responsibilities of the government in the organization and regulation of health care. Depending on the health care system in place, the individual patients or citizens are faced with different responsibilities, liberties, and challenges:

- **PHI**: High patient sovereignty. High responsibility for the individual citizen to protect themselves against health risks and related costs.
- **NHS**: Low patient sovereignty. The government takes care of providing health care services for their residents.
- **SHI**: Medium patient sovereignty. Health insurance is mandatory, and the scope of services may be legally defined; however, to a limited extent there can be freedom of choice, e.g., when it comes to additional, private insurance services.

2. Please differentiate between Health IT availability, adoption, use, impact, and diffusion.

- Health IT **availability**: A technology for the health care sector is in place, e.g., a hospital has bought an electronic health record (EHR) system.

- Health IT **use**: A technology for the health care sector is applied in practice, e.g., the nurses and physicians of a hospital use the EHR system to store patient data.
- Health IT **adoption**: A technology for the health care sector is available and is used in a meaningful way, e.g.,. the EHR system is used to share patient data.
- Health IT **impact**: A technology for the health care sector has an impact, e.g., for the patients: The use of the EHR system increases patient safety because all health care professionals in a hospital have all relevant patient data.
- Health IT **diffusion**: Passive spread of a technology through the health care sector, e.g., a diffusion of 100% would mean that every hospital in a country has an EHR system.

3. International efforts: What are similarities and differences between the Nordic eHealth benchmarking and the efforts from the OECD and the WHO?

Comparison between the Nordic eHealth benchmarking, the OECD ICT benchmarking, and the WHO atlas of eHealth country profiles:

SIMILARITIES	DIFFERENCES
Comparable objectives: monitoring the developments, cross-country learning	Scope of surveyed countries: differences in the number of included countries from eight in the Nordic eHealth Benchmarking to 125 in the WHO atlas.
Data collection via surveys	The OECD and Nordic eHealth benchmarking focus only on high-income countries. The WHO sample is more heterogenous.
Longitudinal approach: continued measurements	Somewhat different emphases
Adjustment of the methods over time	
Aggregated data	

4. Compare and assess the Health IT status between Finland, Germany, and the United States based on the information provided in this chapter.

Finland, Germany, and the United States are countries which differ in size, population, and health care system type. What they have in common is that they are high-income countries which spend a lot on health care. Therefore, Health IT faces quite different environments; however, financial opportunities are at hand.

The international comparison from the OECD [22] indicates that the use of electronic systems in the primary care sector reaches similar levels across Finland, Germany, and the United States; in regard to acute care facilities which exchange results (radiology results or images) with outside organizations, Finland attains better values. This impression corresponds with the information provided in the country-specific examples. Health Information Exchange is a current focus in Germany and the United States, while Finland has moved on to a new challenge: providing meaningful Health IT for their citizens.

References

1. Böhm K, Schmid A, Götze R, Landwehr C, Rothgang H. Five types of OECD healthcare systems: empirical results of a deductive classification. Health Policy. 2013;113(3):258–69. https://doi.org/10.1016/j.healthpol.2013.09.003.
2. OECD. Financing and delivering health care: a comparative analysis of OECD countries. OECD; 1987.
3. Wendt C. Changing healthcare system types. Soc Policy Admin. 2014;48(7):864–82. https://doi.org/10.1111/spol.12061.
4. Paris V, Devaux M, Wei L. Systems institutional characteristics: a survey of 29 OECD countries. OECD Health Working Papers No. 50. https://dx.doi.org/10.1787/5kmfxfq9qbnr-en. OECD; 2010.
5. Villumsen S, Adler-Milstein J, Nøhr C. National monitoring and evaluation of eHealth: a scoping review. JAMIA Open. 2020;222(e1):181. https://doi.org/10.1093/jamiaopen/ooz071.
6. Daim TU, Behkami N, Basoglu N, Kök OM, Hogaboam L. Healthcare technology innovation adoption: electronic health records and other emerging health information technology innovations. Cham: Springer; 2016.
7. Villumsen S, Hardardottir GA, Kangas M, Gilstad H, Brattheim B, Reponen J, et al. Monitoring the amount of practical use of eHealth on National Level by use of log data: lessons learned. Stud Health Technol Inform. 2015;218:138–44.

8. Greenhalgh T, Robert G, MacFarlane F, Bate P, Kyriakidou O. Diffusion of innovations in service organizations: systematic review and recommendations. Milbank Q. 2004;82(4):581–629.

9. Rogers EM. Diffusion of innovations. New York: Free Press; 2003.

10. Barber S, French C, Matthews R, Lovett D, Rollinson T, Husson F, et al. The role of patients and carers in diffusing a health-care innovation: a case study of "my medication passport". Health Expect. 2019;22(4):676–87. https://doi.org/10.1111/hex.12893.

11. Esdar M, Hüsers J, Weiß J-P, Rauch J, Hübner U. Diffusion dynamics of electronic health records: a longitudinal observational study comparing data from hospitals in Germany and the United States. Int J Med Inform. 2019;131:103952. https://doi.org/10.1016/j.ijmedinf.2019.103952.

12. Hüsers J, Hübner U, Esdar M, Ammenwerth E, Hackl WO, Naumann L, Liebe JD. Innovative power of health care organisations affects IT adoption: a bi-National Health IT benchmark comparing Austria and Germany. J Med Syst. 2017;41(2):33. https://doi.org/10.1007/s10916-016-0671-6.

13. Denis J-L, Hébert Y, Langley A, Lozeau D, Louise-Hélene T. Explaining diffusion patterns for complex health care innovations. Health Care Manag Rev. 2002;27(3):60–73.

14. Leviss J. HIT or Miss, 3rd edition: lessons learned from health information technology projects. New York: Productivity Press; 2019.

15. Greenhalgh T, Wherton J, Papoutsi C, Lynch J, Hughes G, A'Court C, et al. Beyond adoption: a new framework for theorizing and evaluating nonadoption, abandonment, and challenges to the scale-up, spread, and sustainability of health and care technologies. J Med Internet Res. 2017;19(11):e367. https://doi.org/10.2196/jmir.8775.

16. Adler-Milstein J, Holmgren AJ, Kralovec P, Worzala C, Searcy T, Patel V. Electronic health record adoption in US hospitals: the emergence of a digital "advanced use" divide. J Am Med Inform Assoc. 2017;24(6):1142–8. https://doi.org/10.1093/jamia/ocx080.

17. Hyppönen H, Faxvaag A, Gilstad H, Hardardottir GA, Jerlvall L, Kangas M, et al. Nordic eHealth indicators: organisation of research, first results and plan for the future. In: Proceedings of the 14th world congress on medical and health informatics. 2013; 192:273–7.

18. Hyppönen H, Koch S, Faxvaag A, Gilstad H, Nohr C, Hardardottir GA, et al. Nordic eHealth benchmarking. Copenhagen: Nordic Council of Ministers; 2017.

19. Hyppönen H, Kangas M, Reponen J, Nøhr C, Villumsen S, Koch S, et al. Nordic eHealth benchmarking. Status 2014. Nordic Council of Ministers; 2015.

20. Adler-Milstein J, Ronchi E, Cohen GR, Winn LAP, Jha AK. Benchmarking health IT among OECD countries: better data for better policy. J Am Med Inform Assoc. 2014;21(1):111–6. https://doi.org/10.1136/amiajnl-2013-001710.

21. OECD. Draft OECD guide to measuring ICTs in the health sector. https://www.oecd.org/health/health-systems/Draft-oecd-guide-to-measuring-icts-in-the-health-sector.pdf. Accessed 15 Apr 2020. OECD; 2015.

22. Zelmer J, Ronchi E, Hyppönen H, Lupiáñez-Villanueva F, Codagnone C, Nøhr C, et al. International health IT benchmarking: learning from cross-country comparisons. J Am Med Inform Assoc. 2017;24(2):371–9. https://doi.org/10.1093/jamia/ocw111.

23. WHO (ed.). Atlas of eHealth country profiles. The use of eHealth in support of universal health coverage. Based on the findings of the third global survey on eHealth 2015. 2015.

24. WHO. Global diffusion of eHealth: making universal health coverage achievable. Report of the third global survey on eHealth. https://www.who.int/goe/publications/global_diffusion/en/. Accessed 18 Apr 2020. WHO; 2016.

25. Yamey G. What are the barriers to scaling up health interventions in low and middle income countries? A qualitative study of academic leaders in implementation science. Glob Health. 2012;8(11)

26. Vehko T, Ruotsalainen S, Hyppönen H. E-health and e-welfare of Finland. Check Point 2018. National Institute for Health and Welfare; 2019. https://www.julkari.fi/handle/10024/138244. Accessed 18 April 2020.

27. Stafford N. Germany is set to introduce e-health cards by 2018. BMJ. 2015;350:h2991. https://doi.org/10.1136/bmj.h2991.

28. Commonwealth Fund. International Health Care System Profiles. https://international.commonwealthfund.org/features/ehrs/. Accessed 11 May 2020.

29. Hübner U, Esdar M, Hüsers J, Liebe JD, Naumann L, Thye J, Weiß, JP. IT-Report Gesundheitswesen: Wie reif ist die Gesundheits-IT aus Anwender-Perspektive? Befragung ärztlicher und pflegerischer Krankenhaus-Direktoren*innen. 2020. Hochschule Osnabrueck. https://www.hs-osnabrueck.de/it-report-gesundheitswesen. Accessed 18 Apr 2020.

30. Naumann L, Esdar M, Ammenwerth E, Baumberger D, Hübner U. Same goals, yet different outcomes: analysing the current state of eHealth adoption and policies in Austria, Germany, and Switzerland using a mixed methods approach. Stud Health Technol Inform. 2019;264:1012–6. https://doi.org/10.3233/SHTI190377.

31. Halamka JD, Tripathi M. The HITECH era in retrospect. N Engl J Med. 2017;377(10):907–9. https://doi.org/10.1056/NEJMp1709851.

32. Adler-Milstein J, Jha AK. Health information exchange among U.S. hospitals: who's in, who's out, and why? Healthc (Amst). 2014;2(1):26–32. https://doi.org/10.1016/j.hjdsi.2013.12.005.

33. Pagliari C, Sloan D, Gregor P, Sullivan F, Detmer D, Kahan JP, et al. What is eHealth (4): a scoping exercise to map the field. J Med Internet Res. 2005;7(1):e9. https://doi.org/10.2196/jmir.7.1.e9.

Nigeria: Interprofessional Health Informatics Collaboration

46

Bilikis J. Oladimeji, Okey Okuzu, and Oluwaseun Olaniran

Learning Objectives
- To introduce readers to Nigeria, a country in Africa and its land, people, climate, etc.
- To understand the Nigerian healthcare system with emphasis on governance, regulation, financing, education, and training of healthcare workers and health outcomes
- To introduce readers to the history, opportunities, and outlook of Informatics and Health IT adoption throughout Nigeria with a case study to show its application to one of the nation's pressing challenges
- To promote the understanding of interprofessional Health Informatics collaboration in Nigeria

Key Terms
- ICT—Information and Communication Technology
- HI—Health Informatics
- NPHCDA—National Primary Health Care Development Agency
- National Health Bill

- National Health Act 2014
- UHC—Universal Healthcare Coverage
- PHC—Primary Health Care
- NHIS—National Health Insurance Scheme
- MDCN—Medical and Dental Council of Nigeria
- HCW—Healthcare Workers
- CHO—Community Health Officers
- CHEW—Community Health Extension Worker
- DHIS2—District Health Information Software
- FMoH—Federal Ministry of Health
- MINPHIS—Made in Nigeria Primary Healthcare Information System
- EWORS—Early Warning Outbreak Recognition System
- DFID—Department for International Development

Introduction

Brief Overview of Nigeria Geography, Wealth, People, Culture, and Languages

Nigeria is a country in Africa located along the coast of the Atlantic Ocean in the South and bordered by Benin, Cameroon, and Niger in the West, East, and North, respectively (see Fig. 46.1). The climate in Nigeria varies across the different regions: equatorial in the south, tropical in the center, and arid in the North. Its

B. J. Oladimeji (✉)
Optum/UHG, Boston, MA, USA
e-mail: bilikis.akindele@optum.com

O. Okuzu
InStrat Global Health Solutions, Montclair, NJ, USA
e-mail: okey@instratghs.com

O. Olaniran
Health Informatics Society of Nigeria,
Columbia, South Carolina, Nigeria

© Springer Nature Switzerland AG 2022
U. H. Hübner et al. (eds.), *Nursing Informatics*, Health Informatics,
https://doi.org/10.1007/978-3-030-91237-6_46

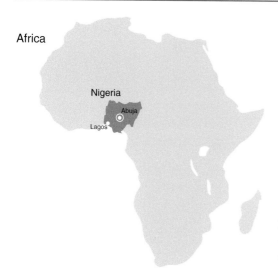

Fig. 46.1 Map of Africa and Nigeria with Abuja (capital) and Lagos (largest, most populated city) (source: own)

vast natural resources include natural gas, petroleum, tin, iron ore, coal, limestone, niobium, lead, zinc, and arable land. Nigeria is home to an estimated 250 ethnic groups [1], with over 500 languages, and the variety of customs and traditions among them gives the country great cultural diversity. The Hausas, Yorubas, and Igbo make up the three largest ethnic groups of Nigeria. There are also the Efik, Ibibio, Annang, and Ijaw among the Southeastern minority populations while the Urhobo-Isoko, Edo, and Itsekiri constitute Nigeria's Midwest minority populations. Nigerian Pidgin is used widely as an unofficial medium of communication across these, especially in the main Nigerian cities where different ethnic groups are bound to interact. Religious groups include Muslim, Christian, and others. The country gained independence from the British colony in 1960 and the influence of colonization is still apparent in its governance and educational system.

With a population of over 200 million people, it is the most populous country in Africa and the United Nations (UN) estimates that Nigeria will have a population of 400 million by 2050. Nigeria is referred to as the "Giant of Africa" because of the size of its economy and population. Nigeria and South Africa make up half of sub-Saharan Africa's gross domestic product

(GDP) [2] and both countries have vied for the position of Africa's largest economy. While there continues to be uncertainties about how the COVID-19 pandemic affect the economies of all countries in the world including Nigeria, data from the Annual GDP for 2019 showed that Nigeria is the largest economy in Africa with a GDP of $476 billion or $402 billion, depending on the rate used [2].

Despite this economic and population advantage, according to a United Nations Development Programme (UNDP) Human Development Report, the Nigeria Human Development Index (HDI) value for 2018 was 0.534, ranking 158 out of 189 countries and territories.

There are also far-reaching inequalities across gender and economic lines. According to the Oxfam Commitment to Reducing Inequality (CRI) Index, Nigeria has the unenviable position of being at the bottom of the Index. Its social spending (on health, education, and social protection) is low, reflected in very poor social outcomes for its citizens. According to the Nigerian National Bureau of Statistics (NBS), youth unemployment and underemployment was 55.4% in Q3 of 2018. In another report about poverty and inequality from September 2018 to October 2019, NBS says 40% of people in Nigeria lived below its poverty line of 137,430 nairas per year which is the equivalent to $1.05/day.

Healthcare Landscape in Nigeria

The healthcare landscape of Nigeria is one with strengths, challenges, and vast opportunities for growth. To highlight this, let us take a quick look at recent health indices:

Health Indices

According to World Bank (https://data.worldbank.org/country/nigeria)

- Physicians (per 1000 people): 0.381 (2018)
- Nursing and midwifery personnel (per 1000 people) : 1.5 (2019)

- Neonatal mortality rate (per 1000 live births): 35.85 (for both sexes) (2019)
- Under-five mortality rate (probability of dying by age 5 per 1000 live births): 117.2 (2019)
- Maternal mortality ratio (per 100,000 live births, modeled estimate): 917 (2017)
- Life expectancy at birth (in years): 54.7 (2019)
- Births attended by skilled health personnel (%): 43.3 (2018)
- Literacy rate among adults aged >= 15 years (%): 62 (2018)
- Poverty headcount ratio (2011 PPP) at $1.90 a day is applicable to 39.1% of the population (2018)

These numbers are disappointing but do not exist in a vacuum. They are a consequence of the various challenges plaguing the Nigerian economy and healthcare system. However, with every challenge comes an opportunity to improve and healthcare informatics and technology can play a role in providing a host of resolutions.

Governance/Level of Health Services

The three tiers of the Nigerian government (Federal, State, and Local) are largely responsible for the provision of healthcare. The University Teaching Hospitals and Federal Medical Centers (tertiary level of care) are maintained by the federal government while the state government oversees various general hospitals (secondary level of care). Dispensaries (primary level of care) are the responsibilities of the local governments. Primary healthcare activities are regulated by the **National Primary Health Care Development Agency (NPHCDA)** which is an arm of the Federal Government. Primary care services in Nigeria are delivered and accessed through primary, secondary, and tertiary health facilities, while in rural areas primary care is mostly situated in governmental **primary health care (PHC)** centers and faith-based clinics [3].

The Nigeria *National Health Bill* [4] provides a framework for the regulation, development, and management of a national health system and sets standards for rendering health services in Nigeria

and other connected matters. The bill was first proposed when Professor Eyitayo Lambo was Minister of Health in 2004 but was passed in 2014 under the presidency of Goodluck Jonathan. The **National Health Act** 2014 (NHA 2014) is the first in the history of the country and continues to maintain the basic focus of the national health policy on PHC as central to providing health for all. The Act creates a basic healthcare provision fund (not less than 1% of federal government consolidated revenue fund) of which 50% was planned to provide essential drugs, vaccines and consumables, and infrastructure; develop human resources; and ensure emergency medical treatment at the PHC level [3].

Apart from Government facilities, privately-owned healthcare centers play a very important role in filling the gaps in the provision of healthcare, in particular for the middle to high socioeconomic class. According to a 2015 BMI Research (now Fitch Solutions Macro Intelligence Solution) report, there were an estimated 3534 hospitals in 2014, of which 950 were in the public sector. These include 54 federal tertiary hospitals comprising 20 teaching hospitals, 22 federal medical centers, three national orthopedic hospitals, the National Eye Centre, the National Ear, Nose, and Throat (ENT, equiv. Otolaryngology) Centre, and seven psychiatric hospitals, which are overseen by the Hospital Services Department of the **Federal Ministry of Health** (**FMoH**). There are also several district hospitals, general hospitals, health centers, and primary care dispensaries. Private hospitals and faith-based organization-owned facilities are also present.

Budget and Healthcare Financing

In Nigeria, revenue for financing the health sector is collected majorly from pooled and unpooled sources [5]. The pooled sources are collected from budgetary allocation, direct and indirect taxation as well as donor funding. However, the unpooled sources contribute to over 70% of total health expenditure (THE). Out-of-Pocket Payments (OPP—both informal or formal direct payments to healthcare providers at the time of service) account for about 90% while payments for medical products (mosquito bed nets, birth control, etc.) are about 10% of the unpooled sources [5]. The recommended GDP percentage to be allocated for healthcare to achieve Universal Healthcare Coverage (UHC) is at least 5% [6]. However, the total expenditure on healthcare as a percentage of GDP in 2017 according to World Bank is 3.756.

Health Insurance

The **National Health Insurance Scheme (NHIS)** was introduced by the Nigerian Federal Government in 2005 to guarantee accessibility to healthcare for Nigerians as a way to enhance universal coverage [5]. The remaining 50% of the Provision Fund from the NHA 2014, described earlier in this chapter, is planned to be disbursed by the NHIS to provide a basic minimum health service to citizens [3]. In 2017, only those employed in the federal formal sector (<5% of the working population) were enrolled [5]. The NHIS only covers 4% of the population which is significantly low [7]. Members who are enrolled in NHIS get to enjoy several benefits and services such as hospital care (maximum of 15 days per year and admission in the general ward), outpatient care, pharmaceutical care (as reflected on the NHIS essential drug list), diagnostic tests per the NHIS diagnostic list, maternal care for up to four life births (per woman); preventive care (immunization, health education, antenatal and postnatal care), eye care, and preventive dental care [8]. Beneficiaries no longer need to pay for the treatment with cash at health centers except for the 10% co-payment for prescription medication [8].

Nine states indicated interest in the scheme (Abia, Enugu, Gombe, Imo, Jigawa, Kaduna, Lagos, Ondo, and Oyo) but only two states (Bauchi and Cross-river) have attempted to enroll their employees in the scheme in 2015 [5]. Despite the promises of the insurance scheme, its implementation and awareness has been marred by inefficiencies. A study conducted in 2018 by Abiola AO et al. showed that 80.7% of the respondents had poor knowledge about the NHIS, only 12.3% of the respondents had registered, and 43.8% of respondents who had not yet registered claimed they did not know where to register [9]; similar findings are observed in other geopolitical zones.

Outside of the NHIS, about 1% of the population is covered by the private insurance plans run by Health Maintenance Organizations (HMOs) and target clients who can afford to pay for the insurance plans which mainly cover primary healthcare and some secondary or tertiary care.

Whereas the NHIS and private insurance have gained sufficient traction in providing coverage to federal public sector workers, their families, and workers of large private organizations, the vast majority of Nigerians are without any form of coverage [10].

The 2018 Nigeria Demographic and Health Survey (NDHS) collected information about specific types of insurance coverage and the percentages of women and men with any health insurance. According to background characteristics, only 3% of women and men aged 15–49 have health insurance [11]. Therefore, an overwhelming majority must be able to cover OOPs or rely on online/offline crowdsourcing or philanthropic gestures, non-governmental organizations (NGOs), and faith-based organizations (FBOs) for healthcare. The ability to afford healthcare services is one of the biggest barriers to care which often forces patients to seek unregulated alternatives such as herbal remedies, hypnosis, etc., sometimes falling victim to deceptions. This many times leads to delayed diagnosis at hospitals and worse care outcomes.

Nigeria remains one of the countries with the highest number of OOP payments for healthcare with expenditures reaching as high as 77.225% paid in cash (World Bank 2017).

Healthcare Education and Interprofessional Collaboration

Education

The regulatory bodies for health care worker (HCW) training in Nigeria are the National

Universities Commission (NUC), **Medical and Dental Council of Nigeria (MDCN)**, and the Nursing and Midwifery Council of Nigeria (NMCN). According to the MDCN, there are 31 fully accredited and six partially accredited medical schools in Nigeria. Nine of the 31 fully accredited medical schools include dental schools, of which seven are fully accredited and two are partially accredited. While the development of medical curricula remains the sole responsibility of the senates of the individual universities, the MDCN and the NUC are mandated to determine the minimum standards of all curricula [12].

The Nigeria FMoH, supported by the United States Agency for International Development (USAID) under the flagship of the Health 20/20 project, developed the Nigeria Undergraduate Medical and Dental Curriculum Template of 2012, from which individual schools could develop their own curriculum *de novo* (begin a new) [13]. Though major revisions to medical/dental curricula are recommended every 5 years, there are lapses in meeting this recommendation by Nigerian medical schools. For example, the revision of the traditional Bachelor of Medicine and Bachelor of Surgery (MBBS) curricula to competency-based curricula (CBME; competency-based medical education) at the College of Medicine, University of Ibadan, took approximately 12 years (2001–2012), in a series of overlapping processes [14].

Some of the medical education shortfalls in the present structure of medical education include old curricula and pedagogical methods, paucity of training programs for educators, inconsistent quality of medical doctors due to lack of standard and unreliable forms of assessment [14]. The Cape Town Declaration of 1995, which was the outcome of the African Regional Conference of the World Health Organization (WHO) and the World Federation for Medical Education (WFME), states that Medical (health sciences) Education Units (MEUs) should be established at every medical school and that mechanisms should be put in place for promoting, coordinating, and evaluating medical education reform. However, very few medical schools in Nigeria have established MEUs [15].

These challenges are also faced when training other HCWs although steps are constantly evolving to address them. Physicians, such as general practitioners and specialist physicians, are trained through accredited medical program and postgraduate programs across the country. In many cases, the medical schools for physician training are co-located or in close proximity to training centers for nurses, pharmacists, laboratory scientists, etc., leading to early collaboration across the interdisciplinary HCWs during training.

Due to the recognition of the great need for PHC services at all levels of care, almost all medical schools are incorporating PHC into the curriculum as required by the National University Commission (NUC) [3]. Since the early 1980s, the government at all levels has invested in the training of the PHC workforce through the Community Health Officers' (CHOs) training program in most teaching hospitals across the country. There are Schools of Nursing and Midwifery that train nurses and midwives located in all states and in the Federal Capital Territory, and Colleges of Health Technology that train other non-clinician PHC workers [3]. It is also important to point out that following the completion of a college degree, there is a mandatory one-year service year known as the National Youth Service Corps which helps to provide care in rural areas of the country. The Corp members are usually assigned work in PHC.

Economic challenges, delayed execution of policies, and lack of adequate funding for the healthcare sector in Nigeria continue to pose a threat to the retention of Nigeria-trained HCWs, especially doctors and nurses. Many doctors and nurses leave Nigeria in high numbers to practice in other countries around the world known as the "Nigerian Medical Brain Drain." Majority of these HCWs immigrate to the USA or the UK, despite the obvious shortage of doctors in the country. Current gaps and HCW shortages, made more apparent by the COVID-19 pandemic, are perpetuating the condition with some countries reportedly relaxing immigration requirements which tend to attract more Nigerian doctors. On another hand, despite the immediate negative impact of these emigrations on HCW availability, the situation brings about some overlooked positives such as remittances, conduct of multiple clinical research, investment, and the creation of employment opportunities and medical missions that provide essential and sometimes advanced diagnostics and treatments to Nigeria, many times for free.

Multiple Disciplines

There are several health disciplines working in the community to provide health services. These include family physicians (FP), public health physicians, general practitioners (GP), nurses and midwives, pharmacy or pharmacy technicians, laboratory technicians, community health extension workers (CHEWs), and voluntary health workers. A variety of medical specialists including traditional (birth attendants and bone setters), alternative patient medicine vendors, and allied health professionals (physiotherapists and social workers) may also be present [3]. Though the leadership of hospitals and healthcare practices/centers sometimes incite rivalry among healthcare providers, for the most part, the different healthcare providers work as a team to deliver care services to patients.

Information and Communication Technology (ICT) Infrastructure in Nigeria: Where Technology Meets Healthcare

The World Bank defined **information and communication technology (ICT)** as the "set of activities that facilitate the processing, transmission, and display of information by electronic means" [16]. The emergence of new technologies brought about by the rapid ICT development from the mid-twentieth century to date has had a tremendous impact on the way the whole world lives, works, and plays [17].

Appropriate software packages for hospitals and health centers were not available locally when healthcare computerization was launched in Nigeria. In response, the Department of Computer Science and Engineering at Obafemi Awolowo University Teaching Hospital

(OAUTH) and the University of Kuopio (now the University of Eastern Finland) established a joint project on health informatics (HI) in 1989. They developed a basic system for in-patient admissions, transfers, and discharges that has been enhanced over the years and later christened the **Made in Nigeria Primary Healthcare Information System (MINPHIS)**. MINPHIS was the first locally developed hospital system in Nigeria. Nigeria's transition into democratic rule in 1999 ushered in a new era of ICT development in the country with the adoption of the National ICT policy which served as the foundation on which the National Information Infrastructure (NII) was built. The policy provided a guide on how technology infrastructures such as the fiber-optic networks and very-small-aperture terminal (VSAT) could be used to make quality education widely available, financially empower citizens, and to provide global opportunities for the citizens to compete. The government further formulated the Nigerian National IT policy (USE IT) in March 2001 with the vision of making Nigeria an IT-capable country and a key player in the Information Society by the year 2005. The National Information Technology Development Agency (NITDA) was established as the implementation agency to develop and regulate the IT sector, in collaboration with the Nigerian Communications Commission (NCC) [18].

In 2006, with support from the UK Department for International Development (**DFID**), through the Partnership for Transforming Health Systems Phase program (PATHS), Nigeria developed the foundational principles for a simple, practicable, and sustainable Health Management Information System. This effort was a precursor to Nigeria's adoption of the **District Health Information Software 2 (DHIS2)** in 2006. DHIS2 is a free and open-source health management data platform used by governments worldwide for health-related projects, including patient health monitoring, improving disease surveillance, and speeding up health data access. DHIS2 was developed by the Health Information Systems Program (HISP) and is supported by the University of Oslo's Department of Informatics.

DHIS2 is the nationally mandated gateway to Nigeria's National Health Management Information System (NHMIS). As such, all health systems that are deployed at the federal or state level in Nigeria are required to demonstrate interoperability with DHIS2.

In recent years, bold steps have been taken by both the government and private sectors to conduct several important sector reforms to improve Nigeria's ICT infrastructure. This has produced far-reaching, low-cost mobile services penetration, thereby creating Africa's largest fixed-line sector with a resultant improvement in the nation's per capita growth performance [19].

In 2018, there were 170 million mobile phone subscriptions in Nigeria and 92.3 million internet users with smartphones accounting for about three-quarters of the Nigerian web traffic. The number of internet users is projected to increase to 187.8 million by 2023 while the current number of smartphone users is projected to increase to more than 140 million by 2025 from the current estimated 25–40 million users. Internet penetration was about 47.1% of the population in 2018 and that figure is projected to hit 84.5% by 2023 [20, 21].

Healthcare providers in Nigeria are still predominantly using paper-based health records. The associated problems of paper-based records such as poor health information management (HIM) capability coupled with the rapid development of IT infrastructure have been a major motivation for the stakeholders in healthcare to increasingly seek for health IT solutions to combat the problems and limitations of paper-based records. In an effort to encourage and coordinate the use of health IT in the management of the nation's healthcare information, the Nigerian government through the FMoH organized the first National Conference on health IT on November 2–4, 2011, where the pathway for the National eHealth Policy and Electronic Health Record (EHR) interoperability was set. Studies have shown that Nigeria's healthcare providers are now deploying more health IT solutions to improve healthcare delivery outcomes [22].

Current Interdisciplinary Focus on Informatics in Nigeria: Training, Collaborations, Associations, and Networks

Interdisciplinary healthcare professionals from medicine, nursing, psychology, psychiatry, etc. come together as a team to collaborate with experts in other professions (engineering, computer science, linguistics, etc.) to find solutions to intricate healthcare challenges. Due to the diversity of their knowledge and training backgrounds, these interprofessional collaborations allow participating individuals to contribute unique viewpoints in providing comprehensive solutions to such challenges. It has been recognized that interdisciplinary collaboration in healthcare could lead to an increase in healthcare productivity with minimum wasted effort in the coordination and delivery of ever-growing myriads of health services, thereby leading to improvement in the quality of patient care [23].

Such collaborations with other fields are being explored to create biomedical engineering training. This interdisciplinary training program was designed to equip low- and middle-income countries' faculty and students with a unique comprehensive hands-on learning experience focused on developing innovative global health technologies. In recent years, Nigerian health professionals have been collaborating more with their ICT counterparts in the use of mobile technologies to improve healthcare delivery [24]. Collaborations in HI among healthcare professionals in Nigeria are focused on comprehending the needs of the stakeholders involved and then applying IT in meeting the needs of those stakeholders [25].

A nationwide study conducted in 2015 on allied healthcare personnel in Nigeria [22] revealed that the vast majority of participants (98.8%) acknowledged the importance and relevance of having IT skills to work in healthcare settings with many expressing their desire for additional IT training with a focus on statistical analysis. Although 8.1% of the respondents possessed some IT skills, there was a gap in IT skills among healthcare personnel. This gap is not compatible with the healthy growth of health IT.

To rectify this anomaly, Nigeria healthcare personnel will need continuous education with a focus on health IT in order to overcome this deficit [22].

As recently as 2010, HI college programs or training did not exist in Nigeria; therefore, most students with an interest in this field at both the undergraduate and postgraduate levels needed to seek additional education outside the country. Students sometimes attend other African schools in Ghana, Ethiopia, South Africa, or go abroad to North America, Europe, and beyond. Observations and past studies have highlighted the challenges facing the practice of HIM in Africa (including Nigeria) to be centered around the quality of professional training, inadequately qualified practitioners, disgruntled practitioners, government's indifference toward the practice, lack of policies, and inadequate technological infrastructure among others [26].

Nigeria's private sector recent investment in health IT is addressing the skills shortage in the area of HI. This is more apparent during the interdisciplinary collaborations in the implementation of health technologies that incorporate training opportunities. Private organizations and associations such as ehealth4everyone, EpidAlert, Oncopadi, PharmAccess Foundation, and the Healthcare Informatics Society of Nigeria (HISN), organize certificate programs, seminars, and conferences to meet some of these needs.

In addition to curricular integration, interdisciplinary training is being encouraged to create a learning environment in which future healthcare professionals can learn to work together to improve healthcare delivery and to better understand the complex and comprehensive nature of disease and treatment as further highlighted in the following case study.

There is increased collaboration among government healthcare agencies like the National Agency for the Control of AIDS (NACA), National Primary Health Care Development Agency (NPHCDA), and non-governmental multinational organizations like Family Health International (FHI) 360 in the use of health IT

resulting in remarkable change initiatives in the healthcare sphere. An example of such an initiative is highlighted in the case study below.

Case Study

Electronic Surveillance of Methanol Poisoning ("Malokun Syndrome") Outbreak in Ondo State, Nigeria

Background

With an estimated population of 3.4 million, a gross domestic product (GDP) of approximately $8 million, and internal revenue of N10.4 billion (approximately $60 million US dollars), Ondo is a mid-sized South Western Nigerian State. In April 2015, residents of Irele local government area (see Fig. 46.2 for a map of the location), approximately 122 km from the state capital, Akure (population of 167,000) residents began to experience severe headaches, followed quickly by blurred vision, loss of sight, convulsions, and death. These symptoms and the quick loss of lives led to widespread panic in the community about a sudden "strange illness." Local traditional leaders immediately tied the outbreak to spiritual forces attributable to the local god, "Malokun." Within just a few days of the emergence of the first symptoms, the number of cases had risen dramatically, resulting in 18 deaths. Local media called the outbreak "more devastating than Ebola."

Rapid Response

The State Governor immediately initiated a rapid response task force including representatives from the World Health Organization (WHO), United Nations Children's Fund (UNICEF), Ondo State Ministry of Health (MoH) epidemiologists, and InStrat Global Health Solutions (InStrat). Working in the operational context of an Emergency Operations Center (EOC), the initial effort to develop an outbreak containment protocol made the determination that "no comprehensive data was available and no disease pattern was identifiable."

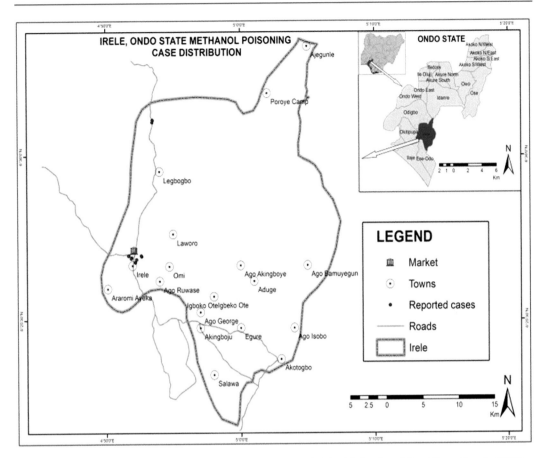

Fig. 46.2 The area of outbreak occurrence. Created by Instrat Global Health Services (Okey Okuzu Founder/CEO)

InStrat, a Nigeria-based health solutions enterprise, was tasked to work with the local members of the WHO team to digitize the epidemiology tools (Line List) for data collection and embed those forms on an electronic disease surveillance platform. This system heralded the introduction of InStrat's **Early Warning Outbreak Recognition System (EWORS)**. EWORS allows electronic capture and analysis of disease data and identifies disease outbreaks based on disease patterns. InStrat deployed EWORS on Android tablet computers and provided ten units to support disease surveillance officers. These officers captured field data electronically from the affected communities and uploaded the information in real time to central servers for aggregation and analysis. Within 36 h, the EOC had not only ruled out any infectious diseases as the cause of the outbreak but identified methanol poisoning as the possible cause. This early identification was subsequently confirmed by toxicity tests on victims. Geospatial data analysis, shown on the map, allowed the isolation of occurrences to local areas which allowed focused disease control activities.

Using real-time data collection, aggregation, and analysis, the Ondo State Government was able to determine the nature of the "unknown" disease outbreak with a high fatality rate, identified the source of the contamination, and controlled the outbreak in less than 2 weeks.

Results A 74.4% case fatality was recorded of the 39 cases line listed. Major presentations of the illness included: Blurring of vision (82.3%), Blindness (82.9%), headache (54.8%), and respiratory distress (41.9%).

Multidisciplinary Contact

The project governance was conducted in the context of the EOC. Under the leadership of the Ondo State MoH, other EOC members included the Ondo State Primary Healthcare Development Board, United Nations International Children's Emergency Fund (UNICEF), National Agency for Food and Drug Administration Control (NAFDAC), National Orientation Agency (NOA), WHO, InStrat, Nigeria Field Epidemiology and Laboratory Training Program (NFELTP) and the Department of State Services (DSS).

InStrat provided daily field reports to the EOC to guide the following response teams: Surveillance; facility case management; advocacy and communications; and burial and toxicology.

Summary

The Nigeria healthcare situation is determined by many factors including its population structure, climate governance, financing, technology, and healthcare worker education/training. Dealing with corruption, adoption of standard training, and health IT/informatics are some of the approaches to ensure better health outcomes for its citizens.

ICT has become ubiquitous across all aspects of human endeavor including business, governance, education, and commerce, just to name a few. ICT has also played a critical role in improving healthcare for individuals and communities by enabling new and more efficient ways of accessing, communicating, and storing information. It has helped to bridge information gaps in the health sector between developing and newly industrial countries as it relates to health professionals and the communities they serve. Through the development of databases and accompanying applications, ICT delivers the capacity to improve health systems and reduce medical errors.

Important drivers of health ICT adoption and proliferation include the rapid adoption of mobile communication technologies. Factors behind mobile technology adoption include increasing availability of mobile and broadband internet; reductions in mobile phone cost, and the proliferation of mobile applications that people use in their everyday lives.

Conclusions and Outlook

In 2015, the FMoH and Federal Ministry of Communication Technology (FMCT) led a multi-sectoral and stakeholder development of the National Health Information and Communication Technology (Health ICT) Strategic Framework. The effort was borne out of recognizing the opportunities that ICT presents to support health systems strengthening and the achievement of health system goals. With UHC as one of its main priorities, the Federal Government of Nigeria articulated the following vision: *"By 2020, health ICT will help enable and deliver universal health coverage in Nigeria."*

As of this writing, Nigeria has arguably transitioned from experimentation and early adoption phases of health ICT, to increasingly scaled implementation of ICT projects toward that 2020 vision. The private sector has played an important role in this transition through entrepreneurial initiatives and public/private partnerships which have resulted in the use of ICT across the spectrum of healthcare delivery services. These service areas include: Electronic Medical Records (EMR) systems that have been adopted at hospitals and now increasingly in primary healthcare facilities (e.g., Helium Health, InStrat); supply chain management (e.g., LMIS, Spoxil); disease surveillance and response (e.g., Surveillance, Outbreak Response Management and Analysis System-SORMAS, EWORS); health worker training (e.g., VTR Mobile); human resource management (e.g., human resource information system (HRIS); telemedicine and/telehealth (e.g., MobiHealth, MDoc); health insurance management (e.g., Care Pay, InStrat); and treatment adherence and appointment reminders (e.g., txtalert). International multilateral organizations such as USAID and the DFID and private sector donors like the Bill and Melinda Gates Foundation and Ford Foundation have provided important catalytic funding for health ICT projects across all stages of investment, from proof of concept to country-wide scaling.

The private sector has embraced technology and health standards at a faster pace and is leading major efforts in the adoption of health IT. The public sector, on the other hand, lags behind in the adoption of informatics but progress is slowly being made. On January 5, 2020, news covered the introduction of the EMR to replace patients' cards and paper files at the Federal Medical Centre and Ebute Metta in Lagos. Aside from privately run facilities such as the Nigerian National Petroleum Corporation Hospital, Paelon Memorial Hospital, Lakeshore Cancer Centre, and Abuja Clinics, other government-owned hospitals and centers using the electronic card to capture patient data are the Federal Medical Centre in Keffi; National Hospital in Abuja; and the University of Maiduguri Teaching Hospital and Federal Medical Centre located in Nguru.

The promise of health ICT, especially in its capacity to support informatics and improved health decision making at both macro (policy) and micro (patient) levels, and at significantly lower costs, has increased Nigeria's odds of attaining its UHC Vision. This has also contributed significantly to Nigeria's progress on the UN Millennium Development Goals.

Useful Resources

1. Nigerian Government website. https://nigeria.gov.ng/
2. Nigeria National Bureau of Statistics. https://www.nigerianstat.gov.ng/
3. United Nations Population Fund. Nigeria Overview—Population. https://www.unfpa.org/data/world-population/NG
4. Health Indices—WHO. https://aho.afro.who.int/ng
5. Nigeria Undergraduate Medical And Dental Curriculum Template, 2012. https://www.hfg-project.org/wp-content/uploads/2015/02/Nigeria-Undergraduate-Medical-and-Dental-Curriculum-Template.pdf
6. Developing Innovative Interdisciplinary Biomedical Engineering Programs in Nigeria: Lessons Learned. Paper ID #17523 ASEE 2016 International Forum New Orleans Louisiana United States. https://oer.ui.edu.ng/sites/default/files/developing-innovative-interdisciplinary-biomedical-engineering-programs-in-nigeria-lessons-learned.pdf
7. Postgraduate Medical Education in Nigeria. http://www.tjogonline.com/article.asp?issn=0189-5117;year=2018;volume=35;issue=1;spage=1;epage=13;aulast=Okonofua
8. Knowledge and attitude toward interdisciplinary team working among obstetricians and gynecologists in teaching hospitals in South East Nigeria. https://www.ncbi.nlm.nih.gov/pmc/articles/PMC4451848/
9. News report on introduction of medical records in government hospitals. https://healthwise.punchng.com/fmc-introduces-e-medical-record-to-replace-paper-cards-files/
10. Nigeria, DFID PATHS2 Mid-term Evaluation Study. https://www.itad.com/project/nigeria-paths2-mid-term-evaluation-study/
11. Characterisation of the Health Information System in Nigeria Report of Findings by XavierBosch-Capblanch et al. https://pdfs.semanticscholar.org/b047/e6119b958c6a4f-65212f5631e6c5eb3e673d.pdf
12. Society for Quality in Health Care. https://sqhn.org/
13. EpidAlert (formerly EbolaAlert). www.epidalert.org
14. PharmAccess Foundation. https://www.pharmaccess.org/nigeria/
15. Mobihealth International. https://mobi-healthinternational.com/
16. Instrat Global Health Solutions. http://instratghs.com/our-services/
17. Surveillance, Outbreak Response Management and Analysis System—SORMAS. http://health.bmz.de/ghpc/case-studies/software_disease_surveillance_outbreak_response/index.html
18. UN Millenium Development Goals. https://www.un.org/millenniumgoals/

Review Questions

1. True or False: The acronym NDHS stands for the Nigeria Demographic and Healthcare Survey

2. Multiple choice: Nigeria is home to approximately how many ethnic groups and languages?
   (a) 150 ethnic groups and 400 languages
   (b) 200 ethnic groups and 450 languages
   (c) 250 ethnic groups and 500 languages
   (d) 300 ethnic groups and 600 languages

3. Multiple choice: Primary care services in Nigeria are delivered through:
   (a) Primary, secondary, and governmental healthcare centers
   (b) Primary, secondary, and faith-based clinics
   (c) Primary, secondary, and tertiary health facilities
   (d) Primary, governmental healthcare centers, and faith-based clinics.

4. Multiple choice: In what year was the NHIS introduced and what percentage of the population is covered?
   (a) 2004 and 1%
   (b) 2005 and 4%
   (c) 2006 and 6%
   (d) 2007 and 7%

5. True or False: The fleeing of nurses and doctors seeking better pay and working conditions abroad is referred to as the Nigerian Medical "brain gain."

Appendix: Answers to Review Questions

1. True or False: The acronym NDHS stands for the Nigeria Demographic and Healthcare Survey.

False: The acronym NDHS stands for the Nigeria Demographic and Health Survey. In 2018, NDHS collected information about specific types of insurance coverage and the percentages of women and men with any type of health insurance.

2. Multiple choice: Nigeria is home to approximately how many ethnic groups and languages?
   (a) 150 ethnic groups and 400 languages
   (b) 200 ethnic groups and 450 languages
   (c) 250 ethnic groups and 500 languages
   (d) 300 ethnic groups and 600 languages

The correct answer is d: Nigeria is home to an estimated 250 ethnic groups, with over 500 languages. The variety of customs and traditions make for great cultural diversity throughout the country.

3. Multiple choice: Primary care services in Nigeria are delivered through:
   (a) Primary, secondary, and governmental healthcare centers
   (b) Primary, secondary, and faith-based clinics
   (c) Primary, secondary, and tertiary health facilities
   (d) Primary, governmental healthcare centers, and faith-based clinics.

The answer is c: Primary, secondary, and tertiary health facilities. These facilities are often not available in rural areas. Rural areas primary care is mostly offered at governmental primary care centers and faith-based clinics.

4. Multiple choice: In what year was the NHIS introduced and what percentage of the population is covered?
   (a) 2004 and 1%
   (b) 2005 and 4%
   (c) 2006 and 6%
   (d) 2007 and 7%

The correct answer is c: The National Health Insurance Scheme (NHIS) was introduced in 2005 and only covers 4% of the population which is significantly low.

5. True or False: The fleeing of nurses and doctors seeking better pay and working conditions abroad is referred to as the Nigerian Medical "brain gain."

False: The fleeing of nurses and doctors seeking better pay and working conditions abroad is referred to as the Nigerian Medical "brain drain." Many doctors and nurses leave Nigeria in high numbers to practice in other countries around the world.

References

1. Encyclopaedia Britannica. https://www.britannica.com/place/Nigeria. Retrieved 4 July 2020.
2. Bloomberg News Nigeria Tops South Africa as the Continent's Biggest Economy. https://www.bloomberg.com/news/articles/2020-03-03/nigeria-now-tops-south-africa-as-the-continent-s-biggest-economy. Retrieved 4 July 2020.
3. Gyuse AN, Ayuk AE, Okeke MC. Facilitators and barriers to effective primary health care in Nigeria. Afr J Prim Health Care Fam Med. 2018;10(1):e1–3.
4. http://publications.universalhealth2030.org/uploads/nigeria_national_health_bill_-_2014_-_complete.pdf. Accessed 11 July 2020.
5. Uzochukwu B, Ughasoro MD, Etiaba E, Okwuosa C, Envuladu E, Onwujekwe OE. Health care financing in Nigeria: implications for achieving universal health coverage. Niger J Clin Pract. 2015;18:437–44. https://doi.org/10.4103/1119-3077.154196.
6. Mcintyre D, Meheus F, Røttingen JA. What level of domestic government health expenditure should we aspire to for universal health coverage? Health Econ Policy Law. 2017;12(2):125–37. https://doi.org/10.1017/S1744133116000414.
7. Onoka CA, Onwujekwe OE, Uzochukwu BS, Ezumah NN. Promoting universal financial protection: constraints and enabling factors in scaling-up coverage with social health insurance in Nigeria. Health Res Policy Syst. 2013;11:20. https://doi.org/10.1186/1478-4505-11-20.
8. Onyedibe KI, Goyit MG, Nnadi NE. An evaluation of the National Health Insurance Scheme (NHIS) in Jos, a north-central Nigerian city. Glob Adv Res J Microbiol. 2012;1(1):005–12.
9. Abiola AO, Ladi-Akinyemi TW, Oyeleye OA, Oyeleke GK, Olowoselu OI, Abdulkareem AT. Knowledge and utilisation of National Health Insurance Scheme among adult patients attending a tertiary health facility in Lagos State, South-Western Nigeria. Afr J Prm Health Care Fam Med. 2019;11(1):a2018. https://doi.org/10.4102/phcfm.v11i1.2018.
10. Okpani AI, Abimbola S. Operationalizing universal health coverage in Nigeria through social health insurance. Niger Med J. 2015;56(5):305–10. https://doi.org/10.4103/0300-1652.170382.
11. 2018 Nigeria Demographic and Health Survey (NDHS). https://www.dhsprogram.com/pubs/pdf/FR359/FR359.pdf. Accessed 7 Nov 2020.
12. Adefuye AO, Adeola AH, Bezuidenhout J. Medical education units: a necessity for quality assurance in health professions education in Nigeria. Afr J Health Professions Educ. 2018;10(1):5–9. https://doi.org/10.7196/AJHPE.2018.v10i1.966.
13. Federal Ministry of Health of Nigeria (Health Systems 20/20 Project). Nigeria Undergraduate Medical and Dental Curriculum Template, 2012. Bethesda, MD: Abt Associates Inc.; 2012.
14. Olopade FE, Adaramoye OA, Raji Y, Fasola AO, Olapade-Olaopa EO. Developing a competency-based medical education curriculum for the core basic medical sciences in an African medical school. Adv Med Educ Pract. 2016;7:389–98. https://doi.org/10.2147/2FAMEP.S100660.
15. Ofoegbu EN, Ozumba BC. Establishment of an office of medical education: Nigeria. Med Educ. 2007;41(5):507. https://doi.org/10.1111/j.1365-2929.2007.02730.x.
16. Are poor countries losing the information revolution? (English). infoDev working paper. Washington, D.C.: World Bank Group. http://documents.worldbank.org/curated/en/600361468762019045/Are-poor-countries-losing-the-information-revolution. Accessed 11 July 2020.
17. Ogunsola LA, Aboyade WA. Information and communication technology in Nigeria: revolution or evolution. J Soc Sci. 2005;11(1):7–14. https://doi.org/10.1080/09718923.2005.11892487.
18. Babalola Y. Nigeria's information infrastructure policy: implications for E-government. Arab J Bus Manag Rev. 2013;2:8–15.
19. Foster, Vivien; Pushak, Nataliya. 2011. Nigeria's infrastructure: a continental perspective. Africa Infrastructure Country Diagnostic; World Bank, Washington, DC; 2011. https://openknowledge.worldbank.org/handle/10986/27257. Accessed 12 July 2020
20. Statista Internet User Metrics. https://www.statista.com/statistics/183849/internet-users-nigeria/. Accessed 12 July 2020
21. Statista Smartphone Users Forecast. https://www.statista.com/statistics/467187/forecast-of-smartphone-users-in-nigeria/. Accessed 12 July 2020
22. Taiwo Adeleke I, Hakeem Lawal A, Adetona Adio R, Adisa AA. Information technology skills and training needs of health information management professionals in Nigeria: a nationwide study. Health Inf Manag. 2015;44(1):30–8. https://doi.org/10.1177/183335831504400104.
23. Iyoke CA, Lawani LO, Ugwu GO, et al. Knowledge and attitude toward interdisciplinary team working among obstetricians and gynecologists in teaching hospitals in South East Nigeria. J Multidiscip Healthc.

2015;8:237–44.   https://doi.org/10.2147/JMDH.
S82969.

24. Asangashi I, MacLeod B, Meremikwu M, Arikpo
    I, Roberge D, Hartsock B, Mboto I. Improving the
    routine HMIS in Nigeria through mobile technology
    for community data collection. J Health Inform Dev
    Countries. 2013;7(1):76–87.

25. Daniel GO, Oyetunde MO. Nursing informatics: a
    key to improving nursing practice in Nigeria. Int J
    Nurs Midwifery. 2013;5(5):90–8.

26. Ojo A. Repositioning health information manage-
    ment practice in Nigeria: suggestions for Africa.
    Health Inf Manag. 2018;47(3):140–4. https://doi.
    org/10.1177/1833358317732008.

Saudi Arabia: Transforming Healthcare with Technology

Taghreed Justinia

Learning Objectives

This chapter is focused on how *vision can drive health care technological transformation* on a national level. Vision is discussed as a main driver for change. 'Transformation' is explored as the theoretical underpinning of the chapter. The case study focuses on the Saudi Arabian experience in transforming its e-Health landscape guided by a national transformation program. This chapter offers insights about what drives digital health transformation, and how this can be led by a national strategy. Readers of this chapter will be able to:

- Explain the difference between change and digital transformation in health care
- Define various drivers for technological transformation in health care
- Describe examples of government-led digital health transformation projects
- Understand how strategic vision can drive digital health transformation
- Understand the national e-Health strategy transformation project in Saudi Arabia and the role of government in defining the vision

Key Terms
- Vision Realization Program
- National Transformation Program
- Transformation
- Change management
- Project management
- e-Health
- Digital health
- Digital transformation
- Digitization

Introduction

Health Care Complexity and Technology

Digital Health Innovations

Adoption of evidence-based digital health innovation promises to revolutionize health by reducing medical errors, improving quality of care, controlling costs, empowering individuals to understand their health care needs, and supporting public health initiatives [1]. Providers and governments have implemented and continue to implement a wide range of clinical and administrative applications, with a belief that digital implementations will offer benefits. Although the specific benefits may vary, the literature overwhelmingly shows that there are substantial advantages to digital health applications, which can have a positive impact on health care practice

T. Justinia (✉)
College of Public Health and Health Informatics,
King Saud bin Abdulaziz University for Health
Sciences & King Abdullah International Medical
Research Center, Jeddah, Saudi Arabia

© Springer Nature Switzerland AG 2022
U. H. Hübner et al. (eds.), *Nursing Informatics*, Health Informatics,
https://doi.org/10.1007/978-3-030-91237-6_47

and delivery, enhancing patient safety, and eventually lowering costs [1].

Health care organizations need to take advantage of the technologies that can improve data flow to meet quality clinical and administrative outcomes, with a clear necessity for the technological infrastructure to support their application [2]. Yet, health care information technology (IT) implementations are not simple, and when these projects are implemented on a larger scale, the associated transformation challenges are exasperated. Couple that with the workings of health care organizations and the complexities can become overwhelming [3]. These infrastructures are known to be complex and continually evolving in their design and deployment. The subsequent assessment of such foundations to meet professional outcomes, and to achieve value for health care organizations through their capability, is equally complicated [4]. Health care leaders must be comfortable with complexity and eager to embrace fast-paced, revolutionary changes. They must be equally prepared to lead in integrated health care environments that harness technology and value data [5]. This data is commonly provided by the health care industry, leading to a new relation of information asymmetry between the health care industry and government [6], which needs to be explored.

Challenges in Digital Health

Despite the well-documented advantages of investing in digital health projects, it is estimated that only one third of health care IT projects achieve success [7], and half of all large-scale IT projects go beyond original budgets by 45%, and 7% over intended time, while delivering 56% less value than predicted [8]. Merely investing in the technology does not ensure its success [9]. It is not surprising then that large-scale IT projects are prone to take too long, are usually more expensive than expected, and, crucially, fail to deliver the expected benefits [8]. Despite considerable investment in digital health, with growing health ecosystems, there are multiple challenges to successfully implementing these solutions. Since many health care systems have recognized the potential of digital health [10], it is crucial for the

health care industry and government to invest in effective strategies for successful implementation. These can be guided by a leading body to ensure the effective delivery of all intended digital health projects, thereby avoiding information irregularity, and achieving the intended outcomes.

Digital Transformation in Health Care

Transformation and Change

'Transformation' has been a frequent theme of government discourse in recent years, but what differentiates transformation from mere change has yet to be adequately explained [11]. Ultimately, a deeper understanding of technology-enabled transformation can help government to better utilize technology [11]. While organizational *change* can be described as examining the current state of affairs, and determining the ideal future situation; organizational *transformation* can be described as completely redefining the current state of affairs. These concepts can be applied to managing technological change and digital transformation in health care. Within this context, we can define *change management* as the process of directing, administering, and managing organizational changes in the health care environment. On the other hand, digital transformation can be defined as the process of integrating digital technology, which results in a transformation that can impact technology, culture, or the health care environment. Both desired situations should be based on the initial organizational vision and strategy.

Many IT health care projects in the public sector are done on a large scale, and usually span a state, a region, or an entire country [3], leading to transformative government [11]. Bannister and Connolly [11] argue that not all technology-driven or -enabled transformation is for the better, and encourage 'transformative governments' to examination the critical transformational impact of technology, and its effect on public sector values. They go on to explain that there is a wide and continuous spectrum between incremental change and transformation, the greater part of which is not transformational [12]. It is therefore important to be clear when using the term *transformation*. One of the criticisms of transformative government is the semantic vagueness of the word *transform*, especially when there may be an improvement but it does not result in a transformation [12]. Commonly, what is claimed to be transformative is largely incremental without any substantial change. In such cases there may be a visible improvement, but it should not be labeled a transformation [11].

Fundamental Drivers for Digital Transformation

There are certain fundamental drivers for transformation, and these include the need to increase revenues or to decrease costs; to become more efficient [13]; to create opportunity, disruption, or innovation; and to realize a strategic vision. Strategic technology trends also have the potential to both create opportunity and drive significant disruption. Technology innovation leaders must evaluate these top trends to determine how combinations of trends can power their innovation strategies [14]. In the Gartner Report, Cearley and Jones [14] list the top 10 strategic technology trends for 2020, and of these the following have the potential to directly drive transformation in the health care ecosystem: (1) *hyper-automation*; (2) *a multi-experience world*; (3) h*uman augmentation*; (4) *distributed cloud services*; (5) *autonomous things*; and (6) *transparency and traceability* (especially relevant for health data).

Another driver for transformation is consumer demand. Consumers are increasingly aware that their personal data is valuable and are demanding control. This includes ownership, value, and privacy of patient data, a much-contended topic. Organizations recognize the increasing risk of securing and managing personal data, and governments are implementing strict legislation and regulatory requirements to address these needs. Disruptive technological solutions such as 'blockchain' have been eyed by many as a possible ways to give back control of valuable patient data to the consumers themselves, with the potential to drive transformation in models of care

[15]. Governments and technology innovation leaders must evaluate the drivers for transformation to determine how combinations of trends can influence their innovation strategies [14], while considering new avenues to drive technological transformation.

Digital Health Reinvention and Digitization

Technology has already transformed many sectors of society and life, including the health care sector, which has resulted in what we call 'digital health.' Digital health can be defined as "the cultural transformation of how disruptive technologies that provide digital and objective data accessible to both caregivers and patients leads to an equal-level doctor-patient relationship with shared decision-making and the democratization of care" [2, p. 1]. The Ministry of Health (MOH) in Saudi Arabia describes *digital health* as "the cost effective and secure use of information and communication technologies and the associated cultural change it induces, to help people manage their health and wellbeing and transform the nature of health care delivery"[16, p. 5].

As part of the MOH e-Health transformation strategy, the terms 'digital reinvention,' 'digitization,' and 'digital transformation' are also used [16]. *Digital reinvention* in health care involves a fundamental reimagining of the way a health care organization engages with patients and other stakeholders to realize patients' ambitions and aspirations. While *digitization* improves efficiency by applying technology to individual resources or processes, *digital transformation* digitizes whole aspects of health care business and *digital reinvention* incorporates digital technologies like never before to deliver health care benefits by applying innovative strategies.

As technological innovations become inseparable from health care, and as health care systems worldwide are becoming financially unstable, a paradigm shift is imminent [2]. Andrews and Thornton [17] identify five challenges that government leaders must tackle in order to successfully implement digital reforms: (1) moving from small changes to transformation; (2) bringing policy and implementation together; (3) tackling

IT legacies; (4) adapting project governance; and (5) building a digitally capable workforce.

Under the term 'digital health,' advanced medical technologies, disruptive innovation, and digital communication have become synonymous with providing best practice health care, with a pressing need for transformation in the basic structure of health care [2]. Meskó and Drobni [2] contend that the practice of medicine must catch up with the rapid progress of the medical technology industry. However, this transition is slowed down by strict regulations; the reluctance of stakeholders in health care to change; and ignoring the importance of cultural changes and the human factor in an increasingly technological world.

Digital Health Innovation and Transparency

Policymakers globally face the challenge of keeping up with rapid innovations, and these trendsetters find it hard to integrate their solutions into overregulated or bureaucratic health care systems. Innovation has the potential to lead to value-based health care, and help make human skills from clinical judgment and experience to creative technical problem-solving. Digital health represents this transformation; however, most of the literature on this issue has focused on the technological instead of the human component, by not taking into consideration, for example, the importance of providing coaching with the technology [2]. It has also been argued that giving a certain disruptive technology alone to a patient has not improved health outcomes [4].

Technology also transforms the way people perceive and manage their health and wellbeing. New technologies are entering health care ecosystems, driven by unconventional actors that transcend geographical, cultural, and regulatory boundaries, thereby disrupting established models of production and delivery [6]. With this increased adoption of technology, the risk of patients turning to an accessible but unregulated technological solution for their health concerns is likely to increase [2]. Consequently, Meskó [2] and colleagues contend that medical professionals and policymakers have a responsibility to involve patients in designing care and decision-making, and guiding them in using regulated digital health technologies.

As digital health has become more integrated in health care structures, the issue of trust and transparency is raised. The one factor that does seem important and which can be greatly facilitated by technology is transparency, which leads to trust. This is why a government-led transformation initiative needs to be transparent to all those affected by the transformation [12]. Bannister and Connolly [12] contend that trust in government can be divided into two broad categories: general trust in the competence of the government to manage the state, and specific trust in the government not to abuse its power. Observing models of successful digital health integration led and governed by trusted governments would provide valuable direction in advancing digital health projects.

Strategic Vision Driving Digital Health Transformation

Strategically Enabling Digital Health

Thompson and Martin [18] clarify that strategies are the means through which organizations seek to achieve objectives and fulfill their mission or purpose, and therefore should not be thought of as having one single definition or perspective. They explain that there are three ways in which the strategies are created: with visionary leadership, from a planning process and adaptively, and incrementally as new decisions are taken in real time. How these translate into a process that can lead to reinvention on a large scale is left to the creativity, skill, and imagination of those leading the strategy, especially when transformation is required and government led.

As with the introduction of any new innovation, the potential benefits may be accompanied by unintended consequences, which reinforces the need for it to be carefully planned, implemented, and monitored. Ricciardi and Pita Barros [19] argue that a framework for the governance of the digital transformation of health services and its impact is vital to effectively stimulating the use of digital health strategies at various levels across health care ecosystems. Although many countries have not yet formulated a concise digital health strategy, it is expected that developments in formulating these strategies will result in better outcomes and in improving overall patient care [19]. Envisioning and establishing health policies that encourage innovation are significantly important in enabling digital health services. The role of government should go beyond merely evaluating, funding, and implementing technologies, and should also lead the adoption of digital health by creating incentives and steering the decentralized development, adoption, and use of these technologies [19]. In other words, the role of government should be to strategically enable and support the adoption of digital health.

The Visioning Process

There is an obvious role for strategic planning in transformation projects, as local authorities have to work within guidelines and budget constraints set by central government to improve efficiencies and to implement any central government requirements [18]. McCarthy [7] explains that establishing and clearly communicating a compelling vision is a critical success factor in creating an effective context for change that is the picture of the desired future state. The more complex the change, the more important it is to reach agreement on the future state. Digital health implementations are complex undertakings. A clear vision motivates and helps focus decisions during the natural stresses of a large project. Common mistakes with future state vision include: (1) not developing a near future state vision, (2) creating the vision but never cascading the message to the front line, (3) not using development of the vision as a process to engage the entire organization, (4) and not sharing the vision [18].

In a good visioning process, leaders take the time to truly think about where the organization is heading, and about what might be possible as opposed to what is. Creating a vision is all about starting a transformational journey with the end in mind. Organizations are increasingly faced with juggling countless transformational initiatives. With a clear vision these initiatives can be aligned with the direction of the organization [7], and when the transformation is carried out on a nationwide level, the visioning process must be aligned with the overarching national vision.

Governing Digital Health Care Transformation

Digital Era Governance Framework

The arrival of digital technology has not removed the complex accountabilities of government. Therefore, the governance of agile projects requires a specialist understanding of how they work [17]. Many digital transformation roles are not well integrated into existing organizational functions, which creates transformation adoption challenges. The absence of a clear mechanism to adopt new ways of working, coupled with the range of stakeholders involved in changes in work culture, creates a chasm that must be closed [20].

Margetts and Dunleavy [21] argue that handling digital change effectively requires a new macro-theory of public sector development, and a radically different mind-set, culture, and characteristic patterns of organizational governance. They explain that the three main themes of Digital Era Governance (DEG) are: organizational and budgetary factors internal to the state apparatus (reintegration); citizen-oriented factors in public services (holism); and influences from the societal adoption and cultural adaptation of technological drivers (digital change). They also explain that making a success of digital government means getting more people to do their business with government online, which means more and better online services [17]. New operating models are therefore needed to ensure that decisions are made in a consistent way, with digitally enabled, system-wide transformation in mind, a task that requires strong leadership [17].

Public and Private Sector Governance

Corydon and Ganesan [22] explain that public sector organizations with the most successful digital capabilities use four enablers to support and accelerate their transformation efforts: (1) their strategies reflect the capabilities and opportunities associated with digital technologies; (2) their governance models and organizational structures are built to handle the new tensions and risks associated with digital capabilities; (3) they recruit and develop workers to manage transformation programs and new capabilities; and (4) they create or acquire technological assets that are suited to the government's emerging digital functions. To further ensure value success in large-scale IT projects, Bloch and Blumberg [8] suggest focusing on managing strategy and stakeholders instead of exclusively concentrating on budget and scheduling, and building effective teams by aligning their incentives with the overall goals of the project.

Strategic management in different sectors such as small and global businesses and the public sector have many differences [18]. The composition of the public sector has changed over recent years and this includes their modus operandi. Many health care services have been privatized, resulting in multiple complementary businesses [18] with their unique regulatory methodologies that are normally accompanied by some form of regulation and government influence. This implies a broader stakeholder engagement that includes deregulated bodies and involvement from the private sector. The trend toward privatization has gathered momentum, and valuable lessons can be learned [18]. Public sector strategy can borrow from private sector practices, which have proven successful in the public health domain. For example, in the United Kingdom (UK), the National Health Service (NHS) works alongside the private health care sector and, although the rules and limits differ, the same consultants operate in both sectors [18].

The public sector also stands to gain from predictive and advanced analytics in defense, social welfare, public safety, and health care. Governments therefore need to set up data sharing systems that bring together data sets from different agencies [22], which can be amalgamated into the wider strategic vision.

Governing Socio-Technical Transition

Digital governance is in its infancy in many organizations. The transition to a mature digital governance model within a longstanding organization is a complex and disruptive journey [20]. Benjamin and Potts [20] explain that it can be challenging when organizations conceptualize digital transformation as a clearly defined change management exercise, rather than a fundamental transformation in how the organization functions.

When evaluating digital health services, many specific governance aspects need to be considered. Governance should play a more active role in the further optimization of both the process of decision-making and the related outcomes. The wider preparation of the health care ecosystem to be able to fully deal with digitization, from education, through financial and regulatory preconditions, to implementation of monitoring systems performance remains important [19]. Governance of digital transformation can be done on a higher and more strategic level when governments take on this role.

When planning and preparing health care professionals for the digital transformation, a good knowledge of these technologies by governments is required [19]. The resulting transformation must be aligned with the organization's work processes, as "people with a good understanding of technology can generate policy ideas that may not have been otherwise apparent" [17, p. 17]. More than understanding how transformations are planned, having a multifaceted approach can be helpful. Frennert [23] emphasizes that the multilevel perspective of socio-technological transition emphasizes that digital transformation is not just the result of the work of scientists and engineers, but is due to multiple actors at different levels. For governments, seeing technological change and digital transformation from a multilevel perspective enables them to understand their potential to change current practices [23] or completely reinvent them.

Digital Transformation and Government: A Global Perspective

Globally, there is a movement toward advancing digital services through government, and this extends to health care in many countries. When digital health is delivered at scale, there needs to be involvement from multiple stakeholders, and government often has a central and guiding role in leading these initiatives. Understanding how governments are planning digital transformation is of utmost importance when preparing for strategic technological transformation [20].

Different countries have sought varying approaches to revamping and modernizing their health care systems. In examining the service standards within governments in Canada, the UK, the US, Australia, and New Zealand, one sees an almost identical set of principles. In the rollout of these various initiatives worldwide, many health technology innovators have referred to these countries' experiences as valuable benchmarks. The implication of this is that those who can draw upon successful case studies from other governments worldwide potentially have a less onerous journey in making the case for change within their own governments. In contrast, those pioneers who blazed their trails generally fought long and painful bureaucratic battles to demonstrate the need for digital transformation [20]. We are now in a position where there are enough cases worldwide to refer to without the need to struggle as first-time-innovators. Sweden is one of these trailblazers that has articulated a discourse, stimulated knowledge, and opened pathways to digital transformation in health care with the 'Swedish e-Health Vision 2025' [23]. Another case is Kaiser Permanente (KP) which at one point was the largest not-for-profit integrated health care delivery system in the United States (US), serving 8.7 million members across eight regions. Similarly, there is Canada's Health Infoway [24], MedCom in Denmark, and in the Middle East, one example is the Saudi Arabian Ministry of National Guard-Health Affairs [25]. There is also the UK's National Program for IT (NPfIT)—an initiative that has been the subject of much contention [3].

While the rate of change is slow, public health systems are nonetheless slowly transforming their method of working to accommodate transformative new technologies in remarkable ways [20]. Governments using existing industry approaches to improve, update, or fundamentally re-design services tend to share common themes: they place a high value on user-centered design, prioritize iteration over the waterfall process, and use set design principles at a macro-organizational level to create consistency and ease of use [17]. These digital transformation teams have a strong focus on end-to-end service design over stop-gap digital solutions. They also use a rhetoric of openness and transparency [11], which is especially critical since health care is more complex in terms of governance [20].

While many governance principles and government initiatives have proven successful, others have been less effective. England's NHS experience when implementing the UK's NPfIT highlights the complexity of bringing contemporary digital design practices into big organizations. England's government pursued an overambitious and unwieldy centralized model without considering how this would impact user satisfaction and confidentiality issues. The UK's NPfIT lacked clear direction, was weak in project management, and had no exit strategy, meaning that the inevitable setbacks of pursuing such an ambitious program quickly turned into system-wide failures [3, 20]. Furthermore, the culture within the government in general was not conducive to swift identification and rectification of strategic or technical errors, citing a lack of clear leadership, a lack of concern for privacy issues, no exit plans and no alternatives, and lack of project management skills [3]. In September 2011, the UK government announced the dismantling of the project, underlining the inappropriateness of a centralized authority making top-down decisions on behalf of local organizations [20].

Acknowledging the previous failure of the top-down approach, the UK government instead called for health IT driven by local decision-making, hoping that the new approach would take a modular angle, allowing NHS organizations to introduce smaller, more manageable change [3, 20]. Later in 2015, a team from the Department of Health, NHS England and NHS

Digital, and contractors from the Government Digital Service (GDS) came together to help develop the new vision for the UK's NHS [20]. This new vision was articulated to be a leader in excellence in health care services. To achieve this, the UK government adopted a zero-tolerance approach, also referred to as the seven no's: (1) no barriers to health and well-being; (2) no avoidable deaths, injury, or illness; (3) no avoidable suffering or pain; (4) no helplessness; (5) no unnecessary waiting or delays; (6) no waste; and (7) no inequality. The vision set out the fundamental objectives and direction of the NHS in the region [26]. It was shared with other public bodies, embedded in local strategy documents, promoted by local champions, and cascaded down to all levels of the workforce [26]. The leadership style of 2015 was based on a new vision that was critical to the success of transformational change [3, 26].

Digital technology can alter choices, assumptions, and strategies that a government makes about its digitization efforts. Corydon and Ganesan [22] describe an approach that governments can use to reimagine their digitization strategies. They suggest considering the opportunities that digital technology creates and then set transformation goals in line with overall government priorities, as in the case of Denmark, which pursued an ambitious digitization strategy between 2011 and 2015 that would move it toward full digital delivery of government services. Designing the digitization strategy to support the broader policy-making agenda helped to speed its execution and led to favorable results [22]. In Sweden, Vision for e-Health 2025 claims to be best in the world at using the opportunities offered by digitization to make it easier to achieve equal health and welfare, and to develop and strengthen their own resources for increased independence and participation of society [23, 27]. Another example is the national e-Health strategy in Saudi Arabia [28], an initiative that was led by government as part of a central strategy to transform all sectors of the nation, including health care.

Information and Communication Technology Market in Saudi Arabia

Saudi Arabia is the region's largest information and communication technology (ICT) market, and ranks 13th globally, with a value of $28.7 billion in 2019 and strong growth in both the consumer and enterprise segments. Supported by a young and tech-savvy population, Saudi Arabia is a market of early technology adopters, with one of the highest social media penetrations in the world. Mobile subscribers stood at 43.8 million in 2019, representing a 129% penetration of the total population. Supported by a 93% Internet user penetration versus the global average of 53%, Saudi Arabia also became the first adopter of commercial 5G technology in the Middle East and North Africa, and the third largest globally—an achievement that is set to boost the adoption of other digitalization trends characterizing the 'Fourth Industrial Revolution.' In parallel, the Kingdom is the 5th G20 country in Internet speed, and jumped 80 places from 105th to 25th in the relevant global rankings, with a 51.8 Mbps average speed. It comes as no surprise that technology adoption in all sectors including health care come at the top of the national agenda [29]. The technological readiness of this country and its infrastructure makes the national e-Health strategy in Saudi Arabia an interesting case study to observe and learn from.

Case Study

Background to Case Study

There are many drivers for technological transformation, and one fundamental driver is strategy and vision. When transformation happens on a national level, there are many lessons to learn. Technology driven by vision can be at the heart of health care transformation. What is witnessed in the case of Saudi Arabia is transformation that is planned and executed to drive a national digital health strategy. The experience is rich, setting the stage for an unprecedented benchmark on a global level. Many lessons can be learnt from this experience, both during the implementation and after the full vision is realized. This case study is focused on how a national vision was the main driver to achieve the e-Health transformation programs in the Kingdom.

Launch of the National Transformation Program

Saudi Arabia adopted a National Transformation Program (NTP), also referred to as 'Vision 2030,' as a roadmap for economic growth and national development. Vision 2030 outlined the Kingdom's general objective to become a world-class model of a successful and pioneering nation. Saudi Arabia aims to achieve its Vision 2030 objectives through three main pillars: a vibrant society, a thriving economy, and an ambitious nation [30]. Saudi Arabia's transformation strategy comprises 96 strategic objectives, governed by a number of Key Performance Indicators (KPIs) that will be achieved through a number of initiatives co-developed and executed by different governmental entities alongside private and non-profit organizations. In order to build the capacity and capabilities required to achieve its ambitious goals, the NTP was launched on June 6, 2016, with Vision Realization Programs (VRP) across 24 government bodies operating in the economic and development sectors in Saudi Arabia in its first year. Its main aim was to develop governmental work and establish the needed infrastructure [30]. The program's strategic objectives are linked to interim targets. The first phase of initiative implementation was launched on April 25, 2016, and was then followed every year by phases involving more public bodies. It focused on achieving governmental operational excellence, improving economic enablers, and enhancing living standards through accelerating the implementation of primary and digital infrastructure projects. It also emphasizes engaging stakeholders in identifying challenges,

co-creating solutions, and implementing the program's initiatives [31].

Governance Model for Achieving Saudi Arabia's Vision 2030

The Council of Ministers entrusted the Council of Economic and Development Affairs (CEDA) with the task of establishing the mechanisms and measures necessary to achieve Saudi Arabia's Vision 2030. The CEDA developed a comprehensive governance model aimed at institutionalizing and enhancing its work, facilitating the coordination of efforts among relevant stakeholders, and effectively following up progress, as outlined in Fig. 47.1 [32]. Support Units were also established with the role of supporting certain government entities with communication activities, finance, budgeting, and performance control, in addition to other bodies supporting Vision 2030 realization efforts. Roles have been dedicated to those units within the Vision 2030 governance activities, like the various VRPs, as well as Vision Realization Offices (VRO) under each execution body like the different ministries. The CEDA set up an effective governance model with the aim of translating Vision 2030 into multiple VRPs working in parallel [32].

Establishing the Vision Realization Office

To ensure a smooth evolution, the VRO for the MOH was established as the main body to foresee the implementation of all elements of Vision 2030 on the ground. The vision of the VRO is to provide a health system that promotes, protects, and restores the health of both individuals and society. The mission of the VRO is to transform the health sector in a gradual, safe, and efficient manner, from the beneficiary's perspective, to ensure that the system is dynamic and technology enabled, as well as fostering both preventive and therapeutic health services for both individuals and the society. The VRO seeks to achieve four key objectives: (1) achieving the objectives of both the 2020 National Transformation Program and

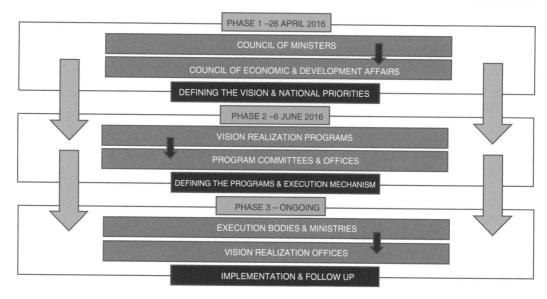

Fig. 47.1 Governance model for achieving Saudi Arabia's Vision 2030

Vision 2030; (2) monitoring transformational initiatives, tracking the progress of implementation plans, and continuously assessing the level of performance and quality; (3) creating a motivating and productive work environment that attracts competent and national talent; and (4) working within the Vision 2030 governance framework to ensure alignment with government [33].

Transforming Health Care in Saudi Arabia

Transform Health Care Theme

There are eight main themes of the Vision 2030 program: (1) Transform Health Care, (2) Improve Living Standards & Safety, (3) Ensure Sustainability of Vital Resources, (4) Social Empowerment & Non-Profit Sector Development, (5) Achieve Government Operational Excellence, (6) Labor Market Accessibility, (7) Contribute to Enabling the Private Sector, and (8) Develop Tourism & National & Heritage Sectors. At the heart of the vision is the goal of completely transforming health care services in Saudi Arabia. The Transform Health Care theme includes easing access to health care services; improving value, quality, and efficiency of health care services;

and promoting prevention of health threats . This theme has three strategic objectives, ten main KPI indicators, 24 KPI sub-indicators, and 70 initiatives. First, it seeks to achieve a vibrant society by restructuring the health sector to become a comprehensive and effective system. Next, it intends to promote public health through the implementation of a new model of care that focuses on prevention and improving society's health awareness. Last, it aims to improve access to health services through optimal coverage, equitable geographical distribution, as well as comprehensive and expanded e-Health services and digital solutions. Under the Transform Health Care theme, e-Health is identified as a key enabler of the health care transformation. Out of the 70 key initiatives under this theme, 12 initiatives are directly related to technology, as outlined in Table 47.1 [16].

MOH Role in Guiding e-Health Strategy Principles

The MOH defines a strategic objective to improve the efficiency and effectiveness of the health care sector through the use of IT and digital transformation. Other sectors of government in Saudi Arabia are also driven by the national strategy, like the Ministry of ICT with a strategic objective

Table 47.1 Transform health care theme initiatives related to technology

Initiative	Description
e-Health	The initiative aims to improve the efficiency of the health care sector through information technology, digital transformation, and utilizing state-of-the-art technologies to ease access to health care (such as tele-medicine and tele-consultations).
Technology Assessment Center	The initiative aims to establish a national center for the assessment of health care technologies, which can then be classified as preventive, diagnostic, therapeutic, rehabilitative, and palliative.
National Health Information Center— cross-cutting e-Health initiatives	The initiative aims to provide an electronic service focused on working with all sectors providing health care services and other related sectors, in order to construct a more coherent system; more integrated health services will enable the beneficiaries to easily access medical services of high quality and security.
National Health Innovation Center	The initiative aims to establish a national center to encourage and foster creativity and innovation in health care.
Establish an electronic tracking system	The initiative aims to establish an e-tracking system for pharmaceuticals so that their distribution can be tracked to ensure their safety and availability within the market.
Technology Development Center	The initiative aims to establish a center of excellence that develops health information systems which can be used in the health care education sector.
Establish the Standard Electronic System	The initiative aims to develop and standardize registration, licensing, inspection, clearance, export, and enforcement procedures for investors in the Saudi Food & Drug Agency (SFDA) in all sectors.
Saudi Center for Appointments and Medical Referrals	The initiative aims to manage medical referrals and the procedures of booking appointments for all patients transferred between health facilities inside and outside the Kingdom, through standard work procedures and through the design of a unified e-system for referrals and appointments.
National Health Referral Plan	The initiative is concerned with the revision of referral systems among health facilities in all sectors to design systems that are compatible with sector priorities.
"HESN" program	The initiative aims to improve public health outcomes and provide an adequate and integrated database that will help to take preventive measures to prevent the outbreak of diseases and epidemics.
National Horizontal Health Records	The initiative aims to establish health records that collect detailed data on procedures for the treatment of predetermined diseases and health conditions by identifying a set of key data for these diseases and collecting them nationally from all health care providers.
National Register of Organ Failure	The initiative aims to use a specialized e-system to register patients with organ failure and organ donors, and develop the necessary procedures for follow-up.

for 2030 to develop the IT sector [31]. In the 2018 updated roadmap to the digital health strategy [16], they explain that the cultural change that they drive will play a significant role in supporting the delivery of digital health vision and in achieving Vision 2030.

The MOH's e-Health strategic framework was designed to guide the development of the e-Health Strategy and five-year roadmap, and ensure alignment with the MOH business strategy and objectives. Aligning the e-Health strategic objectives with the MOH's overarching objectives is expected to provide a strong foundation for achieving clinical and business value and is instrumental to the success of the transformation [28].

Summary

Technology leaders and governments need to develop tools to ensure the overall health success and sustainability of complex health care systems. These tools usually emerge as technology innovations that have the potential to completely transform health care ecosystems. In health care, there are many fundamental drivers for digital transformation. These enablers can include costs, efficiency, opportunity, innovation, consumer demand, strategic technology trends, and/or realizing a strategic vision. Planning and ensuring successful implementation of digital health initiatives requires careful governance frameworks, which are sometimes led by government. Digital health steered by a national government can therefore be viewed as an impetus for transformation that can completely re-envision the delivery of health services. This chapter explains how to successfully implement transformation in overall project success planning, and demonstrates how these concepts were applied in health care technology programs on a national level. For illustration and clarification purposes, a case study is presented about transforming health care in Saudi Arabia and how this transformation was led by a national vision that ultimately transformed into a national e-Health strategy.

Conclusions and Outlook

Transformation as a business concept in health care services involves fundamentally changing the way a health care organization engages with patients and other stakeholders. The differences were dispelled throughout this chapter. Digital health transformation was identified as a guiding theme. Currently, there are many drivers for technological transformation, and two fundamental drivers are strategy and vision. When transformation happens on a national level, there are many lessons to learn. What is witnessed in the Saudi Arabia case study is transformation that is planned and executed to drive a national e-Health strategy. The experience is rich, yet there are still many challenges to overcome before the final vision is realized. What this case study implies is that technology driven by vision can be at the heart of health care transformation, while many more lessons can be learnt after the full vision is realized.

Useful Resources

Websites

1. Saudi Arabia Ministry of Health. Available from: https://www.moh.gov.sa/en/
2. https://www.moh.gov.sa/en/Ministry/nehs/Pages/default.aspx
3. Canada Health Infoway. Available from: https://infoway-inforoute.ca/en/
4. UK NHS Digital. Available from: https://www.gov.uk/government/organisations/nhs-digital
5. Sweden Ministry of Health and Social Affairs. Available from: https://www.government.se/government-of-sweden/ministry-of-health-and-social-affairs/
6. Saudi Arabia National e-Health Strategy MOH. Available from: https://www.moh.gov.sa/en/Ministry/nehs/Pages/default.aspx
7. Saudi Arabia National Transformation Program: Available from: https://vision2030.gov.sa/en/node.
8. Saudi Arabia Vision Realization Office. Available from: https://www.moh.gov.sa/en/Ministry/vro/Pages/default.aspx.

Reports
1. Saudi Arabia National Transformation Program Delivery Plan 2018-2020. Available from: https://vision2030.gov.sa/sites/default/files/attachments/NTP%20English%20Public%20Document_2810.pdf
2. Saudi Arabia Digital Health Strategy Update 2018. Available from: https://www.moh.gov.sa/Ministry/vro/eHealth/Documents/MoH-Digital-Health-Strategy-Update.pdf
3. Corydon, B., V. Ganesan, and M. Lundqvist, *Digital by default: A guide to transforming government.* 2016: McKinsey Center for Government. Available from: https://www.mckinsey.com/business-functions/mckinsey-digital/our-insights/delivering-large-scale-it-projects-on-time-on-budget-and-on-value
4. Bloch, M., S. Blumberg, and J. Laartz, Delivering large-scale IT projects on time, on budget, and on value. McKinsey Quarterly, 2012. 27: p. 2-7. Available from: https://www.mckinsey.com/business-functions/mckinsey-digital/our-insights/delivering-large-scale-it-projects-on-time-on-budget-and-on-value
5. Sweden Ministry of Health and Social Affairs, Vision for e-Health 2025: Common starting points for digitisation of social services and health care. 2016: Stockholm. Available from: https://www.government.se/information-material/2016/08/vision-for-ehealth-2025/
6. Andrews, E., et al., Making a success of digital government. 2016, Institute for Government.

Available from: https://www.instituteforgovernment.org.uk/sites/default/files/publications/IFGJ4942_Digital_Government_Report_10_16%20WEB%20%28a%29.pdf

Review Questions

1. How is digital transformation different from change management?
2. What are some drivers for IT transformation in health care?
3. What role can government have in a visioning process leading to digital health?
4. Case Study: What strategies are recommended by Saudi Arabia's MOH to achieve a national vison toward digital health?

Appendix: Answers to Review Questions

1. How is digital transformation different from change management?

Organizational change is assessing the past, comparing it to the present, and determining the ideal future state from the current business state. Success measurement of change is how much better the future state is from the current state. On the other hand, transformation is redefining what something is. It begins by first assessing the present to the desired future. While organizational change can be described as examining the current state of affairs, and determining the ideal future situation, organizational transformation can be described as completely redefining the current state of affairs. Change management can be defined as the process of directing, administering, and managing organizational changes in the health care environment. On the other hand, digital transformation can be defined as the process of integrating digital technology, which results in a transformation that can impact technology, culture, or the health care environment. Both desired situations should be based on the initial organizational vision and strategy.

2. What are some drivers for IT transformation in health care?

There are fundamental drivers for IT transformation, and these inducers can be to increase revenues or to decrease costs; to become more efficient; to create opportunity, disruption, or innovation; or to realize a strategic vision, which is the enabler that was disused in depth throughout this chapter. Strategic technology trends also have the potential to directly drive transformation in the health care ecosystem. Another driver for transformation is consumer demand. Consumers are increasingly aware that their personal data is valuable and are demanding control. This includes ownership, value, and privacy of patient data, a much contended topic. Organizations recognize the increasing risk of securing and managing personal data, and governments are implementing strict legislation and regulatory requirements to address these needs.

3. What role can government have in a visioning process leading to digital health?

In a good visioning process, leaders take the time to truly think about where the organization is heading, and about what might be possible as opposed to what is. With a clear vision, initiative can be aligned with the direction of the organization, and when the transformation is carried out on a nationwide level, the visioning process must be aligned with the overarching national vision. Envisioning and establishing health policies that encourage innovation are significantly important in enabling digital health services. The role of government should go beyond merely evaluating, funding, and implementing technologies, and should also lead the adoption of digital health by creating incentives and steering the decentralized development, adoption, and use of these technologies. In other words, the role of government should be to strategically enable and support the adoption of digital health.

4. Case Study: What strategies are recommended by Saudi Arabia's MOH to achieve a national vison toward digital health?

In order to ensure appropriate levels of deployment success, and with the many lessons learned throughout the various stages of realizing the national vision toward digital health, the following strategies are recommended by the Saudi Arabia MOH [16, 28]:

- *Outsource Functions*: During the initial years of the program, including maintenance, support, and supplies delivery, with long-term goals of repatriating these services to staff functions.
- *Share Services*: Especially in urban areas were economies of scale can be achieved, and there is potential for clustering of computer data centers.
- *Proactive Setup Techniques*: For new installations such as pre-populating client records via extractions from demographic information, and conversion of existing electronic files.
- *Incentives for e-Health Change Leaders*: Provide extra incentives for the health change leaders, and those employees demonstrating high-proficiency usage of new technology.

References

1. Abdelhak M, Grostick S, Hanken MA. Health information: management of a strategic resource. 4th ed. St. Louis: Elsevier.
2. Meskó B, et al. Digital health is a cultural transformation of traditional healthcare. Mhealth. 2017;3:38.
3. Justinia T. The UK's National Programme for IT: why was it dismantled? Health Serv Manag Res. 2017;30(1):2–9.
4. Williams PA, et al. Improving digital hospital transformation: development of an outcomes-based infrastructure maturity assessment framework. JMIR Med Inform. 2019;7(1):e12465.
5. Rosenberg L. Are healthcare leaders ready for the real revolution? J Behav Health Serv Res. 2012;39(3):215–9.
6. Alami H, Gagnon MP, Fortin JP. Digital health and the challenge of health systems transformation. Mhealth. 2017;3:31.
7. McCarthy C, Eastman D, Garets DE. Effective strategies for change. Chicago: HIMSS; 2014.
8. Bloch M, Blumberg S, Laartz J. Delivering large-scale IT projects on time, on budget, and on value. McKinsey Q. 2012;27:2–7.
9. Protti D. Implementing information for health: even more challenging than expected? 2002 [cited 2016 23 February]. Available from https://www.uvic.ca/hsd/hinf/
10. Tseng J, et al. Catalyzing healthcare transformation with digital health: performance indicators and lessons learned from a digital health innovation group. Healthc (Amst). 2018;6(2):150–5.
11. Bannister F, Connolly R. ICT, public values and transformative government: a framework and programme for research. Gov Inf Q. 2014;31(1):119–28.
12. Bannister F, Connolly R. Trust and transformational government: a proposed framework for research. Gov Inf Q. 2011;28(2):137–47.
13. Kotter JP. Accelerate! Harv Bus Rev. 2012;90(11):44–52.
14. Cearley D et al. Top 10 strategic technology trends for 2020. 2019, Gartner.
15. Justinia T. Blockchain technologies: opportunities for solving real-world problems in healthcare and biomedical sciences. Acta Inform Med. 2019;27(4):284–91.
16. Ministry of Health. Digital Health Strategy. 2018 September 2018 [cited 2020 20 June]. Available from https://www.moh.gov.sa/Ministry/vro/eHealth/Documents/MoH-Digital-Health-Strategy-Update.pdf
17. Andrews E et al. Making a success of digital government. 2016, Institute for Government.
18. Thompson J, Martin F. Strategic Management awareness and change. 5th ed. New York: Thompson Learning; 2005. p. 873.
19. Ricciardi W, et al. How to govern the digital transformation of health services. Eur J Pub Health. 2019;29(Suppl 3):7–12.
20. Benjamin K, Potts HW. Digital transformation in government: lessons for digital health? Digit Health. 2018;4:2055207618759168.
21. Margetts H, Dunleavy P. The second wave of digital-era governance: a quasi-paradigm for government on the web. Philos Trans A Math Phys Eng Sci. 1987;2013(371):20120382.
22. Corydon B, Ganesan V, Lundqvist M. Digital by default: a guide to transforming government. London: McKinsey Center for Government; 2016.
23. Frennert S. Hitting a moving target: digital transformation and welfare technology in Swedish municipal eldercare. Disabil Rehabil Assist Technol. 2019;2019:1–9.
24. Canada Health Infoway. Electronic Health Records 2016 [cited 2020 20 February]. Available from https://www.infoway-inforoute.ca/en/solutions/electronic-medical-records
25. Justinia T. Implementing large-scale healthcare information systems: the technological, managerial and behavioural issues. Germany: Scholars Press; 2014.

26. Hunter DJ, et al. Doing transformational change in the English NHS in the context of "big bang" redisorganisation. J Health Organ Manag. 2015;29(1):10–24.

27. Ministry of Health and Social Affairs. Vision for eHealth 2025: common starting points for digitisation of social services and health care. 2016; Stockholm.

28. National eHealth Strategy-MOH. 2020 [cited 2020 15 January]. Available from https://www.moh.gov.sa/en/Ministry/nehs/Pages/default.aspx.

29. Ministry of Communications & Information Technology. 2020 [cited 2020 10 Jan]. Available from https://www.mcit.gov.sa/en/standard-indicators/99050.

30. Vision 2030. *National Transformation Program Delivery Plan 2018-2020.* 2018 [cited 2020 20 June]. Available from https://vision2030.gov.sa/sites/default/files/attachments/NTP%20English%20Public%20Document_2810.pdf

31. National Transformation Program. 2016 [cited 2020 10 June]. Available from https://vision2030.gov.sa/en/node.

32. National Transformation Program. *Governance Model for Achieving Saudi Arabia's Vision* 2030. 2020 [cited 2020 10 July]. Available from https://vision2030.gov.sa/en/governance

33. Vision Realization Office. 2018 [cited 2020 10 Jan]. Available from https://www.moh.gov.sa/en/Ministry/vro/Pages/default.aspx

Part X

Future Trends in Health Informatics

Emerging Technologies: Data and the Future of Surgery

48

Nadine Hachach-Haram and Jamila S. Karim

Learning Objectives
- Define the role that data plays in surgery and explain how this role is continuously developing.
- Explain the difference between structured and unstructured data.
- Discuss the impact and applications of surgical data science.
- Outline important sources of surgical data and explain how the pool of data assets used in surgery is expanding, particularly with reference to data from imaging and video.
- Explore how the information contained in data can be turned into meaningful, actionable intelligence.
- Define AI and Big Data and explain the potential applications and benefits of AI in surgery.
- Explain how data-led intelligence can best be communicated in the operating room (OR) with specific emphasis on how insights gained from data can be integrated into surgical workflows and deliver real-time guidance during procedures.

Key Terms
- Big Data analytics
- Artificial intelligence
- Machine learning
- Surgical data science
- Artificial neural networks
- Natural Language Processing
- Computer vision
- Augmented reality
- Human-to-human communication
- Operating room
- Surgical services
- Telementoring

Introduction: The Role of Data in Surgery

Like every other commercial, industrial and service sector, healthcare is undergoing rapid digital transformation. It is a process that is already having a significant impact on interventional medicine. In surgery, technological breakthroughs such as minimally invasive techniques, advanced imaging and robotic automation have yielded a wide range of benefits, including improving accuracy and patient outcomes, boosting throughput by reducing the time surgery takes, and laying the foundations for patient-specific planning [1].

The steady progress of digitisation has also had another effect. Digital medical imaging and diagnostic tools, laparoscopic and computer-assisted surgical systems and electronic health records (EHRs) all share one thing in common:

N. Hachach-Haram (✉)
London, UK

J. S. Karim
London, UK

© Springer Nature Switzerland AG 2022
U. H. Hübner et al. (eds.), *Nursing Informatics*, Health Informatics,
https://doi.org/10.1007/978-3-030-91237-6_48

they create and/or contain vast quantities of digital data.

Data has quickly come to be viewed as the most valuable commodity in the emerging global digital economy [2]. But what is data, and why does it matter? In its rawest form, data is the long binary sequences of ones and zeroes, known as bytes, that every computer-based system uses to function. While such a jumble of digits might not look too promising, the value of data stems from the fact that it comprises a record of every process, every exchange, every transaction undertaken by the system in question. Essentially, data is an objective digital record of activity. Analyse that record in the right way and you can reveal statistical patterns which in turn provide insights into systems and processes at a level of accuracy and detail never previously imagined.

As Maier-Hein et al. (2017) suggest, surgical practice has always had something of an "artisanal craft" about it, relying on a certain degree of individuality in the skills and expertise of practitioners. While those talents can and do save lives, relying on the competencies and preferences of individuals also inevitably leads to variation in standards and outcomes [3].

Data, by contrast, offers an objective, evidence-based knowledge source built on robust statistical analysis [1]. Data leaves no room for debate as to which approaches have the best outcomes. Therefore, it has a potentially transformational impact on clinical decision making and planning and can help to optimise workflows, cut waste and reduce costs [3].

However, work needs to be done before surgeons can enjoy the benefits of data-based intelligence. The process of gleaning meaningful statistical insights from long lists of ones and zeros is known as data analytics. Analytics uses special algorithms which in effect 'read' the patterns contained in digital data. But to do this, algorithms (or traditional ones, at least) need data to be in a consistent, organised format.

Unfortunately, the sources of data available in surgery are particularly heterogeneous and complex, originate from various sources and are provided in multiple different formats. Moreover, an estimated 80% of the data available to surgeons is either considered 'unstructured' (not organised enough for a standard algorithm to read it) or exists in a non-digital format altogether (e.g. handwritten clinical notes) [4].

This has significantly impeded the ability for data to truly impact surgery to date. However, it has also triggered interest in developing a surgery-specific approach to data science to resolve these issues [3]. Data science is best understood in the context of so-called Big Data analytics, an umbrella term for a groundbreaking field of analytics which aims to acquire valuable intelligence from large volumes of heterogeneous, unstructured data in rapid time [4]. Before Big Data, analytics was restricted by limitations in the amount and type of data conventional algorithms could work with. This meant spending a lot of time and energy preparing and converting data prior to feeding it through analytics software in manageable chunks. As data volumes have grown exponentially, this has become increasingly unviable.

Surgical data science is an emerging field that aims to provide a common framework for the collection, analysis and modelling of the massive, heterogeneous data resources available within clinical settings [1]. Ultimately, when you consider the volume and variety of data now available to support every clinical decision made (something we'll look at in more depth in the next section), surgeons need help making sense of it all [3]. That help comes in the form of cutting-edge processing technologies being developed under the *Big Data* umbrella [5]. The goal is not to replace human decision making. Rather, Big Data aims to support and augment clinical acumen by laying out robust models based on the full spectrum of information available and by quantifying processes and outcomes, allowing surgeons to measure success step by step along the way.

In terms of applications and benefits, the standout promise of *surgical data science* is improving patient outcomes, for example by using advanced modelling techniques to predict the likelihood of severe complications for each patient [6]. In its 2018 *Future of Surgery* report, the Royal College of Surgeons of England outlined the role that data will play in the evolution of precision medicine, stating that "patients can confidently expect surgery to become gradually less invasive, more accurate, have more predictable outcomes, faster recovery times and lower risk of harm" [7].

By collecting all of the data from individual care pathways and making it available for comparison in national and international databases, *surgical data science* can also deliver significant benefits to service planning, governance and research [6]. The more data there is available, the more accurately and fairly we'll be able to benchmark outcomes of different service providers. In turn, this will lead to a better understanding of the reasons for outcome variations and enable us to minimise them [5]. This can equate to significant efficiency gains based on robust, objective analysis of best practice. For example, the UK's Getting It Right First Time (GIRFT) programme aims to save the National Health Service (NHS) £1.4bn using *Big Data* techniques to identify waste. In surgery, it has already identified the fact that 30,000 bed days could be saved by reducing the average length of stay post appendicectomy down from 3.5 days to 2 days, a figure already achieved by half of Trusts [4].

Over time, the development of large surgical databases and application of *Big Data* techniques will also help to overcome some of the challenges inherent in surgical research, such as recruiting subjects, selection bias and collecting samples. These factors often lead to surgical innovations and new devices being approved for release without undergoing testing at scale [4, 7]. In lieu of clinical trials, *surgical data science* will be able to extrapolate comparisons with existing techniques and technologies, and then refine analysis of outcomes, risks and best practice over time based on 'real life' usage data [5].

Finally, in addition to creating an objective knowledge base for research and guidance, a data science approach can also provide practitioners with valuable feedback in the form of clinical support. Rather than having to rely on memory to recall the latest best practice advice in the midst of surgery (assuming the latest developments have already been released for clinician con-

sumption), *Big Data* tools can 'scrape' available literature for information relevant to the procedure and present it in a targeted way at the appropriate stage of the care pathway [4].

Sourcing Surgical Data

We have already established that the sources for surgical data are incredibly numerous and diverse, to the extent that this may have hindered the development of data-led surgical practice to date [3]. These sources are only expected to multiply further as the digitisation of surgery continues. Although the emergence of *Big Data analytics* promises a practical solution to the heterogeneity of data available in surgery, an important step in the development of *surgical data science* will be to identify and focus efforts on sources that yield the most useful and robust insights.

Let's start by listing some of the main sources of data and information currently available to surgical practitioners. A simple distinction can be drawn between 'external' sources, or data/information that originates outside the clinical setting and exists prior to the commencement of a particular care pathway, and 'internal' sources, which refers to data generated in the process of delivering care within the clinic/hospital.

In the external category, we could list things like surgical databases and registries, clinical trial data, best practice guidelines and regulations. Data of this type forms part of the 'domain knowledge' surgeons use to support decision making, and poses particular challenges around consistency of presentation and interpretation [3]. In a mature system built around *surgical data science*, where data from all individual pathways and procedures is fed into shared registries, we can expect databases (and the analysis of the data they contain) to take a leading role in the modelling of agile, optimised approaches.

In the internal category, data and information is recorded throughout the end-to-end process of assessment, diagnosis, intervention and recovery. This type of data is increasingly created by a dizzying array of technology: diagnostic equipment, medical monitors, advanced imaging technologies, computer-assisted surgical systems and more [1]. Within *the OR alone*, the data being generated by surgical devices is continuously developing in sophistication—ranging from precise positional and ergonomic data available from surgical robots to video feeds and force/pressure measurements generated by laparoscopic systems [5].

Straddling the divide between these external and internal data sources is the EHR. The EHR is undoubtedly an important resource for practitioners as it combines a patient's prior medical history with 'in-progress' data relating to the current care episode. Yet, as widely used as the EHR is across medical care, Vedula and Hager (2017) argue that it "remains an incomplete record of data generated by the care process itself" [6]. This is partly due to the fact that there is still no universal standard that outlines which data points should be captured in the EHR. Fundamentally, due to the unstructured and voluminous nature of some of the data sources involved, the EHR simply cannot capture all of it. For example, a medical imaging report does not encompass all of the data contained by the image itself.

Imaging plays a particularly prevalent role in surgical care pathways. Since the arrival of X-ray, surgeons have reaped the benefits of an ever-expanding array of technologies: computer tomography (CT), ultrasound, magnetic resonance imaging (MRI), positron emission tomography (PET) and other radionuclide techniques, which help them to see into the patient's body in order to make decisions on what needs to be done and how [8]. Medical imaging is most frequently used by surgeons for assessment and diagnostics. However, as demonstrated by the use of X-ray fluoroscopy and ultrasound to guide catheter and needle insertion, imaging also has intraoperative, interventional and therapeutic uses [9]. As technology evolves, the use of imaging as a clinical support tool in *the OR* is becoming increasingly prevalent.

The basic premise of image-guided surgery is straightforward. By creating a workable visual model of the patient's anatomy, images provide a useful reference point for surgeons as they oper-

ate [10]. With the guidance of increasingly sophisticated images, surgeons have been able to improve precision and reduce mistakes. This works best when 'live' images of the patient (as opposed to preoperative images) can be fed back to the surgical team in real time. The archetype for this kind of approach is the use of video cameras in laparoscopy. There are, however, numerous other examples in common use, such as stereotaxy (triangulating coordinates to locate small objects in the body) and advanced angiographic techniques for identifying blood vessels in neurosurgery [11].

Medical images are packed full of information which may well be unavailable from any other source (e.g. what exactly is taking place at the end of the endoscope during a laparoscopic procedure?). From a data science perspective, the data they contain is very much in an unstructured form. Interpretation of the image is left to the individual judgements of surgeons, which, as we have discussed, will inevitably lead to variation and errors. Surgery might be increasingly guided by images, but we are yet to utilise the data that they contain to its full potential.

Let's take video as an example. Video is a much richer source of valuable data than even the most sophisticated of static images—one minute of HD surgical video, for instance, is believed to contain 25 times the data that a single high-resolution CT scan contains [12]. Spearheaded by laparoscopy, which has the advantage of creating video recordings of every procedure as a matter of course, video has started to gain a following as a useful tool for postoperative review, coaching and education. A video recording does, after all, provide a more complete and objectively reliable account of what went on in *the OR* than clinical notes [13]. As such, numerous clinical reviews have linked use of video in this setting to improvements in performance and outcomes through upskilling practitioners, for example by identifying and addressing error-event sequences even in successful procedures where such 'mistakes' would not otherwise be brought to light [14].

This work is undoubtedly beneficial. The current question is whether it could be pushed even further. It has been suggested that video could be used more formally to assess skill competencies against established benchmarks, or even for determining what those benchmarks should be by identifying best practice examples from comparison of videos [14]. Both would depend on having a consistent and robust framework for measuring and interpreting success. The question then is how such assessments should be made. Different individuals are always liable to draw different conclusions about what best practice looks like from observation alone, whether in person or via a video recording. The only way to truly drive consistency and minimise variation in practice would be to link intraoperative performance with a reliable selection of outcome data. This would require that the unstructured data contained in a video recording be made available for interrogation and comparison alongside other data sets.

If intraoperative video can be made subject to robust comparative analysis for the purpose of formal skills/performance assessment, could it also be used more broadly for formal clinical auditing and empirical research? [15] This would likely necessitate 'whole room' recording, rather than a more narrow focus on what takes place at the surgical site, in order to capture the full spectrum of contextual information—the conversations members of the team have, their movements around the room and position at the surgical table, the instruments selected, the procedural sequences followed, the timings, the minutiae of what they do to the patient. That, of course, means yet more complex and diverse data to harness and analyse.

Finally, a further question is whether this kind of deep analysis could be useful not just postoperatively but in real time as well. For example, if a particular recurring set of circumstances or events can be linked to less than optimum outcomes, there is clearly a benefit in using this information after the fact to coach practitioners to make improvements. However, there is even more value in being able to feed back this information during a procedure, to alert surgeons that they are about to repeat an error-event sequence so that they can correct themselves. A precedent for this is the growing trend for telementoring, or

the use of 'live' video links to allow consultants to remotely provide guidance and instruction to colleagues [16]. The question is if and how the purely subjective interpretation of the live video feed by the operator or the observer could be bolstered by a more objective data-led approach.

Getting the Most Out of Surgical Data

When we consider the volumes of data being generated in and around surgical practice and its potential uses and benefits, it is clear that we are only part way along our journey towards a data-led approach to surgery. Yes, there is no shortage of data available, but its complexity and variety means that there is too much for surgeons to be able to fully incorporate and synthesise into their practice for optimal benefit. Not without help, anyway [17].

As the example of video demonstrates (Fig. 48.1), available data sources are likely to provide the most value when the complete 'big picture' is available at once, when data can be subjected to rigorous comparative analysis, and when the insights it contains are available in real time to support practice in *the OR*, not just as a resource for pre-operative planning or postoperative review. This is all beyond the capabilities of the human brain, which is why subjective interpretation of sources like imaging and video alone falls short of extracting the full value from the data available.

Big Data analytics has established the framework for working with massive, complex, heterogeneous data sets of the kind we are faced with in interventional medicine. As interest in how we optimise use of ever-increasing volumes of data comes to the fore, a new generation of analytical approaches is emerging, driven by a futuristic and highly disruptive family of technologies— *Artificial Intelligence (AI)*.

AI is widely expected to have a transformational impact on healthcare over the course of the next decade. It has been predicted that *AI* could help to improve outcomes by 30% to 40% while simultaneously halving costs. In 2018, 97% of

Fig. 48.1 A depiction of how advanced technologies may be used in the future to detect abnormalities, such as polyps

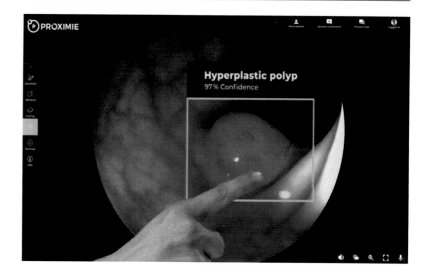

healthcare leaders taking part in one survey agreed that *AI* is "the most reliable path toward equitable, accessible, and affordable healthcare" [18].

So what makes *AI* so special, and how can it help achieve a data-led future for surgery? Let's take a look at four specific *AI* technologies and how they are starting to be applied in the OR and across *surgical services* in general.

Machine Learning

Machine Learning (ML) is a sophisticated analytical approach best known in the field of robotics and 'smart' automation for its ability to 'learn' from and adapt according to patterns observed in data over time, opening the door to machines being able to operate with considerable autonomy from human oversight.

ML offers another quality that makes it particularly useful to surgeons—its deep reading of patterns in data means it can predict future outcomes with a high degree of statistical probability. This is immensely promising for anticipating intraoperative complications such as sepsis, surgical site infections (SSIs) and adverse drug reactions [19]. *ML* is already outperforming traditional threshold-based decision making and more accurately reflecting the high frequency of heterogeneous events. For example, the University of Iowa

Hospital in the United States (US) and associated clinics were able to reduce incidents of SSIs by 74% in 3 years using a similar approach [18].

As a paradigm for how digital systems use data, *ML* has a vast range of potential applications. In surgery, these range from pre-screening patients to predict the likelihood of complications post-operatively to providing real-time analysis in *the OR* of things like workflow management, safety protocols and time efficiency [18].

Artificial Neural Networks

Artificial Neural Networks (ANNs) have very similar capabilities and uses to *ML*, with the key difference being that *ANNs* are designed to handle particularly large and heterogeneous data sets. Modelled on the way a brain works, *ANNs* use a complex array of 'neurons' or individual units to process quantities of data separately before combining and assimilating the findings from each [12]. Like a brain, *ANNs* also learn over time how best to weigh information gleaned from different sources to achieve the optimum conclusion. This is often referred to as *deep learning*.

Given the size and complexity of the data sets that surgical teams have to work with, *ANNs* are viewed as having significant potential in areas such as risk mitigation and delivery of precision care. In one study, an *ANN* predicted in-hospital mortality after open repair of an abdominal aortic aneurysm with an accuracy of 95.4%, using data such as patient history, blood pressure readings and current medications [12]. With that level of insight, more widespread use of *ANNs* will surely lead to more personalised, patient-centric approaches to surgical care. At the same time, *ANNs* offer the breadth and scale to be able to analyse a live video feed of *the OR* in real time, picking out relevant details and patterns that even an expert human observer would be expected to miss in a postoperative review, interpreting that information in light of known risk factors relating to the patient, clinical guidance and its own previous deep learning, and feeding all of this back to the surgical team in the form of recommended next steps.

Natural Language Processing

Natural Language Processing (NLP) addresses the issue that, from a data science perspective, written and spoken language represents unstructured data that is beyond the reach of conventional computer algorithms. Famously used as the cornerstone of smart voice assistants, which effectively let us have conversations with our computers, *NLP* is also widely used to extract information from written texts (or audio recordings), making it available for analysis.

In surgery, as in healthcare as a whole, this is important because of the amount of written text that is still used in EHRs (recall Vedula and Hager's view that EHRs represent only an incomplete record of any care pathway). On this basis, we can assume that any statistical analysis based on EHR data performed prior to NLP has inevitably been incomplete due to the sheer volume of narrative documentation and clinical notes that could not be included.

In one study, *NLP* was able to predict anastomotic leak after colorectal resections with a sensitivity of 100% and specificity of 72% solely from the notes contained in EHRs. This was partly performed by identifying words within the

EHRs that described the state of the patient that linked to known risk factors [12]. By incorporating *ML* techniques, *NLP* tools can also self-improve over time. One consequence of this is that practitioners in the future may be able to record observations in a natural prose style, without choosing codes or pre-programmed stock phrases that are 'visible' to a standard analytics program.

Computer Vision

Finally, *Computer Vision (CV)* does to images what NLP does to written texts or audio recordings—it extracts unstructured data and makes it available for analysis. Given the particular importance of imaging to surgical care pathways, it could be argued that *CV* is the area of *AI* likely to have the biggest impact on surgery.

Combined with *ML* and *ANN* capabilities, there are already numerous examples of how *CV* can be applied across diagnostics, surgical planning, risk management and intraoperative decision making. Kim et al. [17] highlight three areas in particular:

- *CV* has been demonstrated to reduce error rates in the diagnosis of metastatic breast cancer based on the analysis of images of lymph node biopsies, with *ML* tools self-improving differentiation between high-risk and low-risk lesions.
- In wound care, *CV* has the potential to classify and assess the severity of injuries instantaneously with a high degree of accuracy, helping to support timely, responsive planning. One study in Italy has already shown that *CV* can generate robust diagnostic data from a wound image with 94% accuracy.
- The authors describe a 3D visualisation technique proposed for determining etiology and planning surgical interventions for liver disease, and argue for the benefits of applying a similar approach to craniofacial surgery. In craniosynostosis treatment, for example, having a realistic 3D image of the patient's head to work from would allow surgical teams to

plan interventions in precise detail. Furthermore, using *ANNs* would help to predict the likelihood of postoperative complications and recurrence of abnormalities, again within the aim of preparing very specific pathways for each individual patient [17].

CV is also being used to address the problem of depth perception in laparoscopy, which is identified as a leading cause of accidental injury. Because a 2D video feed 'flattens' perspective in a very small area, both human and robotic operatives can misjudge distance. By adding another type of imaging, such as a structured light probe, *CV* can assimilate additional data along with the video feed in order to correct perceptual discrepancies [20].

Significant steps are also being made in developing *CV* tools capable of performing the kind of in-depth data extraction and analysis from video discussed in the last section. One study demonstrated close to 93% accuracy in using *CV* to identify the steps of a sleeve gastrectomy, and subsequently used this knowledge to recognise missteps [12]. Once perfected, this could open the door to real-time intraoperative feedback, alerting practitioners to any missing or unexpected steps based on video analysis of the procedure [18].

Ultimately, *AI* has the potential to help *surgical data science* realise the full value of the entire spectrum of data available. It is likely to be critical to achieving the goals of precision medicine: treating every patient and every case as a unique entity and event, and basing decisions on an appreciation of dynamic competing and correlating factors, moving on from basing diagnosis and treatment on the law of averages applied across a population [17].

Working with Data in the OR

For all the transformational potential of *AI*, there are also challenges. As Lynn (2019) argues, the issue of how data-driven insights are communi-

cated is critical. Communication errors between practitioners already contribute to 60% of adverse events; you don't want to add to that by creating a 'black box' situation where the intelligence presented *by AI* in *the OR* is open to misinterpretation. How can data be communicated effectively so that it is a help and not a hindrance? Or to borrow Lynn's phrase, how do you "cognitively engage a unified patient dataset" when you are concentrating on a complex procedure? [19].

This can be framed as a problem of how we integrate data-led intelligence with surgical workflows. In their analysis of the development of the "*digital operating room*", Koninckx et al. (2013) argue that, over the past 25 years, significant technological developments in operating theatre equipment, medical imaging systems and medical information technology (IT), including EHR, have been poorly coordinated [21]. This has meant that, on more than one occasion, apparent progress in one area of technology has caused significant disruption in others. In their view, one of the objectives of the digital OR should be to achieve full integration of "images, information and workflow". In other words, they want to see equal weight given to how data is captured and how it is made available for use.

Professor Nicolas Padoy, a specialist in medical robotics at the University of Strasbourg in France, has suggested that when *AI* technology is "sufficiently mature", the next phase of development will be to create the right kind of user interfaces in *the OR* [22]. However, it doesn't necessarily follow that focus on the 'presentation layer' of the digital OR stack should only come once surgical *AI* has reached a certain stage of development. Widespread adoption of *AI* in surgery will depend on practitioners being able to use it quickly and intuitively, and therefore see immediate value in it. Moreover, technologies that can fulfil this role are already available.

One of them is *Augmented Reality (AR)*. *AR* is a technology that enhances or augments real-world perception by applying a digital overlay via a mediating screen. So whether you are watching a video stream on a standard device or wearing a piece of equipment like Google Glasses from Microsoft's Hololens, the idea is that you can add extra digital content which blends in seamlessly with what you observe.

Another way to look at *AR* is to see it as bridging the experiential divide between the real world and the digital realm, bringing them together in a single frame of reference. This has the potential to fundamentally change the way that we relate to, understand and use digital content. For example, if I am relying on information from my computer to complete a task—a set of instructions, say—I would normally have to keep switching my focus back and forth from my screen to the task in hand. But with *AR*, I could have the instructions there in front of me, right in my field of vision as I work. This has been demonstrated to improve concentration and application of information [23].

This is of great interest to surgery, which is a cognitively demanding yet fundamentally practical occupation that requires a high degree of skill, concentration and applied knowledge. A good illustration of *AR*'s potential in *the OR* comes from stereotactic neurosurgery, a minimally invasive technique where surgeons use a combination of CT or MRI scan data and a computer tracking system to perform tasks like locating and removing tumours. The challenge for surgeons performing these procedures is that they have traditionally been required to adopt a 'heads up' posture to look at the images on screen while their hands manipulate the instruments. This is cognitively challenging because their focus is effectively on the screen and the representation of what they are doing, not what their hands are actually doing. Our brains rely heavily on visual cues to control and correct complex fine motor manipulation. The disconnect in a neurosurgeon's field of vision between hands and screen may increase stress levels and fatigue, leading to a higher likelihood of error and longer operating times [23, 24].

AR is already being applied to provide a solution. By placing a screen between the surgeon and the patient, the stereotactic guiding images can be accurately superimposed onto a live feed of the patient's anatomy as the surgeon works. By replacing the 'heads up' with a 'see through' posture, surgeons are able to make use of the digital navigation cues in a much more natural way, observing their own motor control and the overlaid digital data in a single field of vision.

AR can be used to deliver supplementary digital input using any of the senses, but it leans heavily towards visual. Again, this is a happy coincidence for surgery because of the prominent role of imaging as a data source. As well as projecting pre-operative images onto the patient's body as an intraoperative guidance tool, another very promising area of research is the way *AR* can be used to visualise composite 3D images put together from multiple data sources by *CV* technology. For example, the Enhanced Vision System for Robotic Surgery (EnViSoRS) addresses the fact that anatomy changes dynamically due to very basic factors like position, heart rate and breathing, which means that preoperative images do not always map exactly to the body the surgeon is working on in *the OR*. These minute discrepancies are believed to be a cause of accidental damage to arteries and veins in robotic laparoscopy. EnViSoRS uses *CV* to create a dynamic 3D model of the 'Safety Area' built from preoperative and intraoperative data, using *AR* to visualise the results even as the model adapts [25].

Data visualisation is another key opportunity *AR* brings to surgery—presenting the full spectrum of data available to the surgeon, not just medical images, in a way that is intuitive, immediate and cognitively easy to assimilate into tasks. Data visualisation might be understood as turning complex, opaque statistical models—the sort of things *AI* algorithms are built to understand—into the kind of accessible visual models that the human brain finds easy to process. With its heavy access of visual augmentation and the fact that it can synthesise models into our natural field of vision as we work, *AR* is a strong candidate for leading the next phase of evolution in data visualisation. In surgery, finding the right format and interface for the rich resources of data available will help to avoid the risk of 'black box' *AI*, and will also mean we don't have to worry unduly about adding advanced data science expertise to the already burgeoning skillsets of surgeons [26].

Finally, we should remember that, even with *AI* taking on an increasingly important role, it will not replace the expertise of individual surgeons. As previously discussed, the value of data in *the OR* lies in how practitioners are able to use it, both within surgical teams and to assist their individual practice. While effective machine-to-human communication will be essential going forward for getting the most out of data in surgery, so will *human-to-human communication*. Data-driven insights must be easy for people to share, discuss, analyse and use together to yield their full impact.

We are already seeing how *AR* can be used to communicate data in various forms and for many different purposes. These include the use of *AR* to support coaching, training and skills development in notoriously challenging fields like neurosurgery, and the ability to draw on AR to support cognition with the visualisation of complex concepts [27]. *AR* is also being used *for telementoring* or remote proctoring, both as a training and education tool and intraoperatively to support delivery. *Telementoring* describes the use of communications technology to allow a senior practitioner to supervise a colleague remotely in real time, whether that involves an expert mentor providing guidance to a trainee carrying out a practice procedure or a specialist guiding a local generalist through a 'live' operation [28, 29]. The key benefits of *telementoring* include removing barriers of time and geography that so often get in the way of the free flow of surgical knowledge and expertise. In theory, remote proctoring means that trainees can be coached by any specialist in the world, improving access to and development of advanced skills. This also helps to ensure that more specialised procedures can be carried out locally by general surgeons, and addresses the chronic issues in distribution of surgical specialists.

The main technological challenge that *telementoring* poses is ensuring that information can be exchanged between remote colleagues in a way that is detailed and cognitively reliable enough to avoid misconceptions and, crucially, protect patient safety. To put it another way, *telementoring* relies on the sound communication of data. To date, most *telementoring* systems have failed to provide a clinically robust solution due to limited annotation capabilities and lack of direct visualisation [29]. These are two issues that *AR* addresses directly. As we have already seen, *AR* is a predominantly visual medium, designed to communicate data in a visualised form within the field of the recipient as they work. This extends to the concept of interactive virtual presence—the idea that a remote specialist can 'beam in' to the OR by having a live feed of gestures and demonstrations overlaid onto the visual field of their colleague, just as if they were standing next to them.

Case Study

Proximie is an *AR*-enhanced video platform developed to support remote collaboration between surgical professionals. Its uses cover training and education, preoperative planning and consultation, intraoperative guidance and support, and postoperative review and coaching.

Clinical reviews have found that use of Proximie as a *telementoring* tool achieves outcomes statistically equivalent to onsite/in-person proctoring. For example, one recent study compared use of Proximie to onsite proctoring in the adoption of an Aquablation system for treating benign prostate enlargement. It concluded that *telementoring* via Proximie can be safely used in the adoption phase of a new robotic technology [30].

In another example, The European Society for Coloproctology (ESCP) wanted to explore ways to remotely support teaching of an emerging colorectal technique called Robotic complete mesocolic excision (CME) across Europe. In particular, the Society wanted to avoid the need for proctors to travel all over the continent to oversee practitioners as they used the robotic system in live procedures.

Proctoring a sophisticated novel procedure like Robotic CME is far from straightforward, even in person. It requires the specialist to communicate an in-depth and complex body of domain knowledge—about the technique, about the procedure, about the technology—in a way that is clear, pertinent and intelligible to the practitioner so they can operate safely. It must be performed whilst taking into account the details of the patient's anatomy, applying data from preoperative imaging, monitoring data from intraoperative sensors, and of course watching the details of what the practitioner is doing and adjusting advice accordingly.

Proximie was used to remotely connect Mr. Danilo Miskovic from St Marks NHS Trust London, one of the expert surgeons nominated by the Society as proctor for the new technique, to Dr. Thalia Petropoulou, an experienced surgeon based in Athens, Greece. Despite the complexities outlined above, Proximie allowed Miskovic to provide real-time virtual support to Petropoulou at a distance of 3000 km in order to ensure that the procedure was performed successfully and without incident (Fig. 48.2).

These use cases demonstrate how AR-enhanced live video can enable data of varying types and from multiple sources to be shared in a free-flowing exchange and be presented in an intuitive, intelligible way. Proximie's ability to facilitate remote virtual presence, enable the digital overlay of sophisticated 3D anatomical images and augment the proctor's view based on real-time data feeds from *OR* systems illustrates how *AR* can make complex data sets accessible, communicable and usable in the *OR* to improve patient outcomes, and how data can be shared usefully over distance (Fig. 48.3).

Case Study Questions to Consider

1. What data sources are being used by the Proximie system to enhance the telementoring experience?

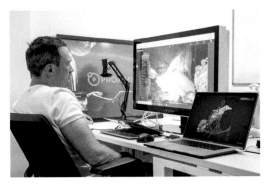

Fig. 48.2 Mr. Miskovic, based in London, remotely proctoring Dr. Petropoulou, who is performing a robotic CME case in Athens

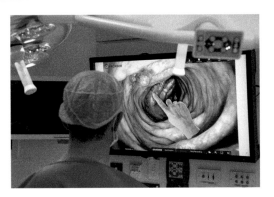

Fig. 48.3 Depiction of a local surgeon being guided by a remote expert using the Proximie system

2. How might surgeons communicate differently when using an AR tool as opposed to performing in-person telementoring?
3. How can AR tools, such as Proximie, be leveraged to address variation in care?

Summary

Data is re-shaping the world we live in and healthcare is anything but immune from its transformational impact. On the contrary, data is already viewed as key to the emergence of an intelligence-led approach to healthcare that will drive massive gains in service efficiencies, patient outcomes and, ultimately, overall population health.

Healthcare is well placed to reap all of the benefits data promises. The ongoing digitisation of medical systems means there is already an enormous resource of data available across the healthcare spectrum. With the right tools and the right expertise, this data can provide a powerful analytical foundation for service planning and administration, oversight of clinical practice, diagnostic decision making and much more.

In this chapter, we explored the impact data is having in our own field of expertise, surgery, and the potential it has to drive further transformation of *surgical services* in the future. We outlined what difference data might make to *surgical services*, before aiming to answer three questions:

- What are the most important sources of surgical data?

- How can surgical practitioners get optimal use of the data available?
- How can the insights gained from data best be communicated in the *operating room*?

In addressing these three questions in turn, we considered the ways in which data is currently captured before, during and after surgery, and which of them promise most for future planning and service delivery. We then moved on to look at the technologies that will allow data to be put to use in the *operating room* (OR) and beyond, looking first at *Artificial Intelligence* (AI) and its role in delivering complex data analytics.

Finally, we also assessed the critical role *Augmented Reality* (AR) could play in communicating data-led intelligence to and between surgical professionals, with a key focus on how complex information gleaned from data can be presented in an intuitive, person-friendly format to support real-time decision making.

Conclusions and Outlook

We remain at an early stage of development of a data-led approach to surgical services. Many of the technologies we have outlined will help us benefit from the full value data has to offer to interventional medicine—the various *AI* examples in particular remain at the proof-of-concept stage. As Vedula and Hager (2017) argue, realisation of a robust, purposeful, effective *surgical data science* will require cultural as well as technological shifts. Practitioners will have to adapt the way they learn, think and work to accommodate the new systems and the new paradigms of knowledge. Whole new ecosystems will have to emerge within the healthcare industry that ensure data products are designed with the specific, exacting needs of surgery in mind, to guarantee efficacy and widespread adoption [6].

These are details to be considered and addressed rather than obstacles that may prevent a data-led transformation of healthcare in the long term. As we have seen, surgery already has all the raw materials it needs for its data revolution. Digitisation continues at pace, and so the already huge volumes of data available keep growing.

Paired with Big Data techniques, predictive analytics and AI, we already know that data delivers enormous value in providing objective clarity and detail on which to base decision making, helping to drive better outcomes, improve efficiency and lower costs. These are advantages that would be welcome by a global healthcare system beset with soaring demand and spiralling costs.

There are various forecasts as to what the data-led surgical services of the future might look like. It is reasonable to expect the emergence of AI-driven clinical systems that are capable of managing everything from macro-level strategic organisation to scheduling and bed allocation. Coupled with the growing role of genetic data in medicine, diagnosis will become increasingly predictive and interventional medicine will shift to a more preventative role [7]. All of this will be paired with the ability to peer into what Kay et al. call the "minutiae" of detail on a case-by-case basis, opening the door to precision medicine and true personalization of care" [17].

Then, of course, there is the matter of surgical automation in the form of sophisticated robotic systems. This is already an advanced trend in surgery and, although closely related, one we feel sits apart from the topics we have discussed in this chapter. Plenty will be written and said about the role of robotic automation in surgery and it will undoubtedly have great value. Equally, the focus of this chapter has been the broader role data will play in supporting the invaluable expertise and talents of practitioners, and perhaps helping people work in new and better ways. That is why we believe that the question of how practitioners can interact with data, and how the insights gained from it are communicated and assimilated, is so important, and why technologies such as *AR* should be considered in conversations about *surgical data science, Big Data* and *AI*.

Review Questions

1. Which of the following is an internal source of data?
   (a) Surgical registry
   (b) X-ray performed on admission
   (c) Clinical trial data
   (d) Best practice guideline

2. What is 'Big Data'?
   (a) A field of analytics which aims to acquire intelligence from small volumes of complex, heterogeneous data in rapid time
   (b) A field of analytics which aims to acquire intelligence from large volumes of heterogeneous, structured data over a prolonged period of time
   (c) A field of analytics which aims to acquire intelligence from large volumes of heterogeneous, unstructured data in rapid time
   (d) A field of analytics which aims to acquire intelligence from large volumes of homogeneous, structured data in rapid time

3. Which of the following statements is correct?
   (a) Most surgical data is presented in a similar format.
   (b) It is estimated that 60% of data available to surgeons is considered unstructured or exists in a non-digital format.
   (c) EHR provides a complete record of data generated by the care process.
   (d) Augmented reality is a technology that enhances real-world perception by applying a digital overlay via a mediating screen.

4. How can Natural Language Processing (NLP) be useful in surgery?
   (a) NLP can help doctors write notes more legibly.
   (b) NLP replaces clinical notes.
   (c) NLP can extract information from written text, making it available for analysis.
   (d) NLP can record notes intraoperatively.

Appendix: Answers to Review Questions

1. Which of the following is an internal source of data?
   (a) Surgical registry
   (b) X-ray performed on admission
   (c) Clinical trial data
   (d) Best practice guideline

An X-ray is created during a patient's care episode and is therefore classed as an internal data source. A surgical registry, clinical data trial and best practice guideline are all external data sources as they have been generated outside of the clinical episode.

2. What is 'Big Data'?
   (a) A field of analytics which aims to acquire intelligence from small volumes of complex, heterogeneous data in rapid time
   (b) A field of analytics which aims to acquire intelligence from large volumes of heterogeneous, structured data over a prolonged period of time
   (c) A field of analytics which aims to acquire intelligence from large volumes of heterogeneous, unstructured data in rapid time
   (d) A field of analytics which aims to acquire intelligence from large volumes of homogeneous, structured data in rapid time

Recall that surgical sources of data are varied and presented in an unstructured, heterogeneous form. 'Big Data' refers to the analysis of this type of data in a short period of time.

3. Which of the following statements is correct?
   (a) Most surgical data is presented in a similar format.
   (b) It is estimated that 60% of data available to surgeons is considered unstructured or exists in a non-digital format.
   (c) EHR provides a complete record of data generated by the care process.
   (d) Augmented reality is a technology that enhances real-world perception by applying a digital overlay via a mediating screen.

Statements a, b and c are false.

4. How can Natural Language Processing (NLP) be useful in surgery?
   (a) NLP can help doctors write notes more legibly.
   (b) NLP replaces clinical notes.
   (c) NLP can extract information from written text, making it available for analysis.
   (d) NLP can record notes intraoperatively.

References

1. Nagy D, Rudas I, Haidegger T. Surgical data science, an emerging field of medicine [conference paper] IEEE 30th Jubilee Neumann Colloquium, 2017 Nov. Online. https://core.ac.uk/download/pdf/148786989.pdf
2. Thirani V, Gupta A. The value of data [internet], The World Economic Forum, 2017 Sep. https://www.weforum.org/agenda/2017/09/the-value-of-data/
3. Maier-Hein L, Vedula S, Speidel S, et al. Surgical data science: enabling next-generation surgery, Nature Biomedical Engineering, 2017 Jan. https://arxiv.org/ftp/arxiv/papers/1701/1701.06482.pdf
4. Gibson J, Dobbs T, Kerstein R, et al. Making the most of big data in surgery, The Future of Surgery [Evidence Paper], Royal College of Surgeons of England, 2018. Online. https://futureofsurgery.rcseng.ac.uk/evidence/gibson-j-a-g-dobbs-t-d-kerstein-r-et-al-making-the-most-of-big-data-in-surgery-improving-outcomes-protecting-patients-and-informing-service-providers-2018
5. Targarona E, Balla A, Batista G. Big data and surgery: the digital revolution continues, Cirugía Española (English Edition), 2018 May, 96(5):247–249. Online. https://www.elsevier.es/en-revista-cirugia-espanola-english-edition%2D%2D436-articulo-big-data-surgery-the-digital-S2173507718300929
6. Vedula S, Hager G. Surgical data science: the new knowledge domain. Innov Surg Sci 2017;2(3):109–21. Online. https://www.ncbi.nlm.nih.gov/pmc/articles/PMC5602563/
7. The future of surgery [internet], Royal College of Surgeons of England, 2018. Online. https://futureofsurgery.rcseng.ac.uk/
8. Elson D, Yang GZ. The principles and role of medical imaging in surgery. In: Athanasiou T, Debas H, Darzi A, editors. Key topics in surgical research and methodology, 2010. Online. https://link.springer.com/chapter/10.1007/978-3-540-71915-1_39#citeas
9. Dunne R, O'Neill A, Tempany C. Imaging tools in human research: focus on image-guided intervention. In: clinical and translational Science. 2nd edn. 2017. pp. 181–190. Online. https://www.sciencedirect.com/science/article/pii/B9780128021019000107
10. Image-guided minimally invasive diagnostic and therapeutic interventional procedures. In: Mathematics and physics of emerging biomedical imaging, 1996 Chapter 12. Online. https://www.ncbi.nlm.nih.gov/books/NBK232483/
11. Khajuria R, Gross B, Du R. Image-guided open cerebrovascular surgery. Neurosurgery. 2015;2015:277–96.
12. Hashimoto D, Rosman G, Rus D, Meireles O. Artificial intelligence in surgery: promises and perils. Ann Surg. 2018 Jul;268(1):70–6.
13. Grenda T, Pradarelli J, Dimick J. Using surgical video to improve technique and skill. Ann Surg. 2016 Jul;264(1):32–3.
14. Bonrath E, Gordon L, Grantcharov T. Characterising 'near miss' events in complex laparoscopic surgery through video analysis. BMJ Qual Saf. 2015 Aug;24(8):516–21.
15. Bezemer J, Cope A, Korkiakangas T, et al. Microanalysis of video from the operating room: an underused approach to patient safety research. BMJ Qual Saf. 2017 June;26:583–7.
16. El-Sabawi B, Magee W. The evolution of surgical telementoring: current applications and future directions. Ann Transl Med. 2016 Oct;4(20):391.
17. Kim Y, Kelley B, Nasser J, Chung K. Implementing precision medicine and artificial intelligence in plastic surgery: concepts and future prospects. Plast Reconstr Surg Glob Open. 2019 Mar;7(3):e2113.
18. Saver C, How will artificial intelligence impact surgical patient care? Part 1 [Internet], OR Manager, 2019 Apr. Online. https://www.ormanager.com/will-artificial-intelligence-impact-surgical-patient-care-part-1/.
19. Lynn L. Artificial intelligence systems for complex decision-making in acute care medicine: a review. Patient Saf Surg. 2019 Feb;13:6.
20. Andersen M. Surgical automation gets more precise vision, Thanks to Multiple Data Sources [Internet]. Robotics Business Review, 2017 Dec. Online. https://www.roboticsbusinessreview.com/health-medical/surgical-automation-gets-precise-vision-data/
21. Koninckx PR, Stepanian A, Adamyan L, et al. The digital operating room and the surgeon. Gynecol Surg. 2013 Feb;10:57–62.
22. Saver C, How will artificial intelligence impact surgical patient care? Part 2 [Internet]. OR Manager, 2019 May. Online. https://www.ormanager.com/will-artificial-intelligence-impact-surgical-patient-care-part-2/
23. Doswell J, Skinner A. Augmenting human cognition with adaptive augmented reality. In: Schmorrow DD, Fidopiastis CM, editors. Foundations of augmented cognition. Advancing human performance and decision-making through adaptive systems, 2014. Online. https://link.springer.com/chapter/10.1007/978-3-319-07527-3_10
24. Khor W, Baker B, Amin K, et al. Augmented and virtual reality in surgery-the digital surgical environment: applications, limitations and legal pitfalls. Ann Transl Med. 2016 Dec;4(23):454.
25. Penza V, Momi E, Enayati N et al. EnViSoRS: enhanced vision system for robotic surgery. a user-defined safety volume tracking to minimize the risk of intraoperative bleeding. Front Robot AI. 2017 May. Online. https://www.frontiersin.org/articles/10.3389/frobt.2017.00015/full
26. Nichols G, Data visualization via VR and AR: how we'll interact with tomorrow's data [Internet]. 2019 March. https://www.zdnet.com/article/data-visualization-via-vr-and-ar-how-well-interact-with-tomorrows-data/
27. Si W, Liao X, Qian Y, et al. Assessing performance of augmented reality-based neurosurgical training. Vis Comput Ind Biomed Art. 2019 July;2:6.
28. Guraya S. Using telementoring and augmented reality in surgical specialties. J Taibah Univ Med Sci. 2019 Mar;14(2):101–2.
29. Rojas-Muñoz E, Andersen D, Cabrera ME, et al. Augmented reality as a medium for improved telementoring. Mil Med. 2019;184(Suppl 1):57–64.
30. Asmar J, Labban M, El Hajj A. Integration of Telementoring during the adoption phase of a novel robotic technology: is a virtual approach virtuous? J Urol. 2020 Apr;203(4).

Daniel Kraft and Shawna Butler

Learning Objectives
- Understand the pace of change (what is new now and what comes next) that will impact the future of nursing and healthcare
- Understand the role of wearables, sensors, connected data, and information across the care continuum
- Understand approaches for integrating connected, digital, and mobile solutions to health promotion, disease prevention, surveillance, clinical care across multiple settings, chronic care, disability management, and virtualized care
- Understand evolutions of convergent technologies and their potential across healthcare
- Understand implications for nursing, public and global health, and ancillary care

Key Terms
- Ambient Sensing
- Artificial Intelligence/Robotics
- Blockchain
- Chatbots
- Computer Vision
- Digital Therapeutics
- Exponential Technologies

- Genomics/Panomics (from Genome, to Microbiome, to Metabalome and beyond)
- IoT (Internet of things)/IoMT (Internet of Medical Things)
- Machine Learning
- Natural Language Processing
- Virtual Care/Telemedicine
- Virtual Reality/Augmented Reality/Extended Reality/Mixed Reality
- Voice in Healthcare
- Voice Recognition
- Wearables, Insideables, Trainables

Introduction

Healthcare is ripe for change and evolution as it enters the fourth industrial age. The rapid advancement of many convergent technologies is enabling a shift from reactive, intermittent 'sick care' to one of real-time, proactive, predictive, personalized, data-driven healthcare.

Nurses already, and will increasingly, leverage technologies to improve and enable public health, patient care (from prevention and health optimization to earlier detection to the management of disease, all the way to ensuring peaceful, dignified death and bereavement), and community health by connecting the dots of social determinants and the evolution of new knowledge via clinical trials, health services research, and a variety of health innovation activities. By using

D. Kraft (✉)
Exponential Medicine & Singularity University,
Mountain View, CA, USA

S. Butler
Radboud University Medical Center,
Nijmegen, The Netherlands

© Springer Nature Switzerland AG 2022
U. H. Hübner et al. (eds.), *Nursing Informatics*, Health Informatics,
https://doi.org/10.1007/978-3-030-91237-6_49

emerging technologies, nurses and others will increasingly be enabled and 'upskilled' to provide care that is available on-demand, asynchronously, and not geographically unbounded.

Embracing the accelerating pace of change and the convergence of technologies available today and emerging in the near future will help innovators from a broad range of disciplines consider new and novel approaches to addressing challenges across the healthcare continuum. Problems that once seemed intractable, too big, or too complex become problems of technology, data, and connectivity.

Enabling the Shift from 'Sick Care' to 'Healthcare'

We live in an increasingly digitized world, automated and enhanced by technologies ranging from mobile computing riding the Internet of things (IoT) to robotics integrating Big Data and artificial intelligence (AI). These and other technologies and enabling platforms that have disrupted entire industries created new ones and fostered the creation of business models that have dramatically impacted and changed our lives, lifestyles, and livelihoods—everything from how we bank, shop, and travel to how we gather information, learn, and consume entertainment. While fields such as AI, Big Data, and robotics have ushered many industries into the 'Fourth Industrial Age,' health and medicine lags behind and often seem confined to the Third or even Second Industrial Age.

Walk into the ward or clinic of many top academic, public, or private hospitals and you will still find clinical workflow and scheduling managed with clipboards, paper sign-out cards, and fax machines, relatively unchanged since the 1980s. Despite the emergence of electronic health records (EHRs), patients and front-desk clerks (and the data flow into EHRs) are still all too often tied to completing repetitious analog paper forms by hand. Many imaging studies, while digitized, are only available when carried by hand across town for a second opinion by the patient on 30-year-old CD-ROM technology. Waiting

rooms live up to their name, with wait times far longer than the average 15-min primary care visit [1] obtained after often waiting weeks to get the appointment. Furthermore, the organization of our institutions remains relatively siloed, from traditionally organized academic departments to the organization chart of pharmaceutical companies that have changed little in the last 50 years.

Our current care models are primarily based and designed on a reactive 'sick care' model that is reliant upon intermittent and episodic data obtained and visible only within traditional clinical interactions and settings, i.e., the outpatient clinic, emergency department, hospital ward, or intensive care unit, and often confined within the records of an institution or health system. Rarely do our school health, dental, pharmacy, or optical care records communicate or connect with other health records. Fortunately, most individuals spend only a fraction of their lives within the brick-and-mortar clinical setting, and thus their real-world data has remained largely invisible and inaccessible to providers and systems.

The intermittent and episodic data obtained during an urgent care or primary care visit (i.e., labs and ECG, vital signs to a review of systems) is often scattered between paper records and electronic medical record systems, which lack interoperability. Even when an engaged patient diligently measures and records their own data at home (i.e., their blood pressure, glucose, or a collection of symptoms), it is often challenging to transmit and share this information with their care providers. This intermittent data from individuals leads to our reactive model, where providers all too often rely on waiting for their patients to present with an urgent condition (i.e., chest pain, stroke, or late-stage cancer).

The potential for many of the existing and emerging technologies covered in this chapter is to shift from 'sick care' to 'healthcare' and increasingly leverage continuous information collected outside of the traditional healthcare setting that can be contextualized and personalized and lead to more proactive insights and information. In a nutshell, this shift could lead to more precise and personalized prevention, and care that is increasingly democratized and available

Fig. 49.1 The future of health from 'sick care' to 'healthcare'

The Future of Health

	Today: System	Future: Person
TIMING	Reactive, sick care	Proactive, preventative, **predictive**
PRECISION	1 size fits all, crude, analog	Personalized, intelligent
MODALITY	Institution-centred	Digi-cal | decentralized
DURATION	Episodic, intermittent, silo'd	Continuous | team
POWER	Provider	People-powered
CURRENCY	Volume, inputs, costs, fee-4-service	Value, outcomes, fee-4-health

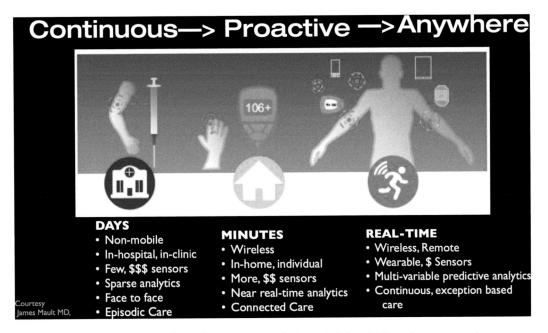

DAYS
- Non-mobile
- In-hospital, in-clinic
- Few, $$$ sensors
- Sparse analytics
- Face to face
- Episodic Care

MINUTES
- Wireless
- In-home, individual
- More, $$ sensors
- Near real-time analytics
- Connected Care

REAL-TIME
- Wireless, Remote
- Wearable, $ Sensors
- Multi-variable predictive analytics
- Continuous, exception based care

Courtesy James Mault MD,

Fig. 49.2 Potential offered by existing and emerging technologies to shift from 'sick care' to 'healthcare'

virtually any time, anywhere at lower costs and with improved outcomes (see Figs. 49.1 and 49.2).

Understanding Accelerating Technologies and Exponential Change

Many of the technologies with a potential to reshape elements of healthcare are advancing rapidly and, in some cases, exponentially, in which the power and potential increase every year at an exponential rate, or the cost drops by half, or both. In contrast with the easy-to-understand progression of linear technologies, exponential technologies advance and accelerate in a non-intuitive and deceptive manner. Taking 30 linear one-meter steps, one can advance 30 meters across a room, but taking 30 exponential steps (doubling the distance with each step) (1, 2, 4, 8, 16, 32, 64…128 meters…) the 15th step would reach 16,384 meters, and by 15 more exponential steps, just over 1 billion meters in a single step, equating to 26 times around the planet on the 30th exponential step.

Another example to illustrate exponential growth is to picture yourself at the uppermost row of a football stadium at 12 noon. A drop of water is placed in the center of the field, doubling every minute. How much time do you have to get out of the stadium dry? And when will you realize that it is urgent? After 6 min, the water fills a thimble. After 45 min, 7% of the stadium is filled. The 'hockey stick' showing the exponential growth arrives just 4 min later at 12.49 pm and fills the entire stadium. In other words, you will have 45 min where it looks as if everything is under control and only 4 min where you rapidly see the remaining 97% of the stadium filled.

The classic example of exponential technology is the advancement of computational power as exemplified by 'Moore's Law' where calculations per second per constant dollar have reliably doubled every 18–24 months, now for over 100 years. Exponentially faster, cheaper, and more powerful chips have enabled the supercomputing potential in our pockets in which our smartphones contain more computing power than a 30M dollar, 5500-pound Cray supercomputer from the mid-1980s. Today's $800 smartphone also has two or three cameras, GPS, cellular, wifi, Bluetooth, a display with over 3 mm pixels, a battery that lasts a day, a compass, a 3-axis gyroscope, speakers, an accelerometer, ambient light and proximity sensors, a barometer, and a microphone. It can record 4 K videos. It can take 8MP photos while recording 4k video.

Convergence

The expensive pile of disparate physical tools in our possession in the 1970s and 1980s (from a video camera to a Walkman, to a GPS navigator, to a flashlight, etc.) has now been 'app'ified' and fits in our pocket through our smart devices. Leveraging Moore's Law, technologies and solutions have been digitized, dematerialized, and in many cases demonetized (approaching free), resulting in the democratization of these technologies and access to their capabilities [2]. What used to require a desktop computer plugged into an electrical outlet now fits on a highly mobile smartphone or even our smart wristwatch. With sensors and video becoming utilized in

healthcare, our increasingly 'medicalized smartphones' now function to provide far more than phone calls. They have become core components of our connected mobile health and medicine.

As indicated in Fig. 49.3, the acceleration of technologies ranging from AI and robotics to synthetic biology, low cost-sequencing, and computation can impact almost every element across the healthcare spectrum. From health, wellness, and prevention to earlier and more accurate forms of diagnosis, to therapies that are much more personalized and less toxic, it could undoubtedly make healthcare more accessible, equitable, affordable, and more powerful.

Exponential small, cheap, connected devices have led to what is often referred to as the Internet of Things (IoT), or in healthcare, the Internet of Medical Things (IoMT), with medical devices and connected homes increasingly riding 5G networks (100X the speed of 4G). These connected technologies, however, have generated a massive wave of data, whether that be from wearables, electronic records, imaging studies, scheduling information, and gene sequencing, to billing and telemedicine data, which is often siloed and disconnected and does not necessarily translate to useful information, knowledge, and actionable insights. A large gap remains between information and knowledge to where the knowledge is transferred and can be readily and regularly applied at the point of care.

Technology alone is not a panacea, of course. Incentives need to be aligned to leverage emergent technology-based solutions, as well as regulatory and payment models. As many healthcare systems transition from 'fee for service' to 'value-based care,' incentives are being aligned to pay for remote patient monitoring and telehealth and rewarding prevention, and are accelerating care from 'hospital to home to phone' and to care and even diagnostic services provided by large pharmacy chains, to virtualized app-based care platforms.

The rapidly evolving paradigm of ever more mobile, connected, and data-driven care is often termed 'Digital Health,' enabled by the following:

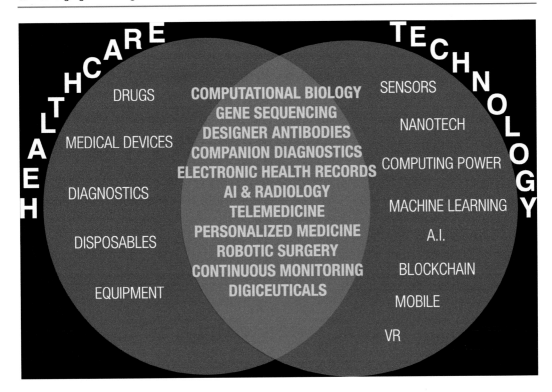

Fig. 49.3 The intersection between healthcare and technology

1. *Sensors*, often IoT-enabled wearable devices that collect data in real time
2. *Mobile apps* that can help integrate and present information and guidance
3. *Telehealth* that can reach patients remotely
4. *AI* that can process the streams of data to glean insights and make data actionable
5. *Robotics and automation* to conduct basic to more advanced services usually performed by humans

In 2020, the Healthcare Information and Management Systems Society (HIMSS) published the following definition of digital health: "Digital health connects and empowers people and populations to manage health and wellness, augmented by accessible and supportive provider teams working within flexible, integrated, interoperable and digitally-enabled care environments that strategically leverage digital tools, technologies and services to transform care delivery" [3].Of course 'Digital' is only one arena of rapid and exponential advancement. The convergence of ever smaller, faster, cheaper, and more powerful technologies and fields includes low-cost genomic sequencing, synthetic biology, augmented and virtual reality, digital manufacturing (3D printing), blockchain drones, robotics, material science, and social networks.

Given that traditional healthcare (pharmaceuticals, medical devices, diagnostics, disposables) needs are now being addressed by technology, it has led to new industries, fields, and careers at the interface ranging from computational biology, telemedicine, robotic surgery, and companion diagnostics. Together, these can help address many of the local pain points and grand challenges nurses, doctors, healthcare professionals, and healthcare systems face worldwide.

New Forms of Measuring and Optimizing Health, Prevention, and Managing Disease

While an individual's genetics certainly play a role in their health, behaviors play a much larger

Fig. 49.4 Wearables—a source of capturing physiologic and behavioral data. (Source: Piwek L, Ellis DA, Andrews S, Joinson A (2016) The Rise of Consumer Health Wearables: Promises and Barriers. PLoS Med 13 (2): e1001953. https://doi.org/10.1371/journal.pmed.1001953; Copyright: © 2016 Piwek et al. This is an open-access article distributed under the terms of the Creative Commons Attribution License, which permits unrestricted use, distribution, and reproduction in any medium, provided the original author and source are credited.)

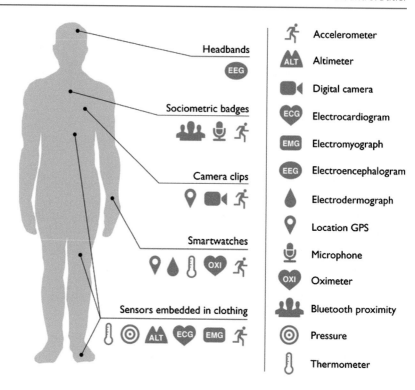

role, particularly risky behaviors including smoking, poor diet, low levels of physical activity, excessive alcohol intake, and insufficient sleep. These behaviors drive the incidence of the top chronic conditions, which account for 80% of total costs for chronic illnesses worldwide.

This section describes various technologies used in measuring and optimizing health, prevention, and managing disease.

Wearables

The era of 'wearables' emerged in late 2009 with the launch of the first Fitbit, a basic wrist-based accelerometer that could track steps. In the decade since there has been an explosion of wearable devices that can measure almost every element of physiology and behavior. These measures also catalyzed the 'Quantified Self' movement [4], the term that embodies self-knowledge through self-tracking. Increasingly, with the advent of platforms like Apple's HealthKit, the data once siloed on Quantified Selfers phones has become connected to the provider's EMR. Though still in the early stages, this promises a new era of 'Quantified Health,' where the

data flows to and from the patient to the providers and care team.

As a source of capturing physiologic and behavioral data (Fig. 49.4), these wearables, ranging from consumer watches to FDA-cleared cardiac monitors, can provide a facile, anytime anywhere means to:

1. Measure digital biomarkers to create objective measurements to help glean insights and to help measure and influence behaviors (i.e., exercise and sleep)
2. Diagnose diagnostics, often blending measures and algorithms

   and for

3. Treatment in the form of 'digital therapeutics'

These quantifying devices go far beyond the wrist-based accelerometer. Modern wearables are now integrating a widening array of sensors and measures to detect heart rate and heart rate variability, and oxygen saturation, and even accurately determine blood pressure [5]. Several groups are pursuing non-invasive continuous glucose monitoring [6]. Form factors (i. e., the overall design and functionality of a computer or piece of electronic hardware) have shrunk connected sensors into 'smart' rings [7], patches to those embedded in clothing like socks (which can detect diabetic ulcers early [8]) to 'underwearables,' embedded in underwear that measure pulse, respiratory status, and movement to facilitate remote patient monitoring (RPM). Stylish 'Smart Belts' have even been sensorized to enable gait analysis and estimate when meals were taken [9].

The insights and resulting 'nudges' generated from wearables to connected scales and blood pressure cuffs, when used effectively, have the potential for the engaged user to help track, optimize, and change behaviors. Sleep tracking and coaching with personalized data and advanced algorithms provide actionable information that will improve sleep health. This is of great utility given the critical role sleep (and poor sleep habits) plays in risk for and recovery from disease and immune function to risks for obesity and many chronic diseases [10]. Sleep apnea can be screened for with various consumer-grade wearables, triggering earlier diagnosis, evaluation, and intervention.

Even simple consumer-grade step counters can be exceedingly helpful in managing and tracking patients and disease progression or recovery (Fig. 49.5). For example, a patient discharged home following a total knee replacement would be expected to progress in the number of daily steps slowly. If a patient is walking less than expected, with daily step counts, distance walked, calories expended, and sedentary time measured out of expected norms based on excessive pain, the care team could be informed and intervene early and proactively [11].

Beyond traditional wearables, the blending of exponential technologies into a variety of form factors has brought additional technologies, such as:

- *Hearables:* From playing music to hearing aids, some versions can track vital signs and provide physiology-based exercise coaching or even assistance to those with cognitive issues or treatment of conditions such as tinnitus [12].
- *Insideables*: These [13] are subcutaneous biosensors that can wirelessly transmit a patient's tissue oxygenation to the swallowable 'PillCam' [14] for visualization of the small bowel. An example is the Profusa Lumi.
- *Breathables:* Leveraging the breath as a biomarker, several academics and startups are developing sensors that analyze the molecules in breath to detect signs of early cancer [15], and metabolic and infectious diseases [16], as well as those that can measure metabolism [17] to determine if the user is burning fats or carbohydrates.

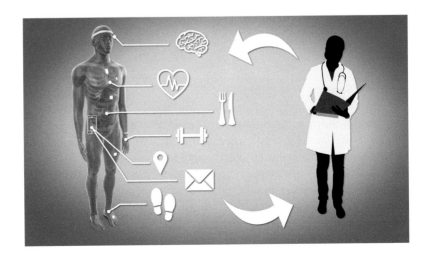

Fig. 49.5 Use of wearable devices in managing and tracking patients and disease progression or recovery

- *Trainables:* These are wearable devices that can both measure and provide direct feedback that can help modify behaviors. An example is the Upright Go device, which measures back posture and provides feedback via a buzz when 'hunched' to help remind the user to address their posture. Several sessions reportedly help improve awareness and correct posture [18].

- *Sweatables:* This involves sweat biomarker analyte detection that can enable health monitoring, from hydration status, and potentially foster on-demand regulation of drugs that can be delivered using integrated wearables if verification between sweat and blood measurements can be validated [19].

Quantifying our Diets

As diet plays such a key role in health and disease, our meals can increasingly be quantified via apps. Pocket-sized spectrophotometers have been developed that can establish the molecular footprint of different foods [20], and Continuous Glucose Monitors (CGM) are becoming common to help diabetic patients manage their disease and understand their individual metabolic response to various foods and activities [21]. 'Output' as measured by connected 'Smart Toilets' may soon, from the privacy of our homes, bring insights into our gastrointestinal health and metabolism [22]. As measures of metabolome, microbiome, genome, diet, and activity levels become cheap and commoditized, there is an emerging field of 'precision nutrition' in which a digital nutritionist will integrate the data to provide personalized, actionable recommendations [23].

Ambient Sensing Technologies

The 'wearable' and related categories summarized above have several disadvantages: the devices generally only work when worn correctly, connected to mobile apps, or when the batteries are charged. A new class of measurement is evolving using remote photoplethysmography imaging (rPPG)—a camera-based solution for non-contact cardiovascular monitoring, proven to be as accurate as traditional PPG devices. This enables off-the-shelf cameras, or those in a smartphone or laptop, to measure heart and respiratory rate, oxygen saturation, and heart rate variability, and even provide an estimation of blood pressure by extracting vital signs using a video taken of the upper cheek region of the face and analyzing it with advanced AI and deep learning algorithms, including computer vision technology and signal processing [24]. Cameras and AI software can also detect movement and behaviors. They can be useful to watch a patient (i.e., detecting a fall), whether in a hospital room or at home, enabling safer 'aging in place.' One startup is leveraging AI with a 'Kepler Night Nurse' to help nurses look after the well-being of patients at night in care facilities with a 40% reduction in caregivers' workload at night and a 99% reduction in false alarms [25].

Voice is also proving to be a useful new biomarker for health and early detection of neurologic diseases like Parkinson's [26] and even a biomarker associated with hospitalization and mortality in heart failure patients [27]. It can also be a biomarker providing insight into mental health (imagine a bipolar patient's voice when depressed or manic).

Even using a passive radio-wave-based home monitor (essentially modified wifi) developed by a team of MIT engineers has been shown to detect behaviors, movement, vitals, sleep cycles, and more [28] with applications including sleep disorders, musculoskeletal disorders, pulmonary disease, and neurological disease.

With increasingly 24/7 collected 'digital exhaust,' many challenges arise, ranging from privacy to data ownership. Access to more patient data does not automatically translate into better care or outcomes. Nurses, physicians, and providers of all varieties are already overwhelmed with EHRs and other charting burdens. The EHR and related components have been well documented to contribute to healthcare professional stress and burn-out. For the emerging era of digital health tools to translate from the 'health and wellness' realm to the medical spectrum, attention needs to be paid to workflow and designing user interfaces that facilitate sharing of accessible information that is digestible, actionable, and aligned with the care provider's incentives. Increasingly, designers appreciate the need to design interfaces that also delight users and gamify the experience to improve provider/user experience while also achieving greater care goals and health outcomes [29].

No nurse or doctor wants to or will log into a myriad array of apps, portals, and data streams generated by a single patient using a range of devices and apps. The launch of platforms like Apple's HealthKit and, more recently (for Android systems), CommonHealth [30] enables patients to integrate data from various connected devices and data sources (i.e., scale, activity monitor, blood pressure cuff, glucometer) via their mobile phones. The data in many healthcare systems can (with patient permission) opt in to connect to the patient's electronic medical record. But what happens next? Is the clinical team responsible for reviewing that data? What insights can be gleaned from consumer wearable data?

The future of patient-generated real-world data is one where millions of patients and their data points will be put in an individualized context for that particular patient and even a specific community. Ongoing trials include Verily (a subsidiary of Google)'s "Project Baseline" whose tagline is "we've mapped the world, now let's map human health," with over 10,000 volunteers sharing their digital data and electronic medical records. The National Institutes of Health has launched the ongoing 'All of Us' trial [31], aiming to enroll 1 million Americans from across diverse geographical, racial, cultural, and socioeconomic backgrounds, to provide a twenty-first-century 'Framingham Trial' at a massive scale.

As insights are gained from crowd-sourced trials like these, 'predictive analytics' can be increasingly applied to leverage multi-streams of data and provide personalized insights. This can offer proactive early warning directly to the patient or collaboration with their care team, similar to how a 'check engine light' works via software that integrates multiple signals from hundreds of sensors within modern cars. Early examples of 'check engine lights' exist, with some current consumer smartwatches able to detect heart rate and notify the wearer if their heart rate is well above expected ranges when the wearer is not moving (sign of potential atrial fibrillation), or to detect if the wearer had a hard fall and hasn't gotten up, and then message family members or caregivers [32].

An individual's wearable and other data can also be used to detect early signs of infectious disease. In the setting of the Covid-19 pandemic, several academic groups have studied the signals from smartwatches to detect disease in patients who may not even exhibit obvious symptoms [33]. Other wearable data analysis and tracking of individuals' 'physiomes' have enabled early detection of Lyme disease and metabolic disorders [34].

Leveraging New Forms of Data, Communication, and Coaching to Impact Behavior Change and Health Outcomes

While information and insights derived from the expanding array of sensors, sources, and powerful analytics can be useful, this does not translate easily to behavior change or other lifestyle modifications that can impact wellness, prevention, or disease management. Digital coaching platforms, whether connecting the user to a human coach (via telemedicine) or via a chatbot to advanced avatar coaching, have demonstrated efficacy. Studies of data and mobile-integrated coaching have shown efficacy in lowering hemoglobin A1c (HbA1c), achieving weight loss [35], and improving mental health with depression and anxiety scores [36].

Health and behavior changes is also a social endeavor. 'Digital behavioral coaching' platforms like those pioneered by Omada Health have demonstrated the positive outcomes in working with patients identified as pre-diabetic via digital coaching and integration with a cohort providing mutual support and also leveraging wearables to track activity and connected scales. Published outcomes have found a 30% decrease in progression to type 2 diabetes, a 16% decrease in the incidence of stroke, and a 13% decrease in the incidence of heart disease [37]. The use of such platforms also translated to cost savings for healthcare systems [38].

Disease-focused platforms focused on diabetic patients have blended continuous glucose monitoring data, coaching, and analytics to lower HbA1c, improve medication adherence, and reduce emergency room visits and hospital admissions [39, 40]. As virtual health coaches expand in their abilities, they will play an increasing role in driving behavior change and as a tool to manage acute and chronic disease, reducing costs while helping minimize clinician burden [41].

Voice Interfaces for Coaching, Health Communication, and Digital Therapeutics

Voice user interfaces (VUI), smart speaker technologies, and virtual assistants like Amazon's Alexa and Google Home are platforms that are increasingly being leveraged for health information [42], coaching, access, and connection to a variety of health services and platforms [43]. These can be used in the home, hospital room, clinic (e.g., for accessing medical records [44]), and even operating room to foster hands-free communication, activating safety checklists and interaction. A growing set of Alexa 'skills' have been built from payors and healthcare systems to digital therapeutic platforms [45].

Augmented, Virtual, and Extended Reality

The convergence of wearable computing and high-speed Internet with graphics and display technologies has brought us augmented reality (AR), virtual reality (VR), mixed reality (MXR), and extended reality (XR). AR/VR is becoming less expensive and more available, with dramatic and surprising use cases across the healthcare continuum, from medical education, facility design, surgical and procedural planning, disaster preparation, and simulation, to VR as a therapeutic modality. VR technology that cost millions

and was only available in academic labs a decade ago has now been consumerized on platforms like HTC Vive and Oculus VR.

Augmented reality (AR) is an interactive experience of a real-world environment where the objects that reside in the real world are enhanced by computer-generated perceptual information, sometimes across multiple sensory modalities, including visual, auditory, haptic, somatosensory, and olfactory [46]. The first generally available AR platform was Google Glass, launched in 2013 and it has continued with Google Glass Enterprise Edition 2 entering production in 2019. While Google Glass was not a consumer success, it has found use in healthcare as a tool to assist the clinician. Augmedix is a startup that has developed an app for Glass allowing clinicians to live-stream the patient visit to reduce electronic health record documentation challenges and improve clinician–doctor interactions. The video stream is passed to remote scribes in Health Insurance Portability and Accountability Act-secure rooms where the doctor–patient interaction is transcribed.

Surgeons have used Google Glass to record hands-free photo and live-streaming video documentation of procedures [47]. Swiss researchers assessed in a randomized controlled trial the adherence of emergency team leaders to the American Heart Association's (AHA) Pediatric Advanced Life Support (PALS) guidelines by adapting and displaying them in Google Glasses during simulation-based pediatric cardiac arrest scenarios [48].

Applications for new mothers and lactation nurses have included an application for hands-free breastfeeding [49]. The Google Glass Breastfeeding app trial allowed mothers to nurse their baby while viewing instructions about common breastfeeding issues or calling a lactation consultant via a secure Google Hangout, who could view the issue through the mother's Google Glass camera and provide coaching.

For addressing children with autism, a Boston-based company called Brain Power created an app to allow children with autism to teach themselves life skills, emotion decoding, eye contact, language, social engagement, conversation skills, and control of behaviors [50].

Healthcare-related applications built for AR and mixed reality expanded dramatically with the launch of Microsoft Hololens [51]. Use cases have included immersive healthcare training (i.e., students learning anatomy via shared healthcare educational holographic experience. Each user interacts with the same shared hologram, individually manipulating as they require. Case Western Reserve University and the Cleveland Clinic partnered with Microsoft to transform the way medical, dental, and nursing students learn about the human body. With holography, students can cut into a virtual, 3D human body to understand the intricacies of and connections among all of its systems. They have also included providing standardized patient experiences for medical education and nurse education and diagnostics training with an ultrasound simulator. Freed from the limits of a 2D environment inside a monitor, healthcare professionals can display, enlarge, and rotate realistic-looking anatomical parts and can witness, in real time, the ultrasound beam as it cuts through the human anatomy. In addition, they have included holographic surgical planning to enable visualization of patient-specific anatomy, as well as navigation platforms to help guide surgical procedures step by step [52].

Virtual reality has evolved beyond video games and into a vast array of interactive, immersive healthcare applications ranging from medical training to use as a therapeutic tool by which the user is able to look around the artificial world, move around in it, and interact with virtual features or items. The following are just a few applications:

- As an educational tool, students can immerse themselves within virtual anatomy and physiology [53], with both normal and pathophysiology as in Stanford's Virtual Heart project [54].
- Procedures can be recorded or live-streamed for real-time viewing by thousands of students around the world, providing an opportunity to democratize medical education [55].

- Interventional training in which users can simulate, learn, and practice procedures, ranging from orthopedic implant surgeries to endoscopy. Studies have validated improvement in participants' overall surgical performance when prepared with VR training [56].

The era of clinical training of 'see one, do one, teach one'... will shift to one of 'Simulate one… Sim one, Sim one...' until you get it right. AR/VR/XR platforms will serve as the equivalent to high-fidelity flight simulators, which train, test, and maintain currency for airline pilots.

VR is also demonstrating its ability to be used as a therapeutic platform:

- Therapeutic VR has emerged as an effective, drug-free tool for pain management in hospitalized patients [57], including great success with analgesic benefit of immersive VR for burn patients [58]
- When VR is utilized as a tool for physical therapy, patients remain more engaged and have improved activities of daily living [59].
- VR can also help develop empathy and enable clinicians to experience the limitations of their patients, for example, macular degeneration [60].

Diagnostics and Monitoring

What about advancement in diagnostics and monitoring? What used to require a full clinic can now fit into a digital doctor's bag, scrub pocket, or the diaper bag of a new parent or backpack of a high school or college student.

Diagnostic tools such as Covid-19 quarantine kits, enabling tracking of oxygen saturation, temperature, and lung sounds, and integrating into virtual visits to provide real-time enhancement of a virtualized physical exam, are becoming increasingly infused with AI and machine learning (ML). This includes a consumer ultrasound, which can bring diagnostics anywhere at very low cost, including being used to evaluate the lungs in suspected Covid-19 patients [61].

Traditional laboratories have transitioned to microfluidic platforms that can enable anyone to obtain measurements from blood or saliva. Many of these diagnostics are leveraging the smartphone and its camera for a 'Medical Selfie.' For example, instead of taking urine to the lab to diagnose a potential urinary tract infection, you can now do this in the privacy of your home. Simply dip the urine dipstick, take a picture with your smartphone camera, send it to the lab, and have results immediately available to your doctor and pharmacy [62].

Similar phone-based approaches are being developed for fast, frequent, cheap, and easy Covid-19 testing [63], while novel approaches to community-level diagnostics are being explored, including NextGen sequencing of sewage for Covid-19, identifying hot spots and predicting outbreaks [64].

There have been tremendous advances in artificial intelligence and machine learning (ML) within the past decade, especially in the application of deep learning to various challenges. These include advanced competitive games (such as Chess and Go), self-driving cars, speech recognition, and intelligent personal assistants. The lens of AI and ML is increasingly being applied to diagnostics as the explosion of data sources is beyond the capacity for the human mind to effectively integrate [65].

Undoubtedly, AI is becoming integral for the clinician and increasingly for the patient to enable 'Self-Care.' The following are just a few examples:

- *Dermatology:* AI-infused mobile apps for dermatology screening allow a patient, nurse, or community health worker to determine if a lesion is a benign mole or a possible melanoma [66].
- *Radiology:* AI is being leveraged in reading everything from a standard chest X-ray to CT scans, MRI, and ultrasound images. In several studies, the AI agents were comparable to or even outperformed experienced radiologists [67].
- *Pathology* is increasingly being digitized as well, and AI + ML will speed up the accuracy

and precision therapy approaches, especially in fields like oncology [68]. AI can also enhance the vision of a gastroenterologist performing a colonoscopy to identify dangerous lesions that might have otherwise been missed [69].

While AI is perceived as a threat by many clinicians, it cannot replace the human touch or empathy. Doctors, nurses, and pharmacists will not be replaced by AI, but clinicians and healthcare systems which do not work collaboratively with AI in the future will be replaced by those which do [70].

Future of Therapy

The onset of the Covid-19 pandemic of 2020 dramatically accelerated the use of virtual visits. Telemedicine visits increased on the order of 1000% in many settings and will never revert to pre-Covid-19 levels as patients and clinicians are discovering the compelling convenience and efficacy. Even before a virtual Zoom or Facetime with a clinician, asynchronous screening and support were provided by ever-smarter chatbots, which can help discern symptoms and help triage problems effectively at a much lower cost. In addition to this comes the virtualization and digital and virtual augmentation to meet the mental health crisis exacerbated by the many economic and other stressors accompanying the pandemic. At the same time, 3D Printing is finding a role in healthcare [71] with newfound applications, from the printing of personalized masks to critical parts of ventilators, leveraged by the growing Maker Community, playing a significant role in the pandemic response, from making face shields and masks to improvising DIY ventilators. The Maker Nurse [72] and Maker Health Programs include the physical space for prototyping tools and materials along with the back-end operating system to bring staff up to speed with making for health. This includes training, integration into operations, and a web platform to connect all health makers and their ongoing projects to communities.

Fig. 49.6 The future of health and medicine at the convergence of many rapidly developing and exponential technologies

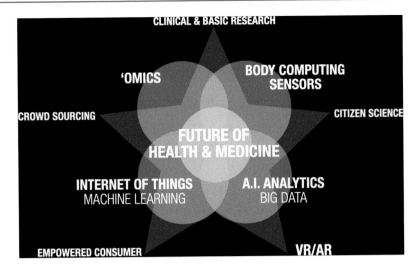

Accelerating Discovery

Altogether, these efforts enable the potential for democratization of health and medicine across the planet and access to information and care that was previously inaccessible. Clinical trials are being reshaped, leveraging smart devices, cloud-based analytic platforms, and collaborators worldwide.

As shown in Fig. 49.6, we are at the convergence of many rapidly developing and exponential technologies that can reshape and scale healthcare in our pandemic age. This includes:

1. Dramatically expanding access to basic healthcare that is increasingly personalized and proactive, leveraging the scale of digital platforms and technologies
2. Using digital connection/empathy and ability to blend virtual and in-person care
3. Leveraging the power of the crowd to share and build better maps that guide our individual health and public health journeys and to develop, validate, and scale more rapidly

Summary

The advances in technology experienced for the past few years have brought us into a completely digitized world, automated and enhanced by technologies ranging from mobile computing riding the Internet of things (IoT) to robotics integrating Big Data and artificial intelligence. Managing one's health today involves an app, a 'smart' device, or a patient portal. The method of delivering healthcare through digitally enabled technologies is moving fast and furiously, creating both opportunities and risks. Nevertheless, the positives outweigh the negatives, and the impact of this technology-driven era provides more analytics, accountability, and accessibility. Embracing the accelerating pace of change and the convergence of technologies available today and emerging in the near future will help innovators from a broad range of disciplines consider new and novel approaches to addressing challenges across the healthcare continuum.

Conclusions and Outlook

Healthcare is set to advance through smart integrations of technology, data, and shared insights, which will enable advancements in prevention, diagnosis, therapy, and public and global health. If we want to move from a 'sick care' system to a 'healthcare' system, current practitioners, academics, and industry leaders need to be aware of what is on the horizon and integrate solutions while re-imagining potentials across the healthcare ecosystem. The future of health depends on all of us.

Useful Resources

1. ExponentialMedicine.com/videos (content/ talk on future of medicine)
2. SeeYouNowPodcast.com
3. Digital.Health
4. Virtual Medicine.org
5. AI-Med.io
6. National Geographic Issue: Future of Medicine https://www.nationalgeographic. com/magazine/2019/01/
7. Internet of Intelligence https://arxiv.org/ abs/1909.08068
8. Deep Medicine (book) by Eric Topol MD
9. VRx: How Virtual Therapeutics Will Revolutionize Medicine (book) by Brennan Spiegel

Review Questions

1. What technologies and solutions can be used today and are likely to be used in 5–10 years?
2. What 'pain points' and challenges might be addressed with emerging technologies?

Appendix: Answers to Review Questions

1. What technologies and solutions can be used today and are likely to be used in 5–10 years?

   Examples include:
   - Internet of things
   - Artificial intelligence
   - Augmented, virtual, and extended Reality
   - Blockchain
   - 3D printing
   - Medical drones
   - Robotics and automation
   - Mobile health
   - Telemedicine and telehealth
   - Wearables
   - Food sensors

2. What 'pain points' and challenges might be addressed with emerging technologies?

   - Traditional healthcare (pharmaceuticals, medical devices, diagnostics, disposables)

needs are now being addressed by emerging technologies, which have in turn created new industries, fields, and careers at the interface of computational biology, telemedicine, robotic surgery, and companion diagnostics. Together, these can help address many of the local pain points and major challenges nurses, doctors, healthcare professionals, and healthcare systems face worldwide.

References

1. https://www.pbs.org/newshour/health/need-15-minutes-doctors-time. Accessed 2021.
2. Diamandis P. The 6 D's 2016. https://www.diamandis.com/blog/the-6ds. Accessed 2020.
3. Snowdon A. HIMSS defines digital health for the global healthcare industry. 2020. https://www.himss.org/news/himss-defines-digital-health-global-healthcare-industry. Accessed 2020.
4. Quantified self. A framework for personal science. 2021. https://quantifiedself.com/. Accessed 2020.
5. Muoio D. Cuffless blood pressure, oxygenation, heart rate monitor receives 510(k) clearance. 2019. https://www.mobihealthnews.com/news/north-america/cuffless-blood-pressure-oxygenation-heart-rate-monitor-receives-510k-clearance. Accessed 2020.
6. Albert H. Gloves aren't just for Covid-19: This one can be used to help diabetes patients. 2020. https://www.forbes.com/sites/helenalbert/2020/06/13/gloves-arent-just-for-covid-19-this-one-can-be-used-to-help-diabetes-patients/?sh=7a16f8af1380. Accessed 2020.
7. Sawh M. Best smart rings: put a ring on it in 2020. 2020. https://www.wareable.com/fashion/best-smart-rings-1340. Accessed 2020.
8. Reyzelman AM, Koelewyn K, Murphy M, Shen X, Yu E, Pillai R, Fu J, Scholten HJ, Ma R. Continuous temperature-monitoring socks for home use in patients with diabetes: observational study. J Med Internet Res. 2018;20:12. https://doi.org/10.2196/12460.
9. WELT. Personalized digital therapeutics for the treatment of diseases with high unmet medical needs. 2020. https://www.weltcorp.com/. Accessed 2020.
10. Bianchi MT. Sleep devices: wearables and nearables, informational and interventional, consumer and clinical. Metab Clin Exp. 2018;84(99–108) https://doi.org/10.1016/j.metabol.2017.10.008.
11. Patterson JT, Wu HH, Chung CC, Bendich I, Barry JJ, Bini SA. Wearable activity sensors and early pain after total joint arthroplasty. Arthroplasty Today. 2020;6(1):68–70.
12. Tinnitracks. 2018. www.tinnitracks.com. Accessed 2020.

13. Profusa. 2020. https://profusa.com/. Accessed 2020.
14. Medtronic. Pillcam SB 3 system. 2020. https://www.medtronic.com/covidien/en-us/products/capsule-endoscopy/pillcam-sb-3-system.html. Accessed 2020.
15. Owlstone medical. A breathalyzer for disease. 2020. https://www.owlstonemedical.com/. Accessed 2020.
16. Blum B. New breath test sniffs out Covid-19 in 30 seconds. 2020. https://www.israel21c.org/breathalyzer-from-israel-a-gamechanger-for-covid-testing/. Accessed 2020.
17. Lumen. 2020. https://www.lumen.me/. Accessed 2020.
18. Elliott AL. The upright go wearable posture device: an evaluation of postural health, improvement of posture, and salivary cortisol fluctuations in college students. University of Mississippi, Honors Theses. 2019. https://egrove.olemiss.edu/hon_thesis/1062
19. Chung M, Fortunato G, Radacsi N. Wearable flexible sweat sensors for healthcare monitoring: a review. J R Soc Interface. 2019; https://doi.org/10.1098/rsif.2019.0217.
20. Perry TS. What happened when we took the SCiO food analyzer grocery shopping. 2017. https://spectrum.ieee.org/. Accessed 2020.
21. Rachal M. Rivalry of the year: Abbott and Dexcom's race to dominate CGM. 2019. https://www.medtech-dive.com/news/rivalry-cgm-abbott-dexcom-glucose-monitoring-dive-award/565923/. Accessed 2020.
22. Armitage H. 'Smart toilet' monitors for signs of disease. 2020. https://med.stanford.edu/news/all-news/2020/04/smart-toilet-monitors-for-signs-of-disease.html. Accessed 2020.
23. Hamideh D, Arellano B, Topol EJ, Steinhubl SR. Your digital nutritionist. Lancet. 2019;5:393. https://doi.org/10.1016/s0140-6736(18)33170-2.
24. Binah AI. A unique mix of signal and AI technologies. 2020. https://binah.ai/technology/. Accessed 2020.
25. Kepler Vision Technology. Improve elderly care with the Kepler night nurse. 2020. https://keplervision.eu/night-nurse/. Accessed 2020.
26. Tracy JM, Özkanca Y, Atkins DC, Ghomi RH. Investigating voice as a biomarker: deep phenotyping methods for early detection of Parkinson's disease. J Biomed Inform. 2020;104:103362. https://doi.org/10.1016/j.jbi.2019.103362.
27. Maor E, Perry D, Mevorach D, Taiblum N, Luz Y, Mazin I, Lerman A, Koren G, Shalev V. Vocal biomarker is associated with hospitalization and mortality among heart failure patients. J Am Heart Assoc. 2020;9:7. https://doi.org/10.1161/jaha.119.013359.
28. MIT Computer Science & Artificial Intelligence Lab. 2020. https://www.csail.mit.edu/. Accessed 2020.
29. Rahemi Z, D'Avolio D, Dunphy LM, Rivera A. Shifting management in healthcare: an integrative review of design thinking. Nurs Manag. 2018;49(12):30–7. https://doi.org/10.1097/01.numa.0000547834.95083.e9.
30. Common Health. 2020. www.commonhealth.org. Accessed 2020.
31. National Institute of Health. All of us research program. 2020. https://AllofUs.nih.gov. Accessed 2020.
32. Apple Newsroom. ECG app and irregular heart rhythm notification available today on Apple watch. 2018. www.apple.com/newsroom/2018/12/ecg-app-and-irregular-heart-rhythm-notification-available-today-on-apple-watch/. Accessed 2020.
33. Mishra T, Wang M, Metwally AA, Bogu GK, Brooks AW, Bahmani A, Alavi A, Celli A, Higgs E, Dagan-Rosenfeld O, Fay B, Kirkpatrick S, Kellogg R, Gibson M, Wang T, Rolnik B, Ganz AB, Li X, Snyder AP. Early detection of COVID-19 using a smartwatch. MedRxiv. 2020. https://doi.org/10.1101/2020.07.06.20147512.
34. Li X, Dunn J, Salins D, Zhou G, Zhou W, Schüssler-Fiorenza RS, Perelman D, Colbert E, Runge R, Rego S, Sonecha R, Datta S, McLaughlin T, Snyder MP. Digital health: tracking physiomes and activity using wearable biosensors reveals useful health-related information. PLoS Biol. 2017. https://doi.org/10.1371/journal.pbio.2001402.
35. Mao AY, Chen C, Magana C, Caballero Barajas K, Olayiwola JN. A mobile phone-based health coaching intervention for weight loss and blood pressure reduction in a national payer population: a retrospective study. JMIR Mhealth Uhealth. 2017;5(6):e80. https://doi.org/10.2196/mhealth.7591.
36. Finn HE, Watson RA. The use of health coaching to improve health outcomes: implications for applied behavior analysis. Psychol Rec. 2017;67:181–7. https://doi.org/10.1007/s40732-017-0241-4.
37. Su W, Chen F, Dall TM, Iacobucci W, Perreault L. Return on investment for digital behavioral counseling in patients with prediabetes and cardiovascular disease. Prev Chronic Dis. 2016;13 https://doi.org/10.5888/pcd13.150357.
38. Chiguluri V, Barthold D, Gumpina R, Castro Sweet C, Pieratt J, Cordier TA, Matanich R, Renda A, Prewitt TD. Virtual diabetes prevention program—effects on medicare advantage health care costs and utilization. Diabetes. 2018;67.
39. Łuczyński W, Głowińska-Olszewska B, Bossowski A. Empowerment in the treatment of diabetes and obesity. J Diabetes Res. 2016. https://doi.org/10.1155/2016/5671492.
40. https://www.rochediabeteshealthconnection.com/. Accessed 2021.
41. Bevilacqua R, Casaccia S, Cortellessa G, Astell A, Lattanzio F, Corsonello A, D'Ascoli P, Paolini S, Di Rosa M, Rossi L, Maranesi E. Coaching through technology: a systematic review into efficacy and effectiveness for the ageing population. Int J Environ Res Public Health. 2020;17(16):5930.
42. Chung AE, Griffin AC, Selezneva D, Gotz D. Health and fitness apps for hands-free, voice-activated assistants. JMIR Mhealth Uhealth. 2018;6(9):e174. https://doi.org/10.2196/mhealth.9705.
43. Cimino JD, Stefanacci RG, Alexa PM. Can you transform healthcare? Manag Healthc Exec. 2020. https://www.managedhealthcareexecutive.com/view/alexa-can-you-transform-healthcare-0. Accessed 2020.

44. Kumah-Crystal YA, Pirtle CJ, Whyte HM, Goode ES, Anders SH, Lehmann CU. Electronic health record interactions through voice: a review. Appl Clin Inform. 2018;9(3):541–52. https://doi.org/10.1055/s-0038-1666844.

45. Jiang R. Introducing new Alexa healthcare skills. 2019. https://developer.amazon.com/en-US/blogs/alexa/alexa-skills-kit/2019/04/introducing-new-alexa-healthcare-skills. Accessed 2020.

46. Huffington Post. The lengthy history of augmented reality. 2016. http://images.huffingtonpost.com/2016-05-13-1463155843-8474094-AR_history_timeline.jpg. Accessed 2020.

47. Trombini V. World's first Google glass assisted surgery was successfully performed: video. 2013. https://www.americaninno.com/boston/worlds-first-google-glass-assisted-surgery-was-successfully-performed-video/. Accessed 2020.

48. Siebert JN, Ehrler F, Gervaix A, Haddad K, Lacroix L, Schrurs P, Sahin A, Lovis C, Manzano S. Adherence to AHA guidelines when adapted for augmented reality glasses for assisted pediatric cardiopulmonary resuscitation: a randomized controlled trial. J Med Internet Res. 2017;19(5) https://doi.org/10.2196/jmir.7379.

49. Papple D. Google glass connects breastfeeding moms with lactation help. 2016. https://www.inquisitr.com/1224638/google-glass-connects-breastfeeding-moms-with-lactation-help/. Accessed 2020.

50. Liu R, Salisbury JP, Vahabzadeh A, Sahin NT. Feasibility of an autism-focused augmented reality smartglasses system for social communication and behavioral coaching. Front Pediatr. 2017;5:145.

51. Microsoft HoloLens. Microsoft HoloLens & mixed reality healthcare industry deck. 2017. http://www.nln.org/docs/default-source/professional-development-programs/health-industry-deck%2D%2D-microsoft-hololens.pdf. Accessed 2020.

52. Vavra P, Roman J, Zonca P, Ihnat P, Nemec M, Kumar J, Habib N, El-Gendi A. Recent development of augmented reality in surgery: a review. J Healthc Eng. 2017;2017:4574172. https://doi.org/10.1155/2017/4574172.

53. Samadbeik M, Yaaghobi D, Bastani P, Abhari S, Rezaee R, Garavand A. The applications of virtual reality technology in medical groups teaching. J Adv Med Educ Prof. 2018;6(3):123–9.

54. Stanford Children's Health. The Stanford virtual heart – revolutionizing education on congenital heart defects. 2017. https://www.stanfordchildrens.org/en/innovation/virtual-reality/stanford-virtual-heart. Accessed 2020.

55. Davis N. Cutting-edge theatre: world's first virtual reality operation goes live. 2016. https://www.theguardian.com/technology/2016/apr/14/cutting-edge-theatre-worlds-first-virtual-reality-operation-goes-live. Accessed 2020.

56. Blumstein G, Zukotynski B, Cevallos N, Ishmael C, Zoller S, Burke Z, Clarkson S, Park H, Bernthal N, SooHoo NF. Randomized trial of a virtual reality tool to teach surgical technique for tibial shaft fracture intramedullary nailing. J Surg Educ. 2020;77(4):969–77. https://doi.org/10.1016/j.jsurg.2020.01.002.

57. Spiegel B, Fuller G, Lopez M, Dupuy T, Noah B, Howard A, Albert M, Tashjian V, Lam R, Ahn J, Dailey F, Rosen BT, Vrahas M, Little M, Garlich J, Dzubur E, IsHak W, Danovitch I. Virtual reality for management of pain in hospitalized patients: a randomized comparative effectiveness trial. PLoS One. 2019;14(8):e0219115. https://doi.org/10.1371/journal.pone.0219115.

58. Sharar SR, Miller W, Teeley A, Soltani M, Hoffman HG, Jensen MP, Patterson DR. Applications of virtual reality for pain management in burn-injured patients. Expert Rev Neurother. 2008;8(11):1667–74. https://doi.org/10.1586/14737175.8.11.1667.

59. Laver KE, Lange B, George S, Deutsch JE, Saposnik G, Crotty M. Virtual reality for stroke rehabilitation. Cochrane Database Syst Rev. 2017;11(11):CD008349. https://doi.org/10.1002/14651858.cd008349.pub4.

60. Dyer E, Swartzlander BJ, Gugliucci MR. Using virtual reality in medical education to teach empathy. J Med Libr Assoc. 2018;106(4):498–500. https://doi.org/10.5195/jmla.2018.518.

61. Sultan LR, Sehgal CM. A review of early experience in lung ultrasound in the diagnosis and management of COVID-19. Ultrasound Med Biol. 2020;46(9):2530–45.

62. Healthy io. Turning the smartphone into a medical device. 2020. https://healthy.io/services/uti-gp/. Accessed 2020.

63. Allam M, Cai S, Ganesh S, Venkatesan M, Doodhwala S, Song Z, Hu T, Kumar A, Heit J, Coskun AF. COVID-19 diagnostics, tools, and prevention. Diagnostics (Basel). 2020;10(6):409. https://doi.org/10.3390/diagnostics10060409.

64. Medema G, Been F, Heijnen L, Petterson S. Implementation of environmental surveillance for SARS-CoV-2 virus to support public health decisions: opportunities and challenges. Curr Opin Environ Sci Health. 2020;17:49–71. https://doi.org/10.1016/j.coesh.2020.09.006.

65. Chan S, Siegel EL. Will machine learning end the viability of radiology as a thriving medical specialty? Br J Radiol. 2019;92(1094):20180416. https://doi.org/10.1259/bjr.20180416.

66. Gomolin A, Netchiporouk E, Gniadecki R, Litvinov IV. Artificial intelligence applications in dermatology: where do we stand? Front Med (Lausanne). 2020;7:100. https://doi.org/10.3389/fmed.2020.00100.

67. Murphy K, Smits H, Knoops AJG, Korst MBJM, Samson T, Scholten ET, Schalekamp S, Schaefer-Prokop CM, Philipsen RHHM, Meijers A, Melendex J, Ginneken BV, Rutten M. COVID-19 on chest radiographs: a multireader evaluation of an artificial intelligence system. Radiology. 2020;296(3):E166–72. https://doi.org/10.1148/radiol.2020201874.

68. Bera K, Schalper KA, Rimm DL, Velcheti V, Madabhushi A. Artificial intelligence in digital pathology - new tools for diagnosis and precision oncology. Nat Rev Clin Oncol. 2019;16(11):703–15. https://doi.org/10.1038/s41571-019-0252-y.

69. Yang YJ, Cho BJ, Lee MJ, Kim JH, Hyun L, Bang CS, Jeong HM, Hong JT, Baik GH. Automated classification of colorectal neoplasms in white-light colonoscopy images via deep learning. J Clin Med. 2020;9(5):1593.

70. McGrow K. Artificial intelligence: essentials for nursing. Nursing. 2019;49(9):46–9. https://doi.org/10.1097/01.nurse.0000577716.57052.8d.

71. Yan Q, Dong H, Su J, Han J, Song B, Wei Q, Shi Y. A review of 3D printing technology for medical applications. Engineering. 2018;4(5):729–42. https://doi.org/10.1016/j.eng.2018.07.021.

72. Maker Nurse. 2019. http://makernurse.com/. Accessed 2020.

Index

© Springer Nature Switzerland AG 2022
U. H. Hübner et al. (eds.), *Nursing Informatics*, Health Informatics,
https://doi.org/10.1007/978-3-030-91237-6

Printed in the United States
by Baker & Taylor Publisher Services